AF413084

ASTHMA AND IMMUNOLOGICAL
DISEASES IN PREGNANCY
AND EARLY INFANCY

LUNG BIOLOGY IN HEALTH AND DISEASE

Executive Editor

Claude Lenfant
Director, National Heart, Lung and Blood Institute
National Institutes of Health
Bethesda, Maryland

ADDITIONAL VOLUMES IN PREPARATION

The opinions expressed in these volumes do not necessarily represent the views of the National Institutes of Health.

ASTHMA AND IMMUNOLOGICAL DISEASES IN PREGNANCY AND EARLY INFANCY

Edited by

Michael Schatz and Robert S. Zeiger

Kaiser Permanente Medical Center
San Diego, California
and
University of California, San Diego, School of Medicine
La Jolla, California

Henry N. Claman

University of Colorado School of Medicine
Denver, Colorado

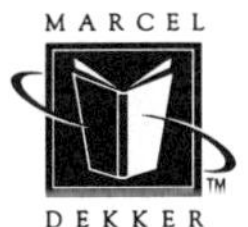

MARCEL DEKKER, INC.   NEW YORK · BASEL · HONG KONG

ISBN 0-8247-0095-3

MARCEL DEKKER, INC.
270 Madison Avenue, New York, New York 10016
http://www.dekker.com

Current printing (last digit):
10 9 8 7 6 5 4 3 2 1

PRINTED IN THE UNITED STATES OF AMERICA

INTRODUCTION

It is much easier to write upon a disease than upon a remedy. The former is in the hands of nature and a faithful observer with an eye to tolerable judgment cannot fail to delineate a likeness; the latter will ever be subject to the whim, the inaccuracy and the blunder of man.

William Withering
An Account of the Foxglove, *1758*

This statement has an element of truth that probably applies to many, if not all, pathological situations. A noteworthy exception is disorders affecting the maternal–fetal relationship. When one considers the complexity of biological reactions and disease manifestations in this symbiotic relationship, it may not be so easy to write about the diseases affecting pregnant women and their unborn babies. Indeed, even in the absence of disease, the interaction between mother and infant is a true immunological *tour de force*, so an immunological disorder affecting the mother presents a formidable challenge. Furthermore, there is increasing evidence that the perinatal period and early infancy are, in part, programmed by the mother–baby interface during pregnancy. Such programming, if triggered by a stimulus or an insult during development, may have a permanent impact.

For all of these reasons, writing about the impact and consequences of immune disorders during pregnancy is not easy. Writing about how to treat these disorders in pregnancy and in early life is not easy either!

The Lung Biology in Health and Disease series has covered a great number of topics from early lung development to the care of the elderly. But, never before has the series discussed the impact of immunological disorders on the pregnant woman, her fetus, and her infant. Therefore, it was a wonderful opportunity when Drs. Schatz, Zeiger, and Claman accepted my invitation to edit this volume. A review of the Table of Contents and the roster of contributors makes it immediately clear that *Asthma and Immunological Diseases in Pregnancy and Early Infancy* is a landmark in the field for what it presents about both the diseases and their remedies.

I believe this volume will indeed improve the quality of medical care and thus the quality of life for pregnant women and for their infants. I am grateful to the editors and the chapter authors for making it possible to include this book in the Lung Biology in Health and Disease series.

Claude Lenfant, M.D.
Bethesda, Maryland

PREFACE

The interface between immunology and pregnancy is usually considered in terms of the apparent paradox that the immunocompetent mother does not immunologically reject her genetically dissimilar fetal allograft. However, the potential clinical overlap between immunology and pregnancy is much broader—there are a number of medical conditions that involve or mimic immunological mechanisms which may affect the pregnant woman or her infant. Included in this group of conditions are asthma and other allergic diseases, immune deficiency states, collagen vascular diseases, and autoimmune conditions.

Our prior work, *Asthma and Allergy in Pregnancy and Early Infancy*, covered asthma and atopic diseases. The current volume updates that work and expands it to include non-atopic immunological diseases. The purpose of this book is to explore in detail the effects of asthma and immunological diseases on pregnancy, the effects of pregnancy on these illnesses, the potential effects of the specific treatments on pregnancy, and the optimal gestational management considering both the well-being of the mother and that of the fetus. Regarding the infant, the book emphasizes prevention, early diagnosis, and natural history, as well as treatment of these conditions.

The first section of the book deals with the relevant physiology of pregnancy, including hormonal changes, pulmonary physiology, immunological changes, and fetal oxygenation and monitoring. The next section explores general therapeutic principles such as psychological care and pharmacological management, and includes gestational safety data on specific relevant medications and medicolegal considerations. The third section discusses specific allergy diagnosis and treatment during pregnancy and describes in detail the relationships to pregnancy and gestational management of specific allergic or related conditions, including rhinitis, anaphylaxis, cutaneous diseases and adverse drug reactions. The next section details the interrelationships between asthma and pregnancy, discusses the diagnosis of gestational asthma, and provides medical and obstetric management guidelines from several perspectives. The fifth section discusses the non-atopic immunological diseases that may complicate pregnancy—systemic lupus erythematosus, rheumatoid arthritis, other connective tissue and autoimmune diseases—as well as HIV infection and other immune deficiency states. This section also explores the current understanding and management of the defined immunological conditions that lead to fetal wastage. The next section covers the development and natural history of allergic diseases in infancy and details the prospects for prevention of these illnesses. The final section describes the diagnosis and management of allergic and immunological diseases during infancy, including the wheezing infant, food hypersensitivity, atopic dermatitis, and immune deficiency.

Pregnancy and early motherhood represents a very special period in a woman's life. However, when this special time is complicated by asthma or allergic or immunological disease, it may be much more difficult. We hope this book will be used to improve the quality of medical care and thus the quality of life for pregnant women and their infants afflicted with asthma, allergies, or other immunological diseases.

Michael Schatz
Robert S. Zeiger
Henry N. Claman

CONTRIBUTORS

Richard S. Abrams, M.D.   Associate Clinical Professor, Department of Medicine and Associate Clinical Professor, Department of Obstetrics and Gynecology, University of Colorado School of Medicine and Rose Medical Center, Denver, Colorado

Bengt Björkstén, M.D., Ph.D.   Professor, Department of Pediatrics, Faculty of Health Sciences, University Hospital, Linköping, Sweden

S. Allan Bock, M.D.   Staff Physician, Department of Pediatrics, National Jewish Medical and Research Center, Denver, Colorado

Walter A. Brown, M.D.   Clinical Professor, Department of Psychiatry and Human Behavior, Brown University School of Medicine, Providence, Rhode Island

Valerian A. Catanzarite, M.D., Ph.D.   Associate Director, Maternal Fetal Medicine, Mary Birch Hospital for Women at Sharp Memorial, San Diego, California

Henry N. Claman, M.D.   Distinguished Professor, Departments of Medicine and Immunology, University of Colorado School of Medicine, Denver, Colorado

Steven L. Clark, M.D.   Professor, Department of Obstetrics and Gynecology, University of Utah School of Medicine and Director, Intermountain Health Care Perinatal Centers, Salt Lake City, Utah

William O. C. M. Cookson   Wellcome Senior Clinical Research Fellow, Nuffield Department of Medicine, John Radcliffe Hospital, Oxford, England

Larry Cousins, M.D.   Director, Maternal Fetal Medicine, Mary Birch Hospital for Women at Sharp Memorial, San Diego, California

Donna S. Dizon-Townson, M.D.   Maternal–Fetal Medicine Fellow, Department of Obstetrics and Gynecology, University of Utah School of Medicine, Salt Lake City, Utah

Mitchell P. Dombrowski, M.D.   Interim Chairman and Chief, Department of Obstetrics and Gynecology, Wayne State University/Hutzel Hospital, Detroit, Michigan

Reuben Falkoff, M.D., Ph.D.   Staff Physician, Department of Allergy and Immunology, Kaiser Permanente Medical Center, San Diego, California

Frederick H. Fern, R.Ph., J.D.   Partner, Lester Schwab Katz & Dwyer, New York, New York

Noah J. Friedman, M.D.   Assistant Clinical Professor, Department of Pediatrics, University of California, San Diego, School of Medicine, La Jolla and Staff Allergist, Kaiser Permanente Medical Center, San Diego, California

Adolfo Gonzalez-Garcia, M.D.   Assistant Professor, Perinatal Division, University of Miami School of Medicine, Miami, Florida

Paul A. Greenberger, M.D.   Professor, Department of Medicine, Division of Allergy–Immunology, Northwestern University Medical School, Chicago, Illinois

Jean A. Hobart, J.D.   Attorney-at-Law, Beverly Hills, California

Clement P. Hoffman, M.D.   Assistant Clinical Professor, Department of Reproductive Medicine, University of California, San Diego, School of Medicine, La Jolla and Kaiser Foundation Hospital, San Diego, California

Gary A. Incaudo, M.D.   Clinical Professor, Department of Medicine, Division of Rheumatology and Allergy, University of California, Davis, School of Medicine, Chico, California

Alan F. Isles, M.B., B.S.(Hons), M.Sc., F.R.A.C.P.   Associate Professor, Department of Respiratory Medicine, Royal Children's Hospital, Brisbane, Queensland, Australia

Elizabeth F. Juniper, M.C.S.P., M.Sc.   Associate Professor, Department of Clinical Epidemiology and Biostatistics, McMaster University Medical Centre, Hamilton, Ontario, Canada

Geeta Khare, M.D.* Consultant, Department of Allergy/Clinical Immunology, University of Colorado School of Medicine, Denver, Colorado

N-I Max Kjellman, M.D. Professor of Pediatric Allergology, Department of Pediatrics, Faculty of Health Sciences, University Hospital, Linköping, Sweden

Armand Lione, Ph.D. Reproductive Toxicology Center and Associated Pharmacologists and Toxicologists, Washington, D.C.

Michael D. Lockshin, M.D. Special Assistant to the Director, Warren Grant Magnuson Clinical Center, National Institutes of Health, Bethesda, Maryland

Allan T. Luskin, M.D. Associate Professor, Departments of Immunology/Microbiology and Medicine, Rush Medical Center, Chicago, Illinois

Helen Mawhinney, M.D., F.R.C.P. Clinical Assistant Professor, Department of Medicine, University of California, Los Angeles, School of Medicine, Los Angeles, California

Michael H. Mellon, M.D. Pediatric Allergist, Department of Allergy, Kaiser Permanente Medical Center, San Diego and Associate Professor, Department of Pediatrics, University of California, San Diego, School of Medicine, La Jolla, California

Joseph F. Mortola, M.D. Director, Division of Reproductive Endocrinology, Department of Obstetrics and Gynecology, Cook County Hospital, Chicago, Illinois

J. Lee Nelson, M.D. Associate Member, Program in Immunogenetics, Fred Hutchinson Cancer Research Center and Associate Professor, Division of Rheumatology, Department of Medicine, The University of Washington School of Medicine, Seattle, Washington

Michael T. Newhouse, M.D., M.Sc., F.R.A.C.P.(C), F.A.C.P., F.C.C.P. Clinical Professor, Department of Medicine, McMaster University and St. Joseph's Hospital, Hamilton, Ontario, Canada

Christopher J. L. Newth, M.B., F.R.C.P.(C), F.R.A.C.P. Professor, Department of Pediatrics, University of Southern California School of Medicine, Children's Hospital of Los Angeles, Los Angeles, California

Christopher P. Orlando, R.Ph., J.D. Attorney, Renzulli, Gainey & Rutherford, New York, New York

Monika E. Østensen, M.D., Ph.D. Professor, Department of Rheumatology, University Hospital of Trondheim, Trondheim, Norway

---

**Current affiliation*: Consultant in Allergy and Clinical Immunology, Pueblo, Colorado

Mary Jo O'Sullivan, M.D.   Professor, Department of Obstetrics and Gynecology, University of Miami School of Medicine, Miami, Florida

Roy Patterson, M.D.   Ernest S. Bazley Professor of Medicine and Chief, Division of Allergy–Immunology, Department of Medicine, Northwestern University Medical School, Chicago, Illinois

Steven W. Rubinstein, M.D.   Assistant Professor, Department of Pediatrics, Lucille Packard Children's Hospital at Stanford, Stanford, California

Hugh A. Sampson, M.D.   Professor, Department of Pediatrics, Johns Hopkins University School of Medicine, Baltimore, Maryland

Frederick M. Schaffer, M.D.   Assistant Professor, Department of Biochemistry and Molecular Biology, Mississippi State University, Starkville, Mississippi

Michael Schatz, M.D.   Staff Allergist, Department of Allergy, Kaiser Permanente Medical Center, San Diego and Clinical Professor, Department of Medicine, University of California, San Diego, School of Medicine, La Jolla, California

Richard I. Schiff, M.D., Ph.D.   Director, Department of Clinical Immunology, Miami Children's Hospital, Miami, Florida

Anthony R. Scialli, M.D.   Associate Professor, Department of Obstetrics and Gynecology, Georgetown University Medical Center and Reproductive Toxicology Center, Washington, D.C.

Gillian M. Shepherd, M.D.   Clinical Associate Professor, Department of Internal Medicine, The New York Hospital–Cornell University Medical Center, New York, New York

Sheldon Laurence Spector, M.D.   Clinical Professor, Department of Medicine, University of California, Los Angeles, School of Medicine, Los Angeles, California

Andrea Bein Stone, M.D.   Assistant Professor, Department of Psychiatry, University of Massachusetts Medical School, Worcester, Massachusetts

Pamela Stratton, M.D.   Special Assistant in Gynecology and Clinical Research, Center for Population Research, Contraceptive Development Branch, National Institute of Child Health and Human Development, Bethesda, Maryland

Claire E. Wainwright, M.R.C.P.(UK), F.R.A.C.P.   Department of Respiratory Medicine, Royal Children's Hospital, Brisbane, Queensland, Australia

Stephen I. Wasserman, M.D.   The Helen M. Ranney Professor and Chairman, Department of Medicine, University of California, San Diego, School of Medicine, La Jolla, California

Gary M. White, M.D.   Department of Dermatology, Kaiser Permanente, San Diego and Assistant Clinical Professor, Department of Dermatology, University of California, San Diego, School of Medicine, La Jolla, California

Robert A. Wise, M.D.   Associate Professor, Division of Pulmonary and Critical Care Medicine, Johns Hopkins University School of Medicine, Baltimore, Maryland

Robert S. Zeiger, M.D., Ph.D.   Chief, Department of Allergy, Kaiser Permanente Medical Center, San Diego and Clinical Professor, Department of Pediatrics, University of California, San Diego, School of Medicine, La Jolla, California

CONTENTS

ASTHMA AND IMMUNOLOGICAL DISEASES IN PREGNANCY AND EARLY INFANCY

Part One

BASIC SCIENCE

1

Hormonal Changes During Normal Pregnancy and Their Consequences

JOSEPH F. MORTOLA

Cook County Hospital
Chicago, Illinois

I. Introduction

Pregnancy is characterized by extensive physiological and anatomical adaptations that maximize the chances for survival of the fetus. These adaptations, which include alterations in every organ system, result primarily from enhanced production of steroid and peptide hormones by the fetal-placental-decidual unit. The level of most of these hormones reached during pregnancy is unparalleled by any other physiological state. The capacity of the mother to tolerate these large increases in hormone levels is dependent on a simultaneous increase in buffering systems and antihormones during pregnancy. While these buffering systems are usually sufficient to prevent the pathological sequelae which may otherwise result from the hormonal excess, an increase in hormone action prevails, particularly in target tissues, which is sufficient to render pregnancy a state of controlled hormone excesses.

II. Progesterone

Progesterone is the hormone most clearly associated with maternal adaptation to pregnancy. It is essential for the maturation of the uterine endometrium into a tissue capable of accepting and facilitating implantation. During the normal menstrual cycle, progesterone is produced by the corpus luteum from the time of ovulation until the time of involution of the corpus luteum just prior to menses. The lifespan of the corpus leuteum is prolonged in pregnancy, and ovarian progesterone production continues until 7–10 weeks gestational age. After 10 weeks, progesterone production is almost exclusively from the placenta. The corpus luteum's capacity to maintain production of progesterone as well as estrogen in early pregnancy is the result of stimulation by placenta-derived human chorionic gonadotropin (hCG). hCG can be detected in the maternal circulation within 1 day of implantation. Circulating hCG is almost entirely derived from a placental source (with the exception of a small production by the pituitary in the nonpregnant state), and thus its detection in serum serves as the basis for modern pregnancy tests (1).

In the corpus luteum, hCG, like luteinizing hormone (LH) produced during the menstrual cycle, induces progesterone synthesis through a series of sequential steps from HDL-cholesterol (2). The synthesis of progesterone in addition to estrogen distinguishes the corpus luteum from the preovulatory follicle from which it arises, in which estrogen predominates as the end product of the steroidogenic pathway. The shift from the estrogen production in the follicular (preovulatory) phase to production of both estrogen and progesterone in the luteal (postovulatory) phase is crucial to maintenance of the normal menstrual cycle. These sequential events are required to prepare the endometrium for implantation of the dividing fertilized egg at the blastocyst stage approximately 7 days after ovulation. Thus, adequate endometrial maturation is dependent on the addition of progesterone to an estrogen-primed endometrium. As a result of progesterone, the glandular component of the endometrium undergoes marked secretory changes and the structural matrix undergoes a characteristic edematous change (3). Progesterone administration without prior estrogen influence produces quite a different effect, with widely spaced glands lined by atrophic cuboidal epithelium (4). Progesterone, therefore, has effects which are dependent on the previous estrogen priming of the uterus. In the case of prolonged progesterone exposure accompanied by sufficient estrogen, such as is seen in pregnancy, the uterine endometrium undergoes even more marked changes, termed decidualization. In this process, stromal cells adopt a distinct polyhedral shape, with clearly delineated borders which are believed to be the result of glycoprotein deposition in the cell membrane (5). Within the glandular epithelial cells, the nuclei become hyperchromatic, assume a polyploid shape, and are surrounded by expanded cytoplasm; these changes are thought to reflect hypersecretory activity. The development of such large hypersecretory cells is referred to as the Arias-Stella reaction, and is considered a characteristic histological marker for pregnancy (6). The actions of progesterone on the uterus which both prepare the endometrium for implantation and maintain the pregnancy once implantation has occurred may be the result not only of progesterone itself but also of a metabolite, 20α-OH-pregn-4-ene-3-one, synthesized within the endometrium (7).

Progesterone has also been implicated in the localized uterine immunosuppression which is required for successful survival of the embryo. Effective immunorejection requires antigen-presenting cells capable of externalizing the immune complex to the cell surface, and subsequent activation and proliferation of specific lymphocyte subsets. Uterine decidua has been shown to contain relatively large numbers of both the macrophages and lymphocytes which would be required for this process (8). Decidua has also been shown to be a source of interleukin-1 (IL-1) (9) and to contain the type II major histocompatibility antigen termed the human leukocyte antigen (HLA-DR) (8), both of which are thought to be integral components of normal immune responsivity (10). Progesterone as well as estrogen have been shown to alter immune function in vivo through the actions on IL-1 (11). While low doses of these hormones stimulate IL-1β mRNA, high doses, such as these achieved in pregnancy, are inhibiting. Thus, hormonal changes in the luteal phase and early pregnancy may inhibit semiallograft rejection of the embryo through suppression of IL-1β, which is obligate for such immunological rejection.

While the most widely recognized effects of progesterone and its metabolites are on endometrial tissue, progesterone is assumed to be largely responsible for many of the marked systemic physiological changes that accompany pregnancy. Progesterone levels increase at least 10-fold between the 6th and 36th weeks of pregnancy (Fig. 1). Progesterone or its metabolites has been shown to decrease vascular responsiveness to angiotensin-II through a prostaglandin-mediated mechanism (12) and thus may contribute to the decreased peripheral vascular resistance seen in pregnancy (13). The decreased total pulmonary vascular resistance of pregnancy has long been postulated to be the result of progesterone action as well (14).

Among the most important adaptive changes in pregnancy is the increased material O_2 uptake which results from increased minute ventilation. This increased ventilatory effort results from a marked increase in tidal volume without a significant change in the respiratory rate (see Chapter 3). The increased tidal volume appears to be a progesterone-mediated event

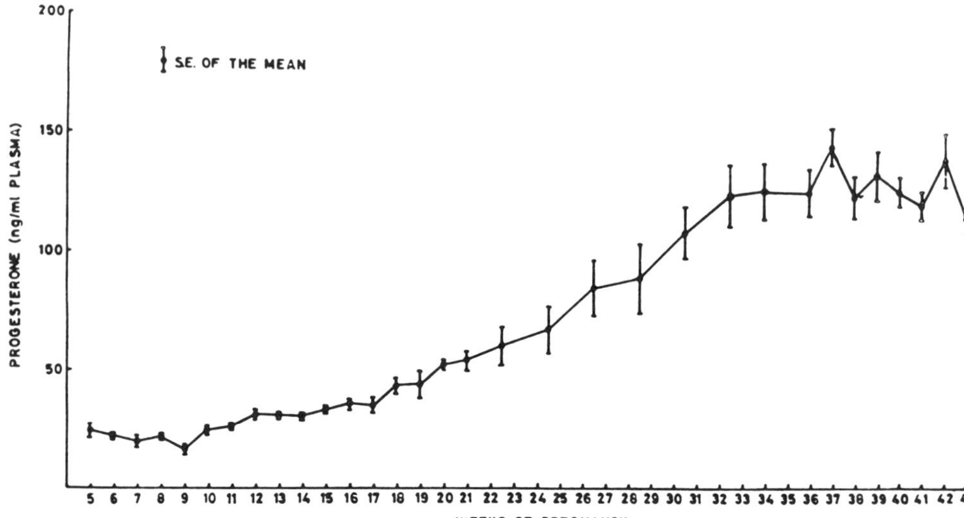

Figure 1 Plasma progesterone levels during normal pregnancy. (Reproduced from Johansson ENB. Acta Endocrinol (Kbh) 1979; 61:607.)

through central nervous system actions of the hormone. Evidence for this hypothesis is afforded by the demonstration that increased respiratory drive results when nonpregnant obese patients who hypoventilate are given a progesterone analog, medroxyprogesterone acetate (15).

In addition to changes in the vascular and pulmonary systems, pregnancy is characterized by a decreased gastrointestinal transit time. This includes both slower gastric emptying and prolonged intestinal transit. These alterations have been hypothesized, but not proven, to be the result of progesterone action. The urinary tract in pregnancy is also characterized by marked changes in architecture. Both hydronephrosis and hydroureter are widely reported. Typically, the hydronephrosis and hydroureter are more marked on the right side (16), suggesting that mechanical compression by the dextrorotated uterus may be a factor. There is evidence, however, that hormonal influences also play a part. Pregnant monkeys with the fetus removed, but the placenta allowed to remain intact, continued to be hydronephrotic (17). Such a result would not be expected if the effect were estrogen dominated, since a majority of the precursor for placental estrogen production is of fetal origin. In contrast, this experiment supports the notion that progesterone may be largely responsible for hydromorphic changes in pregnancy, since progesterone precursors are largely of maternal origin.

Progesterone is among the numerous factors which alter glucose-insulin homeostasis during pregnancy. Progesterone, like estrogen, induces hyperinsulinimea and islet β-cell hypertrophy. However, unlike estrogen, progesterone has not been found to produce hypoglycemia. This suggests a role for progesterone in the hyperinsulinimic-euglycemic state observed during pregnancy, probably as a result of insulin antagonism in peripheral tissues (18,19).

III. Estrogens

The second major class of steroid hormone produced during pregnancy is estrogen. Pregnancy is characterized by a marked increase in both of the estrogens produced in the nonpregnant state, estradiol and estrone (20), as well as the appearance of abundant quantities of a third estrogen, estriol (21), which is produced in only trace amounts in the nonpregnant state (Fig. 2). (A fourth estrogen, estetrol, is also produced in pregnancy, although its quantity is negligible and its interest is only that it is entirely unique to pregnancy, with no measurable amounts found in the serum of nonpregnant women.)

The biosynthesis of estrogen is quite different from that of progesterone. While the placenta is capable of producing large amounts of progesterone from low-density lipoprotein (LDL) precursor of maternal origin, a placental cytochrome P450c17 hydroxylase block renders the production of C-19 steroids (androgen) and C-18 steroids (estrogens) directly from high-density lipoprotein (HDL) precursor impossible in the placenta. As a result, the placenta is almost entirely dependent on the provision of C-19 steroids for estrogen production. The low total estrogen levels in the circulation of women with fetuses which are incapable of adrenal steroid synthesis (such as anancephalics) support the concept that the majority of estrogen precursors are derived from the fetal adrenal (22). The fetal adrenal secretes more than 200 mg of the C-19 compound dehydroepiandrosterone sulfate (DHEA-S) daily, which corresponds to levels 10-fold higher than those of the adult (23). Extensive sulfatase activity in the placenta provides DHEA precursor from DHEA-S which is subsequently converted by 3-β-ol hydroxysteroid dehydrogenase/Δ^4-Δ^5 isomerase to androstenedione. Androstenedione is then rapidly converted to either estrone by aromatase or to estradiol by a two-step process (first to the more potent androgen testosterone and later to estradiol). Thus the large production of DHEA-S by the fetal adrenal serves as an important precursor for the formation of both estrone and estradiol in pregnancy. It is estimated that only 50% of maternal circulating estrone and estradiol at term are derived

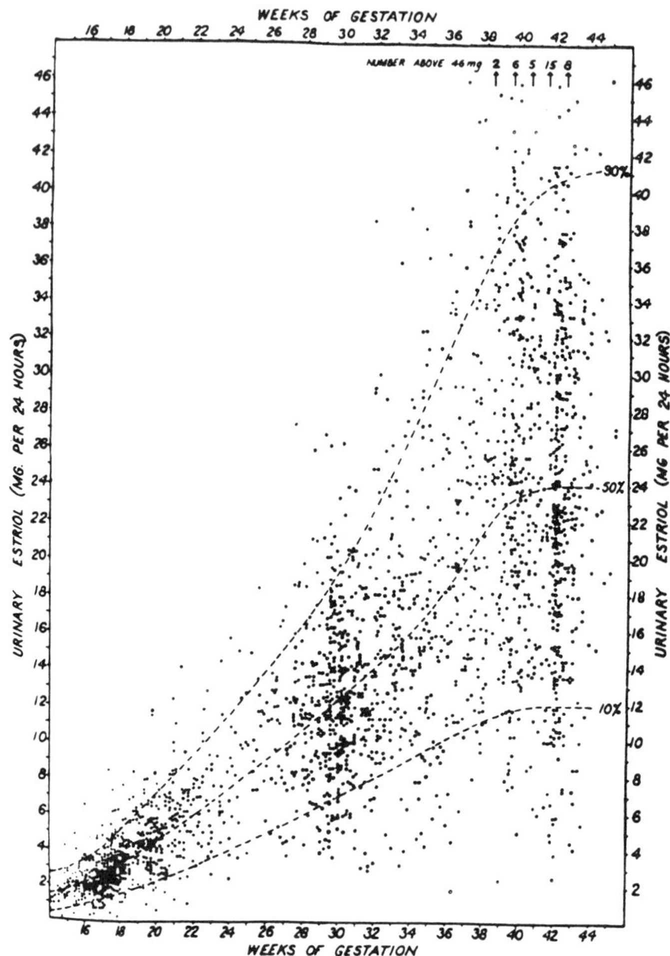

Figure 2 Urinary estriol values from 14 to 44 weeks of pregnancy demonstrating 10%, 50% and 90% percentiles. (From Beischer T, et al., Am J Obstet Gynecol 1969; 103:483.)

from fetal DHEA, with maternal DHEA providing the precursor for the remaining 50%. The fate of most fetal DHEA, however, is not conversion to estrone and estradiol, but rather it is to undergo 16-hydroxylation in the fetal liver and to a lesser extent in the fetal adrenal itself (24). This leads to the product 16-α-OH DHEA, which is converted by the placenta to a series of 16α-hydroxylated variants of the same steroids along the pathway of estradiol production, including 16-α-OH androstenedione, and ending in the production of estriol. At term, more than 90% of estriol is derived from fetal adrenal precursors. Suppression of maternal and fetal adrenal activity by pharmacological doses of either dexamethasone or prednisone (10–20 mg/day) decreases estrone, estradiol, and estriol. However, the greater suppression of estrone and estradiol than of estriol is consistent with the effects of prednisone being primarily on maternal adrenal function (25).

It has been estimated that the potency of estriol is one-tenth the potency of estrone and one one-hundredth the potency of estradiol, the most potent mammalian estrogen in most biological systems. Estriol has a high affinity for the estrogen receptor, but has an inordinately high disassociation constant as well. Thus, it has a poor ability to form a stable hormone–receptor complex necessary for biological action (26). It has been postulated that estriol may in many cases act as more of an antiestrogen than an estrogen, offering some protection against the effects of the extraordinary hyperestrogenic state of pregnancy. Such estrogenic effects include thromboembolic phenomena and perhaps an increased tendency for breast cancer. It has been shown, however, that early age of first pregnancy is protective against breast cancer, perhaps because of a shortening of the time of unopposed estrogen influence (27). Such protection is potentially the result of antiestrogenic effects afforded by estriol, as a result of its ability to compete for the estrogen receptor without initiating biological action. A further protective mechanism may be the ability of estrogens to induce synthesis of sex hormone-binding globulin (SHBG) (28), which then serves to bind estrogen itself as well as androgens.

Despite the availability of these buffering mechanisms to protect against massive hyperestrogenism, pregnancy must be viewed as a hyperestrogenic state. In fact, a complex mechanism is in place to maintain hyperestrogenism, which involves both fetus and placenta. Estrogen itself is a potent inhibitor of the 3β-ol dehydrogenase enzyme (29) and is more potent than any peptide hormone in this regard (30). The inhibition of this enzyme blocks conversion of fetal adrenal precursors to glucocorticoids, mineralocorticoids, and potent sex steroid products. Thus, at the expense of all other steroid hormones, the high estrogen environment produces an abundance of Δ^5 androgens (DHEA and DHEA-S), which the placenta can rapidly and efficiently convert to even more estrogen.

The effects of the hyperestrogenic state on the mother are clear and dramatic. Among the most prominent of these are the cardiovascular adaptations. Blood flow to the uterus increases severalfold, and it appears that the major agonistic actions of estriol, an otherwise very weak estrogen, during pregnancy may be to induce the increased uteroplacental blood flow necessary for oxygenation and nutritional needs of the fetus. These estrogenic effects on the uterine vascular bed have been shown to be mediated through prostaglandins (31). Other estrogenic, though not estriol-induced, cardiovascular alterations are also thought to be prostaglandin mediated. Among these is a decrease in vascular resistance (32). This is in part related to selective dilation of vascular beds, as reflected by a 30–80% increase in renal blood flow (33–35) and an increase in skin perfusion (36). The latter frequently results in an increase in skin temperature and clamminess of the extremities in pregnant women. Vascular spiders and palmer erythema are additional manifestations of increased cutaneous flow. Nasal congestion, which is one of the most persistently bothersome complaints in pregnancy, is also believed to result from increased vascular flow to the nasal mucosa (37). Other mucous membranes, notably the gums, undergo hyperemic changes as well, leading to an increased tendency to bleed during minor trauma. Occasionally a highly vascular lesion of the mouth may develop, called the pregnancy epulis. This regresses spontaneously after delivery.

In addition to vasodilatation and development of a low-resistance uteroplacental vascular bed, pregnancy is marked by dramatic increases in circulating blood volume. Although wide variations have been reported, the best estimate is that a 50% increase in blood volume occurs (38). The increase in blood volume is most pronounced in the first half of pregnancy (39). Based on experimental evidence using estrogen treatment in a variety of non-pregnancy-related conditions, it appears that estrogen may be the key mediator of the hypervolemia (40–42). Several investigators have demonstrated that renin is stimulated by estrogen (43,44). The estrogen-induced increase in renin initiates a cascade of events in which angiotensin-II levels increase, aldosterone increases and, as a result, sodium and water absorption is increased with the net effect of increasing blood volume substantially. Of interest is the well-described resistance of the vasculature of pregnant women to constriction with increased angiotensin-II levels (45). This decreased sensitivity can be reversed by administration of indomethacin or aspirin (46), suggesting a prostaglandin-mediated mechanism.

The increase in the plasma compartment during pregnancy exceeds that of the increase in erythrocyte production, leading to the "physiological anemia of pregnancy." Nonetheless, a 33% increase in red cell mass has been observed (47). The possibility that this may be due to placental lactogen-induced increases in erthropoetin has been suggested based on animal studies (48,49). Leukocytosis in pregnancy has also been seen (50), although the range is highly variable (5,000–12,000 per mm^3).

The expanded circulatory volume resulting from both increased plasma and erythrocytes results in the typical changes in cardiac examination of the pregnant patient (51). These include exaggerated splitting of the first heart sound, a third heart sound, and a systolic murmur in 90% of patients. Soft diastolic murmurs are heard in 19% of patients and a continuous murmur, believed to result from increased breast vasculature, in 10%.

The well-known hypercoagulability of pregnant women is also believed to be the result of estrogen action. During pregnancy, clotting factors, particularly those which are vitamin K-dependent (II, VII, IX, X), are increased. Similar effects are seen with estrogen-containing oral contraceptive pills (52). The hypercoagulability is furthered by an estrogen-mediated decrease in antithromboplastin-III. (53,54). As a result of these changes in the clotting cascade, coupled with a decreased venous return from the stasis produced by a growing uterus, pulmonary embolic events are more common during pregnancy.

IV. Prostaglandins

During pregnancy, circulating levels of prostaglandin E_2 and $F_{2\alpha}$ are unchanged until just prior to the onset of labor. However, with the onset of labor a dramatic rise in both of these prostaglandins occurs (55). Extensive evidence suggests that these prostaglandin changes are essential for the onset of normal labor (56). Both the fetal membranes (amnion and chorion) and uterine decidua have been demonstrated to produce PGE_1 and PGF_2 from arachondonic acid (57–59). It has been suggested that the initiation of labor is the result of decreasing progesterone concentration (60). This fall in progesterone has been proposed to decrease amniotic epithelium production of a specific prostaglandin synthetase inhibitor (61). Earlier in pregnancy, although no clear changes in *circulating* prostaglandins occur, PGE_2 and PGF_2 concentrations in the local area of the uterus are undoubtedly increased. Increased prostaglandin synthesis outside the reproductive system have been postulated based on evidence that estrogen influences prostaglandin synthesis directly (62,63). This may have particular relevance in pulmonary physiology because of the effects of prostaglandins on bronchi.

Prostaglandin mechanisms are also likely to play a role in pregnancy-induced hypertension (PIH), a common and potentially life-threatening complication of pregnancy. The aforementioned resistance of pregnant women to the pressor effects of angiotensin-II, which appears to be prostaglandin mediated, is lost in those women destined to develop PIH, a finding which may occur as early as 10–14 weeks (64). At present, a predominant hypothesis for the development of PIH is a decreased prostacyclin (PGI_2)-to-thromboxane (TXA_2) ratio (Fig. 3). PGI_2 is a potent

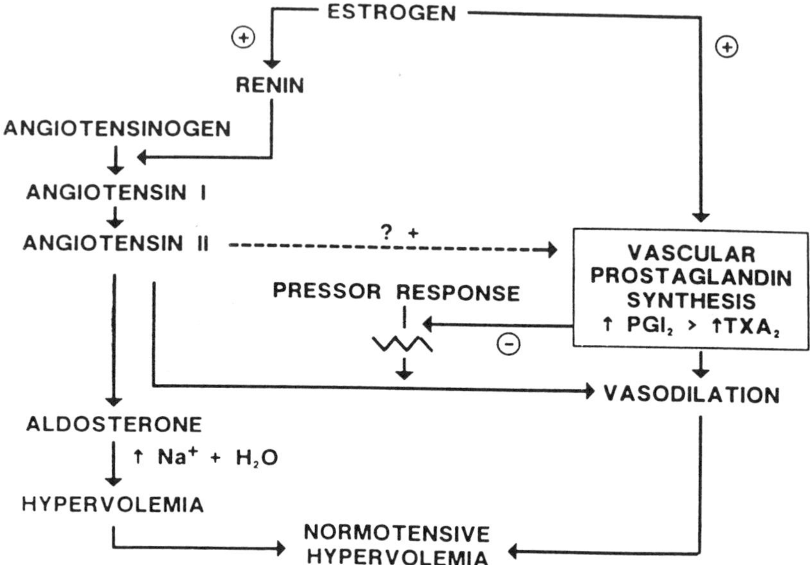

Figure 3 Diagramatic representation of the effects of estrogen on the renin-angiotensin system and vascular prostaglandin synthesis.

vasodilator and TXA_2 a platelet-derived vasoconstrictor. Both PGI_2 and TXA_2 levels are increased in normal pregnancy, although the increase in PGI_2 exceeds that of TXA_2 (65). Several studies have shown a decrease in PGI_2 in PIH as compared with normal pregnancy (66,67). As with the loss of resistance to the pressor effects of angiotensin-II, the decreased prostacyclin levels precede the development of the clinical manifestations of PIH (68). The use of low-dose aspirin has been shown to be able to prevent PIH in high-risk individuals (69,70). When used at low doses, aspirin will decrease TXA_2 selectively, whereas at higher doses inhibition of the true prostaglandins (such as PGI_2) occurs as well (71,72). Thus, use of aspirin in treating PIH should be limited to low-dose regimens.

V. Cortisol and Deoxycorticosterone

In addition to sex steroids, pregnancy is characterized by marked increases in serum cortisol. In 1979, Judziewitsch reported that 9 a.m. cortisol values increased from a nonpregnant range of 4–21 mg/dL to 25–46 mg/dL in the last trimester (73). Despite the increased levels, Carr has shown that the circadian rhythm of cortisol is maintained (74). Although cortisol-binding globulin (CBG) levels triple during pregnancy, an increase in free cortisol has also been reported (75). The increase in cortisol is accompanied by, and perhaps driven by, an increase in ACTH. The magnitude of the increase in cortisol would clearly be sufficient to produce pathological manifestations were it not for the increase in CBG induced by the hyperestrogenism. Thus, a clear buffering mechanism is involved in pregnancy which produces only a moderate increase in free cortisol. Nonetheless, the hypercortisolism is at least one mechanism whereby insulin resistance is induced in pregnancy (76), the others being the result of steroid hormones discussed earlier and of peptide hormones to be discussed later. The effects of the hypercortisolism on immunological function in pregnancy may also be profound. As early as 1938, Hench (77) observed a decrease in symptoms in 43 patients with rheumatoid arthritis and used the hypercortisolism of pregnancy as a rationale for treating nonpregnant patients with cortisone. More recently, however, Unger et al. (78) reported an inverse correlation between pregnancy-associated α_2 globulin levels and symptoms in rheumatoid arthritis patients, suggesting that other factors may be of greater significance when remission is observed.

The elevated cortisol levels in pregnancy are accompanied by elevated circulating corticotropin-releasing hormone (CRH) levels (79) as well as increased placental CRH content (80) as gestation progresses. It is likely that placental CRH stimulates cortisol production through an ACTH-mediated pathway in the fetus as well as the maternal adrenal, and a role for this increased cortisol production in the initiation of parturition has been proposed (81). This interesting possibility awaits further study.

Although normal during the majority of gestation, a dramatic increase in deoxycorticosterone (DOC) levels is found in late gestation. The possibilities include that this arises directly from the fetus or from the conversion of progesterone derived from the placenta (82). In favor of fetal production is the finding that dexamethasone, which suppresses maternal ACTH levels, does not reduce DOC levels. The significance of the higher levels of DOC in late gestation is poorly understood. DOC, as well as progesterone and aldosterone, competitively bind the corticosteroid receptor, albeit with a lower affinity than glucocoroticoids, and may therefore serve as important additional buffers of the hypercortisolemia of pregnancy (83–85).

VI. hCG

Human chorionic gonadotropin (hCG) is a peptide hormone that is essential to maintenance of pregnancy because it is required to stimulate production of estrogen and progesterone. hCG is produced by the embryonic tissue even prior to implantation. Its presence in the maternal circulation is detectable as early as 24 hr after implantation. hCG is structurally homologous and has physiological function similar to luteinizing hormone (LH). Its first action in early pregnancy is to maintain the corpus luteum, which it does more effectively than LH itself, probably because its increased carbohydrate content markedly prolongs its half-life in the circulation. Serum hCG values in the first trimester of pregnancy rise rapidly, from nearly undetectable levels to values exceeding 100,000 mIU/mL. Subsequent to the first trimester, hCG levels decline markedly compared to their first-trimester peak, although they remain several thousandfold greater than in the nonpregnant state (Fig. 4).

In addition to functioning as a gonadotropin in maintenance of the corpus luteum, Jaffe and colleagues (86) have demonstrated that hCG may regulate DHEA production by the fetal zone of the fetal adrenal gland during early gestation, implicating a dual role for the hormone as a corticotropin as well as a gonadotropin. Moreover, hCG has been shown to possess thyrotropin activity as well. hCG is likely to be one mechanism for the increased T4 levels seen in pregnancy (87). Of particular interest has been the suggestion that, like progesterone (88), hCG may have im-

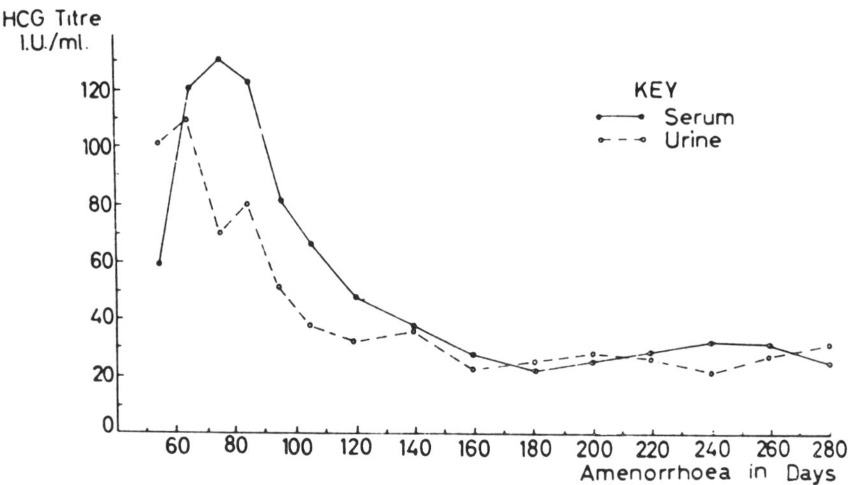

Figure 4 Mean levels of serum and urine chorionic gonadatropin in 600 normal pregnant women. (From Teoh, J Obstet Gynaecol Br Commun 1967; 74:77.)

munosuppressive effects in addition to its endocrine actions (89). Teasdale et al. (90) have shown that hCG inhibits blast cell transformation induced by either phytohemagglutinin or mixed lymphocyte reactions.

VII. Placental Growth Hormones

Human chorionic somatomammotropin (hCS), better known as human placental lactogen (hPL) because of its lactogenic properties in animals (91), is produced in abundant quantities during pregnancy. Until recently, it was considered the sole placental analog of growth hormone (GH), and as a result it has been extensively studied. Circulating concentrations of hCS are directly proportional to placental weight (92), and therefore maternal serum levels rise steadily until the 36th week of gestation (Fig. 5). hCS has been shown to possess similar somatotrophc effects to GH in most animal models, although its biological activity is only 3% or less that of

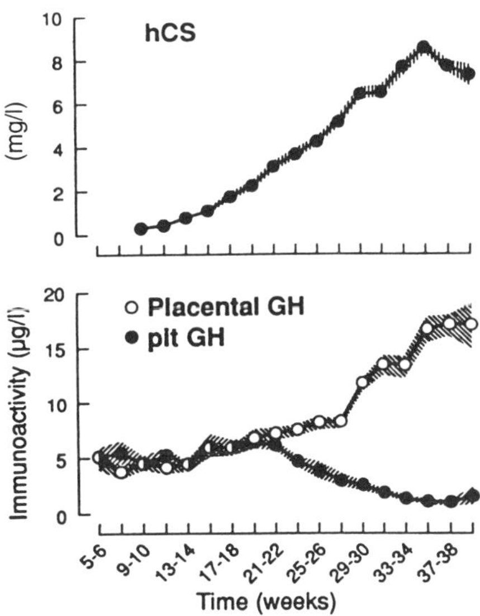

Figure 5 Time course of human placental growth hormone (hPGH) secretion along with its parallelism to human chorionic somatostatin (hCS) and its divergence from that of pituitary growth hormone during pregnancy. (Modified by Yen SSC for Ref. 97.)

GH. hCS is not required for normal pregnancy, since an hCS-deficient patient has been reported to have delivered a normal fetus (93). However, the fact that it does not appear to be essential in a patient with good nutritional health should not be construed to indicate that hCS does not have significant biological effects during normal pregnancy. By the last 4 weeks of pregnancy, mean hCS levels reach 5.4 mg/mL, at least a thousandfold higher than GH levels. In addition to production of hCS, the placenta also produces insulin-like growth factor-1 (IGF-1), providing possible increased potential for hCS action. The extent to which this IGF is buffered by changes in placentally produced IGF-binding protein is not known (94,95).

More recently, two forms of human placental growth hormone (hPGH) distinct from hCS have been identified. Like hCS, hPGH levels increase steadily until term (96). It appears likely that this hPGH suppresses pituitary GH, either directly or via a hypothalamic mechanism, since pituitary GH levels fall throughout pregnancy, independent of changes in IGF-1 (97). Several buffering mechanisms are operative during pregnancy to mitigate the effects of increased GH levels. These include the upregulation of GH-binding protein by estrogen (98), and the increased circulating levels of IGF-binding protein-1 and IGF binding protein-3 to reduce the bioactivity of any GH-induced IGF-1 production that may occur (99).

Largely due to the actions of placental growth hormones (hPGH and hCS), pregnancy has been described by Felig as a "state of accelerated starvation" (100). These hormones confer an insulin-resistant state on pregnancy which is augmented by the anti-insulin actions of estrogen and cortisol as well. Placental levels of hCS are regulated by circulating glucose levels, analogous to the control of pituitary growth hormone. Therefore, in hypoglycemic conditions there is an accelerated release of free fatty acids (accelerated starvation) due to increased hCS levels. In the fed state, when glucose levels increase, the anti-insulin action of hCS serves to maintain higher serum glucose levels. Consequently more glucose is available for transport to the fetus. As a further result of the anti-insulin effects of hCS, pregnancy is characterized by an increase of free fatty acids in excess of the increased total lipids, with no change in the percentage of esterified cholesterol (101).

In pregnancy, therefore, during periods of fasting, there is more ketonuria than in the nonpregnant state. Due to the anti-insulin effect of placental growth hormones (and cortisol), pregnant patients are also prone to the development of gestational diabetes. As expected, in women who develop gestational diabetes, infection has been shown to be more common and more difficult to treat than in nondiabetic pregnancies.

VIII. Thyroid Hormones

In addition to the thyrotropic effect of hCG, the placenta secretes human chorionic thyrotrophin (hCT) and thyrotropin-releasing hormone (TRH). The production of TRH by the placenta is analogous to the placental production of other releasing peptides and inhibiting factors such as CRH, TRH, and somatostatin. As in other systems, a buffering effect to protect against overt hyperthyroidism in pregnancy is present. Although total T_4 levels are increased in pregnancy, a marked increase in thyroid-binding globulin (TBG) is stimulated by estrogen, such that free T_4 and free T_3 levels are normal (102). The increase in TBG is apparent by the marked decrease in T_3 resin uptake (T_3 RU) seen in pregnancy, since T_3 RU serves as an indirect measure of TBG.

IX. Prolactin

The influence of pregnancy on prolactin (PRL), a hormone closely related to hCS and GH, is unique. Estrogen increases pituitary production of prolactin. In the pregnant state prolactin levels reach at least four times the nonpregnant value as a result of hyperestrogenism. This increase is accompanied by a doubling in size of the pituitary gland due to lactotroph hypertrophy. Unlike most hormones of pregnancy, PRL is produced primarily by the fetal membranes rather than the placenta itself. It has been demonstrated to play an osmoregulatory role in amniotic fluid, reminiscent of its primary role in lower vertebrates. The majority of prolactin released into the maternal circulation, however, is of maternal pituitary origin. Again, a buffering mechanism is present. Estrogen, which hypertrophies the lactotroph in preparation for its formidable postpartum task of producing adequate prolactin to stimulate milk production, simultaneously inhibits prolactin action in the breast. It is only after the clearance of estrogen from the circulation which results from placental expulsion at delivery that the effects of hyperprolactmenia are manifest in milk production.

X. Calcitropic Hormones

The need for calcium represents one of the most dramatic requirements of the growing fetus. During pregnancy, 30 g are deposited into the fetus for incorporation into bone. It is expected, then, that specific mechanisms must exist for this transfer. One such mechanism is altered vitamin D metabolism in pregnancy. As in the nonpregnant state, the conversion of vitamin

D_3 to 25-hydroxy vitamin D_3 takes place in the maternal liver. It is the 1-hydroxylation step, however, that is the rate-limiting step in production of the active metabolite 1,25-dihydrocholecalciferol [1,25-$(OH)_2$ D_3]. In pregnancy, 1-hydroxylase is present in the placenta and endometrial decidua as well in the proximal convoluted tubules of the kidney, where it is found in both the pregnant and nonpregnant states. The increased hydroxylation sites as well as the increased availability of the precursor 25-OH D_3 explain the increased levels of vitamin D_3 during pregnancy (103). The twofold rise in circulating levels of vitamin D_3 might be sufficient for the development of toxic manifestations except that a concomitant twofold increase in the buffering hormone, vitamin D_3-binding protein (DBP), is also observed. The effect of the increased vitamin D_3 is primarily to enhance intestinal calcium absorption. PTH levels have also been reported to be somewhat elevated in pregnancy, as has parathyroid hormone-related peptide (PTH-RP) (104). PTH is secreted in response to decreased levels of ionized calcium in the extracellular fluid. The minimal (if any) increase in PTH during pregnancy reflects the careful homeostasis of calcium metabolism. Calcium is obtained from maternal serum for fetal use by an active ATP-dependent calcium pump within the placenta (105). However, the maternal hypocalcemia which may result from such shunting appears to be offset by the increased rate of calcium absorption. Consequently, only a minimal PTH response is noted. This minimal increase in PTH has earned pregnancy the reputation of "physiological hyperparathyroidism." Hypercalcemia, on the other hand, which may result from increased absorption as a result of increased 1,25-vitamin D_3, is compensated for by increased calcitonin. Calcitonin levels have been reported to be increased in pregnancy (106). This may serve as a protective mechanism against the hypercalcemia that would result from both increased absorption and increased bone resorption caused by increased PTH levels.

XI. Summary

From an endocrinological perspective, then, pregnancy appears to be a state of tremendous hormonal excess, providing optimal reserves for the maternal adaptations designed to protect the requirements of the developing fetus. This excess, however, is compensated for by a variety of buffering systems, such as estriol and SHBG for estrogen, TBG for thyroid, and CBG for cortisol. Nonetheless, the hormonal milieu of the pregnant woman is such that in most cases the slight excesses in active hormones that persist over the attempts to buffer them produce profound effects in the mother.

This system of "checked excess" provides both for physiological adaptation in normal circumstances and a reserve for periods of physiological stress. It is clear that many of these hormones exert their influence through second messengers, even in the case of steroids (i.e., prostaglandins). Of particular interest to the field of allergy are the effects of these hormones on prostaglandin synthesis and the immunosuppressive actions of progesterone, cortisol, and perhaps the most crucial regulator of the endocrine events of pregnancy, hCG itself.

References

1. Catt KJ, Dufau ML, Vaitukaitis JL. Appearance of hCG in pregnancy following the initiation of implantation of the blastocyst. J Clin Endocrinol Metab 1975; 40:537–540.
2. Hellig HD, Gattereau D, Lefevre Y, Bolte E. Steroid production from plasma cholesterol: I. Conversion of plasma cholesterol to placental progesterone in humans. J Clin Endocrinol Metab 1975; 30:624–631.
3. Noyes RW, Hertig AT, Rock J. Dating the endometrial biopsy. Fertil Steril 1950; 1:23–25.
4. Roberts DK, Horbelt DV, Powell LC. The ultrastructural response of human endometrium to medroxyprogesterone acetate. Am J Obstet Gynecol 1975; 123:811–818.
5. Wynn RM. Electron microscopy of the developing decidua. Fertil Steril 1965; 16:16–26.
6. Arias-Stella J. Atypical endometrial changes associated with presence of chorionic tissue. Arch Pathol 1968; 58:112–128.
7. Collins JA, Jerkes DM. Progesterone metabolism by proliferative and secretory human endometrium. Am J Obstet Gynecol 1978; 118:179–185.
8. Bulmer JN, Johnson PM. Immunohistological characterization of the decidual leukocytic infiltrate related to endometrial gland epithelium in early human pregnancy. Immunology 1985; 55:35.
9. Romero R, Wu Y-K, Brody DT, Oyarzun E, Duff GW, Durum SK. Human decidua: a source of interleukin-1. Obstet Gynecol 1984; 73:31.
10. Vanue E, Allen P. The basis for the immunoregulatory role of macrophages and other accessory cells. Science 1987; 236:551.
11. Polan ML, Loukides J, Nelson P, Cushing S, Diamond M, Welsh A, Bottomly K. Progesterone and estradiol modulate interleukin 1-β messenger riboneucleic acid levels in cultured human periferal monocytes. J Clin Endocrinol Metab 1989; 69:1200.
12. Gant NF, Worley RJ, Everett RB, MacDonald PC. Control of vascular responsiveness during human pregnancy. Kidney Int 1980; 18:253–258.
13. Metcalfe J, Ueland K. Maternal cardiovascular adjustments to pregnancy. Prog Cardiovasc Dis 1974; 16:363–374.

14. Gee JBL, Packer BS, Millen JE, Robin ED. Pulmonary mechanics during pregnancy. J Clin Invest 1967; 46:945–952.

15. Sutton FD, Zwillich CW, Creagh E, Pierson DJ, Weil JV. Progesterone for the outpatient treatment of Pickwickian syndrome. Ann Intern Med 1975; 83:476–479.

16. Shulman A, Herlinger H. Urinary tract dilation in pregnancy. Br J Radiol 1975; 48:638–645.

17. Van Wegenen G, Jenkins RH. An experimental examination of factors causing ureteral dilation of pregnancy. J Urol 1939; 42:1010–1020.

18. Costrini NV, Kalkoff RK. Relative effects of pregnancy, estradiol and progesterone on plasma insulin and pancreatic islet insulin secretion. J Clin Invest 1971; 50:922–927.

19. Kalkoff RK, Jacobson M, Lemper D. Progesterone, pregnancy and the augmented plasma insulin response. J Clin Endocrinol Metab 1970; 31:24–29.

20. Buster JE, Abraham GE. The applications of steroid hormone radioimmunoassays to clinical obstetrics. Obstet Gynecol 1975; 46:489–499.

21. Goebelsmann U, Chen LC, Saga M, Nakamura RM, Jaffe RB. Plasma concentration and binding protein of oestriol and its conjugates in pregnancy. Acta Endocrinol (Kbh) 1973; 74:592–604.

22. Siiteri PK, MacDonald PC. Placental estrogen biosynthesis during human pregnancy. J Clin Endocrinol Metab 1966; 26:751–761.

23. Madden JD, Gant NF, MacDonald PC. Study of the kinetics of conversion of maternal plasma dehydroisoandrosterone sulfate to 16α-hydroxy-dehydroisoandrosterone sulfate, estradiol and estriol. Am J Obstet Gynecol 1978; 132:392–395.

24. Perez-Palacios G, Perez AE, Jaffe RB. Conversion of pregnenolone $7-\alpha^3$H-sulfate to other Δ^5-3β-0l-hydroxysteroid sulfates by the human fetal adrenal in vitro. J Clin Endocrinol Metab 1965; 28:19–25.

25. Challis J, Patrick J, Richardson B, Tevaarwerk G. Loss of diurnal rhythm in plasma estrone, estradiol and estriol in women treated with glucocorticoids at 34 to 35 weeks gestation. Am J Obstet Gynecol 1981; 139:338–343.

26. Clark JH, Paszko Z, Peck EJ JR. Nuclear binding and retention of the receptor estrogen complex: relationship of the agonistic and antagonistic properties of estriol. Endocrinology 1977; 100:91–96.

27. Korenman SG. Estrogen window hypothesis of the etiology of breast cancer. Lancet 1980; i:700–701.

28. Anderson DC. Sex hormone binding globulin. Clin Endocrinol (Oxf) 1964; 3:69–96.

29. Byrne GC, Perry YS, Winter JSD. Steroid inhibitory effects upon human adrenal 3β-hydroxysteroid dehydrogenase activity. J Clin Endocrinol Metab 1986; 62:413–418.

30. Fujieda K, Faiman C, Feyes FI, Winter JSD. The control of steroidogenesis by human fetal adrenal cells in tissue culture: III. The effects of various hormonal peptides. J Clin Endocrinol Metab 1981; 53:690–693.

31. Resnik R., Brink GW. Modulating effects of prostaglandins on the uterine vascular bed. Gynecol Invest 1977; 8:10.
32. Greiss FC, Anderson SG. Effect of ovarian hormones on the uterine vascular bed. Am J Obstet Gynecol 1970; 107:829–836.
33. Nunlap W. Serial changes in renal hemodynamics during normal human pregnancy. Br J Obstet Gynaecol 1981; 88:1–9.
34. Little B. Water and electrolyte balance during pregnancy. Anaethesiology 1965; 26:400–408.
35. Chesley LC. Renal function changes in normal pregnancy. Clin Obstet Gynecol 1960; 3:349–363.
36. Katz M, Sokal MM. Skin perfusion in pregnancy. Am J Obstet Gynecol 1980; 137:30–33.
37. Fabricant ND. Sexual functions and the nose. Am J Med Sci 1960; 239:498–502.
38. Pritchard JA, Rowland RC. Blood volume changes in pregnancy and the puerperium. III. Whole body and large vessel hematocrits in pregnant and non-pregnant women. Am J Obstet Gynecol 1964; 88:391–395.
39. Lund CJ, Donovan JC. Blood volume during pregnancy. Am J Obstet Gynecol 1967; 98:393–403.
40. Longo LD. Maternal blood volume and cardiac output during pregnancy: a hypothesis of endocrinologic control. Am J Physiol 1983; 245:R720–R729.
41. Friedlander M, Laskey N, Silbert T. Effect of estrogenic substance on blood volume. Endocrinology 1936; 20:329–332.
42. Tapia HR, Johnson CE, Strong CG. Effects of oral contraceptive therapy on the renin-angiotensin system in normotensive and hypertensive women. J Obstet Gynecol 1973; 41:643–649.
43. Crane MG, Heitsch J, Harris JJ, Johns VJ. Jr. Effect of ethinyl estradiol (estinyl) on plasma renin activity. J Clin Endocrinol Metab 1966; 26:1403–1406.
44. Hsueh WA, Luetscher JA, Carlson EJ, Grislis G, Fraze E, McHargue A. Changes in active and inactive renin throughout pregnancy. J Clin Endocrinol Metab 1982; 54:1010–1016.
45. Abdul-Karim R, Assali NS. Pressor response to angiotonin in pregnant and non-pregnant women. Am J Obstet Gynecol 1961; 82:246–251.
46. Everett RB, Worley RJ, MacDonald PC, Gant NF. Effect of prostaglandin synthetase inhibitors on pressor response to angiotensin II in human pregnancy. J Clin Endocrinol Metab 1978; 46:1007–1010.
47. Pritchard JA, Adams RH. Erythrocyte production and destruction during pregnancy. Am J Obstet Gynecol 1960; 79:750–757.
48. Cotes PM, Canning CE, Lind T. Changes in serum immunoreactive erythropoietin during the menstrual cycle and normal pregnancy. Br J Obstet Gynaecol 1983; 90:304–311.
49. Jepson JH, Friesen HG. The mechanism of action of human placental lactogen on erythropoiesis. Br J Haematol 1968; 15:465–471.

50. Efrati P., Presentey B, Margalith M, Rozenszajn L. Leukocytes of normal pregnant women. Obstet Gynecol 1964; 23:429–432.
51. Cutforth R, MacDonald CB. Heart sounds and murmurs in pregnancy. Am Heart J 1966; 71:741–747.
52. Ambrus CM, Niswander KR, Courey NG, Mink IB. Effect of contraceptive drugs on the blood coagulation system. Hematol Rev 1970; 2:163–168.
53. Zuck TF, Bergin JJ, Raymond JM, Dwyre WR. Implications of depressed antithrombin-III activity associated with oral contraceptives. Surg Gynecol Obstet 1971; 133:609–612.
54. Ambrus JL, Ambrus CM, Lillie MA, Browne BJ, Hanson FW, Niswander K., Witul M, Jung OS, Bartfay-Szabo A. Effects of various estrogen treatment schedules on antithrombin-III levels. Res Commun Chem Pathol Pharmacol 1976; 14:543–549.
55. Davidson BJ, Murray RD, Challis JRG, Valenzuela GJ. Estrogen, progesterone, prolactin, prostaglandin E_2, prostaglandin $F_{2\alpha}$, 13, 14-dihydro-15-keto-prostaglandin $F_{2\alpha}$, and 6-keto-prostaglandin $F_{1\alpha}$ gradients across the uterus in labor and not in labor. Am J Obstet Gynecol 1987; 157:54–59.
56. Nelson GH, Fadel HE. Prostaglandins and parturition. Semin Reprod Endocrinol 1985; 3:231–237.
57. Gustavii B. Release of lysosomal acid phosphatase into the cytoplasm of decidual cells before the onset of labor in humans. Br J Obstet Gynaecol 1975; 82:177–182.
58. Schwartz BE, Schultz FM, MacDonald PC, Johnston JM. Initiation of human parturition: III. Fetal membrane content of prostaglandin E_2 and F_2 precursor. Obstet Gynecol 1975; 46:564–570.
59. Curbelo V., Bejar R., Benirschke K., Gluck L. Premature labor: 1. Prostaglandin precursors in human placental membranes. Obstet Gynecol 1981; 57:473–478.
60. Khan-Dawood FS. In vitro conversion of pregnenolone to progesterone in human term placenta and fetal membranes before and after the onset of labor. Am J Obstet Gynecol 1987; 157:1333–1337.
61. Mortimer G, Hunter IC, Stimson WH, Govan ADT. A role for amniotic epithelium in the control of human parturition. Lancet 1985; i:1074–1076.
62. Auletta FJ, Agins H, Scommegna A. Prostaglandin $F_{2\alpha}$ mediation of the inhibitory effect of estrogen on the corpus luteum of the rhesus monkey. Endocrinology 1978; 103:1183–1189.
63. Auletta FJ, Caldwell BV, Speroff L. Estrogen induced luteolysis in the rhesus monkey: reversal with indomethacin. Prostaglandins 1976; 11:745–752.
64. Gant NF, Daley GL, Chand S, Whalley PJ, MacDonald PC. A study of angiotensin II pressor response throughout primagravid pregnancy. J Clin Invest 1973; 52:2682–2689.
65. Fitzgerald DJ, Mayo G, Catella F, Entman SS, Fitzgerald GA. Increased thromboxone biosynthesis in normal pregnancy is mainly derived from platelets. Am J Obstet Gynecol 1987; 157:325–331.

66. Ylikorkala O, Pekonen F, Viinikka L. Renal prostacyclin and thromboxane in normotensive and preeclamptic pregnant women and their infants. J Clin Endocrinol Metab 1987; 63:1307–1312.

67. Goodman RP, Killam AP, Brash AR, Branch RA. Prostacyclin production during normal pregnancy and pregnancy complicated by hypertension. Am J Obstet Gynecol 1982; 142:817–822.

68. Fitzgerald DJ, Entman SS, Mulloy K, Fitzgerald GA. Decreased prostacyclin biosynthesis preceding the clinical manifestations of pregnancy-induced hypertension. Circulation 1987; 75:956–963.

69. Beaufils M, Donsimoni R, Uzan S, Colau JC. Prevention of pre-eclampsia by early antiplatelet therapy. Lancet 1985; ii:240–243.

70. Wallenberg HCS, Dekker GA, Makovitz JW, Rotmans P. Low dose aspirin prevents pregnancy-induced hypertension and preeclampsia in angiotensin-sensitive primigravida. Lancet 1986; i:1–6.

71. Masotti G, Poggesi L, Galanti G, Abbate R, Neri Serneri GG. Differential inhibition of prostaglandin production and platelet aggregation by aspirin. Lancet 1979; ii:1213–1216

72. Ritter JM, Farquhar C, Rodin A, Thom MH. Low dose aspirin treatment in late pregnancy differentially inhibits cyclo-oxygenase in maternal platelets. Prostaglandins 1987; 34:717–721.

73. Judzewitsch R. Thyroid and adrenal function. In: Shearman RP, ed. Reproductive Physiology. 2d ed. Oxford: Blackwell Scientific, 1979.

74. Carr BR, Parker CRP Jr., Madden JD. Maternal plasma adrenocorticotropin and cortisol relationships throughout human pregnancy. Am J Obstet Gynecol 1981; 139:416–422.

75. Nolten WE, Rueckert PA. Elevated free cortisol index in pregnancy: possible regulatory mechanisms. Am J Obstet Gynecol 1981; 139:492–498.

76. Fain JN. Inhibition of glucose transport in fat cells and activation of lipolysis by glucocorticoids. In: Baxter JD, Rousseau GG, eds. Glucocorticoid Hormone Action. New York: Springer-Verlag, 1979:547–560.

77. Hench PG. Ameliorating effect of pregnancy on chronic atrophic (infectious rheumatoid) arthritis, fibrositis and intermittent hydrarthrosis. Proc Mayo Clin 1938; 13:161–168.

78. Unger A, Kay A, Griffin AJ, Panayi GS. Disease activity and pregnancy associated α_2-glycoprotein in rheumatoid arthritis. Br Med J 1983; 286: 750–752.

79. Campbell EA, Linton EA, Wolfe CDA, Scraggs PR, Jones MT, Lowry DJ. Plasma corticotropin-releasing hormone concentrations during pregnancy and parturition. J Clin Endocrinol Metab 1987; 64:1054.

80. Frim DM, Emanuel RL, Robinson BG, Smas CM, Adler GK, Majzoub JN. Characterization and gestational regulation of corticotropin releasing hormone messenger RNA in human placenta. J Clin Invest 1988; 82:287.

81. Robinson BC, Emanuel RL, Frim DM, Majzoub JN. Glucocorticoid stimulates expression of corticotropin-releasing hormone gene in human placenta. Proc Natl Acad Sci USA 1985; 85:5244.

82. Winkel CA, Parker CR Jr, Milewich L, Simpson ER, Gant NF, MacDonald PC. The conversion of plasma progesterone to deoxycorticosterone (DOC) in men, nonpregnant and pregnant women and adrenalectomized subjects: evidence for steroid 21-hydroxylase activity in non-adrenal tissues. J Clin Invest 1980; 66:803–812.

83. Munch A, Brinck-Johnsen T. Specific and nonspecific physiochemical interactions of glucocorticoids and related steroids with rat thymus cells in vitro. J Biol Chem 1968; 10:5556–5565.

84. Bell PA. Agonists, antagonists and models for glucorticoid-receptor interactions. Biochem Soc Trans 1977; 5:639–642.

85. Rousseau GG, Baxter JD, Tomkins GM. Glucocorticoid receptors: relations between steroid binding and biological effects. J Mol Biol 1972; 67:99–115.

86. Seron-Ferre M., Lawrence CC, Jaffe RB. Role of hCG in the regulation of the fetal zone of the human fetal adrenal gland. J Clin Endocrinol Metab 1978; 46:834–837.

87. Nisula BC, Ketlslegers JM. Thyroid stimulating activity and chorionic gonadotropin. J Clin Invest 1974; 54:494–499.

88. Siiteri PK, Febres LE, Clemens LE, Chang RJ, Gondus B, Stites D. Progesterone and the maintenance of pregnancy: is progesterone nature's immunosuppressant? Ann NY Acad Sci 1977; 286:384–397.

89. Carr MC, Stites DP, Fudenberg HH. Cellular aspects of human fetal maternal relationship. II. *In vitro* response of gravida lymphocytes to phytohemagglutinin. Cell Immunol 1973; 8:448–454.

90. Teasdale FE, Adcock EW III, August CS, Cox S, Battaglia FC, Naughton MA. Human chorionic gonadotropin: inhibitory effect on mixed lymphocyte cultures. Gynecol Invest 1973; 4:263–269.

91. Josimovich JB, MacLaren JA. Presence in human placenta and term serum of highly lactogenic substance immunologically related to pituitary growth hormone. Endocrinology 1962; 71:209–220.

92. Selenkow HA, Saxena BM, Dana CL, Emerson K Jr. Measurements and pathologic significance of human placental lactogen. In: Peck A, Fenzi C, eds. The Foeto-Placental Unit. Amsterdam: Excerpta Medica, 1964.

93. Nielsen PV, Pederson H, Karpmann E. Absence of human placental lactogen in an otherwise uneventful pregnancy. Am J Obstet Gynecol 1979; 135: 322–326.

94. Kaistinen R, Kalkkinen N, Huhtala M-L, Seppala M, Bohn H, Rutanen E-M. Placental protein 12 is a decidual protein that binds somatomedin and has an identical N-terminal amino acid sequence with somatomedin binding protein from human amniotic fluid. Endocrinology 1986; 118:1375–1378.

95. Baxter RC, Martin JL, Wood MH. Two immunoreactive binding proteins for insulin-like growth factors in human amniotic fluid: relationship to fetal maturity. J Clin Endocrinol Metab 1987; 65:423–431.

96. Eriksson L, Frankeene F, Eden S, Hennen C, Von Schoultz B. Growth hormone 24-hour serum profiles during pregnancy: lack of pulsatility for the secretion of the placental variant. Br J Obstet Gynaecol 1989; 96:949.

97. Frankeene F, Closset J, Gomez F, Scippo ML, Snel J, Hennen G. The physiology of growth hormone (GHs) in pregnant women and partial characterization of the placental GH variant. J Clin Endocrinol Metab 1988; 66:1771.

98. Blumefield Z, Barkley RJ, Yardin MB, Bradlee JM, Amit T. Growth hormone (GH)-binding protein regulation by estrogen, progesterone and gonadotropins in humans: The effect of ovulation induction, menopausal gonadotropins, GH and gestation. J Clin Endocrinol Metab 1992; 75:1242–1249.

99. Drop SLA, Mortleve DJ, Guyda HJ, Povner BI. Immunoassay of a somatomedin-binding protein from human amniotic fluid: levels in fetal, neonatal and adult serum. J Clin Endocrinol Metab 1984; 59:908.

100. Felig P, Lynch V. Starvation in human pregnancy: hypoglycemia, hypoinsulinemia and hyperketonemia. Science 1970; 170:990–992.

101. Hollingsworth DR. Alterations of maternal metabolism in normal and diabetic pregnancies in insulin-dependent, non insulin dependent and gestational diabetes. Am J Obstet Gynecol 1983; 146:417–429.

102. Dowling JT, Appleton WG, Nicoloff JT. Thyroxine turnover during human pregnancy. J Clin Endocrinol Metab 1967; 27:1749.

103. Weisman Y, Harrell A, Edelstein S. 1–25-dihydroxyvitamin D_3 and 24, 25 dihydroxyvitamin D_3 *in vitro* synthesis by human decidua and placenta. Nature 1979; 281:317–319.

104. Gallagher SJ, Fraser WD, Owens OJ, Dryburgh FJ, Logue FS, Jenkins A, Kennedy J, Bayle IT. Changes in calciotropic hormones and biochemical markers of bone turnover in normal human pregnancy. Eur J Endocrinol 1994; 131:364–374.

105. Fleishman AR. Fetal parathyroid gland and calcium homeostasis. Clin Obstet Gynecol 1980; 25:791–802.

106. Pitkin RM, Reynold WA, Williams GA, Hargis GK. Calcium metabolism in normal pregnancy: a longitudinal study. Am J Ostet Gynecol 1979; 133: 781–790.

2

Fetal Oxygenation, Acid–Base Balance, and Assessment of Well-Being in the Pregnancy Complicated by Asthma or Anaphylaxis

LARRY COUSINS and VALERIAN A. CATANZARITE

Mary Birch Hospital for Women at Sharp Memorial
San Diego, California

I. Introduction

Asthma, the most common chronic respiratory disease seen in pregnant women, affects between 1:80 and 1:200 gravidas (1,2). This overall rate, combined with the 0.2–0.5% prevalence of life-threatening asthma or status asthmaticus in pregnancy (1,3), emphasizes the frequency of risk to which the asthmatic gravida and her fetus may be exposed.

The objectives of this chapter are to review the general issues related to fetal oxygenation, including determinants of uteroplacental-fetal oxygenation and blood flow considerations; to review the impact of alterations in fetal acid–base status on perinatal outcome and methods of assessing fetal well-being; and to recommend an approach to fetal evaluation in pregnancies complicated by asthma or anaphylaxis.

This chapter will not deal in detail with issues addressed elsewhere in this volume that may indirectly influence fetal oxygenation—for example, hormonally induced alterations in respiratory center function, carbon dioxide sensitivity, or bronchial muscular tone; changes in ventilatory mechanics as a result of the enlarging, gravid uterus or alterations in large or small airway function; the natural history of asthma in pregnancy; or the medical management of asthma in pregnancy.

II. Respiratory Gas Exchange

A. Respiratory Gas Transport Between the Atmosphere and the Fetus

The transport of oxygen from the atmosphere to fetal tissues and, conversely, of carbon dioxide from the fetus to the atmosphere, represent a series of steps occurring within the maternal-fetal diad (Fig. 1). If one assumes normal respiratory muscle function, airway dimensions, and ventilatory control mechanisms, there is a volume exchange between the atmosphere and the alveoli that results in alveolar oxygen (Po_2) and carbon dioxide pressures (Pco_2) being maintained within certain limits. The diffusional transfer of oxygen and carbon dioxide across the maternal alveolar membrane is influenced by the Po_2 and Pco_2 gradients between the alveolar lumen and capillaries. Oxygen transport is further influenced by the rate of chemical reaction between oxygen and hemoglobin.

The transport of oxygen from the lungs to the placenta or of carbon dioxide from the placenta to the lungs is controlled, in part, by the blood flow between these organs. Most of the oxygen transported is in the bound state. Oxygen content is determined by Po_2, hemoglobin concentration, and the affinity of hemoglobin for oxygen. At physiological arterial and venous Po_2 (45–105 mmHg), hemoglobin saturations are greater than 75% and, accordingly, the quantity of oxygen per milliliter of blood is roughly equal to the product of oxygen saturation and hemoglobin concentration (4). In contrast to oxygen, carbon dioxide is carried primarily as bicarbonate, with smaller (but significant) amounts carried as dissolved CO_2 and in carbamino compounds.

The rate of transfer of oxygen and carbon dioxide across the placental membrane is influenced by the pressure gradients for these two gases between the villus capillary (fetal compartment) and intervillous space (maternal compartment). The movement of oxygen from the placenta to fetal tissues or carbon dioxide from fetal tissues to the placenta is dependent on blood flow—in a volume sense—and an intact microcirculation. Furthermore, the quantity of oxygen transported from the placenta to fetal tissues is influenced by the hemoglobin concentration and the fetal hemoglobin affinity for oxygen. The oxygen crossing the placenta membrane is equivalent to the sum of the oxygen exiting the placenta through the umbilical venules and the placental utilization of oxygen.

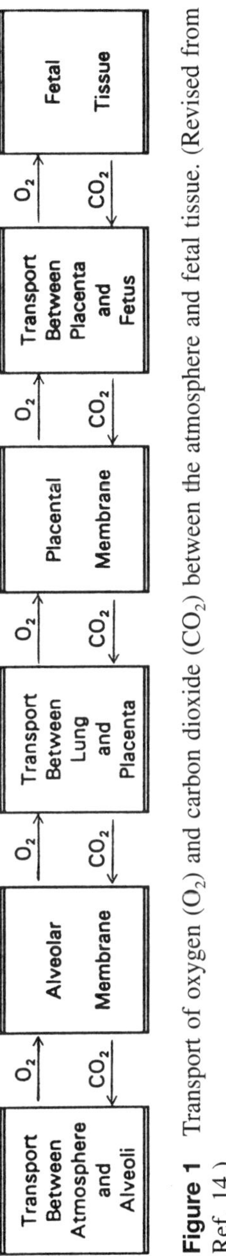

Figure 1 Transport of oxygen (O_2) and carbon dioxide (CO_2) between the atmosphere and fetal tissue. (Revised from Ref. 14.)

The constant uptake of oxygen and production of carbon dioxide within fetal tissue creates relatively low oxygen and high carbon dioxide pressures in and around cells. In the intact organism these oxygen and carbon dioxide pressure gradients from blood to tissues explain the undirectional flow of oxygen to and carbon dioxide from tissues.

To better understand the processes shown in Fig. 1, we should consider how pregnancy or asthma may influence each step.

B.   Minute Ventilation

The most consistently demonstrated physiological respiratory change during pregnancy is an increase in resting ventilation (5) (see also Chapter 3). Prowse and Gaensler reported a 48% increase in minute ventilation in pregnancy (6). Other investigators have reported similar results (reviewed in Ref. 5). The currently accepted explanation for the hyperventilation of pregnancy is respiratory center stimulation by increasing concentrations of progesterone (5).

C.   Diffusing Capacity of the Lung

During early pregnancy, the diffusing capacity of the lung is felt to be generally unchanged or increased over nonpregnant values in the same patient. The diffusing capacity then frequently decreases to a plateau during the latter half of pregnancy, at a level that is equivalent to or slightly less than the nonpregnant level (5). The relative roles of alterations in pulmonary capillary blood volume, membrane diffusing capacity, and changes in maternal hemoglobin concentration on diffusing capacity remain to be clarified.

D.   Oxygen Consumption

Oxygen consumption increases in pregnancy (6–9). The increase in uteroplacental-fetal tissue mass and increased physiological work (cardiac, respiratory, or other) require an increase in oxygen consumption in the normal gravida. Interestingly, it appears that there is a difference in the relative increase in oxygen consumption and minute ventilation. As noted earlier, minute ventilation increases approximately 50% in pregnancy over nonpregnant control levels (6). Furthermore, the increase in minute ventilation peaks well before the increase in oxygen consumption. The same investigators reported a 21% increase in oxygen consumption. Knuttgen and Emerson (7) and Pernoll and associates (8,9) reported a 50% increase in minute ventilation during exercise and a 30–35% increase in oxygen consumption in late pregnancy compared with postpartum measurements.

E. Oxygen Uptake and Ventilation in Labor

Oxygen uptake and minute ventilation are increased in women in labor compared with nonlaboring gravidas (10). Minute ventilation increases from 12 (± 0.7) L/min in early labor to 23 (± 0.2) L/min by the end of second-stage labor (Table 1). A similar, nonlinear increase in oxygen uptake occurs with progression of labor (Table 1). Oxygen uptake is greater during contractions than between contractions. Depending on the duration and strength of a contraction, mean oxygen uptake increases more than twofold, from 281 (± 30) mL/min between contractions to 703 (± 32) mL/min during contractions (10).

F. Arterial Blood Gases and Acid–Base Status

The increase in minute ventilation in pregnancy has been associated with a decrease in alveolar P_{CO_2} (PA_{CO_2}) and arterial P_{CO_2} (Pa_{CO_2}) to the range of 27–32 mmHg (12,13; see also Chapter 3). The increase in the minute ventilation in pregnancy and the resultant relative hypocarbia produce a rise in maternal blood pH. This respiratory alkalosis-induced rise in pH is blunted by increased renal excretion of bicarbonate. The net effects of the respiratory alkalosis and increased renal bicarbonate excretion are a pH in the range of 7.40–7.45, a serum bicarbonate decrease to 18–21 mEq/L, and a base deficit of approximately 3–4 mEq/L (12,13). In a normally

Table 1 Mean ($\pm$ SEM) Oxygen Uptake and Minute Ventilation in the First and Second Stages of Labor

	Oxygen uptake (ml min^{-1} m^{-2})	Minute ventilation (1 min^{-1})
First stage of labor:		
1 cm dilation	145 $\pm$ 18	12 $\pm$ 0.7
5 cm dilation	204 $\pm$ 23	20 $\pm$ 0.3
8 cm dilation	225 $\pm$ 19	21 $\pm$ 0.2
10 cm dilation	259 $\pm$ 27	22 $\pm$ 0.2
Second stage of labor:		
Pelvic floor	266 $\pm$ 23	23 $\pm$ 0.2

Source: Ref. 10.

ventilating gravida, exercise (12) and uterine contractions (10,12) increase minute ventilation and produce a further decrease in Pa_{CO_2}.

G. The Placenta, a Venous Equilibration Exchange Mechanism

To better understand respiratory gas exchange between the maternal and fetal compartments requires an understanding of the exchange mechanism in the human (hemochorial) placenta. The placenta may be thought of as a membrane that separates maternal uterine blood flow and umbilical blood flow. Maternal perfusion of the placenta is by the uterine arteries, which divide into progressively smaller vessels, ultimately ending in the spiral arterioles. These arterial microvessels perfuse the intervillous space and thereby bathe fetal villi. Maternal blood exits the intervillous space by uterine venules that join to form ever-larger venous structures, ultimately exiting the uterus through the uterine veins (primarily) or the venous collaterals of the ovaries, bladder, and vagina. In the fetal circulation, relatively deoxygenated and hypercarbic fetal blood enters the placenta from the umbilical arteries, courses through the villus capillaries, and returns to the fetus through the umbilical vein, oxygenated and eucarbic.

How are these maternal and fetal microcirculations arranged? Possibilities include countercurrent and concurrent models of placental perfusion. In a countercurrent placenta the P_{O_2} of umbilical venous blood tends to equilibrate with the P_{O_2} of maternal arterial blood. As a consequence, in this model umbilical venous P_{O_2} can be higher than uterine venous P_{O_2}. There is no persuasive morphological evidence of a circulatory arrangement within the human placenta whereby the P_{O_2} of fetal venous blood equilibrates with the P_{O_2} of maternal arterial blood (14). The data from humans (10,11) and more extensive data in the rhesus monkey (15) have demonstrated that umbilical venous P_{O_2} may approximate, but does not exceed, uterine venous P_{O_2}. These clinical and experimental data are most consistent with a concurrent model of placental perfusion. A concurrent mechanism, or venous equilibration model (14,16), suggests that umbilical venous P_{O_2} cannot exceed uterine venous P_{O_2}. Umbilical venous P_{O_2} can equilibrate with uterine venous P_{O_2} only if there is no limitation of diffusing capacity across the trophoblastic membrane. The venous equilibration model emphasizes the importance of the uterine venous site as the reference point for understanding umbilical venous blood gas changes.

The surprisingly low P_{O_2} in the oxygenated umbilical venous blood of 30–37 mmHg contrasts with the normal maternal arterial P_{O_2} of 100 mmHg. The fetus tolerates this relatively low P_{O_2} environment by several mechanisms. These include a shift in the oxygen–hemoglobin dissociation curves, which favors oxygen delivery to the fetus, high fetal cardiac output, and a unique distribution of fetal cardiac output. Fetal hemoglobin concentrations are significantly higher than adult blood, 15–18 g/L versus 12–13 g/L. The oxygen–hemoglobin dissociation curve of fetal blood lies to the left of the maternal curve, resulting in relatively high oxygen saturation of umbilical venous blood, despite the low Po_2 (Figure 2). This characteristic of the fetal oxygen–hemoglobin dissociation curve also allows significant desaturation of fetal hemoglobin at the Po_2 levels found in fetal tissues. Lastly, the maximally oxygenated fetal umbilical venous blood is preferentially shunted from the right to left atrium (via the foramen ovale) to vital organs, such as the brain and heart. The less well-oxygenated blood is distributed to lungs, gut, and other vascular beds which are less vital in fetal life.

H. Factors Determining Uterine Venous Oxygen Pressure

Given that the human placenta functions as a concurrent exchanger of respiratory gases, uterine venous Po_2 levels best reflect the Po_2 in fetal oxygenated (umbilical venous) blood. Therefore, it is important to be aware of factors influencing uterine venous Po_2 levels. The primary determinants of uterine venous Po_2 are the oxyhemoglobin dissociation curve of maternal blood and oxygen saturation in uterine venous blood (Table 2). The oxyhemoglobin dissociation curve of maternal blood is influenced by the type of hemoglobin (hemoglobin A, F, S, or other), temperature, 2,3-diphosphoglycerate (2,3-DPG) levels, and pH. Changes in pH shift the oxyhemoglobin dissociation curve (Fig. 2), so that at any given O_2 saturation, the Po_2 is inversely related to pH (i.e., a decrease in pH is associated with an increase in Po_2 and vice versa). Oxygen saturation of uterine ve-

Table 2 Determinants of Uterine Venous Po_2

Oxyhemoglobin dissociation curve:
   Hemoglobin type: A, S, F, etc.
   Temperature
   2,3-diphosphoglycerate (DPG)
   pH
O^2 saturation of uterine venous blood:
   Arterial O^2 saturation
   Uteroplacental blood flow
   O_2 carrying capacity
   Uteroplacental-fetal O_2 consumption

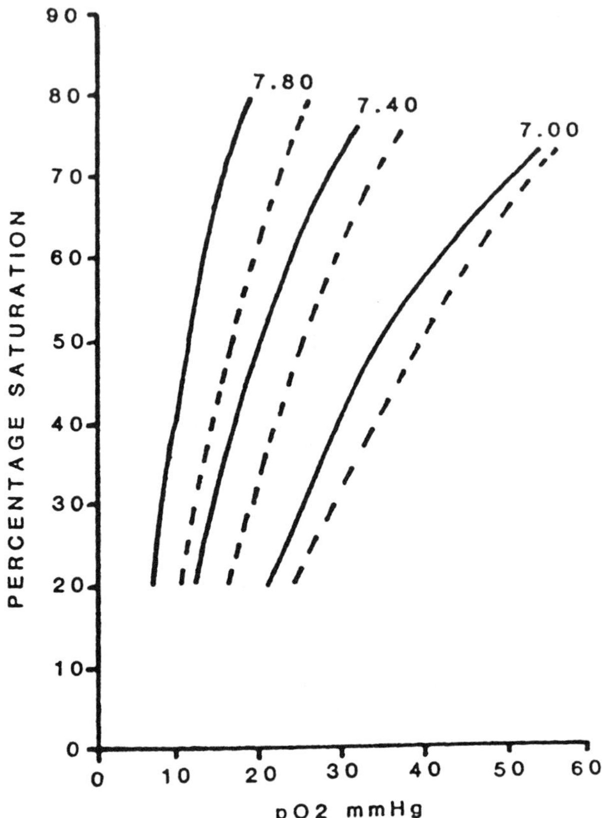

Figure 2 Oxygen dissociation curves of fetal (————) and maternal (– – –) human blood prepared at pH 7.00–7.80 and 38°C. (Revised from Hellegers and Schruefer. Am J Obstet Gynecol 1961.)

nous blood is determined by arterial O_2 saturation, uteroplacental blood flow, oxygen-carrying capacity of maternal blood, and uteroplacental and fetal oxygen consumption.

Therapeutically, the clinician has little influence over the factors influencing the oxyhemoglobin dissociation curve (see Table 2). In contrast, the clinician may influence the factors affecting the oxygenation status of uterine venous blood, and thereby umbilical venous blood and consequently oxygenation of vital fetal organs (brain, heart, etc). Maternal position may influence maternal arterial oxygen tensions. Awe and associates (17), studying 23 nonsmoking, medically uncomplicated gravidas within 6 weeks before delivery, demonstrated that only 1 subject when tested in the sitting position had a P_{O_2} less than 90 mmHg. Among these late pregnant women tested after 15 min in the supine position, 26% had a P_{O_2} less than 90 mmHg (17). The frequency (26%) of modest hypoxemia found in normal, late pregnant, supine gravidas appeared to be prevented by 15° left uterine displacement (13). These investigators studying 20 nonsmoking, medically normal women at 38 weeks gestation in the supine position with 15° left uterine tilt found the arterial P_{O_2} to be 101.8 ± 1.0 mmHg (mean ± SE). This value is remarkably similar to the mean (± SD) of 101.2 (±7.0) mmHg of the late pregnant gravidas sampled by Awe et al. in the sitting position (17). The effect of maternal position on fetal cerebral oxygenation was studied prospectively by Aldrich et al. (18) in 14 uncomplicated term women under epidural anesthesia moved from the left lateral to the supine position. These investigators quantitated changes in fetal cerebral concentrations of oxyhemoglobin, deoxyhemoglobin, cerebral blood volume, and cerebral oxygen saturation using near-infrared spectroscopy. As compared to the left lateral position, the supine position was associated with a significant decrease in the mean (± SD) concentration of fetal cerebral oxyhemoglobin ($1.12 ± 1.0$ μmol 100 g^{-1}, $p < .01$) and a significant decrease in mean (± SD) cerebral oxygen saturation of 8.3 (± 8.8)% ($p < .05$). These changes occurred without any significant change in the mean concentration of deoxyhemoglobin and cerebral blood volume. These maternal position-dependent changes in fetal cerebral oxygenation are consistent with the position-dependent maternal oxygenation changes of Awe and associates (17).

Maternal oxygen therapy can significantly alter maternal arterial and fetal cerebral oxygenation. The oxygen therapy-induced rise in maternal arterial P_{O_2} is accompanied by a small increase in fetal umbilical artery P_{O_2} levels (10). It is important not to conclude from the small umbilical artery P_{O_2} changes with oxygen therapy that maternal oxygen therapy does not benefit the oxygenation status of the fetus. The venous equilibration model of placental exchange and the characteristics of maternal and fetal oxyhemoglobin dissociation curves explain why the change in fetal arterial P_{O_2} with maternal oxygen therapy is numerically small (14). In a gravida with normal P_{O_2}, if oxygen therapy increases her arterial oxygen content 1 mM and there is no appreciable change in uterine blood flow or uterine oxygen consumption, the 1-mM increase in maternal arterial oxygen content would result in approximately a 0.7-mM increase in fetal oxygen content (Fig. 3). Interestingly, and relevant to the pregnant asthmatic patient, maternal oxygen therapy of a gravida who is hypoxic could result in a greater increase in fetal oxygen content than maternal oxygen content (Fig. 4). Recently, maternal oxygen administration (60% FI_{O_2} by ventimask for

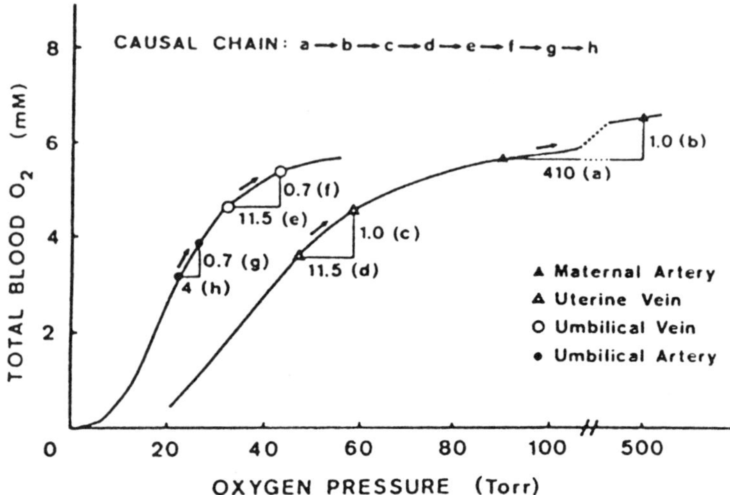

Figure 3 Example of the relationship between oxygen content and Po_2 in maternal and fetal blood before and after maternal inhalation of 100% oxygen (Ref. 14). Numbers shown on graph represent the net change in oxygen pressure (a, d, e, h) and total blood O_2 (b, c, f, g) after maternal oxygen inhalation. The arrows indicate the change in fetal (umbilical) and maternal values along the oxyhemoglobin dissociation curve.

15 min) has been shown using near-infrared spectroscopy to result in a significant increase in mean concentration of fetal cerebral oxyhemoglobin (0.78 ± 0.42 μmol 100 g^{-1} brain tissue), a significant decrease in the mean concentration of deoxyhemoglobin (0.80 ± 0.51 μmol g^{-1}) and an increase in mean cerebral oxygen saturation of 13.6% from 43.9 to 57.3%) (all p values $<.001$) (19). Thus it can be seen that maternal oxygen therapy has the potential to significantly increase fetal oxygen content and, therefore, be especially beneficial in the circumstance in which fetal hypoxia is a direct consequence of maternal hypoxia.

Uteroplacental blood flow is influenced by maternal hydration, cardiac output, and maternal position. Uteroplacental blood flow can be optimized by normalizing hydration and avoiding circumstances that compromise cardiac output or uterine artery compression. An enlarging uterus increases the gravida's predisposition to supine hypotension. This is secondary to venocaval obstruction, venous pooling in the pelvis and lower extremities, decreased cardiac return, and reduced cardiac output. This sequence of events is especially likely in the third trimester. A reduction in cardiac output in the supine position has been convincingly demonstrated

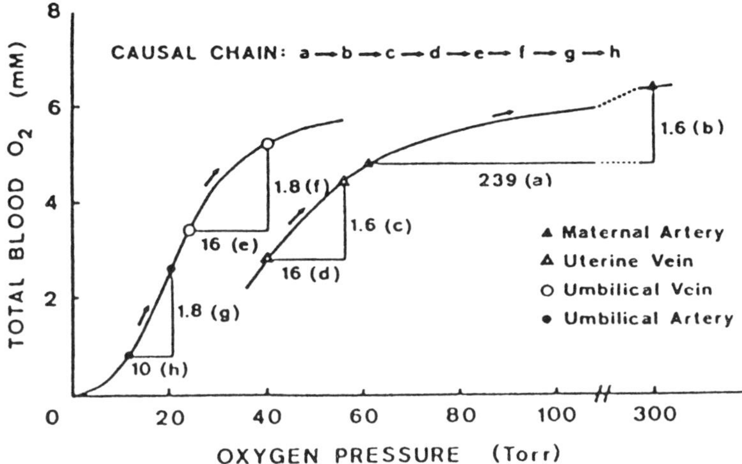

Figure 4 Example of the pronounced effect of oxygen therapy on fetal oxygen content in a case of fetal hypoxia secondary to maternal hypoxia (Ref. 14). See Figure 3 caption for other details.

(20), and such impairment could account for significant reduction in maternal arterial Po_2 (21) and fetal cerebral oxygenation (18).

Steps taken during the antepartum period to ensure a normal maternal hemoglobin will optimize the woman's oxygen-carrying capacity. Maternal anemia (hemoglobin values lower than 10 g/L) should be evaluated and treated.

Fetal hyperglycemia stimulates endogenous insulin secretion, which increases oxygen consumption and may result in hypoxia (reviewed in Ref. 22). It follows that iatrogenic hyperglycemia secondary to bolus infusions of dextrose may increase fetal oxygen consumption. Hyperglycemia, whether spontaneous, as in diabetes, or iatrogenic, should be avoided because it may precipitate fetal hypoxia and acidosis (22).

In summary, maternal venous Po_2 is optimal when the gravida is ventilating normally, afebrile, has a normal hemoglobin level, is normotensive, is euglycemic, and sitting or supine with left uterine displacement. In situations complicated by maternal hypoxia, maternal oxygen therapy should improve uterine venous Po_2, umbilical venous Po_2, and oxygenation of vital fetal organs.

III. Uteroplacental–Fetal Oxygen Utilization

A. Measurement

Oxygen uptake across a vascular bed can be calculated by simultaneously measuring arterial–venous oxygen content differences and blood flow. Application of this rationale, the Fick principle, to the uterine arterial–venous vessels will allow calculation of the combined oxygen utilization of the uterus, placenta, and fetus. The Fick principle, when applied to the umbilical circulation, allows calculation of fetal oxygen uptake. Simultaneous application of these measurements to both the uterine and umbilical circulations allows calculation of oxygen uptake of the uterus, placenta and fetus combined, and the fetus alone. The difference between these two simultaneous measurements would be the oxygen uptake of the uterus and placenta. In the late pregnant, chronically catheterized sheep model, oxygen uptake of the uterus, placenta, and fetus was 9.6 mL min^{-1} kg^{-1} (13). Fetal oxygen uptake was 6.6 mL min^{-1} kg^{-1} (13). Consequently, uteroplacental oxygen uptake was 3.0 mL min^{-1} kg^{-1}. Similarly precise measurements in humans are not available. As pointed out by Meschia (13), extrapolation from nonhuman data should be made cautiously. Among species, differences in body composition (e.g., brain mass and adipose tissue), body temperatures, and growth rates suggest that fetal oxygen uptakes could be remarkably different. Other information, however, indicates that oxygen uptake rates in humans could approximate that in other species. Despite between-species differences in growth, body size, and composition, different species appear to have comparable fetal oxygen uptakes per kilogram of body weight. It is currently possible to obtain maternal arterial, uterine venous, and umbilical arterial and venous samples at the time of caesarean section. Confirmation of human fetal oxygen uptake measurements awaits the availability of a practical method of obtaining simultaneous uterine and umbilical blood flow determinations.

B. Increased Rate of Fetal Metabolism and Placental Reserve

Increased fetal oxygen utilization has been produced in experimental animal models using fetal infusions of norepinephrine and triiodothyronine (23). In the chronically catheterized fetal lamb model, infusions of norepinephrine and triiodothyronine resulted in increased fetal oxygen consumption, without any demonstrable change in placental diffusing capacity or fetal venous and arterial blood gas measurements. The authors concluded that increases in fetal oxygen consumption in the range of 25–30% did not exceed the capacity of the placenta to provide increased oxygen for fetal requirements.

IV. Uteroplacental and Fetal Blood Flow

A. Uterine Blood Flow

The importance of maintaining an adequate and uninterrupted uterine blood flow is emphasized by calculations that suggest that, if uterine blood flow ceases, there is only a 2-min fetal reserve of oxygen (24). The normal 30–50% increase in cardiac output with progression of pregnancy in large part provides for the increase in uterine blood flow that is necessary to nourish and "ventilate" the growing fetal-placental mass. Pathological conditions, such as chronic hypertension, preeclampsia, and other conditions (long-standing diabetes, systemic lupus erythematosus, other collagen vascular disorders), known to affect large and small arterial vessels, may reduce placental perfusion as a result of the vascular changes.

Exaggerated maternal hyperventilation may have a deleterious effect on fetal oxygenation through several mechanisms. One mechanism involves a reduction in uterine blood flow associated with the mechanical effects of hyperventilation. Because both hyperventilation and the resulting hypocarbia may influence uterine blood flow, it had been difficult to sort out the relative contribution of these alterations to fetal acid–base changes, prior to the work of Levinson and associates (15). These investigators constructed an experimental protocol in which they were able to control both P_{CO_2} levels and respiratory rate in chronically catheterized sheep. In hyperventilating pregnant ewes, they demonstrated a reduction in uterine blood flow that was maintained even when maternal P_{CO_2} levels were kept in a eucarbic range. Uterine blood flow returned to normal only when hyperventilation ceased. Although this study seems to have effectively ruled out a direct effect of hypocarbia in reducing uterine blood flow, the precise mechanisms by which hyperventilation reduced uterine blood flow remain to be clarified. Possible mechanisms include a compensatory response to decreased cardiac output that results from the following:

1. A decreased cardiac return secondary to hyperventilation.
2. The decreased venous return associated with hyperventilation may decrease distention of the right and left atria and pulmonary vascular bed. These changes stimulate a sympathetic response that may decrease uterine blood flow (see later section on catecholamine-induced decrease in uterine blood flow).

Other mechanisms linking maternal hyperventilation with reductions in fetal oxygenation include:

1. A left shift in the oxyghemoglobin dissociation curve, resulting in increased affinity of maternal hemoglobin for oxygen and,

therefore, decreased transfer of oxygen from the maternal to the fetal compartment (see Fig. 2).

2. Maternal alkalosis may increase intraplacental shunting, resulting in a mismatching of maternal and fetal circulations (25).
3. To the extent that hyperventilation results in a decrease in cardiac output, there is the potential for a disproportionate reduction in blood flow to the uterine vascular tree.

Uterine blood flow is sensitive to adrenergic stimulation. The first systematic examination of the effect of catecholamines on uterine blood flow was by Robson and Schild (26). They found that uterine arteries of pregnant or spayed cats constricted in response to epinephrine. Subsequently, studies in dogs (27), sheep (28), and rhesus monkeys (29) reported reductions in uterine blood flow with varying maternal infusion regimens of catecholamines. Rosenfeld et al. (28) found that epinephrine infusions into gravid sheep produced 39% reduction in total uterine blood flow. The infusion rates used during the blood flow experiments did not produce a change in maternal blood pressure. The demonstrated reduction in total uterine blood flow was explained by reductions in myometrial, cotyledonary, and endometrial flow. Adamson and associates (29) found, in rhesus monkeys, that epinephrine and norepinephrine infusions to the mother sufficient to raise blood pressure were also associated with increased uterine contractions and decreased uterine blood flow. They concluded that the fetal hypoxia, hypercarbia, and acidosis resulting from catecholamine infusions placed the fetus in double jeopardy of hypoxia and acidosis by directly decreasing uterine blood flow and by increasing uterine activity, which further decrease placental perfusion. An awareness of these adrenergic-induced changes in uterine blood flow is especially relevant to the asthmatic patient, who may be exposed to epinephrine or other catecholamines in the course of her medical treatment.

B. Umbilical Fetal Circulation

Chronic hypoxia may increase erythropoietin levels and, consequently, red blood cell production. A significant increase in hematocrit may be associated with increased viscosity and a compromise in small-vessel perfusion. Umbilical compression is another potential source of reduced fetal perfusion. Umbilical cord compression can occur persistently with fetal entanglement in its umbilical cord (e.g., nuchal cord or with a true knot in the cord), and with oligohydramnios. Whether umbilical compression occurs suddenly or over time, it may result in a reduction in umbilical circulation and consequent impairment of respiratory gas exchange across the placental membrane, hypercarbia, and hypoxia.

V. Relation of Alterations of Maternal Oxygenation to Fetal Oxygenation and Acid–Base Status

The most common cause of maternal hypoxemia in patients with asthma is pulmonary ventilation-perfusion imbalance (30). The absolute or relative hypoxemia that results from the admixture of pulmonary venous effluent from normally ventilated and poorly ventilated areas of lung parenchyma thereby compromises available oxygen perfusing the placenta. Wulf et al. (10) found that a reduction in maternal Po_2 from 92 to 65 mmHg resulted in a reduction in umbilical venous Po_2 from 32 to 26 mmHg. Changes of this degree result in a significant reduction in fetal oxygen content. Even during a mild asthmatic attack, the alterations that occur (decreased Po_2, decreased Pco_2, increased pH, increased respiratory rate) each individually predispose to impaired fetal oxygenation. The mild hypoxemia was addressed in the foregoing. The maternal hyperventilation and decrease in Pco_2 are associated with a decrease in fetal Po_2 levels (10). The rise in maternal pH results in a shift of the oxyhemoglobin dissociation curve to the left and, consequently, to a reduction in the availability of oxygen to the fetus (see Fig. 2). As the severity of an asthmatic attack evolves from mild to moderate (lower Po_2, normal pH, and normal Pco_2) to severe (even lower Po_2, low pH, and hypercarbia), the increased risk to the fetus is proportional to the worsening maternal state (31). If maternal arterial Po_2 falls below 60 mmHg, the fetus is at especially high risk (3).

VI. Effect of Anaphylaxis on the Fetus

Anaphylaxis is problematic in any situation, but especially so during pregnancy (see Chapter 12). This is because both anaphylaxis as well as its treatment have significant implications/risks for the fetus. The clinical features of anaphylaxis that may occur individually or in combination include upper airway obstruction, lower airway (bronchial) constriction, hypotension, and myocardial dysfunction. The maternal and fetal implications of hypoxia, hypercarbia, and hyperventilation, secondary to upper and lower airway obstruction, no doubt explain in part the high mortality rate associated with anaphylactic reactions (32). Maternal hypotension, with or without myocardial dysfunction (e.g., arrhythmias, ischemia), result in a reduction in uterine perfusion. This reduction may be disproportionately large, given that the uterine vasculature is not a protected vascular bed, such as the cerebral or cardiac vasculature.

Epinephrine continues to be the drug of choice for the treatment of anaphylaxis (32). It has retained this position in the treatment armamentarium for anaphylaxis because of its ability to counteract vasodilation, bronchial constriction, and other adverse effects of anaphylactic mediators on target tissues and to inhibit the further release of mediators from mast cells and basophils (32). Treatment of the gravid woman experiencing an anaphylactic reaction is complicated by her pregnancy. Reduction in uterine perfusion that may result from anaphylaxis-induced hypotension may be exaggerated by the profound α-adrenergic effects of epinephrine. Epinephrine-induced uterine vasoconstriction produces decreased uterine perfusion (28,29). Thus, the fetal risk inherent with maternal anaphylaxis may be compounded by α-adrenergic effects of epinephrine on uterine perfusion. This concern led Entman and Moise (33) to suggest that ephedrine, a noncatecholamine adrenergic drug, may be preferable for provision of cardiovascular support in allergic reactions in pregnant women. Ephedrine supports blood pressure by a β-agonist effect of increasing cardiac output. Ephedrine doses of 25–50 mg by intravenous push can be useful in supporting maternal systemic blood pressure without compromising uterine blood flow. Higher doses are associated with an α-adrenergic effect (34).

VII. Fetal Assessment

Fetal compromise occurs uncommonly in mild or in well-controlled asthma, but acute chronic fetal effects may result from severe or poorly controlled asthma. Acute exacerbations of asthma that result in impaired maternal oxygenation may directly impair that of the fetus. If this reaches a critical threshold, fetal distress or death may result. In patients with chronically impaired oxygenation, placental oxygen transfer may be sufficiently restricted to interfere with fetal growth, resulting in long-term effects on the fetus: for example, growth impairment (intrauterine growth retardation, IUGR), which predisposes to fetal distress, fetal death in utero, and neonatal morbidity.

In this section, modalities available for fetal assessment are detailed. In the next, their integration into the obstetrical management of the pregnant asthmatic is described.

A. Gestational Age

Accurate pregnancy dating is a cornerstone of optimal obstetric care. Gestational dating is essential to evaluate fetal growth, to anticipate fetal maturity, and to time obstetrical interventions.

By convention, obstetricians calculate gestational age from the last menstrual period, presuming a regular, 28-day menstrual cycle. In this situation, conception occurs 2 weeks after the first day of the last menstrual period (also 2 weeks before the missed menstrual period). Full-term gestation is considered to be 40 weeks from the last menstrual period. If the cycle length is shorter or longer than 28 days, the estimated date of confinement can be calculated by adding 38 weeks to the ovulation or conception date, if this is known, since ovulation and conception regularly occur 2 weeks before the missed menstrual period. Alternatively, the estimated date of confinement can be calculated by adding 36 weeks to the date of the first missed menstrual period (35).

In the past, the menstrual history and physical examination findings from the first trimester of pregnancy were used in pregnancy dating. However, many women either do not have regular menstrual cycles or do not record them. In particular, women with chronic disease states are prone to menstrual irregularities, which invalidate the use of menstrual dating in gestational age assessment.

Fortunately, ultrasound has become a simple, reliable, and accurate means of dating pregnancy. If fetal measurements from an ultrasound examination fit with the gestational age 7–13 weeks, the error is ± 7 days; if measurements fit with 13–22 weeks, the error is ± 10 days (36). Because biological variation in fetal growth increases with increasing gestational age, particularly during the latter half of gestation, the accuracy of sonography for pregnancy dating decreases as the pregnancy advances. Between 22 and 28 weeks gestation, the accuracy of sonography is ± 2 weeks, and beyond 28 weeks, sonography measurements are less reliable as a predictor of gestational age of (± 21 days). In patients with regular menstrual cycles and a known last period, many obstetricians may use sonography in the 13- to 20-week range to confirm pregnancy dating. If menstrual cycles are irregular or the last period is not accurately known, gestational age assessment by sonography is necessary. Interestingly, sonographic measurements have been shown to predict delivery date as well or better than an optimally accurate menstrual history (37).

B. Fetal Growth

Once the gestational age is established, uterine and sonographic measurements are used for fetal growth assessment. In asthma, IUGR may occur secondary to diminished uteroplacental transfer of oxygen to the fetus. The mechanism is as follows: When the intrauterine environment is suboptimal, the fetal response is to redistribute blood flow to vital organs (i.e., heart, brain, and adrenal glands) (38). The skin, muscles, and gut are relatively hypoperfused. Although this adaptation is useful in protecting the fetus from sudden changes, continued stress of this nature results in an *asym-*

metric growth retardation pattern, in which head growth, and to lesser extent, linear growth of the fetus are relatively spared, whereas abdominal girth, skin thickness, and muscle mass are diminished (39). This asymmetric growth pattern can result in the fetus becoming small for gestational age (SGA), i.e., less than the 10th percentile of weight for gestational age (Fig. 5).

Intrauterine growth retardation represents a significant risk factor for in-utero fetal death, fetal distress during labor, and neonatal morbidity (40).

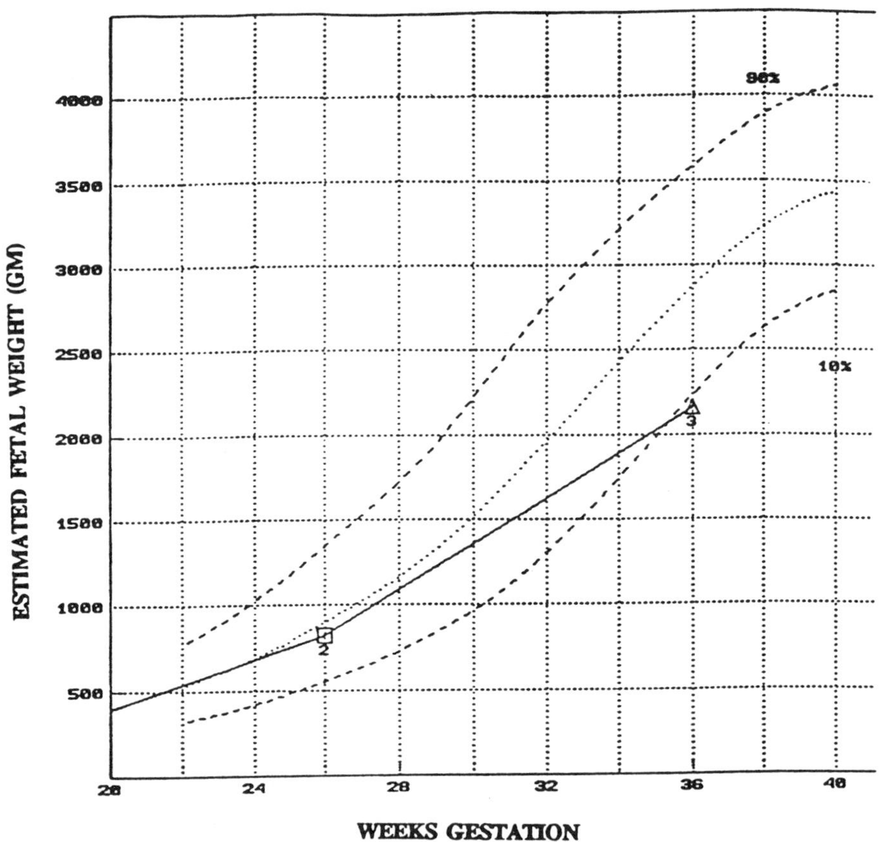

Figure 5 Sonographically estimated fetal weight at 26 and 36 weeks gestation in severely asthmatic patient. At 36 weeks, fetal head and extremity measurements were consistent with 35–36 weeks, while abdominal circumference was consistent with 31.5 weeks.

Thus, it is considered to be an indication for intensive fetal surveillance, and it may be an indication for early delivery (see Chapter 20).

For the low-risk pregnant patient, screening for fetal growth retardation is by serial measurements of the uterine fundal height. Between 20 and 35 weeks gestation, the distance from the symphysis to the top of the fundus, measured in centimeters, matches gestational age within about 2 weeks. If a significant discrepancy between fundal height and gestational age occurs, the more sensitive and specific sonographic assessment is used to assess for fetal growth problems. For the high-risk patient, sonography is used as the screening and confirmatory tool.

Typically, during sonography, the placental location, fetal presentation and position, amniotic fluid volume, and biometry of the fetus are evaluated. Measurements include the biparietal diameter, head circumference, abdominal circumference, and femur length. These individual measurements may be plotted against gestational age to infer patterns of growth disturbance. For example, in asymmetric intrauterine growth retardation, the biparietal diameter and head circumference may fall in the 40th percentile range for gestational age, the femur length at the 20th or 30th percentile, and the abdominal circumference less than the 3rd percentile. Ratios between head and abdominal measurements, and also between femur and abdominal measurements, have also been useful in the diagnosis of IUGR (41). Estimation of fetal weight is available through a number of formulas involving various combinations of biometric parameters (e.g., biparietal diameter and abdominal circumference, head circumference and abdominal circumference, femur length and abdominal circumference) (42). The use of an estimated fetal weight of less than 10th percentile for dates as the diagnostic criterion for IUGR has sensitivity and specificity in the 80–90% range. These levels are comparable with the sensitivity and specificity measurements for any other tested means of detecting IUGR. Fetal weight estimation is the standard in the assessment of fetal growth (43).

In addition to overall estimation of fetal weight, ultrasound and Doppler ultrasound provide the means for inferential assessment of the perfusion of at-risk fetal organ systems. The best-validated tool for such is assessment of amniotic fluid volume. Amniotic fluid is produced continuously during pregnancy by efflux of fluid from the fetal trachea and, quantitatively more important, production of urine. Reduction of renal blood flow, as may occur with redistribution of blood flow in IUGR, results in diminished fetal urine production and, thereby, decreases amniotic fluid volume. The *four-quadrant technique* for assessing amniotic fluid volume during pregnancy has been reproducible and reliable as a screening tool for impaired amniotic fluid production (44). The deepest vertical fluid pocket in each of the four quadrants of the uterus is measured sonographically, and these four measurements are summed to form the *amniotic fluid index* (AFI). An AFI of less than 6 cm is abnormal at any time during the third trimester. Decreased amniotic fluid volume, as assessed by this technique, has been predictive of adverse fetal outcomes, including fetal distress in labor and adverse neonatal outcomes. Decreased amniotic fluid volume occurs commonly in patients with IUGR; however, even in the absence of IUGR, a diminished AFI is a presumptive indicator of chronic uteroplacental insufficiency.

Measurements of blood flow to various fetal organs are now available. Pulse-wave and continuous-wave Doppler techniques have been used to measure systolic and diastolic flow velocity in the intracranial circulation, descending aorta, ductus arteriosus, umbilical cord, and other vascular structures of the fetus. Of these measurements, umbilical flow velocity waveforms have been best studied in relation to pregnancy surveillance. It is clear that elevated placental vascular resistance may reduce diastolic umbilical flow and result in an increased ratio of systolic to diastolic blood flow (S/D ratio) in the umbilical artery. A significantly elevated S/D ratio is suggestive of fetal compromise, even in the absence of IUGR or oligohydramnios. Elevated S/D ratios are considered to be an indicator for intensive fetal surveillance. If diastolic flow ceases, or is reversed, the fetus is at high risk for in-utero death, and delivery is often indicated (45).

C. Relation of Fetal Maturity to Survival

Obstetrical intervention in complicated pregnancies is determined by balancing risks to the fetus from remaining in utero against those of extrauterine life, and balancing these against risks to the mother from intervention. Before about 25 weeks gestation, neonatal survival ex utero is very poor and, thus, if fetal jeopardy is implied, interventions, if any, must be directed toward improving the intrauterine environment. In the recent past, the rate of fetal survival at 25 weeks was about 10% advancing to 60% at 26 weeks gestation, 80% at 28 weeks gestation, and over 90% at 30 weeks gestation (46). More recently, survival statistics have improved further and the incidence of adverse neurological outcomes has decreased as the survival rates have increased (47). In the context of neonatal morbidity and the high rate of abnormal neurological outcomes in very-low-birth-weight babies, obstetric intervention is generally reserved for pregnancies beyond 24–25 weeks gestation.

The threshold for delivery of the fetus, rather than continued in-utero management, declines steadily as gestation advances. Fetal survival and long-term outcome relate well to three factors: fetal weight, condition at delivery, and lung maturity. For the fetus delivered in good condition, with mature lungs, and a weight in excess of 1.8–2 kg, neonatal mortality is virtually nil, and significant morbidity is uncommon.

Fetal weight estimation, as mentioned earlier, is performed by sonographic measurements and application of any of a number of weight-estimation formulas. Lung maturity can be assessed prenatally by measuring surfactant levels in amniotic fluid. The fluid can be obtained invasively by amniocentesis or from a vaginal pool specimen following rupture of the fetal membranes. Amniocentesis is performed by directing a needle, under ultrasound guidance, into the amniotic cavity. In experienced hands, amniocentesis carries minimal risk to the pregnancy.

Several biochemical assessments of lung maturity have been developed (48). The standard test for lung maturity assessment has been the determination of the lecithin/sphingomyelin ratio (L/S) in the fluid, and assay for the presence or absence of phosphatidyl glycerol (PG). A mature lung profile, an L/S ratio higher than 2.0, and the presence of PG predicts that the newborn will not have respiratory distress syndrome. If the L/S ratio is higher than 2.0 in the absence of PG, as long as the patient is not diabetic, the prediction is that the baby will have at worst moderate respiratory disease and short-term ventilator therapy may be required.

The greatest drawback to L/S and PG testing is that the chromatographic laboratory procedure is time consuming and expensive. An automated fetal lung maturity test, the TDX-FLM assay, measures the ratio of total surfactant to albumin. In our laboratory a TDX-FLM test is run before L/S, PG testing. A "mature" result (≥55) is conclusive and precludes the need for L/S, PG testing. If the TDX-FLM does not demonstrate maturity, the full L/S, PG assay is performed (49).

D. Fetal Health

One major goal of fetal surveillance is to prevent stillbirth and fetal distress near the time of delivery. The simplest test of fetal health has been known since ancient times: This is the presence of an actively moving fetus. Both maternal observations and sonographic studies of the fetus confirm that a sleep–wake or activity–inactivity cycle develops in utero as early as 20 weeks gestation. Normally, a fetus will not be inactive for more than 30–45 min at a time. During the third trimester, when intervention for fetal jeopardy would be undertaken, mothers easily perceive fetal movement, and this can be used as a screening test for fetal health. One simple screening tool is to ask patients to count kicks for 1 hr daily; if 10 kicks or discrete movements are not felt during the hour of monitoring, the patient is asked to report for more intensive evaluation (50).

For high-risk patients, or for the patient with an inability to perceive fetal movement, fetal heart rate monitoring is used as a sensitive means of assessment of fetal health in utero. Fetal heart rate accelerations occur regularly in response to fetal movement beyond 28 weeks gestation and are often seen as early as 26 weeks gestation. Empirically, accelerations of the fetal heart rate of 15 beats/min or more (which typically occur during fetal movements) are associated with fetal health in utero. In fact, the presence of such accelerations (*reactive nonstress test*) is associated with a very low rate of fetal death in utero within 3–4 days of testing, as long as the clinical situation is stable and the fetal heart rate tracing is otherwise normal (51).

Although a reactive nonstress test is an excellent predictor of fetal health, the fetus who does not show acceleration is not necessarily compromised. Nonreactive tracings may occur in pregnancies of fewer than 32 weeks, in the fetus with central nervous system anomalies, when the mother has taken sedative-hypnotic drugs or alcohol, or simply, when a prolonged "sleep" state of the fetus is present. There are two alternative means of accessing fetal health in utero in this situation: the biophysical profile (BPP) and the contraction stress test.

The *biophysical profile* consists of a nonstress test, followed by sonographic observation of the fetus for up to 30 min. The biophysical profile test is scored as follows (52):

Amniotic fluid volume: Normal if a pocket at least 2×2 cm is
   present
Fetal tone: Normal if at least one episode of limb or trunk extension
   followed by return to flexion is seen
Limb movement: Normal if at least three discrete movements are seen
Breathing: Normal if at least one episode of breathing lasting at least
   30 sec is seen
Nonstress test: Normal if a reactive fetal heart rate pattern is seen

Each normal observation is scored 2 points, and the sum is added to form the BPP score (range: 0–10). A BPP score of 8 or 10 is highly reassuring for fetal well-being, and the risk of fetal demise within 3–4 days of testing is extremely low. A score of 4–6 is intermediate, and a score of 0 or 2 is indicative of fetal compromise and, usually, delivery is recommended. As with the nonstress test, the BPP is not robust to effects of alcohol or sedative drugs on the mother; fetal tone, limb movements, and breathing movements are absent when such drugs are present.

In the *contraction stress test* (53), the fetal heart rate is continuously monitored while mild uterine contractions are induced, either by means of maternal nipple stimulation or oxytocin infusion. If there are no "late decelerations" of the fetal heart rate following uterine contractions, with a contraction frequency of at least three per 10 min, the contraction stress test is read as "negative," and the chance of fetal death in utero within the next week is extremely low. A tracing showing persistent late decelerations is usually considered an indication for delivery; for tracings showing intermittent late decelerations (late deceleration accompanying less than half of contractions), management is individualized.

Doppler velocimetry, sonographic assessment of the umbilical artery systolic/diastolic blood flow velocity ratio, has proven to be a useful adjunct in some centers, but its role in antenatal testing is still debated (54). Most centers, including our own, use the nonstress test and amniotic fluid volume assessment in assessing fetal well-being in pregnancies at risk for uteroplacental insufficiency. If the NST is reactive and amniotic fluid volume is normal, performing a complete BPP does not improve prediction of fetal health. If the NST is nonreactive or the fluid volume is abnormal, either a contraction stress test or a full BPP is generally done or the patient is delivered.

E. Oxygenation

Fetal oxygenation and acid–base status cannot be monitored directly on a continuous basis in utero. The fetal circulation is intermittently accessible to percutaneous umbilical blood sampling (PUBS). Under ultrasound guidance, a needle may be introduced into the fetal umbilical cord and a blood sample obtained for assessment of acid–base status and oxygenation (55). However, this procedure may be technically difficult (or impossible), depending on fetal and placental position and maternal size. Also, PUBS carries a risk of 2–5% for fetal distress in most series. Because it gives only a single assessment of fetal oxygenation, its use for this purpose is quite limited.

When the intrauterine environment is unstable (i.e., when maternal oxygenation is unstable) or when the fetus is under the stress of uterine activity during labor, continuous fetal heart rate monitoring is indicated. The combination of fetal heart rate accelerations and the absence of late decelerations in response to contractions excludes the possibility of fetal hypoxia or acidosis. For a thorough discussion of the issues of fetal heart rate monitoring, the reader is referred to standard tests (56).

VIII. Obstetrical Management of the Pregnant Asthmatic Patient

The obstetrical management of the pregnant asthmatic patient is also discussed in Chapter 20. Optimally, care of the pregnant asthmatic patient begins with an assessment before conception. At this point, the severity of the patient's asthma and the level of control of asthma can be assessed, and projected risks and interventions during pregnancy can be discussed. The conventional medications used to treat asthma—β-sympathomimetic drugs, corticosteroids, theophylline, and cromolyn—are not contraindicated during pregnancy (see Chapters 8 and 18).

Once the patient becomes pregnant, we perform an ultrasound examination between weeks 16 and 20 of the pregnancy to confirm gestational age and to assess for structural defects of the fetus. For patients with mild or well-controlled asthma, obstetric management is similar to routine pregnancy care. The patient is seen at monthly intervals until 32 weeks, then at 34 and 36 weeks, and weekly until term. Kick counts are recommended to the patient from 26 weeks gestation onward, and the fundal height is measured at each visit. Sonography is performed for these patients only if the fundal height falls behind gestational age or for other obstetrical indications. Routine fetal monitoring is not performed, but is reserved for those patients who have either fetal growth disturbances, as demonstrated by sonography, or abnormal fetal movement.

For the patient with severe or poorly controlled asthma, fetal surveillance is more intensive. We perform sonography for serial assessment of fetal growth at 26 weeks, and then at 4- to 6-week intervals throughout the pregnancy. As long as fetal growth is normal and maternal perception of fetal movement is normal, fetal monitoring is initiated at 32 weeks with twice-weekly nonstress testing. If fetal growth is impaired or if maternal perception of fetal movement is abnormal, fetal heart rate monitoring is initiated earlier, as early as 26 weeks gestation.

In the patient with normal fetal assessment and amniotic fluid volume, the pregnancy is allowed to proceed to term and no other obstetrical interventions are necessary. If intrauterine growth retardation is diagnosed but amniotic fluid volume and nonstress testing remain normal, the pregnancy is generally allowed to proceed. However, if the growth impairment is progressive, early delivery following demonstration of a mature lung profile is often considered.

As mentioned previously, the fetus with reduced amniotic fluid volume is at particular risk for adverse outcomes. For these cases, intensive antenatal surveillance is required, and therapy is individualized; often, oligohydramnios will prompt consideration of early delivery for fetal indications.

When a pregnant patient develops an acute exacerbation of asthma, management of the asthmatic episode per se is as for the nonpregnant patient, with the use of inhaled bronchodilators, corticosteroids, and aminophylline (see Chapter 18). However, careful monitoring of maternal oxygenation, particularly during the third trimester, is essential. Since the placenta is perfused by an admixture of maternal venous and arterial blood, the fetal oxygenation is relatively protected from changes in maternal arterial oxygenation so long as maternal cardiac output and mixed venous oxygenation are maintained. Declines of maternal oxygenation saturation to the 90–92% range ordinarily are not reflected in abnormal fetal heart rate tracings or adverse fetal outcomes. However, if the maternal arterial oxygen saturation falls below the 90% level, continuous fetal monitoring is recommended if intervention on behalf of the fetus would be performed. Furthermore, in such situations, maternal intubation for fetal indications might be required.

Management of labor in the pregnant asthmatic varies little from such management in nonasthmatic women. The stress of labor may occasionally precipitate an exacerbation of asthma, which is medically treated in the usual way. Mabie et al. (57) found that among 200 retrospectively reviewed pregnant asthmatic patients, 12% presented in labor with an asthmatic attack.

One important concern for the pregnant patient in labor, when gastric emptying slows (58), is that oral medications are relatively poorly absorbed. Thus, in the patient with severe asthma or the patient on a regimen of multiple medications, parenteral administration of antiasthmatic medications (e.g., aminophylline) during labor may occasionally be required. Parenteral hydrocortisone (100 mg every 8 hr) is recommended in corticosteroid-dependent patients to prevent asthma exacerbations and to provide steroid coverage for the increased physiological stress of labor and delivery.

Finally, betamimetic drugs, when given systemically, may hamper uterine contractions (59). Although betamimetic drugs are, in fact, used to treat preterm labor because of their uterine-relaxant effect, impaired uterine contractility during term labor is not a commonly encountered clinical problem. When it is encountered, it is usually overcome readily with oxytocin augmentation. None of the usual medications or therapeutic modalities that are used during labor itself are contraindicated in the presence of asthma. Narcotics for pain relief and epidural and spinal anesthesia are well tolerated.

General anesthesia is seldom required in obstetrics today, as regional techniques, such as epidural and spinal anesthesia, are readily available and adequate for caesarean delivery (60). If general anesthesia is required, the technique must be carefully considered. In the nonpregnant asthmatic patient who requires general anesthesia, the anesthesiologist may choose to use a halogenated anesthetic gas as the induction agent to maintain bronchodilatation before intubation. This can be done during pregnancy, but it could have two potential adverse effects. First, the anesthetic agent will reach the fetus and may cause depression at deliver (61). Second and perhaps more important, halogenated anesthetic gases, particularly halothane, are potent relaxants of uterine muscle, and substantial hemorrhage from uterine atony can occur in women anesthetized with halothane (62).

A. Prostaglandins

Prostaglandins (Pg) may be used for labor induction, cervical ripening, or postpartum bleeding. Prostaglandin E and its derivatives relax bronchial smooth muscle, and therefore may safely be used in the pregnant asthmatic. However, prostaglandin F and its derivatives are potent bronchial constrictors and should be used with caution in patients with asthma. Risk versus benefit must be weighed. In our experience, the mild asthmatic seldom develops an exacerbation after treatment for postpartum hemorrhage with the potent $PgF2\alpha$ derivative, Hemabate, which is the standard obstetric drug for severe postpartum uterine atony. We have not treated severe asthmatics with this medication. It may be preferable to use prostaglandin E in this setting—limited data suggest efficacy—but the drug has not been used extensively for uterine atony. Ergonovine derivatives for treatment of postpartum hemorrhage should also be avoided, if possible, in patients with asthma (see Chapter 20).

References

1. Gordon M, Niswander KR, Berendes H, Kantor AG. Fetal morbidity following potentially anoxogenic obstetric conditions. Am J Obstet Gynecol 1970; 106: 421–429.
2. Weinstein AM, Dubin BD, Podleski WK, Spector S, Farr R. Asthma in pregnancy. JAMA 1979; 241:1161–1165.
3. Hernandez E, Angell CS, Johnson JWC. Asthma in pregnancy: current concepts. Obstet Gynecol 1980; 55:739–743.
4. Meschia G. Supply of oxygen to the fetus. J Reprod Med 1979; 23:160–165.
5. Weinberger SE, Weiss ST, Cohen WR, Weiss JW, Johnson TS. Pregnancy and the lung. Am Rev Respir Dis 1980; 121:559–579.
6. Prowse CM, Gaensler EA. Respiratory and acid-base changes during pregnancy. Anesthesiology 1965; 26:381–392.
7. Knuttgen HG, Emerson K. Physiological response to pregnancy at rest and during exercise. J Appl Physiol 1974; 36:549–553.
8. Pernoll ML, Metcalfe J, Kovach PA, Wachtel R, Dunham MJ. Ventilation during rest and exercise in pregnancy and postpartum. Respir Physiol 1975; 25:295–310.

9. Pernoll ML, Metcalfe J, Schlenker TL, Welch JE, Matsumoto JA. Oxygen consumption at rest during exercise in pregnancy. Respir Physiol 1979; 25: 285–293.

10. Wulf KH, Kunzel W, Lehmann V. Clinical aspects of placental gas exchange. In: Longo LD, Bartes H, eds. Respiratory gas exchange and blood flow in the placenta. Proceedings of a symposium in conjunction with XXV International Congress of Physiological Sciences, Hanover, Germany 1971. Bethesda, Md: U.S. Department of Health Education and Welfare, National Institutes of Health, National Institute of Child Health and Human Development, 1972: Publ (NIH) 73-361.

11. Weiner CP. Cordocentesis for diagnostic indications: two years experience. Obstet Gynecol 1987; 70:664.

12. Anderson GH, Walker J. The effect of labor on the maternal blood-gas and acid-base status. J Obstet Gynaecol Br Commonw 1970; 77:289–293.

13. Templeton A, Kelman GR. Maternal blood gases. (Pao_2-Pao_2), physiological shunt and VD/VT in normal pregnancy. Br J Anaesth 1976; 48:1001–1004.

14. Meschia G. Placental respiratory gas exchange in fetal oxygenation. In: Creasy R, Resnik R, eds. Maternal-fetal medicine: principles and practice. 2d ed. Philadelphia: Saunders, 1989:303–313.

15. Levinson G, Shnider S, deLorimier AA, Steffenson JL. Effects of maternal hyperventilation on uterine blood flow and fetal oxygenation and acid-base status. Anesthesiology 1974; 40:340–347.

16. Wilkening RB, Meschia G. Current topic: comparative physiology of placental oxygen transport. Placenta 1992; 13:1–15.

17. Awe RJ, Nicotra MB, Newsom TD, Viles R. Arterial oxygenation in alveolar-arterial gradients in term pregnancy. Obstet Gynecol 1979; 53:182–186.

18. Aldrich CJ, D'Antona D, Spencer JAD, Wyatt JS, Peebles DM, Delpy DT, Reynolds EOR. The effect of maternal posture on fetal cerebral oxygenation during labor. Br J Obstet Gynaecol 1995; 102:14–19.

19. Aldrich CJ, Wyatt JS, Spencer JAD, Reynolds EOR, Delpy DT. The effect of maternal oxygen administration on human fetal cerebral oxygenation measured during labor by near infrared spectroscopy. Br J Obstet Gynaecol 1994; 101:509–513.

20. Lees M, Scott D, Kerr M, Taylor S. The circulatory effects of recumbent postural change in late pregnancy. Clin Sci 1967; 32:453–461.

21. Kelman G, Nunn J, Pryse-Roberts C, Greenbaum R. The influence of cardiac output on arterial oxygenation: a theoretical study. Br J Anaesth 1967; 39: 450–457.

22. Cousins LM. Obstetrical management and fetal surveillance in the pregnant diabetic. In: Brody S, Ueland K, eds. Endocrine Disorders in Pregnancy. Norwalk, CT: Appleton-Century-Crofts, 1989:345–361.

23. Lorijn RHW, Longo LD. Clinical and physiological implications of increased fetal oxygen consumption. Am J Obstet Gynecol 1980; 136:451–457.

24. Longo L, Hill E, Power G. Factors effecting placental oxygen transfer. In: Longo L, Bartes H, eds. Respiratory gas exchange blood flow in the placenta.

Bethesda, Md: Public Health Service, DHEW Publ. (NIH) 73-361, 1972: 345–391.

25. Motoyama E, Rivard G, Acheson F, Cook CD. The effects of changes in maternal pH and Pco_2 on the Po_2 of fetal lambs. Anesthesiology 1967; 28: 891–903.

26. Robson J, Schilid H. Effect of drugs on the blood flow and activity of the uterus. J Physiol 1938; 92:9–22.

27. Ahlquist R, Woodbury R. Influence of drugs in uterine activity upon uterine blood flow. Fed Proc 1947; 6:305–314.

28. Rosenfeld C, Barton M, Meschia G. Effects of epinephrine on distribution of blood flow in the pregnancy ewe. Am J Obstet Gynecol 1976; 124:156–163.

29. Adamson K, Mueller-Heubach E, Myers R. Production of fetal asphyxia in the rhesus monkey by administration of catecholamines to the mother. Am J Obstet Gynecol 1971; 109:248–262.

30. DiMarco AF. Asthma in the pregnant patient: a review. Ann Allergy 1989; 62:527–533.

31. Huff RW. Asthma in pregnancy. Med Clin North Am 1989; 73:653–660.

32. Bochner B, Lichenstein L. Anaphylaxis. N Engl J Med 1991; 324:1895–1901.

33. Entman SS, Moise KJ. Anaphylaxis in pregnancy. South Med J 1984; 77: 402–405.

34. Ladner C, Brinkman C, Weston P, Assali N. Dynamics of uterine circulation in pregnant and nonpregnant sheep. Am J Physiol 1970; 218:257–263.

35. Catanzarite V. Obstetrics and gynecology—antepartum care. In: Rakel R, ed. Conn's Current Therapy. Philadelphia: Saunders, 1991:931–993.

36. Campbell S, Warsof S, Little D, Cooper DJ. Routine ultrasound screening for the prediction of gestational age. Obstet Gynecol 1985; 65:613–620.

37. Geirsson RT. Ultrasound instead of last menstrual period as the basis of gestational age assignment. Ultrasound Obstet Gynecol 1991; 1:212–219.

38. Peeters LLH, Sheldon RE, Jones MD Jr, Makowski EL, Meshia G. Blood flow of fetal organs is a function of arterial oxygen content. Am J Obstet Gynecol 1979; 135:637–646.

39. Crane JP, Kopta MM. Comparative newborn anthropometric data in symmetric versus asymmetric intrauterine growth retardation. Am J Obstet Gynecol 1980; 138:518–522.

40. Hobbins JC, Berkowitz RL, Grannum P. Diagnosis and antepartum management of IUGR. J Reprod Med 1978; 21:319–325.

41. Mintz MC, Landon MB. Sonographic diagnosis of fetal growth disorders. Clin Obstet Gynecol 1988; 31:44–52.

42. Ott WJ, Doyle S, Flamm S. Accurate ultrasonic estimation of fetal weight. Am J Perinatal 1985; 2:178–182.

43. Hadlock FP, Deter RL, Rossavik I. Detection of abnormal fetal growth patterns. In: Athey PA, Hadlock FP, eds. Ultrasound in Obstetrics and Gynecology. 2d ed. St. Louis: Mosby, 1985:60–63.

44. Rutherford SE, Phelan JP, Smith CV, Jacobs N. The four quadrant assessment of amniotic fluid volume: an adjunct to antepartum fetal heart rate testing. Obstet Gynecol 1987; 70:353–653.

45. Rochelson B. The clinical significance of absent end-diastolic velocity in the umbilical artery waveforms. Clin Obstet Gynecol 1989; 32:692–702.

46. Chervenak FA, Berkowitz GS, Thorton J, Kreiss C, Youcha S, Ehrenkranz RA, Hobbins JC, Berkowitz RL. A comparison of sonographic estimation of fetal weight and obstetrically determined gestational age in the prediction of neonatal outcome for the very low-birth weight fetus. Am J Obstet Gynecol 1985; 152:47–50.

47. Hack M, Wright LL, Sharkaran S, et al. Very-low birth-weight outcomes of the National Institute of Child Health and Human Development Neonatal Network, November 1989 to October 1990. Am J Obstet Gynecol 1995; 172: 457–464.

48. Jobe A. Amniotic fluid tests of fetal lung maturity. In: Creasy R, Resnik R, eds. Maternal-Fetal Medicine: Principles and Practice. 2d ed. Philadelphia: Saunders, 1989:426–433.

49. Hagen E, Link JC, Arias F. A comparison of the accuracy of the TDX-FLM assay, lecithin-sphingomyelin ratio and phosphatidyl-glycerol in the prediction of neonatal respiratory distress syndrome. Obstet Gynecol 1993; 82:1004–1008.

50. Moore T, Piaquadio K. A prospective evaluation of fetal movement screening to reduce the incidence of antepartum fetal death. Am J Obstet Gynecol 1989; 160:1075–1080.

51. Rochard F, Schifrin BS, Goupil F, Legrand H, Blottiere J, Sureau C. Non-stressed fetal heart rate monitoring in the antepartum period. Am J Obstet Gynecol 1976; 126:699–706.

52. Manning FA, Morrison I, Lange IR, Harman CR, Chamberlain PF. Fetal assessment based on fetal biophysical profile scoring: experience in 12,620 referred high-risk pregnancies. 1. Perinatal mortality by frequency and etiology. Am J Obstet Gynecol 1985; 151:343–350.

53. Freeman RK. The use of the oxytocin challenge test for antepartum clinical evaluation of uteroplacental respiratory function. Am J Obstet Gynecol 1975; 121:481–489.

54. Alfirevic Z, Neilson JP. Doppler ultrasonography in high-risk pregnancies: systematic review with meta analysis. Am J Obstet Gynecol 1995; 172: 1379–1387.

55. Finberg HJ, Clewell WH. Ultrasound-guided interventions in pregnancy. In: Sander RC, Hill MC, eds. Ultrasound Quarterly. New York: Raven Press, 1990:197–226.

56. Freeman RK, Garite TJ, Nageotte MP, eds. Fetal Heart Rate Monitoring. 2d ed. Baltimore: Williams & Wilkins, 1991.

57. Mabie WC, Barton JR, Wasserstrum N, Sihai B. Clinical observations on asthma in pregnancy. J Mat Fetal Med 1992; 1:45–50.

58. Albright GA, Joyce TH III, Ferguson JE II, Jones MM, eds. Physiology and pharmacology. Physiology of pregnancy. In: Anesthesia in Obstetrics— Maternal, Fetal, and Neonatal Aspects. 2d ed. Woburn, MA: Butterworth, 1986:41–79.
59. Caritis SN, Darby MJ, Chan L. Pharmacologic treatment of preterm labor. Clin Obstet Gynecol 1988; 31:635–651.
60. Shnider SM, Levinson G, eds. Anesthesia for the pregnant patient with asthma. In: Anesthesia for Obstetrics. 2d ed. Baltimore: Williams & Wilkins, 1987:382–391.
61. Shnider SM, Levinson G, eds. Anesthesia for cesarean section. In: Anesthesia for Obstetrics. 2d ed. Baltimore: Williams & Wilkins, 1987:159–178.
62. Gilstrap LC, Hauth JC, Henkins GDJ, Patterson AR. Effect of type of anesthesia on blood loss at caesarean section. Obstet Gynecol 1987; 69:328.

3

Pulmonary Function During Pregnancy

ROBERT A. WISE

Johns Hopkins University School of Medicine
Baltimore, Maryland

I. Introduction

Pregnancy and parturition are accompanied by considerable changes in physiology, which would be expected to have marked effects on lung function. The hormonal milieu is altered, with increased levels of progesterone and estrogens; shifts in the balance of cyclo-oxygenase products; and increased systemic levels of cyclic nucleotides and peptide hormones. The products of conception require increased blood flow to the uterus and placenta; oxygen consumption is increased because of the demands of the fetus as well as the increase in body mass; and there are increases in blood volume and reduction of oncotic pressure which promote tissue edema formation. Over the years, there have been several excellent reviews of the effects of pregnancy on the respiratory system in health and disease (1–3). The remarkable finding from this body of information is how little normal lung function is altered by the normal pregnant condition. The purpose of this chapter is to review what is known about the effects of pregnancy on lung function in normal women, and the body's compensatory mechanisms (Table 1, see page 59). This chapter will also review the way that lung function measurements may be affected by common diseases.

Several different strategies have been employed to study the effect of pregnancy on lung function. Ideally, one would want to follow a cohort of women from the nonpregnant state throughout pregnancy and parturition. This has not been done, presumably because of the inconvenience of selecting a group of women who will soon become pregnant. More commonly, investigators have employed cross-sectional studies of nonsmoking healthy women at various stages of pregnancy and compared them to nonpregnant women. Other investigators have followed women longitudinally throughout pregnancy and compared the pregnant state to the postpartum state. In general, these two types of designs have provided similar results about the effect of pregnancy on lung function.

II. Lung Volumes

Many investigators have reported the effect of pregnancy on static lung volumes. There is little change in static lung volumes with pregnancy (Fig. 1). In a number of studies, the main findings have been an absent or minimal reduction in total lung capacity (TLC), a slight reduction in residual volume (RV), and a small increase or no change in vital capacity (VC)

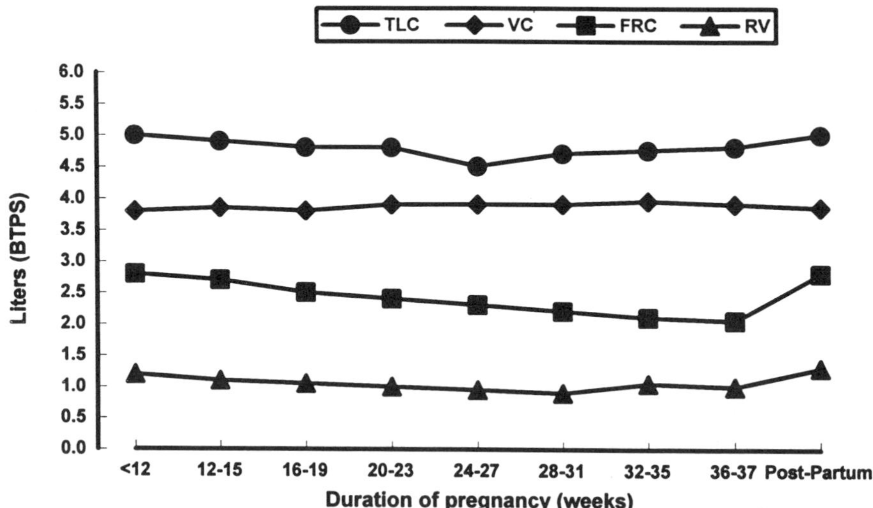

Figure 1 Representative mean changes in lung volumes during pregnancy and postpartum. TLC and VC stay nearly constant. FRC falls progressively throughout pregnancy. RV falls slightly. (Data from Ref. 26.)

(4–12). The most consistent and striking change in static lung volumes with pregnancy is the reduction in end-expiratory lung volume (functional residual capacity, FRC) and expiratory reserve volume (ERV) (13). The reduction in ERV is accompanied by a compensatory increase in inspiratory capacity (IC) so that the VC is preserved. The FRC falls progressively during gestation by about 10–25%, beginning during the second trimester (4). The normal reduction in FRC in the supine position compared to the upright or seated position is accentuated in pregnancy (14,15).

Since FRC represents the unstressed volume of the respiratory system, i.e., the balance of the retractile forces of the lung with the expansive

Table 1 Changes in Lung Functions
with Pregnancy

Measure	Change with pregnancy	
TLC	$\downarrow$	$\leftrightarrow$
VC	$\uparrow$	$\leftrightarrow$
FRC	$\downarrow$	
RV	$\leftrightarrow$	$\downarrow$
Lung compliance	$\leftrightarrow$	
Chest wall compliance	$\downarrow$	
Total respiratory compliance	$\downarrow$	
Pa_{o2}	$\uparrow$	
Pa_{co2}	$\downarrow$	
pH	$\leftrightarrow$	
Minute ventilation	$\uparrow$	
Tidal volume (TV)	$\uparrow$	
Breathing rate (f)	$\leftrightarrow$	
Airway conductance (raw)	$\uparrow$	
Closing volume (CV)	$\uparrow$	$\leftrightarrow$
Closing capacity (CC)	$\leftrightarrow$	
FEV1	$\leftrightarrow$	
MVV	$\leftrightarrow$	
PEFR	$\leftrightarrow$	$\downarrow$
Dl_{co}, rest upright	$\leftrightarrow$	
Dl_{co}, rest supine	$\downarrow$	
Dl_{co}, exercise	$\leftrightarrow$	

Key: $\uparrow$, increase; $\downarrow$, decrease; $\leftrightarrow$, no change. When two symbols are given, it indicates a diversity of findings in different studies. The second symbol represents the most prevalent or most current finding.

forces of the chest wall, a reduction in FRC may be the consequence of an alteration of the pressure–volume relationships of the thorax or the lung. Several studies have shown that the pressure–volume relationships of the lung are not altered during pregnancy in humans (5,16,17). The total respiratory system compliance and the chest wall compliance are, however, decreased during the last trimester of pregnancy (18). In the recumbent position, the chest wall compliance is reduced 38% at term compared to the immediate postpartum state; and the total respiratory system compliance is reduced 25%. The fall in FRC and reduction in respiratory system compliance are likely caused by the mechanical effects of the enlarged uterus compressing the abdominal compartment, since the reduction in FRC is correlated with the increase in end-expiratory gastric pressure, but not with the end-expiratory esophageal pressure (33).

It is quite likely, however, that the hormonal environment of pregnancy induces intrinsic changes to the elastic properties of the rib cage which tend to offset the mechanical effect of the gravid uterus. This is similar to the effects of pregnancy on the elasticity of the pelvic ligaments. In guinea pigs, pregnancy causes a progressive increase in the compliance of the chest wall throughout gestation (19). The increase in chest wall compliance is thought to be caused by substances produced during pregnancy, such as relaxin, a polypeptide hormone which causes dilatation of the cervix and relaxation of the pelvic ligaments (20,21). The notion that pregnancy induces intrinsic changes in the elastic properties of the chest wall in humans is supported by the finding that the subcostal angle increases from 68° to 103° early in pregnancy, before there is direct compression by the uterus. This change persists for months after pregnancy, when the uterus has returned to near-normal size (6,22,23).

The reduction in RV has never been well explained. Since the total lung capacity and vital capacity are preserved, it is not reasonable to account for this finding on the destruction or filling of lung parenchyma. Normally, in older adults, RV is determined by closure of airways, whereas in children and adolescents, RV is determined by the maximal ability of the expiratory muscles to shorten (23). Since the pregnant population consists of older adolescents and young adults, a reduction in RV must be caused either by a reduced tendency of airways to close, or by improved expiratory muscle function. Studies of airway closure using the single-breath nitrogen washout method have not shown any tendency for lower airway closing volumes or closing capacity (10,13,24,25). Thus, it seems inescapable that the reduction in RV must reflect improved expiratory muscle function. Because the abdominal muscles are extended, and the volume of the abdomen is increased, it would be possible for pregnant women to achieve greater expiratory efforts at low lung volumes. The improved expiratory muscle function and ability to achieve low residual volumes of the lung may also be beneficial for generating high abdominal pressures during active labor. Expiratory muscle strength at high lung volumes remains normal or slightly decreased (33).

III. Spirometry and Airflow Mechanics

Forced expiratory spirometry is often used to follow patients with asthma or other obstructive lung diseases. Several investigators have concluded that pregnancy has no significant effect on FEV1 or FEV1/FVC ratio (12,26–29). Slight reductions have been found for peak expiratory flow rates (PEFR), but these may be effort dependent since flow rates at lower lung volumes are not significantly affected by pregnancy (30). Thus, it is appropriate for the clinician to use nonpregnant baseline measures and nonpregnant reference population standards for evaluation of lung function in pregnant women. The clinician should attribute abnormalities of spirometry to concomitant lung disease rather than the pregnancy.

Flow volume loops have been analyzed to evaluate small airway function in pregnant women. The ratio of the maximum expiratory airflow at 50% and 25% of FVC (MEF_{50}/MEF_{25}) can be used to quantify the convexity of the terminal forced expiratory flow-volume curve. A ratio of 3 or less is considered indicative of normal terminal air flow. In nonsmoking normal pregnant women, this ratio is normal, which is taken as an indication that there is no dysfunction of the small airways (10). Although one early study has shown an elevation of the lung volume at which airways close during pregnancy (25), other subsequent studies have shown that pregnant women have a normal closing volume and closing capacity in both the upright and supine positions (10,24).

Airway conductance has been measured with esophageal balloon methods, body plethysmography, and the interrupter method (5,24,27). All of these studies show that airway conductance tends to increase slightly during the course of pregnancy, possibly the result of increased sensitivity to endogenous β-adrenergic stimulation induced by progesterone, or changes in the balance of bronchodilator and bronchoconstrictor prostaglandins (26).

IV. Chest Wall and Abdominal Mechanics

Pregnancy is associated with elevation of the diaphragm approximately 4 cm; an increase in the anterior-posterior and transverse diameter of the lower thorax by 2 cm, and an increase in the circumference of the ribcage by 5 cm (6,33). This elevation of the diaphragm leads to an increase in the area of apposition between the diaphragm and the lateral wall of the rib cage. This area of apposition permits the increase in abdominal pressure that occurs with contraction of the diaphragm to be translated into expansion of the rib cage (31). During pregnancy, the increase in tidal volume is achieved solely by an increase in the excursion of the rib cage while the excursion of the abdomen remains unchanged (32). Thus, the low FRC of pregnancy can be viewed as improving the efficiency of the diaphragm coupling with the rib cage. This contradicts the more traditional classic view, which pregnancy causes restriction of the diaphragm. Although it has been inferred that the compliance of the abdominal compartment (ΔVabd /ΔPga) may be reduced in some patients (32), direct measurements have failed to find any reduction in abdominal compliance (33). Coupled with the finding of increased end-expiratory gastric pressure during pregnancy, this suggests that the most important effect of pregnancy on the abdominal compartment is a reduction of the unstressed volume of the abdomen.

During lower-body water immersion in pregnancy, an increased external hydrostatic pressure is exerted on the abdomen and blood vessels of lower extremities. Although this stress causes a marked reduction in FRC, measurements have shown no change in FVC or FEV1 throughout most of pregnancy (34). The only period during which water immersion causes a fall in FVC and FEV1 is the 25th week of pregnancy, the period of peak plasma volume. This suggests that the reduction of FVC is due to translocation of blood or edema fluid into the thorax rather than restriction of the diaphragm.

V. Ventilation and Gas Exchange

Pregnancy is accompanied by progressive increase in resting minute ventilation (4,11,35–37). This increase in resting minute ventilation is due solely to an increase in tidal volume (TV), with a constant breathing frequency and duty cycle (T_I/T_{Tot}) (33). (Fig. 2) The ratio of wasted ventilation to tidal breathing (V_d/V_t) remains normal during pregnancy (41). Although not all studies are in agreement, the most common finding is that the increase in minute ventilation occurs early in pregnancy, before the end of the first trimester, and stays constant or increases slightly throughout the remainder of pregnancy (38). During pregnancy, the minute ventilation increases 20–40% compared to the postpartum value. In part, this is the response to the increase in metabolic rate and CO_2 production with pregnancy—about 15–20% above nonpregnant resting values. There is an additional augmentation of oxygen consumption and CO_2 production in the

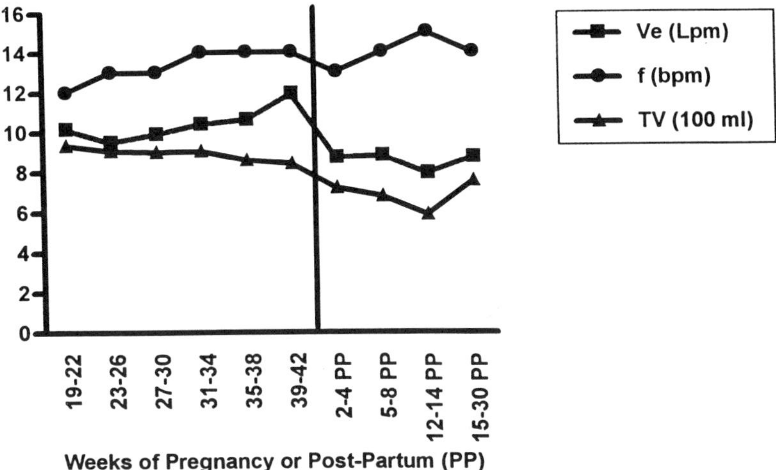

Figure 2 Representative changes in ventilation during pregnancy and postpartum. Minute ventilation (Ve) and tidal volume (TV) are increased throughout pregnancy compared to postpartum. Breathing rate (f) is not different from postpartum values. The vertical line separates pregnancy from postpartum (PP) values. (Data from Ref. 37.)

upright position, increasing from 320 mL/min to 500 mL/min and from 300 to 340 mL/min, respectively (15).

Because the increase in minute ventilation is more than that which is required to clear the excess CO_2 production, the arterial CO_2 falls to 32–34 mmHg from the normal value of 40 mmHg (39). There is renal compensation for the respiratory alkalosis, with excretion of bicarbonate causing a reduction in serum bicarbonate to about 15–20 meq/L from the normal value of 24 meq/L (40–42). This respiratory alkalosis leads to an increased erythrocyte level of 2,3-diphosphoglycerate (2,3-DPG), which causes a rightward shift of the oxyhemoglobin dissociation curve and allows increased oxygen transfer across the placenta (43,44).

The major cause for the increase in minute ventilation is generally considered to be caused by the pregnancy-associated increase in progesterone, which stimulates central respiratory drive. One measure of ventilatory drive, the mean inspiratory flow rate (V_t/T_i), is increased in pregnancy (33). Pregnancy is also accompanied by a 13% increase in the slope and a decrease in the intercept of the CO_2 ventilatory response curve. This increased chemosensitivity remains constant between the first and third trimesters of pregnancy despite increasing metabolic demands of the fetoplacental unit, and returns to normal shortly after delivery (38). In contrast to the CO_2 response, the central respiratory drive, assessed by the immediate response to airway occlusion ($P_{0.1}$), increases progressively during pregnancy, and falls precipitously in the postpartum period. This progressive increase in respiratory drive, despite constant minute ventilation, constant $PaCO_2$, and constant respiratory muscle strength has been interpreted to mean that the effective respiratory impedance is increased throughout the course of pregnancy (33). The increase in respiratory drive correlates with the serum levels of progesterone, which increase during the course of pregnancy (33).

Progesterone has long been established as a respiratory stimulant (45). When administered to men, progesterone increases minute ventilation and increases ventilatory drive measured by the ventilatory response to CO_2 and $P_{0.1}$ occlusion pressure (46–48). It is not clear, however, if progesterone acts through direct stimulation of the respiratory center, or whether it alters the sensitivity to chemostimulation (49). Studies of the cerebrospinal fluid have shown a respiratory alkalosis which is appropriate for the level of arterial respiratory alkalosis, and which is correlated to the progesterone level in arterial blood (50).

Pregnancy has also been associated with an increase in the hypoxic ventilatory response about twice the normal level (51). This occurs despite the respiratory alkalosis which tends to suppress the hypoxic ventilatory response. In contrast to the hypercapnic response, the hypoxic response has not been well correlated with progesterone levels. Animal studies suggest that the increase in sensitivity to hypoxia requires the interaction of progesterone and estrogen (52,53).

The increased alveolar ventilation of pregnancy is associated with an appropriate increase in arterial Po_2 to levels of 100–105 mmHg (40,41,54). The alveolar-arterial oxygen difference is normal in the upright position (38). In some patients, however, the A–a gradient may widen during recumbency (55,56). This is thought to be caused by the reduction in FRC, which allows some airways at the base of the lung to close during portions of tidal breathing (13). It is likely that this phenomenon is more prevalent in patients with elevated airway closing volumes from cigarette smoking or who have a lower FRC because of obesity or polyhydramnios. Because the arterial oxygen tension is near the flat portion of the saturation curve, however, recumbency does not usually cause a significant fall is arterial oxygen saturation (30). Despite the elevation in arterial oxygen tension, the reduction in FRC leads to a reduction in oxygen stores. For this reason, in conjunction with the increased metabolic rate, pregnant patients are particularly prone to arterial oxygen desaturation during breath holding or respiratory depression (57,58).

VI. Diffusing Capacity for Carbon Monoxide

During pregnancy, the blood volume and pulmonary blood flow are increased compared to baseline. While these factors should cause an increase in recruitment of capillary surface area for gas exchange, leading to an increase in diffusing capacity for carbon monoxide (Dco), they are partially offset by the reduction in hemoglobin level that occurs with pregnancy. Thus, most investigators have concluded that there is either no effect or a slight fall of Dco with pregnancy (26,30). Normally, the Dco increases when a person assumes the supine position. This normal increment in Dco in the supine position is absent or diminished in pregnancy (30). One possible explanation for this is that the cardiac output normally rises in the supine position in nonpregnant women, but falls in pregnant women (54). The other possible explanation for the failure to increase Dco in the supine position is that the pulmonary capillary bed is already fully recruited. This second explanation is not likely, however, because the Dco rises normally with exercise in pregnant women (59).

VII. Dyspnea in Pregnancy

Dyspnea, either as a heightened sensation of breathing at rest or a sensation of breathlessness with exercise, is common during pregnancy. About 70–80% of pregnant women report exertional dyspnea by 30 weeks gestation (60–63). The cause for this "physiological" dyspnea has been the subject of considerable speculation. The two general proposed mechanisms are that it is caused either by increased drive to breath or by increased work of breathing. There is no evidence that pregnancy results in increased sensation of dyspnea at the cortical level, although this possibility has not been rigorously tested. The increased drive to breath is generally thought to be caused by elevated progesterone levels. Decreased exercise efficiency from the increased body weight and elevated metabolic rate result in higher requirements for oxygen utilization for a particular level of external work. The increased work of breathing is due to the increased minute ventilation and possibly alterations in the efficiency of the respiratory muscles from the changes in thoraco-abdominal configuration. Other factors which may be postulated to contribute to a sensation of dyspnea in pregnancy include increases in pulmonary blood volume, anemia, or nasal congestion.

The most comprehensive study of the psychophysilogical basis of exertional dyspnea in normal pregnancy has concluded that the sensation of exertional dyspnea in pregnancy can be accounted for by the increase in pleural pressure swings (64). These investigators found that there was no difference in the relationship between pleural pressure swings and tidal volume during pregnancy compared with 3 months postpartum. The subjective rating of breathlessness with exercise was closely linked to the magnitude of the pleural pressure swings, and this relationship was similar in the gravid and postpartum conditions. Although this study needs to be replicated, it suggests that the dyspnea of pregnancy can be accounted for solely by the increase in tidal volume and pleural pressure swings with pregnancy.

Because dyspnea is a common symptom of normal pregnancy, it may be difficult for the health-care provider to distinguish pathological conditions, or to decide when further testing is warranted. Findings that point toward a pathologic cause of dyspnea in pregnancy are shown in Table 2.

VIII. Pulmonary Function in Disease States During Pregnancy

In light of the minor effects of pregnancy on lung function, it can be safely assumed by treating physicians that significant deviations from baseline or from predicted reference values for FVC, FEV1, or Dco represent the effect of concurrent lung disease. Pregnancy can also modulate the progression of several lung diseases because of the hormonal and physical changes which accompany pregnancy. Asthma is treated extensively elsewhere in this text, and will not be discussed here. Other immunologically mediated diseases which are common in young women—in particular, sarcoidosis, systemic lupus erythematosus, and rheumatoid arthritis—have been studied in large populations. Although there is variability, the most common finding is that these inflammatory disorders tend to stabilize or

Table 2 Clinical Findings That Suggest Pathological Dyspnea in Pregnancy

History of cardiac or respiratory disease
Sudden onset or worsening of dyspnea
Respiratory rate greater than 20
Alveolar-arterial oxygen difference greater than 25 mmHg
Arterial P_{co2} less than 30 mmHg
Arterial P_{co2} greater than 35 mmHg
Abnormal spirometry measures (FEV1, FVC, FEV1/FVC)
Abnormal total lung capacity

remit during pregnancy (65–69). This suggests that the increase in steroid hormones during pregnancy or other factors have a mild immunosuppressive effect (70). On the other hand, diseases that are caused by chronic infection, such as tuberculosis or coccidioidomycosis, will often worsen during pregnancy (71–73). Some rare pulmonary disorders, such as lymphangiomyomatosis and familial fibrosing alveolitis, have been anecdotally reported to worsen as a result of pregnancy (74,75). The course of cystic fibrosis, on the other hand, does not seem to be altered by pregnancy (76).

Even with stable lung function, however, the stress of pregnancy with the increased ventilatory drive and demands may worsen already present dyspnea. The increase in cardiac output and systemic blood volume may worsen preexisting pulmonary hypertension (77,78). The work of breathing is increased as a result of the increase in minute ventilation and the decrease in respiratory system compliance. This places women who have chronic respiratory insufficiency from airway, parenchymal, or neuromuscular disease at serious risk for acute respiratory failure (66,79–81). Thus, many believe that the presence of pulmonary hypertension or chronic hypercapnic respiratory failure constitute serious contraindications to pregnancy, and are grounds for recommending therapeutic abortion.

References

1. Fishburne JI. Physiology and disease of the respiratory system in pregnancy. A review. J Reprod Med 1979; 22:177–189.
2. Lapinsky SE, Kruczynski K, Slutsky AS. Critical care in the pregnant patient. Am J Respir Crit Care Med 1995; 152:427–455.
3. Weinberger SE, Weiss ST, Cohen WR, Weiss JW, Johnson TS. Pregnancy and the lung. Am Rev Respir Dis 1980; 121:559–581.
4. Cugell DW, Frank NR, Gaensler EA, Badger TL. Pulmonary function in pregnancy, 1: serial observations in normal women. Am Rev Tuber Pulm Dis 1953; 67:568–589.
5. Gee JBL, Packer BS, Millen JE, Robin ED. Pulmonary mechanics during pregnancy. J Clin Invest 1967; 46:945–952.
6. Thomson KJ, Cohen ME. Studies in the circulation in pregnancy. II. Vital capacity observations in normal pregnant women. Surg Gynecol Obstet 1938; 66:591–603.
7. Gazioglu K, Kaltreider NL, Rosen M, Yu PN. Pulmonary function during pregnancy in normal women and in patients with cardiopulmonary disease. Thorax 1970; 25:445–450.
8. Ihrman K. A clinical and physiological study of pregnancy in a material from northern Sweden; III. Vital capacity and maximal breathing capacity during and after pregnancy. Acta Soc Med Upsalla 1960; 65:147–154.

9. Rubin A, Russo N, Goucher D. The effect of pregnancy upon pulmonary function in normal women. Am J Obstet Gynecol 1956; 72:963–969.

10. Baldwin GR, Moorthi DS, Whelton JA, MacDonell KF. New lung functions and pregnancy. Am J Obstet Gynecol 1977; 127:235–239.

11. Alaily AV, Carrol KB. Pulmonary ventilation in pregnancy. Br J Obstet Gynaecol 1978; 85:518–524.

12. Chhabra S, Nangia V, Ingley KN. Changes in respiratory function tests during pregnancy. Indian J Physiol Pharmacol 1988; 32:56–60.

13. Russell IF, Chambers WA. Closing volume in normal pregnancy. Br J Anaesth 1981; 53:1043–1047.

14. Blair E, Hickham JB. The effect of change in body position on lung volume and intrapulmonary gas mixing in normal subjects. J Clin Invest 1955; 34: 383–389.

15. Schneider KT, Deckardt R. The implication of upright posture on pregnancy. J Perinat Med 1991; 19: 121–131.

16. Pasargiklian R, Brambati B, Robuschi M, Bianco S. Aspetti della funzione respiratoria in gravidanza; 1) Volumi polmonari statici, compliance, ventilazione polmonare e consumo di O2 a riposo durante il secondo trimestre. Minerva Ginecologica 1979; 29:5–12.

17. Pasargiklian R, Brambati B, Robuschi M, Bianco S. Aspetti della funzione respiratoria in gravidanza; 4) volumi statici, compliance ventilazione polmonare e consumo di O2 a riposo durante il terzo trimestre. Minerva Ginecologica 1977; 29:31–38.

18. Marx GF, Murthy PK, Orkin LR. Static compliance before and after vaginal delivery. Br J. Anaesth 1970; 42:1100–1104.

19. Oddoy A, Merker G. Lung mechanics and blood gases in pregnant guinea pigs. Acta Physiol Hung 1987; 70:311–315.

20. Sherwood OD, Downing SJ, Guico-Lamm ML, Hwang JJ, O'Day-Bowman MB, Fields PA. The physiological effects of relaxin during pregnancy: studies in rats and pigs. Oxf Rev Reprod Biol 1993; 15:143–189.

21. Goldsmith LT, Weiss G, Steinetz BG. Relaxin and its role in pregnancy. Endocrinol Metab Clin N Am 1995; 24:171–186.

22. Marx GF, Orkin LR. Physiological changes during pregnancy: a review. Anesthesiology 1958: 19:258.

23. Leith DE, Mead J. Mechanisms determining residual volume of the lungs in normal subjects. J Appl Physiol 1967; 23:221–227.

24. Garrard GS, Littler WA, Redman CW. Closing volume during normal pregnancy. Thorax 1978; 33:488–492.

25. Bevan DR, Holdcroft A, Loh L, MacGregor WG, O'Sullivan JC, Sykes MK. Closing volume and pregnancy. Br Med J 1974; 1(896):13–15.

26. Milne JA. The respiratory response to pregnancy. Postgrad Med J 1979; 55: 318–324.

27. Milne JA, Mills RJ, Howie AD, Pack AI. Large airways function during normal pregnancy. Br J Obstet Gynaecol 1977; 84:448–451.

28. Mokkapatti R, Prasad EC, Venkatraman, Fatima K. Ventilatory functions in pregnancy. Indian J Physiol Pharmacol 1991; 35:237–240.
29. Pasargiklian R, Brambati B, Robuschi M, Bianco. Aspetti della funzione respiratoria in gravidanza; 2) volumi dinamici, resistenza delle vie aeree, curve flusso-volume durante il secondo trimestre. Minerva Ginecologica 1977; 29: 13–20.
30. Norregaard O, Schultz P, Ostergaard A, Dahl R. Lung function and postural changes during pregnancy. Respir Med 1989; 83:467–470.
31. Mead J. Functional significance of the area of apposition of diaphragm to ribcage. Am Rev Respir Dis 1979; 119(suppl):32S.
32. Gilroy RJ, Mangura BT, Lavietes MH. Rib cage and abdominal volume displacements during breathing in pregnancy. Am Rev Respir Dis 1988; 137: 668–672.
33. Contreras G, Gutierrez M, Beroiza T, Fantin A, Oddo H, Villarroel L, Cruz E, Lisboa C. Ventilatory drive and respiratory muscle function in pregnancy. Am Rev Respir Dis 1991; 144:837–841.
34. Berry MJ, McMurray RG, Katz VL. Pulmonary and ventilatory responses to pregnancy, immersion, and exercise. J Appl Physiol 1989; 66:857–862.
35. Rees GB, Pipkin FB, Symonds EM, Patrick JM. A longitudinal study of respiratory changes in normal human pregnancy with cross-sectional data on subjects with pregnancy-induced hypertension. Am J Obstet Gynecol 1990; 162:826–830.
36. Knuttgen HG, Emerson K Jr. Physiological response to pregnancy at rest and during exercise. J Appl Physiol 1974; 36:549–553.
37. Pernoll ML, Metcalfe J, Kovack PA, Wachtel R, Dunham MJ. Ventilation during rest and exercise in pregnancy and postpartum. Respir Physiol 1975; 25:295–310.
38. Liberatore SM, Pistelli R, Patalano F, Moneta E, Incalzi RA, Ciappi G. Respiratory function during pregnancy. Respiration 1984; 46:145–150.
39. Prowse CM, Gaensler EA. Respiratory acid-base changes during pregnancy. Anesthesiology 1965; 26:381–392.
40. Andersen GJ, James GB, Mathers NP, Smith EL, Walker J. The maternal oxygen tension and acid-base status during pregnancy. J Obstet Gynaecol Br Commonw 1969; 76:16–19.
41. Templeton A, Kelman GR. Maternal blood gases, PA_{O_2}-Pa_{O_2}, physiological shunt and V_d/V_t in normal pregnancy. Br J Anaesth 1967; 48:1001–1008.
42. Lucius H, Gablenbeck H, Kleine HO, Fabel H, Bartels H. Respiratory function, buffer system and electrolyte concentrations of blood during human pregnancy. Respir Physiol 1970; 9:311–315.
43. Sherman HF, Scott LM, Rosemurgy AS. Changes affecting the initial evaluation and care of the pregnant trauma victim. J Emerg Med 1990; 8:575–582.
44. Tsai C, De Leeuw NK. Changes in 2,3-diphosphoglycerate during pregnancy and puerperium in normal women and β-thalassemia heterozygous women. Am J Obstet Gynecol 1982; 142:520.

45. Lyons HA, Antonio R. The sensitivity of the respiratory center in pregnancy and after the administration of progesterone. Trans Assoc Am Phys 1959; 72: 173–180.

46. Zwillich CW, Natalino MR, Sutton FD, Weil JV. Effects of progesterone on chemosensitivity in normal men. J Lab Clin Med 1978; 92:262–269.

47. Schoene RB, Pierson DJ, Lakshminarayan S, Shrader DL, Butler J. Effect of medoxyprogesteroneacetate on respiratory drives and occlusion pressure. Bull Eur Physiopathol Respir 1980; 16:645–653.

48. Sutton FD, Zwillich CW, Creagh E, Pierson DJ, Weil JV. Progesterone for outpatient treatment of Pickwickian syndrome. Ann Intern Med 1975; 83: 476–479.

49. Skatrud JB, Dempsey JA, Kaiser DB. Ventilatory response to medoxyprogesterone acetate in normal subjects: time course and mechanism. J Appl Physiol: Respir Environ Exercise Physiol 1978; 44:939–944.

50. Machida H. Influence of progesterone on arterial blood and CSF acid-base balance in women. J Appl Physiol: Respir, Environ, Exercise Physiol 1981; 51:1433–1436.

51. Moore LG, McCullough RE, Weil JV. Increased HVR in pregnancy: relationship to hormonal and metabolic changes. J Appl Physiol 1987; 62:158–163.

52. Hannhart B, Pickett CK, Moore LG. Effects of estrogen and progesterone on carotid body neural output responsiveness to hypoxia. J Appl Physiol 1990; 68:1909–1916.

53. Bayliss DA, Cidlowski JA, Millhorn DE. The stimulation of respiration by progesterone in ovariectomized cat is mediated by an estrogen-dependent hypothalamic mechanism requiring gene expression. Endocrinology 1990; 126: 519–527.

54. Schneider-Affeld F, Kaukel E, Nienstedt K. Lageabhangife Veranderungen von Lungenfunktions und Kreistaufparametern bei graviden Frauen am Geburtstermin. Zeit Geburtsh u Perinat 1983; 187:65–68.

55. Ang CK, Tan TH, Walters WA, Wood C. Postural influence on maternal capillary oxygen and carbon dioxide tensions. Br Med J 1969; 4:201–203.

56. Awe RJ, Nicotra B, Newton TD, Viles R. Arterial oxygenation and alveolar-arterial oxygen gradients in term pregnancy. Obstet Gynecol 1979; 53: 182–186.

57. Schoenfeld A, Ovadia Y, Neri A, Freedman S. Obstructive sleep apnea (OSA)—Implication in maternal-fetal medicine. A hypothesis. Med Hypoth 1989; 30:51–54.

58. Archer GW, Marx GF. Arterial oxygen tension during apnoea in parturient women. Br J Anaesth 1974; 46:358–360.

59. Bedell GN, Adams RW. Pulmonary diffusing capacity during rest and exercise. A study of normal persons and persons with atrial septal defect, pregnancy, and pulmonary disease. J Clin Invest 1962; 41:1908–1914.

60. Gilbert R, Auchincloss JH. Dyspnea of pregnancy; clinical and physiological observations. Am J Med Sci 1966; 252:270–276.

61. Milne J, Howie A, Pack A. Dyspnea during normal pregnancy. Br J Obstet Gynaecol 1978; 85:260–263.
62. Tenholder M, South-Paul J. Dyspnea in pregnancy. Chest 1989; 96:381–388.
63. Zeldis SM. Dyspnea during pregnancy. Distinguishing cardiac from pulmonary causes. Clin Chest Med 1992; 13:567–585.
64. Field SK, Bell SG, Cenaiko DF, Whitelaw WA. Relationship between inspiratory effort and breathlessness in pregnancy. J Appl Physiol 1991; 71: 1897–1902.
65. Dines DE, Banner EA. Sarcoidosis during pregnancy: improvement in pulmonary function. JAMA 1967; 200:726–727.
66. King TE Jr. Restrictive lung disease in pregnancy. Clin Chest Med 1992; 13: 607–622.
67. Noble PW, Lavee AE, Jacobs MM. Respiratory diseases in pregnancy. Obstet Gynecol Clin N Am 1988; 15:391–428.
68. Fortin F, Wallaert B. Interstitial pathology and pregnancy. Rev Mal Respir 1988; 5:275–278.
69. Haynes de Regt R. Sarcoidosis and pregnancy. Obstet Gynecol 1987; 70: 369–372.
70. Barbee RA, Hicks MJ, Grosso D, Sandel C. The maternal immune response in coccidioidomycosis. Is pregnancy a risk factor for serious infection? Chest 1991; 100:709–715.
71. Jacobs RF, Abernathy RS. Management of tuberculosis in pregnancy and the newborn. Clin Perinatol 1988; 15:305–319.
72. Peterson CM, Schuppert K, Kelly PC, Pappagianis D. Coccidioidomycosis and pregnancy. Obstet Gynecol Surv 1993; 48:149–156.
73. Walker MP, Brody CZ, Resnik R. Reactivation of coccidioidomycosis in pregnancy. Obstet Gynecol 1992; 79:815–817.
74. Prichard MG, Musk AW. Adverse effect of pregnancy on familial fibrosing alveolitis. Thorax 1984; 39:319–320.
75. Wahedna I, Cooper S, Williams J, Paterson IC, Britton JR, Tattersfield AE. Relation of pulmonary lymphangio-leiomyomatosis to use of the oral contraceptive pill and fertility in the UK: a national case control study. Thorax 1994; 49:910–914.
76. Canny GJ, Corey M, Livingstone RA, Carpenter S, Green L, Levison H. Pregnancy and cystic fibrosis. Obstet Gynecol 1991; 77:850–853.
77. Roberts NV, Keast PJ. Pulmonary hypertension and pregnancy—a lethal combination. Anaesth Intensive Care 1990; 18:366–374.
78. Baethge BA, Wolf RE. Successful pregnancy with scleroderma renal disease and pulmonary hypertension in a patient using angiotensin converting enzyme inhibitors. Ann Rheum Dis 1989; 48:776–778.

79. Bravo RH, Katz M, Inturrisi M, Cohen NH. Obstetric management of Landry-Guillain-Barre syndrome: a case report. Am J Obstet Gynecol 1982; 142: 714–715.
80. Lalli CM, Raju L. Pregnancy and chronic obstructive pulmonary disease. Chest 1981; 80:759–761.
81. Geisler CF, Bulhler JH, Depp R. Alpha-1-antitrypsin deficiency: severe obstructive lung disease and pregnancy. Obstet Gynecol 1977; 49:31–34.

4

Maternal Immune Function During Pregnancy

REUBEN FALKOFF

Kaiser Permanente Medical Center
San Diego, California

I. Introduction

A great variety of approaches have been applied to the study of immunity during pregnancy. At times dramatic findings have been claimed, and at times these results have been held to be expected, since no immunological event (or nonevent) has been more perplexing than the failure of the mother to reject the fetal allograft. However, the evidence is now overwhelming that the principal reason for the failure of the mother to reject the fetus is the lack of vascular continuity of mother and fetus and their physical separation by a continuous trophoblast layer. There are, of course, many failsafes in the immune system, and suppressive mechanisms at the placental interface may also be of some importance. However, the notion that systemic maternal immunosuppression is necessary for fetal survival is clearly wrong, and any study claiming to find dramatic impairment of immunity must be examined critically given the observation that the vast majority of pregnancies are not complicated by any condition attributable to immunosuppression.

This review will present laboratory findings relevant to an understanding of immunological competence and host defense during pregnancy. In addition, relevant clinical observations will be summarized since these provide clues as to areas of possible immune impairment and place limits on the severity and frequency of these impairments.

II. Humoral Immunity

Humoral immunity is easily studied, since the bottom line is whether or not antibodies of appropriate specificities and classes are found in appropriate amounts following deliberate (immunization) or inadvertent (infectious) exposures. Any change in humoral immunological competence would be manifest as a change in levels of serum immunoglobulins, antigen-specific antibody responses, autoantibodies, or immune complexes.

A. Serum Immunoglobulin Levels

IgG

Numerous studies have found a fall in IgG levels roughly in proportion to the hemodilution of pregnancy (1–4). A longitudinal study found the IgG-to-serum albumin ratio to be almost constant in several specimens for each subject, "which implies that the decrease in IgG class was mainly, if not exclusively, due to hemodilution" (4). All IgG subclasses are transported across the placenta, and although there may be some preferential transport of IgG_1, this does not lead to any change in subclass distribution in maternal blood (5–7).

IgM

IgM levels do not change significantly (1–3); IgM-to-albumin ratios actually increase (4).

IgA

IgA levels either fall slightly or do not change. As with IgM, the ratio to serum albumin actually increases (1–4). Although IgA is not transported across the placenta, increased concentrations of IgA are found in saliva (8); it is not known whether or not a similar increase occurs at other mucosal surfaces.

The failure of IgA and of IgM levels to fall in proportion to the increase in plasma volume during pregnancy suggests a net increase in the amounts of these immunoglobulins. Although it is not clear whether this results from increased production or decreased catabolism, the changes are slight and are not likely to be of clinical significance.

Table 1 Summary of Maternal Immunological Changes in Pregnancy

Parameter	Change during pregnancy
Cell counts	
Total white count	Increase
Neutrophils	Increased
Lymphocytes	No change
Monocytes	Increased
T/B cell ratio	No change
CD4/CD8 ratio	No change
Immunoglobulins	
IgG	Decreased by hemodilution
IgA	No change or minimally decreased
IgM	No change
IgE	No consistent change
Antigen-specific antibodies	No change
Autoantibodies	
Rheumatoid factor	No change
ANA	No change
Antithyroid antibodies	Decreased
Anti-insulin antibodies	Decreased
In-vivo DTH	
Delayed skin test reactivity	No change
Allograft rejection	No change
In-vitro lymphocyte responsiveness	
Mitogens: PHA, Con A, PWM	No change in most studies
Mixed lymphocyte culture	No change
Antigen-induced	Conflicting data
In-vitro cytotoxicity	
T-cell mediated	Little valid data (marginally decreased)
Natural killer cell mediated	30% decrease
Antibody-dependent cell mediated	Conflicting: normal or decreased by 30%
Polymorphonuclear cell function	
Chemotaxis	Slightly decreased
Adherence	Decreased or increased depending on target
Phagocytosis	Unaffected or increased
Reactive oxidative metabolism	Depends on stimulus

IgE

Knobloch (9) reported no statistical difference between serum IgE levels
in pregnant women in the first trimester of pregnancy compared with levels
in different subjects in the third trimester. Amino et al. (2) serially mea-

                                                          Falkoff

sured serum IgE levels during early, mid, and late pregnancy in 10 normal pregnant women and found no significant change in mean levels and no consistent trend toward increasing or decreasing levels. In a study of pregnant asthmatics, Gluck found the levels of IgE to correlate with the activity of the patients' asthma rather than the stage of pregnancy (10), with levels rising, remaining the same, or dropping in equal numbers of patients. In a longitudinal study, Schatz et al. found no significant difference in mean IgE levels in 34 asthmatic women when compared in early, mid, or late pregnancy or 6 weeks postpartum, and IgE levels did not correlate with changes in asthma severity (11). Thus no study has suggested an effect of pregnancy on IgE levels.

B. Antigen-Specific Antibody Responses

Responses to Immunization

Antigen-specific responses to vaccines during pregnancy have been studied in detail. The primary and secondary responses to tetanus toxoid (12–14) and to influenza vaccine (15) have been shown to be normal at all stages of pregnancy, as has the third-trimester response to a group B *Streptococcus* vaccine (16). [A single study found the optimal schedule for immunization to tetanus toxoid to be altered in very late pregnancy, but even this study demonstrated good responsiveness; furthermore, those who received the immunizations latest were also the ones presenting latest and receiving the least prenatal care, so the findings may have been affected by factors other than inherent immunological changes of pregnancy (17)]. In addition, the responses to numerous other vaccines, including pneumococcal, *Hemophilus* influenza, meningococcal, and hepatitis vaccines have all been found to be adequate, but have not been compared directly to the responses of nonpregnant women.

Thus appropriate responses have been demonstrated to both thymus-dependent and thymus-independent vaccine antigens, implying normal B-cell function throughout pregnancy and presumably normal interactions between B cells and all the regulatory cells required in the responses to thymus-dependent antigens. Generally, immunization in pregnancy, including the third trimester, is so reliable that it is now being exploited as a way to increase passive protection for the newborn (18,19).

Responses to Natural Exposures

The levels of preexisting antibodies to herpes simplex, measles, rubella, and influenza A viruses have been followed longitudinally throughout pregnancy. While absolute levels fell 18–48%, when corrected for hemodilution by relating the values to serum albumin concentration, there were only slight declines in the amounts of antibodies directed toward herpes and measles viruses, and the values for rubella and influenza viruses increased slightly (20). In another study, primary infection with rubella during pregnancy resulted in high levels of IgM and IgG, while reinfections led to very high levels of virus-specific IgA (21). Thus, as with immunization, there appear to be no major alterations in antigen-specific antibody responses to viral infections in pregnancy.

C. Autoantibodies

Studies of Unselected or Healthy Women

Sokel et al. (22) found the frequency of the de-novo appearance of red cell autoantibodies to be 1 in 50,000 pregnancies. The data regarding positive antinuclear antibodies (ANAs) is conflicting. Reyes-Lopez et al. (23) found weakly positive ANAs at the same frequency in pregnant and nonpregnant populations, in agreement with the more recent findings of Patton et al. (24), Rosenberg et al. (25), and El-Roeiy et al. (26), who reported the more common autoantibodies as occurring with the same frequencies in pregnant and nonpregnant women. Ailus followed the levels of autoantibodies in 220 women in each trimester and 4–6 months after delivery. Regarding IgG and IgM rheumatoid factors, anticardiolipin antibodies, and anti-ss-DNA antibodies and IgG antithyroglobulin antibodies, "the mean levels of these autoantibodies seemed to reflect changes in the levels of the respective immunoglobulin classes. A clear decline toward term was found in the IgG-class whereas no appreciable change was noted in IgM-class autoantibodies" (4). In a nonlongitudinal study examining the prevalence of non-organ-specific autoantibodies in 203 pregnant and 365 nonpregnant women, Mavridis found anti-ds-DNA and anticardiolipin antibodies to be less frequent in pregnancy (9.4% versus 17.8% of nonpregnant women). In both populations these autoantibodies were "of the IgM class, found in low titers without any clinical importance" (27).

In Patients with Autoimmune Disease or Selected by Virtue of Having Autoantibodies

Several authors have followed autoantibody levels in patients with autoimmune diseases and known autoantibody levels prospectively in pregnancy. Pope et al. (28) found no consistent change in IgM or IgG rheumatoid factors in prospectively followed patients with classic rheumatoid arthritis. Exon et al. (29) found that the levels of anti-insulin antibodies fell in 12 of 13 diabetics; in none of these were the antibodies of any proven clinical significance. Amino (30) found that when antithyroid antibodies were detectable in patients with Graves' disease or autoimmune thyroiditis in early pregnancy, the titers consistently decreased later, only to rise again after delivery; the decrease in titers was often sizable (more than 100-fold). D'Armiento followed the behavior of serum antithyroglobulin antibodies in 6 women without evidence of thyroid disease who had detectable levels when first tested. In all six, the levels fell considerably by term (31).

Interpreting these data in terms of immunoregulatory events is for now impossible; in no case is it understood to what extent these autoantibodies result from an "appropriate" response to antigens (viral, virally modified self-antigens, or altered antigens) as opposed to aberrant immunological reactivity. The data, however, can be summarized as showing de-novo autoantibody formation to be rare in pregnancy, and as showing no consistent effect on the levels of preformed autoantibodies but a significant decrease in the levels of some of those studied to date (antithyroid and anti-insulin antibodies).

For many of the more serious autoimmune disorders (the striking exception being rheumatoid arthritis), a considerable anecdotal literature suggested that pregnancy was dangerous and should be avoided. For most of these disorders, current reviewers either exonerate pregnancy or consider the effects to be so inconsistent that the issue of a pregnancy effect as opposed to random changes cannot be settled.

D. Immune Complexes

Despite earlier reports of the frequent occurrence of circulating immune complexes in normal pregnancies, a detailed study by Pope et al. (32) concluded that they do not occur. Other studies have demonstrated their occurrence but only in a small proportion of pregnancies and at extremely low concentrations (33,34). These latter studies also have suggested that these gestational immune complexes were noncomplement fixing and would therefore have doubtful phlogistic activity.

Despite the failure to find elevated levels of total circulating immune complexes, there have been reports that antigenic components of the syncytiotrophoblast are found in the maternal circulation complexed with maternal antibody directed toward these components. Elevated levels of these antibodies were found frequently in first, and early in some second, but not in subsequent pregnancies (35–37). These immune complexes are of no known significance, and may simply represent an appropriate response to released tissue antigens.

III. Cell-Mediated Immunity

Impairment of cell-mediated immunity (CMI) would be expected to result in an increase in infectious diseases due to viruses, to certain bacteria, and to fungi; to result in the more rapid progression of cancers; to cause delayed graft rejection; and to alter the results of delayed hypersensitivity skin testing. Clinical observations regarding these events in pregnancy will be outlined prior to considering the laboratory studies of CMI in pregnancy, as clinical observations place serious constraints on the significance of the laboratory abnormalities reported.

A. Clinical Observations on CMI

Infectious Diseases

Diverse and constantly evolving infectious agents represent a functional test of immunological competence and of other host defense mechanisms, yet recent texts dedicated to infectious diseases in pregnancy are devoted almost entirely to the effects of maternal infection and it pharmacological treatment on fetal health, since it is rare for pregnancy to have an impact on the course of infections (38,39). Despite this rarity, the evidence that it does occur is presented.

Viral Diseases

Influenza. Influenza is the most common infection that seems to cause greater morbidity in pregnancy, but only particularly virulent strains have been associated with increased risk, and only in the minority of woman who develop influenza pneumonia. Thus, in the pandemic of 1918, the mortality of those pregnant woman ill enough to come to medical attention was 27%, all of whom had developed pneumonia; the mortality of influenza pneumonia increased from 50% to 60% from the first to the third trimester (40). What the mortality from influenzal pneumonia was in the general population is unclear, but it was certainly high, with a record number of 711 deaths in a single day in Philadelphia (41). Because of the uncertainties regarding case selection, other kinds of figures and anecdotes are actually more convincing regarding the morbidity of influenza in pregnancy. Thus, during the Asian flu epidemic of 1957 in New York City, one-quarter of the deaths in patients under 50 years of age were in pregnant woman, the majority of these occurring during the third trimester (42). In Minnesota the same year, one-half of all deaths in women of child-bearing age occurred among those who were pregnant (43). The only fatal case of swine flu resulting from hog exposure among dozens of individuals with serological evidence of infection was in a woman in the 36th week of pregnancy (44). In most years, however, a sizable proportion of pregnant women with influenza proven by seroconversion have no illness severe enough to lead to a clinical diagnosis, and mortality from common influenzal strains has not been demonstrated (45). The extent to which the pregnancy-associated deaths due to infection with virulent strains are due to impaired ability to defend against the influenza virus, as opposed to the inability to survive pneumonia due to increased oxygen requirements and mechanical effects of pregnancy on lung function, is not clear.

Hepatitis.   During an epidemic of non-A non-B hepatitis in Kashmir, a prospective study showed the incidence of hepatitis in pregnant women to be increased sixfold, and the likelihood of a fatal outcome increased from 0% to 44% for women in the third trimester (46). Increased mortality either in the third trimester or at unspecified times in pregnancy has been observed for hepatitis epidemics in India (47), Nepal (48), Burma (49), and Iran (50). These studies were conducted at times that the various agents of non-A non-B hepatitis were not known. A more recent study from Ethiopia found the increased mortality of hepatitis in pregnancy to be almost entirely attributable to hepatitis E. Among 110 consecutive cases of acute hepatitis there were 13 deaths, 9 of these being in pregnant women, the majority of them in the third trimester, and all but one of them due to hepatitis E (51). It is so far unclear whether the fact that increased mortality from hepatitis is not seen in developed countries can be attributed to the rarity of hepatitis E in these countries; it had previously been suggested that the increased morbidity of hepatitis in pregnancy observed in developing countries is due to malnutrition (52).

Herpesviruses.

Herpes simplex virus: Genital herpetic infections are two- to threefold more frequent in the third than in the first trimester (53–55), but the duration of lesions is no longer, asymptomatic shedding and cervical shedding are no more frequent, and the severity of episodes is no worse. Even primary HSV-2 infection in pregnancy is often asymptomatic (56). Young described a case of disseminated HSV-2 associated with primary infection during the 37th week of pregnancy and observed that the only 3 previously reported cases of dissemination in pregnancy had occurred after the 28th week of gestation (57). The rarity of dissemination despite the enormous numbers of women with preexisting infection proves an adequate persistence of preexisting immunity. How much the rarity of dissemination of primary infections can be attributed to adequacy of primary immune responses, a benefit from protective preexisting cross-reactive immunity to HSV-1 (56), or to a relative rarity of primary infections in pregnancy is unknown.

Varicella: Thirty years ago Harris summarized the reported cases of varicella pneumonia. First, second, and third trimester mortality rates were 14%, 29%, and 57% compared with 17% in the reported cases of all adults (58). Even when treated with acyclovir, mortality in pregnancy is substantial; among 21 reported cases of varicella pneumonia in pregnancy treated with acyclovir there were 4 deaths, all of women who had become infected in the third trimester (59). As with influenza, the issue of whether the increased mortality is due to impaired host defence or to altered pulmonary mechanics and oxygen requirements is unknown.

Cytomegalovirus: Urinary excretion and cervical shedding increase 5- to 10-fold between the first and third trimesters (60), but is usually asymptomatic (61). In seropositive women, excretion of virus in the pharynx was not found (62).

Epstein-Barr virus: Antibodies to EB virus early antigen, thought to reflect reactivation of virus, occurred in 55% of pregnant women in contrast with the expected 22–33% (63); this occurred early in pregnancy. In a study of women at parturition, 63% were found to be seropositive for antibodies to the EB early antigens as opposed to 0% of controls (62). In neither study was clinical disease associated with this laboratory evidence of reactivation.

Other Viruses. Pregnancy between 1949 and 1955 in New York City was associated with a 60% increased chance of developing clinical illness with *polio*; however, this increased incidence correlated with maternal age and the number of children in the household and may simply have reflected increased exposure (64). *Measles* is often a serious disease in adults; a review of reported cases of measles in pregnancy suggests a greater likelihood of severe disease and of a fatal outcome (65). An epidemiological approach to this question in Los Angeles County found pregnant women to be three times as likely to be diagnosed as having measles pneumonia and six times as likely to die from measles complications than age-comparable nonpregnant women (66). The authors refer to a 1951 measles epidemic in Greenland, in which mortality in pregnant women was 4.8% as opposed to 1% in nonpregnant women in the same age range. Despite impressive case reports (perhaps reflecting delayed treatment due to pregnancy), *human papillomavirus* does not appear to be more prevalent or to differ in its behavior at any stage of pregnancy (67).

Bacterial Infections

Mycobacterial Infections. Reports regarding the effects of pregnancy on *tuberculosis* in the preantibiotic era were conflicting. There was no lack of anecdotes suggesting pregnancy to be a dangerous period for reactivation and dissemination. In contrast, statistical studies did not verify this. In a typical, mostly preantibiotic study, Rosenbach found no cases of reactivation of disease in 241 pregnancies, and progression of acute disease was documented in only 9% of cases, mostly those with far advanced disease in whom such progression had been occurring prior to pregnancy and in whom it could reasonably have been expected regardless of pregnancy (68). The risk of reactivation of tuberculosis during pregnancy is low enough that the American Thoracic Society recommends that preventive therapy be delayed until after delivery except in the case of those who have been recently infected. Worsening of *leprosy* status with increased concentrations of bacilli in cutaneous smears occurred in 35% of prospectively followed women during pregnancy, with the majority of these women worsening during the third trimester (as opposed to 2% worsening during an unspecified period prior to conception) (69). In addition, downgrading of leprosy, reflecting decreased cell-mediated reactivity, was more common in pregnancy. Conversely, a reversal reaction, reflecting an increase in CMI toward the tuberculoid end of the leprosy scale, is more common in the months after delivery (70).

Intracellular Bacteria. Pregnancy is clearly associated with an increased risk of *listeriosis* (71), but this seems to be due to a favorable environment in the placental tissue rather than to maternal immunological impairment. Recent studies in mice have shown the maternal response to *Listeria* to be normal except in the placental tissues, where the ability to respond was limited (72). "In contrast to the devastating picture shown by infected neonates, maternal manifestations of listeriosis are usually absent or mild (73)," and "the infection is usually self-limited because the nidus of the infection is eliminated with the birth of the infected fetus" (71). Similarly, despite the frequent occurrence of cervical *chlamydial* infections and effects of this on the health of the fetus, there is no evidence of increased problems in the infected women as a result of pregnancy.

Fungal Infections

Coccidiomycosis. In a retrospective study of coccidiomycosis, 12 of 33 cases occurring during pregnancy resulted in disseminated disease and death, including 7 of the 11 patients who contracted the disease during the third trimester (74). Subsequent reviews have confirmed an increased risk of dissemination and mortality in late pregnancy (75,76). A recent tabulation of 109 reported cases of coccidiomycosis in pregnancy reported first thru third trimester rates of dissemination of 19%, 62%, and 79%, with mortality rates of 67%, 63%, and 81% (mostly in the pretreatment era) (77). Other observations document the danger of the third trimester. A person who with intensive treatment survived disseminated disease presented 5 years later at 34 weeks gestation with reactivation of pulmonary disease (77). And in an endemic area only 10 cases of coccidiomycosis could be found among 47,120 pregnancies; those occurring during the first two trimesters did well, but not so for the two who were diagnosed with fulminant disease in the first 10 days postpartum. Both had had respiratory symptoms consistent with infection during the third trimester, and both continued to require treatment 4 years later (78). The demonstration by Drutz that 17-beta-estradiol and progesterone at concentrations found in pregnancy sera stimulate the growth of *Coccidioides immitis* has frequently been cited as evidence that hormonal rather than immunological changes may account for its unique behavior (79), but these effects were relatively minor and would not account for persistent problems postpartum.

Cryptococcosis, Blastomycosis, and Sporotrichosis. These have rarely been reported in pregnancy; Catanzaro has reviewed these reports and concluded that pregnancy does not appear to influence the courses of these diseases (80). Despite this, it is of interest that all 4 case reports of disseminated or active pulmonary blastomycosis were of women who became symptomatic during the third trimester (see Ref. 81 for a report and earlier references). Thus the increased morbidity of coccidiomycosis in pregnancy is either unique among the common fungal infections or the only condition common enough for its risk to be documented.

Summary

In summary, there is epidemiological evidence suggesting that certain viral, bacterial, and fungal infections whose outcomes depend on cell-mediated immune responses may be increased in incidence or severity during pregnancy, particularly during the third trimester. However, increased morbidity is not seen with any of the common infectious diseases, does not occur in a high proportion of infected pregnant women with any infection, and may be due to host alterations that are unrelated to the immune system in some cases.

Cancers and Pregnancy

The most common cancers to occur in pregnant women are those that one finds in women of reproductive age: cervical cancer, breast cancer, hematological malignancies, and malignant melanoma (82).

Cervical Cancer

"Survival is not altered by pregnancy for stage 1B disease" (83).

Breast Cancer

"The prognosis for women with pregnancy-associated breast cancer, stage for stage, is similar to that of women of the same age treated at the same

time period" (84). "However pregnant women are at a higher risk of presenting with advanced disease because pregnancy impedes early cancer
detection (85)."

Hematological Malignancies

Pregnancy has no effect "on either the course or longevity of patients with
Hodgkin's disease" (86). For *non-Hodgkin lymphoma* (NHL), "while in
most cases, clinical remission, amelioration or status quo were predominate
during pregnancy, marked aggravation of symptoms with severe relapse of
NHL occurred postpartum. . . . A number of observations showed a temporary slowdown in the progression of lymphoma during pregnancy which
permitted its completion followed however, by severe acceleration of its
course in the immediate postpartum" (87). "However other investigators
have suggested that pregnancy has no influence on the course of treated
or untreated NHL (88)." "There is no available evidence suggesting that
pregnancy itself alters the incidence, natural history, or the prognosis of
acute leukemia"(89).

Melanoma

"It does not appear that being pregnant before, after, or at the time of
diagnosis of stage I MM influences the 5-year survival rate" (90). "Once
tumor thickness was controlled for, survival rate of women in whom melanoma was diagnosed and treated while they were pregnant did not differ
from that in the other three groups of women" [who had been treated
before any pregnancy, after completing all pregnancies, or between pregnancies (91)].

Thus despite case reports of the rapid progression of tumors in pregnancy, there is no evidence that this occurs more frequently in pregnancy.
Donegan concluded that "for the common cancers, it is difficult to demonstrate that pregnancy materially influences their growth and spread or
has a substantially adverse influence on their inherent curability independent of the patient's age or stage of cancer (92).

Transplantation

Decreased rates of graft rejection would imply impaired CMI. Reports
regarding renal allografts in human pregnancy suffice only to show that
rejection can occur during all trimesters, but for the most part have yet to
analyzed in terms of rejection rates. The exception to this is a survey of
400 pregnant renal transplant patients by Rudolph (93). Serious rejection
episodes occurred in 9% of women, a rate that he felt to be at least as high
as in the nonpregnant state. Subsequent reviewers have noted this to be
strange given the "expectation of immunosuppression" in pregnancy.

There are now numerous reports of pregnancy in recipients of liver and heart transplants; as with renal transplants, they suffice only to show that rejection, even to the point of requiring intensification of immunosuppressive therapy, occurs at all stages of pregnancy.

A study sometimes cited as demonstrating impaired CMI in pregnancy is that of Andresen (94). However, his observation that both first- and second-set skin graft survival were prolonged was based on a study of only 3 pregnant women and was done at a time that the human major histocompatibility antigens were unknown, so the extent of histoincompatibility between donors and recipients was not controlled for. The observations are therefore very tenuous.

Skin Testing for DTH

Studies regarding skin testing for delayed hypersensitivity have suggested either a small or no effect of pregnancy. In one-fourth of the cases studied by Lichtenstein (95), a greater concentration of old tuberculin was needed to obtain a positive response during the third trimester, but in no case did a reactor become nonreactive. Using intermediate-strength purified protein derivative (PPD) (96), Montgomery found no significant change between reactions during and after pregnancy.

In a study of 25,033 tuberculous contacts, 347 who were skin test positive when first tested were pregnant either at that time or when retested 1 year later. Comparing initial with follow-up test results in those who were pregnant at the first, second, or neither time, he found a similar small increase in median diameter of the second test reaction in all groups and no effect of trimester (97). Hawes et al. found no falsely negative skin test reactions to PPD, tetanus toxoid, streptokinase-streptodornase (SKSD), or *Candida albicans* during pregnancy. Although the size of the skin test reactions observed to each antigen were smaller during pregnancy than postpartum, the differences were not statistically significant (98).

B. In Vitro Observations on CMI

T-Cell Surface Markers

Despite one report of decreased levels of T4-positive cells and a decreased T4/T8 ratio in pregnancy (99), numerous workers have found only marginal changes in the numbers of T4- or T8-positive cells (100–110). Although in some of these studies the changes were statistically significant, they were all too slight to be likely to be of biological significance and as many of the studies showed a slight increase in the numbers of T4-positive cells as showed a decrease. Staining T4-positive cells for HLA antigens (which correlate with an activated state), no pregnancy effect was found (Ref. 110, data not presented). Staining T-positive cells for cell-surface antigens believed to correlate with state of memory (naive versus memory cells) or of helper activity for inducer versus suppressor cells also showed no pregnancy effect (110).

Mitogenic Responses

A number of studies have examined in vitro responses to PHA during pregnancy. The proliferative responses to PHA have been reported to be unchanged in several studies (98,111–114) but in some were found to be decreased either throughout pregnancy or, more commonly, prior to the 32nd week (115–119). Many of these studies are uninterpretable, since the data have been presented only as stimulation indices, and this does not allow one to distinguish between decreased proliferation in response to PHA and an increase in the proliferation of unstimulated cells (which has been found in some studies). Most studies were done with mononuclear cell preparations rather than purified lymphocytes. Monocyte numbers are increased substantially in pregnancy (99,100,114,120), with monocyte/lymphocyte ratios peaking during the fourth and fifth months (121). Since monocytes present in increased numbers have been shown to inhibit proliferative responses to mitogens, to allogeneic cells, and to soluble antigens (122–124), it is likely that the reduced PHA responses reported by some workers reflect both the smaller numbers of lymphocytes in their mononuclear cell preparations and the immunomodulatory effect of monocytes. Although one could argue that a decreased response to PHA is important whether or not it is due to monocytes, it is not safe to assume that the ratio of monocytes to lympocytes found in the circulation has any relationship to that in lymphoid or other tissues. Interleukin-2 production in response to PHA has variously been found to be normal in all trimesters (125) or reduced 95% in the third trimester (110). The latter finding is of questionable relevance given the observation that serum Il-2 levels were found to be increased considerably in 61% of pregnant women throughout pregnancy and were in the normal range for most of the others (126) (although the possibility of nonspecificity of the assay with detection of an immunologically cross-reactive pregnancy-associated hormone does not appear to have been considered).

Antigen-Induced Proliferation

The data regarding antigen-induced lymphocyte proliferation during pregnancy is conflicting. Although Hawes (98) found the proliferative responses to SKSD and *Candida* antigens to be slightly augmented throughout pregnancy, Gehrz (112,127) found the responses to these two antigens as well as to tetanus toxoid and CMV to be reduced two- to threefold in the second and third trimesters and to remain depressed until around 90 days postpartum. As with PHA, many studies are somewhat uninterpretable, since the data have been reported only as stimulation indices, and none has controlled for the numbers of monocytes in the mononuclear cell preparations.

Mixed Lymphocyte Reactivity

The ability of mononuclear cells to react in mixed lymphocyte culture is not impaired at any time in pregnancy (113,128,129).

T-Cell Mediated Cytotoxicity

T-cell mediated cytotoxicity is not easily studied. Since the discovery that cytotoxic T cells only recognize antigen when presented by self-MHC molecules, it has become necessary to dismiss the findings of all studies performed with allogeneic target cells. A recent study examined the ability of peripheral blood mononuclear cells to suppress the growth of their own Epstein-Barr virus transformed B cells. A marginal decrease was found which peaked in the first trimester (130).

Natural Killer Cells

When examined by surface marker analysis, morphology, or function, natural killer cells in the circulation are reduced by around 30% either throughout pregnancy or from the second trimester on (108,131). In some studies the numbers of cells capable of binding NK-sensitive targets was normal, but some of the conjugates did not result in target cell lysis (132,133). This defect was reversed by interferon (132), just as the decreased NK activity of pregnancy has been reversed by interferon or IL-2 in less specific assays (134). The importance of natural killer cells in host defense and the relationship between their activity in the blood and in other tissues is unclear. It is also unclear whether the cell types found in peripheral blood which modulate NK activity in in-vitro assays serve such a regulatory purpose in vivo. This is important because monocytes are considerably increased in peripheral blood, and removal of monocytes restores the decreased NK activity of pregnancy to normal levels (135). Despite these reservations, this in-vitro defect is one of the most consistently found anomalies in pregnancy and may turn out to contribute to the more fulminant course seen with certain viral infections in late pregnancy.

Antibody-Dependent Cell-Mediated Cytotoxicity

Antibody-dependent cell-mediated cytotoxicity has been reported to be normal (136) or decreased by one-third (137). As always, the significance of ADCC in vivo, the relationship between the findings in blood to those in tissues, and the clinical importance of a 30% decrease are unknown.

Polymorphonuclear Leukocytes

Pregnancy is accompanied by a progressive leukocytosis (121,138). This leukocytosis is due predominantly to an increase in neutrophils, but while contributing little to the total increase in leukocytes, monocyte counts are increased two- to threefold. Studies regarding neutrophil function in pregnancy are conflicting.

Chemotaxis

There is a 15–30% decrease in the chemotactic response to zymosan-activated serum (139,140) and to fMet-Leu-Phe (140,141) beginning early in pregnancy, but it is not progressive.

Adherence

Adherence to nylon wool was decreased slightly in the third trimester (140), whereas attachment to *Candida albicans* was increased throughout pregnancy, peaking at the fifth to sixth month (142).

Phagocytosis

Phagocytosis of latex particles was found to be unaffected, but phagocytosis of *Candida albicans* increased throughout pregnancy (142). The latter increase may be explained by an increase in Fc and C3b receptors (143).

Reactive Oxidative Metabolism

Superoxide generation was found to be decreased by 35% in response to fMet-Leu-Phe but not in response to phorbol myristic acid (141). However, the production of reactive oxidative metabolites as judged by chemiluminescence was found to increase approximately twofold in response to zymosan (139,143) or polysterene beads (144).

Immunosuppressive Factors

Several authors have referred to a "suppressive" influence of pregnancy sera on proliferative responses to mitogens and allogeneic cells. In fact, one has difficulty finding work that supports such a claim. As emphasized by Baboonian (145), the observations usually interpreted as showing suppression are simply that some pregnancy sera do not support as vigorous a response as that obtained in a pool of sera from nonpregnant women, not that they actively suppress. In one study this failure to support optimal proliferative responses was characteristic of only 15% of sera from primiparous women (146); since individual sera from nonpregnant women were not studied, it is not even clear that the frequency of the failure to support optimal responses is increased in pregnancy. The suboptimal responses observed in selected pregnancy sera have been overcome by the addition of exogenous Il-2 (146,147). Despite the lack of strong evidence for a suppressive effect of pregnancy sera, many studies of pregnancy-associated suppressive factors have been conducted. A number of glycoproteins of fetoplacental origin have been reported to be capable of suppressing lymphocyte responses to PHA or mixed lymphocyte culture. Although HCG has received attention as a possible immunosuppressive factor for more than two decades, work with more purified preparations has questioned whether it is immunosuppressive at all, let alone at physiological concentrations (148,149). No correlation has been found between the "suppressive" effects of pregnancy sera on PHA responses and their content of HCG, HPL, pregnancy-associated plasma protein A, or alpha-fetoprotein (150,151). A better correlation has been found with pregnancy-specific β_1-glycoprotein levels, and physiological levels are said to be suppressive in vitro (152,153). Estradiol receptors have been found on T8-positive but not T4-positive cells (154,155), and progesterone receptors on unspecified lymphocytes in pregnancy, despite the fact that they are not found on lymphocytes from nonpregnant women (156). Like cortisone, estradiol and progesterone have been shown to be immunosuppressive, but at concentrations higher than those attained during pregnancy (157–159). To what extent interactions of these diverse hormones could result in synergistic suppression of immune or inflammatory responses in pregnancy is unknown, but in view of the marginal clinical evidence of immune suppression reviewed above, the in-vivo effects must be limited.

IV. Summary

There is no evidence for a significant alteration of humoral immunity during pregnancy.

In-vivo observations suggest that if there is a defect in cell-mediated immunity, it is either subtle or limited to a minority of clinically relevant antigens. For example, there is no evidence for an impairment in transplantation immunity, there is no change in the clinical course of cancers, and skin test responses for DTH to infectious agents are not significantly affected. Furthermore, the vast majority of infections whose control depends on CMI are dealt with appropriately. However, there is convincing evidence of an altered host response to several viruses, and at least one bacterium (*Mycobacterium leprae*) and at least one fungal pathogen (*Coccidioides immitis*). Marginal decreases in CMI due to T cells, NK cells, and ADC have all been demonstrated in vitro. Although it is difficult to assess the clinical relevance of these minor alterations, they may collectively suffice to account for the altered clinical course of these infections observed in late pregnancy.

References

1. Maroulis GB, Buckley RH, Younger JB. Serum immunoglobulin concentrations during normal pregnancy. Am J Obstet Gynecol 1971; 109:971–976.
2. Amino N, Tanizawa O, Miyai K, Tanaka F, Hayashi C, Kawashima M, Ichihara K. Changes of serum immunoglobulins IgG, IgA, IgM, and IgE during pregnancy. Obstet Gynecol 1978; 52:415–420.
3. Ostensen M, Lundgren R, Husby G, Rekvig OP. Studies on humoral immunity in pregnancy: immunoglobulins, alloantibodies and autoantibodies in healthy pregnant women and in pregnant women with rheumatoid disease. J Clin Lab Immunol 1983; 11:143–147.
4. Ailus KT. A follow-up study of immunoglobulin levels and autoantibodies in an unselected pregnant population. Am J Reprod Immunol 1994; 31:189–196.
5. Malek A, Sager R, Schneider H. Maternal-fetal transport of immunoglobulin G and its subclasses during the third trimester of human pregnancy. Am J Reprod Immunol 1994; 32:8–14.
6. Gasparoni A, Avazini A, Probizer FR, Chirico G, Rondini G, Severi F. IgG subclasses compared in maternal and cord serum and breast milk. Arch Dis Child 1992; 67:41–43.
7. Landor M. Maternal-fetal transfer of immunoglobulins. Ann Allergy 1995; 74:279–283.
8. Widerström L, Bratthall D. Increased IgA levels in saliva during pregnancy. Scand J Dent Res 1984; 92:33–37.
9. Knobloch VV, Jouja V, Sternová H. IgE im Serum von schwangeren Frauen. Zbl Gynäk 1974; 96:1190–1192.
10. Gluck JC, Gluck PA. The effects of pregnancy on asthma: a prospective study, Ann Allergy 1976; 37:164–168.
11. Schatz M, Wasserman S, O'Connor RD, Harden K, Forsythe A, Chilingar L, Hoffman C, Sperling W, Zeiger RS. Distinguishing clinical and biochemical characteristics associated with improvement or deterioration of asthma during pregnancy (abstr). J Allergy Clin Immunol 1985; 75:133.
12. Rao VR, Raman L. Antibody response to tetanus toxoid during pregnancy. Indian J Med Res 1980; 72:840–842.

13. Gill TJ III, Repetti CF, Metlay LA, Rabin BS, Taylor FH, Thompson DS, Cortese AL. Transplacental immunization of the human fetus to tetanus by immunization of the mother. J Clin Invest 1983; 72:987–996.

14. Brabin BJ, Nagel J, Hagenaars AM, Ruitenberg E, van Tilborgh AMJC. The influence of malaria and gestation on the immune response to one and two doses of adsorbed tetanus toxoid in pregnancy. Bull WHO 1984; 62: 919–930.

15. Murray DL, Imagawa DT, Okada DM, St. Geme JW Jr. Antibody response to monovalent A/New Jersey/8/76 influenza vaccine in pregnant women. J Clin Microbiol 1979; 10:184–187.

16. Baker CJ, Rench MA, Edwards MS, Carpenter RJ, Hays BM, Kasper DL. Immunization of pregnant women with a polysaccharide vaccine of group B streptococcus. N Engl J Med 1988; 319:1180–1185.

17. Gini PC, Okafor GO. The response to varied timing and spacing of tetanus toxoid administration in pregnancy. East Afr Med J 1992; 69:157–161.

18. Halsey NA, Klein D. Maternal immunization. Pediatr Infect Dis J 1990; 9: 574–581.

19. Englund JA, Mbawuike IN, Hammill H, Holleman MC, Baxter BD, Glezen WP. Maternal immunization with influenza or tetanus toxoid vaccine for passive antibody protection in young infants. J Infect Dis 1993; 168: 647–656.

20. Baboonian C, Griffiths P. Is pregnancy immunosuppressive? Humoral immunity against viruses. Br J Obstet Gynaecol 1983; 90:1168–1175.

21. Grangeot-Keros L, Nicholas JC, Bricout F, Pillot J. Rubella infection and the fetus (letter). N Engl J Med 1985; 313:1547.

22. Sokol RJ, Hewitt S, Stamps BK. Erythrocyte autoantibodies, autoimmune haemolysis and pregnancy. Vox Sang 1982; 43:169–176.

23. Reyes-López PA, Santos G, Forsbach GN. Absence of ANA in pregnancy (letter). Arthritis Rheum 1980; 23:378.

24. Patton PE, Coulam CB, Bergstralh E. The prevalence of autoantibodies in pregnant and nonpregnant women. Am J Obstet Gynecol 1987; 157: 1345–1350.

25. Rosenberg AM, Bingham MC, Fong KC. Antinuclear antibodies during pregnancy. Obstet Gynecol 1986; 68:560–562.

26. El-Roeiy A, Myers SA, Gleicher N. The prevalence of autoantibodies and lupus anticoagulant in healthy pregnant women. Obstet Gynecol 1990; 75: 390–396.

27. Mavridis AK, Ming LX, Hatzipetrou P, Lentzaris G, Papanikolaou NG, Tzioufas AG, Moutsopoulos HM. Prevalence of non-organ-specific autoantibodies in pregnant and non-pregnant healthy women. Lupus 1992; 1: 141–144.

28. Pope RM, Yoshinoya S, Rutstein J, Persellin RH. Effect of pregnancy on immune complexes and rheumatoid factors in patients with rheumatoid arthritis. Am J Med 1983; 74:973–979.

29. Exon PD, Dixon K, Malins JM. Insulin antibodies in diabetic pregnancy. Lancet 1974; 2:126–128.

30. Amino N, Kuro R, Tanizawa O, Tanaka F, Hayashi C, Kotani K, Kawashima M, Miyai K, Kumahara Y. Changes in serum anti-thyroid antibodies during and after pregnancy in autoimmune thyroid diseases. Clin Exp Immunol 1978; 31:30–37.

31. D'Armiento M, Salabé H, Vetrano G, Scucchia M, Pachì A. Decrease in thyroid antibodies during pregnancy. J Endocrinol Invest 1980; 4:437–438.

32. Pope RM, Yoshinoya S, Persellin RH. The detection of circulating immune complexes and IgG and IgM rheumatoid factors in normal human pregnancy. Am J Reprod Immunol 1982; 2:208–211.

33. Gleicher N, Theofilopoulos AN. Immune complexes and pregnancy. Diag Gynecol Obstet 1980; 2:7–31.

34. Kilpatrick DC, Weston J. A re-examination of the incidence of circulating immune complexes in normal pregnancy. Ann Clin Biochem 1984; 21:105–108.

35. Davies M. The formation of immune complexes in primiparous and multiparous human pregnancies. Immunol Lett 1985; 10:199–205.

36. Davies M. The separation of the antibody and antigen components of immune complexes formed during normal human pregnancy. Immunobiology 1986; 171:180–194.

37. Davies M. Antigenic analysis of immune complexes formed in normal human pregnancy. Clin Exp Immunol 1985; 61:406–415.

38. Gilstrap LC III, Faro S, eds. Infections in Pregnancy. New York: Allan R. Liss, 1990.

39. Gonik B, ed. Viral Diseases in Pregnancy. New York: Springer Verlag, 1994.

40. Harris JW. Influenza occurring in pregnant women: a statistical study of thirteen hundred and fifty cases. JAMA 1919; 72:978–980.

41. Bland PB. Influenza in its relation to pregnancy and labor. Am J Obstet 1919; 79:181–196.

42. Greenberg M, Jacobziner H, Pakter J, Weisl BAG. Maternal mortality in the epidemic of Asian influenza, New York City, 1957. Am J Obstet Gynecol 1958; 76:897–902.

43. Freeman DW, Barno A. Deaths from Asian influenza associated with pregnancy. Am J Obstet Gynecol 1959; 78:1172–1175.

44. McKinney WP, Volkert P, Kaufman J. Fatal swine influenza pneumonia during late pregnancy. Arch Intern Med 1990; 150:213–215.

45. Mullooly JP, Barker WH, Nolan TF. Risk of acute respiratory disease among pregnant women during influenza A epidemics. Public Health Rep 1986; 101:205–211.

46. Khuroo MS, Teli MR, Skidmore S, Sofi MA, Khuroo MI. Incidence and severity of viral hepatitis in pregnancy. Am J Med 1981; 70:252–255.

47. D'Cruz IA, Balani SG, Iyer LS. Infectious hepatitis and pregnancy. Obstet Gynecol 1968; 31:449–455.

48. Kane MA, Bradley DW, Shrestha SM, Maynard JE, Cook EH, Mishra RP, Joshi DD. Epidemic of non-A, non-B hepatitis in Nepal. JAMA 1984; 252: 3140–3145.
49. Maynard JE. Epidemic non-A, non-B hepatitis. Semin Liver Dis 1984; 4: 336–339.
50. Borhanmanesh F, Haghighi P, Hekmat K, Rezaizadeh K, Ghavami AG. Viral hepatitis during pregnancy. Gastroenterology 1973; 64:304–312.
51. Tsega E, Hansson B-G, Krawczynski K, Nordenfelt E. Acute sporadic hepatitis in Ethiopia: causes, risk factors, and effects on pregnancy. Clin Infect Dis 1992; 14:961–965.
52. Snydman DR. Hepatitis in pregnancy. N Engl J Med 1985; 313:1398–1401.
53. Ng ABP, Reagan JW, Yen SSC. Herpes genitalis. Obstet Gynecol 1970; 36: 645–651.
54. Brown ZA, Vontver LA, Benedetti J, Critchlow CW, Hickok DE, Sells CJ, Berry S, Corey L. Genital herpes in pregnancy: risk factors associated with recurrences and asymptomatic viral shedding. Am J Obstet Gynecol 1985; 153:24–30.
55. Harger JH, Amortegui AJ, Meyer MP, Hyg MS, Pazin GJ. Characteristics of recurrent genital herpes simplex infections in pregnant women. Obstet Gynecol 1989; 73:367–372.
56. Boucher FD, Yasukawa LL, Bronzan RN, Hensleigh PA, Arvin AM, Prober CG. A prospective evaluation of primary genital herpes simplex virus type 2 infections acquired during pregnancy. Pediatr Infect Dis J 1990; 9: 499–504.
57. Young EJ, Killam AP, Greene JF Jr. Disseminated herpesvirus infection: association with primary genital herpes in pregnancy. JAMA 1976; 235: 2731–2733.
58. Harris RE, Rhoades ER. Varicella pneumonia complicating pregnancy. Report of a case and review of literature. Obstet Gynecol 1965; 25:734–740.
59. Smego RA, Asperilla MO. Use of acyclovir for varicella pneumonia during pregnancy. Obstet Gynecol 1991; 78:1112–1116.
60. Reynolds DW, Stagno S, Hosty TS, Tiller M, Alford CA Jr. Maternal cytomegalovirus excretion and perinatal infection. N Engl J Med 1973; 289: 1–5.
61. Stagno S, Whitley RJ. Herpesvirus infections of pregnancy. Part 1: Cytomegalovirus and Epstein-Barr virus infections. N Engl J Med 1985; 313: 1270–1274.
62. Sakamoto K, Greally J, Gilfillan RF, Sexton J, Barnabei V, Yetz J, Bechtold T, Seeley JK, O'Dwyer E, Purtilo DT. Epstein-Barr virus in normal pregnant women. Am J Reprod Immunol 1982; 2:217–221.
63. Fleisher G, Bolognese R. Persistent Epstein-Bar virus infection and pregnancy. J Infect Dis 1983; 147:982–986.
64. Siegel M, Greenberg M. Incidence of poliomyelitis in pregnancy. N Engl J Med 1955; 253:841–847.

65. Atmar RI, Englund JA, Hammill H. Complications of measles during pregnancy. Clin Infect Dis 1992; 14:217–226.
66. Eberhart-Phillips JE, Frederick PD, Baron RC, Mascola L. Measles in pregnancy: a descriptive study of 58 cases. Obstet Gynecol 1993; 82:797–801.
67. Kemp EA, Hakenewerth AM, Laurent SL, Gravitt PE, Stoerker J. Human papillomavirus in pregnancy. Obstet Gynecol 1992; 79:649–656.
68. Rosenbach LM, Gangemi CR. Tuberculosis and pregnancy. JAMA 1956; 161:1035–1038.
69. Duncan ME, Pearson JMH, Ridley DS, Melsom R, Bjune G. Pregnancy and leprosy: the consequences of alterations of cell-mediated and humoral immunity during pregnancy and lactation. Int J Lepr 1982; 50:425–435.
70. Duncan ME. An historical and clinical review of the interaction of leprosy and pregnancy: a cycle to be broken. Soc Sci Med 1993; 37:457–472.
71. Gellin G, Broome CV. Listeriosis. JAMA 1989; 261:1313–1320.
72. Redline RW, Lu CY. Specific defects in the anti-Listerial immune response in discrete regions of the murine uterus and placenta account for susceptibility to infection. J Immunol 1988; 140:3947–3955.
73. Boucher M, Yonekura ML. Listeria meningitis during pregnancy. Am J Perinat 1:312–318.
74. Vaughan JE, Ramirez H. Coccidioidomycosis as a complication of pregnancy. Calif Med 1951; 74:121–125.
75. Harris RE. Coccidioidomycosis complicating pregnancy. Obstet Gynecol 1966; 28:401–405.
76. Drutz DJ, Catanzaro A. Coccidioidomycosis. Am Rev Respir Dis 1978; 117:727–771.
77. Walker MPR, Brody CZ, Resnik R. Reactivation of coccidioidomycosis in pregnancy. Obstet Gynecol 1992; 79:815–817.
78. Wack EE, Ampel NM, Galgiani JN, Bronnimann DA. Coccidioidomycosis during pregnancy: an analysis of ten cases among 47,120 pregnancies. Chest 1988; 94:376–379.
79. Drutz DJ, Huppert M, Sun SH, McGuire WL. Human sex hormones stimulate the growth and maturation of *Coccidioides immitis*. Infect Immun 1981; 32:897–907.
80. Catanzaro A. Pulmonary mycosis in pregnant women. Chest 1984; 86(suppl):14S–18S.
81. Daniel L, Salit IE. Blastomycosis during pregnancy. Can Med Assoc J 1984; 131:759–761.
82. Haas JF. Pregnancy in association with a newly diagnosed cancer: a population-based epidemiologic assessment. Int J Cancer 1984; 34:229–235.
83. Hopkins MP, Morley GW. The prognosis and management of cervical cancer associated with pregnancy. Obstet Gynecol 1992; 80:9–13.
84. Petrek JA. Pregnancy-associated breast cancer. Semin Surg Oncol 1991; 7:306–310.

85. Zemlickis D, Lishner M, Degendorfer P, Panzarella T, Burke B, Sutcliffe SB, Koren G. Maternal and fetal outcome after breast cancer in pregnancy. Am J Obstet Gynecol 1992; 166:781–787.

86. Barry RM, Diamond HD, Craver LF. Influence of pregnancy on the course of Hodgkin's disease. Am J Obstet Gynecol 1962; 84:445–454.

87. Ioachim HL, Moroson H. Lymphoma and pregnancy: clinical observations and experimental investigations. Leukemia 1994; 8(suppl 1):S198–S201.

88. Ward FT, Weiss RB. Lymphoma and pregnancy. Semin Oncol 1989; 16: 397–409.

89. Caligiuri MA, Mayer RJ. Pregnancy and leukemia. Semin Oncol 1989; 16: 388–396.

90. Driscoll MS, Grin-Jorgensen CM, Grant-Kels JM. Does pregnancy influence the prognosis of malignant melanoma? J Am Acad Dermatol 1993; 29: 619–630.

91. MacKie RM, Bufalino R, Morabito A, Sutherland C, Cascinelli N for the World Health Organisation Melanoma Programme. Lack of effect of pregnancy on outcome of melanoma. Lancct 1991; 337:653–655.

92. Donegan WL. Cancer and pregnancy, CA-A Cancer Journal for Clinicians 1983; 33:194–214.

93. Rudolph JE, Schweizer RT, Bartus SA. Pregnancy in renal transplant patients: a review. Transplantation 1970; 27:26–29.

94. Andresen RH, Monroe CW. Experimental study of the behavior of adult human skin homografts during pregnancy. A preliminary report. Am J Obstet Gynecol 1962; 84:1096–1103.

95. Lichtenstein MR. Tuberculin reaction in tuberculosis during pregnancy. Am Rev Tuberc 1942; 46:89–92.

96. Montgomery WP, Young RC Jr, Allen MP, Harden KA. The tuberculin test in pregnancy. Am J Obstet Gynecol 1968; 100:829–831.

97. Present PA, Comstock GW. Tuberculin sensitivity in pregnancy. Am Rev Respir Dis 1975; 112:413–416.

98. Hawes CS, Kemp AS, Jones WR, Nccd JA. A longitudinal study of cell-mediated immunity in human pregnancy. J Reprod Immunol 1981; 3: 165–173.

99. Sridama V, Pacini F, Yang S-L, Moawad A, Reilly M, DeGroot LJ. Decreased levels of helper T cells. A possible cause of immunodeficiency in pregnancy. N Engl J Med 1982; 307:352–356.

100. Lucivero G, Selvaggi L, Dell'osso A, Antonaci S, Iannone A, Bettocchi S, Bonomo L. Mononuclear cell subpopulations during normal pregnancy: I. Analysis of cell surface markers using conventional techniques and monoclonal antibodies. Am J Reprod Immunol 1983; 4:142–145.

101. Layward L, Brenchley PEC, Coupes BM, Ellis CM, Pumphrey RSH. Decreased levels of helper T cells in pregnancy (letter). N Engl J Med 1982; 307:1582.

102. Vanderbeeken Y, Vlieghe MP, Delespesse G, Duchateau J. Characterization of immunoregulatory T cells during pregnancy by monoclonal antibodies. Clin Exp Immunol 1982; 48:118–120.
103. Bolis PF, Franchi M, Guaschino S, Sampaolo P, Maccario R. T-Lymphocyte subpopulations in pregnancy. Biol Res Pregnancy Perinatol 1983; 4:107–109.
104. Barnett MA, Learmonth RP, Pihl E, Wood EC. T helper lymphocyte depression in early human pregnancy. J Reprod Immunol 1983; 5:55–57.
105. Cheney RT, Tomaszewski JE, Raab SJ, Zmijewski C, Rowlands DT Jr. Subpopulations of lymphocytes in maternal peripheral blood during pregnancy. J Reprod Immunol 1984; 6:111–120.
106. Canepa S, Horowitz R, Degenne D, Magnin G, Valat C, Bordos P. Correlation of plasma hormone levels and peripheral circulating lymphocyte subpopulations during human pregnancy. Immunol Lett 1984; 8:159–163.
107. Tallon DF, Corcoran DJD, O'Dwyer EM, Greally JF. Circulating lymphocyte subpopulations in pregnancy: a longitudinal study. J Immunol 1984; 132: 1784–1787.
108. Castilla JA, Rueda R, Vargas ML, González-Gómez F, García-Olivares E. Decreased levels of circulating CD4+ T lymphocytes during normal pregnancy. J Reprod Immunol 1989; 15:103–111.
109. Miotti PG, Liomba G, Dallabetta GA, Hoover DR, Chiphangwi JD, Saah AJ. T lymphocyte subsets during and after pregnancy: an analysis in human immunodeficiency virus type 1-infected and -uninfected Malawian mothers. J Infect Dis 1992; 165:1116–1119.
110. Sabahi F, Rola-Plesczcynski M, O'Connell S, Frenkel LD. Qualitative and quantitative analysis of T lymphocytes during normal human pregnancy. Am J Reprod Immunol 1995; 33:381–392.
111. Carr MC, Stites DP, Fudenberg HH. Cellular immune aspects of the human fetal maternal relationship. II. *In vitro* response of gravida lymphocytes to phytohemagglutinin. Cell Immunol 1973; 8:448–454.
112. Gehrz RC, Christianson WR, Linner KM, Conroy MM, McCue SA, Balfour HH Jr. A longitudinal analysis of lymphocyte proliferative responses to mitogens and antigens during human pregnancy. Am J Obstet Gynecol 1981; 140:665–670.
113. Birkeland SA, Kristoffersen K. Cellular immunity in pregnancy: blast transformation and rosette formation of maternal T and B lymphocytes. A cross-section analysis. Clin Exp Immunol 1977; 30:408–412.
114. Plum J, Thiery M, Sabbe L. Distribution of mononuclear cells during pregnancy. Clin Exp Immunol 1978; 31:45–49.
115. Purtilo DT, Hallgren HM, Yunis EJ. Depressed maternal lymphocyte response to phytohemagglutinin in human pregnancy. Lancet 1972; 1:769–771.
116. Tomoda Y, Fuma M, Miwa T, Saiki N, Ishizuka N, Cell-mediated immunity in pregnant women. Gynecol Invest 1976; 7:280–292.
117. Yamamoto T, Hirata H, Taniguchi H, Kawai Y, Uematsu A, Sugiyama Y. Lymphocyte transformation during pregnancy: an analysis using whole-blood culture. Obstet Gynecol 1980; 55:215–219.

118. Kumar A, Madden DL, Nankervis GA. Humoral and cell-mediated immune responses to herpesvirus antigens during pregnancy—a longitudinal study. J Clin Immunol 1984; 4:12–17.

119. Baboonian C, Grundy JE, O'Brien PMS, Griffiths PD. Responses to mitogenic stimulation of lymphocytes taken during and after pregnancy. FEMS Microbiol Immunol 1989; 47:199–209.

120. Bailey K, Herrod HG, Younger R, Shaver D. Functional aspects of T-lymphocyte subsets in pregnancy. Obstet Gynecol 1985; 66:211–215.

121. Valdimarsson H, Mulholland C, Fridriksdottir V, Coleman DV. A longitudinal study of leucocyte blood counts and lymphocyte responses in pregnancy. A marked early increase of monocyte-lymphocyte ratio. Clin Exp Immunol 1983; 53:437–443.

122. Laughter AH, Twomey JJ. Suppression of lymphoproliferation by high concentrations of normal human mononuclear leukocytes. J Immunol 1977; 119: 173–179.

123. Stobo JD. Immunosuppression in man: suppression by macrophages can be mediated by interactions with regulatory T cells. J Immunol 1977; 119: 918–924.

124. Goodwin JS, Webb DR. Regulation of the immune response by prostaglandins. Clin Immun Immunopathol 1980; 15:106–122.

125. Hauser GJ, Bino T, Lidor A, David MD, Zakath V, Spirer Z, Rosenberg H. Immunocompetence in pregnancy: production of interleukin-2 by peripheral blood lymphocytes. Cancer Detection Prevention 1987; 1(suppl):39–42.

126. Favier R, Edelman P, Mary J-Y, Sadoul G, Douay L. Presence of elevated serum interleukin-2 levels in pregnant women (letter). N Engl J Med 1990; 322:270.

127. Gehrz RC, Christianson WR, Linner KM, Conroy MM, McCue SA, Balfour HH Jr. Cytomegalovirus-specific humoral and cellular immune responses in human pregnancy. J Infect Dis 1981; 143:391–395.

128. Bissenden JG, Ling NR, Mackintosh P. Suppression of mixed lymphocyte reactions by pregnancy. Clin Exp Immunol 1980; 39:195–202.

129. Vanderbeeken Y, Vlieghe MP, Duchateau J, Delespesse G. Suppressor T-lymphocytes in pregnancy. Am J Reprod Immunol 1984; 5:20–24.

130. Nakamura N, Miyazaki K, Kitano Y, Fujisaki S, Okamura H. Suppression of cytotoxic T-lymphocyte activity during human pregnancy. J Reprod Immunol 1993; 23:119–130.

131. Iwatani Y, Amino N, Kabutomori O, Kaneda T, Tanizawa O, Miyai K. Peripheral large granular lymphocytes in normal pregnant and postpartum women: decrease in late pregnancy and dynamic change in the puerperium. J Reprod Immunol 1989; 16:165–172.

132. Toder V, Nebel L, Gleicher N. Studies of natural killer cells in pregnancy. I Analysis at the single cell level. J Clin Lab Immunol 1984; 14:123–127.

133. Baley JE, Schacter BZ. Diminished NK activity in pregnant women and neonates. J Immunol 1985; 134:3042–3047.

134. Gonik B, Loftin KC, Tan NS, Crump J. Immune modulation of natural killer cell cytotoxicity against herpes infected target cells in pregnancy. Am J Reprod Immunol 1990; 24:95–98.

135. Higuchi K, Aoki K, Kimbara T, Hosoi N, Yamamoto T, Okada H. Suppression of natural killer cell activity by monocytes following immunotherapy for recurrent spontaneous aborters. Am J Reprod Immunol 1995; 33:221–227.

136. Gonik B, Loo LS, West S, Kohl S. Natural killer cell cytotoxicity and antibody-dependent cellular cytotoxicity to herpes simplex virus-infected cells in human pregnancy. Am J Reprod Immunol 1987; 13:23–26.

137. Asari S, Iwatani Y, Amino N, Tanizawa O, Miyai K. Peripheral K cells in normal human pregnancy: decrease during pregnancy and increase after delivery. J Reprod Immunol 1989; 15:31–37.

138. Andrews WC, Bonsnes RW. The leucocytes during pregnancy. Am J Obstet Gynecol 1951; 61:1129–1135.

139. Björksten B, Söderström T, Damber M-G, von Schoultz B, Strigbrand T. Polymorphonuclear leucocyte function during pregnancy. Scand J Immunol 1978; 8:257–262.

140. Krause PJ, Ingardia CJ, Pontius LT, Malech HL, LoBello TM, Moderazo EG. Host defense during pregnancy: neutrophil chemotaxis and adherence. Am J Obstet Gynecol 1987; 157:274–280.

141. Cotton DJ, Seligmann B, O'Brien WF, Gallin JI. Selective defect in human neutrophil superoxide anion generation elicited by the chemoattractant N-formylmethionylleucylphenylalanine in pregnancy. J Inf Dis 1983; 148:194–199.

142. Barriga C, Rodriguez AB, Ortega E. Increased phagocytic activity of polymorphonuclear leukocytes during pregnancy. Eur J Obstet Gynecol Reprod Biol 1994; 57:43–46.

143. Shibuya T, Izuchi K, Kuroiwa A, Harada H, Kumamoto A, Shirakawa K. Study on nonspecific immunity in pregnant women: II. Effect of hormones on chemiluminescence response of peripheral blood phagocytes. Am J Reprod Immunol 1991; 26:76–81.

144. Selvaraj RJ, Sbarra AJ, Thomas GB, Cetrulo CL, Mitchell GW Jr. A microtechnique for studying chemiluminescence response of phagocytes using whole blood and its application to the evaluation of phagocytes in pregnancy. RES: J Reticuloendothel Soc 1982; 31:3–16.

145. Baboonian C, Grundy JE, Lever AML, Griffiths PD. Effect of pregnancy plasma upon in vitro parameters of cell mediated immunity. FEMS Microbiol Immunol 1989; 47:189–198.

146. Nicholas NS, Panayi GS, Nouri AME. Human pregnancy serum inhibits interleukin-2 production. Clin Exp Immunol 1984; 58:587–595.

147. Domingo CG, Domenech N, Aparicio P, Palomino P. Human pregnancy serum inhibits proliferation of T8-depleted cells and their interleukin-2 synthesis in mixed lymphocyte cultures. J Reprod Immunol 1985; 8:97–110.

148. Gundert D, Merz WE, Hilgenfeldt U, Brossmer R. Inability of highly purified preparations of human chorionic gonadotropin to inhibit the phytohemagglutin-induced stimulation of lymphocytes. FEBS Lett 1975; 53:309–312.

149. Huong H-J. The suppressive effects of human chorionic gonadotropin of various preparations on lymphocyte blastogenesis in vitro. Acta Obst Gynaec Jpn 1981; 33:1062–1070.

150. Papiha SS, Wajner M, Wagstaff TI. Inhibition of lymphocyte transformation by serum from pregnant women: lack of correlation with levels of alpha-feto protein. Biol Neonate 1983; 43:109–117.

151. Bischof P, Lauber K, Girard JP, Herrmann WL, Sizonenko PC. Circulating levels of pregnancy proteins and depression of lymphoblastogenesis during pregnancy. J Lab Clin Immunol 1983; 12:93–98.

152. Harris SJ, Anthony FW, Jones DB, Masson GM. Pregnancy-specific β_1-glycoprotein: effect on lymphocyte proliferation in vitro. J Reprod Immunol 1984; 6:267–270.

153. Majumdar S, Dahiya R, Mapa MK, Gopalan S, Devi PK. Lymphocyte response to PHA in the presence of sera of pregnant women and its correlation with serum levels of placental specific $\beta_1$glycoprotein. Indian J Med Res 1984; 79:502–507.

154. Cohen JHM, Danel L, Cordier G, Saez S, Revillard J-P. Sex steroid receptors in peripheral T cells: absence of androgen receptors and restriction of estrogen receptors to OKT8-positive cells. J Immunol 1983; 131:2767–2771.

155. Stimson WH. Oestrogen and human T lymphocytes: presence of specific receptors in the T suppressor cytotoxic subset. Scand J Immunol 1988; 28: 345–350.

156. Szekeres-Bartho J, Reznikoff-Etievant MF, Varga P, Pichon M-F, Varga Z, Chaouat G. Lymphocytic progesterone receptors in normal and pathological human pregnancy. J Reprod Immunol 1989; 16:239–247.

157. Schiff RI, Mercier D, Buckley RH. Inability of gestational hormones to account for the inhibitory effects of pregnancy plasmas on lymphocyte responses *in vitro*. Cell Immunol 1975; 20:69–80.

158. Skinnider LF, Laxdal V. The effect of progesterone, oestrogens, and hydrocortisone on the mitogenic response of lymphocytes to phytohemagglutinin in pregnant and non-pregnant women. Br J Obstet Gynaecol 1981; 88: 1110–1114.

159. Stites DP, Siiteri PK. Steroids as immunosuppressants in pregnancy. Immunol Rev 1983; 75:117–138.

5

The Immunology of Pregnancy:
The Fetus as Allograft

HENRY N. CLAMAN

University of Colorado School of Medicine
Denver, Colorado

I. Introduction

The subject of this chapter is the immunological paradox of pregnancy. This subject has intrigued immunologists for many years. Simply stated in the form of a question, the paradox becomes: How does it happen that the fetus—half of whose genetic makeup is paternally derived (and thus is foreign to the mother)—can survive to term? Considered as a hemiallograft, its survival for 9 months requires the existence of special mechanisms.

This chapter represents a revision, a shortening, and an updating of *The Immunology of Human Pregnancy* (1). This chapter has been written for physicians, particularly pediatricians and internists, and animal data will be scarce. The field of reproductive immunology is growing very rapidly, so the reference list is representative and not exhaustive. There is considerable controversy in this field.

The paradox has been discussed for some time before 1953. In that year, however, Sir Peter Medawar (not yet a Nobel laureate) gave great conceptual impetus to the subject. He wrote a symposium paper entitled "Some Immunological and Endocrinological Problems Raised by the Ev olution of Viviparity in Vertebrates'' (2). This paper is in a hard-to-find book, yet it was very influential. Medawar gave three reasons why the allogenic fetus is not immunologically damaged or rejected by the mother:

1. The fetus and the mother are anatomically separated.
2. The fetus is antigenically immature, i.e., does not express alloantigens.
3. The mother is immunologically "indolent" or "inert" during pregnancy, and thus would not respond to alloantigens.

Medawar discussed the evidence for and against these statements. He also emphasized the role of cortisone-like hormones which he had shown (in rabbit experiments) greatly influenced graft acceptance and rejection. It is not a criticism of Medawar to point out that he made two major errors—after all, the study of transplantation immunology was itself embryonic in 1953. First, he thought that the fetus was not immunologically recognized by the mother; we know that (in limited ways) it is. Second, he thought adrenocortical hormones were important in preventing rejection of the fetus; we know that (in humans) they are not.

Medawar's interest in the immunology of pregnancy was transmitted to his colleague, Rupert E. Billingham. Billingham, in turn, worked with Alan E. Beer. Because of their efforts, the field expanded. In 1981, Beer and his colleagues expanded the list of reasons why the fetus survives. This list can be considered as an updating of Medawar's three conceptual points. The list embodies several thoughts and mechanisms which were not even considered in 1953 (3).

1. The fetal and maternal blood circulations are completely separate.
2. The uterus is an "immunologically privileged site." That is, the fetus expresses paternal alloantigens but there is "an afferent block" in the pregnant uterus so that these alloantigens do not stimulate the maternal immune system.
3. There is an immunological hiatus at the feto–maternal interface because:
   (a) the fetus does not express paternal alloantigens, or
   (b) these antigens are expressed but "masked."
4. There are endocrinologically determined local inhibitors of alloreactivity.
5. Pregnancy involves the production of immunosuppressive cells or factors, local or systemic, by mother and/or fetus.

These five points are not mutually exclusive. This chapter will review current thinking about them.

II.　The Materno–Fetal Interface

The materno–fetal interface comprises those tissues which develop during pregnancy (considered in this chapter to be intrauterine). The embryo develops within the trophoblastic tissue (also derived from the fertilized ovum). It is the trophoblast which is directly opposed to maternal tissue and blood. The villous trophoblast comprises projections of fetal tissue which reach into the intervillous blood spaces containing maternal blood. The outer layer of the villous trophoblast thus becomes the primary feto–maternal interface, which is bathed by maternal blood which includes mobile parts of the mother's immune system in the form of leukocytes. This outer layer is the syncytiotrophoblast, a continuous covering of non-mitotic tissue. It had previously consisted of individual cells which later matured into an acellular syncytium. Beneath the syncytiotrophoblast is another layer, the cytotrophoblast. This is a sheet of nucleated cells which is more metabolically active than the syncytiotrophoblast. Below the cytotrophoblast is the stroma, a loose connective tissue matrix containing many cell types such as macrophages, lymphocytes, large granular leukocytes (LGLs—see below), fibroblasts, etc.

Extravillous trophoblast tissue also contacts maternal tissue but in a less vascular environment. From it develop the chorion laeve, the chorionic plate, the marginal zone, and the basal plate.

Decidual tissue is the mother's contribution to the placenta. It is a highly cellular and vascular modification of the endometrium at the site of implantation.

III.　Is the Uterus an "Immunologically Privileged Site?"

This question has occupied the thoughts of pregnancy immunologists for some time. Immunologically privileged sites are locales in which the ordinary rules of immunology seem to be in abeyance (4). (For the purpose of this chapter, we are particularly interested in the possible privileged status of allograft rejection mechanisms.) In animal systems, the most studied privileged site is the cheekpouch of the Syrian hamster. Allografts placed there survive. The explanation for this phenomenon is that the pouch lacks lymphatic drainage, and so the afferent limb of the immune recognition is nonfunctional. Another similar area is the anterior chamber of the eye. It is of interest that antigens placed there not only fail to evoke an immune response but also induce antigen-specific suppressor cells at remote sites (5).

Animal experiments provide the major route for exploring this question. One consideration is that the hormonal response which accompanies pregnancy might downregulate immune events in the uterus (even though we have seen in Chapter 4 that pregnancy itself has little suppressive effects on the peripheral immune system in general). Nevertheless, allografts placed within the uterus of hormonally prepared ("pseudo-pregnant") rats are not only rejected in the usual fashion, they also sensitize the host (6). These results indicate that pregnancy hormones do not interfere with either the afferent or efferent limbs of the uterine immune response.

Still, these experiments are very artificial. Grafts placed into the uterine cavity are not the same as a fetus developing within the trophoblast, and exogenous estrogens and progestogens are not equivalent to the hormones made during a natural pregnancy.

More physiological approaches have been tried in the rabbit (7). Naive rabbits had skin allografts placed both on the skin and in the pregnant uterus. The skin grafts were rejected in 7–8 days, as expected, and they also showed the expected degrees of leukocytic infiltration. The uterine grafts, however, had not been rejected by 14 days (which was as long as the experiment was able to be carried out), and these grafts lacked a significant degree of inflammation. Thus, these experiments suggest that the intrauterine environment in the immunologically naive pregnant animals does favor the acceptance of allografts, at least to a degree.

If, however, allografts were placed into the decidua of a rabbit which had been presensitized to the histocompatibility antigens on the graft, the tissue was rejected in 8 days. While these results do not tell us whether the rejection was mediated by T cells or antibodies (or both), they do show that the *expression* of allograft immunity can occur in the pregnant uterus.

In summary, the results in this section indicate that (a) the uterine environment itself is not an immunologically privileged site, (b) primary allograft sensitization and rejection may be blunted in the decidual environment, but (c) previously induced systemic allosensitization can be expressed in the decidual locale.

IV. HLA Expression on the Trophoblast

Because the trophoblast is the critical anatomic interface between fetus and mother, it is crucial to understand whether paternal HLA antigens are expressed there. If somehow it happened that there were no paternal HLA antigens on the trophoblast (in contrast to virtually all other non-rbc tissues), then the paradox might be solved. If there were HLA antigens on the trophoblast, the paradox was still unsolved. The question had quite an unexpected answer.

The first indication that the trophoblast might be immunologically unusual came in 1962, when Simmons and Russell did a clever experiment. They transplanted trophoblast tissue alone or embryonic tissue alone (without trophoblast) into allogeneic mice. Trophoblast tissue survived but the embryos were rejected. They concluded that transplantation antigens were either absent from the trophoblast or were not expressed in immunogenic forms (8).

Histochemical studies (9) using antibodies to class I and class II MHC molecules were also informative. Reagents specific for class II MHC (HLA-DR, DQ, DP) did not stain syncytiotrophoblast anywhere, nor the cytotrophoblast cells in the villous trophoblast. In the stroma beneath, however, both maternal and paternal MHC occur, as expected in embryonic tissue. Thus, there was an immunological "hiatus" ("no-person's land") comprising two layers of tissue (syncytotrophoblast and cytotrophoblast) which make up the interface and where MHC antigens are not expressed. The paradox was not completely solved just yet, because the *extravillous* cytotrophoblast did express class I MHC, but in an unexpected way. That is, these cells were stained with reagents which bound to the nonpolymorphic ("generic") parts of class I MHC (such as β-2 microglobulin and the α-3 region of the alpha chain), but the antibodies did not bind to the paternal-specific part of the MHC. Thus there seemed to be MHC in the trophoblast, but it was different. This new form of class I MHC molecule was called HLA-G, which (together with its relatives, HLA-E and -F) comprised a new family of "nonclassical" class I MHC molecules. The important point is that HLA-G shows little if any polymorphism within humans. Thus, if maternal lymphocytes do touch paternal HLA-G, it will not be recognized as allogeneic (10).

To summarize, at the human feto–maternal interface, the trophoblast tissues which might meet the maternal immune system are either devoid of paternal MHC or express a special nonpolymorphic MHC, that is, HLA-G.

The *nonexpression* of classical HLA class I and II in the trophoblast raises interesting and fundamental biological questions. If these molecules are not expressed when their genes (and sometimes their mRNA) are present, what prevents expression? Recent evidence indicates that trophoblast tissue contains a tissue-specific negative regulatory element (NRE) for classical HLA class I but not for HLA-G (which is therefore expressed) (11). Then, *could* classical HLA antigens be upregulated on the trophoblast under certain conditions—a situation which might occur via inflammation-derived cytokines and which would be deleterious to the continuance of pregnancy? It appears that trophoblast tissue resists MHC upregulation by IFN-γ (12–14).

V. Other Antigens at the Materno–Fetal Interface

Complement-regulatory proteins have been found at the feto–maternal interface. Some time ago, explorations were made of an array of proteins called TLX (trophoblast-lymphocyte crossreactive) (15,16). This system appeared to have some genetic polymorphisms which were invoked to explain part of the immunological paradox of pregnancy. More recently, some of these were found to represent members of the CD46 family, and CD46 is a protein which binds to C3b. This and CD55 (DAF or decay-accelerating factor) are part of a network which seems to control and limit complement activation (17). Thus, although these proteins probably do not act as MHC surrogates, they are extremely interesting because they sug-gest another mechanism of fetal protection, i.e., one in which maternal complement-fixing antibodies against the fetus might be downregulated.

Antigens of several other polymorphic systems occur in the trophoblast. The A and B blood group substances are absent from the trophoblast, but Rh(D) is present (18). The biological significance of the presence of Rh(D) here is not clear, as it is believed that the passage of fetal Rh(D)$^+$ red cells to the Rh(D)$^-$ mother is the pathway for Rh isoimmunization.

VI. Cells in Placental Tissue

The decidual stroma contains a variety of lymphoid and nonlymphoid cells, as one would expect, yet there are special characteristics of some of these cell populations which are not the same as those in corresponding cells elsewhere in the periphery.

Macrophages are abundant in the trophoblast and decidua. They express MHC class II and CD14. They appear capable of carrying out antigen-presenting and proinflammatory functions characteristic of macrophages elsewhere.

T lymphocytes are abundant in human decidua. Unlike T cells in the periphery, most have the $\gamma\delta$ type of T-cell receptor (TcR) rather than the $\alpha\beta$ TcR present in the majority of peripheral T cells. Many decidual T cells are CD56$^+$ and carry the CD45 RO isoform, supposedly typical of "memory" T cells. Decidual T cells are relatively low in the expression of CD3 and CD4 and (to a lesser degree) CD8. They do not respond in mixed leukocyte cultures nor to anti-CD3 but do respond to plant lectin mitogens (19). Altogether, decidual T cells appear to be specially selected and somewhat unresponsive.

The most frequent immune cells found in first-trimester decidual tissues are large cells, called large granular leukocytes (LGLs). These do not appear to be typical macrophages nor lymphocytes nor granulocytes. Instead, they share some characteristics of each of those three lineages. Phenotypically, they are CD2$^+$ CD3$^-$ CD16$^-$ CD45$^+$ CD56$^+$ CD57$^+$ (HNK-1$^+$). They are close to NK cells, but the latter are CD16$^+$ and uterine LGLs are CD16$^-$. Uterine (U)-LGL cells do have NK activity against conventional NK targets, but trophoblast cells seem to be resistant to NK lysis (20). The precise role of U-LGL cells is not clear. As mice without LGLs can go to term, LGL cells are not essential for a successful pregnancy.

VII. Placental Cytokines

Research in the biology of implantation has been rapid and impressive (reviewed in Ref. 21). A number of cytokines and cytokine receptors have been identified in various areas of the placenta. So far, most of the research has been descriptive, and the precise role(s) of any or all cytokines remains to be determined. Some interesting generalizations have emerged, however. IL-1 has been found. IL-2 activity is low in the placenta, and it is interesting that uterine T cells seem to lack CD25, the high-affinity IL-2 receptor. This suggests that T-cell proliferation there may be dampened. Cytokine expression may be compartmentalized. While mRNA for IL-1β and IL-4 were found in both trophoblast layers, that of CSF-1 and TNF-α were found mostly in syncytiotrophoblast and IFN-γ occurred only in cytotrophoblast (22). TNF-α is transcribed and translated by human syncytio- and cytotrophoblast, although its function is unclear (23).

A most provocative generalization was put forth by the late Thomas Wegmann and others. This is that pregnancy involves a "tilt" *toward* TH-2 functions and *away* from TH-1 functions (24). Thus, pregnancy would favor humoral (TH-2) responses toward paternal antigens, and it would result in less cell-mediated (TH-1) responses. As we know that systemic humoral and and cell-mediated capacities are normal (or nearly normal) during pregnancy (see Chapter 4), this situation, if operative, would occur mainly within the uterus. Thus it would represent an interesting example of a localized immunological microcosm. Nevertheless, the appeal of this schema is that it would provide some rationale for a situation in which maternal antibody formation (which is unlikely to harm the fetus) is favored and cell-mediated immunity (which might well be deleterious) is thwarted. Although it is almost certain that the system will not turn out to be that simple, it is a provocative concept—one that is surely stimulating important new experiments and observations.

VIII. Cellular Traffic Across the Feto–Maternal Interface

If there were complete and impenetrable separation of fetal and maternal circulatory system, the job of the pregnancy immunologist would be simpler. In fact, however, although the circulatory systems are independent and largely separate, cells and molecules do cross in both directions.

Trophoblast deportation is a vivid phrase which describes the traffic of both syncytiotrophoblast and cytotrophoblast cells from the fetus into the mother's circulation. The frequency of this phenomenon is not known, but it does occur in many pregnancies. The best estimate of the rate of exit comes from examining uterine vein blood as the deported cells later tend to get trapped in the pulmonary circulation. Therefore, sampling mother's mixed venous blood shows even fewer deportees. The rate of traffic is greater in preeclampsia (25). The possible role of deported cells in either the development of allosensitization or tolerance (should there be stromal cells attached) is unknown.

IX. Fetal Cell Traffic

Fetal erythrocytes can enter the maternal circulation as early as the 10th week of gestation (26). About 30% of women have some circulating fetal red cells during the second and third trimesters. This phenomenon probably accounts for the occasional situation in which Rh isosensitization occurs during the first pregnancy. However, most of the fetal erythrocytes which gain access to maternal blood do so during parturition. Those that do pass survive or not according to the usual ABO relations between mother and fetus.

Maternal erythrocytes do reach the fetal circulation, but the extent and importance of this fact is unclear.

Fetal leukocytes (of particular interest are the lymphocytes) have been detected in small numbers in the maternal circulation, even early in pregnancy (27,28). However, these data have occasional strong criticisms (29). Perhaps it would be best to say that some (but only a few) fetal leukocytes reach the maternal circulation.

X. Immunoglobulin Transfer to the Fetus

It is well known that maternal IgG readily crosses into the fetal circulation. This is not simply a matter of passive diffusion, for two reasons. First, a molecule of similar size, i.e., IgA, does not cross. (Also, IgM, IgD, and IgE do not cross into the fetus.) Second, the level of IgG in fetal blood at term is actually about 10% higher than the maternal level. Both facts are accounted for by a process of facilitated diffusion via FcR receptors for IgG. The facilitated diffusion of IgG provides the fetus with a measure of passive humoral immunity for the first 6–9 months of postuterine life.

There is one important exception to the phenomenon. Maternal antipaternal HLA antibodies (if present) are trapped in the "placental sink." This occurs both because of Fc receptors for immunoglobulins in general and because paternally encoded HLA are present in the stroma of the trophoblast. Thus, these antibodies do not reach the fetus, where they would be able to cause major complement-mediated damage if passage occurred.

Do maternal lymphocytes reach the fetus? This is technically difficult to study, but the concept is of importance, as significant mother-to-fetus lymphocyte traffic raises the possibility of graft-versus-host disease (GVHD). So far, chimerism has been found in the fetus mainly in cases of severe combined immunodeficiency (30). Whether the chimeric state is responsible for the clinical syndrome or is a result of it is as yet unclear.

XI. Maternal Immunological Reactions to the Fetus

A. Maternal Antibodies to Fetal and Placental Antigens

In spite of the apparent immunological nonreactivity which exists at the feto–maternal interface, it has been known since the 1950s that pregnant women can and often do make antibodies to paternal antigens. This fact was recognized by Rose Payne and by Jon van Rood and their colleagues (31,32).

Studies showed that the antibodies were directed against paternal class I and class II antigens, that they were both IgM and IgG, and that they could be detected by leukoagglutinating and leukocytotoxic assays. One puzzle soon emerged and has remained. While the prevalence of these antibodies in groups of women was roughly correlated with the number of pregnancies, it was noted early that many women never made detectable antiparternal antibodies, in spite of repeated pregnancies. In fact, the prevalence of antibodies in multiparas rarely goes above about 50% (33).

Thus, several questions arose. First, what was the route by which fetal tissue bearing paternal class I and II MHC antigens gained access to the maternal immune system? It did not appear to be via recognition at the trophoblast, for the reasons mentioned earlier in this chapter. While the answer is not yet certain, a good candidate is the small number of fetal leukocytes which do gain access to the maternal circulation, either during pregnancy or at delivery. Another (less popular) idea is that during trophoblast deportation, some underlying stroma (carrying classical MHC antigens) is carried along, together with syncytiotrophoblast and cytotrophoblast.

A second question concerns the biological significance of these antibodies in terms of the success or failure of the pregnancy. Certainly it seems that it would be detrimental to the fetus if the antibodies gained access to the fetal circulation. IgM antibodies, of course, would not cross the placenta, but what about IgG? It is quite clear that although the bulk of maternal IgG does reach the fetal circulation, antipaternal IgG is trapped in "the placental sink" via interaction with the HLA antigens themselves. Thus, although maternal antipaternal antibodies do not reach the fetus, one can ask if these antibodies, while not harmful, might actually be helpful in maintaining pregnancy, perhaps by promoting the production of growth factors. After all, the antibodies made by highly multiparous women have been the major source of tissue typing reagents used in histocompatibility laboratories. Thus, the presence of even high titers of these antibodies does not seem to be prejudicial to subsequent pregnancies. Whether they are beneficial remains an open question.

A last question for this section concerns the large percentage of women who apparently do *not* make antipaternal antibodies, in spite of repeated pregnancies with the same partner. One explanation is that these women are simply "nonresponders" (whatever that may mean). A much more intriguing possibility is that these women do indeed make anti-HLA antibodies but these, in turn, are "masked" by anti-anti-HLA antibodies, i.e., by anti-idiotypic antibodies. That this does occur has been shown in elegant experiments by Suciu-Foca and her colleagues (34) and by Torry et al. (35). Again, however, it is not clear how often anti-idiotypes are made, and what fraction of apparently nonresponding women do react in this way.

B. Maternal T-Cell Reactivity to the Fetus

It has been of great interest to determine if maternal T cells specifically recognize paternal antigens on the fetus. Thus, this would represent the T-cell analog of the B-cell and antibody reactivity described above. Meth-

Table 1 Possible Mechanisms by Which the Fetus Escapes Immunologic Recognition by the Mother (in approximate order of importance)

1. Absence of paternal HLA antigens at feto–maternal interface.
   a. Presence of nonpolymorphic HLA-G in special parts of the trophoblast
2. Blunted T-cell activation mechanisms in the decidua
3. Trophoblast resistance to:
   a. Upregulation of class I and class II MHC molecules
   b. Lysis by CTL or NK mechanisms
4. Failure of maternal antipaternal antibodies (when present) to cross the placenta to the fetus
5. Possible presence of anti-idiotypic (anti-anti-HLA) antibodies which might "mask" antipaternal HLA in the mother
6. Relative degree of "immunological privilege" of the trophoblast within the decidua (perhaps related to point 2 above).
7. A general "tilt" of the maternal immune system toward TH_2 functions, away from TH_1 functions (related to points 2, 5, and 6 above)

odologically, the problem is complicated by the fact that everyone appears to have T-cell alloreactivity to everyone else's MHC. So the situation can be stated as follows: Granted that a woman normally has some T-cell alloreactivity to both paternal MHC haplotypes, does she have any more reactivity to the haplotype inherited by the fetus, either during or after the pregnancy? The possible dangers of such a scenario are not difficult to imagine. However, such heightened alloreactivity has not been demonstrated.

XII. Summary

The success of the fetus, considered as an allograft, is vital. It is extremely important to maintain genetic diversity in the population as a whole. Thus, it is not unexpected to find out that there are multiple overlapping "fail-safe" mechanisms designed to make sure that the fetus is not rejected by the maternal immune system. These mechanisms are outlined in Table 1.

References

1. Claman HN. The Immunology of Human Pregnancy. Totowa, NJ: Humana Press, 1993.

2. Medawar PB. Some immunological and endocrinological problems raised by the evolution of viviparity in vertebrates. Symp Soc Exp Biol 1953; 11: 320–338.

3. Beer AE, Quebbeman JF, Ayers JWT, et al. Major histocompatibility complex antigens, maternal and paternal immune responses and chronic habitual abortions in humans. Am J Obstet Gynecol 1981; 141:987–999.

4. Billingham RE, Silvers WK. Immunobiology of Tissue Transplantation. Englewood Cliffs, NJ: Prentice-Hall, 1971.

5. Streilein JW. Tissue barriers, immunosuppressive microenvironments, and privileged sites: the eye's point of view. Reg Immunol 1993; 5:253–268.

6. Beer AE, Billingham RE. Host responses to intra-uterine tissue, cellular and fetal allografts. J Reprod Fertil 1974; 21:59–60.

7. Dodd M, Andrew TA, Coles JS. Functional behavior of skin allografts transplanted to rabbit deciduomata. J Anat 1980; 130:381–390.

8. Simmons RL, Russell PS. Antigenicity of mouse trophoblast. Ann NY Acad Sci 1962; 99:717–732.

9. Faulk WP, Temple A. Distribution of β_2-microglobulin and HLA in chorionic villi of human placentae. Nature 1976; 262:799–802.

10. Schmidt CM, Orr HT. Maternal/fetal interactions: the role of the MHC class I molecule HLA-G. Crit Rev Immunol 1993; 13:207–224.

11. Chiang MH, Main EK. Nuclear regulation of HLA class I genes in human trophoblast. Am J Reprod Immunol 1994; 32:167–172.

12. Hunt JS, Yelavarthi KK, Yangi Y, Fishback JL. Class I major histocompatibility genes in trophoblast cells: studies on expression, regulation and function. In: Chaouat G, Mowbray J, eds. Cellular and Molecular Biology of the Materno-Fetal Relationship. INSERM/J. Libbey Eurotext, 1991:51–59.

13. Hunt JS, Andrews GK, Wood GW. Normal trophoblasts resist induction of class I HLA. J Immunol 1987; 138:2481–2487.

14. Head JR, Drake BL, Zuckerman FA. MHC antigens on trophoblast and their regulations: implications in the maternal-fetal relationship. Am J Reprod Immunol 1987; 15:12–18.

15. McIntyre JA, Faulk WP, Verhulst SJ, Colliver J. Human trophoblast lymphocyte cross-reactive (TLX) antigens define a new alloantigen system. Science 1983; 222:1135–1137.

16. McIntyre JA. In search of trophoblast-lymphocyte crossreactive (TLX) antigens. Am J Reprod Immunol Microbiol 1988; 17:100–110.

17. Johnson PM. Reproductive and maternofetal relations. In: Lachmann PJ, Peters SK, Rosen FS, Walport MJ, eds. Clinical Aspects of Immunology. 5th ed. Boston: Blackwell Scientific, 1993:755–767.

18. Goto S, Nishi H, Tomoda Y. Blood group Rh-D factor in human trophoblast determined by immunofluorescent method. Am J Obstet Gynecol 1980; 137: 707–712.

19. Mincheva-Nilsson L, Hammarstrom S, Hammarstrom M-L. Human decidual leukocytes from early pregnancy contain high numbers of $\gamma\delta^+$ cells and show selective down-regulation of alloreactivity. J Immunol 1992; 149:2203–2211.

20. Chumbley G, King A, Robertson K, Holmes N, Loke YW. Resistance of HLA-G and HLA-A2 transfectants to lysis by decidual NK cells. Cell Immunol 1994; 155:312–322.
21. Cross JC, Werb Z, Fisher SJ. Implantation and the placenta: key pieces of the development puzzle. Science 1944; 266:1508–1518.
22. Haynes MK, Jackson LG, Tuan RS, Shepley KJ, Smith JB. Cytokine production in first trimester chorionic villi: detection of mRNAs and protein products *in vivo*. Cell Immunol 1993; 151:300–308.
23. Yang Y, Yelavarthi KK, Chen H-L, Pace JL, Terranova PF, Hunt JS. Molecular, biochemical, and functional characteristics of tumor necrosis factor-α produced by human placental cytotrophoblastic cells. J Immunol 1993; 150: 5614–5624.
24. Wegmann TG, Lin H, Guilbert L, Mosmann TR. Bidirectional cytokine interactions in the maternal-fetal relationship: is successful pregnancy a T_H2 phenomenon? Immunol Today 1993; 14:353–356.
25. Chua S, Wilkins T, Sargent I, Redman C. Trophoblast deportation in pre-eclamptic pregnancy. Br J Obstet Gynecol 1991; 98:973–979.
26. Price JO, Elias S, Wachtel SS, Klinger K, Dockter M, Tharapel A, Shulman LP, Phillips OP, Meyers CM, Shook D, Simpson JL. Prenatal diagnosis with fetal cells isolated from maternal blood by multiparameter flow cytometry. Am J Obstet Gynecol 1991; 165:1731–1737.
27. Walkanowska J, Conte FA, Grumbach MM. Practical and theoretical implications of fetal/maternal lymphocyte transfer. Lancet 1969; i:1119–1122.
28. Herzenberg LA, Bianchi DW, Schroder J, Cann HM, Iverson GM. Fetal cells in the blood of pregnant women: detection and enrichment by fluorescence-activated cell sorting. Proc Natl Acad Sci USA 1979; 76:1453–1450.
29. Adinolfi M. The maternal-fetal interaction: some controversies and solutions. Exp Clin Immunogenet 1993; 10:103–117.
30. Sargent IL. Maternal and fetal immune responses during pregnancy. Exp Clin Immunogenet 1993; 10:85–102.
31. Payne R, Rolfs MR. Fetomaternal leukocyte incompatibility. J Clin Invest 1956; 37:1756–1763.
32. van Rood JJ, Eernisse JG, van Leeuwen A. Leucocyte antibodies in sera from pregnant women. Nature 1958; 181:1735–1736.
33. Vives J, Gelabert A, Castillo R. HLA antibodies and period of gestation: Decline in frequency of positive sera during last trimester. Tissue Antigens 1976; 7:209–212.
34. Suciu-Foca N, Reed E, Rohowsky C, Kung P, King DW. Anti-idiotypic antibodies to anti-HLA receptors induced by pregnancy. Proc Natl Acad Sci USA 1983; 80:830–834.
35. Torry DS, Faulk WP, McIntyre JA. Regulation of immunity to extraembryonic antigens in human pregnancy. Am J Reprod Immunol 1989; 21:76–81.

Part Two

GENERAL THERAPEUTICS

6

Psychological Changes During Pregnancy: Implications for Medical Care

ANDREA BEIN STONE

University of Massachusetts Medical
   School
Worcester, Massachusetts

WALTER A. BROWN

Brown University School of Medicine
Providence, Rhode Island

I. Introduction

Pregnancy is a psychological as well as a physical event. The physiological and social role changes associated with pregnancy and pregnancy's particular meaning to a woman produce psychological changes. These changes include the mild forgetfulness of pregnancy, the sense of well-being, the "adaptive anxiety" of the third trimester, and the emotional lability of the puerperium. The extent to which these psychological events affect pregnancy outcome and, particularly, the expression of physical illness during pregnancy is unclear. What is clear is that medical care during pregnancy can be usefully informed by awareness of these psychological changes. In this chapter, we will review the changes in anxiety, mood, and cognition that occur throughout pregnancy and the postpartum period, with an emphasis on normal pregnancy. We will also discuss the special experience of pregnant women who suffer from psychiatric disorders, substance abuse, and physical abuse. Finally, we will discuss the effect of these psychological changes on medical care and will suggest diagnostic and therapeutic interventions for clinicians who care for pregnant women.

II. Overview

Early psychoanalytic theories about emotional adjustment during pregnancy emphasized the importance of reproductive function in fulfilling a woman's development. Helene Deutsch saw pregnancy as a psychologically satisfying stage of life when a woman could devote herself entirely to the developing fetus and home life (1). As research on women's attitudes toward pregnancy began to reveal feelings of disappointment, anxiety, and ambivalence, the conflicts associated with pregnancy and its attendant social role changes became more central to theories about the psychology of pregnancy (2). Bibring proposed that the emotional disturbance found during pregnancy reflected a normative crisis that needed to be resolved for women to successfully proceed with adult development (3). For a while, conflict resolution during pregnancy was considered so important that lack of conflict was viewed as pathological. Zajicek explained the limitations of these early formulations:

> Theories about pregnancy and cultural expectations of women's behavior during this period have often been unrealistic and linked more to the generalized attitude towards women prevalent at the time than to the real experiences of pregnant women (2, p. 33).

Finally, as theories became more informed by research findings, the crises and conflicts of pregnancy were seen as part of the adjustment to motherhood and not confined to the 9 months of pregnancy.

Contemporary research has taken two general approaches: (a) large, naturalistic surveys of psychological symptoms during or after pregnancy and (b) studies of the effect of psychological factors on pregnancy outcome. The survey studies find little distress or differences between patients with and without symptoms if the sample population is selected to represent the general population accurately (2,4). Studies of the connection between adverse pregnancy experiences and psychological condition find that women with greater psychological distress during pregnancy have poorer outcomes (e.g., low birth weight) (5).

One consistent finding in pregnancy research is that physiological, social, and historical events all seem to affect the psychological experience (Table 1). Few studies, however, control adequately for these factors. Sociocultural variables, including age, parity, employment, marital status, national origin, and whether the pregnancy was planned, affect psychological processes (2,4). Perceived support from partners or parents is important (4). Psychiatric history, medical problems, and previous pregnancy experience are all meaningful (6). Normal pregnancy phenomena, such as fatigue and changes in appetite and sleep, can confound the assessment of

Table 1 Factors That Affect the
Psychological Experience of
Pregnancy

Age
Parity
Employment status
Marital status
National origin
Planned versus unplanned pregnancy
Perceived social support
Psychiatric history
Medical problems
Previous pregnancy experience

depression. The timing of measurement is also important. The psychological experience of pregnancy varies with trimester and awareness of the fetus. In addition, the influence of positive psychological changes on pregnancy experience and outcome is unknown.

Taking all of these variables into consideration is a monumental task often overlooked in pregnancy research. Studies that consider these variables most conscientiously find that, although many women report some emotional symptoms (e.g., crying) during pregnancy, most do not have disabling psychological difficulties (Table 2). No study has evaluated women before they become pregnant and followed them through pregnancy and the postpartum period. This approach would provide the most accurate data on pregnancy-specific changes.

Most studies have been done on European populations and may not be generalizable to North American women. Since cultural factors, such as expectations for employment after giving birth, have been shown to be relevant to psychological symptoms, the existing data may not be applicable beyond the culture studied. Furthermore, the few relevant pathophysiological studies of the effects of endogenous steroids on the brain

Table 2 Normal Psychological Changes of Pregnancy

Mild, transient, first-trimester anxiety
Third-trimester anxiety that increases as labor and delivery nears
Moderate, brief, first-trimester depression
Mild forgetfulness, confusion, and distractability

and behavior are hindered by an even more obvious limit to generalizability: almost all of them have been done on rats. Notably absent from existing research are studies examining the psychological implications of pregnancy-related alterations in neurotransmission, despite the wide availability of urine and blood tests to evaluate psychiatrically relevant neurochemicals.

III. Anxiety

Mild, transient anxiety is a part of most pregnancies. The infrequency of disabling anxiety symptoms is notable, given the risks of pregnancy and delivery to both the woman and fetus; the uncertainties about the health of the baby and the ability to assume the parental role; and the financial, career, and interpersonal consequences of having a baby.

Although the pathophysiology of anxiety has not been specifically studied during pregnancy, several changes in endocrine function occurring during pregnancy may be pertinent. Progesterone has sufficient sedating and hypnotic properties to have been used as an anesthetic (7). Also, two progesterone metabolites have barbiturate-like modulating properties at γ-aminobutyric acid (GABA) receptors (7). (GABA, an inhibitory neurotransmitter, appears to play a fundamental role in the regulation of anxiety.) Rauramo et al. demonstrated that β-endorphin levels show a more prolonged increase in response to stress in pregnant women than in nonpregnant controls exposed to the same stress (8). These endocrine changes may contribute to the lack of significant anxiety symptoms in most pregnant women, despite the obvious stress of pregnancy. β-endorphin and progesterone's central nervous system activities may enable women to handle the demands accompanying pregnancy without disruptive anxiety symptoms.

Anxiety appears to vary during the course of pregnancy. Some, but not all, researchers have found that women may be most vulnerable to symptoms of anxiety during the first and third trimesters (9,10). Somatic symptoms appear to be associated with anxiety levels (11). The first and third trimesters are usually associated with the most uncomfortable physical symptoms of pregnancy. Third-trimester anxiety may be an adaptive phenomenon (11,12); it appears to increase as delivery nears, may predict a positive-birthing experience (12), and seems to reflect a realistic attitude toward labor and delivery. Third-trimester anxiety alone has not been associated with adverse pregnancy outcome (11).

The consequences of anxiety earlier in pregnancy, especially during the first trimester, are less clear. In a prospective study, Cox and Reading found an increase in anxiety before the onset of complications such as hypertension, intrauterine growth retardation, and edema (13). Other researchers have also found an association between higher anxiety levels early in pregnancy and adverse outcome (11,14). These and other studies of the relation between anxiety and outcome have come under considerable criticism owing to their methodological limitations (5). For example, the clinical relevance of the anxiety levels found in these studies is rarely determined. Robinson et al. found a decrease in maternal anxiety after prenatal testing (15). The "high levels of anxiety" before testing, however, were only at the 70th percentile of anxiety levels for a nonclinical control group. The follow-up levels were at the 28th percentile. Although anxiety fluctuated, it never reached levels sufficient to warrant a diagnosis or cause disability. Lubin et al. also detected changes in anxiety levels during pregnancy, but the pooled means for each trimester were within the normal range for the psychometric instruments employed (9). The use of a control group suggests that, although levels of anxiety change during pregnancy, pregnant women in general have, at most, average levels of anxiety.

Certain women appear to be more at risk for developing symptoms of anxiety during pregnancy (Table 3). Women who were younger, unmarried, and smoked, with lower education levels, financial difficulties, and poor social supports, were more anxious and had babies with a lower gestational age at birth than older women with fewer socioeconomic stressors (14). Previous pregnancy experience affects anxiety as well. Women who have a history of both live births and spontaneous abortion have higher

Table 3 Features Associated with Psychological Difficulties During Pregnancy

Age
Marital status
Marital discord
Smoking
Alcohol or drug abuse
Unemployment
Financial difficulties
Poor social supports
Educational level
Doubts about the pregnancy
History of major mental illness
History of postpartum psychosis
Family history of depression or mania
Physical abuse

anxiety levels than women who have not had spontaneous abortions (9). When more average populations (e.g., married, without a history of miscarriage or significant socioeconomic distress) are studied, anxiety levels are low (15,16).

Some women may experience the first symptoms of a significant anxiety disorder during pregnancy or the postpartum period. One study of women with obsessive-compulsive disorder found that 39% of the women with children had experienced their first symptoms during pregnancy (17). Sichel et al. describe the new onset of obsessive compulsive disorder in 15 puerperial women (18). Symptoms started within the first 3 weeks after delivery and were characterized by severe, intrusive thoughts of harming their infants, without accompanying compulsive behaviors. All women responded to treatment with antidepressants or, in one case, electroconvulsive therapy.

The diverse results from these studies reflect the fundamental difficulty of studying pregnancy and, especially, pregnancy outcome. Physiological, demographic, and personal matters contribute to each variable, and many variables determine outcome. Significant early-pregnancy anxiety might reflect problematic aspects of a woman's life that may be more directly relevant to pregnancy outcome than the emotional symptom. Late-pregnancy anxiety appears to be a productive adaptation to cope with labor, delivery, and impending motherhood.

IV. Mood Changes During Pregnancy

Dysphoric or low mood is the most investigated mood symptom during pregnancy. As with anxiety, there is little consensus concerning the frequency, significance, or cause of this symptom.

All of the steroid hormones have been shown to influence brain activity (19). Estrogen and progestins can alter neurotransmitter synthesis, degradation, release, uptake, and receptor activity (20). In rats, estradiol interacts with both the serotonergic and noradrenergic systems, the leading targets of antidepressant treatment (21,22). The brain structures that contain the greatest concentration of intracellular steroid receptors, the limbic system and the hypothalamus, are probably central to the regulation of mood (20). Therefore, brain exposure to the high levels of circulating hormones of pregnancy might be expected to affect mood.

Progesterone can function as a central nervous system depressant. Estrogens, on the other hand, have been used effectively as antidepressant therapy and to potentiate the action of other antidepressants (23). In most women, oral contraceptives do not produce mood changes. However, one-sixth of women describe an elevation in mood while taking oral contraceptives; other subgroups experience depressed mood. For example, women with a history of premenstrual symptoms complain of more depression while taking high-dose estrogen compounds (24). This suggests that individuals differ in their susceptibility to the mood-altering properties of gonadal steroids.

In a well-designed study of emotional disorders in pregnancy, Kumar and Robsom found that, among women who were not depressed before pregnancy, 10% experienced moderate, brief depressions during the first trimester (6) (see Table 2). Nearly all new cases of depression remitted by the second or third trimester. They found that depressive symptoms were correlated with marital difficulties, doubts about the pregnancy, a previous history of induced abortion, bereavement during pregnancy, preterm delivery, and cigarette smoking. Other researchers have found an association between depressive symptoms and being unmarried, older, and unemployed (25) (see Table 3). Depressed, pregnant women have been found to be more likely to smoke cigarettes, drink alcohol, abuse cocaine and marijuana, and to have less weight gain than nondepressed pregnant women (25).

In contrast with anxiety, psychological factors, such as perceived social support, appear to be more important than demographic variables, such as age or income, in the development of depressive symptoms during pregnancy. Kendell describes the importance of cultural factors in his review of suicide rates during pregnancy (26). He found that the suicide rate among pregnant women is very low and has dropped significantly in the second half of this century. Most of the earlier suicides were among unmarried women. He attributes both the low rate and the drop over the last 40 years to social values. The influence on mood of other psychological factors, such as the desirability of the pregnancy, attitudes toward motherhood, and self-esteem, are unknown and probably differ greatly among women. For example, Zajicek found that women with high self-esteem during pregnancy had lower self-esteem during the first 4 months postpartum; women with medium self-esteem during pregnancy did not change throughout pregnancy and the first year postpartum; and women with low self-esteem during pregnancy had improved self-images between 4 and 14 months postpartum (2).

Most women do not experience serious, lasting depressive symptoms during or after pregnancy. The first trimester appears to be a time of increased symptoms. Psychological factors related to previous pregnancy experiences play a role in the development of symptoms during subsequent pregnancies. Substance abuse may complicate depression during pregnancy.

V. Cognitive Changes

During pregnancy, many women complain of cognitive difficulties, such as forgetfulness, but little systematic investigation has been devoted to this topic (27). Attentional deficits, such as forgetfulness, confusion, and distractability, are consistently found during pregnancy (27–29) (see Table 2). But reasoning and judgment are not impaired (27,30). Condon and Ball found that a pregnant woman's complaints of cognitive impairment were highly correlated with her partner's report (27), but women perceived a greater magnitude of difficulty than did their partners. Poser et al., in a study inspired by one of the author's pregnancy experiences, asked 51 health professionals who had 79 pregnancies to complete a questionnaire about conditions associated with pregnancy (29). Twenty-one women with 28 pregnancies had at least one of four symptoms of cognitive dysfunction: forgetfulness, disorientation, confusion, or reading difficulty. Symptom onset occurred during all three trimesters. They also found that cognitive deficits did not correlate with either depressed mood or sleep disturbance. They termed the cognitive dysfunction a "benign encephalopathy of pregnancy." All cognitive difficulties resolved after delivery.

A psychodynamic explanation for this difficulty comes from the concept of pregnancy as a developmental crisis: Women have trouble thinking because they are unable to resolve their conflicts about having a baby (28). Psychotherapists have noted changes in women's thinking during pregnancy. They have described a "shift toward primary process thinking," meaning that pregnant women appear to use more intuitive than rational mode of thinking (32). Systematic investigations have failed to support these observations (28,30).

Although pathophysiological mechanisms underlying cognitive changes during pregnancy have not been studied, Hampson has found that women's abilities to perform certain cognitive tests vary across the menstrual cycle (31). She found that women performed optimally when estradiol levels were in the midrange. These cognitive differences were not secondary to mood changes. Jarrahi-Zadeh et al. propose that the 2.5-fold increase in corticosteroid levels during pregnancy may be responsible for both mood and cognitive changes (28).

Although it is the least-studied psychological change of pregnancy, pregnant women complain of difficulties with attention and concentration more frequently than they complain of depression or anxiety. These symptoms are independent of mood or sleep difficulties and may be secondary to the central nervous system effects of estradiol or corticosteroids. They remit after pregnancy.

VI. Special Issues

Normal pregnancy does not appear to produce clinically significant emotional disturbance. However, women with psychiatric disorders, substance abuse disorders, and those who are victims of physical abuse are at special psychological risk (see Table 3).

A. Preexisting Psychiatric Disorders

About two-thirds of women with serious psychiatric disorders will have symptoms during pregnancy (33,34). These symptoms may reflect deterioration, improvement, or no change from their prepregnancy state (35). The remaining one-third experience pregnancy as a respite from chronic symptoms. Psychiatric diagnosis and age explain most of this variation (36). Younger women tend to encounter more difficulty during pregnancy than older women with the same diagnoses (36).

Women with psychotic disorders, such as schizophrenia, manic or depressive psychoses, or schizoaffective disorders, often have less difficulty with their psychiatric symptoms during pregnancy; they often require less medication (37), have fewer hospitalizations (38), have lower rates of illness than non-child-bearing control subjects (39), and report improved symptoms (35). Estrogen's antidopaminergic effect may explain this phenomenon (40). In rats, extended estrogen treatment blocks dopamine receptors, as does haloperidol (41). The high levels of estrogen during pregnancy may be "treating" psychotic disorders, allowing women to require less medication, have fewer relapses, and feel better. Psychological and social factors, such as the need to care for a fetus and baby and increased support from family and friends, may play a role in improved mental health for these women as well, but this has not been studied.

Women who suffer from recurrent, nonpsychotic depressive disorders may have depressive episodes during or after pregnancy (42). Those who were younger at the onset of their depressive disorder and who have more severe depressive symptoms before pregnancy are more susceptible to pregnancy-related symptoms than women with later-onset milder disorders (42).

Women with panic attacks may be less symptomatic during pregnancy, with symptoms returning and worsening after delivery, but the course of panic disorder is variable (43). Progesterone's sedative-hypnotic properties may inhibit panic symptoms (7). Women with more severe symptoms may be at greater risk for ongoing symptoms and require continued prophylactic treatment.

There is tremendous individual variation in how pregnancy affects symptoms of preexisting psychiatric disorders that is not explained by demographic factors, personality style, life stressors, or mental health at the time of pregnancy (36). Despite the existence of serious psychiatric symptoms in over two-thirds of these women, most are not evaluated by a psychiatrist during pregnancy (34). The effects of pregnancy on preexisting personality disorders, generalized anxiety disorders, and obsessive-compulsive disorder have not been studied.

B. Nausea and Vomiting

As detailed earlier, women with no previous psychiatric history do not usually suffer from serious psychiatric symptoms during pregnancy. Despite this, the search for psychological components to the diverse experiences of pregnancy continues. Nausea and vomiting during pregnancy have inspired considerable research and speculation on their psychological origins. They have been seen as both normal or pathological, acceptance or rejection of pregnancy, and wholly psychological or wholly physiological (44). In Wolkind and Zajicek's prospective, psychosocial study of 247 pregnant women, they found that nausea and vomiting that leads to dehydration and ketosis and that cannot be explained medically occasionally heralds an underlying eating disorder, such as bulimia nervosa, that would require psychiatric intervention (45). In general, nausea and vomiting during pregnancy appear to be a manifestation of physiological, not psychological processes.

C. Postpartum Disorders

In contrast with pregnancy, the first 3 months postpartum is a time of increased vulnerability to serious psychiatric symptoms, especially psychoses (38,46,47). Since Pitt first described an atypical depression occurring after childbirth, a tremendous volume of medical literature has been devoted to the subject of postpartum depressive symptoms (48). Syndromes as different as emotional lability for a few days after delivery to psychotic disorders have been characterized as "postpartum depression." Postpartum "blues," a mild, transient depressive phenomenon, occurs 2–4 days after delivery in 50–80% of women (49). Postpartum psychotic illness develops in 0.2% of women (49). These two syndromes appear to be specific to the postpartum period. The underlying pathophysiological mechanism may be related to the tremendous drop in estrogen and progesterone that occurs after parturition. The "blues" do not appear to be related to demographic or obstetric variables or to have lasting psychiatric importance (46).

The only obstetric variable associated with postpartum psychosis is primiparity. A personal or family history of affective disorders, especially bipolar disorder, is the single best predictor of postpartum psychosis (46). Women with bipolar illness may have a rate of postpartum recurrences as high as 50% (50). The onset is usually within the first month and often within the first 2 weeks postpartum. The syndrome is characterized by an extremely volatile course. Women may be asymptomatic at one moment and severely disturbed a short time later. Prominent symptoms include agitation, confusion, hallucinations, delusions, disrupted sleep, and occasionally, violent behavior (51). The risk of suicide or infanticide is serious enough to warrant hospitalization or constant observation. The treatment is the same as for any acute psychotic episode. Mood-stabilizing agents, such as lithium, valproic acid, or carbamazepine, may be necessary. Premenstrual relapses and relapses after subsequent pregnancies are common (46,52). A postpartum psychosis may also herald the onset of bipolar illness with recurrences unrelated to pregnancy (53).

The consistent timing of the onset of postpartum psychosis implicates the tremendous drop in reproductive hormones that takes place immediately after delivery. Estrogen is known to modulate dopamine receptor sensitivity (41). The rapid withdrawal of estrogen after delivery may lead to psychotic symptoms in vulnerable individuals owing to supersensitive dopamine receptors (54). Prophylactic, high-dose estrogen treatment beginning within 24 hr of delivery in women with a history of postpartum psychosis has been effective in preventing relapses (51; Sichel DA, personal communication).

Some women will develop other serious psychiatric illnesses for the first time during the postpartum period. Depression, panic disorder, and obsessive-compulsive disorder all have had their onset postpartum (18,46,55,56). Once again, family history or a history of other psychiatric disorders has been associated with the development of these postpartum syndromes.

The significance of moderate to severe nonpsychotic depressive episodes occurring after pregnancy is controversial. These syndromes are characterized by more severe and persistent symptoms than the "blues." Women may be markedly depressed, hopeless, and anhedonic, and have disturbances in appetite and sleep, but they are not psychotic. The onset of symptoms may coincide with the "blues" or may be weeks to months later. The average prevalence rate for postpartum depressive episodes that begin within 3 months of delivery is 12% (46,47). Many women remain symptomatic for more than 6 months. Depressive symptoms during pregnancy, a personal or family history of mood disorder, and marital difficulties, or poor social support may increase the likelihood of a depressive episode occurring at this time. Recent, well-controlled studies have shown that the prevalence rate of nonpsychotic depressive episodes postpartum does not differ from the rate of depressive episodes in well-matched, non-pregnant control subjects (47). The main difference between the child-bearing and the non-child-bearing groups was that postpartum subjects had more severe symptoms when depressed than non-child-bearing women O'Hara suggests "that childbirth and the demands of the postpartum period constitute a non-specific stress which increases the likelihood of a depressive episode in an already vulnerable woman" (46).

D. Substance Abuse

Other than documentation of the negative consequences to the fetus, there is little information about substance abuse during pregnancy. Nevertheless, women do abuse alcohol and drugs during pregnancy (45,57). In a recent evaluation of urine drug screens in low-income clinics serving minority women and private obstetrical settings serving middle-class white women, the incidence of positive drug screens was about 15% in both places (58). Substance abuse has serious negative health consequences for both the fetus and mother. Alcohol and other recreational drugs can be teratogenic (57). Many women substance abusers do not receive adequate antenatal care. Undiagnosed substance abuse poses hazards to the mother and fetus at delivery owing to unanticipated withdrawal syndromes and interactions with both anesthesia and pain management. Women with depressive symptoms and those who are victims of physical abuse or other forms of violence are more likely to abuse substances than other women (25).

E. Physical Abuse

Pregnant women, compared with nonpregnant women, are at increased risk for physical abuse (59). Gelles reported that pregnant women were at greater risk than nonpregnant women for all types of violence: overall, minor, and severe (59). Previous abuse is the best predictor of abuse during pregnancy, although abuse may begin in pregnancy (60,61). Preexisting battering may increase, decrease, or stay the same during pregnancy. Perpetrators are usually male partners, but pregnant adolescents and young adults may be abused by their parents (60). A male partner's substance abuse also predicts a pregnant woman's susceptibility to violent victimization (62).

Nearly half of abused pregnant women report emotional symptoms, especially depression. Many have a history of suicide attempts (60,62). Abused pregnant women are more likely to drink alcohol and smoke cigarettes than are nonabused pregnant women (60). Although there have been no studies looking at physical violence as a specific risk factor for adverse pregnancy outcome, its associations with alcohol abuse, smoking, and suicidality suggest that it increases the likelihood of adverse outcome (63).

F. Special Issues: Conclusions

Women with psychiatric disorders, substance abuse, or physical abuse may have significant psychopathology during pregnancy or in the postpartum period. Although psychotic disorders are often improved during pregnancy, the postpartum period presents a time of increased vulnerability both for women with preexisting conditions and for women with a predisposition to developing major psychiatric disorders.

Depressions that occur postpartum may be more severe than depressions occurring at other times of life. Depressive symptoms during pregnancy often coexist with substance abuse and physical abuse. When left untreated, these instances of serious psychiatric difficulties clearly have a negative effect on mothers and infants. Unfortunately, more often than not, they are undiagnosed and untreated.

VII. Implications for Medical Care

A. Routine Interventions

Most psychological changes during pregnancy are mild and transient. They do not need treatment by a mental health professional. Support, education, allowing a patient to discuss her concerns (ventilation), and providing reassurance are effective approaches for many mild difficulties (Table 4) (64). The challenge for the medical practitioner is to recognize serious symptoms that require further evaluation and care.

Perceived social support and continuing employment have both been associated with less psychological distress during pregnancy. Therefore, the involvement of a woman's partner or parent in her medical care may

Table 4 General Principles for Psychological Management During Pregnancy

Ventilation
Support
Education
Reassurance
Referral to mental health professional when symptoms are severe or prolonged

provide "emotional prophylaxis." Also, unless medically contraindicated, a physician may recommend continued employment during pregnancy for the same purpose.

During pregnancy, most women receive medical care more routinely than at any other time of life. Accordingly, medical practitioners have the opportunity to educate women in a consistent, nonconfrontational way on the health effects of smoking, drinking, substance abuse, noncompliance with prescribed medical regimens, and other health-risk behaviors. Women have been shown to be highly motivated toward behavior change during pregnancy; they decrease both smoking and drinking (65,66). Diagnostic tests, such as ultrasound, that enable a woman to see the fetus, can lead to improved health behaviors (65). These changes can be long term (66).

Reassuring and educating women about the "normal" range of psychological experiences during pregnancy is helpful, even before psychological symptoms have developed. Anxiety (especially in the third trimester), mild, transient depressive symptoms, forgetfulness, and confusion all can be part of the normal pregnancy. These symptoms can be quite distressing if women do not realize that they often accompany pregnancy, are usually transient, and do not reflect any profound, underlying deficiencies. Ultrasound examinations and other genetic testing may decrease anxiety in women who are especially concerned about the well-being of the fetus (15,67). Written instructions for medical treatment may improve compliance with treatment and may help alleviate the frustration and anxiety caused by memory difficulties. Learning to make lists also may help accomplish this (31).

Significant anxiety during the first trimester and depressive symptoms that are persistent require further evaluation. Detailed investigation of a woman's stressors, including financial difficulties, perception of social support, substance abuse, and the presence of physical abuse, may point to the source of a pregnant woman's symptoms. Women with protracted depressive symptoms may require evaluation by a mental health professional (see Table 5).

Certain medical presentations may arise from underlying psychological distress. For example, anxious pregnant patients often present with somatic symptoms that cannot be explained by their medical status (9). Battered women often come to the emergency room with a confusing array of physical symptoms and injuries (60). Alcohol use and cigarette smoking that continue unchanged during pregnancy may suggest underlying depressive pathology or ongoing physical violence (25,62).

Although there are no data on how psychological changes during pregnancy modify asthma or immunological disorders, pregnancy may exacerbate any condition in which symptoms tend to worsen with stress.

Table 5 Reasons for Referral for Psychiatric Evaluation

Suicidal ideas or behavior
Persistent symptoms that do not respond to other interventions
New onset of depressed mood or loss of interest or pleasure that has been present
   for at least 2 weeks and is associated with at least three of the following
   nearly every day during the same 2 weeks:
   Significant weight loss or gain or change in appetite
   Insomnia or hypersomnia
   Observable restlessness or slowing
   Fatigue, low energy
   Feelings of worthlessness or excessive guilt
   Difficulty concentrating, or indecisiveness
   Recurrent thoughts of death or suicide

Source: Adapted from American Psychiatric Association. Diagnostic and Statistical Manual of Mental Disorders. 4th ed. Washington, DC: American Psychiatric Association, 1994.

Schatz et al. have adapted the general principles of psychological management during pregnancy (ventilation, education, support, and reassurance) to this patient population (68). A woman should be given the opportunity to express her fears and concerns about her pregnancy. Education should include information concerning the effects of asthma and immunological diseases on pregnancy and the infant, the effects of pregnancy on asthma and immunological disorders, the effects of medications, and the likelihood of having a baby with asthma or immunological disease. Providing support includes scheduling regular visits and being available to handle unanticipated problems. Applying these principles provides reassurance, as does the knowledge that the medical physician, the obstetrician, and the patient are collaborating to maximize the chances of a good outcome for the woman and her child.

Since the pharmacokinetics of most drugs during pregnancy are unknown, drugs taken during pregnancy may cause unexpected psychological symptoms. A drug's metabolism and effects are altered by gender, blood volume, and circulating hormones (69). If new psychological symptoms develop in a pregnant woman receiving medication, the possibility of a drug-induced side effect should be included in the differential diagnosis.

B. Psychiatric Disorders and Substance Abuse

Women with a history of a previous psychotic episode, manic episode, or major depressive episode, especially one that occurred postpartum, should probably be referred for psychiatric evaluation (45). This permits assessment of baseline mental status and education of the patients about risks of recurrence of symptoms; it establishes a relationship with a psychiatric practitioner and facilitates prophylactic interventions. Women with a family history of major affective illness should be carefully monitored for the development of affective symptoms, especially postpartum.

Women with chronic psychiatric disorders such as schizophrenia, bipolar disorder (manic-depressive illness), or recurrent depression should be referred for psychiatric evaluation if they are not already involved in treatment. They can be safely treated for most symptoms of major mental illness, particularly after the first trimester. Untreated mental illness is distressing to the patient and potentially dangerous. Changes in existing psychiatric medication should be done in consultation with the treating psychiatrist. When necessary, a psychiatric hospitalization may provide the safest means for treating a pregnant woman during the first trimester.

Since the risk of an untreated postpartum psychosis, obsessional disorder, or major depression includes danger to both the mother and infant, all women should be asked about psychological symptoms early in the postpartum period, especially 1–3 weeks postpartum. Any woman who appears to have developed symptoms that are disruptive or interfere with her functioning, even if they wax and wane, should be referred for psychiatric evaluation.

The diagnosis of ongoing substance abuse may be made more difficult to make by the advent of legal prosecution as child abusers of women who use drugs and alcohol during pregnancy. Asking women about substance abuse routinely, establishing an open, nonjudgmental relationship, and education about risks may help uncover substance abuse difficulties. When substance abuse is suspected, the evaluation should include urine testing, especially since many drug abusers use multiple substances. Ideally, treatment should take place in a setting experienced in treating pregnant women, since detoxification is not always safe toward the end of pregnancy.

VIII. Summary

Psychological symptoms cannot be treated if they are unrecognized. Most women experience mild, transient psychological symptoms during pregnancy that respond to support, reassurance, and education. The first trimester has the highest incidence of anxious and depressive symptoms. Reassurance that these symptoms are normal and transient will alleviate associated anxiety. The postpartum period is a time of particular vulnerability to psychological symptoms. Women with persistent, disturbing symptoms should be referred for further evaluation.

Pregnancy provides a unique opportunity for physicians to initiate preventive medical care. Pregnant women are especially motivated for behavior change. Physicians can take advantage of this by providing health education and intervention for alcohol and other substance abuse, cigarette smoking, and physical abuse.

References

1. Deutsch H. The Psychology of Women. New York: Grune & Stratton, 1947.
2. Zajicek E. The experience of being pregnant. In: Wolkind S, Zajicek E, eds. Pregnancy: A Psychological and Social Study. New York: Grune & Stratton, 1981:31–56.
3. Bibring GL. Some consideration of the psychological processes in pregnancy. Psychoanal Study Child 1959; 14:113–121.
4. Nilsson A. Para-natal emotional adjustment: a prospective investigation of 165 women. Acta Psychiatr Scand Suppl 1970; 220:1–61.
5. Istvan J. Stress, anxiety, and birth outcomes: a critical review of the evidence. Psychol Bull 1986; 100:331–348.
6. Kumar R, Robson KM. A prospective study of emotional disorders in child-bearing women. Br J Psychiatry 1984; 144:35–47.
7. Cowley DS, Roy-Byrne PP. Panic disorder during pregnancy. J Psychosom Obstet Gynaecol 1989; 10:193–210.
8. Rauramo I, Salminen K, Laatikainen T. Release of β-endorphin in response to physical exercise in nonpregnant and pregnant women. Acta Obstet Gynecol Scand 1986; 65:609–612.
9. Lubin B, Gardener SH, Roth A. Mood and somatic symptoms during pregnancy. Psychosom Med 1975; 37:136–146.
10. Elliott SA, Watson JP, Brough DI. Mood changes during pregnancy and after the birth of a child. Br J Clin Psychol 1983; 22:295–308.
11. Gorsuch RL, Key MK. Abnormalities of pregnancy as a function of anxiety and life stress. Psychosom Med 1974; 36:352–362.
12. Crowe K, von Baeyer C. Predictors of a positive childbirth experience. Birth 1989; 16:59–63.
13. Cox DN, Reading AE. Fluctuations in state anxiety over the course of pregnancy and the relationship to outcome. J Psychosom Obstet Gyneacol 1989; 10:71–78.
14. Pagel MD, Smilkstein G, Regen H, Montano D. Psychosocial influences on newborn outcomes: a controlled prospective study. Soc Sci Med 1990; 30:597–604.
15. Robinson GE, Garner DM, Olmsted MP, Shime J, Hutton EM, Crawford BM. Anxiety reduction after chorionic villus sampling and genetic amniocentesis Am J Obstet Gynecol 1988; 159:953–956.

16. Reading AE, Cox DN. The effects of ultrasound examination on maternal anxiety levels. J Behav Med 1982; 5:237–247.
17. Neziroglu F, Anemone R, Yaryura-Tobias JA. Onset of obsessive-compulsive disorder in pregnancy. Am J Psychiatry 1992; 149:947–95.
18. Sichel DA, Cohen LS, Dimmock JA, Rosenbaum JF. Postpartum obsessive compulsive disorder: a case series. J Clin Psychiatry 54:156–159.
19. Pfaff DW, McEwen BS. Actions of estrogens and progestins on nerve cells. Science 1983; 219:808–814.
20. McEwen BS. Gonadal and adrenal steroids and the brain: implications for depression. In: Halbreich U, ed. Hormones and Depression. New York: Raven Press, 1987:239–253.
21. Biegon A, McEwen BS. Modulation by estradiol of serotonin$_1$ receptors in brain. J Neurosci 1982; 2:199–205.
22. Sar M, Stumpf WE. Central noradrenergic neurones concentrate ^{3}H-oestradiol. Nature 1981; 289:500–502.
23. Duman KS, Enna SJ. On the relationship between hormones, depression and neurotransmitter receptor responses to antidepressants. In: Halbreich U, ed. Hormones and Depression. New York: Raven Press, 1987:279–296.
24. Glick ID, Quitkin FM, Bennett SE. The influence of estrogens, progestins and oral contraceptives on depression. In: Halbreich U, ed. Hormones and Depression. New York: Raven Press, 1987:339–356.
25. Zuckerman B, Amaro H, Bauchner H, Cabral H. Depressive symptoms during pregnancy: relationship to poor health behaviors. Am J Obstet Gynecol 1989; 160:1107–1111.
26. Kendell RE. Suicide in pregnancy and the puerperium. Br Med J 1991; 302:126–127.
27. Condon JT, Ball SB. Altered psychological functioning in pregnant women: an empirical investigation. J Psychosom Obstet Gynaecol 1989; 10:211–220.
28. Jarrahi-Zadeh A, Kane FJ, Van De Castle RL, Lachenbruck PA, Ewing JA. Emotional and cognitive changes in pregnancy and early puerperium. Br J Psychiatry 1969; 115:797–805.
29. Poser CM, Kassirer MR, Peyser JM. Benign encephalopathy of pregnancy. Acta Neurol Scand 1986; 73:39–43.
30. Bailey LA, Bailey BJ. The psychological experience of pregnancy. Int J Psychiatry Med 1986; 16:263–274.
31. Hampson E. Estrogen-related variations in human spatial and articulatory-motor skills. Psychoneuroendocrinology 1990; 15:97–111.
32. Condon JT. Altered cognitive functioning in pregnant women: a shift towards primary process thinking. Br J Med Psychol 1987; 60:329–334.
33. Zajicek E. Psychiatric problems during pregnancy. In Wolkind S, Zajicek E, eds. Pregnancy: A Psychological and Social Study. New York: Grune & Stratton, 1981:57–73.
34. McNeil TF, Kaij L, Malmquist-Larsson A. women with nonorganic psychosis: mental disturbance during pregnancy. Acta Psychiatr Scand 1984; 70:127–139.

35. McNeil TF, Kaij L, Malmquist-Larsson A. Women with nonorganic psychosis: pregnancy's effect on mental health during pregnancy. Acta Psychiatr Scand 1984; 70:140–148.

36. McNeil TF, Kaij L, Malmquist-Larsson A. Women with nonorganic psychosis: factors associated with pregnancy's effect on mental health. Acta Psychiatr Scand 1984: 70:209–219.

37. Krener P, Simmons MK, Hansen RL, Treat JN. Effect of pregnancy on psychosis: life circumstances and psychiatric symptoms. Int J Psychiatry Med 1989; 19:65–84.

38. Pugh TF, Jerath BK, Schmidt WM, Reed RB. Rates of mental disease related to childbearing. N Engl J Med 1963; 268:1224–1228.

39. Paffenbarger RS, Epidemiological aspects of mental illness associated with childbearing. In: Brockington IF, Kumar R, eds. Motherhood and Mental Illness. New York: Grune & Stratton, 1982; 19–36.

40. Euvrard C, Oberlander C, Boissier JR. Antidopaminergic effect of estrogens at the striatal level. J Pharmacol Exp Ther 1980; 214:179–185.

41. Di Paolo T, Poyet P, Labrie F. Effect of chronic estradiol and haloperidol treatment on striatal dopamine receptors. Eur J Pharmacol 1981; 73:105–106.

42. Frank E, Kufper DJ, Jacob M, Blumenthal SJ, Jarrett DB. Pregnancy-related affective episodes among women with recurrent depression. Am J Psychiatry 1987; 144:288–293.

43. Cohen LS, Sichel DA, Dimmock JA, Rosenbaum JF. Impact of pregnancy on panic disorder: a case series. J Clin Psychiatry 1994; 55:284–288.

44. Wolkind S. Nausea and vomiting of pregnancy. In: Wolkind S, Zajicek E, eds. Pregnancy: A Psychological and Social Study. New York: Grune & Stratton, 1981:75–88.

45. Oppenheim GB. Psychological disorders in pregnancy. In: Priest RB, ed. Psychological Disorders in Obstetrics and Gynaecology. London: Butterworths, 1984:93–146.

46. O'Hara MW. Postpartum "blues," depression, and psychosis: a review. J Psychosom Obstet Gynecol 1987; 7:205–227.

47. O'Hara MW, Zekoski EM, Philipps LH, Wright EJ. A controlled prospective study of postpartum mood disorders: comparison of childbearing and non-childbearing women. J Abnormal Psychol 1990; 99:3–15.

48. Pitt B. "Atypical" depression following childbirth. Br J Psychiatry 1968; 114:1325–1335.

49. Harding JJ. Postpartum psychiatric disorders: a review. Compr Psychiatry 1989; 30:109–112.

50. Reich T, Winokur G. Postpartum psychosis in patients with manic-depressive disease. J Nerv Ment Dis 1970; 151:60–68.

51. Hamilton JA. Postpartum psychiatric syndromes. Psychiatr Clin N Am 1989; 12:89–103.

52. Brockington IF, Kelly A, Hall P, Deakin W. Premenstrual relapse of puerperal psycosis. J Affective Disord 1988; 14:287–292.

53. Akiskal HS, Walker P, Puzantian VR, Kind D, Rosenthal TL, Dranon M. Bipolar outcome in the course of depressive illness. J Affective Disord 1983; 5:115–128.

54. Seeman MV. Interaction of sex, age, and neuroleptic dose. Compr Psychiatry 1983; 24:125–128.

55. Metz A, Sichel DA, Goff DC. Postpartum panic disorder. J Clin Psychiatry 1988; 49:278–279.

56. Sichel DA, Cohen LS, Driscoll J, Rosenbaum JF. Postpartum onset of obsessive compulsive disorder. Psychosomatics 1993; 34:277–279.

57. Brockington IF, Kumar R. Drug addiction and psychotropic drug treatment during pregnancy and lactation. In: Brockington IF, Kumar R, eds. Motherhood and Mental Illness. New York: Grune & Stratton, 1982:239–255.

58. Chasnoff IJ, Barrett ME, Landress HJ. [Letter]. N Engl J Med 1990; 322:1202.

59. Gelles RJ. Violence and pregnancy: are pregnant women at greater risk of abuse? J Marriage Fam 1988; 50:841–847.

60. Hillard PJA. Physical abuse in pregnancy. Obstet Gynecol 1985; 66:185–190.

61. Helton AS, McFarlane J, Anderson ET. Battered and pregnant: a prevalence study. Am J Public Health 1987; 77:1337–1339.

62. Amaro H, Fried LE, Cabral H, Zuckerman B. Violence during pregnancy and substance use. Am J Public Health 1990; 80:575–579.

63. Newberger EH, Barker SE, Leiberman ES, McCormick MC, Yllo K, Gary LT, Schechter S. Abuse of pregnant women and adverse birth outcome: current knowledge and implications for practice. JAMA 1992; 267:2370–2372.

64. Brown WA. Psychological care during pregnancy and the postpartum period. New York: Raven Press, 1979.

65. Reading AE, Campbell S, Cox DN, Sledmere CM. Health beliefs and health care behaviour in pregnancy. Psychol Med 1982; 12:379–383.

66. Fingerhut LA, Kleinmen JC, Kendrick JS. Smoking before, during and after pregnancy. Am J Public Health 1990; 80:541–544.

67. Reading AE, Cox DN. The effects of ultrasound examination on maternal anxiety levels. J Behav Med 1982; 5:237–247.

68. Schatz M, Hoffman CP, Zeiger RS, Falkoff R, Macy E, Mellon M. The course and management of asthma and allergic diseases during pregnancy. In: Middleton E, Reed CE, Ellis EF, Adkinson NF, Yunginger JW, Busse WW, eds. Allergy: Principles and Practice. 4th ed. St. Louis: Mosby, 1993:1310.

69. Kato R. Sex-related differences in drug metabolism. Drug Metab Rev 1974; 31–32.

7

Use of Medication During Pregnancy and Lactation: General Considerations

RICHARD S. ABRAMS

University of Colorado School of Medicine
and Rose Medical Center
Denver, Colorado

CLEMENT P. HOFFMAN

University of California, San Diego, School
  of Medicine, La Jolla
and Kaiser Foundation Hospital
San Diego, California

I. Introduction

Less than a generation ago, physicians reassured expectant mothers that their fetuses enjoyed complete protection within the uterus. Tragic experiences with substances such as thalidomide and alcohol have now swung public perception to the commonly held belief that nothing is safe to take during pregnancy, thus relegating pregnant women to the status of "therapeutic orphans." Few clinical settings dramatize the delicate balance between risk and benefit better than pregnancy. Even though it appears that most drugs do not harm the developing fetus, a small number of drugs clearly do increase the risk of fetal anomalies, and our knowledge of which additional drugs pose some degree of risk must be considered incomplete. The use of any drug during pregnancy should be presumed to carry some small degree of risk. The physician must balance this risk against the need to keep the mother healthy. Obviously, the fetus is also going to benefit if the mother maintains adequate placental perfusion and oxygenation. These risks and benefits require careful communication between health care professional and patient. Indications for the use of any drug during pregnancy must be carefully considered, ideally before conception.

Medical conditions such as asthma can jeopardize the health of both mother and fetus (see Chapter 15). When drug therapy is indicated, it is important to use drugs as effectively as possible. Medications must be given in effective doses, and patients should be monitored for therapeutic effect. Whenever possible, drugs with which there has been some experience in pregnancy should be used. Fortunately, a broad range of medication with substantial track records of safety are available for treatment of asthma and allergies. Patients must be encouraged to actively participate in their own medical care by providing them with a clear understanding of their medical disorder and its effect on pregnancy, what is known and not known about the proposed treatment, possible alternatives to drug therapy, and continuing access to care to assess effectiveness and any adverse consequences.

Clearly, choosing appropriate drug therapy for pregnant women with asthma and allergies must include an understanding of altered pharmacokinetics during gestation and an appreciation for the general principles of developmental toxicity in the fetus. This chapter briefly highlights current knowledge about drug therapy and human reproduction. Information about drug therapy for the management of specific allergic and immunological conditions will be discussed in subsequent chapters.

A. Major Causes of Human Developmental Defects

Developmental defects in humans are broadly divided into those resulting from known genetic causes, approximately 20%; chromosomal aberrations, 3–5%; environmental causes (drugs, chemicals, infections, maternal metabolic imbalance, and radiation), 4–6%; and unknown causes, 65–70%. Thus the cause of most congenital anomalies remains unknown. These unknown causes of birth defects may include unrecognized complex interactions among drugs, chemicals, other environmental factors, and genetic causes—the so-called multifactorial etiology.

While there are over a thousand chemicals which are teratogenic in animals (1), a relatively small group of medications are generally accepted to have proven teratogenic risks in human pregnancy. These include thalidomide, diethylstilbestrol, androgens, folic acid antagonists, alkylating agents, penicillamine, ethanol, anticonvulsants, iodides, lithium, aminoglycocides, tetracycline, warfarin, the retinoids isotretinoin and etretinate, and the angiotensin-converting enzyme inhibitors.

It is important to realize that the standing of agents on this list may be subject to change. Lithium, in the 1970s, for example, was thought to have a relative risk ratio of 400 for Epstein's anomaly of the heart, based on a registry of voluntarily submitted cases. Two subsequent controlled epidemiological cohort studies suggest that the risk is much lower—a relative risk of 1.5 and 3.0 for all congenital anomalies and 1.2 and 1.7 for cardiac malformations (2). The addition of the retinoids to the list has been relatively recent; these are potent teratogens (3). The angiotensin-converting enzyme inhibitors, used to treat hypertension, are now strongly linked by case reports and epidemiological work to a pattern of fetal hypotension, anuria-oligohydramnios, growth retardation, renal tubular dysplasia, and hypocalvaria (4–6).

B. Evaluating Drug Risk

Perhaps the greatest impediment to ensuring the safety of drugs during pregnancy is the inability to test them prospectively in humans. For obvious practical and ethical reasons, experimental animals are used to test pharmaceutic products before obtaining Food and Drug Administration (FDA) approval. Animal studies have the advantage of allowing evaluation of many subjects over short generation times, avoiding unnecessary human exposure and providing the ability to test one variable at a time. With the exception of coumarin-type anticoagulants, almost every chemical known to be teratogenic in humans is also teratogenic in one or more laboratory species. It thus appears that positive animal teratology studies are at least suggestive of human potential harm. The more animal species in which a compound is teratogenic, the more likely it is to have a human effect, although possibly not the same effect as in animals (7). Conversely, negative animal studies are reassuring relative to the drug's potential for human teratogenecity. Clinicians should definitely not ignore developmental toxicity tests in animals merely because laboratory rats are not like humans. Unfortunately, animal models are far from perfect. It must be remembered that before its release in the 1950s, thalidomide was tested in rats and mice and determined to be free of teratogenic effects. Only later did testing reveal anomalies in monkeys and rabbits (8).

Other sources of information on the reproductive safety of drugs include case reports and epidemiological studies. Case reports of variable detail and quality are submitted by clinicians to registries and for journal publication. Their major benefit is to identify rare events. Case reports provided the first awareness of teratogenesis following maternal use of thalidomide. One limitation of case reports is that they cannot establish the incidence of pregnancy risk. The other disadvantage is that many chemicals have been implicated as teratogens, only to be exonerated by further study. In fact, most such hypotheses are wrong. The coincidental occurrence of an environmental exposure in a pregnant woman and congenital anomalies in her child is very common, especially if the exposure or the defect or both are relatively common (9). Initial reports have led to unjustified incrimination of useful medications, including Bendectin, oral contraceptive hormones, diazepam, and vaginal spermicides (10). These agents have not been linked to anomalies by subsequent careful epidemiological studies. The case of Bendectin was especially egregious. Bendectin was an extremely useful medication for the treatment of nausea in pregnancy. It is probably the most studied drug in pregnancy and there is little, if any, evidence that it is a teratogen. Nonetheless, Bendectin was the subject of excessive litigation. Although Merrell-Dow was able successfully to defend most of the lawsuits, the company voluntarily removed the product from the marketplace in 1983 (11).

The epidemiological techniques of case-controlled studies and cohort studies are often used to further explore possible links between drugs and adverse reproductive outcome. Case-controlled studies begin with a specific outcome and examine medical records for exposure to a drug. Records of a control group of nonaffected children are searched to arrive at an odds ratio for a drug producing a specific effect. Confidence intervals should be presented to indicate whether a relationship is statistically significant. Such retrospective studies are always fraught with potential bias from the researcher, as well as recall bias of any interviewees. Moreover, these studies often require numerous subjects to achieve meaningful confidence intervals.

Cohort studies are the opposite of case-controlled studies. They begin with a group of subjects exposed to a drug and a control group of nonexposed subjects. These groups are both followed prospectively to determine the frequency of adverse outcomes and to calculate a risk ratio. If an adverse outcome is rare, cohort studies need even more subjects than are required for case-controlled studies.

Another consideration in epidemiological studies is that the maternal condition may be partly responsible for an increased adverse outcome in the pregnancy. For example, it is known that maternal hypertension itself causes intrauterine growth retardation; it may be difficult to sort out what additional effect an antihypertensive agent might have. Similarly, patients with seizure disorders generally have an increased risk of congenital anomalies even if they do not use antiseizure medicines. It may be hard to ascertain the additional risk of an antiseizure medication in a given study group.

Epidemiological studies of drug risks during pregnancy have clearly grown in importance. It is essential, however, to remember the pitfalls in interpreting them and to be cautious in advising patients on the basis of studies that purport to show only weak associations between exposures and adverse pregnancy outcomes. Unknown or inadequately accounted for confounding variables can easily produce artifactual small effects. It is far less likely that confounding variables account for large effects (12).

C. Food and Drug Administration's Use-in-Pregnancy Ratings

The FDA has established categories for the use of drugs during pregnancy (Table 1), which are described in the *Physicians Desk Reference* (13) as follows: these "categories are based on the degree to which available information has ruled out risk to the fetus, balanced against the drug's potential benefits to the patient. Ratings range from A for drugs that have been tested for teratogenicity under controlled conditions without showing evidence of damage to the fetus, to D and X for drugs that are definitely teratogenic. The D rating is generally reserved for drugs with no safe alternatives. The X rating means there is absolutely no reason to risk using the drug during pregnancy." This classification attempts to address a very complex problem. Most drugs are assigned to categories B and C, where safety cannot be assured. The rating system does not apply to adverse effects of drugs during breast feeding.

A study that compared the FDA categories with data from the Teratogen Information System (TERIS) found a lack of correlation between the two classification systems (14).

Table 1 Key to FDA Use-in-Pregnancy Ratings

Category	Interpretation
A	Controlled studies show no risk. Adequate, well-controlled studies in pregnant women have failed to demonstrate risk to the fetus.
B	No evidence of risk in humans. Either animal findings show risk, but human findings do not; or, if no adequate human studies have been done, animal findings are negative.
C	Risk cannot be ruled out. Human studies are lacking, and animal studies are either positive for fetal risk, or lacking as well. However, potential benefits may justify the potential risk.
D	Positive evidence of risk. Investigational or postmarketing data show risk to the fetus. Nevertheless, potential benefits may outweigh the potential risk.
X	Contraindicated in pregnancy. Studies in animals or humans, or investigational or postmarketing reports have shown fetal risk that clearly outweighs any possible benefit to the patient.

II. Developmental Toxicity of Drugs

A. Teratogens

In the past, the primary focus in teratology was the causation of a physical malformation. A teratogen is now more broadly defined as an agent that can induce a range of abnormal development, including complete pregnancy loss (often before the pregnancy is recognized), structural abnormalities, growth alterations, and long-term functional defects involving learning and behavioral skills.

Friedman states that assessment of an agent's teratogenicity can be made on the basis of reproducability and consistency of available clinical, epidemiological, and animal data. The observed associations should make biological sense. The exposure should produce a consistent effect on a structure at the appropriate gestational time. Usually, a dose-response relationship will be apparent. Ideally, a causal effect would be strongly supported if a definite cellular mechanism could be established (9), although this has not generally been possible at the current level of knowledge.

Recent advances in the basic biological sciences are being brought to bear on studying the mechanisms of normal and abnormal reproductive development and on understanding the pharmacokinetics and pharmacodynamics of chemical agents in pregnancy, both in animal and ultimately in human models. A current program sponsored by the National Institute of Environmental Health Sciences and the U.S. Environmental Protection Agency will bring together molecular and cellular biologists and embryologists, developmental toxicologists, and human embryologists to integrate their research efforts in this field (15). As our knowledge improves, we may learn better to what degree drugs and chemicals contribute to the estimated 65–70% of birth defects where the cause is yet unknown.

B. Malformations

Malformations constitute structural abnormalities of prenatal origin that are present at birth and that seriously interfere with viability or physical well-being. A major malformation is defined as one that is incompatible with survival or that requires major surgery for correction, such as cleft palate or congenital heart disease. Numerous studies have concluded that approximately 3% of all newborn children are affected by major malformations. Inclusion of minor malformations, such as ear tags or extra digits, increases the overall malformation rate to approximately 7–10%. This figure constitutes the so-called background incidence of malformations. To understand the additional risk of malformation after exposure to a drug or chemical, the background incidence of anomalies in the general population must always be considered.

C. Abnormal Growth

It is now clear that important development continues beyond the classic teratogenic period of the first trimester. After organogenesis until term, the fetus undergoes significant growth, and adverse effects of drugs during this time can result in abnormalities of fetal growth. In humans, agents known to cause generalized intrauterine growth retardation include cigarette smoke, warfarin, phenytoin, heroin, methadone, and trimethadione.

D. Functional Impairment

Maturation of organ systems, especially the central nervous system, also occurs after the first trimester. It is now known that medications or chemicals administered during pregnancy may produce long-term neurological or neurobehavioral effects. Examples of human behavioral effects of antenatal toxicity include hyperactivity, brief attention span, and temper outbursts observed in offspring of narcotic-addicted mothers; mental retardation in the offspring of women exposed to anticonvulsants, alcohol, and lead; and the severely abnormal reflexes seen in children born to mothers who ingested methyl mercury (16). Long-term deficits involving learning ability and social skills will undoubtedly prove much more difficult to ascertain than traditional, physically obvious birth defects.

III. Principles of Teratogenesis

Whether or not a drug or chemical can potentially cause abnormal fetal development is governed by several fundamental principles of teratogenesis. Schardein (16) illustrated these principles by the following axiom: "a teratogenic response depends upon the administration of a specific treatment of a particular dose to a genetically susceptible species when the embryos are in a susceptible stage of development."

A. Species Variability

The current basis for evaluating drug risk use during pregnancy relies largely on extrapolation of data from animal studies to humans. Unfortunately, not all species are equally susceptible or sensitive to teratogenic effects of a drug or chemical. A study by Jelovsek et al. demonstrated that 75% of positive human teratogens can be predicted on the basis of animal studies alone (7). However, false negative results in this study remained high, reaching 25%.

Human experience reminds us of the fallibility of animal studies. The thalidomide experience was discussed previously. Conversely, certain strains of mice are extremely sensitive to substances that have not been shown to cause adverse effects in humans. For example, in mice, corticosteroids cause cleft lip, but there is no evidence to suggest that therapeutic does of corticosteroids produce any congenital anomalies in humans (8). Some species variability can be explained on the basis of genetic factors. However, variable teratogenicity occurs even within litters of genetically homogeneous inbred animals. Other factors that may account for differing effects in strain susceptibility include maternal parity and weight, fetal weight, number of young, placental transfer, rate of drug metabolism, fetal and maternal production of hormones, use of vitamin supplements, and environmental factors such as diet, season, and temperature.

B. Dose and Timing Relationships

The effect of most teratogens lies within a narrow range between that which will kill the fetus and that which will have no discernible effect. Within that range, most teratogens demonstrate a quantitative correlation between embryopathy and the dose of the agent. Such a dose-response relationship has been repeatedly demonstrated in animal models. For example, the number of fetuses affected with cleft palate in a litter of mice can be predicted by the dose of corticosteroid given at a critical period of gestation. The threshold dose for teratogens is that dose below which a defect will not occur. Presumably, this is because the developing cells or organs can compensate for or repair the injury up to a certain point.

Another important variable is duration of treatment. In general, exposure to a greater quantity of the agent should increase the likelihood of abnormalities (17). Paradoxically, however, short-term dosage schedules can cause a greater insult to the developing embryo than extended administration, provided that the agent is given for a sufficient time before the vulnerable window. This effect is probably explained by induction or activation of maternal enzyme systems which detoxify and eliminate the drug (16). The frequency of administration can also be an important variable. The exact molecular structure of the chemical can be critical, with even the slightest alteration making an all-or-none difference in teratogenic effects (16).

The vehicle, carrier, or suspending agent, either by delaying absorption or by prolonging blood concentrations of a drug or chemical, may also be a confounding factor in determining embryopathy (16). Finally, drug interactions may influence teratogenicity. For example, cyclophosphamide and fluorouracil given individually to rats produce malformations in frequencies of 26% and 10%, respectively. Given together, however in the same doses, they produce malformations in 100% of the offspring (16).

C. Periods of Gestation

Preorganogenesis

Our knowledge of the mechanisms by which teratogens actually cause alterations is minimal. Until recently, it has been assumed that most developmental defects of organ systems were induced by exposure to chemical or physical agents during the window of vulnerability of organogenesis. Most authorities felt that the preorganogenesis period was a safe time in terms of drug exposure. During this time, it has been felt that the cells of the blastula and early gastrula are totipotential, and can replace damaged cells without loss of capacity for normal development. However, there is now mounting animal model evidence that exposure to teratogens prior to organ formation can lead to damage to the conceptus which is revealed during organogenesis (15). Intrauterine growth retardation, that is, a fetal effect (see below), has been observed in the offspring of pregnant rabbits given a combination of ethanol, nicotine, caffeine, sodium salicylates, and dichlorodiphenyltrichloroethane (DDT) during preimplantation (18). There is also information that prepregnancy exposure to agents in the human mother can affect pregnancy development. The Centers for Disease Control recommend maternal preconception folate therapy to reduce the risk of neural tube defects (19). This benefit has been demonstrated empirically; the cellular mechanism for this protection has yet to be determined.

Preorganogenesis damage in animal models can be demonstrated during the perifertilization, preimplantation, and early postimplantation periods. The hypothesis to explain this effect is that certain chemicals may cause or protect against subtle derangements in the early activation of the developmental genes which orchestrate cellular imprinting, lineage specification, recognition, interaction, migration, and differentiation (15). At least theoretically, it is possible that prefertilization exposure of gametes in either the male or the female to teratogens could alter the genetic material, leading to birth defects. Authors have started to call for more investigation into these areas, especially with regard to gathering data on paternal exposure (20–22).

Organogenesis

Until more is known about very early pregnancy teratogenesis, we must still consider the time of greatest teratogenetic potential to occur in the period during which organ development occurs. The classic teratogenetic period in humans occurs from 4 weeks through 10 weeks after the last menstrual period. It is important to notice the difference between menstrual age and embryonic age. Menstrual age includes a phathom time frame of 2 weeks from the first day of menstruation until conception. Menstrual age is less precise than embryonic age because of the variability of actual ovulation timing, but it is a well-established landmark in clinical practice that is frequently used in journals and texts.

During organogenesis, major activities include rapid, high-fidelity cellular proliferation, selective necrosis of unneeded cells, biosynthesis, cellular differentiation, tissue interaction, and movement and association of specific groups of cells. Abnormal development may follow from interference with any of these processes (23). To cause a defect, the timing of the specific teratogen exposure must coincide with the timing of the target organ formation. For example, an agent capable of causing a neural tube defect will not take effect if given after the closure of the neural tube.

In recent years, it has become apparent that there can be delayed effects of drugs given during pregnancy. The concept of long-term latency was illustrated by the discovery that female fetuses exposed to diethylstilbestrol (DES) are at an increased risk for adenocarcinoma of the vagina, not discovered until after puberty (17). Nor have male offspring been spared the long-term effects of DES, including epididymal cysts, hypotrophic testes, capsular induration, and pathological semen. Attention must also be paid to long-lasting drugs in the maternal serum. It is known that etretinate, an agent for psoriasis treatment, has caused congenital malformations up to a year after the mother discontinued the drug. Serum levels of the drug have been detected over 2 years after discontinuation (24).

Fetal Development

The fetal period from approximately 10 weeks after the last menstrual period until term is characterized by growth and functional maturation of the fetus. Adverse drug effects during this period of gestation tend to result in abnormalities of intrauterine growth and brain function. Emerging interests in behavioral teratology has focused on the period of fetal development. Functional maturation of liver, kidney, lung, gonads, and other organs may also be affected during this period of gestation. Some agents may cause later damage to organ systems that began normal development in organogenesis. Examples include limb reduction defects due to fetal vascular disruption, such as caused by cocaine exposure (3), and eye and brain defects caused by maternal coumarin use (17). Cases of dysmorphic development of the fetal kidney, with cystic dilatation of developing nephrons, have been reported with indomethacin (25).

Perinatal Period

There has been a rapid increase in the use of medications during the immediate perinatal period. Drugs used during this time may have profound maternal effects in addition to their effects on the fetus and the newborn's immediate adjustment to extrauterine life. Since the neonate metabolizes and clears drugs slowly, effects of maternally administered drugs may last for several hours or days during a time when the neonate must make major cardiorespiratory adjustments and become metabolically independent.

Prevention of preterm labor has become a major goal of obstetricians. Beta-adrenergic receptor agonists such as ritadrine and terbutaline can effectively cause uterine smooth muscle relaxation. These agents do not compromise placental blood flow, but do cause a wide variety of maternal side effects, including tachycardia, arrhythmias, increased cardiac output, hypotension, hyperglycemia, and hypokalemia. There is a risk of pulmonary edema as well (26). Neonatal defects include hypoglycemia and hypokalemia (26).

Indomethacin, a prostaglandin synthetase inhibitor, blocks prostaglandin-mediated uterine contractility and is also employed to treat premature labor. Potential fetal risks have limited the use of indomethacin as a first-line tocolytic agent. Indomethacin can cause constriction of the fetal ductus arteriosis, which can lead to pulmonary hypertension and cariomyopathy. Indomethacin can also cause decreased fetal renal blood flow, leading to oligohydramnios, and in more serious instances, fetal renal failure after third-trimester exposure (25,26). Maternal renal impairment has been reported as well (27). It has been recommended that these risks can be minimized by limiting the dose of indomethacin to 200 mg/day and limiting the course of treatment to a maximum of 48 hr (25).

Birth may also mean sudden discontinuation of transplacentally acquired drugs. It is now well recognized that the newborn may suffer withdrawal symptoms from maternally ingested narcotics (3).

The principle of treating or protecting the fetus by administering medications to the mother has been well established. Agents include antimicrobials for syphilis and toxoplasmosis, Rhogam at 28 weeks to prevent Rh isoimmunization, betamethasone to induce more rapid fetal lung maturation, antiarrhythmic drugs for abnormalities in fetal cardiac rhythm, and ampicillin for group B streptococcus prophylaxis in labor (28). New therapeutic agents will certainly become available. A clinical trial is currently investigating the addition of intravenous thyrotropin-releasing hormone along with corticosteroids to mothers with threatened preterm labor to enhance fetal lung maturation (28). More recently, the use of zuvidene for HIV-positive mothers to prevent HIV transmission to the fetus has been recommended (29).

IV. Pharmacokinetic Alterations During Pregnancy

A. Absorption

Gastric emptying time during gestation has been demonstrated to diminish from an average of 50 min in nonpregnant individuals to between 80 and 130 min (30). The clinical significance of this change would be expected to be a delay in the attainment of peak drug concentrations. Small-intestinal transit time is also prolonged, but the clinical significance of this observation remains poorly understood. There is little clinical information about the absorption of drugs in pregnant women.

Pregnancy-associated changes in drug absorption are not confined to the gastrointestinal tract. Because of increases in respiratory minute volume, alterations have been demonstrated in the absorption of drugs administered as volatile gases (anesthetic agents) and as aerosols (bronchodilators) (31). It might be anticipated that highly lipid-soluble anesthetic agents would be absorbed and cleared more rapidly during pregnancy. Moreover, an increase might be expected to occur in the absorption rate of inhaled bronchodilators during pregnancy.

B. Distribution

After absorption, drugs distribute into body fluids and tissues. Changes in blood volume, tissue perfusion, drug lipid solubility, and protein binding affect drug distribution and the rate at which equilibrium between tissue and plasma concentration is achieved. During pregnancy, plasma volume increases by approximately 50% (32), and cardiac output by 35–50% (33). Total body water increases by 8 L, or more if edema is present. The implications of this physiological increase in volume include lower plasma concentration after a given dose of a drug, and a decrease in drug elimination (i.e., a prolonged half-life) unless there is a simultaneous increase in drug metabolism or excretion.

Distribution of any drug also depends on its lipid solubility and the total body fat content. The property of lipid solubility allows drugs to cross biological barriers, such as cell membranes, the blood–brain barrier, and the placenta, whereas highly water-soluble drugs usually cross such membranes poorly. Total body fat increases during pregnancy by 3–4 kg (31).

Thus, not only will fat-soluble drugs have an increased volume of distribution, but increased serum lipids may compete for protein-binding sites, leading to a greater fraction of unbound drug.

Protein binding also plays a major role in the pharmacokinetics of gestation. Plasma albumin concentration falls approximately 10 g/L by the third trimester. The effect of this decrease is particularly significant for highly protein-bound acidic drugs. Since only the unbound fraction of a drug is biologically active, reduced binding capacity may change the ratio of unbound/bound drug and alter the therapeutic effect. Alterations in protein binding must be considered when interpreting the clinical significance of plasma measurements of highly protein-bound drugs.

C. Excretion and Metabolism

There is a 50% increase in glomerular filtration rate during pregnancy, which results in a creatinine clearance of 150–200 mL/min, compared with approximately 100 mL/min in nongravid individuals. By 26 weeks' gestation, renal plasma flow increases by 80%. It then decreases gradually until term, but remains 60% higher than in nonpregnant women (34). The result of these changes is increased clearance of drugs excreted by the kidneys.

Water-soluble drugs are excreted mainly unchanged by the kidneys, but lipid-soluble drugs must be metabolized by the liver before they are excreted in bile or urine. Pregnancy increases the rate of hepatic metabolism through a greater concentration of progesterone, which enhances the activity of hepatic microsomal oxidation (35). For drugs that require hepatic metabolism, the net effect is a decrease in plasma drug concentration relative to dose.

The complex interrelation of drug distribution and elimination can be illustrated by the fate of theophylline. Studies have demonstrated that the volume of distribution of theophylline increases as gestation progresses. Moreover, clearance is reduced approximately 20–50%, and its half-life is prolonged by about 30% (36–38). These pharmacokinetic changes during pregnancy may result in increased plasma theophylline concentration during the third trimester, with the potential for clinical drug toxicity. For those patients for whom theophylline is indicated in pregnancy, theophylline serum concentrations should be followed frequently.

As a practical matter, most drugs studied have an overall net decrease in steady-state serum concentrations during pregnancy. This includes anticonvulsants, digoxin, lithium, and many antibiotics, specifically ampicillin, cephalosporins, clindamycin, erythromycin, kanamycin, amikacin, tobramycin, nitrofurantoin, and sulfamethoxazole-trimethoprim (39). Iron ically, although the obvious maneuver in terms of risk management would seem to be to use lower doses of medication in pregnancy, larger doses may actually be indicated to achieve efficacy.

D. Placental Passage of Drugs

The properties of drugs that permit them to be absorbed and to distribute across biological membranes also allow them to cross the placenta. There is, in fact, no "placental barrier" to most medications, as was once believed. The question, therefore, should not be whether a drug crosses the placenta, but rather what concentration it achieves in the fetus. Differences in steady-state drug concentrations reflect factors such as molecular weight, lipid solubility, ionization, and protein binding. Most drugs are simple chemical compounds of low molecular weight that easily diffuse across the placenta. Chemicals of molecular weight less than 100 will readily cross biological membranes, regardless of their lipid solubility, whereas those of molecular weights over 1000 generally do not cross the placenta, even if they are highly lipid-soluble. Insulin and heparin, for instance, do not cross the placenta at all.

Differences in pH between maternal blood (pH 7.35–7.40) and fetal blood (pH 7.20–7.25) can lead to unequal drug concentrations in the two compartments. Nonionized molecules cross biological membranes more readily than ionized molecules. Drugs that are weak bases, with pK_a values near blood pH, are mainly nonionized, and therefore easily cross the placenta. After crossing the placenta, weak bases become more acidic in fetal blood; accordingly, the concentration of nonionized drug diminishes in the fetal compartment. This mechanism is commonly referred to as ion trapping. In contrast to weak bases, ion trapping induced from fetal to maternal circulations is likely to occur with weak acids (39).

The degree of protein binding is another determinant of a drug's ability to cross the placenta. Throughout pregnancy, there is a gradual decrease in the concentration of maternal albumin and an increase in fetal concentrations. Since only the free fraction of a drug crosses the placenta, highly protein-bound drugs (e.g., dicloxacillin, 96%) achieve higher maternal concentrations, whereas the least protein-bound drugs (e.g., digoxin, ampicillin, 20%) reach high concentrations in the fetus and amniotic fluid (39). Another factor is that fetal protein binding may differ from maternal protein binding.

Placental transfusion can be summarized by stating that the fetus receives unbound, nonionized, lipid-soluble molecules of a lower molecular weight. Of course, most drugs fulfill these criteria, since it is these very properties that allow them to cross all biological membranes.

E. Intermediate Metabolites

It is now recognized that many adverse fetal effects result not from parent drugs, but from their metabolism to more active or toxic compounds. Oxidative intermediates, such as epoxides, are highly reactive and capable of binding covalently to embryonic or fetal nucleic acids, which at critical periods of growth are theoretically capable of disrupting normal development.

The metabolism of thalidomide to a toxic metabolite only in certain species, including humans, has been proposed as the explanation for why the drug causes birth defects in some animals and not others (40). The well-known teratogenicity of several anticonvulsant medications has now been linked to toxic intermediary metabolites produced during the biotransformation of the parent compound. Drug combinations may be potentially even more toxic. Some epidemiological data suggest that when combinations of anticonvulsant drugs (e.g., phenytoin, carbamazine) that form oxidative metabolites are administered together during pregnancy, the risk of an adverse outcome is approximately eight times as high as with single-drug therapy (41). One study suggested that enzymatic markers exist that permit determination of which fetuses are at increased risk for congenital malformations induced by anticonvulsant medications (42).

V. Drugs and Lactation

With the capability to detect minute concentrations of drugs, it has been shown that virtually all maternally ingested drugs will enter breast milk, usually in amounts less than 2% of the maternal dose (43). The ability of any drug to enter breast milk depends on its molecular size, binding to milk proteins, lipid solubility, and ionization.

The molecular size of most drugs is not an impediment to passage into breast milk. All but the very largest molecules, such as insulin and heparin, are able to cross the alveolar acini in the mammary gland. Only the fraction of drug that is not protein-bound can leave the maternal circulation and enter breast milk. Thus, drugs that are highly protein-bound are less likely to enter breast milk when compared with drugs that are less protein-bound (44). Lipid solubility is also important for the concentration of drugs in breast milk. Highly lipid-soluble drugs enter breast milk to a greater extent than less lipid-soluble drugs. Finally, drug ionization must be considered. The average pH of breast milk is 7.08, which is lower than that of maternal blood. Therefore, the pK_a of a drug will affect the amount that enters breast milk. Weak acids are likely to be ionized in the maternal circulation, thereby reducing their transfer into breast milk. Weak bases are likely to be nonionized in maternal circulation, increasing both their lipid solubility and passage into milk. Once reaching the relatively acidic milk, weak bases will be ionized, leading to ion trapping in the milk (45).

Drug transfer from breast milk to the neonate from the GI tract is also governed by many factors, and the serum levels depend on the balance of absorption, distribution, metabolism, and excretion, all of which may differ from adult processes. The field has not been well studied pharmacologically.

Relatively few drugs are felt to be absolutely contraindicated in breast feeding, primarily on theoretical grounds rather than solid data. These include antineoplastic agents, histamine H2 receptor antagonists, methimazole and thiouracil used for hyperthyroidism, phenindione used as an anticoagulant (warfarin and dicumarol may be used), ergotamine for migraine treatment, gold salts, and bromocriptine (45). The use of specific asthma and allergy medications during breast feeding is discussed in Chapter 8.

VI. Risk Counseling

We have seen that the use of any drug during pregnancy entails acceptance of some small degree of risk. Equally important is the understanding that failure to treat an important medical problem may jeopardize the health of both a mother and her unborn child. These risks require careful communication between physician and patient.

The indications for any prescribed medication must be clearly explained and alternatives to pharmacological therapy considered. The potential effects of the drug on both mother and fetus need to be considered. Important background information essential for counseling includes known teratogenic risks of a particular drug, drug dose, and gestational age at exposure. Since the specific response of the conceptus will depend on genetic factors, in addition to dose-dependent pharmacological effects, information about genetic background should be included. Taking a careful family history may identify individuals at unusually high risk. For example, a family history of neural tube defects, congenital heart disease, or other birth defect suggests that the risk of any drug may be theoretically greater than it might be for the general population. Although this increased risk may not be quantifiable, its theoretical presence may influence decisions, and patients must be aware that they are accepting higher than average risks.

Three common scenarios will help illustrate the kinds of problems encountered while counseling patients about the use of medications during pregnancy (46). First, the most frequently asked question is: "Is any medication safe to take during pregnancy?" Patients should be counseled that, technically, drugs are not determined to be safe. Some have been proved harmful, and others are presumed to be safe when no evidence of harm can be demonstrated. The difference is subtle, but it means that no drug can be guaranteed to be 100% safe. The best approach to this problem is for the physician to obtain all the information available about the particular drug and, then, help the patient decide if the drug is necessary. Detailed reference texts are available for this purpose (1,16,47). Computer databases can be easily accessed, such as TERIS and REPROTOX. Regional teratology services, often at medical schools, can be helpful. Studies mentioned in the *Physicians Desk Reference* should be reviewed with the understanding that they may include unpublished, non-peer-reviewed studies. It is important to remind patients that even if a drug is in no way teratogenic, 3% of the women who take it will be expected to have a baby with a significant abnormality. This risk constitutes the background incidence of birth defects in the general population.

A second commonly asked question is: "Since I took this drug before I knew I was pregnant, should I terminate the pregnancy?" It is unreasonable either to reassure the patient that no risk is associated with the drug or, conversely, to recommend termination of a pregnancy solely because of exposure to a drug about which only limited information is available. Once an attempt has been made to gather all current information about the known risks of a drug, patients must play an active role in the decision process. They should also be informed that contemporary techniques of prenatal diagnosis can be effectively employed before 20 weeks' gestation to detect most major congenital anomalies. These techniques include triple marker maternal serum screening, high-resolution ultrasonography, and, where indicated, amniocentesis.

Finally, we are often confronted by a woman who has given birth to an infant with an anomaly who asks: "Did any of the medications I took cause the birth defect?" Implicit in this question is the assignment of responsibility to oneself or one's physician. We need not be reminded of the medico-legal implications of this question. Discussions need to be open and direct. Counseling requires an understanding of the process of disbelief, anger, and guilt that characterizes parents' adaptations to this crisis. It will be useful to help parents understand the basic principles of teratology and to remind them of the relatively brief period of gestation during which the fetus is most vulnerable to a teratogen. They should be reminded that all of the major organ systems have been formed before the completion of the first trimester. Therefore, it is generally true that exposure to a drug during the second or third trimester is unlikely to cause a major structural defect.

A complete examination by an expert in dysmorphology may often provide a clue to the cause of a major anomaly that would otherwise be overlooked. It is always appropriate to obtain an autopsy in cases of intrauterine fetal death or neonatal death. The findings may have significant bearing on the patient's perception and plans for future pregnancy. It is also important to schedule a counseling session a month or more after the birth of an anomalous child or a neonatal death. This allows family members to voice their concerns and ask questions that may affect future family planning. At this time, it is also essential to explore the effect of the tragic event on the psychological health of each member of the family.

References

1. Shepard TH. Catalog of Teratogenic Agents. Baltimore: Johns Hopkins Press, 1992.
2. Cohen LS, Friedman JM, Jefferson JW, Johnson EM, Weiner ML: A reevaluation of risk of in utero exposure to lithium. JAMA 1994; 271:146–150.
3. Cunningham FG, MacDonald PC, Gant NFG, Leveno KJ, Gilstrap LC III, eds. Drugs and medications during pregnancy. In: Williams Obstetrics, 19th ed. Norwalk, CT: Appleton & Lange, 1993: 959–980.
4. Jones KL. Effects of therapeutic, diagnostic, and environmental agents. In: Creasy RK, Resnik R, eds. Maternal Fetal Medicine. Philadelphia: Saunders, 1994.
5. Piper JM, Ray WA, Rosa FW. Pregnancy outcome following exposure to angiotensin-converting enzyme inhibitors. Obstet Gynecol 1992; 80:429–432.
6. Pryde PG, Sedman AB, Nugent CE, Barr M. Angiotensin-converting enzyme inhibitor fetopathy. J Am Soc Nephrol 1993; 3:1575–1582.
7. Jelovsek FR, Mattison DR, Chen JJ. Prediction of risk for human developmental toxicity: how important are animal studies for hazard identification? Obstet Gynecol 1989; 74:624–636.
8. Blake DA, Niebyl JR. Requirements and limitations in reproductive and teratogenic risk assessment. In Niebyl JR, ed. Drug Use in Pregnancy. Philadelphia: Lee & Febiger, 1988.
9. Friedman JM, Polifka JE. Teratogenic Effects of Drugs A Resource for Clinicians. Baltimore: Johns Hopkins University Press, 1994.
10. Koren G. Teratogenic drugs and chemicals in humans. In: Koren G, ed. Maternal-Fetal Toxicology. A Clinician's Guide. New York: Marcel Dekker, 1990.
11. Leeder JS, Spielberg SP. Teratogenicity and litigation. In: Koren G, ed. Maternal-Fetal Toxicology. A Clinician's Guide. New York: Marcel Dekker, 1990.
12. Angell M. The interpretation of epidemiologic studies. N Engl J Med 1990; 323:823–825.

13. Physicians Desk Reference. Montvale, NJ: Medical Economics Data Production Company, 1995.
14. Friedman JM, Little BB, Brent RL, Cordero JF, Hanson JW, Shepard TH. Potential human teratogenicity of frequently prescribed drugs. Obstet Gynecol 1990; 75:594–599.
15. Kimmel CA, Generoso WM, Thomas RD, Bakshi KS. Contemporary issues in toxicology: a new frontier in understanding the mechanisms of developmental abnormalities. Toxicol Appl Pharmacol 1993; 119:159–165.
16. Schardein JL. Chemically Induced Birth Defects. New York: Marcel Dekker, 1985.
17. Little BB, Gilstrap LC III. Human teratology principles. In: Gilstrap LC III, Little BB, eds. Drugs and Pregnancy. New York: Elsevier, 1992.
18. Fabro S, McLachlan A, Dames NM. Chemical exposure of embryos during the preimplantation stages of pregnancy; mortality rate and intrauterine development. Am J Obstet Gynecol 1984; 148:929–938.
19. From the Centers for Disease Control and Prevention. Recommendations for use of folic acid to reduce number of spina bifida cases and other neural tube defects. JAMA 1993; 269(10):1233, 1236–1238.
20. Colie C. Male mediated teratogenesis. Reprod Toxicol Rev 1993; 7:3–9.
21. Davis DL, Friedler G, Mattison D, Morris R. Male-mediated teratogenesis and other reproductive effects: biologic and epidemiologic findings and a plea for clinical research. Reprod Toxicol 1992; 6:289–292.
22. Soyka LF, Joffe JM. Male-mediated drug effects on offspring. Prog Clin Biol Res 1980; 36:49–66.
23. Kurzel RB, Cetrulo CL. Chemical teratogenesis and reproductive failure. Obstet Gynecol Surv 1985; 40:397–424.
24. Geiger JM, Baudin M, Saurat JH. Teratogenic risk with etretinate and acitretin treatment. Dermatology 1994; 189:109–116.
25. Van der Heijden BJ, Carlus C, Narcy F, Bavoux F, Delezoide AL, Gubler MC. Persistent anuria, neonatal death, and renal microcystic lesions after prenatal exposure to indamethacin. Am J Obstet Gynecol 1994; 171:617–623.
26. Caritis SN, Kuller JA, Watt-Morse ML. Pharmacologic options for treating preterm labor. In: Rayburn WF, Zuspan FP, eds. Drug Therapy in Obstetrics and Gynecology. St. Louis: Mosby Year Book, 1992.
27. Walker MPR, Cantrell CJ. Maternal renal impairment after indomethacin tocolysis. J Perinatol 1993; 13:461–463.
28. Rayburn WF. Drugs for fetal therapy. In: Rayburn WF, Zuspan FP, eds. Drug Therapy in Obstetrics and Gynecology. St. Louis: Mosby Year Book, 1992.
29. Zidovudine for the prevention of HIV transmission from mother to infant. Morbid Mortal Wkly Rep 1994; 43:285–287.
30. Krauer B, Krauer F, Hytten FE. Pregnancy and its effect on drug handling. In: Lind T, Singer A, eds. Current Reviews in Obstetrics and Gynecology. Edinburgh: Churchill-Livingstone, 1984.
31. Jeffries WS, Bochner F. The effect of pregnancy on drug pharmacokinetics. Med J Austral 1988; 149:675–677.

32. Pirani BKK, Campbell DM, MacGillivray I. Plasma volume in normal first pregnancy. J Obstet Gynaecol Br Commonw 1973; 80:884–887.

33. Duvekot JJ, Peeters LH. Maternal cardiovascular hemodynamic adaptation to pregnancy. Obstet Gynecol Surv 1994; 49(suppl):S1–S14.

34. Dunlop W. Serial changes in renal haemodynamics during normal human pregnancy. Br J Obstet Gynaecol 1981; 88:1–9.

35. Davis M, Simmons CJ, Dordoni B, Maxwell JD. Induction of hepatic enzymes during normal human pregnancy. J Obstet Gynaecol Br Commonw 1973; 80: 690–694.

36. Carter BL, Driscoll CE, Smith CD. Theophylline clearance during pregnancy. Obstet Gynecol 1986: 68:555–559.

37. Frederiksen MC, Ruo TI, Chow MJ, Atkinson AJ Jr. Theophylline pharmacokinetics in pregnancy. Clin Pharmacol Ther 1986; 40:321–328.

38. Gardner MJ, Schatz M, Cousins L, Zeiger R, Middleton E, Jusko WJ. Longitudinal effects of pregnancy on pharmacokinetics of theophylline. Eur J Clin Pharmacol 1987; 31:289–295.

39. Koren G. Changes in drug disposition in pregnancy and their clinical implications. In: Koren G, ed. Maternal-Fetal Toxicology. A Clinician's Guide. New York: Marcel Dekker, 1990.

40. Gordon GB, Spielberg SP, Blake DA, Balasubramanian V. Thalidomide teratogenesis: evidence for a toxic arene oxide metabolite. Proc Natl Acad Sci USA 1981; 78:2545–2548.

41. Lindhout D, Hoppener RJ, Meinardi H. Teratogenicity of antiepileptic drug combinations with special emphasis on epoxidation (of carbamazepine). Epilepsia 1984; 25:77–83.

42. Buehler BA, Delimont D, van Waes M, Finneli RH. Prenatal prediction of risk of the fetal hydantoin syndrome. N Engl J Med 1990; 322:1567–1572.

43. Rivera-Calimlim L. The significance of drugs in breast milk. Clin Perinatol 1987; 14:51–70.

44. Gardner DK. Drugs in breast milk. In: Rayburn WF, Zuspan FP, eds. Drug Therapy in Obstetrics and Gynecology. St. Louis: Mosby Year Book, 1992.

45. Rieder MJ. Drugs and breastfeeding. In: Koren G, ed. Maternal-Fetal Toxicology. A Clinician's Guide. New York: Marcel Dekker, 1990: 63–85.

46. Coustan DR, Carpenter W. The use of medications in pregnancy. Med Times 1984; 112:45–51.

47. Briggs GG, Fresman RK, Yaffe SJ. Drugs in Pregnancy and Lactation. Baltimore: Williams & Wilkins, 1994.

8

Pregnancy Effects of Specific Medications Used to Treat Asthma and Immunological Diseases

ANTHONY R. SCIALLI

Georgetown University Medical Center
and Reproductive Toxicology Center
Washington, DC

ARMAND LIONE

Reproductive Toxicology Center
and Associated Pharmacologists and
  Toxicologists
Washington, DC

The adverse effects of inadequately treated asthma during pregnancy are discussed elsewhere in this volume. In spite of these clear risks, there is often great concern on the part of both patients and health care providers that the use of medication in women who are pregnant or who may become pregnant will impair normal embryonic development. In fact, it has been estimated that only 1% of birth defects can be attributed to drug exposure (1); however, cases of embryopathy and fetopathy from isotretinon and angiotensin-converting enzyme inhibitors are recent examples of adverse outcomes associated with commonly used agents. Concerns about hurting the baby have led to a therapeutic nihilism resulting in the withholding even of medications important for the health of the mother–baby dyad. Our goal in this chapter is to present data on the pregnancy effects of medications, to permit practitioners to develop a greater level of comfort when treating pregnant women, and to aid in counseling patients about the therapeutic decisions that are being made to restore or maintain their health.

I. Developmental Toxicology

The study of the effects of drugs and other chemicals on pregnancy outcome has enabled us to understand some of the ways in which adverse pregnancy outcome can be induced. Although a thorough discussion of principles of developmental toxicology is beyond the scope of this chapter and can be found elsewhere (2), some general principles will be useful in understanding the drug summaries that follow.

A. Adverse Outcome Is More Than Birth Defects

Although limbless babies captured the attention of the public in the thalidomide episode of the 1960s, other manifestations of developmental toxicity are also important. For example, intellectual, motor, or behavioral abnormalities induced by central nervous system toxicants can be devastating, as witnessed in pregnancies exposed to sufficient doses of ionizing radiation, ethanol, or methyl mercury.

Adverse developmental effects include, besides gross structural malformations, alterations in function (a kind of malformation on a tissue, cell, or molecular level), death of the conceptus (miscarriage or stillbirth), and growth impairment. In addition, transplacental carcinogenesis is a concern for some agents, although to date only one drug (diethylstilbestrol) has been documented to have such properties in humans.

B. Adverse Pregnancy Outcome Is Not Unusual

Approximately 30% of recognized pregnancies miscarry, birth defects occur in 3–8% of children, and mental retardation is diagnosed in about 1% of children. This burden of adverse outcome in the general population imposes a difficulty in counseling women who are exposed to agents during pregnancy: It is not possible to say whether or not the pregnancy will be normal, only whether or not the exposure is likely to produce an increase in adverse outcome. In addition, when an adverse outcome occurs in a pregnancy in which drug exposure has occurred, it is natural to believe that an exposure must have caused the problem, even though the best evidence may be that the abnormality would have occurred anyway and that the exposure was incidental.

C. There Are Statistical Limitations to Estimating Risk

It is common to hear people conclude that we should not give medications to pregnant women because we can never be "sure" that a medication is safe, yet the concept of safety is one that carries substantial statistical baggage. A drug would be considered safe if it does not cause an increase in the incidence of adverse outcomes, but it is clear that with empiric data, we can only detect increases of a certain magnitude. If, for example, 1000 pregnant women take a drug and if 30 of them have a baby with a birth defect, the 3% incidence of defects (which is the expected population rate) does not exclude the possibility that 1 or 2 of the malformations was causally associated with the exposure. More sophisticated work, as discussed below, must be done to exclude the likelihood of such an association.

In some instances, the identification of an exposure that produces adverse outcome is simple. For example, if isotretinoin is used early in pregnancy, an adverse outcome (miscarriage or birth defects) occurs much of the time. In other cases, it may be difficult to identify an association. Pregnancy exposure to valproic acid, an anticonvulsant, increases the incidence of spina bifida from about 0.1% to about 1%, a 10-fold increase but an increase that required hundreds of exposed embryos to detect. For many drugs, published human pregnancy information, if it exists at all, consists of perhaps a few dozen exposures, and people are correct to wonder whether such information, *by itself*, is an indicator of safety.

All of therapeutics involves similar uncertainty issues. If an infant with otitis media is given amoxicillin, parents and physicians do not spend a lot of time worrying that the drug will interfere with brain development or might cause a cancer to develop in later life. Of the children exposed, however, a few will experience abnormalities in brain development and a substantial proportion will develop a cancer at some time in their lives. Why do we believe that these events are independent of amoxicillin exposure? Do we have large-scale studies excluding with certainty the possibility of amoxicillin-induced brain dysfunction or cancer?

In fact, when we make a therapeutic decision that a drug is "safe," we often do not have such large-scale studies: We base our belief on empiric data and theoretical considerations about drug action. In order to conclude that a drug is toxic, we require certain elements of causation. If there is sufficient reason to believe that enough of the elements of causation do not apply, we conclude that there is no association between the drug and the putative toxicity, even if we have not ruled out all statistical possibility of an association.

II. Elements of Causation

Causation is a statistical concept that implies an increased likelihood of an outcome if a causative factor is present. We do not require that the outcome always follows the cause, only that it does so more often than if the cause is not present. We believe that cigarette smoking causes lung cancer because lung cancer is more likely to occur in smokers than in nonsmokers. The fact that not all smokers get lung cancer and the fact that some nonsmokers get lung cancer does not dissuade us from our view of causation. It is also useful in causation to be able to invoke a mechanism or a series of events that lead from the cause to the effect.

In considering the evidence for causation, we evaluate several elements to decide how strongly we feel about a possible cause–effect relationship. Not all of these elements need to be present for a causal relationship to be concluded, although the larger the number that are present, the more convincing is the case for causation.

A. Strength of the Association

The more evident the increased incidence of the effect, the better is the case for causation. For example, it is widely believed that growth failure, microcephaly, mental retardation, and facial defects are caused by prenatal exposure to high doses of ethanol, because 20–40% of women who drink heavily during pregnancy have affected children. It is less widely accepted that ingestion of lithium during pregnancy increases congenital heart disease, because the outcome occurs in only perhaps 1% or so of exposed children.

B. Consistency of the Association

Demonstration of an increased incidence of an effect after a putative cause is applied should be possible in different populations during different time periods. The link between thalidomide and limb defects, for example, was made independently in Germany and in Australia. An increase in congenital heart defects in children exposed antenatally to lithium has not been found in all studies, calling into question the causal nature of the association. In some cases, the appearance of new studies with results contrary to older studies reverses thinking in the field. At one time, diazepam was believed to be a cause of cleft palate in humans; however, there has been sufficient failure to confirm the association that a causal relationship is no longer accepted.

C. Biologic Plausibility

A causal association ought to make sense. The relationship between cigarette smoking and intrauterine growth restriction is plausible because impairment of oxygen exchange by carboxyhemoglobin and nicotine-associated vascular abnormalities would be expected to result in fetal growth restriction. The association between cytotoxic drugs and developmental toxicity is plausible because excessive cell death is believed to be an important mediator of abnormal embryo development.

The suggestion that amoxicillin might cause future cancer development is biologically implausible because amoxicillin does not have properties that we associate with cancer-inducing or cancer-promoting agents. Amoxicillin also does not have properties that are associated with agents producing developmental toxicity, which is one of the reasons we feel comfortable giving this drug during pregnancy.

D. Appropriate Timing of Exposure and Response

We expect events to occur in a certain order, with a sensible temporal relationship. The causal relationship between cigarette smoking and cancer would be weak if a person were diagnosed with cancer one day after smoking her first cigarette, because we think of cancer as requiring time to be induced. In embryology, we recognize a sequence of developmental events and we ask putative causal relationships to be consistent with this sequence of events. We would find it unlikely that an exposure at 20 gestational weeks would be responsible for a cleft palate or that an exposure at 6 weeks would cause isolated mental retardation.

E. Gradient of Response

It is considered axiomatic in developmental toxicity that effects are proportional to the amount of exposure to a causative agent. Responses are expected to vary from zero (that is, no increase in adverse outcome) as the exposure to an agent is raised from a low level. It is believed that for all developmentally toxic agents, there is a dose below which there is no toxicity. It is also believed that for all agents, there is a dose at which toxicity will occur, although this toxic dose may be very high and may be associated with substantial toxicity to the mother. For example, if we give enough penicillin to a pregnant woman, she will convulse and die and her fetus will also die. This kind of "developmental toxicity" is not clinically relevant, however, because we do not use penicillin in such high doses, and so we think of penicillin as being "safe" for use in pregnancy.

The belief in the existence of a gradient of response for all agents translates very practically into one of the most important tenets of clinical developmental toxicology: The question to be answered is not whether a drug is or is not a developmental toxicant, but whether it will increase toxicity when used therapeutically.

It would be toxicologically inappropriate to posit a cause–effect relationship in which a gradient of response did not occur. For example, we know that x-ray exposures of 50 rad or more during pregnancy are associated with an increased incidence of microcephaly and mental impairment in the offspring. A woman exposed to 50 mrad should not be expected to have the same potential for an adverse outcome, and in fact, such an exposure is not associated with any increase in adverse effects. Because most diagnostic radiology procedures involve exposures much closer to 50 mrad than to 50 rad, it is misleading to think of x-rays as "teratogenic;" it is not the x-ray itself that is toxic, rather it is the high x-ray *exposure* that can be toxic.

F. Experimental Models

The existence of an experimental model of toxicity is an important element to be considered in deciding about causal relationships. There are few, if any, instances of toxicity that are particular to intact human beings; that is, experimental models using experimental animals or in-vitro systems can be developed to simulate human response to toxicants. Although we are accustomed to thinking of human beings as special in many ways, the response of our tissues to foreign chemicals is often similar to the response of analogous tissues of other organisms. If a putative cause-and-effect relationship cannot be reproduced in an experimental system, there ought to be considerable doubt about whether the relationship is truly causal.

In developmental toxicology, experimental models do not always produce the same response as is seen in humans. Valproic acid exposure in humans increases the incidence of spina bifida, whereas in mice, exencephaly, another kind of neural tube defect, is more commonly seen. It is also not necessarily the case that all species will have similar sensitivities to drugs. Mice are more sensitive to all-*trans*-retinoic acid (a drug marketed as Retin-A) than to 13-*cis*-retinoic acid (isotretinoin; Accutane); this difference is due to differences in the manner in which mice handle these two isomers.

It is the use of experimental models that has produced the most mistrust of drug information in developmental toxicology. As will be seen from the agent summaries that follow, most of the data consist of information obtained in experimental animals. It is important, then, to evaluate what these data can help us learn.

III. Using Experimental Animal Data

Because we are interested in discovering whether a drug might increase adverse pregnancy outcome even to a small extent, we should not feel very comfortably relying entirely on a relatively small number of case reports in pregnant women. As we have discussed, the lack of an observed increase in birth defects among the offspring of a few dozen exposed women would not exclude a 10-fold increase in the incidence of spina bifida. To some extent, this problem of the *power* of a human pregnancy study can be addressed with an animal study in which high doses of an agent are used in an attempt to bring out the ability of a drug to disrupt development. To be sure, power is an issue in animal studies as well as in human studies. A typical developmental toxicology experiment will contain 20 pregnant animals in each dose group. For rodents, each pregnant animal may have 15 pups or so, giving the possibility of 300 offspring to be evaluated at each dose.* It will not be possible, therefore, to detect very small increases in birth defects or even large increases in very unusual birth defects, but it is hoped that by using high doses, enough offspring will be affected in a manner that permits the agent to be flagged as a potential problem.

Animal studies also include the use of different dose groups, permitting a gradient of response to be investigated. The presence of a relationship between dose and response is an important element in the evaluation of animal study results. The selection of doses is not entirely an arbitrary matter. It is customary to use three doses, as well as to use a control group. Of the three doses, the lowest is generally similar to the dose anticipated to be used in humans, or a low-order multiple of the human dose. The highest dose is one that produces some degree of maternal toxicity. The middle dose is between the low and the high dose, often logarithmically equally spaced between the two.

The use of a maternally toxic dose guarantees that a dose with a biologic effect for the species under study has been selected; in other words, the adult animal is used as a kind of dosimeter to guarantee that dose selection is not way below a relevant range for that species. Under ideal circumstances, the maternal toxicity consists of a small reduction in the rate of pregnancy weight gain and is not anticipated to make a large impact on fetal well being; however, there are many instances in which maternal toxicity in an experiment is substantial. Under such circum-

---

*These offspring do not constitute independent observations, because there is an important litter effect for many toxicants; that is, members of the same litter are more likely to respond in a similar manner than are members of different litters.

stances, it is not surprising that fetal well-being is adversely affected. When offspring are adversely affected only at a dose that produces significant maternal toxicity, it is sometimes difficult to know whether the effects on the conceptus are due only to the maternal toxicity or to independent adverse effects of the agent on embryo development. In such instances, the kind of toxicity may give a clue; for example, a small reduction in litter weight is plausibly related to poor maternal weight gain, while an increase in a birth defect that is not ordinarily seen in the species under study is less plausibly related to minimal maternal toxicity.

Because of species differences in drug handling, it is helpful to have pharmacokinetic information relevant to the species under study. For example, if a drug is extensively bioactivated by humans, it is helpful to use test animals that bioactivate the drug in the same manner. Pharmacokinetic information may be available for recently introduced agents, but older studies were often performed without such detailed knowledge. It has been customary to perform pregnancy studies with at least two species, one of which is not a rodent. It is hoped that at least one of the two species will handle the drug in a manner sufficiently similar to humans to be predictive.

Does this system of testing work to protect humans? Thus far, the answer is a qualified yes. There are no agents that produce developmental toxicity in humans that would not be predicted by current methods of animal testing. Even thalidomide, widely rumored to be "negative" in animal studies, produces an unequivocal response in rabbits, the most commonly used nonrodent test species. In fact, animal testing appears if anything to have the problem of being overly protective: Far more agents are known to produce developmental toxicity in animals than produce developmental toxicity in humans. In large measure this is an issue of dose, because the high doses used in animal studies may not be relevant to doses used clinically.

How are animal studies to be interpreted, then, in the agent summaries that follow? There is no hard-and-fast rule, but there are suggested guidelines.

> If the embryo is much more sensitive to toxicity than the adult, the agent should be regarded with concern. An example is trimethadione, an anticonvulsant that produces a high incidence of birth defects in mice at doses well below those that produce toxicity in the mother. Trimethadione use by humans has also been associated with an increase in birth defects (3).
>
> If developmental toxicity is not seen even at doses that produce maternal toxicity in two species, the agent is unlikely to produce developmental toxicity with human pregnancy exposure. Such a con-

clusion is most tenable if details of absorption, biotransformation, and mechanism of drug action are understood. Reassuring animal studies are often used to increase the confidence in human studies that show no increase in adverse pregnancy outcome associated with an exposure.

Mechanisms of developmental toxicity in animal studies may be helpful in evaluating human risk. The observation that retinoids inhibit neural crest cell migration in experimental animals was useful in predicting isotretinoin-associated anomalies in exposed human pregnancies. Constriction of the fetal ductus arteriosus and mesenteric circulation in experimental animals exposed to nonsteroidal antiinflammatory agents appears to be predictive of a similar response in the human.

In some instances, a large amount of experience with a class of compounds in experimental animal studies increased confidence that an unexpected mechanism of toxicity is not being overlooked. Salicylates are a class of agent that has been particularly well studied in experimental animals.

For any given agent, it is unlikely that a single study will be sufficient to be reassuring; however, in many instances the full data set can be used to reach the conclusion that safety has been adequately demonstrated. Therapeutic decisions of necessity involve considering the potential for toxicity to all sites, whether kidney, lung, liver, or embryo. Developmental toxicity can be predicted with about the same precision as other kinds of toxicity. The lack of a guaranteed exclusion of all possible risk should not paralyze the practitioner with regard to developmental effects any more than with regard to other target organs that might be adversely affected by drug use.

IV. Case Reports and Human Epidemiologic Studies

Case reports typically involve one or a few births in which an adverse outcome in a pregnancy was found to occur following a defined prenatal drug exposure. Case reports give no information about the putative causal nature of an association and are unable to estimate the magnitude of any increase in risk associated with an exposure. Controlled epidemiologic studies, on the other hand, collect data from many pregnancies that include an exposure or an outcome of interest and can be used to estimate the likelihood that an agent increases the risk of adverse developmental outcome. If a pattern can be detected among reported defects, it may be possible to identify a specific event in development that is altered by the presence of a drug. A classic example of the successful use of this approach is the identification of thalidomide as a teratogen based on an increase in the incidence of phocomelia in Germany (4) and Australia (5). Research data eventually demonstrated that thalidomide had to be taken by a mother before limb development was complete in order to produce limb abnormalities (6).

A detailed discussion of the use of case reports and epidemiologic methods to uncover associations between various drugs and the incidence of birth defects is available elsewhere (2,7). One epidemiologic study that has provided preliminary data on a large variety of drugs, including the older antihistamines, is the National Collaborative Perinatal Project (NCPP; Ref. 8). In the early 1970s, this multicenter project enrolled more than 50,000 pregnant women in the United States and collected a history from each women that included the drugs used prior to enrollment and throughout the remainder of gestation. After delivery, the incidence of abnormalities in this population was correlated with reported drug exposures. To control for the random occurrence of birth defects in the general population, the number and type of defects in the drug-exposed pregnancies were compared with the defects reported in all other pregnancies in the study that did not include exposure to the same compound. Drug exposures were defined prospectively in this study (women were asked about their exposures before knowing the outcome of their pregnancy), but the control groups used for making comparisons (other women in the study who used other drugs) did not necessarily include women of comparable age, parity, and other factors that ideally would be accounted for in suitable controls. Because a large number of exposures and a large number of outcomes were evaluated, many associations were likely to have arisen by chance alone; such associations should be viewed only as hypothesis-generating and not as definitive. Conversely, because many exposures occurred in small numbers of women, failure to find an association with an adverse outcome may have been due simply to insufficient power to identify a small increase in isolated abnormalities.

V. Antihistamines

Antihistamines first became available in the late 1940s, with the introduction of diphenhydramine (9). There are now nearly two dozen antihistamines that are effective for the treatment of allergic diseases that are marketed in the United States (see Table 1). These agents have been incorporated into hundreds of prescription and nonprescription products. Because some of them—diphenhydramine and pyrilene are notable examples—have significant hypnotic effects, certain antihistamines are also

Table 1 Animal Teratogenicity Testing of Antihistamines (H_1 blockers) Used for Allergic Diseases

Compound	Animal	Dose[a]	Comment	Reference
Ethanolamines				
Diphenhydramine	Mouse	ND[b]	Decreased fetal weight/survival	10
	Rat	24	No defects	11
	Rabbit	24	No defects	11
Dimenhydrinate[c]	Rat	45	No defects	12
Carbinoxamine	Mouse	600	Decreased fetal survival	13
	Rat	750	Decreased fetal weight	13
Clemastine	Rat	312	No defects	Insert[d]
	Rabbit	188	No defects	Insert[d]
Diphenylpyraline	Rat	37.5 mg/kg/day[e]	No defects	14
Doxylamine	Rat	1,500	No defects	15
	Rabbit	1,500	No defects	15
	Rat	12,000	Decreased fetal weight/survival	16
Phenyltoloxamine			No data	
Alkylamines				
Brompheniramine			No data	
Chlorpheniramine	Mouse	650	No defects	10
Pheniramine			No data	
Triprolidine	Rat	125	No defects	Insert[d]
	Rabbit	125	No defects	Insert[d]
Acrivastine			No data	
Ethylenediamines				
Antazoline			No data	
Methapyrilene	Rat	ND[b]	No defects	14
Pyrilamine	Mouse	ND[b]	No defects	10
	Rat	ND[b]	No defects	17
Tripelennamine	Rat	12	Behavioral effects (given with pentazocine)	18
Piperidines				
Astemizole	Rat	200	No defects	Insert[d]
	Rabbit	200	No defects	Insert[d]
Azatadine	Rat	12.5	No defects	Insert[d]
	Rabbit	25	No defects	Insert[d]

Table 1 Continued

Compound	Animal	Dose[a]	Comment	Reference
Terfenadine	Unstated	125	No defects	Insert[d]
	Rat	300	No defects	19
	Rabbit	500	No defects	19
Phenothiazine-like				
Cyproheptadine	Rat	165	No defects, islet toxicity	20,21
	Rat	750	Visceral defects	22
	Rat	450	Visceral and limb defects	23
Trimeprazine			No data	
Loratadine	Rat	Not stated	No defects	Insert[d]
	Rabbit	Not stated	No defects	Insert[d]
Phenindamine			No data	

[a]Expressed as multiple of the maximum recommended human dose on a mg/kg basis.
[b]ND = not determinable.
[c]Dimenhydrinate is the chlorotheophylline salt of diphenhydramine.
[d]Unpublished information from the package insert.
[e]Administered dose; human dose not available.

found in over-the-counter (OTC) sleeping aids. The newest antihistamines, such as terfenadine, astemizole, and loratadine, are characterized as being distinctly nonsedating, since they have been pharmacologically designed not to gain entry into the central nervous system. Among the antihistamines that are piperazine and phenothiazine derivatives, buclizine, cyclizine, meclizine, and promethazine are used primarily as antiemetics and will not be discussed here.

A. Animal Studies

Table 1 summarizes the available animal studies that have investigated the teratogenicity and embryotoxicity of the antihistamines in question. Despite the availability of some antihistamines for as long as 50 years, few animal investigations were found for most agents, and none for eight of the listed antihistamines.

In general, however, there were few indications that any of the tested antihistamines were likely to produce adverse effects on developing fetuses at doses below those that cause maternal toxicity. The most commonly reported effects produced by these agents included reductions of fetal weight and number of surviving fetuses, as well as skeletal variations, which are all effects that commonly accompany the maternally toxic effects of high doses of many agents (2).

The ethylenediamine derivatives, pyrilamine, methapyrilene, and tripelennamine, have been scrutinized as possible genotoxicants or carcinogens. Tripelennamine was weakly genotoxic in cultured human hepatocytes (24). Pyrilamine had genotoxic effects in a number of test systems (25). Methapyriline is the most intensely studied member of this group. This antihistamine has been shown to be a hepatic carcinogen in rats but not in other animals and appears to operate through a nongenotoxic mechanism (26). Some tests have shown methapyrilene to be mutagenic (25,27), and one report found this drug to increase the methylation of hepatocyte DNA (28), but the majority of studies have not identified methapyrilene genotoxicity (29–32). One paper suggested that hepatic carcinogenicity was secondary to cytotoxicity and subsequent regeneration rather than to a genotoxic mechanism (24). Methapyrilene is no longer in clinical use but remains of interest to the extent that its toxicity may reflect that of other agents of this class.

Among the few provocative findings in Table 1 are the rat studies that suggest that prenatal cyproheptadine exposure may have diabetogenic effects (20,21). Cyproheptadine is undistinguished as an antihistamine and an unlikely choice for routine use, since it is more likely than other antihistamines to have side effects due to its serotonin antagonist actions. The toxicity to fetal pancreatic cells in rats was demonstrated at doses clearly below the maternally toxic level (20,21). Unlike other insulin-depleting compounds, such as alloxan and streptozotocin, cyproheptadine is likely to be distributed to the fetal pancreas in quantities sufficient to produce cell damage (33). Although these observations are a focus for concern, as we will discuss next, comparable fetal effects have not been reported in human pregnancies.

B. Human Reports

The NCPP included pregnancies with exposure to an assortment of antihistamines, including diphenhydramine, doxylamine, phenyltoloxamine, pheniramine, chlorpheniramine, brompheniramine, pyrilamine, tripelennamine, hydroxyzine, and promethazine. Since embryogenesis was viewed as being completed in the first trimester, drug exposures were categorized as occurring either during the first 4 months of gestation or at any time during gestation. For the majority of agents, no increased risk of major or minor abnormalities was uncovered (8). The only antihistamines that were seemingly associated with elevated risks were chlorpheniramine, brompheniramine, pheniramine, and pyrilamine.

Small but statistically significant associations were seen between maternal use of chlorpheniramine during the first four lunar months of pregnancy and inguinal hernia and eye or ear anomalies among exposed infants (8). In later epidemiologic studies, however, no increase in the frequency of these or other congenital anomalies was observed among more than 275 infants born to women who took chlorpheniramine during the first trimester of pregnancy (34), suggesting that the NCPP findings may have arisen by chance.

The NCPP also reported a slightly increased frequency of congenital anomalies among the children of 65 women who took brompheniramine during the first four lunar months of pregnancy. An analysis of this finding showed that the anomalies in question were mild defects that occurred with widely varying rates at participating institutions. These data did not seem indicative of a clear adverse drug effect (8). The NCPP also reported an association between the use of pheniramine during the first 4 months of pregnancy and a possible increase in respiratory tract abnormalities in exposed offspring (8). Although we would expect some consistency of adverse effects from similar compounds, this observation differs from the associations found for the related compounds chlorpheniramine and brompheniramine.

Jaffe et al. (35) reported on a child who was born with a limb defect after a prenatal exposure to pyrilamine during the fourth week of gestation. In contrast to this isolated observation, however, the NCPP identified 121 pregnancies that included first-trimester exposures to pyrilamine without a significant increase in the incidence of major or minor malformations (8). A total of 392 gestational exposures to pyrilamine were identified among women who used this antihistamine at some time during pregnancy. In this group, one possible association with malformations was detected: Of the 12 offspring with a detectable malformation, 6 involved benign tumors.

One study has reported that maternal use of antihistamines (agents and doses not specified) during the 2 weeks preceding premature delivery was associated with an increased risk of retrolental fibroplasia (36). The incidence of this condition was 22% (19 of 86) in infants exposed to antihistamines and 11% (324 of 2940) in infants not exposed. Collaborative data to support this association and a plausible biologic mechanism are not currently available.

Data from another epidemiologic report, based on a very small number of cases, suggested a possible association between the use of antihistamines and the increased incidence of pyloric stenosis (37). Although two additional epidemiologic observations, based on only 16 cases of pyloric stenosis (38,39), provided suggestive data supportive of this association, the absence of subsequent reports on this topic suggests that an association between antihistamine use and the incidence of pyloric stenosis has not been found in the analysis of data from larger populations.

In retrospective studies of drug use during pregnancy, mothers are asked about prenatal drug use after delivery, when they know their child is normal or has been born with a defect. It is difficult to control for bias in data collected retrospectively, since the outcome of a pregnancy may influence the intensity and accuracy of recall (2). In a retrospective study, Saxén (40) found that first-trimester use of diphenhydramine was more common among 599 children born with oral clefts (20 exposures) than among 590 controls without clefts (6 exposures). In contrast, however, no significant increase in the incidence of major or minor malformations was uncovered in the NCPP, which analyzed the outcomes of 595 births that included first-trimester use of diphenhydramine, and 2948 pregnancies that included the use of this drug at some time during pregnancy (8). Data from another study indicated that significantly fewer infants with malformations were exposed to antihistamines while in utero than were controls (41). At the time of this study (1971), diphenhydramine was the second most commonly used antihistamine in the study population.

C. Fetal and Neonatal Toxicity

The placental transfer of diphenhydramine and several other antihistamines has been demonstrated, and a comparable fetal distribution in humans is likely for all members of this class of drugs. Diphenhydramine withdrawal has been reported in one infant who was exposed in utero (42). In this report, generalized tremulousness and diarrhea began on the fifth day of life of an infant whose mother had taken 150 mg/day of diphenhydramine throughout pregnancy. The infant was treated with phenobarbital until the symptoms disappeared.

In the fetal lamb, low fetal diphenhydramine concentrations produced sedative effects, including reduced REM sleep and fetal breathing activity. Higher drug levels caused transient vigorous breathing activity, hypoxemia, acidemia, tachycardia, and an increased transitional electrocorticographic pattern. Moreover, fetal CNS effects were seen at plasma concentrations of the drug below those associated with sedation in adult humans (43). The effect of this dose on the ewe was not made clear. However, during the diphenhydramine infusions, no evidence for the convulsive and seizure activity described in children subjected to diphenhydramine overdose was observed.

There is concern that the physiologic role of histamine in the fetus may be compromised by these agents. Histamine, for example, is felt to be important in the cardiovascular response to stress in the newborn. Also, infants and young children may convulse when given antihistamines, raising the concern that third-trimester use of these drugs may cause adverse nonmalforming effects that have yet to be characterized. Diphenhydramine has been shown to competitively antagonize histamine-induced contractions in venous smooth muscle of placental tissue in humans (44).

The use of hydroxyzine as a sedative during labor and delivery has been considered effective and relatively safe (8,45). Like many sedatives, hydroxyzine can decrease the response rate of the fetal heart, but this effect has not been associated with clinical significance in terms of fetal well-being (46). One case of neonatal withdrawal syndrome was associated with hydroxyzine after maternal use of this compound as an antipruritic throughout pregnancy. This pregnancy also included prenatal exposure to phenobarbital during the 3 weeks before delivery (47). Respiratory depression in the neonate is a theoretical consequence of hydroxyzine administration to the laboring woman. This problem would not be amenable to treatment with an opioid antagonist such as naloxone.

There are conflicting reports on the incidence of neonatal respiratory depression following the administration of promethazine during labor (48–51). Although the majority of the available reports have not detected this effect (49–51), the possible induction of respiratory depression in the neonate cannot be completely dismissed. A warning from one manufacturer of promethazine has informed physicians that this drug was shown to depress respiratory mechanisms in normal infants (52) and should not be administered to children less than 2 years of age (53). This warning was sufficient to induce one clinician to suggest that the use of promethazine during labor be discontinued, particularly when the fetus is at risk of hypoxia (53). The use of promethazine during labor may impair platelet aggregation in the mother, and more so in the newborn (54,55). While this effect has not been associated with significant clinical bleeding problems, the degree of platelet impairment is comparable with that seen in other disorders associated with excessive bleeding.

D. Use During Lactation

Although some antihistamines have been classified as compatible with breast feeding by the American Academy of Pediatrics (56) and the WHO Working Group on drugs and human lactation (57), there are theoretical and clinical concerns that conflict with these recommendations (58). Because of their anticholinergic effects, antihistamines may, in theory, reduce milk production. If a patient should choose to continue her use of antihistamines while breast feeding, efforts may be made to minimize neonatal exposure by taking the dose immediately after nursing, to maximize the time between drug ingestion and the next feeding.

Measurement of milk concentrations of terfenadine are very low, and it has been estimated that a nursing infant would ingest less than 0.5% of the maternal weight-adjusted dose from this source (59). Such a small dose would not be expected to produce toxicity in the newborn.

VI. Glucocorticoids

Cortisone and its congeners are commonly used anti-inflammatory agents that have produced considerable concern because of adverse effects on rodent and rabbit embryonic development. Cleft palate has been produced by cortisone, beclomethasone, betamethasone, dexamethasone, prednisone, prednisolone, methylprednisolone, and triamcinolone (60–73). In a comparison of the glucocorticoids, triamcinolone was found to be 200 times as potent as cortisone in producing palatal clefting in mice (60). The high potency of triamcinolone was also shown in avian teratology experiments in which scale and feather development were inhibited by triamcinolone with 10,000 times the potency of cortisone (74).

Glucocorticoid-associated palatal clefting in rodents is receptor-mediated and is characterized by delay in elevation of the palatal shelves and inhibition of lysosome-mediated breakdown of the epithelium of the shelves at the point of contact (75). It is not clear that these mechanisms of toxicity occur with glucocorticoid exposure in primates. Triamcinolone will produce CNS and craniofacial abnormalities (including cleft palate) in nonhuman primates; however, inhibition of normal cartilage formation appears to be the most important mediator of craniofacial abnormalities in these animals (76–81).

Human pregnancies exposed to glucocorticoids have not been found to be at increased risk of structural malformations (8,82–91). Concern has been expressed that the number of pregnancies exposed in the first trimester may not be sufficient to exclude a small increase in risk of palatal clefting, although the combined reports include more than 1100 exposed pregnancies. In addition, in mice there is a common receptor for phenytoin and cortisone that appears to mediate the teratogenic effect of both agents (92), and phenytoin exposure of human embryos increases the incidence of cleft palate. Based on the nonhuman primate experiments with triamcinolone, cited above, it appears likely that if glucocorticoids increase the risk of cleft palate in humans, high doses may be necessary before such toxicity is seen.

Isolated case reports of anomalies in newborns after glucocorticoid-exposed pregnancies have appeared (reviewed by Schardein, Ref. 93). There were no patterns of malformations suggestive of a medication-associated birth defect syndrome. The possibility exists, however, that case reports of congenital cataracts and of immunosuppression are causally related to maternal glucocorticoid use (94,95), because these adverse effects are noted on occasion in association with the use of glucocorticoids at any time in postnatal life. Immunosuppression does not appear to be at all common in neonates exposed antenatally to these agents (96).

Data from animal and human experience suggest that glucocorticoids retard fetal growth and may increase the incidence of low birth weight (84,97–99). In many instances, the decreased fetal growth may have been associated with the underlying condition for which the medication was given, because these medications are often used for collagen-vascular and renal disease. In at least two studies, however, the underlying disorder was unlikely to have been involved. In one (97), glucocorticoids were given to women with fertility problems under the assumption that their pregnancy outcome would be improved. Similar women who were not so treated were used as controls. A clinically modest but significant decrease in mean birth weight was demonstrated in the treated group. The second study (99) found a decrease in birth weight among women treated with glucocorticoids to prevent rejection of renal transplants; in these women, transplant function and blood pressure were essentially normal and not likely to have had a significant impact on fetal growth. There is also a case report of a pregnant woman who used triamcinolone, 40 mg/day, for atopic dermatitis from 12 to 29 weeks' gestation, whose baby showed severe intrauterine growth retardation (100).

Early third-trimester glucocorticoid treatment of pregnant women at risk for premature delivery has been used for many years to decrease the incidence and severity of respiratory distress syndrome of the neonate. Such regimens were actively endorsed by a National Institutes of Health expert panel in 1995 (101). Betamethasone and dexamethasone are the agents most commonly used, and considerable published experience supporting the lack of toxicity of these agents has appeared (102–108). Although the general view is that steroid therapy for threatened prematurity is without undue risk, some investigators have expressed concern about possible drug-associated increases in neonatal blood pressure (109), retinopathy of prematurity (110,111), or gastrointestinal perforation (112) with fetal or neonatal treatment. Betamethasone has also been found to produce transient, mild constriction of the fetal ductus arteriosus when administered antenatally to the mother (113).

Glucocorticoids enter breast milk in small amounts (114–116). The amount of prednisolone, for example, absorbed by a nursing infant is inconsequential compared to the infant's endogenous cortisol production (116). These agents are considered by the American Academy of Pediatrics (56) to be compatible with breast feeding.

There are no clear comparative data to guide the choice of glucocorticoid for use in pregnant women. Among oral agents, prednisone has been used most commonly, although late-pregnancy use of dexamethasone is also common. Parenteral agents that have been used with some frequency include betamethasone, methylprednisolone, and hydrocortisone. Beclomethasone is the inhaled agent with which there is the greatest published pregnancy experience, including two reports that comprise 101 exposed pregnancies (83,84). Due to the greater potency of triamcinolone in animal studies, there has been reluctance to recommend this agent for use during pregnancy; however, potency considerations should be controlled by the lower doses of triamcinolone delivered by inhalation cannisters. There are no published data on flunisolide.

VII. Sympathomimetics

Drugs with adrenergic effects are often discussed as having alpha- or beta-sympathomimetic activity. Alpha-adrenergics are often used as vasoconstrictors (e.g., decongestants), and beta-adrenergics are used as smooth muscle relaxants (e.g., bronchodilators). Some drugs (e.g., epinephrine) have mixed alpha and beta effects.

A. Oxymetazoline

Oxymetazoline is an alpha-adrenergic agonist used in nonprescription nasal decongestants. Nasal congestion is common during pregnancy, and there is concern that unrestricted self-medication with oxymetazoline may lead to overdosage. The excessive use of an oxymetazoline nasal spray was reported to have produced bradycardia and hypotension in an elderly patient (117) and a diverse group of adverse reactions in young children, including sedation, epileptiform events, and insomnia (118).

Uterine blood vessels contain alpha-adrenergic receptors, which are capable of causing constriction when stimulated. Normally, these vessels are maximally dilated (119). Phenylephrine in a dose equivalent to the content of one "cold" tablet has been shown to decrease uterine blood flow by 40% in pregnant sheep (120). In these animals, the uterine vascular bed is substantially more responsive to the vasoconstrictive effects of alpha-agonists than the overall systemic vasculature (121). A single dose of a 0.05% oxymetazoline nasal spray did not significantly alter blood flow velocity, measured by Doppler ultrasound, in the uterine arcuate artery, fetal aorta, or umbilical artery in 12 healthy pregnancies (122). The conclusion of this study was that use of recommended doses of oxymetazoline was without apparent adverse effect; however, the findings could not be extended to conditions under which absorption might be enhanced, such as rhinitis, or pregnancies complicated by conditions such as uteroplacental insufficiency. In one case report, the excessive use of an oxymetazoline nasal spray by a woman in her 41st week of pregnancy was associated with a nonreactive nonstress test and late decelerations in fetal heart rate, suggesting that uterine perfusion may have been impaired (123).

B. Phenylephrine

Phenylephrine is an alpha-adrenergic that has been used in the treatment of glaucoma and as a pressor as well as in cold medications as a decongestant. Application of this agent to the chorioallantoic membrane of the chick embryo produces hemorrhagic lesions (124), an effect consistent with the vasoconstrictive properties of the drug. Phenylephrine use during pregnancy was identified in case-control studies as associated with congenital heart defects in the offspring (125,126). Information on a large number of exposures was sought, and some of these exposures may have been associated with adverse outcomes by virtue of the "fishing expedition" nature of the investigation. The National Collaborative Perinatal Project (NCPP) included more than 4000 women exposed to this agent during pregnancy, 1249 of whom were exposed during the first four lunar months (8). Possible associations were found between first-trimester exposure and ear and eye defects, syndactyly, and clubfoot, and between pregnancy use in general and hip dislocation, musculoskeletal deformities, and umbilical hernia. In contrast with the previous studies, an increased incidence of heart defects was not found. The associations identified in this study were based on the appearance of small numbers of children with malformations. For example, for abnormalities associated with first-trimester exposure to phenylephrine, the largest group consisted of 8 children with eye and ear defects. The exploratory nature of the NCPP has been discussed above as requiring confirmation of an associations because of the large number of comparisons that were made.

Perhaps of greater concern than the NCPP report is the potential for phenylephrine, and other alpha-adrenergic agonists, to induce maternal hypertension and to reduce uterine blood flow at doses comparable to those used in therapy. Uterine blood vessels contain alpha-adrenergic receptors, which cause constriction when stimulated. These vessels are maximally dilated during normal pregnancy (119). A dose of phenylephrine equivalent to one cold tablet has been shown to decrease uterine blood flow by 40% in pregnant sheep (120). The sheep uterine vascular bed is substantially more responsive to the vasoconstrictive effects of alpha-agonists than the overall systemic vasculature (121), and sensitivity to phenylephrine vasoconstriction increases during pregnancy in the sheep model (127). Because of their vasoconstrictive effects, phenylephrine and the related agent, phenylpropanolamine, can produce a rapid increase of diastolic blood pressure at doses only two to three times their recommended therapeutic dose (128,129). In contrast, the decongestant, pseudoephedrine, requires a dose greater than four times its therapeutic dose to affect blood pressure. Because of this more favorable toxic/therapeutic dose ratio, pseudoephedrine is recommended over other alpha-adrenergic drugs for use during pregnancy.

C. Phenylpropanolamine

Phenylpropanolamine is used in nonprescription cold pills and diet pills. Experimental animal studies on phenylpropanolamine have not been located. The National Collaborative Perinatal Project found a possible association between use of this agent during the first 4 months of pregnancy and hypospadias, eye and ear malformations, polydactyly, and pectus excavatum (8). The number of malformations in this study was small (7 cases in the largest of the groups), and the fishing expedition nature of this project does not permit the conclusion that phenylpropanolamine caused these abnormalities. A retrospective study with a similar design did not find an association between phenylpropanolamine use during pregnancy and an increased incidence of birth defects (34). A case-control study of gastroschisis found no association with pregnancy use of phenylpropanolamine; there were 76 affected children in the case group (130).

As noted above, phenylephrine decreases uterine blood flow in sheep (120). Although phenylpropanolamine has not been investigated in this model, the similarity of this drug to phenylephrine makes uterine vasoconstriction a matter of potential concern.

Myocardial injury (131) and intracranial hemorrhage (132,133) have been associated with the use of recommended doses of phenylpropanolamine. One case of intracerebral hemorrhage occurred in a patient 3 weeks after childbirth (133). This patient had used phenylpropanolamine as a dieting aid without incident for an extended period before pregnancy. The hypertensive effects of phenylpropanolamine may be particularly problematic for patients with preexisting hypertension or those using medications that may enhance the effects of phenylpropanolamine, such as monoamine oxidase inhibitors (128). Phenylpropanolamine can produce a rapid increase of diastolic blood pressure at doses not much above recommended therapeutic dose (128,129). In contrast to phenylpropanolamine, pseudoephedrine will not increase blood pressure until more than four times the therapeutic dose is used (128). Because of this more favorable therapeutic index, pseudoephedrine is preferred when a decongestant is recommended during pregnancy.

The use of phenylpropanolamine as a diet aid during pregnancy is inappropriate in the light of clinical observation that it lacks effectiveness for this indication (134), and the recommendation that weight loss not be undertaken during pregnancy.

D. Pseudoephedrine

Pseudoephedrine is a sympathomimetic used as a decongestant. We have not located animal developmental toxicology studies of this compound. There is a case report describing a woman who consumed 480–840 mL per day of a cough syrup that contained pseudoephedrine throughout pregnancy. Daily drug intake from this source was 5 g pseudoephedrine, 16.8 g guaifenesin, 1.68 g dextromethorphan, and 79.8 mL ethanol. The infant had features of fetal alcohol syndrome, and displayed irritability, tremors, and hypertonicity (135). It is difficult to implicate pseudoephedrine as a cause of this child's abnormalities, and available data on this and related sympathomimetic amines do not suggest that they increase the incidence of human congenital anomalies (8,136). A case-control study involving the recall of first-trimester medications found an elevated relative risk (3.2, 95% CI 1.3–7.7) of gastroschisis among users of pseudoephedrine (130). This risk estimate was derived from the reports of medication use of only 9 mothers and involved recall of drug use as long as 14 months previously. The investigators did not determine the possible doses or timing of the use of this or other drugs.

Pseudoephedrine has mixed alpha- and beta-agonist properties. Although the alpha-agonist phenylephrine has been associated with the impairment of uterine blood flow in sheep (120,121), ephedrine, an optical isomer of pseudoephedrine, does not reduce intervillous blood flow (137,138). In women, a single 60-mg dose of pseudoephedrine did not significantly alter maternal blood pressure or blood flow velocities in the uterine or fetal circulation (139).

The dose of pseudoephedrine that will alter blood pressure is about four times the therapeutic dose. This therapeutic index is higher for pseudoephedrine than for other alpha-adrenergic decongestants (128). Pseudo-ephedrine is therefore the preferred decongestant for use during pregnancy.

Use of a long-acting pseudoephedrine (120 mg) for 7 days before a nonstress test was reported in a single case report to be associated with an elevated baseline fetal heart rate of 175–185 beats/min with decreased variability (140). One day after the drug was discontinued, the fetal heart rate was in the normal range. No adverse effects on the outcome of the pregnancy were detected.

Pseudoephedrine is found in breast milk. The milk:plasma ratio for this agent is approximately 2.5, indicating the drug is concentrated in milk (141). Calculations from the available data indicate that a nursing neonate may ingest between 0.6% and 3.0% of the maternal dose (57,141). The use of this drug during lactation has not been associated with adverse effects in exposed newborns. The American Academy of Pediatrics considers pseudoephedrine compatible with breast feeding (56), and the WHO Working Group on human lactation concluded that the occasional use of pseudoephedrine during lactation would probably be safe (57).

E. Epinephrine

Epinephrine (adrenaline) is an endogenous sympathomimetic catecholamine. Direct injection of rat fetuses with $1-50$ μg of epinephrine on day 17 of gestation, which is just prior to term, produced an increase in limb defects (142). Administration of similar doses to rabbit fetuses on days 18–22 (just after midpregnancy) induced hemorrhage, edema, and necrosis of the distal extremities (124). The injection of pregnant mice with epinephrine produced a 14% frequency of cleft palate (143). In the chick embryo, direct application of epinephrine to the chorioallantoic membrane produces a variety of abnormalities, including hemorrhages of the head, skin, and extremities (144) and malformation of the cardiovascular system (145). The latter have been attributed to catecholamine-induced dysrhythmias that are blocked by metoprolol (146). There is concern that epinephrine administration during pregnancy will decrease uterine perfusion. In a pregnant sheep model, a 34.5% reduction in cotyledonary uterine blood flow occurred after a dose of epinephrine that did not alter blood pressure (147). Although uterine perfusion was decreased under these circumstances, the extraction of oxygen per unit of blood increased, resulting in no net decrease in oxygen delivery to the uterus and its contents (148). In pregnant monkeys, administration of epinephrine and norepinephrine produced an increase in uterine muscular activity (although epinephrine also had relaxant effects) and produced uterine vasoconstriction associated with impaired fetal gas exchange (149). The dose of epinephrine used in this study (0.5–20 μg/kg/min for 1–8 min) also resulted in an increase in maternal blood pressure.

Epinephrine crosses the human placenta (150). The National Collaborative Perinatal Project found a significant association between first-trimester exposure to epinephrine and an increased risk of major and minor malformations (8). The only specific malformation associated with epinephrine was inguinal hernia. The fishing expedition nature of this study does not permit the conclusion that epinephrine was causally related to these abnormalities. In a study on 259 pregnant asthmatics who used inhaled beta-sympathomimetics, 180 of whom used these agents during the first trimester, there was no increase in congenital anomalies or adverse perinatal outcome attributable to the therapy (151). Although few of these women used epinephrine (most used metaproterenol), the report is reassuring about agents of this class.

F. Ephedrine

Ephedrine is a sympathomimetic agent used in cold, allergy, and asthma preparations and in the treatment of hypotension after spinal or epidural block. Even small doses produce cardiovascular anomalies in the chick (152). This teratogenic effect was potentiated by caffeine (153), an observation that may be relevant to the presence of theophylline, a related methylxanthine, in some ephedrine-containing asthma medications.

There is a case report of a human abortus with a major congenital heart defect that was exposed at embryo day 30 to ephedrine, theophylline, and phenobarbital (154), but isolated case reports give no information on whether the exposure may have played a role in the identified abnormalities. The National Collaborative Perinatal Project was unable to identify an association between ephedrine exposure in the first trimester and an increase in any kind of birth defect (8). This report included 373 exposed pregnancies. A case-control study of gastroschisis was conducted to evaluate the possible association of this disorder with medications; no such association was found for ephedrine (130).

Ephedrine may be given to treat or avoid hypotension associated with epidural analgesia or with anaphylactic reactions during late pregnancy (137,138,155–157). Administration during labor has been reported to increase fetal heart rate and beat-to-beat variability (158,159); this exposure is not associated with adverse fetal effects (137,138,157,158). Ephedrine does not alter intervillous blood flow (137,138); however, some investigators found an unacceptably high incidence of maternal hypertension when ephedrine was given prophylactically before spinal anesthesia, and a potential for adverse effects on fetal circulation if general anesthesia was also administered (160–162).

There is a single report of a baby with disturbed behavior who was exposed through breast milk to ephedrine and to an antihistamine. The child's symptoms resolved when nursing was discontinued (163). It is not known whether the infant's behavioral problems were due to maternal use of ephedrine.

G. Isoproterenol

Isoproterenol (isoprenaline; Isuprel) is the isopropyl analog of epinephrine. Injection into chick eggs produces cardiomegaly, coronary artery maldevelopment, fatty degeneration of cardiac muscle, ventricular septal defect, aortic arch anomalies, and hypoplasia of right-sided heart structures (164–168). The induction of cardiovascular abnormalities in the chick can be prevented by pretreatment with beta-blocking agents (165–167). Catecholamine-induced alterations in blood flow in the embryonic cardiovascular system may be responsible for isoproterenol-associated developmental abnormalities in the chick (168,169). Isoproterenol also causes hepatotoxicity and limb malformations in a small percentage of chick embryos (170,171).

Teratogenic effects have also been noted after administration of isoproterenol to mice (172) and hamsters (173). Rats and rabbits appear to be less sensitive to malforming effects of this drug, although hemodynamic alterations in pregnant animals and fetuses can be shown in many experimental species (174–181). The National Collaborative Perinatal Project included only 31 women who used this agent during the first trimester. No increase in birth defects was shown (8). In a study on 259 pregnant asthmatics who used inhaled beta-sympathomimetics, 180 of whom used these agents during the first trimester, there was no increase in congenital anomalies or adverse perinatal outcome attributable to the therapy (151). Although few of these women used isoproterenol (most used metaproterenol), the report is reassuring about agents of this class.

Isoproterenol decreases uterine muscle contractility in animals and humans (182–184). This agent is not used to treat preterm labor, however, because side effects in the mother and perhaps the fetus are more problematic than those of more selective beta-agonists such as terbutaline.

H. Metaproterenol

Metaproterenol (orciprenaline), a selective β_2-adrenergic agent, is used orally or by inhalation in the treatment of asthma. It also has been given intravenously to treat premature labor and to decrease uterine contractions in the face of fetal bradycardia during parturition. Teratology experiments in mice, rats, and rhesus monkeys have not associated metaproterenol with teratogenic activity at high doses, although embryotoxicity (skeletal ossification delays) may occur (185,186). In mice, metaproterenol administration to the pregnant animal is associated with an increase in serum corticosterone and consequent induction of cleft palate in the offspring (187). This mechanism of teratogenicity would not be expected to apply to humans. Rabbit studies have produced conflicting results ranging from the induction of multiple defects (186) to no discernable effects on the offspring (188). A third rabbit study examined effects on aortic arch structures, particularly the ductus arteriosus, and found no anomalies attributable to metaproterenol treatment of the doe (176).

A study of 259 women with asthma who used inhaled bronchodilators (primarily metaproterenol) during pregnancy showed no significant increase in the incidence of perinatal mortality, congenital malformations, preterm births, low-birth-weight infants, labor/delivery complications, or postpartum bleeding (151). An increased incidence of maternal hypertension and transient tachypnea of the neonate were observed in the women using inhaled bronchodilators, but these outcomes seemed more clearly associated with the severity of the mother's asthmatic condition than with the use of bronchodilators. A long-term follow-up of infants who were exposed to a related beta-agonist (ritodrine) in utero during the third trimester did not uncover any association with harmful effects (189).

Like other beta-agonists, metaproterenol in sufficient doses will cause a variety of side effects in the mother, including tachycardia, hyperglycemia, nervousness, and tremor (190–192). Similar symptoms also may be found in exposed neonates.

I. Albuterol

Albuterol (salbutamol) is a beta-sympathomimetic used in the treatment of asthma. This agent has also been used to inhibit preterm labor. In one preliminary report, teratogenic effects were found when albuterol was administered to pregnant mice, but similar effects were not found in rats or rabbits (193). Published experience with albuterol in early pregnancy is limited. No abnormalities were found in the offspring of three women who received albuterol continuously, beginning in the second trimester (194–196). In a study on 259 pregnant asthmatics who used inhaled beta-sympathomimetics, 180 of whom used these agents during the first trimester, there was no increase in congenital anomalies or adverse perinatal outcome attributable to the therapy (151). Although few of these women used albuterol (most used metaproterenol), the report is reassuring about agents of this class.

There is a great deal of published experience with the use of albuterol as a tocolytic agent in late pregnancy (197–206). Typically, albuterol increases maternal cyclic-AMP, glycogenolysis, lipolysis, and insulin levels, but decreases serum potassium levels. The overall effects on the circulatory system include an increase in heart rate and a drop in blood pressure. Although these effects are more prominent in the mother, the fetus may show similar responses. By contrast, inhaled albuterol at recommended doses did not appear to affect maternal blood pressure, heart rate, or Doppler flow velocity studies of the uterine and fetal central circulation (207).

In contrast to the use of intravenous albuterol, clinical studies have found that no significant increase in the length of gestation was associated with the chronic oral administration of albuterol (206,208). One newborn with chronic intrauterine exposure to albuterol had a significant elevation of growth hormone levels (209). Long-term adverse effects in the offspring, including alterations in growth, have not been noted with beta-sympathomimetics as a group (189,210–212).

J. Terbutaline

Terbutaline is a sympathomimetic drug with predominantly β_2 activity. In addition to its use for asthma, it is popular for the treatment of preterm labor (210,213–217). According to the manufacturer (Geigy Pharmaceuticals, Ardsley, NY), reproductive studies in rats and rabbits were negative at maternal doses more than 1000 times the recommended human dose. As is the case for sympathomimetic amines in general, terbutaline produces an increase in cardiovascular malformations in chick embryos (218), an effect ameliorated by coadministration of a beta-blocking drug.

Tocolytic doses of terbutaline are associated with maternal and fetal side effects similar to those seen with other agents in this class, including hyperglycemia, cardiovascular complications, reversible uterine atony, non-diabetic ketoacidosis, and pulmonary edema in the gravida, and a reactive postnatal hypoglycemia in the neonate (216,217,219–224). Terbutaline tocolytic therapy may be associated with ketoacidosis and insulin resistance in women with diabetes (225), and with impaired glucose tolerance in nondiabetic pregnant women (226).

Because of its uterine relaxant effect, terbutaline has been used to relieve fetal bradycardia associated with labor (192,227–229). Terbutaline has been demonstrated to preserve or increase uterine blood flow (230–232).

Fetal exposure to terbutaline has been associated with decreased umbilical vascular resistance (233). Concern has been raised that this effect may be associated with a shunting of blood to other vascular beds and may actually decrease placental blood flow, but such concerns have yet to be confirmed. There has been a single case report of tricuspid regurgitation and cardiac failure in an infant born after prolonged subcutaneous terbutaline tocolysis (234). Biopsy of the right ventricle showed myocardial necrosis consistent with catecholamine excess. There is no information on how often such a complication may occur in association with terbutaline therapy during pregnancy.

Terbutaline is excreted in breast milk, and milk:plasma ratios between 1.4 and 2.9 have been reported. Peak milk concentrations were found 4 hr after asthmatic mothers used this drug (235,236). Approximately 0.7% of the maternal dose may be ingested by the suckling neonate (57). No symptoms of adrenergic stimulation have been observed in exposed infants. The WHO Working Group on human lactation (57) and the American Academy of Pediatrics (54) classified terbutaline as compatible with breast feeding.

K. Isoetharine

Isoetharine is a sympathomimetic amine with predominant β_2 activity. We have been unable to locate published references on possible reproductive effects of this agent, but isoetharine has structural and pharmacologic similarity to terbutaline, and reproductive effects of the two agents may also be similar.

L. Biltolterol

Bitolterol is a β_2-adrenergic drug used by inhalation for asthma. Bitolterol is metabolized by lung esterases to colterol, the active bronchodilator. According to the manufacturer (Winthrop, New York, NY), inhalation of radiolabeled bitolterol was followed by detection of small amounts of label in blood and urine, suggesting that colterol or its metabolites are absorbed from the lung. We have not found published studies on reproductive effects of bitolterol. Studies by the manufacturer were reported not to show teratogenicity in rats and rabbits. A small increase in incidence of cleft palate was seen in mice receiving subcutaneous injections of high-dose bitolterol.

M. Pirbuterol

Pirbuterol, a beta-sympathomimetic, is an analog of albuterol. Administration of pirbuterol at 300 mg/kg/day to pregnant rats and rabbits did not result in an increase in birth defects in the offspring (237). The highest dose was associated with fetal growth impairment in the rats and with abortion in some of the rabbits.

N. Salmeterol

Salmeterol is a beta-adrenergic agonist. We have been unable to locate published references on the reproductive effects of this albuterol analog. According to the manufacturer (Allen & Hanburys, Research Triangle Park, NC), this agent did not produce adverse effects on pregnancy outcome in rats exposed to 160 times the human dose on a surface-area basis. In one strain of rabbit, cleft palate and skeletal abnormalities in the offspring were associated with pregnancy exposures greater than 12 times the area-under-the-curve estimates for human therapy. These effects were not seen in a less sensitive strain of rabbit at up to 1600 times the human dose on a surface-area basis and are believed to be due to nonspecific beta-adrenergic effects in the sensitive rabbit strain.

VIII. Mast Cell Stabilizers

A. Cromolyn

Cromolyn is used to prevent bronchospasm by stabilizing mast cells and inhibiting the release of inflammatory mediators. Less than 10% of an inhaled dose of cromolyn is believed to be absorbed systemically (238).

In mice, rats, and rabbits, injections of cromolyn or closely related compounds did not produce fetal malformations (239). The incidence of congenital defects was not significantly elevated in 296 births that included the use of cromolyn during all or part of pregnancy (240). No information was located on the transfer of cromolyn across the placenta or its excretion into breast milk.

B. Nedocromil

Nedocromil is an anti-inflammatory agent and mast cell stabilizer used by inhalation in the treatment of allergy and asthma. No adverse reproductive effects were noted in rats and rabbits given 800 times the human therapeutic dose (241).

IX. Methylxanthines

A. Theophylline

Theophylline is a methylxanthine stimulant that occurs naturally in teas and cocoa. It has a variety of drug uses in its purified form, including bronchodilation. In pregnant mice, theophylline administration produced cleft palate and digit defects (242,243). In rat experiments, however, similar teratogenic effects were not observed (244–246). In mice and rats, the no observable adverse effect level (NOAEL) for developmental toxicity was approximately 10- to 30-fold greater than doses required to maintain clinically useful serum levels of theophylline (246). High doses of theophylline, administered chronically, did produce adverse effects on reproduction in male and female rodents (247), but it is questionable whether data from such high-dose studies are applicable to the human use of this compound. In cultured cells, the induction of sister chromatid exchange and chromosomal breakage were significantly elevated by concentrations of theophylline that correspond to serum levels obtained clinically (248).

Theophylline has been used commonly in the treatment of asthma and chronic obstructive pulmonary disease, and numerous pregnancies have included exposure to this agent without an observable increase in congenital defects (249–252). Also, epidemiologic studies have not found evidence that prenatal theophylline increases the risk of malformations or stillbirth (8,253). A collection of case reports has described three pregnant asthmatics who used theophylline and other drugs throughout gestation and gave birth to offspring with cardiovascular anomalies (254). Case reports are not able to provide information on a possible cause-and-effect relationship between theophylline and adverse pregnancy outcome.

The potential toxicity of theophylline to the mother, fetus, and neonate is of concern in the clinical use of this drug. The volume of distribution of theophylline increases in pregnancy, but the renal clearance of this drug may decrease (255–257). These changes make it difficult to predict how pregnancy may alter the dose requirements of an individual woman. Thus, serum theophylline levels should be used to guide therapy. Theophylline readily crosses the placenta (258–262), and concentrations in the fetus are likely to be equal to or slightly higher than those in the mother (260,261). Theophylline is metabolized to caffeine in the fetal liver (263,264).

Theophylline intoxication, including jitteriness, tachycardia, and vomiting, has been reported in newborns who were exposed prenatally (258,259). Generally, these symptoms have been associated with neonatal blood theophylline levels of more than 10 μg/mL (260,261). Therapeutic levels in adults are often maintained between 8 and 20 μg/mL (262), and it should be anticipated that the newborn will show drug effects if these guidelines for nonpregnant adults are used. In one case, exposure to theophylline throughout gestation resulted in severe apneic spells in a newborn, requiring therapy with theophylline until the spells resolved (260). Because of alterations in protein binding of theophylline during pregnancy, maternal levels of 8–12 μg/mL are likely to be effective and will produce less neonatal toxicity. These lower levels have been recommended by the National Asthma Education Program (265). Theophylline and other methylxanthines can depress lipid synthesis in developing neural systems, raising the concern that theophylline exposure during gestation may induce neurologic deficits in some offspring (266). Normal neurologic development has been reported in infants treated with theophylline for apnea at 9 through 27 months of age (267,268).

Theophylline appears in breast milk (257,269–271). A milk:plasma ratio of 0.73 has been reported (271). Theophylline, administered orally at a dose of 1 mg/kg/day, did not significantly affect the milk volume and composition or the growth of rat pups (272,273). Although less than 1% of the maternal dose of theophylline may be transferred to the neonate (269,270), increased sensitivity to this drug may produce toxic effects in the newborn, including vomiting, feeding difficulties, jitteriness, and cardiac arrhythmias. Some clinicians suggest that breast feeding women nurse their infants just before ingesting their regular dose of theophylline, in order to minimize neonatal exposure to the drug (274).

B. Aminophylline

Aminophylline is a methylxanthine composed of theophylline and ethylenediamine. In pregnant rats, high doses of aminophylline increased the incidence of digit deformities in the offspring (275). Reports on human experience with this drug have not noted a measurable increase in birth defects in exposed pregnancies (8,37). Data from a rabbit model suggest that aminophylline treatment during pregnancy increased fetal pulmonary phospholipids and decreased the incidence of the respiratory distress syndrome of prematurity (276); however, agreement with this conclusion is not universal (277). Improved pulmonary function in preterm rabbits after maternal antepartum treatment with aminophylline has been attributed to accelerated fetal body growth and improved postnatal regulation of breathing rather than to an increase in surfactant phospholipids (278). A comparison between glucocorticoids and aminophylline on the induction of fetal lung maturity in preterm human pregnancy suggested that aminophylline may also be useful for this indication (279).

The smooth muscle relaxant effect of aminophylline extends also to the uterus (280). When tested as a tocolytic agent, aminophylline has been shown to inhibit uterine muscle contractions (281), but not all studies have found it effective (282). Aminophylline crosses the placenta readily, and cord blood levels of the drug are similar to levels in maternal blood (261). Signs of methylxanthine toxicity may occur in the newborn, including jitteriness and a possible withdrawal syndrome (260). Methylxanthines are present in breast milk and may theoretically affect the nursling (271).

X. Anticholinergics

A. Atropine

Atropine is an anticholinergic agent that can be used as a bronchodilator, although systemic side effects from this medication detract from its usefulness. It has been given by oral inhalation for the short-term treatment and prevention of bronchospasm, but atropine formulations for this purpose are no longer available in the United States. Animal experiments have not suggested that atropine readily induces congenital abnormalities. In rats, chicks, or dogs, relatively high doses of atropine did not cause developmental abnormalities (283–285). When atropine was administered to pregnant mice on day 9 of gestation, an increase in skeletal abnormalities was detected, but these may have resulted from the maternal toxicity of the atropine, and not by a selective teratogenic mechanism (286). An attempt to reproduce these findings was not successful (287).

Although atropine readily crosses the human placenta (288,289) and may alter fetal heart rate (290) or inhibit fetal breathing (291), human pregnancy exposure to this drug has not been associated with adverse developmental effects or significant fetotoxicity (8,37). Adverse effects also have not been noted when the drug is given shortly before delivery (292–294).

Although the elimination of atropine is reduced in children below 2 years of age, atropine exposures through breast milk have not been widely associated with neonatal toxicity (295). The American Academy of Pediatrics considers the use of atropine compatible with breast feeding (56).

B. Ipratropium

Ipratropium is *n*-isopropylatropine, a quaternary ammonium anticholinergic used as a bronchodilator. Systemic anticholinergic effects of inhaled ipratropium are infrequent (296). The manufacturer (Boehringer Ingelheim, Ridgefield, CT) has reported negative reproductive studies in mice, rats, and rabbits, and negative teratogenicity studies in rats and rabbits at doses several hundred to several thousand times the recommended human dose. Published teratology studies have also been negative in rats and rabbits (297,298). We have been unable to locate references on possible reproductive effects of this agent in humans; however, the potential for developmental hazard associated with maternal inhalation therapy is believed to be low.

XI. Antibiotics

Various antibiotics are used to treat sinus or pulmonary infections. We will review the major classes of available antibiotics. Whenever possible, commonly used agents with a long history of safe use in pregnancy are preferred to newer agents.

A. Penicillins

Penicillins have been formulated with a variety of substituents added onto the fundamental beta-lactam-thiazolidine nucleus. Benzylpenicillin (penicillin G) and phenoxymethylpenicillin (penicillin V) are two of the oldest and most commonly used derivatives. Ampicillin and amoxicillin are widely used aminopenicillins. High-dose animal experiments in mice, rats, and rabbits did not reveal adverse reproductive effects (299–302). One study reported an increase in limb defects in rats after high-dose maternal treatment with ampicillin (303), but this has not been supported by subsequent reports.

The pharmacokinetics of the penicillins during pregnancy have been studied in detail (304–307), and the placental transfer of these antibiotics has been well characterized (304–308). Penicillins accumulate in amniotic fluid in large amounts during maternal ingestion (306). This is caused by fetal urinary excretion of the antibiotic into the amniotic fluid, which continues until the mother stops ingesting the drug. Thereafter, the fetus gradually reabsorbs the antibiotic (probably by swallowing the amniotic fluid) and clears the drug by passage across the placenta to the mother. No adverse fetal effects have been associated with this process. In general, the use of penicillins during pregnancy has not been shown to measurably increase the incidence of congenital anomalies (8,309), and these agents are regarded as antimicrobials of choice for the treatment of susceptible infections during pregnancy.

All penicillins may produce anaphylaxis during pregnancy or immediately postpartum (310) (see Chapter 12). If anaphylaxis is severe and uncontrolled, it may compromise the placental circulation, and cause fetal damage or death (311).

Penicillins are excreted into breast milk in small amounts (312,313). This exposure is unlikely to have detectable effects in the newborn, but possible alterations in bowel function or abnormal results in tests for an occult infection may occur. Also, this exposure to penicillins may be sufficient to cause allergic sensitization in the infant.

B. Cephalosporins

The cephalosporins are a large group of semisynthetic antibiotics that are structurally and pharmacologically related to penicillins. Cephalosporins are generally divided into three groups based on their spectra of activity. As representative of the first-, second-, and third-generation cephalosporins we will consider cephalexin, cefaclor, and cefixime.

Cephalexin is well absorbed after oral administration and readily crosses the placenta (314,315); cord blood levels after maternal ingestion of the drug at term are about one-third those found in the maternal serum (315). This drug was not teratogenic when tested in rats and mice (316,317). Use of cephalexin during human pregnancy without adverse consequences has been described (314,318–320).

Cefaclor was not teratogenic when tested in rats, mice, rabbits, or ferrets at up to 2 g/kg/day (321–323). We have been unable to locate human studies on reproductive effects of this agent. Cephalexin and cefaclor pass into breast milk in small amounts (324,325). Although breast milk concentrations are low, changes in the bacterial flora of the infant gastrointestinal tract may occur if a mother takes any of these antibiotic while nursing. This is not considered a contraindication to nursing. Although data were not available on the milk levels of these drugs after repeated maternal use, the WHO Working Group on human lactation concluded that the use of cephalexin and cefaclor by nursing mothers is probably safe (57).

Cefixime was evaluated for developmental effects in animal studies performed by the manufacturer (Lederle Laboratories, Wayne, NJ). When given to pregnant mice and rats in doses up to 400 times the human dose, this agent did not produce adverse fetal effects. Also, doses of cefixime up to 125 times the human dose did not impair fertility or the reproductive performance of rats (238). We have not located references on possible human reproductive effects of this agent. Studies in rats indicate that cefixime is capable of crossing the placenta and of entering breast milk; however, the levels found in the offspring after exposure by either route are very low (326).

Cefuroxime was not teratogenic when tested in mice and rabbits (327,328). There is a negative teratology study in the Russian literature, available in abstract only; however, the animal used is not specified (329). In humans, cefuroxime crosses the third-trimester placenta (330–332). Adverse effects have not been reported in association with the clinical use of cefuroxime; however, we have not been able to locate controlled studies on possible human reproductive effects of this agent.

C. Clavulanate

Clavulanate is a beta-lactam that inhibits the activity of bacterial beta-lactamases on coadministered antibiotics, and extends their effectiveness. The administration of clavulanic acid with amoxicillin did not produce teratogenic effects in rats and pigs (333–335). The administration of this combination to 80 women with bacteriuria of pregnancy was not associated with detectable adverse effects in the exposed offspring (320). The principal maternal side effect of amoxicillin-clavulanic acid was vaginal irritation or discharge, which may have been caused by an overgrowth of *Candida* or other opportunistic organisms (320).

In a study using perfused human placental cotyledons, clavulanic acid could not be documented to cross the placenta (336). This was believed by the authors to be due to insensitivity of their assay rather than to lack of placental transfer.

D. Erythromycin

Erythromycin is a macrolide antibiotic. In one rat teratology study, erythromycin increased the incidence of urogenital abnormalities (337). No consistent pattern of defects has been evident in human case reports on newborns exposed in utero to erythromycin (35,338). In the 79 pregnancies with first-trimester exposure to this antibiotic and 230 exposures at any time during pregnancy identified in the National Collaborative Perinatal Project, no relationship to major or minor malformations was identified (8). Although erythromycin does cross the placenta in small quantities (339–341), maternal dosing with this antibiotic has not proven effective in treating fetal infection (342).

The estolate ester of erythromycin has been associated with a relatively high incidence of subclinical, reversible hepatotoxicity when used during pregnancy (343); therefore, the use of other derivatives of erythromycin is preferred.

Erythromycin is found into the breast milk in small quantities (344). This antibiotic was classified as compatible with breast feeding by the American Academy of Pediatrics (56). The WHO Working Group on drugs and human lactation also concluded that the use of this drug for a short (1-week) period during breast feeding is probably safe (57). There was no information on longer-term use.

E. Clarithromycin

Clarithromycin (Biaxin) is 6-*O*-methylerythromycin, a macrolide antibiotic, structurally similar to erythromycin. According to the manufacturer (Abbott, Abbott Park, IL), two studies in one rat strain showed an increase in cardiovascular abnormalities in the offspring after maternal administration of 150 mg/kg/day. Four earlier studies at a higher dose in a different strain of rats had not shown cardiovascular or other congenital abnormalities. In mice, the administration of much higher doses (500 and 1000 mg/kg/day) increased the incidence of cleft palate. In rabbits, the intravenous administration of a dose 17 times less than the maximum human oral daily dose caused an increased incidence of fetal loss. An oral dose of 70 mg/kg/day caused fetal growth retardation in monkeys. At 150 mg/kg/day, maternal toxicity and embryonic loss occurred in monkeys.

The production of defects and fetal loss at these very high doses does not indicate that clarithromycin will necessarily produce adverse pregnancy outcome under clinically relevant conditions; however, the manufacturer's data stand in sharp contrast to the clinical impression of safety of erythromycin. It is possible that clarithromycin is more toxic during development than its parent compound, erythromycin. On the basis of the animal data reported by the manufacturer, clarithromycin has been granted a special product warning label by the U.S. Food and Drug Administration that states it "should not be used in pregnant women except in clinical circumstances where no alternative therapy is appropriate." At present there is an abstract reporting 34 pregnancies exposed to clarithromycin without an apparent increase in adverse outcome (459).

Clarithromycin and its 14-hydroxy-metabolite can be found in human breast milk (345). The manufacturer also reports finding that clarithromycin was excreted in the milk of lactating animals. In the human subjects, the mean peak concentrations of clarithromycin and 14-hydroxy-clarithromycin in breast milk were about 25% and 75%, respectively, of the corresponding serum concentrations. Because of its considerable concentrations in breast milk, clarithromycin was recommended for the treatment of puerperal mastitis. The safety of nursing while using this antibiotic was not investigated.

F. Azithromycin

Azithromycin is a macrolide antibiotic derived from erythromycin. It is concentrated in prostatic tissue and in the female genital tract (346). There are two reports on the use of azithromycin for chlamydia infections in 31 pregnant women, but gestational age at the time of treatment and descriptions of the outcomes of the exposed pregnancies were not mentioned

(347,348). According to the manufacturer (Pfizer Labs, New York, NY), administration to pregnant rats and mice at maternally toxic doses (200 mg/kg/day) did not produce evidence of developmental toxicity.

Azithromycin appears in milk. After ingestions of 500 mg/day, a woman had breast milk levels that increased in time, reaching 2.8 μg/mL (349). The authors of the report concluded that azithromycin accumulates in milk; however, maternal serum levels were not included in the report. The calculated dose to the infant was less than 0.5 mg/day and was not expected to be a clinically significant exposure.

G. Tetracyclines

Tetracyclines are a group of antimicrobials that were commonly used during pregnancy after first being introduced in the 1950s (350), but recognition of their toxicity to bone and staining of developing teeth greatly curtailed their use. Administration of tetracyclines in the second or third trimester of pregnancy was shown to cause staining of the teeth of the child and up to a 40% depression of bone growth, especially of the fibula in preterm pregnancies (351–353). The antimicrobial action of the tetracyclines is produced by selective inhibition of protein synthesis in susceptible organisms.

Animal data on the developmental effects of the tetracyclines have not been consistent. Exposure of gestating rats to tetracycline was shown in one study to result in an increase in cleft palate and limb abnormalities (354); however, three other studies did not find any teratogenic effects of this agent in rats (355–357), and a fourth showed only an increased incidence of hydroureter in exposed animals (12). Oxytetracycline was not teratogenic mice, rats, and rabbits (358,359), but it did produce an increase in congenital defects in dogs (360). There have been a small number of studies suggesting that tetracycline treatment of pregnant rats caused abnormal development of lymphatic and thymic tissues (361,362). This raises the possibility of altered immunoregulation related to antenatal drug exposure. Staining of the cornea and lens of the eye has also been observed in rat fetuses exposed to tetracycline (363), and congenital cataract has been reported in 4 children with antenatal or lactational exposure to tetracyclines (364); however, there are no controlled clinical data to indicate whether there is a causal association between maternal use of tetracycline and congenital eye disease.

The National Collaborative Perinatal Project (8) was not able to identify the tetracyclines as causes of major birth defects. Possible associations with minor defects were suggested; however, the small number of cases (most of which involved inguinal hernia as the only defect) and the exploratory nature of the study do not permit causation to be inferred. Tetracycline given intravenously may result in hepatic necrosis in pregnant women (365,366). Many women reported to have developed this complication had been treated for pyelonephritis, and it is possible that renal impairment is a contributor to this toxic effect. The mobilization of tetracycline from bone during pregnancy has been suggested as a possible toxic mechanism for some cases of fatty liver during pregnancy (367). This scenario would be possible among women who had been treated chronically with tetracycline for dermatologic conditions (357).

Tetracycline is excreted into breast milk in small amounts. The milk: plasma ratios have been reported to range from 0.25 to 1.5 (350,368,369). Serum levels of breast-fed infants exposed to maternal tetracycline in their milk were too low for measurement (350). The American Academy of Pediatrics classified tetracycline as compatible with breast feeding (56). The WHO Working Group on human lactation noted that the risk to the infant appears low when the antibiotic is used for 7–10 days (57). Other antibiotics are preferable for longer periods of therapy during lactation.

H. Sulfamethoxazole

Sulfamethoxazole is a sulfonamide antibacterial that has been administered in combination with trimethoprim in the oral treatment of urinary tract infections, chronic bronchitis, and gonorrhea (370). Much concern regarding the administration of this drug combination in pregnant women has focused on the folate antagonist in the mixture, trimethoprim (see below).

Like other sulfonamides, sulfamethoxazole can cross the placenta in humans (370,371), and shares the potential problems of this class of antimicrobials, including the induction of idiosyncratic sulfa reactions and the displacement of other compounds from plasma proteins. In the fetus and newborn, sulfamethoxazole may theoretically displace bilirubin from plasma-binding sites and may cause kernicterus to develop at lower bilirubin levels. This concern, although theoretical, is the predominant reason for withholding sulfonamide therapy in the third trimester of pregnancy. An increase in human birth defects has not been associated with this group of drugs (8,372–374). The number of human cases studies available for sulfamethoxazole and other sulfonamides is still small, however. Animal data suggest that sulfonamides can increase the incidence of malformations in some species (375,376).

Sulfamethoxazole and other sulfonamides are excreted into breast milk (377,378). Exposure to this group of anti-infectives should be avoided in premature infants and in infants with hyperbilirubinemia or glucose-6-phosphate dehydrogenase deficiency. Except for the preceding conditions, the American Academy of Pediatrics classified various sulfonamides, including the structurally similar compound, sulfisoxazole, as compatible with breast feeding (56).

I. Trimethoprim

Trimethoprim is used as an antimicrobial agent. It is structurally similar to folic acid and is believed to act as a folic acid antagonist. Although trimethoprim is available for use as a single agent, it is commonly administered in combination with a sulfonamide (see above), because together they produce a superior antimicrobial effect. A concern that trimethoprim may limit the availability of folic acid to the fetus and impair normal growth provides the basis for avoiding the use of this drug during pregnancy (379,380).

Trimethoprim is readily transferred across the placenta to the fetus (370,371). During organogenesis in rats, high doses of trimethoprim and sulfamethoxazole caused an increase in cleft palate, micrognathia, and limb shortening (381). Similar doses of sulfamethoxazole alone were not embryotoxic.

There are reports on several hundred woman successfully exposed to trimethoprim during pregnancy (372,373,382–385). In the one exposed infant born with birth defects, the pattern of defects seen—mental and growth retardation and craniofacial malformations—was consistent with the Niikawa-Kuroki syndrome (386). In mice, trimethoprim coadministration increases the incidence of valproic acid-induced neural tube defects (387). The authors of this study recommended that the use of trimethoprim be avoided in epileptic women treated during pregnancy with valproic acid.

Trimethoprim is excreted in breast milk (388,389). No adverse effects have been observed in exposed infants (388), and trimethoprim use has been classified as compatible with breast feeding (56,389).

XII. Expectorants and Antitussives

A. Iodides

Iodine is a nonmetallic halogen element. It is usually encountered as I_2, which is composed of two identical atoms, with no ionic charge. The single, negatively charged ion is termed iodide. Iodine has been used as a disinfectant of drinking water. Various iodide salts have been used as expectorants and as topical antiseptics during pregnancy. Although there is a report indicating that there may be significant differences in the bioavailability of iodine and iodide (390), both species will be considered here interchangeably.

Iodine can be readily transferred to the fetus (391), and chronic maternal exposure to iodine-containing medications has produced hypothyroidism and goiter in offspring (391,392). If large enough, goiter may cause tracheal compression and asphyxiation. A majority of the reported fatalities due to iodine intoxication resulted from the use of iodine-containing expectorants during pregnancy. An analysis of these cases suggested that cardiomegaly may also be associated with excessive iodine exposure during gestation (392). The American Academy of Pediatrics has classified the use of iodide expectorants as contraindicated during pregnancy (393). In contrast, the administration of iodine for several days before maternal thyroid surgery has not been associated with fetal hypothyroidism or goiter (394–396).

Iodine is readily transferred to breast milk (397,398). In one case report, a mother who had used a povidone-iodine vaginal gel for 6 days without douching became concerned when she noted an iodine odor coming from her 7-month-old breastfed baby. Serum and urine iodine levels in the newborn were elevated but no signs of thyroid dysfunction were detected in the baby (388). Based on these observations, the repeated or routine use of iodine-containing products is not recommended during pregnancy or lactation (393,397–401).

B. Guaifenesin

Guaifenesin is used as an expectorant. The FDA Panel on Cough and Cold Products classified this compound as an effective expectorant in patients with chronic bronchitis; however, the small study used as the basis for this classification has not yet been published in a refereed journal (402). Other studies have not produced data that indicate this agent is effective as an expectorant (403,404). Kuhn et al. (404) did not find that guaifenesin significantly reduced cough frequency; it only decreased sputum thickness in the subjective reports made by patients with colds. The dose of guaifenesin used in this study was approximately two times higher than that recommended by the manufacturer (405).

We have not located experimental animal studies on the developmental effects of this agent. Among 197 pregnancies exposed to guaifenesin during the first trimester, the National Collaborative Perinatal Project found an increased incidence of inguinal hernias (8). No significant association was identified in the same study when pregnancy outcomes were evaluated after exposures anytime during gestation. A separate study involving 241 women exposed to guaifenesin during the first trimester did not identify an increase in congenital defects (34).

C. Dextromethorphan

Dextromethorphan is the *d*-isomer of the opioid, levorphanol. It is not active as an analgesic, and retains only the antitussive properties of these agents. It is commonly used in nonprescription cough medicines.

We have not located experimental animal developmental toxicity studies of dextromethorphan. The National Collaborative Perinatal Project identified 300 women who had used dextromethorphan during the first 4 months of pregnancy. No detectable increase in anomalies was identified in this population (8). A cohort study involving 59 women who used dextromethorphan during the first trimester did not find an association with congenital defects (34).

D. Codeine

Codeine is a narcotic analgesic that is widely used as an antitussive. Codeine administration to pregnant hamsters and mice has been associated with skeletal abnormalities, but this may be related to the narcotic effects of this agent and altered food intake (406,407). A more recent study did not find a significant increase in anomalies in the offspring of treated hamsters and mice; rather, developmental toxicity was manifest as a decrease in fetal body weight, occurring at 10 mg/kg/day in the hamsters, which was the more sensitive species (408). No increase in congenital anomalies was shown when codeine was administered to pregnant rats or rabbits (409). At the top dose in the rat study (120 mg/kg/day), maternal toxicity occurred and was associated with reduced fetal weight and increased resorptions. The top dose in the rabbit study (30 mg/kg/day) did not produce adverse effects on the pregnant animals or the offspring.

In a case-control study of 141 infants with cardiac malformations, no association with first-trimester use of codeine was uncovered (410). In retrospective studies of human pregnancies that included first-trimester use of codeine, a variety of anomalies has been identified, including respiratory tract malformation, pyloric stenosis, inguinal hernia, cardiac and circulatory system defects, and cleft lip and palate (8,125,411,412). The lack of a consistent pattern of defects argues against a causative relation to the drug exposure.

In women who have regularly taken codeine-containing medications in the days prior to delivery, some exposed neonates have manifested codeine withdrawal, characterized by tremor, jitteriness, diarrhea, and poor feeding (413,414). If administered during labor, codeine can produce respiratory depression in the newborn, which can be treated with naloxone.

Small amounts of codeine and its metabolite, morphine, are transferred to breast milk (415,416). If maternal dose is less than 240 mg/day, the quantity of these compounds ingested by a suckling infant is probably so low that breast feeding is not contraindicated (56,416).

XIII. Desensitization ("Allergy Shots")

Allergy shots desensitize by exposing susceptible subjects to small doses of allergens. Most of these allergens are environmental, and it may be assumed that all pregnant women are exposed to many such allergens. No specific allergens have been shown to be causes of abnormal pregnancy outcome in humans. Published studies have not demonstrated an increase in the incidence of birth defects in women receiving allergy shots (33,417–422). Desensitization to a penicillin allergy has been used successfully during pregnancy to permit the use of this drug for the treatment of syphilis (423).

A possible complication of desensitization regimens is anaphylaxis, which, when severe, can be associated with hypotension and decreased uterine perfusion (see Chapter 12). For this reason, some allergists prefer not to institute or increase desensitization programs during pregnancy.

XIV. Influenza Vaccine

Influenza is a respiratory tract infection caused by a variety of myxoviruses. The influenza vaccine contains inactivated virus. One case report describes a baby born with severe brain abnormalities after a pregnancy in which the mother was vaccinated at 6 weeks postconception (424). The authors believed that the timing of vaccination might implicate it in the development of the brain abnormalities. There have been two studies that include, in total, 245 women vaccinated just before or during pregnancy. No adverse outcomes were attributable to the vaccine (425,426). The Advisory Committee on Immunization Practices of the Centers for Disease Control classified this vaccine as safe to administer during pregnancy to women with medical conditions that increase their risk of complications from influenza (427,428). The American College of Obstetricians and Gynecologists supports this recommendation (429).

XV. Analgesics/Antipyretics

Many OTC "cold" medications contain an analgesic such as aspirin, ibuprofen, or acetaminophen (paracetamol). Of these agents, acetaminophen is considered the analgesic/antipyretic of choice for use during pregnancy. Like aspirin and ibuprofen, acetaminophen appears to produce its analgesic and antipyretic effects by inhibiting prostaglandin synthesis in the central nervous system. Acetaminophen and its metabolites cause genotoxic effects in several test systems (430,431). An increased incidence of sister-chromatid exchanges and chromatid breaks were found in peripheral lymphocytes of human subjects (432). Among the proposed mechanisms for these genotoxic effects are the binding of acetaminophen to DNA or the inhibition of replicative DNA synthesis (433). Human lymphocytes may be uniquely sensitive to the effects of acetaminophen (432), and it is not clear at this time that these data have any clinical relevance. This drug did not increase developmental abnormalities in mice or rats (434–436).

As would be expected, there are a sizeable number of human case reports of malformed babies being born after use of this widely available analgesic (437,438–442). Many of these cases also include exposures to a large number of other agents. In addition, the lack of uniformity of abnormalities among these cases make less likely their association with a single causative agent. The National Collaborative Perinatal Project did not find an association between use of acetaminophen during pregnancy and increased risk of congenital anomalies (8). A retrospective study on congenital heart disease did not find an association between this group of abnormalities and maternal acetaminophen use during pregnancy (126). No significant increase in malformations was identified in 697 women who had first-trimester exposure to acetaminophen, with and without codeine (34). A case-control surveillance program focused on first-trimester drug use and gastroschisis reported a "nonsignificant elevation" of relative risk [RR = 1.7; 95% CI (1.0–2.9)] for pregnancies including acetaminophen use (130).

There has been concern about the possible embryotoxicity of acetaminophen. In one case report, a continuous, high-dose regimen of acetaminophen was associated with severe maternal anemia and fatal kidney disease in the newborn (443). Although hepatotoxicity of this drug appears to be less in young animals than in adults (444), there has been at least one case report of a human stillbirth with evidence of hepatotoxicity after maternal ingestion of 30 g of acetaminophen in a 24-hr period (445). Cases of acetaminophen overdose during pregnancy with normal outcomes for the offspring have also been reported (446–451,460).

The observation that other prostaglandin synthetase inhibitors have been associated with neonatal hemorrhage, inhibition of labor, and premature closure of the ductus arteriosus has raised concern about the use of acetaminophen therapy near term. However, these complications have not been documented in human pregnancies exposed to acetaminophen.

Table 2 Drugs for Asthma and
Associated Conditions Preferred for Use
During Pregnancy

Class	Specific drug
Anti-inflammatory	Cromolyn
	Beclomethasone
	Prednisone
Bronchodilator	Inhaled β_2-agonist
	Theophylline
Antihistamine	Chlorpheniramine
	Tripelennamine
Decongestant	Pseudoephedrine
	Oxymetazoline
Cough	Guaifenesin
	Dextromethorphan
Antibiotics	Amoxicillin

One study on neonatal intracranial hemorrhage found a significant association with maternal aspirin use but not with use of acetaminophen (452). Studies in rats (453) and in sheep (454) have demonstrated that acetaminophen, like aspirin, can be associated with premature closure of the ductus arteriosus.

One small study on the use of acetaminophen for pain relief during interruption of pregnancy with mifepristone and the prostaglandin sulprostone found that multiparous women given acetaminophen reported more intense pain than the placebo group (455). The investigators suggested that acetaminophen be included with the existing contraindication of nonsteroidal anti-inflammatory drugs during this form of pregnancy termination.

Acetaminophen is excreted in breast milk in small amounts (456,457). Available estimates suggest that a suckling infant would ingest a maximum of 4% of the weight-adjusted maternal dose, which corresponds to about 4% of the single therapeutic dose that is used in infants (57). In one case report, a 2-month-old infant whose mother was receiving acetaminophen repeatedly developed a rash when her mother was challenged with acetaminophen (458). No similar reports of adverse effects in exposed infants were located. The WHO Working Group on drugs and human lactation concluded that the use of this drug during breast feeding is safe (57).

XVI. Summary

The importance of adequate therapy of serious illness during pregnancy makes it necessary to use available experimental animal and human data to make a determination of the acceptability of particular medications. Proof that a medication is 100% without risk of adverse effect is not practical or necessary during pregnancy any more than it is in other clinical settings. Based on the data available for the agents presented in this chapter, the National Asthma Education Program Working Group on Asthma and Pregnancy (265) has recommended certain drugs as "preferred" for use during pregnancy (Table 2). Pharmacologic management of specific allergic and immunologic illnesses during pregnancy is discussed elsewhere in this volume.

References

1. Czeizel A, Racz J. Evaluation of drug intake during pregnancy in the Hungarian Case-Control Surveillance of Congenital Anomalies. Teratology 1990; 42:505–512.
2. Scialli AR. A Clinical Guide to Reproductive and Developmental Toxicology. Boca Raton, FL: CRC Press, 1992.
3. German J, Kowal A, Ehlers KH. Trimethadione and human teratogenesis. Teratology 1980; 3:349–362.
4. Lenz W. Thalidomide and congenital abnormalities. Lancet 1962; 1:271.
5. McBride WG. Thalidomide and congenital abnormalities. Lancet 1961; 2: 1358.
6. Lenz W. Discussion. In: Robson JM, Sullivan SM, Smith RL, eds. Embryopathic Activity of Drugs. Boston: Little, Brown, 1965:182–185.
7. Lione A. The use of available data sets to define the safety of occupational chemical exposures during pregnancy. Semin Perniat 1993; 17:28–36.
8. Heinonen OP, Slone D, Shapiro S. Birth Defects and Drugs in Pregnancy. Littleton, MA: Publishing Sciences Group, 1977.
9. Lowe ER. The antihistamine properties of Benadryl, beta-dimethylaminoethyl benzhydryl ether hydrochlorides. J Pharmacol Exp Ther 1946; 86:229–238.
10. Naranjo P, Naranjo E. Embryotoxic effects of antihistamines. Arzneim Forsch 1968; 18:188–195.
11. Schardein JL, Hentz DL, Petrere JA, Kurtz SM. Teratogenesis studies with diphenhydramine HCl. Toxicol Appl Pharmacol 1971; 18:971–976.
12. McColl JD, Globus M, Robinson S. Effect of some therapeutic agents on the developing rat fetus. Toxicol Appl Pharmacol 1965; 7:409–417.

13. Maruyama H, Yoshida S. Pharmacology of a new antihistamine, carbinoxamine diphenyldisulfonate. 2. Toxicity and influences on fetuses. J Med Soc Toho Univ 1968; 15:367–374.

14. King CTG, Weaver SA, Narrod SA. Antihistamines and teratogenicity in the rat. J Pharmacol Exp Ther 1965; 147:391–398.

15. Gibson JP, Staples RE, Larson EJ, et al. Teratology and reproduction studies with an antinauseant. Toxicol Appl Pharmacol 1968; 13:439–447.

16. Tyl RW, Price CJ, Marr MC, Kimmel CA. Developmental toxicity evaluation of Bendectin in CD rats. Teratology 1988; 37:539–552.

17. Bovet-Nitti F, Bignami G, Bovet D. Antihistamine drugs on rat pregnancy: effects of pyrilamine and meclizine. Life Sci 1963; 2:303–310.

18. Driscoll CD, Meyer LS, Riley EP. Behavioral and developmental effects of prenatal exposure to pentazocine and tripelennamine combinations. Neurobehav Toxicol Teratol 1986; 8:605–613.

19. Gibson JP, Staples RE, Larson EJ, Kuhn WL, Holtkamp DE, Newberne JW. Teratology and reproduction studies with an antinauseant. Toxicol Appl Pharmacol 1968; 13:439–447.

20. Chow SA, Fischer LJ. Alterations in rat pancreatic B-cell function induced by prenatal exposure to cyproheptadine. Diabetes 1984; 33:572–575.

21. Chow SA, Fischer LJ. Susceptibility of fetal rat endocrine pancreas to the diabetogenic action of cyproheptadine. Toxicol Appl Pharmacol 1986; 84: 264–277.

22. de la Fuente M, Alia M. The teratogenicity in two generations of Wistar rats. Arch Int Pharmacodyn Ther 1982; 257:168–176.

23. Druga A, Nyitray M, Magyar B. Teratogenicity of cyproheptadine chlorhydrate and possible mode of action in Wistar rats. Teratology 1988; 38:17A.

24. Robbiano L, Gazzaniga GM, Martelli A, Pino A, Brambilla G. DNA-damaging activity of tripelennamine in primary cultures of human hepatocytes. Mutat Res 1986; 173:229–232.

25. Turner NT, Woolley JL Jr, Hozier JC, Sawyer JR, Clive D. Methapyrilene is a genotoxic carcinogen: studies on methapyrilene and pyrilamine in the L5178Y/TK +/− mouse lymphoma assay. Mutat Res 1987; 189:285–297.

26. Lijinsky W, Yamashita K. Lack of binding of methapyrilene and similar antihistamines to rat liver DNA examined by 32P postlabeling. Cancer Res 1988; 48:6475–6477.

27. Ashby J, Callander RD, Paton D, Zeiger E, Ratpan F. Weak and unexpected mutagenicity to *Salmonella* of the rat hepatocarcinogen methapyrilene. Environ Mol Mutagen 1988; 12:243–252.

28. Hernandez L, Allen PT, Poirier LA, Lijinsky W. S-adenosylmethionine, S-adenosylhomocysteine and DNA analogs. Carcinogenesis 1989; 10:557–562.

29. Steinmetz KL, Tyson CK, Meierhenry EF, Spalding JW, Mirsalis JC. Examination of genotoxicity, toxicity and morphologic alterations in hepatocytes following in vivo or in vitro exposure to methapyrilene. Carcinogenesis 1988; 9:959–963.

30. Kammerer RC, Froines JR, Price T: Mutagenicity studies of selected antihistamines, their metabolites and products of nitrosation. Food Chem Toxicol 1986; 24:981–985.

31. Casciano DA, Schol HM. Methapyrilene is inactive in the hepatocyte-mediated Chinese hamster ovary/hypoxanthine-guanine phosphoribosyl transferase mutation assay. Cancer Lett 1984; 21:337–341.

32. Iype PT, Ray-Chaudhuri R, Lijinsky W, Kelley SP. Inability of methapyrilene to induce sister chromatid exchanges in vitro and in vivo. Cancer Res 1982; 42:4614–4618.

33. Hucker HB, Balleto AJ, Stauffer SC, Zacchei AG, Arison BH. Physiological disposition and urinary metabolites of cyproheptadine in the dog, rat and cat. Drug Metab Dispos 1974; 2:406–415.

34. Aselton P, Jick H, Milunsky A, Hunter JR, Stergachis A. First-trimester drug use and congenital disorders. Obstet Gynecol 1985; 65:451–455.

35. Jaffe P, Liberman MM, McFayden I, Valman HB. Incidence of congenital limb-reduction deformities. Lancet 1975; 1:526–527.

36. Zierler S, Purohit D. Prenatal antihistamine exposure and retrolental fibroplasia. Am J Epidemiol 1986; 123:192–196.

37. Mellin GW. Drugs in the first trimester of pregnancy and the fetal life of *Homo sapiens*. Am J Obstet Gynecol 1964; 90:1169–1180.

38. Eskenazi B, Bracken MB: Re: Pyloric stenosis and maternal antihistamine exposure at Group Health Cooperative. Am J Epidemiol 1985; 122:196–197.

39. Aselton P, Jick H. Re: Pyloric stenosis and maternal antihistamine exposure at Group Health Cooperative. Am J Epidemiol 1985; 122:197.

40. Saxén I. Cleft palate and maternal diphenhydramine intake. Lancet 1974; 1: 407–408.

41. Nelson MM, Forfar JO. Associations between drugs administered during pregnancy and congenital abnormalities of the fetus. Br Med J 1971; 1: 523–527.

42. Parkin DE. Probable Benadryl withdrawal manifestations in a newborn infant. J Pediatr 1974; 85:580.

43. Rurak D, Yoo S, Kwan E, Taylor S, et al. Effects of diphenhydramine in the fetal lamb after maternal or fetal administration. J Pharmacol Exp Ther 1988; 247:271–278.

44. Reviriego J, Fernandez-Alfonso M, Marin J. Actions of vasoactive drugs on human placental vascular smooth muscle. Gen Pharmac 1990; 21:719–727.

45. Zsigmond EK, Paterson RL. Double-blind evaluation of hydroxyzine hydrochloride in obstetric anesthesia. Anesth Analg 1967; 46:275.

46. Petrie RH, Yeh S, Murata Y, Paul RH, Hon EH, Barron BA, Johnson RJ. The effect of drugs on fetal heart rate variability. Am J Obstet Gynecol 1978; 130:294–299.

47. Prenner BM. Neonatal withdrawal syndrome associated with hydroxyzine hydrochloride. Am J Dis Child 1977; 131:529.

48. Crawford JS, as quoted by Moya F, Thorndike V. The effects of drugs used in labor on the fetus and newborn. Clin Pharmacol Ther 1963; 4:628–653.

49. Powe CE, Kiem IM, Fromhagen C, Cavanagh D. Propiomazine hydrochloride in obstetrical analgesia. JAMA 1962; 181:290–294.
50. Potts CR, Ullery JC. Maternal and fetal effects of obstetric analgesia. Am J Obstet Gynecol 1961; 81:1252–1259.
51. Carroll JJ, Moir RS. Use of promethazine (Phenergan) hydrochloride in obstetrics. JAMA 1958; 168:2218–2224.
52. Kahn A, Hasaerts D, Blum D. Phenothiazine-induced sleep apneas in normal infants. Pediatrics 1985; 75:844–847.
53. Hall PF. Use of promethazine (Phenergan) in labour. Can Med Assoc J 1987; 136:690–691.
54. Corby DG, Shulman I. The effects of antenatal drug administration on aggregation of platelets of newborn infants. J Pediatr 1971; 79:307–313.
55. Whaun JM, Smith GR, Sochor VA. Effect of prenatal drug administration on maternal and neonatal platelet aggregation and PF4 release. Haemostasis 1980; 9:226–237.
56. Committee on Drugs, American Academy of Pediatrics. The transfer of drugs and other chemicals into human breast milk. Pediatrics 1994; 93:137–150.
57. Bennet PN, ed. Drugs and Human Lactation. Amsterdam: Elsevier, 1988.
58. American Hospital Formulary Service: Antihistamines. In: McEvoy GK, ed. Drug Information 94. Bethesda, MD: American Society of Hospital Pharmacists, 1994:5.
59. Lucas BD Jr, Purdy CY, Scarim SK, Benjamin S, Abel SR, Hilleman DE. Terfenadine pharmacokinetics in breast milk in lactating women. Clin Pharmacol Ther 1995; 57:398–402.
60. Walker BE. Cleft palate produced in mice by human-equivalent dosage with triamcinolone. Science 1965; 149:862–863.
61. Walker BE. Induction of cleft palate in rabbits by several glucocorticoids. Proc Soc Exp Biol Med 1967; 125:1281–1284.
62. Walker B. Induction of cleft palate in rats with antiinflammatory drugs. Teratology 1971; 4:39–42.
63. Pinsky L, DiGeorge AM. Cleft palate in the mouse: a teratogenic index of glucocorticoid potency. Science 1965; 147:402–403.
64. Shah RM, Kilistoff A. Cleft palate induction in hamster fetuses by glucocorticoid hormones and their synthetic analogues. J Embryol Exp Morphol 1976; 36:101–108.
65. Baxter H, Fraser FC. Production of congenital defects in offspring of female mice treated with cortisone. McGill Med J 1950; 19:245–249.
66. Buresh JJ, Urban TJ. The teratogenic effect of the steroid nucleus in the rat. J Dent Res 1970; 43:548–554.
67. Fainstat T. Cortisone induced cleft palate in rabbits. Endocrinology 1954; 55:502–508.
68. Wilson JG, Fradkin R, Schumacher HJ. Influence of drug pretreatment on the effectiveness of known teratogenic agents. Teratology 1970; 3:210–211.

69. Esaki K, Izumiyama K, Yasuda R. Effects of inhalant administration of beclomethasone diproprionate on reproduction in mice. CIEA Preclin Rep 1976; 2:213–222.
70. Oguru Y, Kiyohara A, Miyagawa A, Imamura S, Koyama K, Hara T. Pharmacologic and toxicologic studies on beclomethasone diproprionate. Yamaguchi Igaku 1970; 19:65–86.
71. Yamada T, Nakano M, Ichihashi T. Fetal concentration after topical application of betamethasone 17,21-diproprionate (S-3440) ointment and teratogenesis in mice and rabbits. Oyo Yakuri (Pharmacometrics) 1981; 21: 645–655.
72. Mosier HD, Dearden LC, Jansons RA, Roberts RC. Disproportionate growth of organs and body weight following glucocorticoid treatment of the rat fetus. Dev Pharmacol Ther 1982; 4:89–105.
73. Ishimura K, Honda Y, Neda K, Ishikawa I, et al. Teratological studies on betamethasone 17-benzoate (MS-1112) II. Teratogenicity test in rabbits. Oyo Yakuri 1975; 10:685–694.
74. Fisher CJ, Sawyer RH. A comparison of hydrocortisone and triamcinolone inhibition of scale and feather development. Teratology 1986; 33:37–45.
75. Larsson KS. Studies on the closure of the secondary palate. IV. Autoradiographic and histochemical studies of mouse embryos from cortisone-treated mothers. Acta Morphol Neurol Scand 1962; 4:369–386.
76. Hendrickx AG, Sawyer RH, Terrell TG, Osburn BI, Henrickson RV, Steffek AL. Teratogenic effects of triamcinolone on the skeletal and lymphoid systems in nonhuman primates. Fed Proc 1975; 34:1661–1665.
77. Hendrickx AG, Pellegrini M, Tarara R, Parker R, Silverman S, Steffek AJ. Craniofacial and central nervous system malformations induced by triamcinolone acetonide in non-human primates. 1. General teratogenicity. Teratology 1980; 22:103–114.
78. Parker RM, Hendrickx AG. Craniofacial and central nervous system malformations induced by triamcinolone acetonide in nonhuman primates. 2. Craniofacial pathogenesis. Teratology 1983; 28:35–44.
79. Tarara RP, Cordy DR, Hendrickx AG. Central nervous system malformations induced by triamcinolone acetonide in nonhuman primates: pathology. Teratology 1989; 39:75–84.
80. Jerome CP, Hendrickx AG. Comparative teratogenicity of triamcinolone acetonide and dexamethasone in the Rhesus monkey (*Macaca mulatta*). J Med Primatol 1988; 17:195–203.
81. Hendrickx AG, Tarara RP. Triamcinolone acetonide-induced meningocele and meningoencephalocele in rhesus monkeys. Am J Pathol 1990; 136: 725–727.
82. Fine LG. Systemic lupus erythematosus in pregnancy. Ann Intern Med 1981; 94:667–677.
83. Greenberger PA, Patterson R. Beclomethasone diproprionate for severe asthma during pregnancy. Ann Intern Med 1983; 98:478–480.

84. Fitzsimons R, Greenberger PA, Patterson R. Outcome of pregnancy in women requiring corticosteroids for severe asthma. J Allergy Clin Immunol 1986; 78:349–353.

85. Yackel DB, Kempers RD, McConahey WM. Adrenocorticosteroid therapy in pregnancy. Am J Obstet Gynecol 1966; 96:985–989.

86. Walsh SD, Clark FR. Pregnancy in patients on long-term corticosteroid therapy. Scot Med J 1967; 12:302–306.

87. Cargnino P, Morelli P, Gouvernet P, Arnaud A, Charpin J. [Risks of prolonged corticotherapy during pregnancy]. Mars Med J 1971; 108:661–663.

88. Richards IDG. A retrospective enquiry into possible teratogenic effects of drugs in pregnancy. In: Klingberg MA, Abramovici A, Chemke J, eds. Drugs and Fetal Development. New York: Plenum Press, 1972:441–455.

89. Schatz M, Patterson R, Zeitz S, O'Rourke J, Melam H. Corticosteroid therapy for the pregnant asthmatic patient. JAMA 1975; 234:804–807.

90. Kullander S, Källén B. A prospective study of drugs and pregnancy. 3. Hormones. Acta Obstet Gynecol Scand 1976; 55:221–224.

91. Ricke PS, Elliott JP, Freeman RK. Use of corticosteroids in pregnancy-induced hypertension. Obstet Gynecol 1980; 55:206–210.

92. Katsumata M, Gupta C, Goldman AS. Glucocorticoid receptor IB: mediator of anti-inflammatory and teratogenic functions of both glucocorticoids and phenytoin. Arch Biochem Biophys 1985;243:385–395.

93. Schardein JL. Chemically induced birth defects. New York: Marcel Dekker, 1993:310–311.

94. Kraus AM. Congenital cataract and maternal steroid ingestion. J Pediatr Ophthalmol 1975; 12:107.

95. Cote CJ, Meuwissen HJ, Pickering RJ. Effects on the neonate of prednisone and azathioprine administered to the mother during pregnancy. J Pediatr 1974; 85:324–328.

96. Cederqvist LL, Merkatz IR, Litwin SD. Fetal immunoglobin synthesis following maternal immunosuppression. Am J Obstet Gynecol 1977; 129:687–690.

97. Reinisch JM, Simon NG, Karow WG, Gandelman R. Prenatal exposure to prednisone in humans and animals retards intrauterine growth. Science 1978; 202:436–438.

98. Scott JR. Fetal growth retardation associated with maternal administration of immunosuppressive drugs. Am J Obstet Gynecol 1977; 128:668–676.

99. Pirson Y, Van Lierde M, Ghysen J, et al. Retardation of fetal growth in patients receiving immunosuppressive therapy. N Engl J Med 1985; 313:328.

100. Katz VL, Thorpe M Jr, Bowes WA Jr. Severe symmetric intrauterine growth retardation associated with the topical use of triamcinolone. Am J Obstet Gynecol 1990; 162:396–397.

101. NIH Consensus Development Panel. Effect of corticosteroids for fetal maturation on perinatal outcomes. JAMA 1995; 273:413–418.

102. Sumi SM, Truog WE 3d, Kessler DM. Maternal corticosteroid therapy and the fetal brain in experimental hyaline membrane disease. Pediatr Res 1984; 18:440–444.

103. Morales WJ, O'Brien WF, Angel JL, Knuppel RA, Sawai S. Fetal lung maturation: the combined use of corticosteroids and thyrotropin-releasing hormone. Obstet Gynecol 1989; 73:111–116.

104. Collaborative Group on Antenatal Steroid Therapy. Effects of antenatal dexamethasone administration on the infant: long-term follow-up. J Pediatr 1984; 104:259–267.

105. Avery ME. The argument for prenatal administration of dexamethasone to prevent respiratory distress syndrome. J Pediatr 1984; 104:240.

106. Schmidt PL, Sims ME, Strassner HT, et al. Effect of antepartum glucocorticoid administration upon neonatal respiratory distress syndrome and perinatal infection. Am J Obstet Gynecol 1984; 148:1781–1786.

107. Benesova O, Pavlik A. Perinatal treatment with glucocorticoids and the risk of maldevelopment of the brain. Neuropharmacology 1989; 28:89–97.

108. Collaborative Dexamethasone Trial Group. Dexamethasone therapy in neonatal chronic lung disease: an international placebo-controlled trial. Pediatrics 1991; 88:421–427.

109. Greenough A, Emery EF, Gamsu HR. Dexamethasone and hypertension in preterm infants. Eur J Pediatr 1992; 151:134–135.

110. Ehrenkranz RA. Steroids, chronic lung disease, and retinopathy of prematurity. Pediatrics 1992; 90:646–647.

111. Batton DG, Roberts C, Trese M, Maisels MJ. Severe retinopathy of prematurity and steroid exposure. Pediatrics 1992; 90:534–536.

112. Ng PC, Brownlee KG, Dear PR. Gastroduodenal perforation in preterm babies treated with dexamethasone for bronchopulmonary dysplasia. Arch Dis Child 1991; 66:1164–1166.

113. Wasserstrum N, Huhta JC, Mari G, et al. Betamethasone and the human fetal ductus arteriosus. Obstet Gynecol 1989; 74:897–900.

114. Katz FH, Duncan BR. Entry of prednisone into human milk. N Engl J Med 1975; 293:1154.

115. McKenzie SA, Selley JA, Agnew JE. Secretion of prednisolone into breast milk. Arch Dis Child 1975; 50:894–896.

116. Ost L, Wettrell G, Bjorkhem I, Rane A. Prednisolone excretion in human milk. J Pediatr 1985; 106:1008–1011.

117. Glazener F, Blake K, Gradman M. Bradycardia, hypotension, and near-syncope associated with Afrin (oxymetazoline) nasal spray. New Engl J Med 1983; 309:731.

118. Soderman P, Sahlberg D, Wiholm BE. CNS reactions to nose drops in small children. Lancet 1984; 1:573.

119. Smith NT, Corbascio AN. The use and misuse of pressor agents. Anesthesiology 1970; 33:58–101.

120. Cottle MKW, Van Petten GR, van Muyden P. Effects of pheylephrine and sodium salicylate on maternal and fetal cardiovascular indices and blood oxygenation in sheep. Am J Obstet Gynecol 1982; 143:170–176.

121. Magness RR, Rosenfeld CR. Systemic and uterine responses to alpha-adrenergic stimulation in pregnant and nonpregnant ewes. Am J Obstet Gynecol 1986; 155:897–904.

122. Rayburn WF, Anderson JC, Smith CV, Appel LL, Davis SA. Uterine and fetal Doppler flow changes from a single dose of a long-acting intranasal decongestant. Obstet Gynecol 1990; 76:180–182.

123. Baxi LV, Gindoff PR, Pregenzer, Parras MK. Fetal heart rate changes following maternal administration of a nasal decongestant. Am J Obstet Gynecol 1985; 153:799–800.

124. Gatling RR. The effect of sympathomimetic agents on the chick embryo. Am J Pathol 1962; 40:113–127.

125. Rothman KJ, Fyler DC, Goldblatt A, Kreidberg MB. Exogenous hormones and other drug exposures of children with congenital heart disease. Am J Epidemiol 1979; 109:433–439.

126. Zierler S, Rothman KJ. Congenital heart disease in relation to maternal use of Bendectin and other drugs in early pregnancy. N Engl J Med 1985; 313: 347–352.

127. McLaughlin MK, Keve TM, Cooke R. Vascular catecholamine sensitivity during pregnancy in the ewe. Am J Obstet Gynecol 1989; 160:47–53.

128. Pental P. Toxicity of over-the-counter stimulants. JAMA 1984; 252: 1898–1903.

129. Horowitz JD, Lang WJ, Howes LG, et al. Hypertensive responses induced by phenylpropanolamine in anorectic and decongestant preparations. Lancet 1980; 1:60–61.

130. Werler MM, Mitchell AA, Shapiro S. First trimester maternal medication use in relation to gastroschisis. Teratology 1992; 45:361–367.

131. Pentel PR, Mikel FL, Zavoral JH. Myocardial injury after phenylpropanolamine ingestion. Br Heart J 1982; 47:51–54.

132. Kase CS, Foster TE, Reed JE, Spatz EL, Girgis GN. Intracerebral hemorrhage and phenylpropanolamine use. Neurology 1987; 37:399–404.

133. Maher LM. Postpartum intracranial hemorrhage and phenylpropanolamine use. Neurology 1987; 37:1686.

134. Anonymous. Phenylpropanolamine for weight reduction. Med Lett 1984; 26: 55–56.

135. Chasnoff IJ, Diggs G. Fetal alcohol effects and maternal cough syrup abuse. Am J Dis Child 1981; 135:968.

136. Nishimura K, Tanimura T. Clinical Aspect of the Teratogenicity of Drugs. New York: Elsevier Excerpta Medica, 1976.

137. Hollmen AI, Jouppila R, Albright GA, Jouppila P, Vierola H, Koivula A. Intervillous blood flow during caesarean section with prophylactic ephedrine and epidural anaesthesia. Acta Anaesth Scand 1984; 28:396–400.

138. Hollmen AI, Jouppila R, Jouppila P. Regional anaesthesia and uterine blood flow. Ann Chir Gynaecol 1984; 73:149–152.

139. Smith CV, Rauburn WF, Anderson JC, Duckworth AF, Appel LL. Effect of a single dose of oral pseudoephedrine on uterine and fetal doppler blood flow. Obstet Gynecol 1990; 76:803–806.

140. Anastasio GD, Harston PR. Fetal tachycardia associated with maternal use of pseudoephedrine, an over-the-counter oral decongestant. J Am Board Fam Pract 1992; 5:527–528.

141. Findlay JWA, Butz RF, Sailstad JM, Warren JT, Welch RM. Pseudoephedrine and triprolidine in plasma and breast milk of nursing mothers. Br J Clin Pharmacol 1984; 18:901–906.

142. Jost A. Degénerescence des extremités du foetus de rat provoquée par l'adrenaline. CR Acad Sci (Paris) 1953; 236:1510–1512.

143. Loevy H, Roth BF. Induced cleft palate development in mice: comparison between the effect of epinephrine and cortisone. Anat Rec 1968; 160:386.

144. Gatling RR. The effect of sympathomimetic agents on the chick embryo. Am J Pathol 1962; 40:113–127.

145. Hodach RJ, Gilbert EF, Fallon FJ. Aortic arch anomalies associated with administration of epinephrine in chick embryos. Teratology 1974; 9:203–210.

146. Rajala GM, Kolesari GL, Khulmann RS, Schnitzler HJ. Ventricular blood pressure and cardiac output changes in epinephrine- and metoprolol-treated chick embryos. Teratology 1988; 38:291–296.

147. Rosenfeld CR, Barton MD, Meschia G. Effects of epinephrine on distribution of blood flow in the pregnant ewe. Am J Obstet Gynecol 1976; 124:156–163.

148. Clapp JF 3d. Effect of epinephrine infusion on maternal and uterine oxygen uptake in the pregnant ewe. Am J Obstet Gynecol 1979; 133:208–212.

149. Adamsons K, Mueller-Heubach E, Myers RE. Production of fetal asphyxia in the rhesus monkey by administration of catecholamines to the mother. Am J Obstet Gynecol 1971; 109:248–262.

150. Morgan CD, Sandler M, Panigel M. Placental transfer of catecholamines in vitro and in vivo. Am J Obstet Gynecol 1972; 112:1068–1075.

151. Schatz M, Zeiger RS, Harden KM, Hoffman CP, Forsythe AB, Chilingar LM, Preco RP, Benenson AS, Sperling WL, Saunders BS, Kagnoff MC. The safety of inhaled (beta)-agonist bronchodilators during pregnancy. J Allergy Clin Immunol 1988; 82:686–695.

152. Nishikawa T, Bruyere HJ Jr, Takagi Y, Gilbert EF, Uno H. Cardiovascular teratogenicity of ephedrine in chick embryos. Toxicol Lett 1985; 29:59–63.

153. Nishikawa T, Bruyere HJ, Jr, Gilbert EF, Takagi Y, et al. Potentiating effects of caffeine on the cardiovascular teratogenicity of ephedrine in chick embryos. Toxicol Lett 1985; 29:65–68.

154. Matsuoka R, Gilbert EF, Bruyere H Jr, Opitz JM. An aborted human fetus with truncus arteriosus communis—possible teratogenic effect of Tedral. Heart Vessels 1985; 1:176–178.

155. Hughes SC, Ward MG, Levinson G, Shnider SM, Wright RG, Gruenke LD, Craig JC. Placental transfer of ephedrine does not affect neonatal outcome. Anesthesiology 1985; 63:217–219.

156. Entman SS, Moise KJ. Anaphylaxis in pregnancy. South Med J 1984; 77: 402.

157. Stalder JB, Suppan P, Ditesheim PJ, Meyer S. [Cesarean section under peridural anesthesia and hypotension: value of preventative intravenous ephedrine]. Rev Med Suisse Romande 1983; 103:867–870.

158. Wright RG, Shnider SM, Levinson G, Rolbin SH, Parer JT. The effect of maternal administration of ephedrine on fetal heart rate and variability. Obstet Gynecol 1981; 57:734–738.

159. Cherala SR, Mehta D, Greene R. Ephedrine as a marker of intravascular injection in laboring parturients. Reg Anesth 1990; 15:15–18.

160. Rolbin SH, Cole AFD, Hew EM, Pllard A, Virgint S. Prophylactic intramuscular ephedrine before epidural anaesthesia for caesarean section: efficacy and actions on the foetus and newborn. Can Anaesth Soc J 1982; 29: 148–153.

161. Kang YG, Abouleish E, Caritis S. Prophylactic intravenous ephedrine infusion during spinal anaesthesia for caesarean section. Anesth Analg 1982; 61: 839–842.

162. Rout CC, Rocke DA, Brijball R, Koovarjee RV. Prophylactic intramuscular ephedrine prior to caesarean section. Anaesth Intensive Care 1992; 20: 448–452.

163. Mortimer EA Jr. Drug toxicity from breast milk? Pediatrics 1977; 60: 780–781.

164. Dusek J, Ostadal B. Ultrastructure of isoproterenol-induced myocardial damage in chick embryos. Physiol Bohemoslov 1985; 34:297–302.

165. Ostadal B, Janatova T, Krause EG, Prelouch V, Dusek J. Different effect of propranolol and verapamil on isoprenaline-induced changes in the chick embryo heart. Physiol Bohemoslov 1987; 36:301–311.

166. Janatova T, Pelouch V, Ostadal B, Krause EG. The effect of oxidized isoprenaline on the chick embryonic heart. Can J Physiol Pharmacol 1986; 64: 897–903.

167. Kuhlmann RS, Kolesari GL, Kalbfleisch JH. Reduction of catecholamine-induced cardiovascular malformations in the chick embryo with metoprolol. Teratology 1983; 28:9–14.

168. Cheung MO, Gilbert EF, Bruyere HJ Jr, Ishikawa S, Hodach RJ. Chronotropism and blood flow patterns following teratogenic doses of catecholamines in 5-day-old chick embryos. Teratology 1977; 16:327–343.

169. Clark EB, Hu N, Dooley JB. The effect of isoproterenol on cardiovascular function in the stage 24 chick embryo. Teratology 1985; 31:41–47.

170. Dusek J, Ostadal B. Isoproterenol-induced damage to the liver of chick embryos. Physiol Bohemoslov 1984; 33:67–73.

171. Bruyere HJ Jr, Fallon JF, Gilbert EF. External malformations in chick embryos following concomitant administration of methylxanthines and beta-

adrenomimetic agents. I. Gross pathologic features. Teratology 1983; 28: 257–269.

172. Robson JM, ed. Embryopathic Activity of Drugs. Boston: Little Brown, 1965:110.

173. Geber WF. Comparative teratogenicity of isoproterenol and trypan blue in the fetal hamster. Proc Soc Exp Biol Med 1969; 130:1168–1170.

174. Jones-Price C, Ledoux TA, Reel JR, Wolkowski-Tyl R, Langhoff-Paschke L. Teratologic evaluation of isoproterenol hydrochloride (CAS No. 51-30-9) in CD rats. Govt Rep Announcements & Index. Issue 9, 1983.

175. Vogin EE, Goldhamer RE, Scheimberg J, Carson S. Teratology studies in rats and rabbits exposed to an isoproterenol aerosol. Toxicol Apply Pharmacol 1970; 16:374–381.

176. Hollingsworth RL, Scott WJ Jr, Woodard MW, Woodard G. Fetal rabbit ductus arteriosus assessed in a teratologic study on isoproterenol and metaproterenol. Toxicol Appl Pharmacol 1971; 18:231–234.

177. Robkin MA, Shepard TH, Dyer DC, Guntheroth WG. Autonomic receptors of the early rat embryo heart: growth and development. Proc Soc Exp Biol Med 1976; 151:799–803.

178. Tweed WA, Davies JM, Alexander F, Csorba T, Weber S. Effects of isoproterenol-induced tachycardia on myocardial blood flow and glycogen in the fetal lamb. Biol Neonate 1987; 52:104–114.

179. Van de Walle AF, Martin CB Jr. Effect of isoproterenol on uterine blood flow and cardiac output distribution in pregnant guinea pigs. Am J Obstet Gynecol 1985; 152:1058–1062.

180. Macdonald AA, Colenbrander B, Wensing CJ. Effects of adrenergic agonists and antagonists on the blood pressure and heart rate of the pig fetus. Res Vet Sci 1984; 36:61–65.

181. Iwasaki T, Takino Y, Suzuki T. Effects of isoproterenol on the developing heart in rats. Jpn Circ J 1990; 54:109–116.

182. Legrand C, Maltier JP, Benghan-Eyene Y. Rat myometrial adrenergic receptors in late pregnancy. Biol Reprod 1987; 37:641–650.

183. Maruta K, Mizoguchi Y, Osa T. Changes in action potential and beta-adrenergic effects of the circular muscle of postpartum rat uterus. Jpn J Physiol 1985; 35:567–579.

184. Ke R, Vohra M, Casper R. Prolonged inhibition of human myometrial contractility by intermittent isoproterenol. Am J Obstet Gynecol 1984; 149: 841–844.

185. Banerjee BN, Woodard G. Teratologic evaluation of metaproterenol in the rhesus monkey (*Macaca mulatta*). Tox Appl Pharmacol 1971; 20:562–564.

186. Rx Bulletin. Orciprenaline sulphate 1971; 2:25–28.

187. Iida H, Kast A, Tsunenari Y, Asakura M. Corticosterone induction of cleft palate in mice dosed with orciprenaline sulfate. Teratology 1988; 38:15–27.

188. Matsuo A, Kast A, Tsunenari Y. Teratology study with orciprenaline sulfate in rabbits. Arzneim Forsch Drug Resch 1982; 32:808–810.

189. Freysz H, Willard D, Lehr A, Messer J, Boog G. A long term evaluation of infants who received a beta-mimetic drug while in utero. J Perinat Med 1977; 5:94–99.

190. Baillie P, Meehan FP, Tyack AJ. Treatment of premature labour with orciprenaline. Br Med J 1970; 4:154–155.

191. Zilianti M, Aller J. Action of orciprenaline on uterine contractility during labor, maternal cardiovascular system, fetal heart rate, and acid-base balance. Am J Obstet Gynecol 1971; 109:1073–1079.

192. Mendez-Bauer C, Shekarloo A, Cook V, Freese U. Treatment of acute intrapartum fetal distress by $beta_2$-sympathomimetics. Am J Obstet Gynecol 1987; 156:638–642.

193. Szabo KT, Difebbo ME, Kang YJ. Effects of several beta-receptor agonists on fetal development in various species of laboratory animals: preliminary report. Teratology 1975; 12:336–337.

194. Lind T, Godfrey KA, Gerrard J, Bryson MR. Continuous salbutamol infusion over 17 weeks to pre-empt premature labour. Lancet 1980; 2:1165–1166.

195. Addis GJ. Long-term salbutamol infusion to prevent premature labour. Lancet 1981; 1:42–43.

196. Edmonds DK, Letchworth AT. Prophylactic oral salbutalmol to prevent premature labour. Lancet 1982; 1:1310–1311.

197. Grummerus M. The management of premature labor with salbutamol. Acta Obstet Gynecol Scand 1981; 60:375–377.

198. Hastwell G, Halloway CP, Taylor TLO. A study of 208 patients in premature labor treated with orally administered salbutamol. Med J Austral 1978; 1: 465–469.

199. Korda AR, Lyneham RC, Jones WR. The treatment of premature labor with intravenously administered salbutamol. Med J Austral 1974; 1:744–746.

200. Liggins GC, Vaghan GS. Intravenous infusion of salbutamol in the management of premature labor. J Obstet Gynaecol Br Commonw 1973; 80:29–33.

201. Ng KH, Sen DK. Hypotension with intravenous salbutamol in premature labour. Br Med J 1974; 3:257.

202. Pincus R. Salbutamol infusion for premature labour—the Australian trials experience. Austral NZ Obstet Gynaecol 1981; 21:1–4.

203. Thomas DJB, Dove AF, Alberti KG. Metabolic effects of salbutamol infusion during premature labour. Br J Obstet Gynaecol 1977; 84:497–499.

204. Lunell NO, Joelsson I, Larsson A, Persson B. The immediate effect of a beta-adrenergic agonist (salbutamol) on carbohydrate and lipid metabolism during the third trimester of pregnancy. Acta Obstet Gynecol Scand 1977; 56:475–478.

205. Wager J, Fredholm BB, Lunell NO, Persson B. Metabolic and circulatory effects of oral albutamol in the third trimester of pregnancy in diabetic and non-diabetic women. Br J Obstet Gynaecol 1981; 88:352–361.

206. Gummerus M, Halonen O. Prophylactic long-term oral tocolysis of multiple pregnancies. Br J Obstet Gynaecol 1987; 94:249–251.

207. Rayburn WF, Atkinson BD, Gilbert K, Turnbull GL. Short-term effects of inhaled albuterol on maternal and fetal circulations. Am J Obstet Gynecol 1994; 171:770–773.
208. Ashworth MF, Spooner SF, Verkuyl DA, Waterman R, Ashurst HM. Failure to prevent preterm labour and delivery in twin pregnancy using prophylactic oral salbutamol. Br J Obstet Gynaecol 1990; 97:878–882.
209. Desgranges MF, Moutquin JM, Peloquin A. Effects of maternal oral salbutamol therapy on neonatal endocrine status at birth. Obstet Gynecol 1987; 69:582–584.
210. Wallace RL, Caldwell DL, Ansbacher R, Otterson WN. Inhibition of premature labor by terbutaline. Obstet Gynecol 1978; 51:387–392.
211. Hadders-Algra M, Touwen BC, Huisjes HJ. Long-term follow-up of children prenatally exposed to ritodrine. Br J Obstet Gynaecol 1986; 93:156–159.
212. Polowczyk D, Tejani N, Lauersen N, Siddiq F. Evaluation of seven-to-nine-year old children exposed to ritodrine in utero. Obstet Gynecol 1984; 64:485–489.
213. Haller DL. The use of terbutaline for premature labor. Drug Intell Clin Pharm 1980; 14:757–764.
214. Stubblefield PG, Heyl PS. Treatment of premature labor with subcutaneous terbutaline. Obstet Gynecol 1982; 59:457–462.
215. Beall MH, Edgar BW, Paul RH, Smith-Wallace T. A comparison of ritodrine, terbutaline, and magnesium sulfate for the suppression of preterm labor. Am J Obstet Gynecol 1985; 153:854–859.
216. Kosasa TS, Nakayama RT, Hale RW, Rinzler GS, Freitas CA. Ritodrine and terbutaline compared for the treatment of preterm labor. Acta Obstet Gynecol Scand 1985; 64:421–426.
217. Ingemarsson I. Bengtsson B. A five-year experience with terbutaline for preterm labor: low rate of severe side effects. Obstet Gynecol 1985; 66:176–180.
218. Lenselink DR, Kuhlmann RS, Lawrence JM, Kolesari GL. Cardiovascular teratogenicity of terbutaline and ritodrine in the chick embryo. Am J Obstet Gynecol 1994; 171:501–506.
219. Katz M, Robertson PA, Creasy RK. Cardiovascular complications associated with terbutaline treatment for preterm labor. Am J Obstet Gynecol 1981; 139:605–608.
220. Brown MS. Does terbutaline cause uterine atony and increase intraoperative blood loss? Am J Obstet Gynecol 1989; 161:259.
221. Patriarco MS. Does terbutaline cause uterine atony and increase intraoperative blood loss? Am J Obstet Gynecol 1989; 161:259.
222. Roth AC, Milsom I, Forssman L, Ekman LG, Hedner T. Effects of intravenous terbutaline on maternal circulation and fetal heart activity. Acta Obstet Gynecol Scand 1990; 69:223–228.
223. Bernstein IM, Catalano PM. Ketoacidosis in pregnancy associated with the parenteral administration of terbutaline and betamethasone. J Reprod Med 1990; 35:818–820.

224. Epstein MF, Nicholls E, Stubblefield PG. Neonatal hypoglycemia after beta-sympathomimetic tocolytic therapy. J Pediatr 1979; 94:449–453.

225. Tibaldi JM, Lorber DL, Nerenberg A. Diabetic ketoacidosis and insulin resistance with subcutaneous terbutaline infusion: a case report. Am J Obstet Gynecol 1990; 163:509–510.

226. Main EK, Main DM, Gabbe SG. Chronic oral terbutaline tocolytic therapy is associated with maternal glucose intolerance. Am J Obstet Gynecol 1987; 157:644–647.

227. Patriarco MS, Viechnicki BM, Hutchinson TA, Klasko SK, Yeh SY. A study on intrauterine fetal resuscitation with terbutaline. Am J Obstet Gynecol 1987; 157:384–387.

228. Ingemarsson I, Bengtsson B. Single injection of terbutaline in term labor. I. Effect on fetal pH in cases with prolonged bradycardia. Am J Obstet Gynecol 1985; 153:859–865.

229. Shekarloo A, Mendez-Bauer C, Cook V, Freese U. Terbutaline (intravenous bolus) for the treatment of acute intrapartum fetal distress. Am J Obstet Gynecol 1989; 160:615–818.

230. Akerlund M, Anderson KE. Effects of terbutaline on human myometrial activity and endometrial blood flow. Obstet Gynecol 1976; 47:529–535.

231. Akerlund M, Bengtsson LP, Carter AM. A technique for monitoring endometrial or decidual blood flow with an intrauterine thermistor probe. Acta Obstet Gynecol Sand 1975; 54:469–477.

232. Csakany MG, Bagdany S, Viltay P, Birtalan I, Torok M, Gati I. The effect of Bricanyl on placental circulation in late toxaemia of pregnancy. Ther Hung 1982; 30:138–140.

233. Wright JW, Patterson RM, Ridgway LE 3d, Berkus MD. Effect of tocolytic agents on fetal umbilical velocimetry. Am J Obstet Gynecol 1990; 163: 748–750.

234. Fletcher SE, Fyfe DA, Case CL, Wiles HB, Upshur JK, Newman RB. Myocardial necrosis in a newborn after long-term maternal subcutaneous terbutaline infusion for suppression of preterm labor. Am J Obstet Gynecol 1991; 165:1401–1404.

235. Lonnerholm G, Lindstrom B. Terbutaline excretion into breast milk. Br J Clin Pharmacol 1982; 13:729–730.

236. Boreus LO, de Chateau PU. Terbutaline in breast milk. Br J Clin Pharmacol 1982; 13:731–732.

237. Sakai T, Owaki Y, Noguchi Y. Reproduction studies of pirbuterol hydrochloride. Yakuri to Chiro 1980; 8:731–743, cited in Shepard TH. Catalog of Teratogenic Agents. Baltimore, MD: Johns Hopkins University Press, 1992: 320.

238. American Society of Hospital Pharmacists, McEvoy GK, et al., eds. Bethesda, MD: American Hospital Formulary Service Drug Information 94; 1994:2440.

239. Cox JSG, Beach JE, Blair AM, et al. Disodium cromoglycate (Intal). Adv Drug Res 1970; 5:115–196.

240. Wilson J. Use of sodium cromoglycate during pregnancy. J Pharm Med 1982; 8:45–51.

241. Clark B, Clarke AJ, Bamford DG, Greenwood B. Nedocromil sodium preclinical safety evaluation studies: a preliminary report. Eur J Resp Dis 1986; 69[147 suppl]:248–251.

242. Fujii T, Nishimura H. Teratogenic actions of some methylated xanthines in mice. Okajimas Folia Anat Jpn 1969; 46:167–175.

243. Tucci SM, Skalko RG. The teratogenic effects of theophylline in mice. Toxicol Lett 1978; 1:337–341.

244. Maren TH, Ellison AC. The teratological effect of certain thiadiazoles related to acetazolamide, with a note on sulfanilamide and thiazide diuretics. Johns Hopkins Med J 1972; 130:95–104.

245. Fujii T, Kondo M, Matsuzaka Y. Rat fetal edema by methylated xanthines. Teratology 1972; 6:106.

246. Lindstrom P, Morrissey RE, George JD, Price CJ, Marr MC, Kimmel CA, Schwetz BA. The developmental toxicity of orally administered theophylline in rats and mice. Fundam Appl Toxicol 1990; 14:167–178.

247. Morrissey RE, Collins JJ, Lamb JC 4th, Manus AG, Gulati DK. Reproductive effects of theophylline in mice and rats. Fundam Appl Toxicol 1988; 10: 525–536.

248. Day P, Shalaby Z, Cohen MM, Wasserman SS, Schwartz S. Effects of theophylline on chromosomal breakage and sister-chromatid exchange. Mutat Res 1989; 224:409–413.

249. Greenberger P, Patterson R. Safety of therapy for allergic symptoms during pregnancy. Ann Intern Med 1978; 89:234–237.

250. Hernandez E, Angell CS, Johnson JW. Asthma in pregnancy: current concepts. Obstet Gynecol 1980; 55:739–743.

251. Lalli CM, Raju L. Pregnancy and chronic obstructive pulmonary disease. Chest 1981; 80:759–761.

252. Turner ES, Greenberger PA, Patterson R. Management of the pregnant asthmatic patient. Ann Intern Med 1980; 93:905–918.

253. Neff RK, Leviton A. Maternal theophylline consumption and the risk of stillbirth. Chest 1990; 97:1266–1267.

254. Park JM, Schmer V, Myers TL. Cardiovascular anomalies associated with prenatal exposure to theophylline. South Med J 1990; 83:1487–1488.

255. Carter BL, Driscoll CE, Smith GD. Theophylline clearance during pregnancy. Obstet Gynecol 1986; 68:555–559.

256. Frederiksen MC, Ruo TI, Chow MJ, Atkinson AJ Jr. Theophylline pharmacokinetics in pregnancy. Clin Pharmacol Ther 1986; 40:321–328.

257. Gardner MJ, Schatz M, Cousins L, Zieger R, Middleton E, Jusko WJ. Longitudinal effects of pregnancy on the pharmacokinetics of theophylline. Eur J Clin Pharmacol 1987; 31:289–295.

258. Arwood LL, Dasta JF, Friedman C. Placental transfer of theophylline: two case reports. Pediatrics 1979; 63:844–846.

259. Yeh TF, Pildes RS. Transplacental aminophylline toxicity in a neonate. Lancet 1977; 1:910.
260. Horowitz DA, Jablonski W, Mehta KA. Apnea associated with theophylline withdrawal in a term neonate. Am J Dis Child 1982; 136:73–74.
261. Ron M, Hochner-Celnikier D, Menczel J, Palti Z, Kidroni G. Maternal-fetal transfer of aminophylline. Acta Obstet Gynecol Scand 1984; 63:217–218.
262. Labovitz E, Spector S. Placental theophylline transfer in pregnant asthmatics. JAMA 1982; 247:786–788.
263. Aranda JV, Louridas AT, Vitullo BB, Thom P, Aldridge A, Haber R. Metabolism of theophylline to caffeine in human fetal liver. Science 1979; 206: 1319–1321.
264. Bory C, Baltassat P, Porthault M, Bethenod M, Frederich A, Aranda JV. Metabolism of theophylline to caffeine in premature newborn infants. J Pediat 1979; 94:988–993.
265. National Asthma Education Program. Management of asthma during pregnancy. Bethesda, MD: National Institutes of Health Publication No. 93-3279, 1993.
266. Volpe JJ. Effects of methylxanthines on lipid synthesis in developing neural systems. Semin Perinatol 1981; 5:395–405.
267. Aranda JV, Dupone C. Metabolic effects of methylxanthines in premature infants. J Pediatr 1976; 89:833–834.
268. Nelson RM, Resnick MB, Holstrum WJ, Eitzman DV. Developmental outcome of premature infants treated with theophylline. Dev Pharmacol Ther 1980; 1:274–280.
269. Yurchak AM, Jusko WJ. Theophylline secretion into breast milk. Pediatrics 1976; 57:518–525.
270. Stec GP, Greenberger P, Ruo TI. Kinetics of theophylline transfer to breast milk. Clin Pharmacol Ther 1980; 28:404–408.
271. Berlin CM. Excretion of methylxanthines in human milk. Semin Perinatol 1981; 5:389–394.
272. Hart AD, Grimble RF. Effect of methylxanthines on lactational performance of rats. Ann Nutr Metab 1990; 34:297–302.
273. Hart AD, Grimble RF. Effect of methylxanthines on milk volume and composition, and growth of rat pups. Br J Nutr 1990; 64:339–350.
274. Berkowitz RL, Coustan DR, Mochizuki TK. Handbook for Prescribing Medications During Pregnancy. 2d ed. Boston: Little, Brown, 1986:283.
275. Georges A, Denef J. Les anomalies digitale: manifestations teratogèniques des dérivés xanthique chez le rat. Arch Int Pharmacodyn Ther 1968; 172: 219–222.
276. Patterson CE, Davis KS, Beckman DE, Rhoades RA. Fatty acid synthesis in the fetal lung: relationship to surfactant lipids. Biochem Biophys Acta 1986; 878:110–126.
277. Landers S. Effect of aminophylline and caffeine on total and surfactant phospholipid in fetal rabbit lung. Am Rev Resp Dis 1984; 130:204–208.

278. Cosmi EV, Saitto C, Barbati A, Del Bolgia F, Di Renzo GC, Grossmann G, Lachmann B, Robertson B. Effect of aminophylline on lung maturation in preterm rabbit fetuses. Am J Obstet Gynecol 1986; 154:436–439.

279. Granati B, Grella PV, Pettenazzo A, Di Lenardo L, Rubaltelli FF. The prevention of respiratory distress syndrome in premature infants: efficacy of antenatal aminophylline treatment versus prenatal glucocorticoid administration. Pediatr Pharmacol 1984; 4:21–24.

280. Laifer SA, Ghodgaonkar RB, Zacur HA, Dubin NH. The effect of aminophylline on uterine smooth muscle contractility and prostaglandin production in the pregnant rat uterus in vitro. Am J Obstet Gynecol 1986; 155:212–215.

281. Melis GB, Fruzzetti F, Strigini F, Barale E, Capriello P, Baisi F, Cipolloni C, Fioretti P. Aminophylline treatment of preterm labor. Acta Eur Fertil 1984; 15:357–361.

282. Lipshitz J. Uterine and cardiovascular effects of aminophylline. Am J Obstet Gynecol 1978; 131:716–718.

283. Back KC, Newberne JW, Weaver LC. A toxicopathologic study of endobenzyline bromide, a new cholinergic blocking agent. Toxicol Appl Pharmacol 1961; 3:422–430.

284. Maeda H, Yasuda M. Induction of digital malformations in rat fetuses by combined administration of papaverine hydrochloride and atropine sulfate. Teratology 1979; 20:157.

285. Beuker ED, Platner WS. Effect of cholinergic drugs on development of chick embryo. Proc Soc Exp Biol Med 1956; 91:539–543.

286. Arcuri PA, Gautieri RF. Morphine-induced fetal malformations: III. Possible mechanisms of action. J Pharm Sci 1973; 62:1616–1634.

287. Zellers JE. Influence of atropine and diphenhydramine on the teratogenic capability of codeine in CF-1 mice. Diss Absts Int 1979; B:39:5870.

288. Kivalo I, Saarikoski S. Placental transmission of atropine at full-term pregnancy. Br J Anaesth 1977; 49:1017–1021.

289. Kanto J, Virtanen R, Iisalo E, Maenpaa K, Liukko P. Placental transfer and pharmacokinetics of atropine after a single maternal intravenous administration. Acta Anaesth Scand 1981; 25:85–88.

290. Onnen I, Barrier G, d'Athis Ph, Sureau C, Olive G. Placental transfer of atropine at the end of pregnancy. Eur J Clin Pharmacol 1979; 15:443–446.

291. Roodenburg PJ, Wladimiroff JW, Van Weering HK. Effect of maternal intravenous administration of atropine (0.5 mg) on fetal breathing and heart pattern. Contr Gynec Obstet 1979; 6:92–97.

292. Abboud T, Raya J, Sadri S, Grobler N, Stine L, Miller F. Fetal and maternal cardiovascular effects of atropine and glycopyrolate. Anesth Analg 1983; 62: 426–430.

293. Diaz DM, Diaz SF, Marx GF. Cardiovascular effects of glycopyrrolate and belladonna derivatives in obstetric patients. Bull NY Acad Med 1980; 56: 245–248.

294. Janz D, Fuchs U. Are anti-epileptic drugs harmful when give during pregnancy? Ger Med Mon 1964; 9:20–22.

295. Stewart JJ. Gastrointestinal drugs. In: Wilson JT, ed. Drugs in Breast Milk. Balgowlah, Australia: ADIS Press, 1981:65–71.
296. Anderson WM. Hemodynamic and non-bronchial effects of ipratropium bromide. Am J Med 1986; 81:45–53.
297. Nishimura M, Kast A, Tsunenari Y. Reproduction studies of ipratropium bromide (SCH 1000) on rats and rabbits. Iyakuhin Kenkyu 1978; 9:393–416.
298. Niggeschulze A, Palmer AK. [Reproductive toxicological investigations with ipratropium bromide]. Arzneimittelforschung 1976; 26:989–992.
299. Boucher D, Delost P. Development post-natal des descendents issues de mères traitées de la pénicilline au cours de la gestion chez la souris. CR Soc Biol (Paris) 1964; 158:528–532.
300. Brown DM, Harper KH, Palmer AK, Tesh SA. Effects of antibiotics upon pregnancy in the rabbit. Toxicol Appl Pharmacol 1968; 12:295.
301. Bachev S, Petrova L, Voicheva V, Shishkova M, Kolev N. Experimental studies on the teratogenic effect, acute and chronic toxicity of ampicillin. Suvrem Med 1974; 25:28–32.
302. Korzhova VV, Lisitsyna NT, Mikhailova EG. Effect of ampicillin and oxacillin on fetal and neonatal development. Bull Exp Med (USSR) 1981; 91: 169–170.
303. Nishimura H, Tanimura T. Clinical Aspects of the Teratogenicity of Drugs. Amsterdam: Excerpta Medica, 1976:231.
304. Philipson A. Pharmacokinetics of ampicillin during pregnancy. J Infect Dis 1977; 136:370–376.
305. Bray RE, Boe RW, Johnson WL. Transfer of ampicillin into fetus and amniotic fluid from maternal plasma in late pregnancy. Am J Obstet Gynecol 1966; 96:9328–9342. .
306. Hutter A, Parks J. The transmission of penicillin through the placenta. A preliminary report. Am J Obstet Gynecol 1945; 49:663–665.
307. Woltz J, Zintel H. The transmission of penicillin to the previable fetus. JAMA 1946; 131:969–970.
308. Wasz-Hockert O, Nummi S, Vuopala S, Jarvinen PA. Transplacental passage of azidocillin, ampicillin, and penicillin G during early and late pregnancy. Acat Paediatr Scand 1970; 206(suppl):109–110.
309. Ravid R, Toaff R. On the possible teratogenicity of antibiotic drugs administered during pregnancy—a prospective study. In: Klingber M, et al., eds. Drugs and Fetal Development. New York: Plenum Press, 1972:505–510.
310. Gallagher JS. Anaphylaxis in pregnancy. Obstet Gynecol 1988; 71:491–493.
311. Kosim H. Intrauterine fetal death as a result of anaphylactic reaction to penicillin in a pregnant woman. Dapim Refuiim 1959; 18:136–137.
312. Green HJ, Burkhart B, Hobby GL. Excretion of penicillin in human milk following parturition. Am J Obstet Gynecol 1946; 51:732–733.
313. Branebjerg PE, Heisterberg L. Blood and milk concentrations of ampicillin in mothers treated with pivampicillin and in their infants. J Perinat Med 1987; 15:555–558.

314. Paterson ML, Henderson A, Lunan CB, McGurk S. Transplacental transfer of cephalexin. Clin Med 1972; 79:23–24.
315. Creatsas G, Pavlatos M, Lolis D, Kaskarelis D. A study of the kinetics of cephapirin and cephalexin in pregnancy. Curr Med Res Opin 1980; 7:43–46.
316. Aoyama T, Furuoka R, Hasegawa N, Nemoto K. Teratologic studies of cephalexin in mice and rats. Oyo Yakuri 1969; 3:249–263.
317. Welles JS, Froman RO, Gibson WR, Owen NV, Anderson RC. Toxicology and pharmacology of cephalexin in laboratory animals. Antimicrob Agents Chemother 1968; 8:489–496.
318. ChuChen K, Sabeti S. L'évaluation clinique de la cephalexin orale. Int J Clin Pharmacol 1970; 2(suppl):124–128.
319. Mizuno S, Metsuda S, Mori S. Clinical evaluation of cephalexin in obstetrics and gynaecology. Proc Symp Clin Evaluation of Cephalexin, Royal Society of Medicine, London, 1969.
320. Pedler SJ, Bint AJ. Comparative study of amoxicillin-clavulanic acid and cephalexin in the treatment of bacteriuria during pregnancy. Antimicrob Agents Chemother 1985; 27:508–510.
321. Markham JK, Hanasono GK, Adams ER, Owen NV. Reproduction studies on cefaclor (Lilly cephalosporin 99638) in four species. Toxicol Appl Pharmacol 1978; 45:292.
322. Nomura A, Furuhashi T, Ikeya E, Sawaki A, Nakayoshi H. Reproduction study of cefaclor. I. Teratological study in mice, rats, and rabbits. Chemotherapy 1979; 27(suppl 7):846–864.
323. Furuhashi T, Nomura A, Uehara M, Komuro E, Nakayoshi H. Reproduction studies on cefaclor (CCl) 2. Fertility study and perinatal study in rats. Chemotherapy 1979; 27:865–880.
324. Kafetzis DA, Siafas CA, Georgakopoulos PA, Papadatos CJ. Passage of cephalosporins and amoxicillin into the breast milk. Acta Paediatr Scand 1981; 70:285–288.
325. Takase A. Clinical and laboratory studies of cefaclor in the field of obstetrics and gynecology. Chemotherapy (Tokyo) 1979; 27(suppl):666–671.
326. Halperin-Walega E, Batra VK, Tonelli AP, Barr A, Yacobi A. Disposition of cefixime in the pregnant and lactating rat. Transfer to the fetus and nursing pup. Drug Metab Dispos 1988; 16:130–134.
327. Capel-Edwards K, Atkinson RM, Pratt DA. Toxicological studies on cefuroxime sodium. Toxicology 1979; 13:1–5.
328. Furuhashi T, Nomura A, Ikeya E, Nakazawa M. Teratological studies on cefuroxime in rabbits. Chemotherapy 1979; 27:273–279.
329. Skosyreva AM, Akhtamova ZM, Golovanova IV, Yavorskaya AN. [Effect of cefuroxime on embryonic and fetal development in an experiment]. Antibiot Med Biotekhnol 1986; 31:277–280.
330. Craft I, Mulliger BM, Kennedy MR. Placental transfer of cefuroxime. Br J Obstet Gynaecol 1981; 88:141–145.
331. de Leeuw JW, Roumen FJME, Bouckaert PXJM, Cremers HMHG, Vree TB. Achievement of therapeutic concentrations of cefuroxime in early preterm

gestations with premature rupture of the membranes. Obstet Gynecol 1993; 81:255–260.

332. Holt DE, Fisk NM, Spencer JA. Transplacental transfer of cefuroxime in uncomplicated pregnancies and those complicated by hydrops or changes in amniotic fluid volume. Arch Dis Child 1993; 68:54–57.

333. Baldwin JA, Schardein JL, Kashima Y. Reproduction studies of BRL 14151K and BRL 25000. Teratology and peri- and postnatal studies in rats. Chemotherapy 1983; 31:238–262.

334. Hirakawa T, Suzuki T, Sano Y, Kamata T, Nakamura M. Reproduction studies in rats. Chemotherapy 1983; 31:263–272.

335. James PA, Hardy TL, Koshima Y. Reproduction studies of BRL 25000. Teratology studies in the pig. Chemotherapy 1983; 31:274–279.

336. Fortunato SJ, Bawdon RE, Swan KF, Bryant EC, Sobhi S. Transfer of Timentin (ticarcillin and clavulanic acid) across the in vitro perfused human placenta: comparison with other agents. Am J Obstet Gynecol 1992; 167: 1595–1599.

337. Takaya M. [Teratogenic effects of antibiotics]. J Osaka City Med 1965; 14: 107–115.

338. Liban E, Abramovici A. Fetal membrane adhesions and congenital malformations. In: Klingberg MA, Abramovici A, Chemke J, eds. Drugs and Fetal Development. New York: Plenum Press, 1972:337–350.

339. Kiefer L, Rubin A, McCoy JB, Foltz EL. The placental transfer of erythromycin. Am J Obstet Gynecol 1955; 69:174–177.

340. Philipson A, Sabath LD, Charles D. Transplacental passage of erythromycin and clindamycin. N Engl J Med 1973; 288:1219–1220.

341. Rothman K, Pochi P. Use of oral and topical agents for acne in pregnancy. J Am Acad Dermatol 1988; 16:431–442.

342. Fenton LJ, Light LJ. Congenital syphilis after maternal treatment with erythromycin. Obstet Gynecol 1976; 47:492–494.

343. McCormack WM, George H, Donner A, Kodgis LF, Alpert S. Hepatotoxicity of erythromycin estolate during pregnancy. Antimicrob Agents Chemother 1977; 12:630–635.

344. Matsuda T. Transfer of antibiotics into maternal milk. Biol Res Pregnancy Perinatol 1984; 5:57–60.

345. Sedlmayr T, Peters F, Raasch W, Kees F. [Clarithromycin, a new macrolide antibiotic. Effectiveness in puerperal infections and pharmacokinetics in breast milk] Geburtshilfe Frauenheilkd 1993; 53:488–491.

346. Krohn K. Gynaecological tissue levels of azithromycin. Eur J Clin Microbiol Infect Dis 1991; 10:864–868.

347. Edwards M, Rainwater K, Carter S, Williamson F, Newman R. Comparison of azithromycin and erythromycin for *Chlamydia* cervicitis in pregnancy. Am J Obstet Gynecol 1994; 170:419.

348. Bush MR, Rosa C. Azithromycin and erythromycin in the treatment of cervical chlamydial infection during pregnancy. Obstet Gynecol 1994; 84: 61–63.

349. Kelsey JJ, Moser LR, Jennings JC, Munger MA. Presence of azithromycin breast milk concentrations: a case report. Am J Obstet Gynecol 1994; 170: 1375–1376.

350. Posner AC, Konicoff NG, Prigot A. Tetracycline in obstetric infections. In: Antibiotics Annual, 1954–55. New York: Medical Encyclopedia, 1956: 345–348.

351. Rendle-Short TJ. Tetracycline in teeth and bone. Lancet 1962; 1:1188.

352. Kline AH, Blattner RJ, Lunin M. Transplacental effect of tetracyclines on teeth. JAMA 1964; 188:178–180.

353. Kutscher AH, Zegarelli EV, Tovell HM, Hochberg B, Hauptman J. Discoloration of deciduous teeth induced by administrations of tetracycline antepartum. Am J Obstet Gynecol 1966; 96:291–292.

354. Fillippi B. Antibiotics and congenital malformations: evaluation of the teratogenicity of antibiotics, in Woollam DHM, ed. Advances in Teratology. Vol 2. New York: Academic Press, 1967:237–256.

355. Bevelander G, Cohlan SQ. The effect on the rat fetus of transplacentally acquired tetracyclinc. Biol Nconate 1962; 4:365–370.

356. Hurley LS, Tuchmann-Duplessis H. Influence de la tetracycline sur la développement pré- et post-natal du rat. CR Acad Sci (Paris) 1963; 257: 302–304.

357. Cohlan SQ. Drugs and pregnancy. Prog Clin Biol Res 1980; 44:77–96.

358. Mela V, Filippi B. Una carenza vitaminica insorta nel corso di un trattamento antibiotico puo avere effetto teratogeno. Minerva Med 1957; 48:2459–2462.

359. Morrissey RE, Tyl RW, Price CJ, Ledoux TA, Reel JR, Paschke LL, Marr MC, Kimmel CA. The developmental toxicity of orally administered oxytetracycline in rats and mice. Fundam Appl Toxicol 1986; 7:434–443.

360. Savini EC, Moulin MA, Herrou MF. Effets teratogènes de l'oxytetracycline. Therapie 1968; 23:1247–1260.

361. Savitskaia TN. [Features of the structure of the mesenteric and tracheobronchial lymph nodes in rat offspring after exposure to tetracycline]. Arkh Anat Gistol Embriol 1984; 87:66–72.

362. Petrova TB. [Structure of the thymus gland of the rat in the prenatal and early postnatal periods of development after exposure to tetracycline during the period of fetogenesis]. Arkh Anat Gistol Embriol 1984; 87:61–66.

363. Krejci L. Eye changes due to systemic use of tetracycline in pregnancy. Ophthal Res 1980; 12:73–77.

364. Harley JD, Farrar JF, Gray JB, Dunlop IC. Aromatic drugs and congenital cataracts. Lancet 1964; 1:472–473.

365. Schultz JC, Adamson JS Jr, Workman WW, Normal TD. Fatal liver disease after intravenous administration of tetracycline in high dosage. N Engl J Med 1963; 269:999–1004.

366. Allen ES, Brown WE. Hepatic toxicity of tetracycline in pregnancy. Am J Obstet Gynecol 1966; 95:12–18.

367. Wenk RE, Gebhardt FC, Bhagavan BS, Lustgarten JA, McCarthy EF. Tetracycline-associated fatty liver of pregnancy, including possible pregnancy

risk after chronic dermatologic use of tetracycline. J Reprod Med 1981; 26: 135–141.

368. Knowles JA. Drugs in milk. Pediatr Curr 1972; 21:28–32.

369. Graf VH, Reimann S. Untersuchungen uber die knozentration von pyrroli-dono-methyl-tetracycline in der muttermilch. Dtsch Med Wochenschr 1959; 84:1694.

370. Ylikorkala O, Sjostedt E, Jarvnen PA, Tikkanen R, Raines T. Trimethoprim-sulfonamide combination administered orally and intravaginally in the 1st trimester of pregnancy: its absorption into serum and transfer to amniotic fluid. Acta Obstet Gynecol Scand 1974; 52:229–234.

371. Reid DWJ, Caille G, Kaufmann NR. Maternal and transplacental kinetics of trimethoprim and sulfamethoxazole, separately and in combination. Can Med Assoc J 1975; 112:67S–72S.

372. Williams JD, Brumfitt W, Condie AP, Reeves DS. The treatment of bacteriuria in pregnant women with sulphamethoxazole and trimethoprim. Postgrad Med J 1969; 45(suppl):71–76.

373. Brumfitt W, Pursell R. Trimethoprim/sulfamethoxazole in the treatment of bacteriuria in women. J Infect Dis 1973; 128(suppl):S657–S663.

374. Czeizel A. A case-control analysis of the teratogenic effects of co-trimoxazole. Reprod Toxicol 1990; 4:305–313.

375. Bass AD, Yntema CL, Hammond WS, Frazer MI. Mechanism by which sulfadiazine affects the survival of the mammalian embryo. J Pharmacol Exp Ther 1951; 101:362–367.

376. Kato T, Kitigawa S. Production of congenital anomalies in fetuses of rats and mice with various sulfonamides. Congen Anom 1973; 13:7–15.

377. Hepburn JS, Paxson NF, Rogers AN. Secretion of ingested sulfanilamide in breast milk and in the urine of the nursing infant. Arch Pediatr 1942; 59: 413–418.

378. Stewart HL, Pratt JP. Sulfanilamide excretion in human breast milk and effect on breast-fed babies. JAMA 1940; 111:1456–1458.

379. McEwen LM. Trimethoprim/sulfamethoxazole mixture in pregnancy. Br Med J 1971; 4:490–491.

380. Smithells RW. Co-trimoxazole in pregnancy. Lancet 1983; 2:1142.

381. Helm F, Kretzschmar R, Leuschner F, Neumann W. Untersuchungen uber den Einfluss der Kombination SulfamoxolTrimethoprim (CN3123) and Fertilitat und Embryonalentwicklung an Ratten und Kaninchen. Arzneim Forsch 1976; 26:643–651.

382. Ochoa AG. Trimethoprim and sulfamethoxazole in pregnancy. JAMA 1971; 217:1244.

383. Brumfitt W, Pursell R. Double-blind trial to compare ampicillin, cephalexin, co-trimoxazole, and trimethoprim in treatment of urinary infection. Br Med J 1972; 2:673–676.

384. Bailey RR. Single-dose antibacterial treatment for bacteriuria in pregnancy. Drugs 1984; 27:183–186.

385. Colley DP, Kay J, Gibson GT. Study of the use in pregnancy of co-trimoxazole sulfamethizole. Austral J Pharm 1982; 63:570–575.

386. Koutras A, Fisher S. Niikawa-Kuroki syndrome: a new malformation syndrome of postnatal dwarfism, mental retardation, unusual face and protruding ears. J Pediatr 1982; 101:417–419.

387. Elmazar MM, Nau H. Trimethoprim potentiates valproic acid-induced neural tube defects (NTDs) in mice. Reprod Toxicol 1993; 7:249–254.

388. Arnauld R, Soutoul JH, Gallier J, Borderon JC, Borderon E. A study of the passage of trimethoprim into the maternal milk. Quest Med 1972; 25:959–964.

389. Miller RD, Salter AJ. The passage of trimethoprim/sulpha-methoxazole into breast milk and its significance. In Daikos GK, ed. Progress in Chemotherapy, Proc 8th International Congress of Chemotherapy, Athens, 1973. Athens: Hellenic Society for Chemotherapy, 1974:687–691.

390. Thrall KD, Bull RJ. Differences in the distribution of iodine and iodide in the Sprague-Dawley rat. Fundam Appl Toxicol 1990; 15:75–81.

391. Wolff J. Iodide goiter and the pharmacologic effects of excess iodide. Am J Med 1969; 47:101–124.

392. Mehta PS, Mehta SJ, Vorherr H. Congenital iodide goiter and hypothyroidism: a review. Obstet Gynecol Surv 1983; 38:237–247.

393. Committee on Drugs, American Academy of Pediatrics. Adverse reactions to iodide therapy of asthma and other pulmonary diseases. Pediatrics 1982; 57:272–274.

394. Herbst AL, Selenkow HA. Hyperthyroidism during pregnancy. N Engl J Med 1965; 273:627–633.

395. Selenkow HA, Herbst Al. Hyperthyroidism during pregnancy. N Engl J Med 1966; 274:165–166.

396. Pritchard JA, MacDonald PC, Gant NF. Williams Obstetrics. 17th ed. Norwalk, CT: Appleton-Century-Crofts, 1985:605.

397. l'Allemand D, Gruters A, Heidemann P, Schurnbrand P. Iodine-induced alteration of thyroid function in newborn infants after prenatal and perinatal exposure to povidone iodine. J Pediatr 1983; 102:935–938.

398. Postellon DC, Aronow R. Iodine in mother's milk. JAMA 1982; 247:463.

399. Vorherr H, Vorherr UF, Mehta P, Ulrich JA, Messer RH. Vaginal absorption of povidone-iodine. JAMA 1980; 244:2628–2629.

400. Danziger Y, Pertzelan A, Mimouni M. Transient congenital hypothyroidism after topical iodine in pregnancy and lactation. Arch Dis Child 1987; 62:295–296.

401. Jacobson JM, Hankins GV, Young RL, Hauth JC. Changes in thyroid function and serum iodine levels after prepartum use of a povidone-iodine vaginal lubricant. J Reprod Med 1984; 29:98–100.

402. Anonymous. Expectorant drug products for over-the-counter human use; final monograph. Fed Reg Feb. 28, 1989: 8494–8509.

403. Hirsch SR, Viernes PF, Kory RC. The expectorant effect of glyceryl guaiacolate in patients with chronic bronchitis. A controlled in vitro and in vivo study. Chest 1973; 63:9–14.

404. Kuhn JJ, Hendley JO, Adams KF, Clark JW, Gwaltney JM Jr. Antitussive effects of guaifenesin in young adults with natural colds. Chest 1982; 82: 713–718.

405. Hendley JO, Gwaltney JM. Antitussive effect of guaifenesin. Chest 1983; 84:118–119.

406. Geber WF, Schramm LC. Comparative teratogenicity of morphine, heroin, and methadone in the hamster. Pharmacologist 1975; 11:248.

407. Zellers JE, Gautieri RF. Evaluation of teratogenic potential of codeine sulfate in CF-1 mice. J Pharm Sci 1977; 66:1727–1731.

408. Williams J, Price CJ, Sleet RB, George JD, Marr MC, Kimmel CA, Morrissey RE. Codeine: developmental toxicity in hamsters and mice. Fundam Appl Toxicol 1991; 16:401–413.

409. Lehmann VH. [Teratologic studies in rabbits and rats with the morphine derivative codeine]. Arznein Forsch 1976; 26:551–554.

410. Shaw GM, Malcoe LH, Swan SH, Cummins SK, Schulman J, Harris JA. Risks for congenital cardiac anomalies relative to selected maternal exposures during early pregnancy. Teratology 1990; 41:590.

411. Bracken MB, Holford TR. Exposure to prescribed drugs in pregnancy and association with congenital malformations. Obstet Gynecol 1981; 58:336–344.

412. Saxén I. Associations between oral clefts and drugs taken during pregnancy. Int J Epidemiol 1975; 4:37–44.

413. Van Leeuwen G, Guthrie R, Stange F. Narcotic withdrawal reaction in a newborn infant due to codeine. Pediatrics 1965; 36:635–636.

414. Mangurten HH, Benawra R. Neonatal codeine withdrawal in infants of nonaddicted mothers. Pediatrics 1980; 65:159–160.

415. Horning MG, Stillwell WG, Nowlin J, Lertratanangkoon K, Stillwell RN, Hill RM. Identification and quantification of drugs and drug metabolites in human breast milk using GC-MS-COM methods. Mod Probl Paediatr 1975; 15:73–79.

416. Meny RG, Naumburg EG, Alger LS, Brill-Miller JL, Brown S. Codeine and the breastfed neonate. J Hum Lact 1993; 9:237–240.

417. Chester SW. Pregnancy and the treatment of hay fever, allergic rhinitis, and pollen asthma. Ann Allergy 1950; 8:772–798.

418. Derbes VJ, Sodeman WA. Reciprocal influence of bronchial asthma and pregnancy. Am J Med 1946; 1:367–375.

419. Jensen K. Pregnancy and allergic diseases. Acta Allergol 1953; 6:44.

420. Maietta AL. The management of the allergic patient during pregnancy. Ann Allergy 1955; 13:516–522.

421. Metzger WJ, Turner E, Patterson R. The safety of immunotherapy during pregnancy. J Allergy Clin Immunol 1978; 61:268–272.

422. Schaefer G, Silverman F. Pregnancy complicated by asthma. Am J Obstet Gynecol 1961; 82:182–189.

423. Ziaya PR, Hankins GD, Gilstrap LC III, Halsey AB. Intravenous penicillin desensitization and treatment during pregnancy. JAMA 1986; 256: 2561–1562.

424. Sarnat HB, Rybak G, Kotagal S, Blair JD. Cerebral embryopathy in late first trimester: possible association with swine influenza vaccine. Teratology 1979; 20:93–99.

425. Deinard AS, Ogburn P Jr. A/NJ/8/76 influenza vaccination program: effects on maternal health and pregnancy outcome. Am J Obstet Gynecol 1981; 140:240–245.

426. Sumaya CV, Gibbs RS. Immunization of pregnant women with influenza A/New Jersey/76 virus vaccine: reactogenicity and immunogenicity in mother and infant. J Infect Dis 1979; 140:141–146.

427. Advisory Committee on Immunization Practices, Centers for Disease Control: Prevention and control of influenza. Morbid Mortal Weekly Rep 1988; 37:361–373.

428. Sterner G, Grandien M, Enocksson E. Pregnant women with acute respiratory illness at term. Scand J Infect Dis Suppl 1990; 71:19–26.

429. American College of Obstetricians and Gynecologists. ACOG Technical Bulletin No. 160, October 1991.

430. Dybing E, Holme JA, Gordon WP, Soederlund EJ, Dahlin DC, Nelson SD. Genotoxicity studies with paracetamol. Mutat Res 1984; 138:21–32.

431. Hongslo JK, Christensen T, Brunborg G, Bjornstad C, Holme JA. Genotoxic effects of paracetamol in V79 Chinese hamster cells. Mutat Res 1988; 204: 333–341.

432. Hongslo JK, Brogger A, Bjorge C, Holme JA. Increased frequency of sister-chromatid exchange and chromatid breaks in lymphocytes after treatment of human volunteers with therapeutic doses of paracetamol. Mutat Res 1991; 261:1–8.

433. Hongslo JK, Björge C, Schwarze PE, Brögger A, Mann G, Thelander L, Holme JA. Paracetamol inhibits replicative DNA synthesis and induces sister chromatid exchange and chromosomal aberrations by inhibition of ribonucleotide reductase. Mutagenesis 1990; 5:475–480.

434. Wright HN. Chronic toxicity studies of analgesic and antipyretic drugs and congeners. Toxicol Appl Pharmacol 1967; 11:280–292.

435. Reel JR, Lawton AD, Lamb JC 4th. Reproductive toxicity evaluation of acetaminophen in Swiss CD-1 mice using a continuous breeding protocol. Fundam Appl Toxicol 1992; 18:233–239.

436. Lubawy WC, Burriss Garret RJ. Effects of aspirin and acetaminophen on fetal and placental growth in rats. J Pharm Sci 1977; 66:111–113.

437. Williams DA, Weiss T, Wade E, Dignan P. Prune perineum syndrome: report of a second case. Teratology 1983; 28:145–148.

438. Golden SM, Perman KI. Bilateral clinical anophthalmia: drugs as potential factors. South Med J 1980; 73:1404–1407.

439. General Practitioner Clinical Trials. Drugs in pregnancy survey. Practitioner 1963; 191:775–780.

440. Opitz JM, Grosse FR, Haneberg B. Congenital effects of bromism? Lancet 1972; 1:91–92.

441. McNeil JR. The possible teratogenic effect of salicylates on the developing fetus. Brief summary of eight suggestive cases. Clin Pediatr 1973; 12: 347–350.

442. Golden NL, King KC, Sokol RJ. Propoxyphene and acetaminophen. Possible effects on the fetus. Clin Pediatr 1982; 21:752–754.

443. Char VC, Chandra R, Fletcher AB, Avery GB. Polyhydramnios and neonatal renal failure—a possible association with maternal acetaminophen ingestion. J Pediatr 1975; 86:638–639.

444. Mancini RE, Sonawane BR, Yaffe SJ. Developmental susceptibility to acetaminophen toxicity. Res Commun Chem Pathol Pharmacol 1983; 27:603–606.

445. Haibach H, Akhter JE, Muscato MS, Cary PL, Hoffman MF. Acetaminophen overdose with fetal demise. Am J Clin Pathol 1984; 82:240–242.

446. Roberts I, Robinson MJ, Mughal MZ, Ratcliffe JF, Prescott LF. Paracetamol metabolites in the neonate following maternal overdose. Br J Clin Pharmacol 1984; 18:201–206.

447. Byer AJ, Traylor TR, Semmer JR. Acetaminophen overdose in the third trimester of pregnancy. JAMA 1982; 247:3114–3115.

448. Stokes IM. Paracetamol overdose in the second trimester of pregnancy. Case report. Br J Obstet Gynaecol 1984; 91:286–288.

449. Ludmir J, Main DM, Landon MB, Gabbe SG. Maternal acetaminophen overdose at 15 weeks of gestation. Obstet Gynecol 1986; 67:750–751.

450. Riggs BS, Bronstein AC, Kulig K, Archer PG, Rumack BH. Acute acetaminophen overdosage during pregnancy. Obstet Gynecol 1989; 74:247–253.

451. Rosevear SK, Hope PL. Favourable neonatal outcome following maternal paracetamol overdose and severe fetal distress. Case report. Br J Obstet Gynaecol 1979; 96:491–493.

452. Rumack CM, Guggenheim MA, Rumack BH, Peterson RG, Johnson ML, Braithwaite WR. Neonatal intracranial hemorrhage and maternal use of aspirin. Obstet Gynecol 1981; 58:52S–56S.

453. Momma K, Takeuchi H. Constriction of fetal ductus arteriosus by nonsteroidal anti-inflammatory drugs. Prostaglandins 1983; 26:631–643.

454. Peterson RG. Consequences associated with nonnarcotic analgesics in the fetus and newborn. Fed Proc 1985; 44:2309–2312.

455. Weber B, Fontan JE. Acetaminophen as a pain enhancer during voluntary interruption of pregnancy with mifepristone and sulprostone. Eur J Clin Pharmacol 1990; 39:609.

456. Bitzen P-O, Gustafsson B, Jostell KG, Melander A, Wahlin-Boll E. Excretion of paracetamol in human breast milk. Eur J Clin Pharmacol 1981; 20: 123–125.

457. Berlin Jr CM, Yaffe SJ, Ragni M. Disposition of acetaminophen in milk, saliva, and plasma of lactating women. Pediatr Pharmacol 1980; 1:135–141.
458. Matheson I, Lunde PKM, Notarianni LJ. Infant rash caused by paracetamol in breast milk? Pediatrics 1985; 76:651–652.
459. Schick B, Hom M, Librizzi R, Donnenfeld A. Pregnancy outcome following exposure to clarithromycin. Reprod Toxicol 1996; 10:162.
460. McElhatton PR, Sullivan FM, Volans GN. Paracetamol overdosage in pregnancy. Analysis of the outcomes of 300 cases referred to the teratology information service. Reprod Toxicol 1997; 11:85–94.

9

Medical/Legal Aspects of Prescribing During Pregnancy

FREDERICK H. FERN

Lester Schwab Katz & Dwyer
New York, New York

JEAN A. HOBART

Attorney-at-Law
Beverly Hills, California

CHRISTOPHER P. ORLANDO

Renzulli, Gainey & Rutherford
New York, New York

I. Introduction

Few personal injuries are so emotion-laden as those of a defective newborn. Birth defects trigger feelings of surprise, guilt, and disappointment following an event that has been joyfully anticipated as a celebration of life. In times past, parents could be expected to adjust to their child's abnormality, recognizing the blessings of life in whatever form and accepting the additional responsibilities that their new child's special needs might present. In today's litigious environment, however, shattered expectations can cause tough questions to be asked: What went wrong? Who is to blame? And, inevitably, is somebody legally liable? The frequency of drug use during pregnancy, and the knowledge that some drugs are teratogens, may focus attention on a drug used by a mother as the possible cause of a newborn's injury.

If it can be shown with a reasonable degree of scientific certainty that a drug ingested by a pregnant woman caused harm to the fetus, then the logical conclusion is that the harm could have been avoided through noningestion of the drug. The question then becomes whether ingestion of the drug would have been prevented if somebody along the drug distribution chain had made a better decision about exposing the fetus to the risk of harm. Recent litigation has examined the decisions made by drug manufacturers, physicians, and pregnant women concerning fetal exposure to risk. Since a fetus is in no position to avoid exposure to risk, that body of litigation has queried to what degree drug manufacturers, physicians, and pregnant women owe a duty to a fetus to avoid exposure of the fetus to an unreasonable risk of harm. The responsibility of the physician to prevent drug-induced birth defects can only be evaluated within the framework of the totality of responsibility, which includes the pharmaceutical manufacturer as well as the patient, and possibly others.

II. Characterizing a Legal Action on Behalf of a Fetus

A. Types of Actions

In 1946, *Bonbrest v. Katz* (1) held that a child born alive may recover for injuries suffered before birth if the fetus was viable at the time of injury. This rule, or variants of it, has now been adopted in all jurisdictions (2). Recent litigation has expanded on the *Bonbrest* rule, and has become complex, both conceptually and semantically. Distinctions are based on whether the lawsuit is brought on behalf of the parents or child, and on whether the child was born healthy or impaired.

A "wrongful pregnancy" action is brought by the parents of a healthy, but unplanned child, where the complaint alleges preconception negligence by a physician, pharmaceutical manufacturer, or pharmacist regarding a contraceptive procedure or medication that did not work (3). In a "wrongful birth" case, the parents of a deformed or handicapped child are suing for alleged postconception negligence of a physician or other party whose failure to act prevented the parents from exercising their option to terminate the pregnancy (4). A "wrongful life" claim is brought by or on behalf of a child who suffers an impairment. This action is difficult to distinguish from the parents' wrongful birth claim, because it also alleges that the parents were prevented from terminating the pregnancy (5). Wrongful life claims have been virtually unanimously rejected by courts, due to the difficulty of rationally determining whether the plaintiff has suffered a legally cognizable injury by being born, when the action which allegedly should have occurred would have resulted in no life at all. Courts have steered away from a theory that assumes nonexistence is desirable (6).

Acceptance of the wrongful life theory in a drug-induced birth defect case first occurred in *Harbeson v. Parke-Davis, Inc.* (7), the court overcoming reservations expressed in the previous cases. In an analysis of this case, Furrow used the phrase "diminished life" (8), which he had coined earlier (9). The concept of diminished life, as suggested by Furrow, relates to the difference between a defective child who claims that it would be better not to have been born because accurate genetic counseling would have led to an abortion, as opposed to a defective child who claims that it would be better to have been born without the defect because counseling regarding teratogenicity would have led to a drug not being used by the mother. In the case of the first child, the defendant's alleged negligence is passive, it being a failure to act to prevent the birth of a child whose defect was not caused by the defendant. In the case of the second child, the defendant's alleged negligence is active. By distributing or prescribing a drug without an adequate warning, the action of the defendant has caused the child's defect. Because damages are clear and the value of life is not questioned, diminished life as a theory of recovery is free of pragmatic and policy concerns that attend the wrongful life action. Thus, a court need not decide whether nonexistence is better than impaired existence.

B. Fetal Rights

Legal recognition of the fetus as an entity with its own rights occurred first in property law, where the fetus was given the status of a person solely for the purpose of inheritance and subject to the condition that it later be born alive (10). The live birth requirement has also been incorporated into criminal statutes, many of which recognize fetal existence but impose criminal penalties for harm to the fetus only after the victim has been born (11). Adherence to a live birth requirement limits the right of a fetus because there is no recognition of the fetus as separate from the woman prior to birth. In this regard, the early cases in property law and criminal law are more a recognition of the woman's rights during pregnancy than of fetal rights.

A perspective on fetal rights that is consistent with medical principles and that helps clarify duties to the fetus in a drug exposure situation was proposed by Capron within the context of genetic counseling (12). Capron argues that a fetus has the right to have its parents decide what is in its best interests. If one accepts this argument, then effectively the fetus is placed on equal footing with other patients who must have a decision made for them because they lack the capacity to make the decision themselves. Exposure to a drug involves possible benefits and possible detriments that must be weighed when making a decision. Applying Capron's logic to a fetal drug exposure case, it becomes a fetal right to have a decision regarding use of a possibly teratogenic drug made in such a way that consideration is given to the potential detriment to the fetus in light of all relevant factors.

Presumably, the person best able to consider fetal risks is the woman who carries the fetus. Only she can hazard a guess as to how life will be for the child if it is born with an impairment, given the variability of family situations and parenting skills. But her decision can only be as sound as the information she is given, and adequate information must be given by the manufacturer to the physician, who can help the woman understand the information and appreciate its significance to her and her fetus. Where the potential benefit to the woman is slight and the potential harm to the child is great, a logical extension of fetal rights is to impose a duty on physicians to consider fetal risk carefully prior to prescribing, and not to prescribe the drug if fetal risk outweighs maternal benefit.

III. Food and Drug Administration Regulation

A. Teratogenicity Testing

The recognition of a teratogenic agent in humans is often difficult. Traditional methods of testing drug safety, using clinical trials to compare the incidence of an adverse effect in exposed and unexposed populations, are severely limited in teratogenicity testing for moral reasons. The result is that the most reliable data come either from animal experiments in which agents are administered at high doses throughout the period of organogenesis, or from epidemiological surveys of women who usually have had low-dose exposure at unknown time periods and frequencies.

The regulatory guidelines for animal reproductive studies issued by the Food and Drug Administration (FDA) have become standard as a screen for teratogenicity (13). Two test species are used, most frequently the rat and rabbit. Pregnant females are dosed daily with the test compound during organogenesis and are killed prior to birth of the offspring. The uterus is removed, and fetuses are examined for external, visual, and skeletal anomalies. Different dosages are administered, and a "no observable effect level" is determined. This dose is then divided by a safety factor to determine a safe dose for humans. Unfortunately, while animal tests may reveal teratogenic activity, they do not necessarily correlate well with risks in humans (14).

After a drug has been marketed for a period of time, it may be possible to use epidemiological methods to examine a relationship between exposure and outcome in humans. Using prospective cohort studies or retrospective case-control studies, statistical analysis may be used to determine whether chance alone or the background incidence rate can be ruled out as the reason for an association between exposure and outcome. Only after a significant period of human exposure can there be sufficient data on which to base a conclusion that a drug poses no appreciable risk of harm to the human fetus. In the interim, the high degree of scientific uncertainty justifies extreme caution in the prescribing of newly marketed drugs.

B. Teratogenicity Information

The acquisition of scientific information serves little purpose unless the information is conveyed in an orderly and understandable fashion to those who need the information to make decisions. In an effort to increase the amount of information available concerning teratogenicity and to standardize the way the information is expressed to facilitate comparisons, the FDA has adopted a letter-coded categorization of drugs based on their risk to the fetus (15). The letters A, B, C, D, and X are used, with the fetal risk increasing as the letter goes farther down the alphabet (i.e., A equals least risk, X equals the highest risk). This system applies only to prescription drugs, so it is included in the labeling directed to the physician, not the patient.

A survey of the 100 most frequently prescribed products disclosed that only 59 conform to the letter-code system (16). The majority of letter-coded products were labeled as category C, which signifies that "Either studies in animals have revealed adverse effects on the fetus (teratogenic or embryological or other) and there are no controlled studies in women, or studies in women and animals are not available. Drugs should be given only if the potential benefit justifies the potential risk to the fetus" (17). Another 22 drugs did not follow the letter-coded system, but carried a statement along the lines of "Safety for use in pregnancy has not been established. This drug should be given only if the potential benefit outweighs the potential harm to the fetus" (18).

Ambiguous warnings, such as those presented by the drugs in category C and the 22 minimally labeled drugs, disclose no hard data about fetal risk, but they admonish that this risk should be balanced against the benefit prior to prescribing. Such warnings place the physician in a quandary. How can the uncertainty of fetal risk be balanced against the certainty of maternal benefit? A caution that discloses no useful information, but instructs that informed decisions should be made, encourages overly conservative decisions. The decision to use a drug carries with it potential responsibility for having caused a birth defect should one occur. Making decisions based on known risk is difficult enough; good decisions based on unexplained uncertainty are impossible.

IV. Responsibility to the Fetus

A. The Manufacturer

Traditionally, the law has recognized that the duty owed by the drug manufacturer to the patient is to disclose known or knowable information about drug risks to the physician but not directly to the patient. This prescription drug rule has been criticized generally (19) and specifically with regard to teratogenicity (20). The criticism focused on the responsibility to protect the patient's right to know about material risks. In an attempt to protect the patient, a comprehensive program of direct-to-patient warnings was adopted by the FDA in 1980 but was later rescinded (21). Civil litigation that would modify the prescription drug rule has not been warmly received (22). The problem of inadequate information is a very real one in the area of teratogenicity, where studies indicate that pregnant women want to know the probability that a drug may have adverse fetal effects, but they are not receiving the information (23). Under such circumstances, responsible maternal decision making is not possible.

As the best expert on its own drug, a manufacturer should also be the best source of information. This means not only that reasonable and state-of-the-art scientific methods be used to obtain information, but also that the information be conveyed on a timely basis to those who need it to make a decision about drug risks. Physicians know the characteristics of their patients, but must rely on manufacturers for information about drug products. Labeling directed to the physician might be made more useful if it had a separate section designated as "fetal toxicity information for the patient," in which specific language was used to describe what is known about teratogenicity and what is reported or suspected but not yet confirmed. Vague admonitions in drug labeling to consider poorly characterized and ill-defined risks place a high degree of responsibility on the shoulders of the physician, without effectively equipping the physician to meet the responsibility. Pharmaceutical manufacturers must attempt to ascertain all relevant information about teratogenic effects and effectively disseminate that knowledge to the medical community.

B. The Physician

For those drugs that are recognized teratogens or fetal toxins, the physician's responsibility is clear: Don't prescribe such drugs during pregnancy.

But there are several complicating factors. Conception does not immediately cause the occurrence of physiological or psychological changes, so a fertile and sexually active woman faces the constant possibility of being pregnant and not knowing it. The physician has the responsibility of helping a patient during child-bearing years manage this problem through contraceptive advice and if possible by recommending a waiting period before initiating drug therapy, to either confirm or rule out pregnancy. When a patient contemplates using a drug that is of benefit to her but potentially harmful to the fetus, she has a right to know the character of the risk. This involves not only the simple disclosure of information by the physician, but also provision of the opportunity for reflection and assistance in reaching a decision (24).

A far greater problem is presented by drugs that are suspected but unconfirmed teratogens. It has been suggested that physicians feel particularly uncomfortable dealing with uncertainty in obstetrics (25). A physician admitting to a patient that the teratogenic risk of a recommended drug is unknown is difficult because it concedes fallibility. Physicians are unlikely to admit to patients that: (a) they are acting with uncertainty; (b) there are multiple decision strategies under scrutiny, ranging from high risk-averse ones to less risk-averse ones; (c) physicians prefer a strategy that focuses on fetal risk and preventing it; and (d) this strategy may decrease maternal benefit or increase maternal risk (26). Yet the physician's disclosure responsibility is to assist the patient in understanding the information that is available, limited though it may be. No matter what a pharmaceutical manufacturer may do to increase the availability of information, the manufacturer cannot write a warning directed to each individual patient. Only the physician knows the unique characteristics of the patient's lifestyle, education level, and values, and must tailor the consultation accordingly. It is the physician who can disclose risk-related information and then instruct the patient on the decision-making strategies and options available.

A pregnant woman may make a decision with which her physician disagrees. This will most likely occur when another physician has prescribed medication for a woman who then becomes pregnant and continues using the medication contrary to her obstetrician's advice. It is foreseeable that a woman who is using medication would disregard her physician's advice to avoid pregnancy. Under such circumstances, the physician may attempt to coerce the woman into adopting rational behavior either through counseling (You don't want to do anything that might hurt your baby, do you?) or by eliminating the availability of the medication, refusing to prescribe it or canceling previously authorized refills. But patient behavior is not irrational simply because it is contrary to what the physician believes is correct. The physician's responsibility is to inform and assist with a decision; once an informed decision is made by the patient, the physician's responsibility is to treat the patient within the parameters of that decision.

C. The Pregnant Woman

A pregnant woman has a responsibility to manage her medication use in a way that accounts for the risks and benefits of drugs both to herself and to the fetus she carries. A woman's responsibility not to cause harm to a fetus, once she has foregone the exercise of her legal right to terminate the pregnancy, must impose certain limitations on her freedom of action. In deciding whether a woman acted improperly by exposing her fetus to an unreasonable risk of harm, it is necessary to evaluate both the magnitude and probability of harm to the fetus posed by hazard exposure and the magnitude and probability of harm to the woman posed by hazard avoidance. Invariably this analysis will occur after the risk to the fetus has materialized, so care must be taken not to overemphasize the reality of fetal harm; for when the woman made her decision, the harm was a theoretical probability and not yet a reality. The result of the analysis will be a comparison of the woman's actual behavior with that of the "reasonable pregnant woman."

Because the relationship between mother and fetus is unique among interpersonal relationships, the standard for reasonable maternal conduct requires unique analysis. Cherniak develops a realistic model of maternal liability for prenatal injury, limited entirely to gross negligence (27). Within this model, for there to be liability, a conscious disregard for the welfare of the fetus would have to be proved. Only if it could be shown that the woman knew or should have known that her conduct created a substantial risk of serious harm to the fetus, and the cost to her of avoiding the risk was minimal, would liability attach. The focus is on the woman's actual or constructive knowledge and on her responsibility to consider the risk to the fetus as well as the risk to herself prior to engaging in risk behavior. Thus the ingestion of potentially teratogenic medication would not be actionable unless the woman knew or should have known that there was the possibility of harm to the fetus and she disregarded that knowledge in deciding to use the drug for her benefit. A pregnant woman who has considered fetal risk, has used a drug, and has given birth to a defective child has not acted unreasonably unless the risk is so frequent and so severe that it would be clearly deemed unacceptable when compared with the usual and customary behavior of other pregnant women.

V. Lessons from Litigation

A. Manufacturer Liability

One of the earliest legal opinions to establish the manufacturer's responsibility in a fetal harm case is *Woodill v. Parke-Davis* (28). The parents of a minor child sought to recover damages for injuries suffered in utero, the injuries having allegedly been caused by the drug Pitocin. The issue of primary concern was whether, in an action seeking to hold a defendant manufacturer liable for failure to warn of a danger attendant to the use of the drug, the plaintiff must allege and prove that the defendant actually knew, or should have known, of the danger. The court held that the imposition of a knowledge requirement is a proper limitation to place on a manufacturer's liability predicated upon a failure to warn of a danger inherent in a product. The reasoning of *Woodill* was reinforced and updated in *Brown v. Superior Court* (29). In this case brought by a number of DES daughters, the court rejected the plaintiff's assertion that a drug manufacturer should be held liable for failure to warn of risks inherent in a drug even though it did not know and could not have known, by the application of scientific knowledge available at the time of distribution, that the drug could produce the undesirable side effects suffered by the plaintiff. In essence, this approach relieves the drug manufacturer of the burden of the scientific uncertainty that accompanies the distribution of an as yet undocumented teratogen. Yet if the manufacturer does not bear the burden of uncertainty, then that burden must shift to the physician and the patient.

B. Physician Liability

The case of *Harbeson v. Parke-Davis, Inc.* (30) considers the level of knowledge required of physicians when prescribing drugs and when advising patients regarding the use of drugs during pregnancy. When Dilantin was prescribed for Mrs. Harbeson, none of the doctors knew that the drug could cause fetal hydantoin syndrome (FSH). The lower court found that a search of the medical literature would have revealed several articles regarding the correlation of Dilantin and FSH. In addition, there was evidence that the warning in the *Physician's Desk Reference* (PDR) was sufficient to put physicians on notice as to the effect of the drug. The court held that it was not unreasonable to expect the doctors in this case to discover the risk.

The *Harbeson* case next considered whether the risks Dilantin posed to the fetus were material. The court applied a two-step test of materiality incorporating an objective standard. The first step is to define the existence and nature of the risk and its likelihood of occurrence. The second step is to decide whether the probability of that type of harm is a risk which a reasonable patient would consider in deciding on treatment. The court referred to expert testimony presented at trial and agreed that this testimony satisfied the first step in the materiality test. The court also concluded that a reasonable patient would have considered the risk of teratogenicity in deciding on treatment. Therefore, the appeals court upheld the finding by the district court that the risks posed by Dilantin were material, noting that the goal of risk disclosure is to make the patient an active participant in the decision-making process. If a risk is material, then it must be disclosed to the patient.

In the unusual case of *Roberts v. Patel* (31), the court was asked to decide whether the fetus, as well as the mother, is a patient. The facts of this case disclose that, while the natural mother was in labor, the defendant physicians advised that the labor should be temporarily halted by the use of alcohol and another drug. Allegedly as the result of this treatment, the child suffered permanent spastic quadriplegia. A lawsuit was initiated by the adoptive mother of the child, but the natural mother was not a party to the lawsuit. The defendant argued that the only duty of disclosure owed was to the natural mother, and that the lawsuit should be dismissed because she was not involved in the legal action. The court rejected this argument, citing a line of Illinois fetal rights cases, and concluded:

> In light of the strong Illinois policy favoring protection of a fetus, and in light of Illinois' recognition of a protectable interest in the fetus in ordinary malpractice claims, even prior to conception, we hold that [the] mother's physicians owed a duty of informed disclosure not only to [the] mother, but to [the child] as well; in this situation the physician had two patients (32).

Obviously, recognizing a duty of disclosure to a fetus is one thing, while a realistic way of meeting the duty is an entirely separate matter. In the ensuing discussion, the court indicated that, while there is a duty of disclosure to the fetus, this duty can be met by informing the woman of the risks to the fetus.

Thus, when a physician treats a pregnant woman, there are in reality two patients being treated, and both patients may bring an action against the physician based on informed consent. The guide for disclosure is materiality, the presumption being that individuals have a right to determine what shall be done with their bodies. Teratogenicity would appear to be of such a significant character that if teratogenic potential is disclosed to the physician by the manufacturer, it likewise must be disclosed by the physician to the patient. While theoretically possible, it is difficult to imagine a pregnant woman who would not want to consider the possibility of fetal harm when deciding whether or not to use a drug.

C. Maternal Liability

The only reported legal opinion squarely on point as to the civil liability of a pregnant woman to her fetus is *Grodin v. Grodin* (33). In this case a child, through his father, appealed from a judgment dismissing his mother as a defendant in a lawsuit brought by him. The child had developed brown and discolored teeth as a result of his mother's ingestion of tetracycline during pregnancy. He alleged negligence of his mother in failing to seek proper medical care, failing to request that her physician perform a pregnancy test, and failing to inform her physician that she was taking tetracycline. The lower court granted judgment for the mother, based on parent–child tort immunity, which prevents a child from suing a parent.

The Appellate Court ruled that parent–child immunity had largely been overruled, but that an exception remained within which the exercise of reasonable parental discretion still shielded a parent from a lawsuit brought by a child. The *Grodin* court acknowledged that a woman's decision to continue taking drugs during pregnancy is an exercise of her discretion, therefore it should be immunized from litigation. But the court also held that the reasonableness of that exercise of discretion is subject to litigation, and the judgment for the mother was reversed, with the case remanded for a determination of the reasonableness of the alleged negligent conduct. However, the court provided no indication of the parameters for determining the standard of a reasonable pregnant woman.

VI. Legal Standards for Causation

A. Causation Defined

The term "proximate cause" is most often used to describe the combination of causation issues that need to be addressed prior to the imposition of legal liability on the defendant (34). This combination may be divided into two distinct components: (a) causation in fact, and (b) causation in law. Causation in fact, sometimes referred to as "but for" causation, determines whether there is a connection between the defendant's conduct and the injury—namely, that the injury would not have occurred but for the defendant's conduct (35). Causation in law, also referred to as legal causation, determines whether the connection is sufficiently substantial that the law will hold the defendant responsible for his injury-causing conduct (36). This latter determination is a policy decision made by courts, not the jury, based on the evidence set forth in the case. As one court noted, "Proximate cause is designed not only to allow recovery for damages incurred because of another's act, but also to define such limits on recovery as are economically and socially desirable (37).

The threshold issue of causation in fact, specifically whether the defendant caused the plaintiff's injury, is usually a question of fact which is decided by the jury (38). In drug-induced birth defects litigation, the relationship between the defendant's product and the injury is often fiercely disputed, because the mechanism of the injury may not be patent, if present at all. Although definite proof of causation in fact may be impossible to obtain (39), the law requires that it be established by a "preponderance of the evidence" as in all other civil litigation (40). In other words, the plaintiff must show that exposure to the product was more likely than not the cause of the injury (41). Causation may be proved by a sufficient quantum of circumstantial evidence. If the plaintiff merely demonstrates that the drug was a possible cause, he or she has failed to prove causation. As stated by the court in *Holbrook v. Rose* (42), the "proof must be sufficient to tilt the balance from 'possibility' to 'probability'" (43).

In order to prove causation in fact, most courts require a two-step approach (44). The first step requires the plaintiff to prove that the agent can and does cause birth defects. This is referred to as a general causation. The second step requires proof that the agent caused the birth anomaly in the particular plaintiff. This is known as specific causation. Causation "requires a complex series of inferences drawn from scientific experiment and observation and statistical comparisons" (45). Mere temporal association is not sufficient to establish causation (46). Failure to prove general causation is often fatal to establishing causation in the particular case (47). However, courts may permit cases to be decided by the jury based solely on evidence of specific causation in very limited circumstances (48).

B. Opposing Experts

Expert testimony is crucial in linking plaintiff's injury to the defendant's product. Today, experts in a multitude of fields may testify on the complex medical and scientific issues involved in a drug-induced birth defect case. For example, parties may consult and/or call as expert or fact witnesses, diverse specialists such as geneticists, teratologists, developmental toxicologists, embryologists, biostatisticians, dysmorphologists, epidemiologists, toxicologists, and physicians from various disciplines. Often the primary responsibility of the expert witnesses is to testify that the defendant's product was or was not the cause in fact of the birth anomaly, and this testimony must be based on a reasonable degree of medical certainty (49). In order for the defendant to be found liable, this testimony must persuade the jury that the product more likely than not caused the injury (50).

Often, the medical and scientific communities have not determined a causal relationship between exposure to the defendant's product and birth defects. In these cases, the jury, generally composed of ordinary citizens with no medical or scientific background, are asked to decide whether a causal link exists between the defendant's product and the birth defects (51). Additionally, jury decisions on the issue of causation may be unduly influenced by scientific opinion testimony of experts, which may neither be generally accepted in the medical and scientific communities nor derived by the scientific method and supported by appropriate validation (52).

In most cases, both sides present testimony from expert witnesses to support their position, and such testimony often is diametrically opposed. One court eloquently articulated the problem regarding proof of causation by expert witnesses in Bendectin birth defect cases by stating:

> The expert witnesses on each side are often the same, from case to case, and even when different the scientific conclusions and theories are based on the same or similar statistical studies and scientific experiments. The cases are variations on a theme, somewhat like an orchestra which travels to different music halls, substituting musicians from time to time but playing essentially the same repertoire (53).

This observation illustrates the issue of determining whether the persons retained and presented to testify by either side are true experts in their respective fields or merely "hired guns," who will present an opinion without any supporting scientific basis (54). To mitigate this problem, federal courts have the authority to appoint and take testimony from a court-appointed expert who is in theory unbiased, whose testimony is admitted into evidence to assist the court in its search for truth (55). However, attorneys typically resist this route, due to strategic and cost considerations, while courts have not appointed experts on a widespread scale (56).

As discussed in greater detail later, most courts will closely examine the scientific reasoning and basis of the opinions proffered by expert witnesses in reaching their conclusions, so to avoid the potential of improper causation determinations by the jury (57).

C. Minimum Requisites for Admissibility

Historically, expert testimony was not admissible unless it reflected an opinion which the scientific community had generally accepted (58). This "general acceptance" standard was first formulated in *Frye v. United States* (59). There, the court excluded testimony based on the results of a polygraph test and enunciated the standard for the admissibility of scientific evidence based on novel theories or techniques as follows:

> [W]hile courts will go a long way in admitting expert testimony deducted from a well-recognized scientific principle or discovery, the thing from which

> the deduction is made must be sufficiently established to have gained general
> acceptance in the particular field in which it belongs (60).

Therefore, under the precedent of Frye, the opinions of expert witnesses as to causation must be based on principles "sufficiently established to have gained general acceptance in the particular field in which it belongs"; otherwise, the evidence is merely speculation and cannot form the basis of a verdict (61). In discussing some advantages of *Frye*, one court noted:

> [B]ecause neither judge nor jury may be able to separate "junk science" from good science, *Frye* helps guarantee "that reliability will be assessed by those in the best position to do so: members of the relevant scientific field who can dispassionately study and test the new theory" (62).

The court also conceded that *Frye* has significant shortcomings. For example, new discoveries which have direct experimental and clinical support may not be immediately accepted within the scientific community and, thus, would be inadmissible (63). Additionally, "generally accepted scientific theory is not always correct" (64).

Although *Frye* was followed for many years in both federal and state courts, it fell into disfavor at approximately the same time the Federal Rules of Evidence were adopted. These rules authorize the admission of expert testimony in federal court, so long as the testimony is rendered by a qualified expert and is helpful to the trier of fact (65). Many courts thus abandoned the general acceptance standard of *Frye* in ascertaining whether a scientific hypothesis was proven or merely one expert's opinion (66), and looked instead to whether the testimony was helpful (67). Consequently, relaxation of the traditional barriers to opinion testimony permitted an increase in the quantity of expert testimony allowed to be presented to a jury (68). Courts recognized that controlling the expert testimony presented to a jury had become a difficult problem under the more relaxed Federal Rules of Evidence and began to exercise greater control over its admissibility (69). Commentators also urged the courts to admit opinions of expert witnesses only when the conclusions are based on credible, reliable medical and scientific data (70).

In 1993, the Supreme Court of the United States addressed the admissibility of expert scientific evidence in the landmark case of *Daubert v. Merrell Dow Pharmaceuticals, Inc.* (71). In *Daubert*, plaintiffs sought to introduce expert testimony that their mothers' ingestion of Bendectin during pregnancy caused their birth defects (72). Although epidemiological studies failed to establish the causal link, plaintiffs' experts claimed that there was a connection based on in-vitro and in-vivo testing, on studies of the chemical structure of Bendectin, and on reanalysis of earlier published epidemiological studies. Relying on *Frye*, the trial court found that the principle underlying the experts' opinions was not sufficiently established to have general acceptance in the field to which it belongs, and held that the testimony was inadmissible. The Ninth Circuit Court of Appeals affirmed the trial court's decision to exclude the evidence.

In reversing the lower courts' decisions, the Supreme Court held that the standard articulated in *Frye* was superseded by the enactment of the Federal Rules of Evidence, which provide the exclusive governing standard for the admissibility of scientific evidence in federal courts (73). The Supreme Court noted that Rule 702 "clearly contemplates some degree of regulation of the subjects and theories about which an expert may testify" (74). To be admissible under Rule 702, expert scientific testimony must concern "scientific knowledge" that will "assist the trier of fact to understand or determine a fact in issue." Although the testimony need not be known to a certainty, the Supreme Court recognized, ". . . in order to qualify as 'scientific knowledge,' an inference or assertion must be derived by the scientific method. Proposed testimony must be supported by appropriate validation—i.e., 'good grounds,' based on what is known" (75).

Based on its analysis of the Federal Rules of Evidence, the Supreme Court held that the trial court must make "a preliminary assessment of whether the reasoning or methodology underlying the testimony is scientifically valid and of whether that reasoning or methodology properly can be applied to the facts in issue" (76). Thus, the trial court must examine the proposed expert scientific testimony to ensure, by a preponderance of the evidence (77), that it is both reliable and relevant to the issues in the case. In determining whether the proposed scientific testimony is reliable (i.e., the first prong of *Daubert*), the Supreme Court set forth the following factors that could be examined by the trial court:

1. Whether the theory or technique can be (and has been) tested
2. Whether the theory or technique has been subjected to peer review and publication
3. The known or potential error rate of the theory or technique
4. Whether the theory or technique is generally accepted as reliable by the relevant scientific community (78)

However, the foregoing list of factors does not constitute a "definitive checklist or test"; rather, it simply highlights several factors that are common to proper scientific methods (79). Subsequent legal precedent has also recognized that these factors are not "equally applicable (or applicable at all) in every case" (80).

Under the relevancy analysis (i.e., the second prong of *Daubert*), the Supreme Court held, "Rule 702's 'helpfulness' standard requires a valid scientific connection to the pertinent inquiry as a precondition to admissibility" (81). To be admissible, the proposed testimony must assist the jury to determine or understand an issue of fact in the case. Consequently, " '[e]xpert testimony which does not relate to any issue in the case is not relevant and, ergo, non-helpful' " (82). In light of its ruling, the Supreme Court remanded the case to the Ninth Circuit to determine the admissibility of plaintiffs' expert testimony under the new standard.

Applying the two-prong test articulated by the Supreme Court, the Ninth Circuit reconsidered its earlier decision, and held that plaintiffs' expert testimony was inadmissible (83). The court held that proposed expert testimony failed to satisfy the first prong of the admissibility standard (i.e., reliability). In analyzing the admissibility of the testimony, the court noted that it must determine whether the expert's opinion amounted to " 'scientific knowledge,' constitutes 'good science,' and was 'derived by the scientific method' " (84). Thus, the party presenting the expert must show that the expert's findings are based on sound science, which requires some objective, independent validation of the expert's methodology (85). The court explained that a pivotal consideration for admissibility is whether the testimony is derived from proper scientific method:

> One very significant fact to be considered is whether the experts are proposing to testify about matters growing naturally and directly out of research they have conducted independent of the litigation, or whether they have developed their opinions expressly for purposes of testifying. . . . [I]n determining whether proposed expert testimony amounts to good science, we may not ignore the fact that a scientist's normal workplace is the lab or the field, not the courtroom or the lawyer's office (86).

The court noted that the principal ways to show that the evidence satisfies the reliability requirement are to establish "that an expert's proffered testimony grows out of pre-litigation research or that the expert's research has been subjected to peer review" (87). If neither is possible, the proponent of the expert scientific testimony may attempt to show reliability through the testimony of its own experts, who "must explain precisely how they went about reaching their conclusions and point to some objective source—a learned treatise, the policy statement of a professional association, a published article in a reputable scientific journal or the like—to show that they have followed the scientific method, as it is practiced by (at least) a recognized minority of scientists in their field" (88).

After analyzing the evidence, the Ninth Circuit found that none of plaintiff's experts had based their opinions on preexisting or independent research. Nor had their opinions and research been published (other than in court decisions) and/or subject to peer review. Finally, plaintiffs failed to offer any evidence regarding the methodologies employed by the experts to arrive at their respective opinions, aside from the expert's own unadorned assertions that their methodology comported with standard scientific procedures. Thus, plaintiffs failed to establish that the expert testimony had sufficient indicia of reliability to be admissible.

The Ninth Circuit also concluded that plaintiffs could not satisfy the second prong of *Daubert* (i.e., relevancy or the "fit" of the evidence), which requires the proffered evidence have a "valid scientific connection to the pertinent inquiry" (89). Under this prong, there must be a "fit" between the proffered scientific testimony and an issue in the case; otherwise, the evidence is not relevant (90). The relevancy or "fit" of the evidence is determined by the "pertinent inquiry," namely, causation of plaintiff's birth defects. The court framed this inquiry as follows:

> [W]hat plaintiffs must prove is not that Bendectin causes some birth defects, but that it caused *their* birth defects. To show this, plaintiffs' experts would have had to testify either that Bendectin actually caused plaintiff's injuries (which they could not say) or that Bendectin more than doubled the likelihood of limb reduction birth defects (which they did not say) (91).

The Ninth Circuit then found that plaintiffs could not augment the expert's substantive testimony as to causation, because any tailoring of the experts' conclusions at this stage would "fatally undermine any attempt to show that these findings were 'derived by the scientific method'" (92). Hence, plaintiffs' attempts to cure the relevancy problems in the expert testimony undermined the reliability of this evidence. This illustrates how the two prongs of *Daubert*, reliability and relevancy, work in tandem to screen questionable science from the courtroom.

Daubert has made a significant impact in limiting the admissibility of "junk science" (93) in product liability and toxic tort actions in federal courts. Trial courts are fulfilling the Supreme Court's mandate to act as "gatekeepers" by strictly scrutinizing the admissibility of expert scientific testimony before it is submitted to the jury (94). Once courts are satisfied that the proposed expert testimony is legally reliable and relevant, the jury must decide between the competing opinions. Numerous state courts also have adopted *Daubert*, although many still apply the *Frye* general acceptance standard, or some variation thereof (95). In sum, courts will continue to scrutinize "scientific" opinions under *Frye* and *Daubert*, and exclude expert testimony if it is not based on scientifically valid evidence.

VII. Proven, Possible, and Unlikely Teratogens

Determining the teratogenicity of an agent in humans is extremely difficult. Many scientific and ethical limitations exist in establishing by statistical significance this devastating characteristic of an agent. Proof of teratogenicity was simplified in thalidomide cases by the unique, dramatic, and rare phocomelic effects it caused when taken by women during their early weeks of pregnancy (96). However, this type of definitive causal link has not been duplicated with any scientific certainty between other agents and any given birth defect (97). Additionally, most teratologists agree with Karnofsky's principle, which states that any agent can be shown to be teratogenic in animals provided sufficient quantities are administered at the appropriate time (98). This principle further complicates the study of teratogenicity.

Dr. Thomas Shepard, one of the leading experts in the area of human teratogenicity, has written extensively on the subject. From different sources Dr. Shepard has prepared an amalgamation of criteria to determine whether an agent has human teratogenic potential. These criteria are listed in Table 1. Further, from information known to date, Dr. Shepard has compiled lists of proven, possible, and unlikely teratogens which are considered

Table 1 Amalgamation of Criteria for Proof of Human Teratogenicity

1. Proven exposure to agent at critical times(s) in prenatal development (prescriptions, physician's records, dates).
2. Consistent findings by two or more epidemiologic studies of high quality:
    (a) Control of confounding factors
    (b) Sufficient numbers
    (c) Exclusion of positive and negative bias factors
    (d) Prospective studies, if possible
    (e) Relative risk of six or more (?)
3. Careful delineation of the clinical cases. A specific defect or syndrome, if present, is very helpful.
4. Rare environmental exposure associated with rare defect. Probably three or more cases (examples: oral anticoagulants, methimazole and scalp defects (?), and heart block and maternal rheumatism).
5. Teratogenicity in experimental animals important but not essential (i.e., oral anticoagulants as exception).
6. The association should make biological sense.
7. Proof in an experimental system that the agent acts in an unaltered state. Important information for prevention.

Note: Items 1, 2, and 3 or 1, 3, and 4 are essential criteria. Items 5, 6, and 7 are helpful, but not essential.
Source: Shepard TH. Catalog of Teratogenic Agents. 7th ed. Baltimore, MD: Johns Hopkins University Press, 1992:xxii.

the standard reference for the scientific, medical, and legal communities. Dr. Shepard's compilation of the proven human teratogens appears in Table 2, and possible or unlikely human teratogens in Table 3 (99).

These tables are not considered an inclusive catalog of all the human teratogens which exist in our modern world. Many compounds presently utilized by society have little or no information regarding teratogenicity. New agents which are continuously being developed are added to this roll. With the enormous number of compounds and ethical considerations which preclude testing on human subjects, it is easy to comprehend the immense task researchers face in determining whether products have teratogenic potential. However, the lists provided by Dr. Shepard and other researchers

Table 2　Teratogenic Agents in Human Beings

RADIATION	DRUGS AND ENVIRONMENTAL CHEMICALS
Atomic weapons	Aminopterin and methylaminopterin
Radioiodine	Androgenic hormones
Therapeutic	Busulfan
INFECTIONS	Captopril (renal failure)
Cytomegalovirus (CMV)	Chlorobiphenyls
Herpes virus hominis?I&II	Cocaine
Parvovirus B-19 (Erythema infectiosum)	Coumarin anticoagulants
Rubella virus	Cyclophosphamide
Syphilis	Diethylstilbestrol
Toxoplasmosis	Diphenylhydantoin
Venezuelan equine encephalitis virus	Enaldpril (renal failure)
MATERNAL METABOLIC IMBALANCE	Etretinate
Alcoholism	Iodide and goiter
Cretinism, endemic	Lithium
Diabetes	Mercury, organic
Folic acid deficiency	Methimazole and scalp defects
Hyperthermia	Penicillamine
Phenylketonuria	13-*cis*-Retinoic acid (isotretinoin and Accutane)
Rheumatic disease and congenital heart block	Tetracyclines
Virilizing tumors	Thalidomide
	Trimethadione
	Valproic acid

Source: Shepard TH. Catalog of Teratogenic Agents. 7th ed. Baltimore, MD: John Hopkins University Press, 1992:xxii.

Table 3 Possible and Unlikely Teratogens

POSSIBLE TERATOGENS	UNLIKELY TERATOGENS
?Binge drinking	Agent Orange
?Carbamazepine	Anesthetics
?Chorionic villus sampling, early	Aspartame
?Cigarette smoking	Aspirin (but aspirin in the 2nd half of
?Disulfiram	pregnancy may increase cerebral
?Ergotamine	hemorrhage during delivery)
?High Vitamin A	Bendectin (antinauseant)
?Lead	Birth control pills
?Primidone	Illicit drugs (marihuana, LSD)
?Streptomycin	Metronidazole (Flagyl)
?Toluene abuse	Oral Contraceptives
?Varicella virus	Rubella vaccine
?Zinc deficiency	Spermicides
	Video display screens

Source: Shepard TH. Catalog of Teratogenic Agents. 7th ed. Baltimore, MD: John Hopkins University Press, 1992:xxiii.

serve as guidelines for the physician in assessing questions of teratogenicity and will grow as more scientific research is devoted to this vital assignment (100).

VIII. Prescribing During Pregnancy

A. Goals

Clearly, the intention of any physician in managing a pregnant patient is to achieve a healthy mother and a healthy baby (101). A primary goal of prescribing during pregnancy should be to maintain the mother's health in order to provide a healthy environment for the developing fetus (102). Also, an important consideration in prescribing should be to minimize the risk to the fetus from the medications selected to treat the mother (103). An obstacle to this aim is that many medications possess an unknown teratogenic risk (104). In order to overcome this obstacle, it is essential for the physician to obtain accurate and up-to-date information regarding the potential teratogenicity of medications being prescribed.

The medical community learned a very valuable lesson from the thalidomide experience of the 1960s: Drugs of low toxicity in an adult can present a formidable hazard to a fetus (105). The thalidomide tragedy made an indelible impression on public perception concerning the deleterious effects on a fetus which can result from maternal exposure to medications during pregnancy (106). This heightened awareness has increased the pressure and liability potential on pharmaceutical manufacturers and medical professionals, especially those physicians treating women during childbearing years (107). When medications are prescribed during pregnancy, patients expect their physicians to know that the drugs will not be harmful to the fetus (108). In turn, physicians expect to receive sufficiently reliable information concerning the potential teratogenicity of medications from pharmaceutical manufacturers, governmental agencies, and the scientific community.

The medical profession's need for practical information to meet this expectancy is well recognized. However, some argue that this essential information is not being readily or adequately provided to physicians (109). When the information is available, it is often contradictory or confusing (110). Some of the confusion is due to the lack of reliable data on the reproductive toxicology of a drug (111). Dissemination of available information is at worst imprecise or at best not systematic (112). A more precise and structured method of reporting and providing information about a drug's teratogenic potential to physicians is required in order to provide practical data for the prescriber on which to base clinical decisions.

Human epidemiological studies, whether prospective or retrospective, are the most reliable means of evaluating teratogenicity and causation (113). Because of state-of-the-art limitations or ethical considerations, human data are not always available to determine causation. Further, reproductive toxicology studies seem to convey protection to the pharmaceutical manufacturer or render political protection to the regulatory body such as the FDA rather than produce valuable information for the practitioner (114). Finally, the complex issue of causation makes it extremely difficult to interpret information alleging a link between the medication and the risk to the fetus in definitive scientific terms (115). These barriers need to be removed to enable an informed decision by the practitioner regarding prescribing practices for the pregnant patient.

B. Practical Considerations for the Practitioner When Prescribing During Pregnancy

The expanding complexity and potential for legal liability associated with prescribing medications to a pregnant patient may encourage many physicians to engage in "therapeutic nihilism" (116). Although this stance may invoke sympathy due to the inadequacy of good teratogenic information available to the practitioner, taken together with the current litigious nature of our society, abstaining from prescribing may endanger the health and welfare of both the mother and fetus (117). Pharmacological intervention may be necessary to control a variety of serious medical conditions from which the pregnant patient may suffer, such as diabetes, asthma, epilepsy, and hypertension. Fortunately, medicolegal risks associated with prescribing to a pregnant patient may be diminished, though not eliminated, by adhering to reasonable prescribing procedures.

By instituting sensible, well-informed policies with respect to decisions regarding prescribing, most physicians can avoid being accused of or actually causing harm to the fetus (118). The following nine points are general practical considerations which all practitioners treating patients during child-bearing years should consider, before prescribing medications (119).

1. Consult with all female patients of reproductive age who suffer from medical disorders and are taking medications before they conceive. Refer them to or encourage them to seek counseling before embarking on planned pregnancies.

2. Evaluate the need for any drug being prescribed during pregnancy and give careful consideration to alternate modalities of treatment. Document this process in the patient's medical records.

3. Scrutinize all drug regimens in pregnant patients to determine how careful therapeutics and good control can minimize risks. Utilize the lowest therapeutic dose possible, as fetal risk is likely increased with increased dosage.

4. Prescribe medications which have been widely used by practitioners in pregnancy for years or which have a clearer safety record in human and/or animal data, in preference to medications possessing insufficient teratogenicity information or those recently introduced onto the market.

5. Communicate with patients effectively. Studies have shown that decisions whether to sue the physician are often decided on the basis of prior communications between the patient and the physician (120). Patients are more hesitant to sue a physician whom they like or with whom they have a good rapport.

6. Document, Document, Document! A note should be entered into the patient's medical record briefly summarizing the communication between the physician and the patient. The physician should ensure that the patient understands the information being conveyed and provide an opportunity for the patient to ask any questions that arise. The note should reflect the patient's understanding as well as the final outcome of the discussion. The phy-

sician should write the note contemporaneously or soon after the consultation session.

7. Never guarantee an outcome of a pregnancy. Truthfully and factually discuss the incidence of malformations with women who are concerned.

8. If the patient is on drug therapy when she becomes pregnant, arrange for a consultation with either a geneticist, medical teratologist, dysmorphologist, high-risk obstetrician, or perinatologist. The physician should ensure that the specialists document their discussions with the patient. The option of a therapeutic abortion should be presented, if deemed necessary.

9. Maintain a file on all drugs or family of drugs which are regularly prescribed for or ingested by pregnant patients, including all over-the-counter medications that have known adverse effects, not just prescription pharmaceuticals. State-of-the-art knowledge concerning medications may bc obtaincd from a variety of authoritative sources, as discussed below. Copies of this information should be placed into the patient's file to demonstrate that the physician was familiar with the product(s) and made an informed decision regarding the use of the product(s) during pregnancy. Also, this material may be used in communicating with the patient.

There is no guarantee that a physician will not be sued or even found liable for injury to a fetus if he or she follows these guidelines. However, the guidelines serve as excellent prophylactic measures to avoid harm to the mother and/or fetus, and to protect against the potential of legal liability. At the very least, a physician following these simple suggestions should possess a more defensible position as opposed to one who cannot demonstrate a reasonable prescribing process for his or her pregnant patients.

C. Sources of Information

The acquisition of the latest accurate information concerning the teratogenicity of medications is one of the most challenging tasks facing the medical practitioner treating pregnant patients. Fortunately, the computer revolution has enabled the development of sophisticated databases from which information regarding teratogenicity may be retrieved by the physician. Computers located in a private physician's office or home may be linked to national or international sources of drug information which can provide the latest scientific information on medications. This information may be most beneficial in making prescribing decisions in pregnant patients. Additional avenues of information are being developed and improved in order to facilitate the exchange of information between researchers and clinicians.

The following are some of the potential sources where information on drugs to be prescribed during pregnancy can be found (121).

Package labeling. The FDA has developed letter-coded pregnancy risk categories for prescription medications (122) in order to facilitate comparisons of medications. The attributes and limitations of this system have been discussed previously.

Pharmacists. Pharmacists possess an extensive knowledge of medications, including teratogenic information. They maintain patient drug profiles as well as a large volume of reference materials concerning the pharmacology and teratogenicity of medications. Additionally, a major responsibility of the profession of pharmacy is communicating information about medications to other health care professionals and patients (123).

Peer-review publications. Primary medical and scientific journals publish articles by physicians and researchers regarding the teratogenicity of agents. Although these publications provide the latest information available, a physician may find the tasks of reading all of the journal articles, interpreting the data, and utilizing the data in his or her own practice too time-consuming, and not worth the time invested.

Newsletters. This format provides a physician with a comprehensive yet simplified discussion on a variety of medical topics. The tasks associated with reviewing and summarizing peer-review publications is assumed by the publisher of the newsletter. Consequently, a physician receives up-to-date information without the burden of extensive literature searches and reading primary material. Two newsletters providing valuable information on medications are *The Medical Letter on Drugs and Therapeutics* and *Reproductive Toxicology.*

Textbooks and compendia. Several excellent textbooks and compendia are available on teratogenicity and serve as reference works. *The Handbook of Teratology* (Wilson & Frazier, New York: Plenum Press, 1977), *The Catalog of Teratogenic Agents* (Shepard, 7th ed. Baltimore, MD: Johns Hopkins University Press, 1992), and *Chemically Induced Birth Defects* (Schardein, 1985) serve as valuable resource materials that provide a broad knowledge base. However, a major limitation of this medium is the significant time lapse before publication. Information contained in textbooks may become outdated before publication or shortly thereafter. Therefore, textbooks should not be the sole source of medical information.

Computer-assisted services. As the computer revolution continues to grow, more information is becoming available to the medical community. Computers have enabled the storage of large volumes of data regarding teratogenicity of medications and permit easy access to such information. A physician may contact various services, such as the Reproductive Toxicology Center, or the Arizona Teratogen Information Program, which will assist in answering reproductive issues. Also, computerized medical databases, such as Reprotox, the first computerized database on the reproductive effects of chemical and physical agents, and TERIS, which provides summaries and ratings on risk levels, are excellent sources to evaluate teratogenic risk.

Drug information centers. Many hospitals and schools of pharmacy operate drug information centers which provide answers to a variety of medication questions. These centers possess extensive medical references and are usually staffed by specially trained experts on drug information. Health care professionals as well as patients frequently utilize these centers to obtain practical information on medications.

IX. Conclusion

Efforts directed toward reducing fetal exposure to unreasonable teratogenic risk has as its central focus the generation, dissemination, and responsible use of information relating to reproductive toxicology and teratogenicity. Manufacturers generate or obtain information through scientific research and disseminate it through product labeling. Physicians further disseminate the information by interpreting its significance for a particular patient, and encouraging rational decisions by explaining the risks and benefits of drug use for a patient. Pregnant women use the information to weigh the pros and cons of drug therapy, including risks and benefits to the fetus. Despite best efforts by all involved birth anomalies are inevitable, though careful consideration of available information and effective therapeutic management can help reduce the incidence of drug-induced birth defects.

Notes and References

1. 65 F.Supp. 138 (D.D.C. 1946).
2. *Huskey v. Smith*, 265 So.2d 596 (Ala. 1972).

3. See *Hartke v. McKelwav*, 526 F.Supp. 97 (D.D.C. 1981), *cert. denied*, 464 U.S. 983 (1983).

4. See *Turoin v. Sortini*, 643 P.2d 954 (Cal. 1980).

5. See *Curlender v. Bio-Sciences Laboratories*, 165 Cal. Rptr. 337 (App. 1980).

6. Morreim. The concept of harm reconceived: a different look at wrongful life. Law & Philosophy 1988; 7:3.

7. 66 P.2d 483 (Wash. 1984).

8. Furrow. Impaired children and tort remedies: the emergence of a consensus. Law, Medicine & Health Care 1983; 11:148.

9. Furrow. Diminished lives and malpractice: courts stalled in transition. Law, Medicine & Health Care 1982; 10:100.

10. See, e.g., *Medlock v. Brown*, 136 S.E. 551 (Ga. 1927); *Christian v. Carter*, 137 S.E. 596 (N.C. 1927).

11. See, e.g., *People v. Greer*, 402 N.E.2d 203 (Ill. 1980); *Keeler v. Superior Court*, 470 P.2d 617 (Cal 1970).

12. Capron. Tort liability in genetic counseling. Columbia Law Rev 1979; 79: 618.

13. Palmer. Regulatory requirements for reproductive toxicology: theory and practice. In: Kimmel C, Buelki-Sam J, eds. Developmental Toxicology. 1981.

14. Brown and Fabro. The value of animal teratogenicity testing for predicting human risk. Clinical Obstet Gynecol 1983; 26:467.

15. 21 C.F.R. # 201.57 (1988).

16. Brushwood. Drug induced birth defects: difficult decisions and shared responsibility. W FA Law Rev 1988; 91:51.

17. 21 C.F.R. § 201.57(f)(6) (1988).

18. Brushwood. Drug induced birth defects: difficult decisions and shared responsibility. W Va Law Rev 1988; 91:51.

19. Gilhooley. Learned intermediaries, prescription drugs, and patient information. St. Louis U Law J 1986; 30:633.

20. See Comment, Drugs during pregnancy: dangerous business—the continued movement to provide adequate warnings for the consumer. Neb Law Rev 1983; 62:526.

21. 46 Fed. Reg. 13,193 (1981).

22. Schwartz. Consumer warnings for oral contraceptives: a new exception to the prescription drug rule. Food Drug Cosmetic Law J 1986; 41:241.

23. Brackbill, McManus, Doering, Tobinson. Exposure to drugs with possible adverse effects during pregnancy & birth. Birth 1982; 9:165.

24. Katz. The Silent World of Doctor and Patient. New York: The Free Press, 1984.

25. Rhoden. Informed consent in obstetrics: some special problems. W N Engl Law Rev 1987; 9:67.

26. Ibid at 72.

27. Cherniak. Recovery for prenatal injuries: the right of a child against its mother. Suffolk U Law Rev 1976; 10:582, 607.

28. 402 N.E.2d 194 (Ill. 1980).

29. 751 P.2d 470 (Cal. 1988).

30. 746 F.2d 517 (9th Cir. 1984).

31. 620 F.Supp. 323 (N.D.Ill. 1985).

32. 620 F.Supp. at 326.

33. 301 N.W.2d 869 (Mich. 1980).

34. Woodside. Special problems of birth defect litigation. In: Vinson DE, Slaughter AH, eds. Products Liability: Pharmaceutical Drug Cases. New York: McGraw-Hill, 1988:221, 222.

35. Woodside. Special problems of birth defect litigation. In: Vinson DE, Slaughter AH, eds. Products Liability: Pharmaceutical Drug Cases. New York: McGraw-Hill, 1988:221, 222.

36. Woodside. Special problems of birth defect litigation. In: Vinson DE, Slaughter AH, eds. Products Liability: Pharmaceutical Drug Cases. New York: McGraw-Hill, 1988:221, 222.

37. *Klages v. General Ordinance Equipment Corp.*, 240 Pa. Super. 356, 373, 367 A.2d 304, 313 (Pa. Super. 1976).

38. See, e.g., *Wade-Greaux v. Whitehall Laboratories, Inc.*, 874 F.Supp. 1441, 1448 (D.C. V.I. 1994) (requiring plaintiff's experts to address both general and specific causation); *In re Agent Orange Product Liability Litigation*, 597 F.Supp. 740 (E.D.N.Y 1984); *Lawson v. G.D. Searle & Co.*, 64 111.2d 543, 356 N.E.2d 779 (1976).

39. See *Grinnell v. Charles Pfizer & Co.*, 274 Cal.App. 424, 79 Cal.Rptr. 369 (1969); *Marder v. G.D. Searle & Co.*, 630 F.Supp. 1087 (D.Md. 1986).

40. Prosser. Law of Torts. 5th ed. §41. St. Paul: West Publishing, 1984.

41. Prosser. Law of Torts. 5th ed. §41. St. Paul: West Publishing, 1984.

42. 458 S.W.2d 155 (Ky. Ct. App. 1970).

43. 458 S.W.2d 155 (Ky.Ct.App. 1970). See also *Lynch v. Merrell-National Laboratories*, 830 F.2d 1190 (1st Cir. 1987); *Orth v. Emerson Elec. Co., White-Rodgers Div.*, 980 F.2d 632 (10th Cir. 1992); *Anderson v. Whittaker Corp.*, 894 F.2d 804 (6th Cir. 1990); *Calhoun v. Honda Motor Co., Ltd.*, 738 F.2d 126 (6th Cir. 1984).

44. See, e.g., *Wade-Greaux v. Whitehall Laboratories, Inc.*, 874 F.Supp. 1441, 1448 (D.C. V.I. 1994) (requiring plaintiff's experts to address both general and specific causation); *In re Agent Orange Product Liability Litigation*, 597 F. Supp. 740 (E.D.N.Y. 1984); *Lawson v. G.D. Searle & Co.*, 64 111.2d 543, 356 N.E.2d 779 (1976).

45. *Turpin v. Merrell Dow Pharmaceuticals, Inc.*, 959 F.2d 1349, 1350 (6th Cir. 1992).

46. *In re Richardson-Merrell, Inc.*, 624 F.Supp. 1212. 1228-29 (S.D. Ohio 1985).

47. See e.g., *Muniz Nunez v. American Home Products Corp.*, 582 F.Supp 459 (D.P.R. 1984).

48. See e.g., *Basko v. Sterling Drug*, 416 F.2d 417 (2d Cir. 1969).

49. See e.g., *LeMaire v. U.S.*, 826 F.2d 949, 954 (10th Cir. 1987).

50. See e.g., *Turpin v. Merrell Dow Pharmaceuticals, Inc.*, 959 F.2d 1349, 1350 (6th Cir. 1992).

51. See Weinstein, Improving expert testimony. U Rich Law Rev 1986; 20:473, 491–492, n.71. Austrian. Expert evidence in toxic tort litigation. For The Defense Feb. 1989:17.

52. *Daubert v. Merrell Dow Pharmaceuticals, Inc.*, 113 S.Ct. 2786, 2795 (1993).

53. *Turpin v. Merrell Dow Pharmaceuticals, Inc.*, 959 F.2d at 1351.

54. See *Turpin v. Merrell Dow Pharmaceuticals, Inc.*, 959 F.2d at 1352 (close judicial analysis necessary, since expert witnesses are not always "unbiased scientists").

55. See Federal Rules of Evidence 706. The court-appointed expert is compensated by the parties as the court directs, pursuant to subdivision (b).

56. As reported in Weinstein's Evidence 3:706-3 and 706-4 (Matthew Bender, 1996), during the hearings on adoption of Rule 706 concern was expressed by an attorney association that court-appointed experts would be biased in medical malpractice cases, as the court would most likely appoint a local physician who would be reticent to testify adversely against a local practitioner. These concerns were acknowledged in Rule 706's accompanying Notes of Advisory Committee on Proposed Rules ("The practice of shopping for experts, the venality of some experts, and the reluctance of many experts to involve themselves in litigations, have been matters of deep concern. . . . While experience indicates that actual appointment is a relatively infrequent occurrence, the assumption may be made that the availability of the procedure in itself decreases the need for resorting to it").

57. See e.g., *Cadarian v. Merrell Dow Pharmaceuticals, Inc.*, 745 F.Supp. 409 (E.D. Mich. 1989).

58. Gass. Using the Frye rule to control expert testimony abuse. For The Defense Feb. 1989:23.

59. 293 F.2d 1013 (D.C. Cir. 1923).

60. 293 F.2d 1013, 1014 (D.C. Cir. 1923).

61. See *Puhl v. Milwaukee Automobile Insurance Co.*, 8 Wis.2d 343, 9 N.W.2d 163 (1959).

62. *State v. Bible*, 175 Ariz. 549, 858 P.2d 1152, 1181 (1993).

63. *State v. Bible*, 175 Ariz. 549, 858 P.2d 1152, 1181 (1993).

64. *State v. Bible*, 175 Ariz. 549, 858 P.2d 1152, 1181 (1993).

65. See Federal Rules of Evidence 702, 703, and 705. Rule 702 states: "If scientific, technical or other specialized knowledge will assist the trier of fact to understand the evidence or determine a fact in issue, a witness qualified as an expert by knowledge, skill, experience, training or education, may testify thereto in the form of an opinion or otherwise."

66. Gass. Using the Frye rule to control expert testimony abuse. For The Defense Feb. 1989:23.

67. *Daubert v. Merrell Dow Pharmaceuticals, Inc.*, 113 S.Ct. 2786, 2793, fn. 5 (1993).

68. *Daubert v. Merrell Dow Pharmaceuticals, Inc.*, 113 S.Ct. at 2794.

69. Austrian. Expert evidence in toxic tort litigation. For The Defense Feb 1989: 17. See, e.g., *In re Air Crash Disaster at New Orleans, Louisiana*, 795 F.2d

1230 (5th Cir. 1986); *Richardson v. Richardson-Merrell, Inc.*, 857 F.2d 823 (D.C. Cir. 1988), *cert. denied*, 493 U.S. 882 (1989).

70. See Davis, Ivie, Hernandez. Special problems of birth defect litigation. In: Vinson DE, Slaughter AH, eds. Products Liability: Pharmaceutical Drug Cases. New York: McGraw-Hill, 1988:655, 681. Shelton. The need for scientific data in chemical exposure litigation. For The Defense Dec 1988:18.

71. *Daubert v. Merrell Dow Pharmaceuticals, Inc.*, 113 S.Ct. 2786, 2795 (1993).

72. The pharmaceutical Benedictin was prescribed for morning sickness to approximately 17.5 million pregnant women in the United States, and to over 30 million women worldwide, between 1957 and 1982, when the manufacturer, Merrell Dow, took the drug off the U.S. market despite continued approval from the Food and Drug Administration. *Turpin v. Merrell Dow Pharmaceuticals, Inc.*, 959 F.2d 1349, 1350 (6th Cir. 1992); U.S. Department of Health and Human Services News, No. P80-45 (Oct. 7, 1980).

73. The Supreme Court's decision in *Daubert* deals solely with the Federal Rules of Evidence and is not binding on state courts, even though many states have enacted evidentiary rules that are identical to the federal rules.

74. *Daubert v. Merrell Dow Pharmaceuticals, Inc.*, 113 S.Ct. 2786, 2795 (1993).

75. *Daubert v. Merrell Dow Pharmaceuticals, Inc.*, 113 S.Ct. at 2795 (1993).

76. *Daubert v. Merrell Dow Pharmaceuticals, Inc.*, 113 S.Ct. at 2796 (1993).

77. *Daubert v. Merrell Dow Pharmaceuticals, Inc.*, 113 S.Ct. at 2796 fn. 10.

78. *Daubert v. Merrell Dow Pharmaceuticals, Inc.*, 113 S.Ct. at 2796-2797.

79. *Daubert v. Merrell Dow Pharmaceuticals, Inc.*, 113 S.Ct. at 2796 (1993).

80. *Daubert v. Merrell Dow Pharmaceuticals, Inc.*, 43 F.3d 1311, 1317 (9th Cir. 1995).

81. *Daubert v. Merrell Dow Pharmaceuticals, Inc.*, 113 S.Ct. at 2786, 2796 (1993).

82. *Daubert v. Merrell Dow Pharmaceuticals, Inc.*, 113 S.Ct. at 2795 (1993).

83. *Daubert v. Merrell Dow Pharmaceuticals, Inc.*, 43 F.3d 1311 (9th Cir. 1995).

84. *Daubert v. Merrell Dow Pharmaceuticals, Inc.*, 43 F.3d at 1315.

85. *Daubert v. Merrell Dow Pharmaceuticals, Inc.*, 43 F.3d at 1316.

86. *Daubert v. Merrell Dow Pharmaceuticals, Inc.*, 43 F.3d at 1317.

87. *Daubert v. Merrell Dow Pharmaceuticals, Inc.*, 43 F.3d at 1318.

88. *Daubert v. Merrell Dow Pharmaceuticals, Inc.*, 43 F.3d at 1318-1319.

89. *Daubert v. Merrell Dow Pharmaceuticals, Inc.*, 43 F.3d at 1320; *Daubert v. Merrell Dow Pharmaceuticals, Inc.*, 113 S.Ct. at 2796.

90. *Daubert v. Merrell Dow Pharmaceuticals, Inc.*, 43 F.3d at 1321, fn. 17.

91. *Daubert v. Merrell Dow Pharmaceuticals, Inc.*, 43 F.3d at 1321-1322.

92. *Daubert v. Merrell Dow Pharmaceuticals, Inc.*, 43 F.3d at 1321-1322.

93. See Huber PW. Galileo's Revenge: Junk Science in the Courtroom. United States: Basic Books, 1991. Describes how bad science is caused by the practice of expert-shopping.

94. See, e.g., *In Re Paoli Railroad Yard PCB Litigation* (Paoli, Il), 35 F.3d 717 (3rd Cir. 1994); *Merrell Dow Pharmaceuticals, Inc. v. Havner*, 907 S.W.2d 535 (Tex.Ct. App. 1995) *review granted*; *Wade-Greaux v. Whitehall Labo-*

ratories, Inc. 874 F.Supp. 1441, 1448 (D.C. V.I. 1994); *Byrnes v. Honda Motor Co., Ltd.,* 887 F.Supp. 279 (S.D.Fla. 1994); *Stanczyk v. Black & Decker, Inc.,* 836 F.Supp. 565 (N.D.Ill. 1993).

95. As of November 1, 1996, states which have adopted *Daubert* are: Arkansas, *Jones v. State,* 862 S.W.2d 242 (Ark. 1993); Delaware, *Nelson v. State,* 628 A.2d 69 (Del. 1993); Kentucky, *Cecil v. Commonwealth,* 888 S.W.2d 669 (Ky. 1994); Kansas, *State v. Hill,* 895 P.2d 1238, 1245-47 (Kan. 1995); North Dakota, *City of Fargo v. McLaughlin,* 512 N.W.2d 700 (N.D. 1994); Kentucky, *Tungate v. Commonwealth,* 1994 KY App LEXIS 148 (Dec. 16, 1994); Louisiana, *State v. Foret,* 628 So.2d 1116 (La. 1993); Montana, *State v. Moore,* 885 P.2d 407, 51 Mont. St. Rep. 1151 (1994), and *Hart-Albin Co. v. McLees, Inc.,* 870 P.2d 51 (Mont. 1994); New Mexico, *State v. Anderson,* 118 N.M. 284 (1994); Texas, *E. I. DuPont De Nemours v. Robinson,* 38 S. Ct. J. 852 (Tex. 1995); West Virginia, *Mayhorn v. Logan Medical Foundation,* 454 S.E. 2d 87 (1994), and *Wilt v. Buracker,* 443 S.E.2d 196 (W. Va. 1993) *cert. denied,* 114 S.Ct. 2137 (1994); Iowa, *Hutchison v. American Family Mutual Insurance,* 514 N.W. 882 (Iowa 1994); South Dakota, *State v. Hofer,* 512 N.W.2d 482, 484 (S.D. 1994); Wyoming, *Springfield v. State,* 1993 Wyo. Lexis 149 (Wy. 1993).

The following states have sited *Daubert* with approval but have not formally adopted it: Massachusetts, *Commonwealth v. Lanigan,* 419 Mass. 1526, 641 N.E.2d 1324 (1994) (while not *expressly* adopting it, the court approved of its reasoning); Ohio, *Ault v. Jasko,* 70 Ohio St.3d 114, 637 N.E.2d 870 (1994); Virginia, *Cotton v. Commonwealth,* 19 Va.App. 306, 451 S.E.2d 673 (1994); Illinois, *Dotto v. Okan,* 646 N.E.2d 1277, 1279 (Ill. App. Ct. 1995); Minnesota, *Barna v. Commissioner of Public Safety,* 508 N.W.2d 220 (Minn. App. 1993); Delaware, *Nelson v. State,* 628 A.2d 69 (1993); Washington, *State v. Jones,* 71 Wash. App. 798, 863 P.2d 85 (1993) (noting that *Frye* had been overturned in the federal courts, the tone indicates hope that Washington Supreme Court would soon follow suit); Hawaii, *State v. Maelega,* 907 P.2d 758 (1995); Idaho, *State v. Parkinson,* 909 P.2d 647 (1996); Maine, *Green v. Cessna Aircraft Co.,* 673 A.2d 216 (Me. 1996), and *State v. Williams,* 388 A.2d 500 (Me. 1978); North Carolina, *State v. Goode,* 341 N.C. 513 (1995); Oregon, *State v. O'Key,* 899 P.2d 663 (1995) (although the court relied upon the reasoning in *Daubert,* it held that "*Daubert* is not binding on the states" and is thus merely persuasive); South Carolina, *State v. Dinkins,* 462 S.E.2d 59 (1995) (the court based its reasoning upon *Daubert* having superseded the *Frye* test); Vermont, *State v. Brooks,* 643 A.2d 226, 229 (Vt. 1993).

The following states continue to apply *Frye* or some variation thereof: California, *People v. Leahy,* 8 Cal. 4th 587, 34 Cal. Rptr. 2d 663 (1994); Florida, *Toro v. State,* 642 So. 2d 78, 19 Fla. Law W.D. 1843 (Fla. App. 1994); Maryland, *Keene Corp. v. Hall,* 96 Md. App. 644, 626 A.2d 997 (Md.App. 1993); Missouri, *State v. Davis,* 860 S.W.2d 369 (Mo. Ct. App. 1993); Nebraska, *State v. Carter,* 246 Neb. 953, 524 N.W.2d 763 (1994); New York, *People v. Wesley,* 83 N.Y.2d 417, 633 N.E.2d 451, 611 N.Y.S.2d 97 (1994); Colorado, *Lindsey v. People,* 892 P. 2d 281 (Colo. 1995), but see

Public Service Co. of Colorado v. Willows Water Dist., 856 P.2d 829 (Colo. 1993) (*Frye* still the law in some circumstances); Georgia, *Orkin Exterminating Co. v. McIntosh*, 215 Ga.App. 587 (1994), see also, *Harper v. State*, 249 Ga.App. 519 (1982); Indiana, *Harrison v. State*, 644 N.E.2d 1243 (1995) (agreeing with the reasoning as promulgated in *Daubert*, that a judge exercises more control over experts than over lay witnesses, while maintaining the *Frye* standard), and see also *Cornett v. State*, 450 N.E.2d 498 (Ind. 1983) (applying *Frye* to the admissibility of DNA typing evidence in lieu of a 702 analysis); New Hampshire, *State v. Cressey*, 628 A.2d 696 (N.H 1993); New Jersey, *Bahrle v. Exxon*, 652 A.2d 192 (1995), and see also *State v. Spann*, 130 N.J. 484 (1993) (holding the *Frye* test is applicable in New Jersey); Wisconsin, *State v. Donner*, 192 Wis.2d 305 (1995) (noting that before *Daubert*, the *Frye* test was not the law in Wisconsin, the court relied upon *Daubert* to the extent that *Daubert* and Wisconsin law coincide), and see also *State v. Walstad*, 119 Wis.2d 483 (1984); Connecticut, *State v. Borrelli*, 227 Conn. 153 (1993) (stating *Daubert* "has cast some doubt on the continued viability of the *Frye* test. We need not however address the issue here."), and see also *State v. Hassan*, 205 Conn. 485 (1987) (adopting the *Frye* test); Michigan, *People v. McMillan*, 213 Mich.App. 134 (1995) (holding that until the Supreme Court of Michigan overrules or modifies the *Frye* test, the court is bound to continue to follow *Frye*), and see also *People v. Davis*, 343 Mich. 348 (1955) (adopting *Frye*); Alaska, *Harmon v. State*, 908 P.2d 434 (1995) (the court noted that "it's entirely possible that the supreme court would re-evaluate its position in light of the United States Supreme Court's decision in *Daubert*" but has not yet done so); Pennsylvania, *Commonwealth v. Crews*, 640 A.2d 395 (Pa. 1994) (stating "Whether or not the rationale of *Daubert* will supersede or modify the *Frye* test in Pennsylvania is left to another day"), and see also *Commonwealth v. Topa*, 471 Pa. 223 (1997) (Pennsylvania adopted the *Frye* test).

The following states have acknowledged *Daubert* but have failed to address whether the state would adopt or reject *Daubert*: Nevada, *Nevada Employment Security Department v. Holmes*, 914 P.2d 611 (1996) (referred to *Daubert* in dicta, only to establish that there are "no certainties in science"), and see *Santillanes v. State*, 765 P.2d 1147 (1988) (Nevada currently maintains a relevancy standard which is similar to *Daubert*); Rhode Island, *Soares v. Vestal*, 632 A.2d 647 (1993) (stating: "In this matter we need not reach the issues presented by *Daubert* . . . but we expect that the issues it raises in relation to Rule 702 will be addressed in due course."), and see also *State v. Wheeler*, 496 A.2d 1382 (R.I. 1985) (finding expert testimony in that state to be historically based upon the helpfulness of the evidence); Arizona, *State v. Bible*, 858 P.2d 1152 (Ariz. 1993), *cert. denied*, 114 S.Ct. 1578 (1994); Oklahoma, *Taylor v. State*, 889 P.2d 319 (Okla. App. 1995); Utah, *Dikeou v. Osborn*, 247 Utah Ad. Rep. 9, 881 P.2d 943 (1994) (Citing without approval, but not rejecting *Daubert*).

<ol start="96">
<li>Davis, Ivie, Hernandez, supra note 70 at 655.</li>
<li>Shepard, Human Teratology. In: Wilson, Fraser, eds. Handbook of Teratology. New York: Plenum Press, 1977:313.</li>
</ol>

260   Fern et al.

98. Shepard. Human Teratogenicity. Adv Pediatr 1986; 225, 227.
99. Shepard. Human Teratology. In: Wilson, Fraser, eds. Handbook of Teratology. New York: Plenum Press, 1977:237, 257.
100. See generally: Briggs. Drugs in pregnancy and lactation. In: Young LY, Koda-Kimble MA, eds. Applied Therapeutics: The Clinical Use of Drugs. 1988:1541, 1547 (table on the effect of drugs on the fetus/neonate); Drug interactions and adverse drug reactions. In: AMA Drug Evaluations. 5th ed., Philadelphia: W.B. Saunders, 1983:17, 34–40 [hereinafter Drug Interactions] (table on adverse drug reactions in pregnancy).
101. Hawkins. Prescribing in pregnancy. In: Hawkins HF, ed. Drugs and Pregnancy. Edinburgh: Churchill Livingstone, 1983:41.
102. *Id.*
103. *Id.* at 42. See also Turner, Milstein. Drug-induced diseases. In: Dipiro JT, et al., eds. Pharmacotherapy: A Pathophysiological Approach. 1989:64.
104. See McCombs. Pregnancy. In: Dipiro JT, et al., eds. Pharmacotherapy: A Pathophysiological Approach. 1989:49.
105. Scialli. A Clinical Guide to Reproductive and Developmental Toxicology. Boca Raton: CRC Press, 1992:231–254.
106. Stewart. Adverse drug reactions. In: Gennaro, AR, ed. Remington's Pharmaceutical Sciences. 18th ed. 1990:1340.
107. Scialli, *supra* note 105.
108. *Id.*
109. *Id.*
110. See Schwartz. The obstetrician's view. In: Schwartz RH, Yaffe SJ, eds. Drugs and Chemical Risks to the Newborn. 1979:153–156. Drug Interactions, *supra* note 17 at 33.
111. Scialli, *supra* note 105.
112. See Smithells. The challenge of teratology. Teratology 1980; 22:77.
113. Davis, *supra* note 70 at 667.
114. Hawkins, *supra* note 101 at 41.
115. *Id.*
116. Drug Interactions, *supra* note 100 at 33.
117. *Id.*; Hawkins, *supra* note 101 at 46.
118. Hawkins, *supra* note 101 at 46.
119. *Id.* See also Brent. Medicolegal Aspects of Teratology. In: Sever JL, Brent RL, eds. Teratogen Update: Environmentally Induced Birth Defect Risks. 1986:203, 209–210.
120. See, generally, Hickson et al. Factors that prompted families to file medical malpractice claims following perinatal injuries. JAMA 1992; 267:1359 (families expressed dissatisfaction with physician-patient communication).
121. Scialli, *supra* note 105. See also Shepard, *supra* note 99 at 256; Wexler. Information Resources in Toxicology. 1982.
122. See *supra* text accompanying notes 15.
123. See Molzon, What kinds of patient counseling are required? Am Pharm 1992; NS32(3):50.

Part Three

ALLERGIC DISEASES

10

Allergy Diagnosis, Environmental Control, and Immunotherapy During Pregnancy

HELEN MAWHINNEY and SHELDON LAURENCE SPECTOR

University of California, Los Angeles, School of Medicine
Los Angeles, California

I. Introduction

Atopic disorders, including asthma, are among the most common medical conditions to complicate pregnancy. Asthma occurs in 1–4% of pregnancies (1), and its frequency can be expected to increase as the frequency of asthma in the general population increases. The aim of medical management during pregnancy is to reduce asthma symptoms, consequently maintaining an optimal supply of oxygen to the fetus, while using the lowest possible doses of those medications least potentially harmful to either mother or fetus. Careful allergy assessment, strict adherence to allergen avoidance programs, and proper use of allergen immunotherapy can result in a substantial decrease in the need for asthma medication during pregnancy. Recent studies have shown that proper management of asthma during pregnancy can minimize complications such as prematurity, low birth weight, and perinatal mortality (2).

Numerous factors have been recognized as possible asthma triggers, but for asthmatic women in their child-bearing years, inhaled allergens are among the most common. A recent study showed that 85% of patients with asthma had positive immediate skin tests to common inhalant allergens (3).

Allergy sensitization to at least one allergen occurred in 92% of asthma patients under 45 years of age, by contrast with 48% of patients over 60 years of age (3). Similarly, another study found that 70% of patients presenting to an emergency room with asthma showed evidence of sensitization to common allergens, with allergy as a major risk factor in patients under 50 years of age (4). These data emphasize the importance of allergic diagnosis, environmental control of allergens, and appropriate allergy immunotherapy in both pregnant women and those wishing to become so.

Published guidelines for the management of asthma are regularly updated as our understanding of the pathophysiology of asthma increases and experience with newer medications is gained. In general, the management of the pregnant asthmatic should not differ substantially from the currently recommended guidelines for the treatment of the nonpregnant patient (5). There may, however, be a difference in emphasis in those patients in whom allergy is thought to be playing a significant role. Thus allergen avoidance and immunotherapy can both be used to enhance control of asthma symptoms, while decreasing the need for asthma medications. Both aspects of management are recommended in a recent report entitled *Management of Asthma in Pregnancy*, published by the National Heart, Blood, and Lung Institute (6).

This same report emphasizes the fact that undertreatment of asthma is the major problem in the management of asthma in pregnancy today (6). This is occurring despite the fact that the majority of medications used in the treatment of asthma have been shown to be safe in pregnancy. Many women are wisely concerned about using any medication in pregnancy. Self-limitation of medication use for this reason may be a major cause for the undertreatment of asthma in pregnancy. Consequently, the ideal time to optimize the nonpharmacological treatment of asthma with resultant lifelong benefits may be during early pregnancy—or better yet, before conception.

II. Allergy Diagnosis in Pregnancy

Several questions can be asked regarding allergies and asthma in the recognition of allergy in asthmatic subjects. First, is the patient an atopic subject? The allergic or atopic individual may well have a personal and family history of allergic rhinitis, allergic conjunctivitis, atopic eczema, or asthma. Atopic patients frequently have high total or specific serum IgE levels, and eosinophilia may be present in the blood or elsewhere, e.g., in nasal secretions. A screening panel of immediate-type hypersensitivity skin tests can serve the dual purpose of confirming the diagnosis of allergy while also demonstrating the relevant allergens.

Second, what is the evidence that allergy is an asthma trigger? Two recent investigations looked at the relationship between outdoor aeroallergens and the development of acute seasonal asthma. One study examined the patterns of skin test reactivity in adult asthmatic patients who presented to an emergency room with acute asthma during the spring season (7). Of 59 patients, 92% were allergic to grass pollen. This study further demonstrated that episodes of asthma correlated closely with high grass pollen counts. A second study involved 11 adult asthmatic patients who presented with acute respiratory arrest during the summer and fall seasons (8). In all these patients, asthma attacks occurred while *Alternaria* spore levels were significantly elevated; 91% of the patients had a positive skin test to *Alternaria*.

House dust mite allergens have also been increasingly implicated as asthma triggers and most commonly result in perennial symptoms. A threshold concentration of 10 μg of a major mite allergen (*Der p* 1) per gram of dust has been associated with an increased risk of wheezing in patients who show evidence of sensitivity to house dust mite (9). In another study of children hospitalized because of asthma symptoms, 60% of the children were found to have positive skin tests to house dust mite allergens, and were consistently exposed to significant amounts of *Der p* 1 in their homes (10).

In the United States, cats and dogs are the most common household pets, and both serve as important asthma triggers. It has been suggested that a level of 8 μg of the major cat antigen (*Fel d* 1) per gram of dust is a risk factor for acute asthma (11). On the other hand, a threshold concentration has not been demonstrated for the major dog allergen. Homes with cats often have levels of *Fel d* 1 that exceed the threshold level for asthma symptoms (12). Surprisingly, pet-free homes, schools, and other public places may also have levels of cat and dog allergens that are capable of triggering asthma symptoms (13). It is probable that these animal allergens are carried on clothing into public buildings and pet-free homes (14).

Cockroach allergen has recently been recognized as a common indoor allergen, especially in urban areas (3). Although the major cockroach antigen (*Bla g* II) is predominantly identified in kitchens, it has also been found in large quantities in bedroom carpeting, living room furniture, and bedding (15).

These studies strongly suggest that a positive allergy skin test together with a consistent clinical history is sufficient to implicate that allergen as a significant asthma trigger. Bronchial provocation is rarely required in the diagnosis of allergic asthma, and is certainly not indicated in pregnancy.

In the individual patient, immediate-type hypersensitivity skin testing is the most useful method of determining which substances act as allergens for the individual subject. Scratch or prick tests to inhalant allergens carry little risk of anaphylaxis, and under carefully controlled conditions are considered to be safe in pregnancy (16,17). Nevertheless, they should only be performed if the results are expected to have substantial and immediate therapeutic implications (17). Intradermal skin tests carry a higher risk of anaphylaxis, and should probably not be used in pregnancy. Food allergens have little relevance to asthma in most pregnant individuals, and testing with these allergens should not be carried out unless there is a specific clinical indication. Skin testing with a potent food allergen which might cause an anaphylactic reaction, e.g., peanut, is not recommended. Testing for specific IgE in the serum, e.g., RAST testing, can be helpful. In general, however, these tests are considered to be less sensitive and more expensive than skin tests. They are nevertheless useful in certain circumstances. The most usual indications for serum specific IgE testing are extensive skin disease or dermatographism, which make skin testing unreliable, or a history of anaphylaxis, which might make skin testing more dangerous. Occasionally, specific IgE tests may be helpful if a patient is reluctant to stop taking an antihistamine or tranquilizer or does not wish to delay allergy testing for the 6–8 weeks necessary for the effect of a medication such as astemizole to wear off. Some authors, however, disagree with this philosophy and believe that allergy skin testing should be avoided during pregnancy and in-vitro testing should be used instead (18).

III. Environmental Control of Asthma

The value of allergen avoidance in the management of asthma can never be underestimated, but attention to detail is frequently necessary if environmental control measures are to be successful. An essential prerequisite is a clear definition of the allergens involved. It is hard to justify advising patients to undertake the required measures without a positive skin test or specific IgE result, especially if such measures are costly. Table 1 lists the allergens to which exposure can be avoided or considerably diminished.

A. House Dust Mites

House dust mites are extremely common indoor allergens, and can be found throughout the world. Dust mite numbers within homes are most strongly related to temperature and relative humidity (19), with optimal conditions for growth being 75–80% relative humidity and 25–30°C temperature (20). Accordingly, mite numbers increase during the summer

Table 1 Allergens to Which
Exposure Can Be Avoided
or Diminished

House dust mite
Pollens
Animal danders
Molds
Cockroach

months in areas where the summer humidity is high. Other factors which can be associated with increased concentrations of house dust mites include poor building ventilation (19), older buildings (19), old mattresses (21), and homes on the first floor (22). The highest level of house dust mite allergens is found in dust from mattresses, carpets, upholstered furniture, pillows, and bed covers (22). It has been suggested that feathers and goose down promote higher mite numbers, but this finding was refuted by a recent study that showed no difference between feather and foam pillows (22).

A number of studies have demonstrated that effective control of house dust mite allergen levels in the home can decrease symptoms of asthma and bronchial hyperresponsiveness (22). There are five commonly applied methods of approaching house dust mite allergen control (Table 2):

Table 2 Environmental Control of House Dust Mite

Alterations in bedding
    Wash bed linens weekly in hot water (130°F).
    Encase pillows, mattresses, and box springs in allergen-proof covers.
    Replace quilts and comforters with washable blankets or encase in allergen-
    proof covers.
Vacuum cleaning
    Use a vacuum cleaner equipped with a HEPA filter.
    Asthmatic patients should avoid vacuuming.
Removal of carpets
Air control systems
    Reduce humidity by using air conditioning, a ventilation system, or a
      dehumidifier.
    Use a HEPA filter in the bedroom.
Denaturing agents
    Use agents such as tannic acid and DMS on carpets and upholstered furniture.

1. Alterations in bedding, such as encasing mattresses and pillows in allergen-proof covers and washing bed linens at higher temperatures
2. Vacuum cleaning
3. Removal of carpets
4. Use of air control systems such as air conditioners, ventilation systems, and air purifiers
5. Use of acaricidal and denaturing agents

Alterations in Bedding

Since some of the highest levels of house dust mite allergens are found in mattresses, pillows, bed covers, and bedroom carpets, alterations to bedding and the way in which it is handled can effectively reduce house dust mite allergen concentrations. Hot water (greater than 58°C, or approximately 130°F) effectively denatures house dust mite allergens, whereas cold water washing does not (23). Consequently, washing of bedding in hot water is recommended. Both Velux and cotton blankets can be readily washed at this temperature but other types of blankets are best avoided. Since quilts and comforters usually cannot be washed in hot water, they may be dry cleaned using perchloroethylene. This procedure has been shown to remove 98% of house dust mite allergens (24). Pillows, mattresses, and box springs should be encased in barrier covers. While vinyl and plastic may be used if necessary, they are unpleasant to sleep on and, if possible, covers made from a microporous fabric that allows the passage of water vapor but excludes mites and their allergens should be used. When placed over a mattress, this type of cover reduces levels of house dust mite allergen by 98% (25). Such covers also serve as a useful alternative to dry cleaning quilts and comforters. The comforter can be encased in a cover made of the same microporous fabric, and in turn covered with one of the many attractive duvet covers available. Only this outer cover needs to be washed regularly. It is usually recommended that washing of bed linen be carried out at least every 10 days, and that barrier covers be vacuumed when the outer covers are changed. Washable cotton or Velux blankets may only require washing on a monthly basis.

Vacuum Cleaning

Intensive vacuum cleaning can remove significant amounts of dust from carpets, and tends to diminish the house dust mite allergen reservoir. Conventional vacuum cleaners often emit aerosolized, respirable particles when used, but this effect is usually short-lived (26). Vacuum cleaners may be equipped with HEPA filters, and have been shown to reduce total mite allergens from vacuumed areas by up to 50–85% (27). If the patient is unable to afford this relatively expensive type of vacuum, it may be helpful to run a HEPA filter on a high setting during and for some time after cleaning with a conventional vacuum. House dust mite allergens are highly water-soluble, and it was originally expected that vacuum cleaning after wetting of the carpet might be effective. However, this type of cleaning has been shown to result in increased house dust mite numbers, probably due to the additional moisture (28). It is important to remember that live house dust mites cling tightly to carpet fibers and can replenish the mite allergen reservoir very quickly under appropriate conditions. For this reason, vacuum cleaning can never be relied upon as the sole means of controlling house dust mite exposure.

Removal of Carpets

Since carpets are a major reservoir of house dust mite allergen, and since methods to reduce the amounts of this allergen are cumbersome and not always successful, the ideal solution is for the patient with asthma to remove the carpets in the home, and replace them with wooden or vinyl flooring. Carpets laid on concrete present a particular problem, since the increased humidity resulting from the nonporous concrete increases the house dust mite load, yet replacing the carpet involves laying replacement flooring. This is an ideal which cannot always be reached, especially by those who live in rental property, but where it is feasible it should be highly recommended.

Air Control Systems

A variety of air control systems have had variable success in reducing house dust mite allergen levels or improving asthma symptoms. Air conditioning can lower mite allergen concentrations and the amount of house dust mite by up to 80% by reducing relative humidity in areas with humid summers. This effect has probably been achieved by reducing both relative humidity and air temperature (29). In newer buildings, mechanical exhaust and supply ventilation systems have also reduced house dust mite allergen levels, again most probably by a reduction in relative humidity (30).

High-efficiency particulate air filters (HEPA) have demonstrated clinical benefits in some studies, particularly when the filters are placed in close proximity to the faces of the patients while in bed (31). Conversely, controlled studies of electrostatic air filters have demonstrated that these machines have no more effect than a placebo (31). Negative ionizers were shown in one study to reduce airborne mite allergen concentrations, but there were no beneficial effects on asthma symptoms (32). Positive ionizers have not proven helpful and might cause an irritant effect on the airways of some asthmatic patients. Consequently, the HEPA filtration systems are usually recommended for allergy sufferers.

Use of Acaricidal and Denaturing Agents

A variety of acaricidal and denaturing agents have recently been tested for control of house dust mite allergen in the home. Benzyl benzoate and liquid nitrogen were recently compared, and neither significantly reduced mite allergen levels when applied to carpet, mattresses, or furniture (33). Two controlled trials of the effect of benzyl benzoate on mite allergen concentration have recently been carried out. Neither study showed significant differences from control groups (34,35). Alternatively, tannic acid is a protein denaturing agent that can be applied easily to carpets and upholstered furniture as a 3% solution (Allergy Control Solution, Allergy Control Products, Ridgefield, CT; Allersearch ACD, Allersearch Laboratories, Oakhurst, NJ) and allowed to remain in contact with the carpet or furniture for 4 hr, followed by thorough vacuuming. When used in this way, tannic acid reduced major mite allergens by 70–90% (36). Alcohol-based purified benzyltannate complex (Allersearch DMS) has been shown to have both acaricidal and allergen denaturing properties. When treated with this compound, mite allergen concentrations were reduced in 81% of carpets, but only 56% of soft furnishings such as draperies (37). There is little reason to believe that these latter two preparations pose any hazard to the pregnant woman or her fetus. Tannic acid, benzyl alcohol, and ethanol are all naturally occurring substances which frequently occur as food ingredients, as in tea, beer, and wine. (Tea may contain as much as 60% tannates.) In addition, after tannic acid solution has been applied to carpets or furniture and allowed to dry, only about 1% of the amount applied remains unbound to allergens and other proteins and is readily removed by vacuuming (personal communication, Allersearch Laboratories). A reasonable precaution might be to have someone other than the pregnant mother carry out these treatments.

B. Pollen Allergens (Table 3)

Outdoor aeroallergens such as pollens can be avoided by staying indoors, with doors and windows closed, as much as possible during the relevant season. Air conditioning, especially with a built-in HEPA filtration system, can be of considerable benefit. Otherwise, a room air filter, as discussed above, may be helpful, especially since pollen allergens, unlike house dust mite allergens, usually remain airborne. Because grass and ragweed counts reach their peak around mid-day, sensitized subjects should limit their time

Table 3 Environmental Control of Exposure to Pollen Allergens

---

Keep windows and doors closed when pollen counts are high.
Use air conditioning or a HEPA filter when pollen counts are high.
Stay indoors during the middle of the day and afternoon, when pollen counts are highest.
Exercise in the early morning, when pollen counts are low.

---

out of doors during these hours and exercise in the early morning, when pollen counts are lowest.

C. Animal Danders

Cats and dogs are by far the most common sources of animal dander in the home. As with house dust mite, a number of different means may be used to control or diminish exposure to animal danders in the home (Table 4).

The optimal method of avoiding exposure to animal dander is to remove the pet from the home or at least to limit its access to certain parts of the house. This needs to be followed by aggressive cleaning measures. It may take 4–6 months to reduce allergen levels in settled dust to levels comparable with pet-free homes (38). The same situation arises, for example, when a family including an individual allergic to cat moves to a new home where the prior owners had a cat. The removal of residual allergen may be accelerated by improving ventilation and by removing

Table 4 Environmental Control of Animal Danders

Avoid or diminish contact with the animal.
    Remove the animal from the home or limit its access.
    Keep the pet out of the bedroom.
Decrease air-borne allergens.
    Close heating ducts to the bedroom.
    Use a HEPA filter in rooms to which the pet has access.
Decrease allergen shedding by washing cats weekly.
Remove residual allergens.
    Use aggressive cleaning measures, including the use of protein denaturing agents on remaining carpets and upholstery.
    Remove carpets and upholstery.
    Use ventilation and HEPA filtration.

---

large reservoirs of animal allergen, such as carpets and upholstered furniture. Tannic acid and Allersearch DMS have been shown to reduce levels of cat allergen significantly (36,37). Steam cleaning has not proven helpful in removing animal allergens (38) and, as with house dust mite allergen, conventional vacuum cleaners may leak dust and dander and actually result in increased airborne allergen levels (39). The modified vacuum cleaners introduced for control of house dust mite allergens may be helpful in this situation.

Many patients are unwilling to get rid of their pets, but some degree of avoidance is still possible. The pet's access to particular rooms, especially bedrooms, should be forbidden. In addition, closing forced-air ventilation ducts may help to reduce the allergen load in those rooms. HEPA filters can also be helpful, since some animal allergens, notably cat allergen, bind to particles that remain suspended in the air for long periods of time. Since one of the major cat allergens is present primarily in saliva and is deposited on the cat's hair as the cat washes itself, regular washing of the cat at monthly intervals may be beneficial (40). For those who doubt that it is possible to wash a cat, success in this respect has usually been achieved by introducing the cat to washing while it is still a small kitten. One study, however, did not confirm the usefulness of this procedure (41).

D. Molds (Table 5)

Aspergillus and *Penicillium* species are the most common indoor fungi. They occur most often in areas of water damage in the home. Patients should be instructed to identify areas of water leakage, especially beneath carpeting or above the ceiling and have it fixed promptly. Other areas which may harbor molds are bathroom showers, tiles and floors, cupboards be-

Table 5 Environmental Control of Molds

Outdoor molds
    Keep windows and doors closed when mold counts are high.
    Use air conditioning or a HEPA filter when mold counts are high.
    Stay indoors when mold counts are highest.
Indoor molds
    Repair any areas of water leakage.
    Keep bathrooms, kitchens, and basements well ventilated.
    Clean bathrooms, kitchens, and basements regularly.
    Use cleaning products which inhibit mold growth.
    Use dehumidifiers in dampness-prone areas.

neath sinks, and damp closets and basements. In these areas cleaning with substances that inhibit mold growth is helpful.

E. Cockroaches (Table 6)

Increased household cleanliness, especially in the kitchen, is the best answer to the eradication of cockroach antigen. Unfortunately, the presence of cockroaches often represents poverty and poor housing conditions, often in older buildings and frequently with landlords who are reluctant to upgrade their properties.

It is important that the physician should be aware of how incomprehensible, intimidating, complicated, or expensive the measures required for environmental allergen control, especially for house dust mite control, may seem to the patient. For this reason, leaflets on allergen control should never be handed to a patient without full explanation and discussion. For example, it is helpful when discussing house dust mite control to point out to the patient that she spends a substantial part of each 24 hr in her bedroom, and so it should be the focus of her efforts. In the same way, her bed should the first place to start. Allergen-proof mattress and pillow covers may seem expensive to some patients, but they need to be seen as an investment that will provide considerable relief of symptoms with minimal maintenance over many years. Our personal experience has been that when we made allergen-proof covers, etc., available for purchase in our office, their use by patients increased considerably. When allergy control measures are fully explained, prioritized, and necessary compromises agreed upon, patient compliance with environmental control measures will be considerably enhanced.

IV. Allergy Immunotherapy

Allergen immunotherapy has been used in the treatment of asthma for many years. For much of this time, treatment was on an empirical basis,

Table 6 Environmental Control of Cockroaches

Improve housing stock.
Keep kitchen clean and free from food debris at all times.
Use insecticide sprays or "bombs" (asthmatics should avoid contact with these products).
Use cockroach traps.

and in the past there was meager evidence that it was beneficial to asthma patients by comparison with patients with allergic rhinitis or conjunctivitis. Recent controlled studies, however, have demonstrated that immunotherapy reduces asthma symptoms caused by house dust mites, cat dander, *Alternaria* and *Cladosporium* molds, and grass, birch tree, and ragweed pollens (42).

Since it is nearly impossible to prevent asthma symptoms caused by exposure to pollens and outdoor molds through avoidance measures alone, patients who are sensitive to these allergens are good candidates for immunotherapy and often demonstrate excellent responses (43).

Immunotherapy with mite allergens has been studied extensively. Certain patient characteristics appear to correlate with a good outcome, namely, youth (between 5 and 50 years of age), forced expiratory volume in 1 sec (FEV$_1$) greater than 70% of predicted, and absence of aspirin sensitivity or chronic sinusitis (44).

In the case of both seasonal pollen allergy and house dust mite allergy, immunotherapy appears to be more effective when given for longer periods of time (44). It would appear that treatment for at least 3 years is necessary. However, in areas such as California, where patients are frequently allergic to multiple pollen allergens, there may be considerable merit in advising the patient to remain on immunotherapy injections every 4–6 weeks rather than stopping and having a recurrence of symptoms requiring reinitiation of immunotherapy. This approach may not be recommended for everyone, but it can be particularly useful in an individual who has a "petering out" effect when the usual immunotherapy injection is delayed.

Allergen immunotherapy can be a safe and effective therapy for the pregnant asthmatic. However, systemic reactions occur in approximately 0.5% of all patients undergoing allergen-specific immunotherapy (45). Acute bronchospasm appears to be more common in patients with seasonal asthma than in those with allergic rhinitis (46). In addition, bronchospasm induced by immunotherapy is more likely to occur if the FEV$_1$ is below 70% of predicted and in patients undergoing immunotherapy with mite allergen extract by comparison to pollen extracts (42).

The risk of having a systemic reaction to allergen immunotherapy is no greater during pregnancy than in the nonpregnant patient (47). However, the major problem is that a systemic reaction may result in increased uterine contractility, which may occasionally result in spontaneous miscarriage (48). The recently published Practice Parameters for the Diagnosis and Treatment of Asthma recommends that patients who are on maintenance immunotherapy without difficulty may remain at their current level of treatment (49). Patients on maintenance immunotherapy who have shown any tendency to develop local or systemic reactions should probably have their immunotherapy dosage decreased somewhat during pregnancy (49). Some authorities disagree with this approach and believe that the maintenance dose should always be decreased, to further reduce the risk of anaphylaxis (18). If the patient is on an increasing immunotherapy schedule and becomes pregnant, no further increase in the immunotherapy dose should be given, because many patients are more vulnerable to systemic reactions while the allergen dose is being increased. Ideally, the time to consider immunotherapy for control of asthma in pregnancy is during the period of time when a women is considering becoming pregnant, but has not yet taken any steps to do so. During this preconception period it may be possible to start the patient on immunotherapy and reach satisfactory maintenance levels before she becomes pregnant.

V. Conclusion

In conclusion, it must never be forgotten by either the physician or the patient that a prime concern in the management of the pregnant asthmatic is the well being of the fetus, which requires adequate oxygenation at all times. Women with asthma should be warned about deliberate self-restriction of asthma medication during pregnancy, and the physician should seize the opportunity to introduce or reemphasize the benefits of both allergen avoidance measures and allergen immunotherapy as means of reducing medication requirements.

References

1. Guidelines for the diagnosis and management of asthma. National Heart, Lung and Blood Institute National Asthma Education Program. Expert Panel Report. January 1991.
2. Schatz M, Hoffman C. Interrelationships between asthma and pregnancy: clinical and mechanistic considerations. Clin Rev Allergy 1987; 5:301–315.
3. Kang BC, Johnson JJ, Veres-Thorner C. Atopic profile of inner-city asthma with a comparative analysis on the cockroach-sensitive and ragweed-sensitive subgroups. J Clin Immunol 1993; 92:802–811.
4. Pollart SM, Chapman MD, Fiocco GP, Rose G, Platts-Mills TAE. Epidemiology of acute asthma: IgE antibodies to common inhalant allergens as a risk factor for emergency room visits. J Allergy Immunol 1989; 83:875–882.
5. Schaefer G, Silverman F. Pregnancy complicated by asthma. Am J Gynecol 1961; 82:182–189.

6. Report of the Working Group on Asthma in Pregnancy. National Asthma Education Program. National Heart, Lung and Blood Institutes. NIH Publication No. 93-3279. 1993.

7. Pollart SM, Reid MJ, Fling JA, Chapman MD, Platts-Mills TAE. Epidemiology of emergency room asthma in Northern California: association with IgE antibody to rye grass pollen. J Allergy Clin Immunol 1988; 82:224–230.

8. O'Hollaren MT, Yunginger JW, Offord KP, Somers MJ, O'Connel EJ, Ballard DJ, Sax MI. Exposure to an aeroallergen as a precipitating factor in respiratory arrest in young patients with asthma. N Engl J Med 1991; 324:359–363.

9. Platts-Mills TAE, Hayden ML, Chapman M, Wilkins R. Seasonal variation in dust mite and grass pollen allergens in dust from the houses of patients with asthma J Allergy Clin Immunol 1987; 79:781–791.

10. Sporik R, Platts-Mills TAE, Cogswell JJ. Exposure to house dust mite allergen of children admitted to hospital with asthma. Clin Exp Allergy 1993; 23: 740–746.

11. Woodfolk JA, Luczynska CM, Blay FD, Chapman MD, Platts-Mills TAE. Cat allergy. Ann Allergy 1992; 69:273–275.

12. Van der Brembt X, Charpin D, Haddi D, DeMata P, Vervloat D. Cat removal. Fel d I levels in mattresses. J Allergy Clin Immunol 1991; 87:595–596.

13. Munirak M, Inarsson R, Schou C, Dreborg SKG. Allergens in school dust: 1. The amount of major cat allergen (Fel d I) and dog (Can f I). Allergens in dust from Swedish schools is high enough to probably cause perennial symptoms in most children with asthma who are sensitized to cat and dog. J Allergy Clin Immunol 1993; 91:1067–1074.

14. Enberg RN, Shamie SM, McCullough J, Ownby DR. Ubiquitous presence of cat allergen in cat-free buildings: probable dispersal from human clothing. Ann Allergy 1993; 70:471–474.

15. Gelber LE, Seltzer LH, Bouzourkis JH, Pollart SM, Chapman MD, Platts-Mills TAE. Sensitization and exposure to indoor allergens as risk factors for asthma among patients presenting to hospital. Am Rev Respir Dis 1993; 147: 573–578.

16. Bernstein IL, Storms WW. Practice parameters for allergy diagnostic testing. Ann Asthma Allergy Immunol 1995; 75:543–625.

17. Spector SL, Nicklas RA. Practice parameters for the diagnosis and treatment of asthma. V. Diagnosis and evaluation. J Allergy Clin Immunol (suppl) 1995; 96:732–748.

18. Schatz M, Hoffman CP, Zeiger RS, Falcoff R, Macy E, Mellon M. The course and management of asthma and allergic diseases during pregnancy. In: Middleton E, Reed CE, Ellis EF, Atkinson NF, Yuninger JW, Busse WW, eds. Allergy Principles and Practice. 4th ed. St Louis: Mosby/Year Book, 1993: 1301–1342.

19. Harving H, Korsgaard KJ, Dahl R. House dust mites and associated environmental conditions in Danish homes. Allergy 1993; 48:106–109.

20. Warner JA. Creating optimal conditions for the house dust mite. Clin Exp Allergy 1994; 24:207–209.

21. Kuehr J, Fischer T, Carnaus W, Meinert R, Barth R, Schraub S, Daschner A, Urbanek R, Foster J. Natural variation in light antigen density in house dust and relationship to residential factors. Clin Exp Allergy 1994; 24:229–237.

22. Collof NG, Ayres J, Carswell F, Howarth PH, Merrett TG, Mitchell EB, Walshaw NJ, Warner JO, Warner JA, Woodcock AA. The control of allergens of house dust mites and domestic pets: a position paper. Clin Exp Allergy 1992; 22 (suppl):1–28.

23. Andersen A, Rosen J. House dust mite *Dermaphagoides pteronyssinus* and its allergens: effects of washing. Allergy 1989; 44:396–400.

24. Vandenhove T, Soler M, Birnbaum J, Charpin D, Vervloet D. Effect of dry cleaning on mite allergen levels in blankets. Allergy 1993; 48:264–266.

25. Wickman M, Nordvall SL, Pershagen G, Korsgaard J, Johansen H, Sundell J. Mite allergens during 18 months of intervention. Allergy 1994; 49:114–119.

26. Kalra S, Owen SJ, Hepworth J, Woodcock A. Air-borne house dust mite allergen after vacuum cleaning (letter). Lancet 1990; 336:449.

27. Munir AKM, Ainarsson R, Drebrog SKG. Vacuum cleaning decreases levels of mite allergens in house dust. Pediatr Allergy Immunol 1993; 4:136–143.

28. Wasserman DPJ. Effectiveness of vacuum cleaning and wet cleaning in reducing house dust mites, fungi and mite allergen in a cotton carpet: a case study. Exp Appl Acarol 1988; 4:53–62.

29. Lintner TJ, Brame KA. The effects of season, climate and air-conditioning on the prevalence of *Dermatophagoides* mite allergens in household dust. J Allergy Clin Immunol 1993; 91:862–867.

30. Wickman M, Emenius G, Egmar AC, Axelson G, Pershagen G. Reduced mite allergen levels in dwellings with mechanical exhaust and supply ventilation. Clin Exp Allergy 1994; 24:109–114.

31. Nelson HS, Hirsch R, Ohman JL, Platts-Mills TAE, Reed CE, Solomon WR. Recommendations for the use of residential air-cleaning devices in the treatment of allergic respiratory diseases. J Allergy Clin Immunol 1988; 92: 661–669.

32. Warner JA, Marchant JL, Warner JO. Double blind trial of ionizers in children with asthma sensitive to the house dust mite. Thorax 1993; 48:330–333.

33. Kalra S, Crank P, Hepworth J, Pickering CAC, Woodcock AA. Concentrations of the domestic house dust mite allergen *Der p* I after treatment with solidified benzyl benzoate (Acarosan) or liquid nitrogen. Thorax 1993; 48:10–13.

34. Dietemann A, Bessot JC, Hoyet C, Ott M, Verot A, Pauli G. A double blind, placebo controlled trial of solidified benzyl benzoate applied in dwellings of asthmatic patients sensitive to mites: clinical efficacy and effect on mite allergens. J Allergy Clin Immunol 1993; 91:738–746.

35. Huss RW, Huss K, Squire EN, Carpenter GB, Smith LJ, Salata K, Hershey BA. Mite allergen control with acaricide fails. J Allergy Clin Immunol 1994; 94:27–32.

36. Woodfolk JA, Hayden ML, Miller JD, Rose G, Chapman MD, Platts-Mills TAE. Chemical treatment of carpets to reduce allergen: a detailed study of

the effects of tannic acid on indoor allergens. J Allergy Clin Immunol 1994; 94:19–26.

37. Warner JA, Marchant JL, Warner O, Allergen avoidance in the homes of asthmatic children: the effect of Allersearch DMS. Clin Exp Allergy 1993; 23:279–286.

38. Wood RA, Chapman DM, Adkinson NF, Eggleston PA. The effect of cat removal on allergen content in household dust samples. J Allergy Clin Immunol 1989; 83:730–734.

39. Woodfolk JA, Luczynska CM, de Blay F, Chapman MD, Platts-Mills TAE. The effect of vacuum cleaners on the concentration and particle size distribution of air-borne cat allergen. J Allergy Clin Immunol 1993; 91:829–837.

40. De Blay F, Chapman MD, Platts-Mills TAE. Air-borne cat allergen (*Fel d* I): environmental control with the cat *in situ.* Am Rev Resp Dis 1991; 143: 1334–1339.

41. Klucka CV, Ownby DR, Green I, Zoratti E. Cat shedding of *Fel d* 1 is not reduced by washing, Allerpet/C Spray or acepromazine. J Allergy Clin Immunol 1995; 95:1164–1171.

42. Bousquet J, Francois MB. Specific Immunotherapy in asthma: is it effective? J Allergy Clin Immunol 1994; 94:1–11.

43. Bousquet J, Becker WM, Hejjaoui A, Chanal I, Lebel B, Dhivert H, Michel FB. Clinical and immunological reactivity of patients allergic to grass pollens and to multiple pollen species: II. Efficacy of a double-blind, placebo-controlled specific immunotherapy with standardized extracts. J Allergy Clin Immunol 1991; 88:43–53.

44. Bousquet J, Hejjaoui A, Clauzel AM, Guerin B, Dhivert H, Skassa-Brociek W, Michel FB. Immunotherapy with a standardized *Dermatophagoides pteronyssinus* extract: II. Prediction of efficacy of immunotherapy. J Allergy Clin Immunol 1988; 82:971–977.

45. Matloff SM, Bailit IW, Parks P, Madden N, Greineder DK. Systemic reactions to immunotherapy. Allergy Proc 1993; 14:347–350.

46. Hejjaoui A, Ferrando R, Dhivert H, Michel FB, Bousquet J. Systemic reactions occurring during immunotherapy with standardized pollen extracts. J Allergy Clin Immunol 1992; 89:923–933.

47. Metzger WJ, Turner E, Paterson R. Safety of immunotherapy during pregnancy. J Allergy Clin Immunol 1978; 61:268.

48. Francis N. Abortion after grass pollen injection. J Allergy 1941; 12:559.

49. Spector SL, Nicklas RA. Practice parameters for the diagnosis and treatment of asthma. VII. Special conditions. J Allergy Clin Immunol (suppl) 1995; 96: 821–870.

11

The Diagnosis and Treatment of Rhinosinusitis During Pregnancy and Lactation

GARY A. INCAUDO

University of California, Davis, School of Medicine
Chico, California

I. Introduction

Upper-airway congestive symptoms during pregnancy have been recognized since the turn of the century, yet relatively little has been written concerning this problem despite its frequency and occasional severity (1). Among randomly selected pregnancies, as many as 30% of patients will report substantial symptoms of rhinitis, and this figure may be higher among patients with preexisting atopic disease (2,3). Furthermore, the diagnosis of sinusitis in pregnancy may be as high as 1.5%, which represents a sixfold increase over the frequency observed in a nonpregnant population (4). There is understandable reluctance on the part of physicians caring for pregnant patients to employ the modalities commonly used in the diagnosis and management of rhinitis, because of fetal risk factors, the time-limited nature of pregnancy, and the litiginous propensity of any fetal mishap. Nevertheless, the impact that rhinitis may have on the pregnant mother's eating, sleeping, and emotional well-being, or by worsening associated conditions such as sinusitis and asthma, suggest that rhinitis during pregnancy should be actively evaluated and treated.

II. Nasal Physiology in Pregnancy

In the normal nasal airway, optimal mucosal secretion and nasal patency
depend on a fine balance between adrenergic and cholinergic stimuli.
Alpha-adrenergic stimulation causes vasoconstriction and increases nasal
patency. In contrast, cholinergic stimulation induces both hypersecretion
and vasodilatation, giving rise to stuffiness and rhinorrhea. Factors which
affect this autonomic balance include body cooling, exercise, change in
body position, emotional disturbance, and atmospheric conditions.

The nose functions principally to air-condition the more delicate
lower airway. The nose strives to maintain inspired air at 32°C., 98% relative humidity, and free of dust and foreign vapors. Most water-soluble
gases and particles greater than 10 μm are wholly filtered in the nose.
Particles trapped in the mucociliary escalator mechanism are cleared every
10–15 min. This same escalator is one of the essential factors in promoting
sterility within the paranasal sinuses, despite heavy bacterial colonization
within the nasal passages.

The nasal mucosa of the pregnant female differs histologically from
the nonpregnant state. This differentiation is the result of the direct and
indirect effects of pregnancy-associated hormones on the nasal lining, although the exact mechanism remains obscure. As early as 1956, Henderson
made the observation that the columnar epithelium of the nose is subject
to hormonal influence in a manner similar to the uterine cervical surface
(5). In 1982, Toppozada et al., using electron microscopy (EM) and histochemical assays, demonstrated mucous gland hyperactivity, increased
mucopolysaccharide in the ground substance, and increase phagocytic activity in the nasal mucosa of asymptomatic pregnant women (6). Excessive
autonomic activity was not felt to be present based on cholinesterase activity measurements in these studies, in contrast to earlier, animal-derived
data suggesting that hormonal influences may be the source (7).

The rise in endogenous hormones, especially estrogens, has been indirectly incriminated as the source of the upper respiratory changes seen
in pregnancy. Primate studies have linked estrogens to nasal mucosal swelling as well as perivascular edema (8). Similarly, Toppozada found highly
comparable histological changes in estrogen/progesterone contraceptive
users, strengthening the idea of a hormonal role (9). However, Bende could
find no differences quantitatively in serum levels of estradiol, progesterone,
or vasoactive intestinal polypeptide in pregnant patients with rhinometri-
cally documented nasal congestion and a pregnant, symptom-free control
group. He suggested that if hormonal influences are involved, changes in
end-organ responsiveness may be the cause (10).

The increased incidence of nasal mucosal hyperemia, epistaxis, hypersecretion, and edema during pregnancy has been suggested as indirect evidence that hormonally induced nasal vascular pooling and hypersecretion do indeed exist (11). Circulating blood volume increase 40% during pregnancy, peaking during the last trimester. This volume change could lead to increased nasal vascular pooling, edema, and resultant increased nasal airflow resistance. Schatz and Zeiger have postulated that progesterone-induced nasal vascular smooth muscle relaxation could aggravate this nasal vascular pooling effect, although no confirmation of such a pooling effect exists (12).

Alterations in nasal mucous have been documented as a result of hormonal influences. Henderson has described the formation of large ferns appearing cyclically during ovulation and disappearing premenstrually in human nasal mucous (13). Toppozada et al., using ultrastructural and histochemical studies, have demonstrated an increased level of activity of the nasal mucosal glands during pregnancy (6). This same group also demonstrated similar changes with the administration of estrogen/progesterone contraceptives (9). However, in contradiction to such a consistent unifying physiological concept, Schatz and Zeiger described 348 pregnant asthmatic women with preexisting rhinitis, 15% of whom experienced improvement in their nasal symptoms during pregnancy, often in association with improvement in their asthma (12). These authors have hypothesized that, since free serum cortisol rises during pregnancy, those women who experience improvement in eosinophilic rhinitis and asthma are demonstrating an increased glucocorticosteroid effect due to an inordinately increased free cortisol level, an increased number or affinity of respiratory glucocorticoid receptors, or a decreased competitive antagonism by other pregnancy hormones such as progesterone, deoxycorticosterone, and aldosterone (14). Perhaps, a distinct but variable end-organ responsiveness to normally circulating hormones occurs during pregnancy, which explains these conflicting data. Such a hypothesis, however, has yet to be demonstrated.

In examining the nasal mucosa of pregnant women complaining of nasal congestion, EM and histochemical changes compatible with allergic disease have been described. Suggestions as to the origins of this finding are varied and ill-defined. Placental proteins, fetal proteins, or endogenous hapten were all incriminated as potential antigens in allergic pregnant women. As early as 1903, Roseman and Anderson demonstrated that guinea pigs could be sensitized to extracts of placental proteins (15). Specific immunological reactions to endogenous hormones also have been incriminated by some authors but discounted by others (16–18). The origin of these histological findings may lie simply in the enhancement of a pre-existing atopic state. Both Schatz and Mabry have noted that most women with clinically significant rhinitis during pregnancy have had preexisting nasal symptoms (19,20).

III. Nasal Pathophysiology During the Childbearing Years

Factors of importance that upset the normal physiology of the nose do so by means of either disrupting air flow or interrupting mucociliary clearance. Common causes of a dysfunctional nose pertinent to pregnancy are viral infections, allergic reactions to inhalant aeroallergens, chronic ambient air pollution, anatomical deformities obstructing air and mucous flow, abuse of topical vasoconstrictive drugs, and bacterial infections of the paranasal sinuses.

Common viral infections induce direct tissue damage to the nasal mucosa with resultant inflammation and its consequences. Some indirect consequences of viral invasion are nasal mucosal hyperactivity through alteration in receptor responsiveness and impaired nasal mucociliary clearance. Secondary bacterial invasion is enhanced in these circumstances, especially from the heavily colonized nasal cavity to the paranasal sinuses.

IgE emerged in the 1960s as the mediator of classic allergic reactions. IgE-producing cells are located in the respiratory and gastrointestinal tracts. Upon appropriate stimulation in the susceptible host, homocytotropic, antigen-specific IgE antibodies are produced and fixed to mast cells and circulating basophils. The "classic" allergic response has grown increasingly complex with the realization of late and delayed reactions being common accompaniments. Foxen et al. and Capel believed that nasal allergy was exacerbated or initiated by pregnancy (21,22). A more recent study failed to demonstrate any consistent change in serum IgE during pregnancy (23). The precise influence of pregnancy on each of the complex immunological steps involved in the allergic reaction has yet to be described adequately.

Cigarette smoke, formaldehyde, ozone, and sulfur dioxide are important air pollutants capable of provoking rhinitis symptoms, especially in the hyperreactive airway. Although this has not yet been fully verified, it is likely that various environmental pollutants and chemicals are capable of nonspecifically stimulating the sensory nerves and the nerve terminals of the autonomic nervous system as well as the mast cells and epithelial cells to produce nasal hyperactivity. The increasing frequency with which women smoke, the increasing use of synthetic materials, the increasing incidence of women in the workplace, and the generally deteriorating ambient air quality in our cities are all relevant issues during the child-bearing age.

Anatomical findings such as septal deflections, polyps, and turbinate hypertrophy all serve as potential sources of nasal obstruction in this age group. The degree of obstruction induced will vary according to the extent and location of the anatomic blockage. Turbinate hypertrophy and polyps generally represent the end product of more severe nasal disease. A thorough investigation should ensue in light of these physical findings. Boggy, pale turbinates with clear mucoid discharge generally represent the eosinophilic forms of rhinitis, of which IgE-mediated disease is the most common example.

The actual extent and mechanisms responsible for the increased incidence of bacterial respiratory infections during pregnancy remain uncertain. Although there is a depression of maternal cell-mediated immunity during pregnancy, most authors believe that this is a selective process and not profound enough to account for such a format of infection (23,24). Furthermore, the majority of evidence supports normally functioning humoral maternal immunity during gestation (23) (see Chapter 4). There are, as yet, no direct immunological reasons to explain the observed increased incidence of infectious respiratory diseases during pregnancy. Impaired mucosal hygiene induced by edema and hypersecretion remains a postulated source, although a local immune defect of the nose and sinuses or reduced local inflammatory cell function has not been effectively ruled out.

Limited clinical observations have been made concerning bacterial rhinosinusitis in pregnancy. The organisms do not appear to be different from those found in the nonpregnant state. In one study the peak onset was the second trimester (25). This same study revealed that the classic symptoms and signs of sinusitis were absent in nearly half of the women studied with documented purulent sinusitis during pregnancy. Even in the nonpregnant state, sinusitis can be notoriously subtle in its clinical presentation, with very little in the patient history or physical findings to support a firm diagnosis (26). Considering the sixfold-increased frequency of sinusitis in pregnancy, a high degree of suspicion must be kept in mind in any pregnancy marked by persistent rhinitis of unknown cause.

Complaints of ear congestion, fullness, or stuffiness are frequently encountered during pregnancy. The responsible pathology is usually limited to these conditions: (a) acute or subacute otitis media, commonly complicated by purulent rhinosinusitis; (b) serous otitis media, usually following an episode of rhinosinusitis or a viral upper respiratory infection (URI); (c) eustachian tube obstruction, usually due to an underlying rhinitis state; or (d) patulous eustachian tubes. This latter condition, although not unique to pregnancy, is found most commonly during pregnancy. Clinical clues to this disorder are aggravation of symptoms in the upright position, by exercise, and by nervousness, as well as a sense of disturbed hearing due to autophony. The frequency of onset of patulous eustachian tubes increases with each trimester and typically resolves postpartum (27). Derkay described 20 pregnant volunteers with symptoms of eustachian tube dysfunction, 80% of whom had demonstrable eustachian tube abnormalities by functional testing. Nineteen percent, or 3 of 16, demonstrated patulous eustachian tubes as evidenced by impedance variation synchronous with respiration (28). Hormonal factors may be significantly correlated with this disorder, as evidenced by its frequency both in pregnancy and in women who take birth control pills, but a direct cause-and-effect relationship remains to be established (29,30). The differentiation of patulous eustachian tubes from the other disorders of the middle ear space mentioned above is important in that systemic or topical decongestants aggravate and antibiotics have very little effect on this clinical problem.

IV. Diagnostic Approach

Several published reports suggest that allergic rhinitis, bacterial rhinosinusitis, and rhinitis medicamentosa are most common causes of rhinitis during pregnancy (Table 1) (2,20). Rhinitis medicamentosa has been cited as being common, due to a logical preference that pregnant women and their physicians have for topical versus systemic medications to relieve nasal symptoms. Structural abnormalities, eosinophilic nonallergic rhinitis, and nasal polyps are also occasionally seen in pregnant women. Much less common is the syndrome of "vasomotor rhinitis of pregnancy." Nasal con-

Table 1 Differential Diagnoses
of Rhinitis in Pregnancy

Allergic rhinitis[a]
Bacterial rhinosinusitis[a]
Rhinitis medicamentosa[a]
"Vasomotor rhinitis"
Structural nasal obstruction
Eosinophilic nonallergic rhinitis
Nasal polyposis

[a]Most common.

gestion from vasomotor instability develops most prominently in the second and third trimesters in this disorder and usually disappears within 5 days postpartum, although any accompanying eustachian tube dysfunction may persist for 4–10 weeks (31,32). Schatz and Zeiger have subcategorized gestational rhinitis which is not classifiable to any known disorder into two overlapping, nonallergic, noninfectious, noneosinophilic forms which they term "nonspecific postnasal drip" and "vasomotor rhinitis." They feel that the former is a gestational hormonal effect on nasal mucous, whereas the latter, more "stuffy" disorder represents the nasal vascular effects described previously (12). It is the knowledge of these prevalent etiologies of rhinitis in pregnancy that allows the physician to dictate a logical, direct, and cost-effective diagnostic scheme.

A. History and Physical Examination

The combination of a carefully obtained history and physical exam commonly suggests the etiology of rhinitis in pregnancy (Table 1). The features of the clinical history that are most important to an accurate diagnosis are the presence of itching, sneezing, and runny nose suggesting eosinophilic disease (typically allergic in etiology), unilateral nasal obstruction suggesting a structural cause, anosmia suggesting sinusitis and/or polyposis, and purulent mucous discharge suggesting infection. Clinically nonspecific nasal congestion with or without prominent postnasal drainage may be all that is elicited historically and may be an expression of any of the above clinical problems, including the nonspecific rhinitis associated with the hormonal effects of pregnancy. It is important to remember that most rhinitis states in pregnancy are expressions of problems present in the nonpregnant state.

The examination of the nasal passage in nonspecific postnasal drip and vasomotor rhinitis of pregnancy is rarely revealing, other than a general bogginess of the turbinates, which may be slightly pale in color. In contrast, the allergic nose is typically very boggy, pale and watery in appearance and, when combined with the history of itching and paroxysmal sneezing, such a finding confirms the diagnosis of IgE-mediated disease and will immediately direct treatment. Examination of the mucosal lining of the nose in acute and subacute sinus disease typically reveals an irregular, bright red appearance. Adult patients with acute sinusitis will commonly have mucopus in the nares or the nasopharynx unless drainage is impeded or intermittent due to swelling of the turbinates. Dehydration of nasal secretions after airway heating and cooling, often enhanced by the inhibition of ciliary clearing by inflammatory mediators, may lead to purulent-appearing crusts throughout the nasal vestibule. Such a finding in conjunction with generalized nasal erythema may serve as the only physical suggestion of purulent sinus disease.

Under the best circumstances, only a small portion of the nasal surface area can be seen through a nasal speculum. Even the anterior tip of the middle turbinate, displaced posteriorly, may be obscured by the swollen inferior turbinate. Decongesting with a topical alpha-adrenergic agonist spray such as oxymetazoline is helpful in visualizing the anterior tip of the middle turbinate and the middle meatus. The positioning of the nasal septum relative to the middle turbinate and the patency of the meatal drainage tract can be better appreciated in the decongested nose. Furthermore, decongesting may help visualize pus or polyps emanating directly from the middle meatus.

Direct visualization of the middle turbinate and middle meatus, enhanced by decongesting, can also help in identifying potential structural causes of sinus disease. For example, a nasal polyp may extrude anteriorly from the middle meatus and be readily visible. However, differentiating a nasal polyp from a turbinate can be a source of confusion when examining the nose with a nasal speculum or otoscope. Probing the structure in question with a blunt instrument, the examining physician will find that a polyp is soft, pliable, and without sensation, in contrast to a turbinate, which has a firm cartilaginous undersurface and is sensitive to touch. More direct visualization of the nasal passage with a fiber-optic rhinoscope is the most definitive way of making this distinction. Skilled observers may appreciate potential sources of sinus disease arising from the configuration of the middle turbinate. For example, an enlarged middle turbinate from migration of anterior ethmoid aircells into the turbinate structure (concha bullosae) may be appreciated by simple anterior nasal exam. A septal deviation may be seen compressing the middle turbinate and lateralizing its position, resulting in a compromise in middle meatal drainage. The pale, watery, hyperplastic appearance of the middle turbinate in chronic allergic disease may be a distinguishing insight into the pathophysiology of a particular sinusitis problem.

Palpation of the affected sinus in search of tenderness is a poor indicator of underlying sinus infection. If the inflammation extends beyond the confines of the sinus, there may be pain and swelling of the adjacent tissues. The so-called Potts puffy tumor of acute frontal sinusitis, as well as periorbital cellulitis or proptosis from ethmoid disease, are examples of such disease extension. In maxillary sinusitis, examination and palpation of the upper molars may be important, since infection may spread from an infected tooth directly into the maxillary antrum and vice versa.

B. Nasal Cytology

Nasal cytology is generally underutilized but extremely helpful in many cases. The presence of eosinophils in the nasal mucosa or secretions is strong circumstantial evidence for an allergic etiology and directs ancillary investigative procedures and treatment. However, eosinophilia in nasal secretions is less specific in adults than in children, since secretory eosinophilia may be found in patients with nasal polyposis, nonallergic rhinitis with eosinophilia (NARES), or chronic "intrinsic" asthma with no evidence of significant IgE-mediated involvement. As a corollary, the absence of nasal eosinophilia does not exclude the diagnosis of underlying allergic disease. If verification of allergic disease or the identification of a potential allergen would be useful for formulating avoidance instructions or directing treatment, in-vitro methodology such as selective radioallergosorbent (RAST) or ELISA testing is preferable. Routine skin testing during pregnancy is not recommended because of the remote risk of anaphylaxis and subsequent adverse fetal effects (33–35).

The history of purulent nasal discharge, facial pain or discomfort, and nasal cytology demonstrating neutrophils with phagocytized bacteria in the nasal mucous strongly suggest purulent rhinosinusitis, even when mucopus cannot be demonstrated on physical exam. In bacterial sinusitis, nasal cytology may show a predominance of neutrophils with intracellular bacteria suggestive of active phagocytosis. Studies by Wilson, Jalowayski, and Hamburger in 55 patients (35 children and 20 adults), comparing nasal cytology with sinus x-rays, revealed a 79% correlation when there was more than one neutrophil per high-power field or smear. The correlation improved to 90% if the nasal cytology revealed more than six neutrophils per high-power field and there were bacteria present (36). Specificity and sensitivity was 0.79 in this investigation. The sampling of the nasal mucosa was from the inferior turbinate with a Rhinoprobe and stained with modified Wright-Giemsa. Gill and Neiburger, using nasal secretions discharged into wax paper, examined 300 children and adults, correlating the results of sinus radiographs with the number of neutrophils per high-power field. These authors demonstrated an 86% sensitivity and 40% specificity when more than five neutrophils per high-power field was used as the distinguishing criterion for a positive sinus radiograph (37).

The presence of polymorphonuclear leukocytes by themselves is not as useful. Neutrophilia without intracellular bacteria can be seen in viral respiratory infection or after exposure to mucosal irritants at home or in the workplace. The presence of small amounts of bacteria and neutrophils may be normal in nasal secretions from infancy through adulthood. The major pitfall in the procedure is failure to sample sufficiently posterior on the inferior turbinate and/or sampling secretions only. The primary disadvantage of exclusively using nasal cytology to diagnose sinusitis is the 11–14% false negative readings obtained using plain sinus radiographs as the standard, which, in itself, has limitations. Most authors still conclude that large numbers of neutrophils and bacteria when viewed on a Wright-Giemsa stain of nasal secretions, especially if obtained by scraping the medial portion of the inferior turbinate, most likely represents the presence of true purulent sinus disease (38). More definitive studies using maxillary antral puncture and CT scanning as reference procedures are needed to clarify the place of nasal cytology in the diagnosis of sinusitis.

C. Sinus Radiology

Rhinitis unaccompanied by any of these "classic" findings may still be based on sinus disease. The diagnosis of sinusitis will escape detection in this circumstance unless a sinus radiograph and/or maxillary antral puncture and culture are pursued. Limited sinus radiographs should be considered when necessary for confirmation when the diagnosis is obscure and the patient is not responding to conservative measures (39). Although physicians are rightfully cautious about ordering radiographs during pregnancy, the threshold dose of pelvic radiation exposure for induction of a congenital defect is considered to be 10 rad, more than 1000-fold greater than the amount of radiation received from routine diagnostic radiological studies (40).

Nevertheless, sinus radiographs should be used judiciously and interpreted with caution, since doubt has been cast on the utility of conventional x-rays to define the presence or absence of sinusitis, both in terms of overestimating and underestimating disease. In a study by McAlister et al., comparing simultaneously obtained plain sinus radiographs and CT scans in children and young adults during a posttreatment period for recurrent chronic sinus disease, the authors found that 75% of the patients had findings on plain radiographs which did not correlate with those on CT scans (41). Approximately 45% of the patients had normal findings on conventional radiographs of at least one sinus, with the corresponding sinus being abnormal on the CT scan. Conversely, approximately 35% of the patients had an abnormality on plain radiographs which proved normal on simultaneous CT scanning. The interpretation of plain sinus radiographs poses many problems to the examining physician. The sloping contours of the maxillary sinus may appear on the Waters view as mucosal thickening. A hypoplastic maxillary sinus will appear as opacification in plain radiography. The appearance on the Caldwell view of partial ethmoidal clouding or opacification can be caused by superimposed ethmoidal air cells, slight rotation, nasal secretions, and mild mucous membrane thickening. A small sphenoid sinus may appear partially opacified on lateral sinus radiographs. The maxillary sinuses appear to be the "best" sinuses to study by conventional radiography. Still, in comparison to CT scanning, small amounts of mucosal thickening can be missed even in these areas, and the frequency of false "positive" and false "negative" interpretations is not insignificant (42). Furthermore, if the theory that the ethmoid sinuses are the focal point of chronic or recurrent sinus disease proves correct, the use of plain radiography in the clinical evaluation of the extent and site of sinusitis is open to question (43).

D. A-Mode Ultrasonography

A-mode ultrasonography is a readily available tool to the obstetrician which can be used to evaluate the presence or absence of sinusitis. A-mode ultrasonography has been suggested as a safe and efficacious screening modality for sinus pathology (44,45). In 1980, Roventa, from Finland, reported a statistically significant correlation between the presence of mucosal thickening on plain sinus radiographs and on ultrasonic imaging (46). Antral puncture proven fluid within the maxillary sinus also correlated very well with ultrasound echo findings in this study. Jannert et al., from Sweden, using antral puncture data, demonstrated equally encouraging ultrasound correlations (47). However, this was not reproduced in another Swedish study by Berg et al., nor in an English study by Pfleiderer et al. (48,49).

Experience in the United States with A-mode ultrasonography and maxillary antral disease was also encouraging at first (50,51). Subsequent studies soon dampened enthusiasm. Rohr et al. (52) and Druce et al. (53), studying adults with maxillary sinus disease, found the specificity of A-mode ultrasonography to range from 93% to 61%, respectively. However, the diagnostic sensitivity in both of these studies was unacceptably low, varying from 61% down to 29% in the first investigation, depending on which commercial instrument was used, and 34% in the second study cited. Shapiro et al., studying mostly pediatric patients with allergic rhinitis who had signs and symptoms suggestive of sinus disease, found equally discouraging data (54). Correlating A-mode ultrasonography with a Waters view of the paranasal sinus, these authors found the technique to be lacking in sensitivity and specificity. Wald et al. (55) and Burger (56) came to similar conclusions that A-mode ultrasound is typically diagnostic when complete opacification of the maxillary antrum is present and not particularly useful for the more common mucoperiosteal swelling seen in sinus disease.

A-mode ultrasonography may still have a place in evaluation of the obstetric patient with rhinitis. Rhinitis of pregnancy and rhinosinusitis during pregnancy may be difficult to differentiate, a problem enhanced by a justifiable reluctance to use ionizing radiation in pregnancy for diagnostic purposes. Since ultrasonography is typically a part of routine obstetric practices, the use of A-mode ultrasound may represent a cost-effective (and safe) approach to the diagnosis and monitoring of sinus disease in the pregnant population, as long as the limitations inherent with this technique are recognized.

E. Therapeutic Trial

In the end, a therapeutic trial of carefully selected broad spectrum antibiotics may be pursued as an initial diagnostic approach to the resistant case of rhinitis in pregnancy, even when there are no other clinical findings to suggest sinusitis. However, prolonged antibiotic therapy is not justifiable without confirmatory studies such as radiographic or ultrasound imaging, endoscopic nasal exam, or antral puncture analysis.

V. Pharmacological Treatment of Rhinitis

A. General Considerations

In choosing among drug therapy options during pregnancy, efficacy must be considered along with risk of inducing adverse effects on fetal survival or development (57,58). Most medicines taken by or administered to pregnant women cross the placenta and into the blood of the fetus. Since the fetus cannot process medicines as the mother can, and since some medicines may affect normal development of the fetus, medicines that cross the placenta may have negative and unpredictable effects on the fetus and newborn (see Chapter 7). In 1979, the Food and Drug Administration (FDA) mandated that the package insert for all drugs approved after November 1, 1980, must (a) include all available information about the teratogenic and nonteratogenic effects of the drug during pregnancy and (b) classify the drug regarding its apparent fetal risk (Table 2). No rhinitis medication labeled since 1980 meets the requirements for pregnancy category A: "Adequate and well-controlled studies in pregnant women have failed to demonstrate a risk to the fetus in the first trimester and there is no evidence of a risk in later trimesters" (59). This classification represents a major problem for the physician in choosing a drug during pregnancy, in that no rhinitis medication can be considered "safe" on the basis of "adequate and controlled clinical trials," and such trials are likely never to be done (60). One way to manage pregnant patients with rhinitis in a

Table 2 FDA Pregnancy Classification of Drugs

Category A:	Controlled studies in women fail to demonstrate a risk to the fetus in the first trimester (and there is no evidence of a risk in later trimesters), and the possibility of fetal harm appears remote.
Category B:	Either animal-reproduction studies have not demonstrated a fetal risk but there are no controlled studies in pregnant women or animal-reproduction studies have shown an adverse effect (other than a decrease in fertility) that was not confirmed in controlled studies in women in the first trimester (and there is no evidence of a risk in later trimesters).
Category C:	Either studies in animals have revealed adverse effects on the fetus (teratogenic or embryocidal, or other) and there are no controlled studies in women or studies in women and animals are not available. Drugs should be given only if the potential benefits justifies the potential risk to the fetus.
Category D:	There is positive evidence of human fetal risk, but the benefits from use in pregnant women may be acceptable despite the risk (e.g., if the drug is needed in a life-threatening situation or for serious disease for which safer drugs cannot be used or are ineffective).
Category X:	Studies in animals or human beings have demonstrated fetal abnormalities, or there is evidence of fetal risk based on human experience, or both, and the risk of the use of the drug in pregnant women clearly outweighs any possible benefit. The drug is contraindicated in women who are or may become pregnant.

medico-legal risk-free environment is to refuse to be responsible for their treatment during pregnancy. A more reasonable choice is to emphasize nonpharmacological approaches such as humidification, avoidance of irritants and/or allergens, and applying a judicious amount of tolerance to symptoms as long as sinusitis has not intervened and the mother is resting comfortably at night. Once medication is deemed necessary for symptoms that cannot be controlled by conservative modalities, the decision should be discussed with the patient, referencing its benefits, risks, and alternatives. The discussion should be carefully documented in the medical record, along with a statement as to the patient's consent.

The transfer of maternally ingested medications into breast milk has been extensively reviewed for some medications, with tables presented giving the milk:plasma ratio. However, not all the medications used in the treatment of rhinitis are mentioned (60–62). Nearly all drugs pass into the breast milk. Drugs traverse into maternal milk primarily by passive diffusion. The concentration achieved will be dependent not only on the concentration gradient but also on the intrinsic lipid solubility of the drug, the degree of ionization, and the amount of binding to protein and other cellular constituents. This fact, however, does not presuppose an adverse effect on the newborn, since may drugs will have already been inactivated, remain unabsorbed, or be destroyed in the infant's gut. The newborn, especially if premature, may be more sensitive to the negative effects of certain therapeutic agents because of a greater blood–brain barrier permeability, poorer enzyme-conjugating capacity, diminished protein-binding capability, and decreased glomerular filtration rate. In general, if a drug is released for use in infancy, it can be safely administered to the lactating mother. Due to a lag time before a drug appears in breast milk, it may be best for the nursing mother to try to take short-acting formulations and use them 15 min after nursing and 3–4 hr before the next feeding to minimize breast milk concentrations of the drug in question (63).

The information available regarding the safety of drugs used in the treatment of rhinitis during pregnancy is derived from three major studies and from sporadic case reports or small series describing the outcome of using a given drug in pregnancy. The first major work, and still the most quoted, was the Collaborative Perinatal Project (CPP), which involved 50,282 women studied at 12 centers from 1959 to 1965 (64). "Standardized relative risk" values were derived using the ratio of malformation rates in exposed to nonexposed mother–child pairs. A relative risk greater than 1.5 was considered suggestive of a cause-and-effect relationship. However, despite the large number of women examined, this study suffered from the fact that the number of mothers exposed to any single therapeutic agent was small, creating a problem in defining true toxicity or safety to the satisfaction of all. Furthermore, many newer drugs are being used for rhinitis, such as topically applied cromolyn, beclomethasone, flunisolide, triamcinolone, budesonide, and fluticasone and the orally administered nonsedative H1-selective antihistamines terfenadine, astemizole, and loratadine, which were not included in the CPP. Because of the complexities in analyzing the data from the CPP, the authors warn that "none of the associations . . . should be regarded as anything more than hypothesis requiring independent confirmation" and also that "influences of causality based solely on our data are not appropriate" (64,65).

A second investigation analyzed pharmacy records of 6837 pregnant women who delivered between July 1977 and December 1979. Termed the Group Health Co-operative (GHC) study, it equated prescriptions filled as long as 3 months prior to conception with drug exposure and evaluated pregnancy outcomes. This approach has drawn criticism and clouded the interpretive value of the data (12).

The third major investigation was a surveillance study by Franz Rosa, M.D., of the Division of Epidemiology and Surveillance, Center for Drugs and Biologics, U.S. Food and Drug Administration, of 229,101 pregnant Michigan Medicaid recipients conducted between 1985 and 1992. This study relates the use of 250 drugs consumed during the first trimester to pregnancy outcome and is cited as "personal communication" in *Drugs in Pregnancy and Lactation*, by Gerald G. Briggs et al. (60). Although this study stands as valuable information about possible associations of many drugs and fetal abnormalities in humans, the authors emphasize that independent confirmation is needed from other studies before these associations transcend from hypothesis to fact.

Data on the reproductive effects of specific medications during pregnancy is discussed in Chapter 8. The following sections highlight certain benefit–risk considerations regarding the gestational use of medications for rhinosinusitis. The treatment, during pregnancy, for the most common specific types of rhinitis is summarized in Table 3.

B. Decongestants

For the occasional episode of nasal congestion which may be interfering with sleep, oxymetazoline HCL drops or spray used as minimally as pos-

Table 3 "Safest" Treatment Choices for Common Rhinological Problems in Pregnancy

Type	Nonpharmacological choices	Pharmacological choices
Allergic rhinoconjunctivitis	Avoidance of antigens; continue successful immunotherapy	Topical cromolyn Na; tripelennamine $+/-$ pseudoephedrine; beclomethasone (topical)
Bacterial rhinosinusitis	Nasal irrigation; sinus irrigation for resistant cases	Topical oxymetazoline for <6 days; antibiotics × 2–3 weeks
Rhinitis medicamentosa	Discontinue topical vasoconstrictors	Pseudoephedrine $+/-$ tripelennamine; Beclomethasone (topical)
Vasomotor rhinitis	Nasal irrigation; exercise	Pseudoephedrine $+/-$ tripelennamine; topical oxymetazoline for <6 days (caution re: rhinitis medicamentosa)

sible may suffice. It should be emphasized that the uterine blood vessels have only alpha-adrenergic rectors. It is therefore theoretically possible that the use of an alpha-adrenergic agent, oxymetazoline, could cause reduction of uterine blood flow and induce fetal hypoxia and bradycardia. Late fetal heart rate deceleration and fetal acidosis were described in a 20-year-old, 41-week gestational mother who overdosed on oxymetazoline (24 sprays of 0.05% oxymetazoline in a 15.5-hr interval) (66). However, Rayburn et al. were unable to demonstrate any adverse effects on the maternal and fetal circulations during a period of 2 hr after a single dose of oxymetazoline to 12 women between 27 and 39 weeks' gestation (67). These investigators concluded that the use of oxymetazoline is safe when administered at the prescribed dose and frequency (every 12 hr).

The risk of rhinitis medicamentosa with continued use of this agent beyond 3–5 days should be emphasized. Although there may be little or no appreciable absorption of topical oxymetazoline at recommended doses, overdose of topically applied imidazolines (e.g., Afrin, Neo-Synephrine II) carries the additional risk of maternal hypertension followed by rebound hypotension and shock (68).

Should nasal obstruction require further therapy, pseudoephedrine (pregnancy category B), 30–60 mg every 6 hr or 120-mg time-release capsule every 12 hr, can be considered. Sympathomimetic amines are teratogenic in some animal species, but human teratogenicity has not been demonstrated despite widespread use (69). A study of 6837 maternal–infant pairs demonstrated a less than expected incidence of malformations with the use of pseudoephedrine in conjunction with brompheniramine (70). All other alpha-adrenergic agonists studied by the CPP (epinephrine, phenylephrine, phenylpropanolamine) were associated with significantly increased risks of fetal malformation. For the sympathomimetic class of drugs as a whole, an association was found between first-trimester use and minor malformations (not life-threatening or major cosmetic defects), inguinal hernia, and talipes equino-varus.

The only specific data available concerning the use of decongestants during lactation concerns pseudoephedrine. Findlay investigated two mothers using pseudoephedrine in combination with triprolidine. The milk: plasma ratios at 1, 3, and 12 hr after drug ingestion were 3.3, 3.9, and 2.6, with only 0.25–0.33 mg of pseudoephedrine base excreted in 1000 mL of breast milk (71). There appears to be no adverse risk to the administration of topical oxymetazoline and oral pseudoephedrine at prescribed dosages during lactation.

C. Antihistamines

Patients with known eosinophilic allergic or nonallergic rhinitis accompanied by prominent sneezing and rhinorrhea may benefit from antihistamine therapy. Tripelennamine, 25–50 mg PRN every 6 hr to a maximum of 200 mg/day can be recommended as the "safest" antihistamine for use during pregnancy, based on available studies and the "antiquity" of this drug. Since antihistamines have little or no effect on nasal congestion, many patients will benefit from the addition of pseudoephedrine to this treatment plan after the first trimester. If intolerance or tachyphylaxis intervenes, other antihistamines may be considered, but the risk/benefit ratio must be carefully considered, since the data are particularly unclear. The CPP reported statistically significant associations between brompheniramine and total congenital malformations, while chlorpheniramine was associated with an increased risk of ear and eye malformations and inguinal hernia for first-trimester exposure (72). A later study by Jick et al. did not substantiate this finding with brompheniramine (70). An increased risk with diphenhydramine was also noted in the CPP and extended specifically to cleft lip and palate in a Finnish study (73). Animal teratogenicity in several species treated with hydroxyzine prompted particular concern for this drug, with additional suggestive risk emerging from the CPP data (74). However, no unusual congenital malformation prevalence was seen in another study of 74 women given hydroxyzine in the first trimester for gestational nausea and vomiting (75). Reassurance is suggested by data of Nelson and Forfar, who found significantly less antihistamine use in a group of mothers of infants with congenital malformations compared to matched controls (76). However, taken together, these data suggest that if H-1 antihistamines other than tripelennamine are needed during pregnancy, they are best used after the first 4 lunar months only.

The regular maternal use of antihistamines just prior to or at the time of delivery poses a further set of potential clinical problems. The use of antihistamines in general during the last 2 weeks of pregnancy has been associated with an increased risk of retrolental fibroplasia in premature infants with a birth weight less than 1750 g (77). Parkin described a 5-day-old infant with tremulousness and diarrhea following the maternal ingestion of 150 mg of diphenhydramine daily throughout pregnancy (78). Another mother was reported who used 400 mg of hydroxyzine daily throughout her pregnancy and gave birth to an infant who demonstrated a transient narcotic-like withdrawal symptom complex (79). These data suggest that the regular maternal ingestion of antihistamines, especially in high dosages, should be terminated as soon as possible prior to delivery in an attempt to minimize neonatal withdrawal risk, or avoided altogether in women at risk for delivery of very-low-birth-weight infants.

Some adverse effects might be expected from breast milk containing maternally ingested antihistamines. This has, in fact, rarely proven to be the case (80). A report incriminating clemastine as the cause of drowsiness and irritability in a nursing 10-week-old infant has been recently published (81). Clemastine concentrations in breast milk were 25–30% of the maternal serum values, but none could be detected in the infant's serum. The infant in this report showed resolution of symptoms within 24 hr following drug termination. Another case report of a 3-month-old who developed irritability, excessive crying, and disturbed sleeping patterns while the mother was ingesting 6 mg of dexbrompheniramine and 120 mg of *d*-isoephedrine (82). The symptoms resolved within 12 hr after breast feeding was stopped.

The trend in antihistamine research is being directed toward the development of highly selective, nonsedative drugs which reportedly do not cross the blood–brain barrier. Of the therapeutic agents currently available in the United States, terfenadine and astemizole currently carry a pregnancy category C rating, while loratadine carries a category B rating. Terfenadine, a frequently used nonsedating antihistamine worldwide, has not demonstrated abnormalities or adverse fetal effects in animal studies, and there are no case reports linking this agent with adverse outcomes in humans (83). It may be important to note that cetirizine, a newly developed H-1 selective antihistamine released in the United States and widely available worldwide, is metabolic product of hydroxyzine, a antihistamine whose safety in pregnancy has been a subject of controversy noted earlier.

D. Cromolyn Sodium

Animal and human data suggest that cromolyn sodium (pregnancy category B) is safe in pregnancy, although there are no pregnancy data specifically on intranasal or ophthalmic use. Several points should be emphasized in considering the use of cromolyn sodium in pregnancy for allergic rhino-conjunctivitis. First, animal studies have not shown any harmful effects on the fetus at nontoxic maternal doses (84). Second, very little systemic absorption of cromolyn is seen with topical application. Finally, Wilson has reported a 1.35% congenital malformation rate among 296 asthmatic women who used cromolyn for asthma throughout their pregnancy, which is well within the expected frequency seen within the general pregnant population (85). For women with allergic rhinoconjunctivitis, we feel that intranasal and/or ophthalmic cromolyn sodium may be considered a treatment of choice. There are no published data on the safety of this drug during lactation, but there appear to be no contraindications to its use.

E. Corticosteroids

Animal studies have suggested that corticosteroids may have adverse effects on the developing fetus when taken systemically. Particular attention has been paid to cleft palate, although intrauterine growth retardation, placental insufficiency, fetal resorption, and spontaneous abortion have also been described (86,87). The overall data concerning the use of systematic corticosteroids during human pregnancy is not so ominous. In fact, a large body of data on humans published in the past 25 years has not confirmed the fears generated by animal studies. Even though the controversy persists, the topical use of poorly absorbed or "first-pass-metabolized" derivatives such as beclomethasone (pregnancy category C) for eosinophilic rhinitis during pregnancy, especially after the first trimester, seems justified. Due to their high topical potency and metabolic characteristics, very little if any of these drugs would be expected to reach the fetus during maternal intranasal use, but no specific information is available. In addition, the apparent safety of inhaled beclomethasone in the management of asthma during pregnancy suggests that the intranasal route of this drug also should be safe (88,89). For patients with significantly symptomatic nasal polyposis or eosinophilic rhinitis who are not responsive to antihistamine-decongestants or nasal cromolyn, the above considerations suggest that intranasal beclomethasone can be utilized.

Occasionally, oral corticosteroids may be necessary for severe nasal polyps or eosinophilic nonallergenic rhinitis that do not respond to the above modalities. Prednisone and prednisolone appear to pose very little risk to the developing fetus. Ideally, the oral forms should be withheld until after the first 4 lunar months if the clinical condition warrants such a delay.

With the exception of extremely high parenteral dosages in status asthmaticus, the use of corticosteroids in lactating mothers poses no substantial threat in the infant. A 50-mg dose of prednisone in the lactating mother would transfer to the neonate less than 20% of its daily physiological corticosteroid requirement (90). It is not known whether beclomethasone or other topically applied corticosteroids are excreted into the breast milk.

VI. Immunological Management

Allergy diagnosis, avoidance measures, and immunotherapy are discussed in detail in Chapter 10. For the pregnant patient with known allergic disease, allergen avoidance is particularly important. Avoiding known allergens, when possible, will not only improve maternal well-being, it will also minimize need for pharmacological intervention. If all pertinent allergens have not been identified prior to the pregnancy, identification of the offending agents may be of benefit. Because skin testing with potent antigens may be associated with systematic reactions, and since abortions and other adverse fetal effects have been associated with anaphylaxis (see Chapter 12), skin testing should be replaced with in-vitro methods, such as RAST tests, to identify pertinent allergens (91,92). Historical information will usually suggest if house dust, mold, animal dander, or pollen are involved. Avoidance instructions can be given empirically in these circumstances. However, in selected, cases, especially when dealing with indoor animals, selected RAST testing may be necessary to demonstrate the need for more vigorous avoidance maneuvers.

Using similar reasoning, the initiation of immunotherapy during pregnancy should be avoided (93). However, aside from the risk of systemic reactions, most authors recommend that allergen immunotherapy may be continued in patients who have experienced clinical benefit and who have not experienced systemic reactions (94). Consideration should be given to lowering the maintenance dosage routinely, to minimize the chance of a systemic reaction.

VII. Treatment of Sinusitis

A. General Considerations

The mainstay of treatment for presumed bacterial sinusitis is antimicrobial drugs, possibly combined with adjunctive therapy. Adjunctive therapy includes topical or oral decongestants, nasal saline mist or irrigation, and topical corticosteroids. A culture and sensitivity of infected material from the sinus involved would normally direct antibiotic selection, but random nasal swabs have shown unreliable correlation with cultures obtained by direct sinus puncture (95). Since sinus aspiration is not usually indicated as first-step therapy, empirical antibiotic selection is indicated. A detailed review of the history, physical examination, and severity can direct initial antibiotic selection. The microbiology of sinusitis can be suggested by (a) the duration of illness (Table 4), (b) type of acquisition (nosocomial or community), (c) particular sinus involvement, (d) age of patient, (e) dental history, and (f) immunocompetence. Numerous new antibiotics have flooded our formularies, making empirical antibiotic selection confusing and their injudicious use of clinical concern for potential development of

Table 4 Organisms Most Likely to Be Found in Sinusitis

Acute	Subacute	Acute recurrence of chronic Dx	Nosocomial
S. pneumoniae			⟶
H. influenzae			⟶
M. catarrhalis			⟶
S. pyogenes			⟶
	S. aureus		⟶
	Anaerobes		⟶
		Other gram-negative organisms	⟶
			Fungal

increasing bacterial resistance. Their safety in pregnancy raises an additional level of complexity to the therapeutic decision-making process.

The microbiology of acute and subacute sinusitis has been well defined (Table 4), and the importance of certain bacterial species has not changed appreciably during the past several decades. However, when choosing an antibiotic for treatment, certain points demand review. Some bacterial species have changed their susceptibility to antimicrobial agents, and some newer organisms, such as *Chlamydia*, have been occasionally isolated. *Streptococcus pneumoniae* (30–40% of isolates), *Hemophilus influenzae* (about 20%), and *Moraxella catarrhalis* (about 20%), however, remain the most common pathogens in acute and subacute community-acquired sinusitis in adults, although a variety of additional bacterial and viral isolates have been observed (group A streptococci, group C streptococci, streptococci viridins, peptostreptococci, other *Moraxella* species, and *Eikenella corrodens*) in isolated studies (96). Mixed anaerobic infections have occasionally been seen in adults, possibly of dental origin. Even *Staph. aureus*, rarely implicated in acute community-acquired maxillary sinusitis, can be seen in up to 29% of cultures from sphenoid sinusitis (97). Finally, *Chlamydia pneumoniae* (strain TWAR) has been recently recognized as an important respiratory pathogen. Fungal sinus infections are seen more frequently in patients with diabetes mellitus. A variety of gram-negative bacteria and fungal agents have caused recalcitrant sinusitis in AIDS patients, along with such unusual organisms as *Legionella* and *Acanthamoeba* (98,99). *H. influenzae* and *S. pneumoniae*, however, remain the common bacterial isolates in acute sinusitis, even in these unique clinical settings.

Knowledge of antibiotic resistance patterns within each community are important in antibiotic selection. *H. influenzae* organisms have been found to produce beta-lactamase in 5–30% of isolates, resulting in resistance to the penicillins and some cephalosporins. Seventy-five percent of *Moraxella branhemella* isolates, particularly common among preschool children, produce beta-lactamase. Penicillin resistance even among *S. pneumoniae* has increased alarmingly, from a 4–5% incidence in 1988 to 20% incidence in 1992 secondary to their production of altered penicillin-binding proteins. These penicillin-resistant strains may also be resistant to cephalosporins, with the level of resistance varying according to the drug as indicated by their respective MICs (100).

With a knowledge of the pathogens most likely to cause acute and subacute sinusitis, one must ask which antibiotics would be logical choices based on safety, the likely flora, as well as resistance patterns within each individual community. With the variety of new antibiotics available, a review of their pharmacodynamic properties, antimicrobial spectra, and toxicities is presented. This information will allow a sensible and cost-effective approach for the treatment of acute, subacute, and chronic sinusitis in pregnancy and lactation to be formulated.

B. Antibiotics

Beta-Lactam Antibiotics

Standard initial therapy for acute sinusitis has been ampicillin or amoxicillin because their spectrum of activity covers the major organisms responsible for acute sinusitis in most clinical settings. Gastric acid destroys ampicillin but not amoxicillin, which, with its TID dosage schedule, improves compliance and makes this the more ideal agent to achieve adequate blood levels of drug. These drugs are not effective against most staphylococcal infections, *M. catarrhalis*, and some *H. influenzae* species because of the high frequency of beta-lactamase production among these organisms.

The addition of the beta-lactamase inhibitor, clavulanate potassium, to amoxicillin (Augmentin) extends the spectrum of antimicrobial activity to include more species, such as *H. influenzae* (beta-lactamase resistant), *Moraxella catarrhalis*, *Escherichia coli*, *Bacteroides fragilis*, and other anaeorbes. It is also active against staphylococci that produce lactamase but are not methicillin resistant. Clavulanic acid carries a category B FDA rating, with no evidence of teratogenicity in mice, rats, and pigs. There are limited published reports concerning the use of amoxicillin/clavulanate for various nonsinusitis infections in pregnancy, with no adverse effects being observed (101,102). Although amoxacillin-clavulanate may be a superior combination for the treatment of bacterial sinusitis, its use during pregnancy should be reserved for resistant infections with suspected beta-lactamase-producing bacteria.

Cephalosporins (pregnancy category B) and other beta-lactams (carbecephems, i.e., loracarbef) have the same mechanism of action as penicillin (inhibition of cell-wall synthesis). The oral cephalosporins can be divided into generations according to their spectrum of biological activity. Generally speaking, first-generation cephalosporins are most active against gram-positive bacteria and third-generation compounds have better gram-negative coverage. In general, first-generation cephalosporins should not be used in the treatment of sinusitis because of their limited bacteriological coverage. Cefaclor (Ceclor), one of the earliest second-generation cephalosporins, has activity against both beta-lactamase-positive and beta-lactamase-negative strains of *H. influenzae*. However, sporadic resistance has been noted. Cefaclor has been demonstrated to be less active against *H. influenzae* than amoxicillin-clavulanic acid and trimethoprim/sulfamethoxazole in susceptibility studies (103). In contrast, cefuroxime axetil (Ceftin) and cefprozil (Cefzil) exhibit excellent activity against the organisms most frequently responsible for acute and subacute sinusitis, including *H. influenzae* and *M. catarrhalis*. Loracarbef (Lorabid), a beta-lactam compound with a carbacephem nucleus that improves chemical stability, is equivalent to other second-generation cephalosporins in its bacteriological spectrum.

There is a suggestion of an association between selected cephalosporins and total birth defects, cardiovascular defects, and oral clefts, but other factors, such as maternal disease, concurrent drug use, and chance may be involved. In the surveillance study of Michigan Medicaid recipients involving 229,101 completed pregnancies, positive associations were observed with cephalexin (3613 newborns exposed), cefaclor (1325 newborns exposed), and cephradine (339 exposures), but not cefadroxil (722 exposures) or cefuroxime (143 exposures) (60). We know of no similar data for loracarbef or cefprozil. These contrasting data suggest that cephalosporins should be used with caution, if at all, during the first trimester of pregnancy until further information is available. Although these drugs clearly cross the placenta and distribute in fetal tissue, there are no data to suggest that cephalosporins cannot be used after the first trimester if amoxacillin or erythromycin is contraindicated or unsuccessful.

Cephalosporins are excreted in breast milk in low concentrations. Although these drugs do not appear to be toxic to the infant directly, there is a general lack of sufficient information to make consistent recommendations. The problem of modification of bowel flora and interference with the interpretation of culture results in the event of a fever evaluation in the infant is a potential problem for all broad-spectrum antibiotics.

Macrolides

Erythromycin (pregnancy category B) is commonly mentioned as an alternative drug in the treatment of sinusitis in the penicillin-allergic patient. Erythromycin is widely utilized to treat upper and lower respiratory infections. It has a broad spectrum of antimicrobial activity, including *S. pneumoniae*, *M. catarrhalis*, *Mycoplasma pneumoniae*, *Chlamydia* species and some *S. aureus* and anaerobes. Unfortunately, erythromycin exhibits variable activity against *H. influenzae*, is inactive against some *M. catarrhalis*, and *S. pneumoniae* and staphylococci are rapidly developing resistance to its activity (104). Nevertheless, in pregnancy and lactation, erythromycin still appears as a reasonable alternative.

Azithromycin and clarithromycin expand the spectrum of erythromycin and have better gastrointestinal tolerance. Clarithromycin is active against *S. pneumoniae*, *M. pneumoniae*, and methicillin-sensitive *S. aureus*. It has in-vitro activity against *M. catarrhalis*, *Legionella* species, and *Chlamydia pneumoniae*. It is more effective against *H. influenzae* than erythromycin. The spectrum of activity of azithromycin exceeds that of clarithromycin. Not only does it cover typical sinusitis pathogens such as *S. pneumoniae*, *H. influenzae* (four- to eightfold more active than clarithromycin against *H. influenzae*), and *M. catarrhalis*, it also has activity against *Mycoplasma* species, *Legionella* species, and enhanced activity against *Chlamydia* (105). Its in-vitro activity also includes anaerobes such as peptostreptococci, *Clostridium perfringes*, *C. difficile*, and some members of the *B. fragilis* group. Unfortunately, as with erythromycin, heavy clinical use has resulted in rapid emergence of resistance, and many of the erythromycin-resistant organisms are becoming cross-resistant to clarithromycin and azithromycin (106). Furthermore, animal studies have not been reassuring (see Chapter 8), and there remains insufficient human experience to recommend these alternative macrolides during pregnancy and lactation.

Since decreased serum levels of penicillins, cephalosporins, and erythromycin have been observed in pharmacokinetic studies of pregnant women, larger dosages of these drugs are recommended (107). Dosages of 500 mg three times each day of amoxacillin, amoxicillin-clavulanate, erythromycin, and cefacor and 250–500 mg twice daily of cefuroxime are reasonable for gestational bacterial rhinosinusitis.

Fluroquinolones

Ciprofloxacin (Cipro) and ofloxacin (Floxin) are the two most useful agents in upper respiratory infections, and lomefloxacin (Maxaquin) has recently appeared in the U.S. market. However, because of arthropathy in immature animals, this class of drug is contraindicated in pregnancy and lactation (108).

Sulfonamide Combinations

The combination of trimethoprim and sulfamethoxazole (pregnancy category C) (TMP/SMX) acts by interfering with folate metabolism and nucleic acid synthesis of susceptible microorganisms. TMP/SMX may be bactericidal for some organisms, whereas either drug alone may be bacteriostatic. This synergistic effect may be observed even when organisms are resistant to one agent or the other. Erythromycin is the other drug commonly combined with a sulfonamide.

The spectrum of in-vitro activity of sulfonamide combinations tends to be broad and includes the commonly isolated pathogens of sinusitis, *S. pneumoniae*, *H. influenzae* (including beta-lactamase producing), and *M. catarrhalis*, but not other streptococcal species. TMP/SMX also is active against *S. aureus*, gram-negative bacilli, especially the Enterobacteriaceae (*E. coli*, *Klebsiella*, and *Proteus*), *Neisseria meningitidis*, and some anaerobes, although clinical efficacy is not established. *Pseudomonas aeruginosa* is resistant. The newly emerging penicillin-resistant *Streptococcus pneumoniae* are often equally resistant to non-beta-lactam antibiotics such as TMP/SMX and erythromycin, with incidences as high as 20% and 50%, respectively, in children with otitis media (109,110).

There is reason for concern in using these medications during pregnancy. TMP/SMX has been associated with an increased risk of congenital defects, but the data are conflicting (60,111). The use of TMP/SMX and other sulfonamide combinations outside the first trimester and not near term does not appear to pose a significant risk. However, sulfonamides compete with bilirubin for binding to plasma albumin. After birth, the newborn no longer has the benefit of placental circulation to clear free bilirubin, and kernicterus may result, especially in the premature infant.

A similar concern carries over into breast feeding, where these drugs are best avoided in ill, stressed, or premature infants and in infants with glucose-6-phosphate dehydrogenase deficiency or hyperbilirubinemia. In healthy term infants, sulfonamides, trimethoprim, and erythromycin pose no risk when breast feeding, other than the general concerns for all antibiotics posed earlier (112).

Tetracyclines

Tetracyclines (pregnancy category D) are effective in vitro against a great variety of bacteria including gram-positive, gram-negative, aerobic bacteria, anaerobic bacteria, mycoplasma, chlamydia, legionella, and some protozoa. Doxycycline and minocycline (second-generation agents) are more active, in general, than the parent compound against a variety of organisms. Doxycycline has some activity against *B. fragilis*, while minocycline has improved activity against *S. aureus*. In general, however, the tetracyclines are not recommended for treatment of streptococcal or staphylococcal infections because of an observed rate of resistance. Up to 15% of strains of *S. pneumoniae* and 10% of group A streptococci are not sensitive to tetracycline (113,114).

Tetracyclines should be avoided in pregnancy due to adverse effects on fetal teeth and bones, maternal liver toxicity, and congenital and miscellaneous defects observed with heightened frequency (115,116). However, tetracycline is excreted into breast milk in low concentrations. Although the possibility for inhibition of bone growth and staining of teeth exists, the potential is remote enough for the Academy of Pediatrics to consider tetracycline compatible with breast feeding (112).

Choice of Antibiotics in Sinusitis Treatment

Concerns over the frequency of beta-lactamase-producing *H. influenzae* and *M. catarrhalis* and the emergence of antibiotic-resistant organisms in all clinical forms of sinusitis have prompted many physicians to use liberally the broadest-spectrum antibiotic available. However, given the available safety data, it can be argued that, since the overall rate of spontaneous clinical recovery from acute sinusitis is high (40–45%) and not all organisms found in acute sinusitis are beta-lactamase producers, there is no reason to deviate from the usual initial empirical treatment with amoxicillin (or erythromycin with or without a sulfonamide in truly penicillin-allergic patients) for community acquired disease during pregnancy and lactation. Erythromycin and the tetracyclines, if used alone, miss a large percentage of *H. influenzae*, and TMP/SMX should not be used alone if infection with group A streptococcus is suspected or proven. Furthermore, there is a growing concern that the liberal use of the most broad-spectrum antibiotics available induces the emergence of resistant organisms with increasingly greater frequency.

Guidelines for selecting an alternative to amoxicillin or the other drugs listed above would include (a) no clinical response within 3–5 days of initiating antibiotic treatment, (b) a clinical history of early recurrences or treatment failures of acute sinusitis following amoxicillin therapy, (c) a patient with a history of frequent courses of multiple antibiotics, and (d) a high incidence of beta-lactamase-producing organisms in the community. Under these circumstances an alternative, more broad-spectrum antibiotic should be chosen.

Amoxicillin-clavulanate is the broad-spectrum antibiotic of choice based on its safety in pregnancy and activity against potential beta-lactamase pathogens. TMP/SMX can be used as an alternative second-line drug provided that prior treatment included coverage for group A streptococcus and that other restrictions during pregnancy and lactation previously discussed are considered. Cefaclor or cufuroxime would be other reasonable second-line alternatives, ideally after the first trimester.

Alternative and often more costly second-line regimens, some with broader antimicrobial coverage, include the newer cephalosporins and macrolide agents and possibly the fluroquinolones. Clinical efficacy studies have been performed utilizing these drugs and have shown them to be effective. However, there is enough adverse animal and human data in pregnancy not to permit a recommendation for use. Furthermore, many of the studies suggesting benefit and safety suffer from small numbers of patients and commonly revealed these drugs to be no more effective than amoxicillin or amoxicillin-clavulanate.

C. Adjunctive Measures

The efficacy of topical or oral sympathomimetic decongestants, topical or oral corticosteroids, and mucolytics in the treatment of sinusitis has not been established. Since oxymetazoline appears safe at recommended dosages, its short-term use in sinusitis during pregnancy seems reasonable. However, additional adjunctive medications other than antibiotics should be discouraged. An exception would be the concurrent use of antihistamines and/or topical cromolyn sodium or corticosteroids if the treating physician is convinced that allergic nasal disease is contributing to the sinusitis state.

Nasal irrigation methods deserve mention as a useful nonpharmacological modality in the treatment of sinusitis during pregnancy. This can take the form of a topically applied nasal saline mist available over the counter, or tepid physiological saline washed through the nose using either a bulb syringe, ear syringe, or more vigorously with a Water Pik and special nasal adapter. In the case of severe maxillary sinusitis that does not respond to antibiotic therapy, maxillary antral puncture can be helpful both as a therapeutic modality and for culture purposes.

VIII. Conclusion

The symptomatic human respiratory nasal mucosa in pregnancy represents a challenge to the physician both in terms of its diagnosis and therapy. Although there are several unique influences of pregnancy which may adversely affect nasal mucosa, there is growing recognition that most symptomatic nasal problems are, in fact, exaggerated expressions of known diagnostic entities in the nonpregnant state. In approaching gestational rhinitis, emphasis should be placed on making an accurate diagnosis so that specific and, therefore, limited medicinal intervention can be used. At the same time, the physician should keep in mind that there is morbidity associated with ignoring this clinical problem altogether. Particular attention should be placed on the diagnosis and treatment of sinusitis, which may have a unique tendency for occurrence during pregnancy. Subtleties in clinical symptomatology and reluctance to use radiographs make sinusitis a particularly elusive diagnosis. Specialty consultation with otolaryngology and/or allergy may, at times, be necessary in the symptomatic pregnant woman before an accurate diagnosis and successful therapeutic recommendation can be made.

The medical-legal atmosphere in the United States today unfortunately suggests that absolute safety for the fetus can only be guaranteed by practicing therapeutic nihilism for all women from puberty to menopause. For those physicians choosing to take up this therapeutic challenge, emphasis should be placed on making the appropriate diagnosis so that therapy can be directed as accurately yet as safely as necessary to achieve the desired therapeutic outcome. Some guidelines have been presented to assist the physician in choosing the "safest" form of therapy for the rhinological entities which commonly occur during pregnancy (Table 3). In the individual clinical situation, management decisions must be made only after establishing an exact clinical diagnosis and giving full consideration to the therapeutic risks, benefits, and alternatives. Moreover, the physician's interpretation of the benefit–risk ratio and the therapeutic decisions based thereon must be fully explained to and approved by the pregnant patient and documented in the patient's record.

Note Added in Proof

Two recent studies concerning the safety of the newer H1 selective nonsedative or low-sedative antihistamines have been published. Both studies evolved from The Motherrisk Program from the Hospital for Sick Children and the Departments of Pediatrics, Pharmacology, Pharmacy, and Medicine at the University of Toronto. Pastuszak Schick and colleagues reported 114 women who used astemizole during different stages of pregnancy (117). Two major malformations occuring in the astemizole treated group (hypospadias and spina bifida occulta) compared to two major malformations in the parallel control group. In the second study, Einarson, Bailey, and colleagues prospectively followed 53 women exposed to hydroxyzine and 39 women exposed to citirizine during pregnancy. No significant difference was found in pregnancy outcome and rates of major or minor congenital malformations in the drug treated groups compared to a control group (118).

References

1. MacKinzie JN. The physiological and pathological relations between the nose and the sexual appearance of man. Alienst and Neurol 1898; 19: 219–239.
2. Mabry RL. Intranasal steroid injection during pregnancy. South Med J 1980; 73:1176–1179.
3. Mabry RL. Rhinitis of pregnancy. South Med J 1986; 79:965–971.
4. Sorri M, Bortikanen-Sorri AL, Karja J. Rhinitis during pregnancy. Rhinology 1980; 18:83–86.
5. Henderson ID. Cyclical changes in female mucous. J Clin Endocrinol 1956; 16:905–909.
6. Toppozada H, Michaels L, Toppazada M, El-Ghazzawi I, Talaat M, Elwany S. The human respiratory nasal mucosa in pregnancy. J Laryngol Otol 1982; 96:613–626.
7. Reynolds SRM, Foster FI. Acetylcholine-equivalent content of the nasal mucosa in rabbits and cats, before and after administration of estrogen. Am J Physiol 1940; 131:422–425.
8. Taylor M. An experimental study of the influence of the endocrine system on the nasal respiratory mucosa. J Laryngol Otol 1961; 75:972–979.
9. Toppozada H, Toppozada M, El-Ghazzawi I, Elwany S. The human respiratory nasal mucosa in females using contraceptive pills. J Laryngol Otol 1984; 98:43–51.
10. Bende M, Hallgarde U, Sjogren C, Uvnas-Moberg K. Nasal congestion during pregnancy. Clin Otolaryngol 1989; 14:385–387.
11. Schatz M, Hoffman CP, Zeiger RS, Falkoff R, Mellon M. The course and management of asthma and allergic diseases during pregnancy. In: Middleton E Jr, Reed CE, Ellis EF, Adkinson NF Jr, Yunginger JW, eds. Allergy: Principles and Practice. 3d ed. St. Louis: Mosby, 1988:1093–1155.
12. Schatz M, Zeiger RS. Diagnosis and management of rhinitis during pregnancy. Allergy Proc 1988; 9:545–554.
13. Henderson ID. Cyclical changes in female nasal mucous. J Clin Endocrinol 1956; 16:905–909.
14. Schatz M, Hoffman C. Interrelationships between asthma and pregnancy. Clin Rev Allergy 1987; 5:301–315.
15. Urabach E, Gottiab PM. In: Allergy. 2d ed. New York: Grune & Stratton, 1946:128, 861.

16. Flarer F, Serri IF, Cotton DWK. Proceedings of the XIV International Congress of Dermatology. Amsterdam, Excerpta Medica and New York: American Elsevier, 1974:853.

17. Zondeck B, Bromberg YM. Endocrine allergy—clinical reactions of allergy to endogenous hormones and their treatment. J Obstet Gynecol Br Emp 1947; 54:1–19.

18. Helmy AM, El-Ghazzawi IF, Mandour MA, Shehata MA. The effect of oestrogen on the nasal respiratory mucosa. J Laryngol Otol 1975; 39:1229–1241.

19. Schatz M. Asthma and rhinitis of pregnancy: who's at risk? J Respir Dis 1986; 7:14–15.

20. Mabry RL. Rhinitis of pregnancy. South Med J 1986; 79:965–971.

21. Foxen EH, Preston TD, Lack JA. The assessment of nasal airflow: a review of past and present methods. J Laryngol Otol 1971; 85:811–825.

22. Capel LH. Recent Advances in Otolaryngology. London: Churchill-Livingstone, 1973:235.

23. Falkoff R. Maternal immunologic changes during pregnancy: a critical appraisal. Clin Rev Allergy 1987; 5:287–300.

24. Dzhabbarov KK, Muminov AI. Characteristics of the course and treatment of inflammatory nasal and paranasal sinus disease in pregnancy. Vestn Otorinolaringol Sept-Dec 1993; (5–6):42–45.

25. Sorri M, Bortikanen-Sorri AL, Karja J. Rhinitis during pregnancy. Rhinology 1980; 18:83–86.

26. Incaudo GA, Gershwin ME, Nagy SM. The pathophysiology and treatment of sinusitis. Allergol et Immunopathol 1986; 14:423–434.

27. Bluestone CD. Assessment of eustachian tube function. In: Jerger J, ed. Manual of Impedance Audiometry. Dobbs Ferry, NY: American Electromedics Corp., 1975.

28. Derkay CS. Eustachian tube and nasal function during pregnancy: a prospective study. Otolaryn-Head and Neck Surg 1988; 99:558–566.

29. Plate S, Johnsen NJ, Pedersen SN, Thomsen KA. The frequency of patulous eustachian tubes in pregnancy. Clin Otolaryngol 1979; 4:393–400.

30. Pulec JL. Diseases of the eustachian tube. In: Paparella MM, Shumrick DA, eds. Otolaryngology. 2d ed. Philadelphia: Saunders, 1983:1410–1411.

31. Mohun M. Incidence of vasomotor rhinitis during pregnancy. Arch Otolaryngol 1943; 37:699–709.

32. Derkay CS. Eustachian tube and nasal function during pregnancy: a prospective study. Otolaryn-Head and Neck Surg 1988; 99:558–566.

33. Entman SS, Moise KJ. Anaphylaxis in pregnancy. South Med J 1984; 77:402.

34. Erasmsu C, Blackwood W, Wilson J. Infantile multicystic encephalomalacia after maternal bee sting anaphylaxis during pregnancy. Arch Dis Child 1982; 57:785–787.

35. Klein VR, Harris AP, Abraham RA, Neibyl JR. Fetal distress during a maternal systemic allergic reaction. Obstet Gynecol 1984; 64(suppl):15s–17s.

36. Wilson NW, Jalowayski AA, Hamburger RN. A comparison of nasal cytology with sinus x-rays for the diagnosis of sinusitis. Am J Rhinol 1988; 2: 55–59.

37. Gill FF, Neiburger JB. The role of nasal cytology in the diagnosis of chronic sinusitis. Am J Rhinol 1989; 3:13–15.

38. Meltzer EO, Jalowayski AA. Nasal cytology in clinical practice. Am J Rhinol 1988; 2:47–54.

39. Swartz HM, Reichling BA. Hazards of radiation exposure for pregnant women. JAMA 1978; 239:1907–1908.

40. Jones KL, Chernoff GF. Environmental influences on fetal development: effects of chemical and environmental agents. In: Creasy RK, ed. Maternal and Fetal Medicine. Philadelphia: Saunders, 1984.

41. McAlister WH, Lusk R, Muntz HR. Comparison of plain radiographs and coronal CT scans in infants and children with recurrent sinusitis. Am J Roentgenol 1989; 153:1259–1264.

42. Calhoun KH, Waggenspack GA, Simpson CB, Hokanson JA, Bailey BJ. CT evaluation of the paranasal sinuses in symptomatic and asymptomatic populations. Otolaryngol-Head Neck Surg 1991; 104:480–483.

43. Andrew WK, Swart JG. Fallibility of sinus radiographs in domonstrating ethmoid sinusitis. S Afr Med J 1987; 72:158.

44. Landman MD. Ultrasound screening for sinus disease. Otolaryngol-Head Neck Surg 1986; 94:157–154.

45. Shapiro G, Furukawa C, Pierson W, Gilbertson E, Bierman CW. Blinded comparison of maxillary sinus radiography and ultrasound for diagnosis of sinusitis. J Allergy Clin Immunol 1986; 77:59–64.

46. Revonta M. Ultrasound in the diagnosis of maxillary and frontal sinusitis. Acta Otolaryngol (Stockh) 1980; 370:1–54.

47. Jannert M, Andreasson L, Holmer NG, Lorinc P. Ultrasonic examination of the paranasal sinuses. Acta Otolaryngol 1982; 389(suppl):1–52.

48. Berg O, Carenfelt C. Etiological diagnosis in sinusitis: ultrasonography as clinical component. Laryngoscope 1985; 95:851–853.

49. Pfleidrer AG, Drake-Lee AB, Lowe D. Ultrasound of the sinuses: a worthwhile procedure? A comparison of ultrasound and radiography in predicting the findings of proof puncture on the maxillary sinuses. Clin Otolaryngol 1984; 9:335–339.

50. Isaacson S, Edell SL. A-mode ultrasound evaluation of maxillary sinusitis. ORL 1978; 86:231–235.

51. Landman MD. Ultrasound screening for sinus disease. Otolaryngol Head-Neck Surg 1986; 94:157–164.

52. Rohr AS, Spector SL, Siegel SC, Katz RM, Rachelefsky GS. Correlation between A-mode ultrasound and radiography in the diagnosis of maxillary sinusitis. J Allergy Clin Immunol 1986; 78:58–61.

53. Druce HM, Rutledge J. Chronic sinusitis and rhinitis. Am J Rhinol 1989; 3: 163–166.

54. Shapiro GG, Furukawa CT, Pierson WE, Gilbertson E, Bierman CW. Blinded comparison of maxillary sinus radiography and ultrasound for diagnosis of sinusitis. J Allergy Clin Immunol 1986; 77:59–64.

55. Wald ER, Milmoe GJ, Bowen A, Ledesma-Medina J, Salamon N, Bluestone CD. N Engl J Med 1981; 304:749–754.

56. Berger W, Weiss J. A comparison of A-mode ultrasound and x-ray for screening of maxillary sinus disease (abstr). J Allergy Clin Immunol 1985; 75:187.

57. Hill RM, Tennyson LM. The effect of maternal allergy medications on the fetus. Immunol Allergy Prac 1985; 7:80–91.

58. Greenberg F. The potential teratogenicity of allergy and asthma treatment in pregnancy. Immunol Allergy Prac 1985; 7:4–9.

59. Specific requirements on content and format of labelling for human prescription drugs, Fed Reg 1979; 44:37462.

60. Briggs GG, Freeman RK, Yaffe SJ. Drugs in Pregnancy and Lactation. Baltimore: Williams & Wilkins, 1986:xxi.

61. Gardner DK, Rayburn WF. Drugs in breast milk. In: Rayburn WF, Zuspan FP, eds. Drug Therapy in Obstetrics and Gynecology. Norwalk, CT: Appleton-Century-Crofts, 1982.

62. Lawrence RA. Drugs and breast feeding. Semin Perinatol 1979; 3:271–279.

63. Catz CS, Giacoia GP. Drugs and breast milk. Ped Clin N Am 1972; 19:151–162.

64. Heinonen OP, Slone D, Shapiro S. Birth Defects and Drugs in Pregnancy. Littleton, MA: P.S.G. Publishing, 1977.

65. Slone D, Shapiro S. Drugs and pregnancy (letter), Ann Intern Med 1979; 90:275.

66. Baxi LV, Gindoff PR, Pregenzer GJ, Parras MK. Fetal heart rate changes following maternal administration of a nasal decongestant. Am J Obstet Gynecol 1985; 153:799–800.

67. Rayburn WF, Anderson JC, Smith CV, Appel LL, Davis SA. Uterine and fetal doppler flow changes from a single dose of a long-acting intranasal decongestant. Obstet Gynecol 1990; 76:180–182.

68. Ballen JC, ed. American Medical Association Drug Evaluation. Chicago: American Medical Association, 1980.

69. Nishimura H, Tanimura T. Clinical Aspects of the Teratogenicity of Drugs. Amsterdam: Excerpta Medica, 1976:231.

70. Jick H, Holmes LB, Hunter JR, Madsen S, Stergachis A. First trimester drug use and congenital disorders. JAMA 1981; 246:343–346.

71. Findlay JWA, Butz RF, Sailstad JM, Warren JT, Welch RM. Pseudoephedrine and triprolidine in plasma and breast milk of nursing mothers. Br J Clin Pharmacol 1984; 18:901–906.

72. Slone D, Shapiro S. Drugs and pregnancy (letter). Ann Intern Med 1979; 90:275.

73. Saxin I. Cleft palate and maternal diphenhydramine intake (letter). Lancet 1974; 1:407.

74. King CTG, Howell J. Teratogenic effects of buclizine and hydroxyzine in the rat and chlorcaydizine in the mouse. Am J Obstet Gynecol 1966; 95: 109.

75. Erez S, Schifrin BS, Dirim O. Double-blind evaluation of hydroxyzine as an antiemetic in pregnancy. J Reprod Med 1971; 7:57–61.

76. Nelson MM, Forfar JO. Association between drugs administered during pregnancy and congenital abnormalities of the fetus. Br Med J 1971; 1:523–527.

77. Zierler S, Purohit D. Prenatal antihistamine exposure and retrolental fibroplasia. Am J Epidemiol 1986; 123:192–196.

78. Parkin DE. Probable benedryl withdrawal manifestation in a newborn infant. J Ped 1974; 85:580.

79. Prenner BM. Neonatal withdrawal syndrome associated with hydroxyzine hydrochloride. Am J Dis Child 1977; 131:529.

80. White GT, White MK. Breast feeding and drugs in human milk. Vet Hum Toxicol 1980; 22(suppl):1–11.

81. Kok THHG, Taitz LS, Bennett MJ, Holt DW. Drowsiness due to clemastine transmitted in breast milk (letter). Lancet 1982; 1:914.

82. Mortimer EA Jr. Drug toxicity from breast milk? Pediatrics 1977; 60: 780–781.

83. Gibson JP, Huffman KW, Newborne JW. Preclinical safety studies with terfenedine. Arzneimittelforschung 1982; 22:1179–1184. As cited in Shepard TH. Catalog of Teratogenic Agents. 6th ed. Baltimore: Johns Hopkins University Press, 1989:599.

84. Dykes MHM. Evaluation of an anti-asthmatic agent cromolyn sodium (Aarane, Intal), JAMA 1974; 227:1061–1072.

85. Wilson J. Utilisation du cromoglycate de sodium au cours de la grossesse. Acta Therapeutica 1982; 8(suppl):45.

86. Blackburn WR, Kaplan HS, McKay DG. Morphologic changes in the developing rat placenta following prednisolone administration. Am J Obstet Gynecol 1965; 92:234–236.

87. Fraser FC, Watter BE, Fainstat JD. The experimental production of cleft palate with cortisone and other hormones. J Cell Comp Physiol 1954; 43(suppl 1):237–245.

88. Mawhinney H, Spector SL. Optimum management of asthma in pregnancy. Drugs 1986; 32:178–187.

89. Greenberger PA, Patterson R. Beclomethasone diproprionate for severe asthma during pregnancy. Ann Intern Med 1983; 98:478–481.

90. Hill RM, Tennyson LM. The lactating allergic patient: which drugs cause concern for the infant? Immunol Allergy Prac 1984; 6:221–227.

91. Schatz M, Hoffman CP, Zeiger RS, Falkoff R, Mellon M. The course and management of asthma and allergic disease during pregnancy. In: Middleton E Jr, Reed CE, Ellis EF, Adkinson NF Jr, Yunginger JW, eds. Allergy: Principles and Practice. 4th ed. St. Louis: Mosby, 1993:1301–1342.

92. Francis N. Abortion after grass pollen injection. J Allergy 1941; 12:559–565.

93. Greenberger PA Pregnancy and asthma. Chest 1985; 87 (suppl):85s–87s.

94. Metzger WJ, Turner E, Patterson R. The safety of immunotherapy during pregnancy. J Allergy Clin Immunol 1978; 61:268–271.
95. Gwaltney JM, Sydnor A, Sande MA. Etiology and antimicrobial treatment of acute sinusitis. Ann Otol Rhinol Laryngol 1981; 90(suppl 84):68.
96. Wald ER. Sinusitis. Ped Rev 1993; 14:345–351.
97. Lew D, Southwick FS, Montgomery WW, Weber AL, Baker AS. Sphenoid sinusitis. N Engl J Med 1983; 309:1149–1154.
98. Schlanger G, Lutwick LI, Kurzman M. Sinusitis caused by *Legionella pneumophilia* in a patient with the acquired immunodeficiency syndrome. Am J Med 1984; 77:952.
99. Gonzalez MM, Gould E, Dickinson G, Martinez AJ, Visvesvara G, Cleary TJ, Hensley GT. Acquired immunodeficiency syndrome associated with acanthamoeba infection and other opportunistic organisms. Arch Pathol Lab Med 1986; 110(8):749–751.
100. Thornsberry C, Brown SD, Yee C, Bouchillon SK, Marler JK, Rich T. Increasing penicillin resistance in streptococcus pneumoniae in the U.S. Infect Med 1990; 1(suppl):15–24.
101. Matsuda S. Augmenten treatment in obstetrics and gynaecology. In: Leigh DA, Robinson OPW, eds. Augmentin: Proceedings of an International Symposium, Montreux, Switzerland, July 1981. Amsterdam: Excerpta Medica 1982:179–191.
102. Pedler SJ, Bint AJ. Comparative study of amoxicillin-clavulanic acid and cephalexin in the treatment of bacteriuria during pregnancy. Antimicrob Agents Chemother 1985; 27:508–510.
103. Faden H, Doern G, Wolf J, Blocker M. Antimicrobial susceptibility of nasopharyngeal isolates of potential pathogens recovered from infants before antibiotic therapy: implications for the management of otitis media. Pediatr Infect Dis J 1994; 13:609–612.
104. Helin I., Andreasson L, Jannert M, Petterson H. Acute sinusitis in children—results of different therapeutic regimens. Helv Pediat Acta 1982; 37:83–90.
105. Hardy DJ, Hensey DM, Beyer JM, Vojtko C, McDonald EJ, Fernander PB. Comparative in vitro activities of new 14-, 15- and 16-membered macrolides. Antimicrob Agents Chemother 1988; 32:1710–1719.
106. Moellering R. Introduction: revolutionary changes in the macrolide and azalide antibiotics. Am J Med 1991; 91(suppl 3A):3A-1S–3A-4S.
107. Philipson A. Pharmacokinetics of antibiotics in pregnancy and labour. Clin Pharmacokinet 1979; 4:297–309.
108. Product information. Cipro. Bayer Corp. West Haven, CT, 1995.
109. Faden H, Doern G, Wolf J, Blocker M. Antimicrobial susceptibility of naspharyngeal isolates of potential pathogens recovered from infants before antibiotic therapy: implications for the management of otitis media. Pediatr Infect Dis J 1994; 13:609–612.

110. Nelson CT, Mason EO, Kaplan SL. Activity of oral antibiotics in middle ear and sinus infections caused by penicillin-resistant *Streptococcus pneumoniae*: implications for treatment. Pediatr Infect Dis J 1994; 13:585–589.

111. Ochoa AG. Trimethoprim and sulfamethoxazole in pregnancy. JAMA 1971; 217:1244.

112. Committee on Drugs, American Academy of Pediatrics. The transfer of drugs and other chemicals into human milk. Pediatrics 1994; 93:137–150.

113. Daley CL, Sande M. The runny nose. Infection of the paranasal sinuses. Infect Dis Clin N Am 1988; 2:131–147.

114. Coonan KM, Kaplan EL. In vitro susceptibility of recent North American Group A streptococcal isolates to eleven oral antibiotics. Pediatr Infect Dis J 1994; 13:630–635.

115. Holt GR, Mabry RL. ENT medications in pregnancy. Otolaryngol-Head Neck Surg. 1983; 91:338–341.

116. Schwerz RH. Considerations of antibiotic therapy during pregnancy. Obstet Gynegol 1981(suppl); 58:955–956.

117. Pastuszak A, Schick B, D'alimonte D, Donnenfeld A, Koren G. The safety of astemizole in pregnancy. J Allergy Clin Immunol 1996; 98:748–750.

118. Einarson A, Bailey B, Jung G, Spizzirri D, Baille M, Koren G. Prospective controlled study of hydroxyzine and citirizine in pregnancy. Annals Allergy, Asthma & Immunol 1997; 78:183–186.

12

Anaphylaxis in Pregnancy

STEPHEN I. WASSERMAN

University of California, San Diego, School of Medicine
La Jolla, California

I. Introduction

Anaphylaxis is a true allergic emergency. Fatalities from anaphylaxis have
been demonstrated to occur within minutes, and it is the obligation of the
physician to be prepared to both recognize and treat this clinical situation.
Obviously, in pregnancy there is an increased importance, in that not only
the patient, but also the fetus, is at risk. The purpose of this chapter is to
review understanding of this important clinical entity, to define the unique
pathophysiological mechanisms in pregnancy that are relevant to anaphylaxis, and to identify the best modalities for treatment to preserve maternal
and fetal well-being.

II. Definition

Anaphylaxis is the most critical of allergic emergencies. It may reach its
peak within minutes and can prove fatal despite rapid treatment (1). Anaphylaxis is the best term to describe the clinical syndrome, regardless of
immune mechanism. Its nonspecific manifestations include flushing, pru-

ritus, a metallic taste in the mouth, and a sense of impending doom, symptoms which may then be rapidly followed by tissue specific changes. These may be cutaneous; respiratory; upper (laryngeal edema) or lower airway obstruction; gastrointestinal; nausea, vomiting, abdominal cramping, and diarrhea; and cardiovascular manifestations—dysrhythmia, hypoperfusion, third-space vascular loss, hypotension, and collapse. Of particular import in pregnancy is uterine contraction. These signs and symptoms may occur together or alone.

III. Epidemiology

Exposure determines anaphylactic expression, and age, race, sex, or occupation are important only if they influence exposure patterns. Pregnancy may, for example, predispose to exposure to latex antigen or medications such as oxytocin. Only imprecise statistics for anaphylaxis exist. It is estimated that approximately one of every 2700 hospitalized patients has suffered from an anaphylactic reaction (2), with reactions to hymenoptera envenomation, radiographic contrast dye exposures, and general anesthetic agents being most prevalent. The case rate for fatal anaphylaxis is uncertain, but is cited to be 0.002% for penicillin and 0.001% for hymenoptera (3). Atopy may not place individuals at higher risk of anaphylactic reactions, but once sensitized, atopic individuals (particularly those with asthma) may be at greater risk for severe anaphylaxis and death.

IV. Etiological Mechanisms (Table 1)

A. Immunoglobulin E-Mediated Anaphylaxis

For many agents, the participation of IgE antibody has been proved or appears highly likely, as identified through the use of appropriate skin or blood (radioallergosorbent technique, RAST) testing to identify antigen-specific IgE. Of particular importance are antibiotics, including penicillin and other β-lactam antibiotics, with sulfanamides also being an important cause of anaphylactic reactions. Foreign proteins, such as therapeutic agents (horse serum, murine monoclonal antibodies), hymenoptera venom, latex, various enzymes, and immunotherapy extracts are important causes of IgE-mediated anaphylaxis. Peanuts, eggs, shellfish, and nuts are the most important foods causing anaphylaxis. Several therapeutic and diagnostic agents, including general anesthetics, muscle-relaxing agents, and synthetic hormones such as oxytocin and progesterone (6) all have caused IgE-mediated anaphylactic episodes in pregnant patients (4–9).

Table 1 Mechanisms of Anaphylaxis

A. IgE-mediated agents
1. Antibiotics
2. Foreign proteins
3. Other therapeutic agents (e.g., allergen extracts, vaccines, muscle relaxants)
4. Foods
B. Immune complexes/complement-mediated events
1. Blood or blood products
2. Aggregated proteins
C. Modulators of arachidonic acid metabolism
1. Nonsteroidal anti-inflammatory drugs
D. Agents which directly degranulate mast cells and basophils
1. Opiates
2. Radiocontrast media
3. Dextran
E. Exercise
F. Idiopathic

B. Immune Complex-Mediated Anaphylaxis

The administration of blood and blood products, particularly those that contain immunoglobulin A (IgA), may induce immune complex-mediated anaphylactic episodes, presumably, but not always, through the release of mast cell-activating anaphylatoxins during the consumption of complement (10,11). Immune complexes are formed in patients who have generated IgG antibodies to IgA. Other aggregated proteins, particularly aggregated immunoglobulins, can also induce this syndrome.

C. Altered Arachidonic Acid Metabolism

Hypersensitivity reactions to aspirin and other nonsteroidal anti-inflammatory agents (NSAIDs) are generally easily separable from anaphylaxis, but severe episodes or those which include urticaria may be difficult to distinguish. In general, reactions to nonsteroidal anti-inflammatory agents develop slowly, tend to be manifest primarily by profuse rhinorrhea, nasal obstruction and asthma, and occur most often in patients with pre-existing rhinitis and asthma (12). In some instances, severe and rapidly progressive reactions leading to collapse may occur. NSAIDs inhibit the cyclooxygenase enzymes COX 1 and COX 2, and their relative potency in inducing this syndrome is related to their potency in inhibiting prostaglandin synthesis. The production of excessive amounts of sulfidopeptide leukotrienes, either as mediators or markers, is a feature of this disorder (13).

D. Agents That Directly Degranulate Mast Cells and Basophils

Anaphylactic reactions to a number of therapeutic agents have been shown to be due to the ability of these compounds, in the absence of specific antibody, to release histamine (and other important mediators) from peripheral blood basophils or mast cells. Opiates (14), neuropeptides, highly charged compounds, plasma expanders, and radiocontrast media (15,16) can cause such responses. Because these reactions are not due to antibody, they are unpredictable upon reexposure. With radiocontrast media, risk is highest with intravenous use; in those who reacted previously, a recurrence rate of approximately 30% may be expected.

E. Exercise Anaphylaxis

In some persons, exercise (17), including the physical work of labor and delivery (18), may directly precipitate anaphylaxis. This anaphylactic reaction may occur after eating and, occasionally, only after eating a specific food. In the latter, IgE-mediated food allergy has been demonstrated (19).

F. Idiopathic Anaphylaxis

In some patients who experience recurrent episodes of anaphylaxis, no inciting cause can be identified, despite rigorous and thorough analysis, justifying the diagnosis of idiopathic anaphylaxis (20). Most of these patients are atopic and many respond poorly to usual therapies for anaphylaxis.

V. Clinical and Pathophysiological Findings

The onset, duration, and manifestations of anaphylaxis vary immensely among patients. Involvement of the airway and cardiovascular systems is of primary importance to mortality, with most fatal cases due to respiratory complications and a significant minority to cardiovascular collapse. Symptoms usually occur within minutes of exposure to the causative agent, and anaphylaxis rarely occurs more than 1 hr after exposure to the eliciting stimulus.

Laryngeal edema causes obstruction of the upper airway, with swallowing difficulties and hoarseness, and may cause total asphyxia. Obstruction of the lower airway (asthma) is noted most often in individuals with underlying asthma, but may occur in the absence of such history and often does so in the absence of upper airway obstruction.

Nausea, vomiting, diarrhea, and cramping abdominal pain may accompany anaphylaxis induced by any route, but most often with ingested allergens.

Reproductive system reactions, including uterine cramping may be of special importance in the pregnant individual. However, miscarriage has only rarely been reported from uterine activation as a consequence of anaphylaxis (21).

Of obvious great importance is cardiovascular collapse, which may be due to depressed myocardial function, arrhythmia, hypoxia, or loss of intravascular volume. The known consequences of diminished uterine blood flow to fetal well-being make this of critical importance in pregnancy. Myocardial infarction, as well as diminished myocardial performance, also occur in anaphylaxis.

In rare instances, the first manifestation of anaphylaxis may be loss of consciousness. Death may occur within minutes or may be delayed for days to weeks and occurs as a consequence of hypoxia and hypotension. Although logical, it is unproven that the later the onset of the reaction, the less severe. Biphasic anaphylactic reactions, with severe early manifestations, followed by spontaneous recovery and then a recrudescence has been described (22), but the clinical relevance has been questioned (23).

VI. Pathological and Laboratory Manifestations of Anaphylaxis

There are no pathognomonic changes which can unequivocally identify anaphylaxis. In many fatal cases, laryngeal edema, visceral congestion, pulmonary edema, hyperinflation, and intraalveolar hemorrhage are identified, accompanied by urticaria and angioedema. Increased bronchial secretions and vascular congestion with eosinophil infiltration of the airway and spleen has been reported. Obstruction of the upper airway due to edema is seen in a majority of fatalities, while vascular collapse leaves no marks. Occasionally, myocardial infarction either as a direct effect of anaphylaxis or as a secondary manifestation of hypotension may be seen.

The clinical laboratory can be helpful in the evaluation of patients with anaphylaxis. Airway obstruction can be identified through pulmonary functional assessment, and chest radiographs may demonstrate hyperinflation. Hemoconcentration and elevated hematocrit accompany intravascular volume depletion. Defects in coagulation, perhaps due to mast cell heparin release, are reported. Serum enzymes and electrocardiographic manifestations reflective of myocardial injury may be evident in patients suffering this consequence. Other electrocardiographic manifestations of anaphylaxis include superventricular tachyarrhythmias, T-wave abnormalities, bundle branch block, and intraventricular conduction delays. Elevations in plasma and urinary histamine and in serum or plasma tryptase, a mast cell-specific enzyme, have been reported (24,25). As tryptase has a serum half-life of 1–2 hr, it is the most useful available marker of anaphylaxis.

VII.   Diagnosis and Differential Diagnosis of Anaphylaxis

Because of its rapid onset and severe manifestations, anaphylaxis is usually easily identified. When flushing, premonitory signs and symptoms of pruritus and a sense of oppression and fear on the part of the patient, and an associated event such as an ingestion or injection occur together, the diagnosis should be obvious. The presence of tachycardia, hypotension, upper and lower respiratory obstruction, and other accompanying symptoms such as abdominal discomfort, vomiting, cramping, urticaria, and angioedema are all helpful to the astute clinician. Obviously, the setting in which anaphylaxis occurs is often associated with a number of other potential disorders, making the differential diagnosis of syncope, collapse, hypotension, flushing, and other overlapping syndromes crucial.

The most common mimic of anaphylaxis is vasovagal syncope. The entity occurs after a stressful, painful event such as an injection, and collapse under these circumstances may easily be confused with anaphylaxis. In general, the patient suffering vasovagal collapse is pale, cool, and notes nausea before fainting, but does not flush or itch or manifest respiratory difficulty. Symptoms are rapidly reversed by recumbency. Associated events, including diaphoresis, bradycardia, and a slow pulse and a generally well-maintained blood pressure, differentiate it from anaphylaxis. In some patients, hyperventilation after a stressful or painful event may cause breathlessness and fainting.

Flushing disorders, including those due to alcohol ingestion, occurring during the post/perimenopausal period and those associated with mastocytosis and carcinoid syndrome may be confused with anaphylaxis. Hereditary angioedema, particularly laryngeal edema may, in rare instances, be confused with anaphylaxis. However, the kinetics of this disorder, its hereditary nature, and the absence of urticaria or hypotension should identify it. Patients with globus hystericus (lump in the throat) have chronic, persistent, nonprogressive symptoms associated with no anatomic abnormalities in the pharynx or hypopharynx. Serum sickness should not be confused with anaphylaxis because of its delay in onset and its manifestations, primarily of fever, lymphadenopathy, arthralgia, urticaria, and occasionally nephritis. Physical urticarias, particularly severe episodes of cholinergic or cold urticaria, could be mistaken for anaphylaxis. Severe cholinergic urticaria can mimic exercise-induced anaphylaxis; in cold urticaria, collapse following immersion in cold water could also be confusing. These entities may be diagnosed through physical challenges once the patient has recovered. Other causes of acute collapse, including pulmonary embolism, seizure disorder, cardiac dysrhythmia, myocardial infarction, cerebral vascular accident, and even unsuspected trauma must be recognized and differentiated from anaphylactic collapse.

The diagnosis and differential diagnosis of anaphylaxis may be supported in-vivo or in-vitro tests, including assessment of antigen-specific IgE, as well as physical and other environmental challenges. Application of an ice cube to the forearm or exercise in a warm environment can identify cold and cholinergic urticaria, respectively. Urticaria pigmentosa may be identified by a thorough skin examination, biopsy, or with other tests (such as technetium bone scans). The finding of metabolites of serotonin in the urine may identify carcinoid syndrome. Computed tomography, electrocardiography, echocardiography, ventilation-perfusion scanning, and/or pulmonary angiography should be used as indicated to clarify pulmonary embolism, cerebrovascular accident, myocardial infarction, or cardiac dysrhythmia.

VIII. Pathogenic Mechanisms in Anaphylaxis

Although the immunopharmacological pathways responsible for the mast cell and its constituent mediators are critically important to the manifestations of anaphylaxis, these mediators are, to some degree, also dependent on additional cascades initiated by the inciting agent. IgE-mediated processes, in which IgE bound to high-affinity Fc receptors on mast cells and basophils is cross-linked by antigen, transmit signals eventuating in mediator generation and release. No common features can be discerned to predict the likelihood of IgE reactivity to any particular agent. Mast cells and basophils generate vasoactive-spasmogenic mediators, active enzymes, proteoglycans, and chemoattractant factors. The vasoactive and spasmogenic mediators appear to be critically important to the expression of anaphylaxis. Preformed in this category in the mast cell and basophil is histamine, while the sulfidopeptide leukotrienes (LTC4, D4, and E4), platelet-activating factor, and adenosine may be generated as well.

Histamine is found in blood or urine in human anaphylactic episodes, and histamine injection into humans (26) induces a metallic taste, urticaria, angioedema, flushing, hypotension, headache, and vomiting. Histamine can also augment permeability and induce third-space fluid accumulation and intravascular volume loss. Histamine can diminish coronary blood flow, exacerbating hypotension, and cause cardiac dysrhythmias. The sulfidopeptide leukotrienes, platelet-activating factor, and adenosine also cause many of these same manifestations, particularly intravascular fluid depletion, hypotension, and diminished cardiac output. Although the neutral protease, tryptase, has been a useful marker for identifying anaphylaxis, no direct role for this enzyme has been established in anaphylaxis. Mast cell heparin has been implicated in some of the hemostatic defects seen in anaphylaxis.

The pathway(s) by which non-IgE-mediated anaphylaxis occurs remains largely unexplained. The generation of C3a and C5a by immune complexes are thought to be responsible for directly affecting vascular and respiratory smooth muscle, and activating mast cells to release histamine, and is assumed to be the mechanism whereby anaphylaxis is engendered during reactions to immune complexes.

IX. Considerations in Pregnancy

As noted above, anaphylaxis in the pregnant patient is of particular importance because two individuals are at risk. A unique clinical event in anaphylaxis that is of importance in the pregnant patient is uterine cramping, which may mimic impending delivery; however, miscarriage is not a common complication of anaphylaxis. The fall in uterine blood flow which may occur during cardiovascular collapse may be of particular importance to fetal well-being. Other important clinical points in anaphylaxis in the pregnant patient relate to the unique medications to which such patients are exposed. Obviously, most drugs are avoided during pregnancy. However, oxytocin, which may be used to induce labor, has been associated with mast cell degranulation (4), and some hormonal therapies, including progesterone (7), have been reported to cause IgE-mediated allergic events. In addition, many of the drugs and exposures associated with surgical procedures, such as episiotomy or caesarean section, can induce anaphylaxis. The operating room is a particularly difficult setting in which to evaluate anaphylaxis, because patients are often intubated and sedated, making a clear history difficult to obtain. In this setting, patients are often exposed to a wide variety of agents, including antibiotics, muscle relaxants, opiates, neuromuscular blocking drugs, and latex, and plasma expanders and protamine may also be administered in special circumstances. Many of the clinical clues of impending anaphylaxis are not available in the operating room, and the first sign of anaphylaxis may be hypotension or difficulty ventilating an unconscious patient. Obviously, management of the airway and blood pressure may be facilitated in the operating room because patient often has already been intubated and is receiving intravenous fluids. Postoperative analysis of the causative agents requires a very careful examination of the medical records, evaluation of prior interactions with similar compounds, and supplemental skin testing when available. Highest on the list of suspected agents in this setting would be latex, neuromuscular blocking agents, and antibiotics. Obviously, the history of anaphylaxis during a prior operative procedure in a pregnant patient requires full investigation, and if an etiology cannot be identified, it is essential that if an operative procedure is required (i.e., caesarian section), different classes of agents are utilized to reduce the risk of repeat anaphylaxis. In this setting, the anesthesiologist must be made aware of this prior history and all personnel prepared to deal with an anaphylactic event.

X. Management of the Patient with Anaphylaxis

The management of pregnant patients with anaphylaxis is identical to that of the population as a whole. The acute episode requires understanding of pathophysiology and therapeutic options, the prevention of future anaphylactic episodes requires knowledge of the principles of prevention, identifying causative agents, counseling patients, and community education. Strategies useful to prevent anaphylaxis in high-risk patients requiring encounters with eliciting agents are essential.

A detailed protocol for the medical management of anaphylaxis is described in Table 2. Effective treatment is immensely assisted by the rapid recognition of anaphylaxis symptomatology. Delay in therapy, particularly in the use of epinephrine, is associated with increased mortality (27). The patient should be placed in the left lateral decubitus position. A blood pressure of at least 90 mmHg should be maintained. The treatment of choice in anaphylaxis is epinephrine, and although it may decrease uterine blood flow via an α-adrenergic effect, its unique benefits in anaphylaxis outweigh its potential risks. It must be remembered that fetal distress may accompany anaphylaxis, which may lead to central nervous system abnormalities and even fetal or neonatal death if inadequately treated (28–30). Thus, aqueous epinephrine at a 1:1000 concentration, 0.3–0.5 mL should be immediately administered through the intramuscular or subcutaneous route. This can be repeated every 10–30 min as tolerated and required. Although some physicians advocate the use of intravenous epinephrine, its use has been associated with myocardial infarction and death, and it should

Table 2 Kaiser Permanente Severe Anaphylaxis Protocol

Modify as desired, cross off nonapplicable orders.
 1. Call physician STAT.
 2. P,R, BP every 5 min or every 2 min if BP <90 mmHg.
 3. Patient wt.____ kg.
 4. O_2 at 6 L/min by nasal cannula.
 5. If systolic BP <90 mmHg, use Trendelenburg's position, place patient on left side and ECG monitor.
 6. Continue tourniquet, if reaction secondary to injection, skin test, or sting.
 7. Continue epinephrine (1:1000), 0.3 mL IM in deltoid, repeat every 10 min if reaction persists. In addition, give either half or equivalent dose into site of skin test injection or sting.
 8. Start IV with 18–or 19-gauge needle or intercath, infuse Ringer's lactate; start wide open then check with physician for rate or volume (may require 3 to 10 L).

Consider:
 9. Benadryl (diphenhydramine hydrochloride; 50 mg/mL): 1 mL IV piggyback in 50 mL over 5 min.
 10. Methylprednisolone (125 mg/2 mL) 2 mL in 50 mL IV piggyback over 5 min. Don't mix with Benadryl.
 11. If wheezing, use albuteral (5 mg/mh), 0.5 mL added to 2 mL saline and nebulize; or albuterol, metered-dose inhaler, 6 puffs over 10 min.
 12. If symptoms persist, ranitidine (50 mg/2 mL) 2 mL in 50 mL IV piggback infused in 5 min.
 13. If systolic BP less than 90 mmHg and pulse less than 60/min, give atropine (1 mg/10 mL) 5 mL IV push, may repeat 10 mL if necessary in 5 to 10 min.
 14. If still hypotensive, or hypotension recurs, use maintenance epinephrine; add 1 mL epinephrine (1:1000) to 10 mL saline and infuse over 10 min. Consider repeating if still hypotensive, perfusing immediately after previous dose.
 15. If still hypotensive, or hypotension recurs, use maintenance epinephrine: 1 mL epinephrine (1:1000) in 250 mL D_5 W (4 μg/mL) and infuse at 15 mL/hr (1 μg/min). Titrate every 5 min to maintain systolic BP $\geq$90 mmHg. Maximum dose 60 mL/hr = 4 μg/min.
 16. If still hypotensive, discontinue maintenance epinephrine and infuse dopamine (400 mg/5 mL): mix 5 mL with 250 mL IV solution (1.6 mg/mL) and start infusion at 0.15 × ____ kg (4 μg/kg/min) = ____ mL/hr to maintain systolic BP $\geq$90 mmHg. Titrate every 5 min to maintain systolic BP $\geq$90 mmHg (usual maximum dose 5 × infusion rate = 20 μg/kg min).
 17. If ventricular dysrhythmia occurs, use lidocaine (100 mg/5 mL) acutely: 0.05 × ____ kg = ____ mL IV bolus which may be repeated in 5 min. Consider twice the dose in 15 min if necessary.
 18. If dysrhythmia persists, lidocaine (2 g/50 mL) maintenance dosage: add 50 mL to 500 mL, D_5 W, and start infusion at 30 mL/hr (2 mg/min).
 19. Consider glucagon if patient on β-blocker and anaphylaxis persists. Add 1 mL glucagon diluting solution to glucagon vial and infuse 0.5 mL IV push. May repeat if necessary.
 20. If wheezing persists and patient is on no previous theophylline for past 24 hr,give bolus of aminophylline (500 mg/20 mL) 0.2 × ____ kg = ____ mL IV in 50 mL solution over 20 min.

Source: Modified from Schatz M, Zeiger RS. Allergic diseases. In Gleicher N, ed. Medical Therapy in Pregnancy, 2d ed. East Norwalk, CT: Appleton-Lange, 1992:435.

be reserved for individuals in extremis despite the use of subcutaneous epinephrine. If it must be used intravenously, the 1:1000 concentration of epinephrine should be diluted a further 10- to 100-fold, and administered slowly. If the cause of anaphylaxis has been an injected drug or venom, a portion of the epinephrine should be injected directly into the local site in an attempt to delay absorption of the inciting agent.

Some clinicians favor the use of ephedrine as a first line of treatment to minimize the effects of epinephrine on uterine blood flow (30,31). This may be tried initially if the clinical situation permits, but it has been reported to be less effective than epinephrine in the treatment of anaphylaxis in pregnancy (30,31).

Parenteral diphenhydramine (50 mg intramuscularly or intravenously) should generally be administered for persistent symptoms. Should airway obstruction persist, maintenance of the airway, either through mechanical intubation, or tracheostomy, if necessary, must be undertaken. Should lower airway obstruction (i.e., bronchospasm) be identified, oxygen administration and the administration of theophylline or inhaled β-adrenergic agonists may be useful.

Vascular collapse from third-space loss or fall of effective peripheral resistance should be treated not only with epinephrine, but also by intravenous fluids. Other modalities that have been demonstrated to be useful in some instances of anaphylaxis include combined use of H_1 and H_2 antihistamines in the treatment of prolonged or severe hypotension. Repeated large doses of glucocorticoids, such as 125 mg of methylprednisolone (Solu-Medrol) intravenously, may be helpful, although this has never been conclusively demonstrated. A recent issue has been the recognition of anaphylaxis in patients receiving β-adrenergic blocking agents. Such drugs limit the effectiveness of β-adrenergic agonists and may make the treatment of anaphylaxis quite difficult. Patients who are receiving β-adrenergic blocking drugs should be counseled regarding the difficulting of treating anaphylaxis, and their physician should be aware of the use of such drugs before administering any agent, particularly those with a high incidence of including anaphylaxis. Some advocate the use of glucagon to reverse β-adrenergic blockade in the anaphylactic setting, although the utility of this maneuver is based on isolated case reports (32). Others suggest use of B_1 and B_2 agonists (lacking α-adrenergic effects) titrated to clinical effect in the β-adrenergic-blocked patient.

XI. Prevention

Any physician who has had the responsibility of caring for a patient experiencing anaphylaxis appreciates the need for its prevention. Nothing can completely eliminate the risk of anaphylaxis; however, it is possible to diminish it. Physicians must obtain a complete allergic history and identify the agents which may have previously caused anaphylaxis in their patient. Physicians should be aware of cross-reacting agents (for example, banana, avocado, and chestnut commonly cross-react with latex) and hidden sources of the known inciting agent. If possible, the patient should be tested for sensitivity, preferably in vitro, to solidify clinical impressions. Clearly, patients should eliminate causative antigens from their environment (at home, work, school, hobby, and play). No drugs should be used without clear cause. If feasible, drugs should be administered by the oral route, and patients should be observed for at least a half-hour thereafter. These simple procedures should give the greatest degree of protection to patients at risk of anaphylaxis. Although it is clear that patients may suffer life-threatening or even fatal anaphylaxis as the first manifestation of allergy to a compound, in many patients prior premonitory symptoms indicate sensitization. Eliciting such a history may be life saving.

Three maneuvers, desensitization, immunotherapy, and premedication, are available to the physician in situations in which a sensitized patient must receive an allergen for important diagnostic or therapeutic reasons. Desensitization, the incremental administration of a known drug or agent to which the patient is sensitive, has been demonstrated to permit patients to receive life-saving therapeutic agents in the face of anaphylactic reactivity. The technique requires a clear-cut diagnosis of allergic sensitization and a prior history of anaphylactic reaction to the agent. Desensitization has risks, and systemic or even fatal reactions may occur. Efficacy of this strategy has been shown with penicillin and other beta-lactam antibiotics (33), and for NSAIDs (34), and is best performed by the oral route. Its mechanism may be due to a short-term inability of mediator-releasing cells to respond to the specific antigen. Desensitization provides protection only for the episode in question. If repeat uses of the eliciting agent are required, repeated desensitization maneuvers are necessary. Because of its risk, desensitization should be performed in an environment where emergency medical treatment is immediately available, and only for the administration of life-saving treatments (e.g., the use of penicillin for syphilis in pregnancy, or in a patient with acute bacterial endocarditis to an organism exquisitely sensitive to penicillin). Numerous published protocols exist for desensitization, most achieving desired results over 4–8 hr.

In contrast to the acute, but transient, effects of desensitization, immunotherapy has proven useful in providing long-term protection against anaphylactic reactivity, especially in patients who are sensitive to hymenoptera. In this technique, increasing amounts of antigen are administered over a period of several years. Protection is conferred only after a period of months to years, due to altered T-cell reactivity, diminished antigen-specific IgE production, and increased production of antigen-specific IgG "blocking" antibody.

Premedication is another option for the physician to prevent anaphylactic manifestations when patients must be exposed to an agent to which they are sensitive. This technique is useful in permitting the use of radiocontrast media in patients who have previously experienced adverse reactions to them. A change to low-ionic-strength contrast media and the combined administration of an H_1 antagonist, a glucocorticoid, and a β-agonist have been demonstrated to markedly diminish the incidence of anaphylaxis (35). The use of such a premedication regimen for other agents has not been as well studied and cannot routinely be recommended.

All patients known to be anaphylactically sensitive should receive clear instructions as to how best avoid the allergen(s) to which they are sensitive. This includes education about the various forms that these antigens and cross-reacting compounds may take, the ecology of the insects to which they may be sensitive, and the various unsuspected sources of food antigens. Anaphylactically sensitive persons should carry pertinent medical information on their persons. Immunizations should be kept up to date so that use of heterologous antiserum will not be necessary, and if possible, they should avoid treatment with β-adrenergic-blocking drugs. Importantly, anaphylactically sensitive patients should carry on their persons, at all times, a preloaded syringe of epinephrine.

Angiotensin-converting enzyme inhibitor drugs (ACE inhibitors) are increasingly popular in the treatment of congestive heart failure and hypertension, but are implicated in the direct induction of cough and angioedema and may exacerbate anaphylaxis (36). No modifications in the treatment protocols for anaphylaxis has been suggested for patients taking such agents.

XII. Prognosis

In general, anaphylaxis is rapidly responsive to the administration of adrenaline and fluids, and both mother and fetus do well (28). In the case of severe prolonged hypotension, maternal and fetal death can occur. Unfortunately, severe prolonged hypotension may lead to abnormalities in the fetus, despite the recovery of the mother (29,30). For these reasons, the recognition and prompt treatment of anaphylaxis is essential. The rapid institution of treatment is an essential cornerstone of the therapy, but despite recognition and intervention, death has been reported even in well-staffed, prepared hospital facilities.

References

1. James LP, Austen KF. Fatal systemic anaphylaxis in man. N Engl J Med 1964; 270:597–603.
2. Metcalfe DD. Acute anaphylaxis and urticaria in children and adults. In: Schochet AL, ed. Clinical Management of Urticaria and Anaphylaxis. New York: Marcel Dekker, 1992: 70–96.
3. Idsoe O, Gruthe T, Wilcox RR, et al. Nature and extent of penicillin side reactions with particular references to fatalities from anaphylactic shock. Bull World Health Org 1968; 38:159–188.
4. Kawarabyashi T, Narisawa Y, Nakimura K, et al. Anaphylactoid reaction to oxytocin during cesarian section. Gynecol and Obstet Inv 1988; 25:277–279.
5. Baldo BA, Fisher M, Harle D. Allergy to thiopentone. Clin Rev Allergy 1991; 9:295–307.
6. Vervloet D. Allergy to muscle relaxants and related compounds. Clin Allergy 1985; 5:501–508.
7. Meggs W, Peskovitz O, Metcalfe D, et al. Progesterone sensitivity as a cause of recurrent anaphylaxis. N Engl J Med 1984; 311:1236–1238.
8. Lavent J, Malat R, Smiejan JM, et al. Latex hypersensitivity after natural delivery. J Allergy Clin Immunol 1992; 88:779–780.
9. Turjanmaa K, Reunala T, Turmala R, et al. Allergy to latex gloves: unusual complication during deliver. Br Med J 1988; 297:1029.
10. Vyas GN, Perkins HA, Feudenberg HH. Anaphylactoid transfusion reactions associated with anti-IgA. Lancet 1968; 2:312–315.
11. Burks AW, Sampson H, Buckley RH. Anaphylactic reactions after gamma globulin administration in patients with hypogammaglobulinemia. Detection of IgE antibodies to IgA. N Engl J Med 1986; 314:560.
12. Chafee FH, Settipane G. Aspirin intolerance: I. Frequency in an allergic population. J Allergy Clin Immun 1974; 53:193–199.
13. Jurgens U, Christianson SC, Stevenson DD, Zurow BL. Arachidonic acid metabolism in monocytes of aspirin-sensitive asthmatic patients before and after oral aspirin challenge. J Allergy Clin Immunol 1992; 90:636.
14. Flacke JW, Flacke WE, Bloom B, et al. Histamine release by four narcotics: a double blind study in humans. Anesth Analgesia 1987; 66:723–730.
15. Lieberman P. Anaphylactoid reactions to radiocontrast material. Immunol Allergy Clin NA 1992; 12:649.

16. Brash RC, Rockoff SD, Kuhn C, et al. Contrast media as histamine liberators: II. Histamine release into venous plasma during intravenous pyelography in man. Invest Rad 1970; 6:510–513.

17. Horan RF, Sheffer AL. Exercise-induced anaphylaxis. Immunol Allergy Clin NA 1992; 12:559.

18. Smith HS, Hare M, Hoggarth C, et al. Delivery as a cause of exercise-induced anaphylactoid reaction: case report. Br J Obstet Gynecol 1985; 82:1196–1198.

19. Silverstein SR, Frommer DA, Dobozin B, et al. Celery-dependent exercise-induced anaphylaxis. J Emerg Med 1986; 4:195.

20. Patterson R, Hogan MB, Yarnold PR, Harris KE. Idiopathic anaphylaxis. Arch Intern Med 1995; 155:869.

21. Francis N. Abortion after grass pollen injection. J Allergy 1941; 12:559–563.

22. Stark BJ, Sullivan TJ. Biphasic and prolonged anaphylaxis. J Allergy Clin Immunol 1986; 78:76–83.

23. Douglas DM, Sukenick E, Andrade P, Brown JS. Biphasic systemic anaphylaxis; an inpatient and outpatient study. J Allergy Clin Immunol 1994; 93: 977–985.

24. Smith PL, Kagey-Sobotka A, Bleeker ER, Traystman R, Kaplan AP, Gralnick H, Valentine MD, Perlmutt S, Lichtenstein LM. Physiologic manifestations of human anaphylaxis. J Clin Invest 1980; 66:1072.

25. Schwartz LB, Yunginger JW, Miller J, Bokhari R, Dull D. Time course of appearance and disappearance of human mast cell tryptase in the circulation after anaphylaxis. J Clin Invest 1989; 83:1551.

26. Holgate ST, Robinson C, Church MK. Mediators of immediate hypersensitivity. In: Middleton E, Reed CE, Ellis EF, et al. eds. Allergy Principals and Practice. 4th ed. St. Louis: Mosby, 1993:267–301.

27. Sampson HA, Mendelson L, Rosen JP. Fatal and near-fatal anaphylactic reactions to food in children and adolescents. N Engl J Med 1992; 327:380–384.

28. Klein VR, Harris AD, Abraham RA, Niebyl JR. Fetal distress during a maternal systemic allergic reaction. Obstet Gynecol 1984; 64 (suppl):155–175.

29. Erasmus C, Blackwood W, Wilson J. Infantile multicystic encephalomalacia after maternal bee sting anaphylaxis during pregnancy. Arch Dis Child 1982; 57:785–787.

30. Entman SS, Maise KJ. Anaphylaxis in pregnancy. South Med J 1984; 77:402.

31. Gallagher JS. Anaphylaxis in pregnancy. Obstet Gynecol 1988; 71:491–493.

32. Zaloga GP, Delacey W, Holmboe E, et al. Glucagon reversal of hypotension in a case of anaphylactic shock. Ann Intern Med 1986; 105:65.

33. Sullivan TJ, Yecies LD, Shatz GS, et al. Desensitization of patients allergic to penicillin using orally administered beta-lactam antibiotics. J Allergy Clin Immunol 1982; 69:275.

34. Sweet JM, Stevenson DD, Simon RA, Mathison DA. Long-term effects of aspirin desensitization: treatment for aspirin-sensitive rhinosinusitis-asthma. J Allergy Clin Immunol 1990; 85:59.

35. Greenberger PA, Patterson R, Rodin TC. Two pretreatment regimens for high-risk patients receiving radiographic contrast media. J Allergy Clin Immunol 1984; 74:540.
36. Verresen L, Waer M, Vanrenterghem Y, et al. Angiotensin-converting enzyme inhibitors and anaphylactic reactions to high-flux membrane dialysis. Lancet 1990; 336:1360.

13

Cutaneous Diseases During Pregnancy

GARY M. WHITE and ROBERT S. ZEIGER

Kaiser Permanente Medical Center, San Diego
and University of California, San Diego, School of Medicine
La Jolla, California

I. Introduction

This chapter describes various skin changes which occur in the pregnant woman. It is clinically oriented, with an emphasis on diagnosis and treatment. It will first briefly describe the characteristic cutaneous changes that occur during pregnancy. Then it will give a general approach to itching in the pregnant woman. Next it will discuss the specific pregnancy-related dermatoses in greater detail. Finally, two common atopic cutaneous disorders (urticaria-angioedema and atopic dermatitis), a rare serious systemic disorder with dermatological manifestations (hereditary angioedema), and miscellaneous cutaneous immunological disorders will be highlighted. An understanding of these conditions will aid the concerned clinician in the care of pregnant women suffering from these maladies.

In this era of managed care, the question, "Does this patient need to be referred to dermatology?" may arise with regard to some of the diseases discussed here. In general, the pigmentary, vascular, and other characteristic changes that commonly occur in the skin of a pregnant woman (as described in Section II) do not necessitate referral. Most do not require intervention, and the treatment approach described for melasma postpartum is entirely adequate. On the other hand, it is usually prudent to refer in the setting of a changing or otherwise atypical pigmented lesion for further evaluation and possible excisional biopsy. Pruritus is so common in pregnancy that referral of every patient for this condition would be overly burdensome. It is hoped that the algorithmic approach to such a patient as described in Section III will help the nondermatologist identify the most common causes and effect a cure. Referral should then be made if the pruritus is treatment-resistant and/or the cause remains unknown. The diagnosis and treatment of cholestasis of pregnancy usually occurs outside of dermatology. Finally, each and every patient who is known or suspected to have either pemphigoid gestationis or impetigo herpetiformis should be managed jointly by the dermatologist and obstetrician.

II. Cutaneous Changes in Pregnancy

A. Pigmentation

Darkening of the skin is common during pregnancy and may affect the areolae, genitalia, groin, and axilla. A linear streak running vertically along the midline of the abdomen from the symphysis pubis to the xyphoid process is characteristic of linea nigra (Fig. 1). Resolution of most of these changes postpartum is expected, and no treatment is necessary.

Large, uniformly hyperpigmented, symmetric patches on the face, especially the forehead, temples, upper lip, and cheeks, is called melasma (Fig. 2). It seems to result from a combination of elevated female hormones and the sun. Sun protection during pregnancy will help minimize these changes. For melasma that is slow to fade after delivery, application *post-partum* of hydroquinone (e.g., 3–4% cream or gel topically, BID) and tretinoin (e.g., 0.025% gel applied topically qHS) for 4–6 months along with daily use of a sunscreen is appropriate.

Multiple nevomelanocytic nevi may appear during pregnancy, and preexisting moles may grow or change (Fig. 3). For example, nevi studied prospectively in familial atypical mole syndrome showed a much higher proclivity to change during pregnancy (1). There is no convincing data, however, that a pregnant woman is at increased risk for melanoma. As is true for any patient, a pigmented lesion with two or more of the ABCD criteria (*Asymmetric* shape, irregular *Border*, multiple *Colors*, *Diameter* > 6 mm) should be evaluated histologically, preferably after the lesion is completely excised. Many patients will complain of the growth of pedunculated, fleshy tags. These lesions are invariably benign and are best removed postpartum. It should be emphasised to the patient that it is the large, flat, dark brown or black moles that are most worrisome.

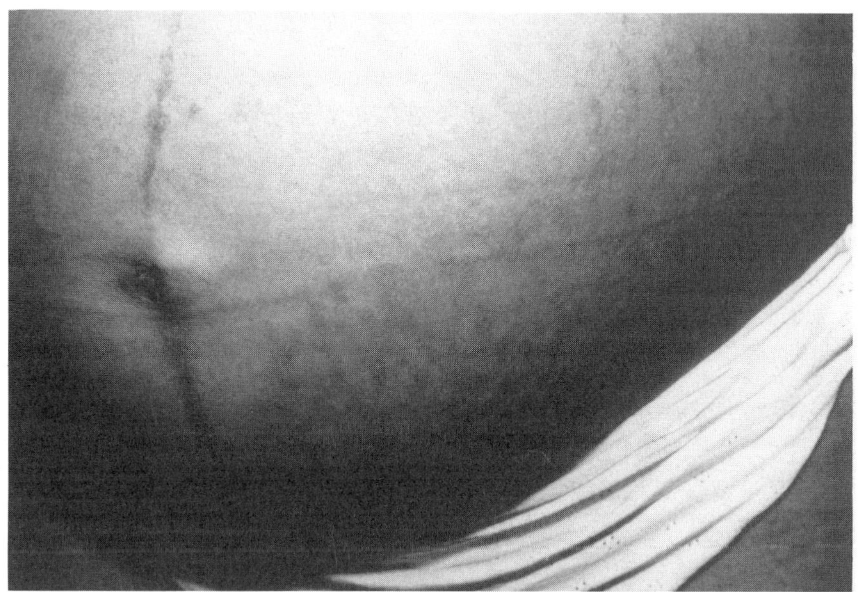

Figure 1 Linea nigra. A linear pigmented line runs vertically along the abdomen.

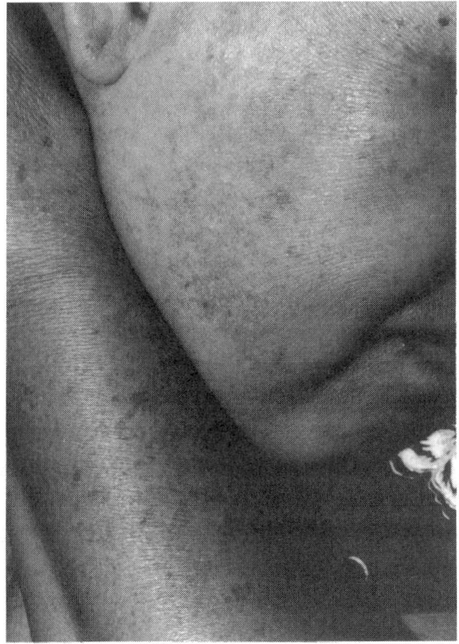

Figure 2 Melasma. Photodistributed pigmented patches seen on the right cheek and left arm.

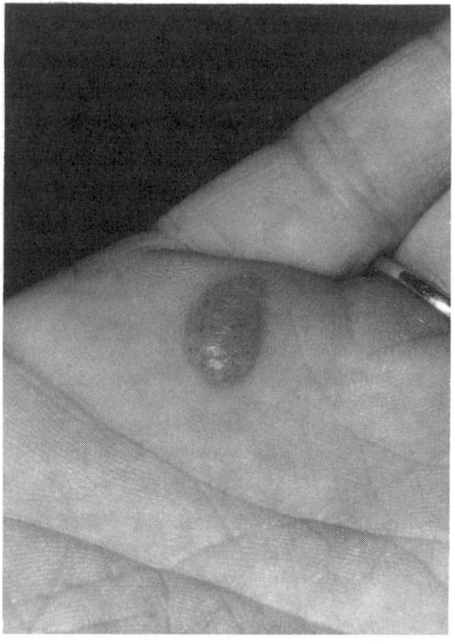

Figure 3   Nevus. A flat, histologically benign mole became raised and itchy during pregnancy.

B.   Vasculature

Palmar erythema is one of the manifestations of the increased vascularity that occurs in pregnancy. A solitary, growing, red, vascular papulonodule that bleeds easily most likely represents a pyogenic granuloma (Fig. 4). It may be shave-biopsied followed by curettage and electrodesiccation for both diagnosis and treatment. Recurrence after treatment is not uncommon. If this occurs, simple excision is usually effective. Arcades of telangiectasias eminating from a central vascular papule reminiscent of a spider's web is characteristic of the spider telangiectasia. It often remits after delivery. If it does not, light electrocautery of the central arteriole is usually adequate treatment.

C.   Other

Mechanical factors may cause stretching of the skin, inducing striae distensae, also known as striae gravidarum. They appear as multiple, linear, atrophic, pink, red, or purplish lesions on the abdomen. The breasts may

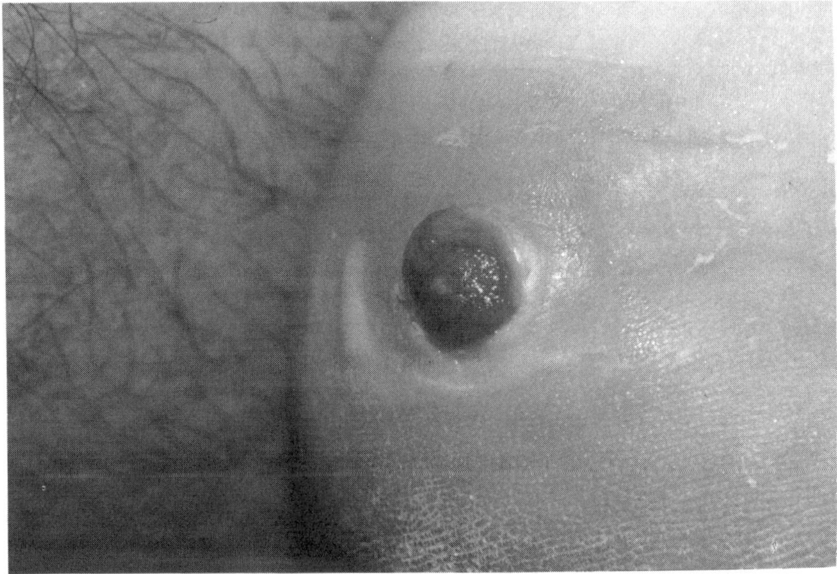

Figure 4 Pyogenic granuloma. A friable, intermittently bleeding, growing papulonodule on the heel.

be affected during lactation. Although many remedies abound, no treatment has been proven effective.

A mild frontoparietal recession and/or thinning of the hair occurs postpartum and is presumed to be a type of telogen effluvium. This disease, which is common postpartum but may occur approximately 2–3 months after virtually any major stress on the body, causes uniform shedding of a significant portion of hairs as new hairs replace them at the root. Patient education and reassurance is needed, as regrowth is expected.

III. Pruritus: General Aspects (Table 1)

As many as 18% of pregnant women will develop pruritus during pregnancy (2). The most important first step when faced with such a patient is to examine the skin for specific changes. The web spaces and wrists should be examined for the burrows of scabies (Fig. 5), and a mineral oil examination done if indicated (Fig. 6). The shins are a common place for the dry, white, scaly changes of xerosis (Fig. 7). The trunk and extremities should be examined for the red, scaly, eczematous changes of asteatotic

Table 1 Non-Pregnancy-Related Causes of Pruritis

Disease	Clinical findings	Confirmatory test	Treatment
Scabies	Diffuse itching ·Family members affected Burrows in web spaces/wrists	Mineral oil preparation shows mites, eggs, and/or feces under microscopic exam	Permethrin 5% overnight from the neck down for family. Precipitated sulfur for pregnant woman
Xerosis	Dry, cracked skin, often whitish, ashy, or fine scaly, particularly on the shins	Excessive bathing history	Heavy cream or ointment applied immediately after bathing daily
Eczema	Occurs often with xerosis, but skin areas are often reddened and inflammed Nummular eczema is round, red, and scaly	Excessive bathing history Atopy history frequent	Medium-potency topical steroid initially followed by above therapy for xerosis
Folliculitis	Multiple erythematous papules, some with surrounding pustules	Bacterial culture	Oral antibiotics as directed by culture

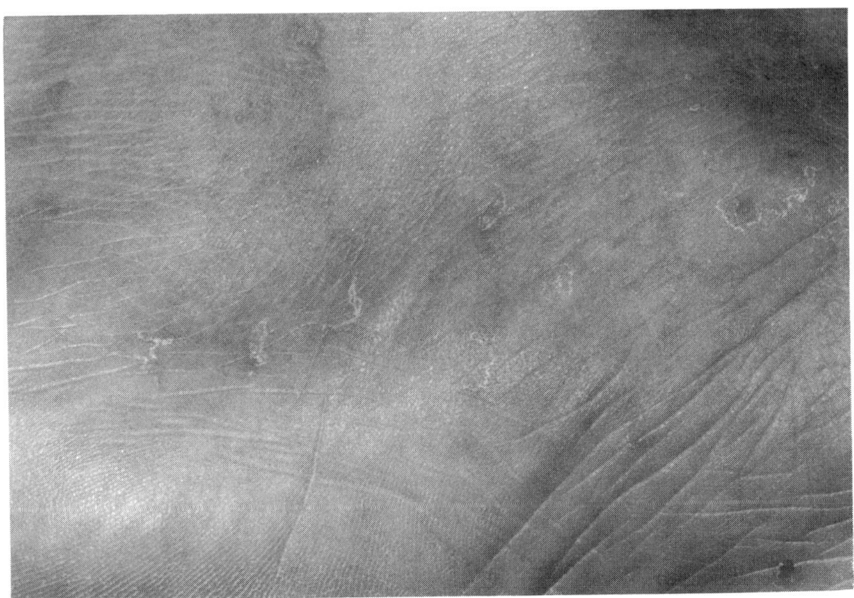

Figure 5 Scabies. Linear, serpiginous scales on the inner foot are the classic burrows of scabies.

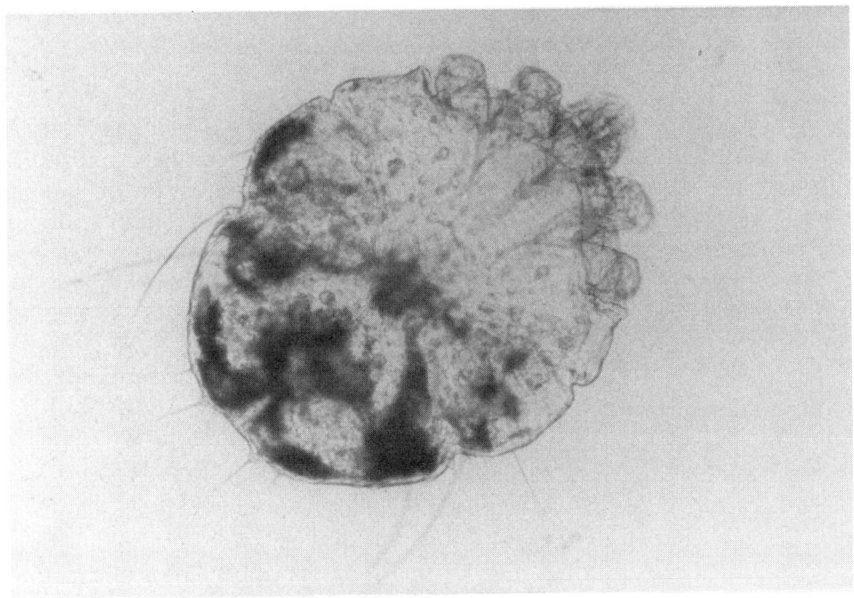

Figure 6 Scabies. Mineral oil examination shows the mite, confirming the diagnosis.

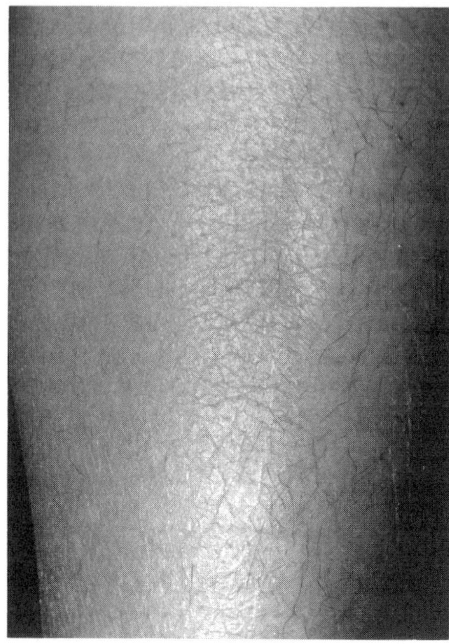

Figure 7 Xerosis. The anterior shins are a common area for the dry, cracked changes of xerosis.

eczema (Fig. 8). Pustules and 3- to 7-mm red, urticarial papules may signal a bacterial folliculitis. (It should also be remembered that bacterial folliculitis may be a primary occurrence or a secondary infection of another process, especially when that process is pruritic and excoriated.) Utilizing this approach, common entities which may occur coincidentally during pregnancy can be excluded.

The specific dermatoses of pregnancy, discussed in the next section, though uncommon, should be considered in the context of pruritus (Table 2). Pruritic urticarial papules and plaques of pregnancy (PUPPP) (Figs. 9 and 10) tend to occur in primigravidas, often begins in the stria of the abdomen, and spreads to the rest of the trunk and extremities. Pemphigoid gestationis (also known as herpes gestationis) (Figs. 11–13) typically presents as pruritic urticarial plaques which rapidly progress to vesicles and bulla. Finally, impetigo herpetiformis is a disease characterized by hundreds of uniform, sterile pustules located at the periphery of erythematous plaques (Fig. 14).

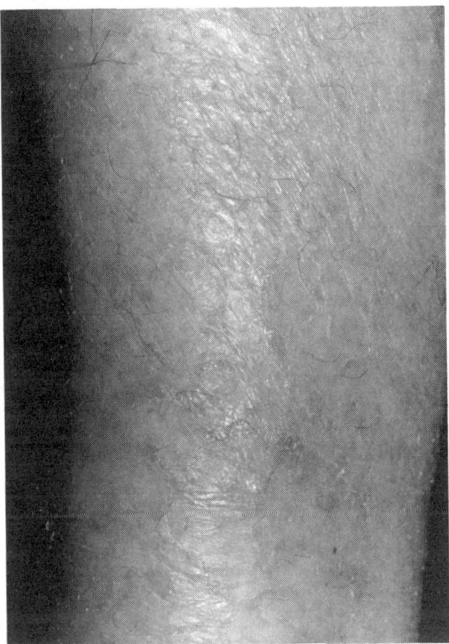

Figure 8 Asteatotic eczema. When the skin gets excessively dry, eczematous changes may occur, signaled by redness and inflammation.

If no specific rash or obvious cause of the itching is found and the patient is in the second half of pregnancy, serum transaminases and/or total biliary salts (postprandial optimal) may be obtained, as a small percentage of patients may have cholestasis. Finally, if no obvious cause of pruritus is found in the absence of significant skin changes, the working diagnosis of idiopathic pruritus may be used. If nonspecific erythematous papules and/or scattered sterile pustules are present, one may use the broad and poorly defined term, polymorphic eruption of pregnancy.

If the diagnosis is in doubt and/or a workup is in progress, one may temporize with regard to treatment by asking the patient to apply an emollient cream (not a lotion) after the bath or shower and at one other time during the day. If this fails to control the itch, an antihistamine such as pyribenzamine, followed, if unsuccessful, with hydroxyzine, diphenhydramine or chlorpheniramine, should be prescribed. It should be emphasized that an antihistamine's main benefit in the pruritic patient is via its ability to induce drowsiness. Nonsedating antihistamines have no role, owing to

Table 2 Dermatoses of Pregnancy

Parameter	PUPPP	Pemphigoid gestationis	Impetigo herpetiformis	Pruritis gravidarum
Prevalence	0.5%	0.002%	Very rare	0.02–2.4%
Onset	Third trimester	Second, third trimesters or postpartum	Second half of pregnancy	Second half of pregnancy
Gravidity predilection	Primigravidas	Multigravidas	None	None
Clinical lesions	Urticarial papules and plaques	Urticarial plaques, vesicles, and large bullae	Many sterile pustules on reddened plaques	Pruritus No primary lesion
Immunofluorescence	Negative	Positive for C_3 ± for IgG	Negative	Negative
Treatment	Topical steroids Antihistamines	Prednisone (40 mg/day to start, tapering as able); may require boost prior to possible postpartum flare	Prednisone (1 mg/kg/day); monitor fetal/maternal serum calcium	Emollients, if these fail, cholestryramine, ursodeoxycholic acid or rarely, dexamethasone
Complications	None Greater twinning	Frequent low-birth-weight and "small for date" infants; 5–10% of infants develop transient lesions	Maternal: hypocalcemia, tetany, delirium, seizures; Fetal: placental insufficiency, stillbirths, perinatal death	Fetal: distress, premature delivery, and perinatal mortality Greater twinning?
Postpartum prognosis	Clearing with rare recurrences	Flares and recurrences common	Clears but recurrences common	Clears but recurrences common

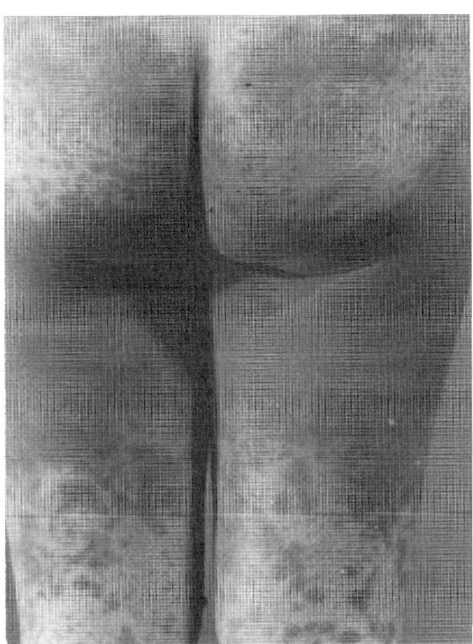

Figure 9 Pruritic urticarial papules and plaques of pregnancy: typical lesions on buttocks and thighs.

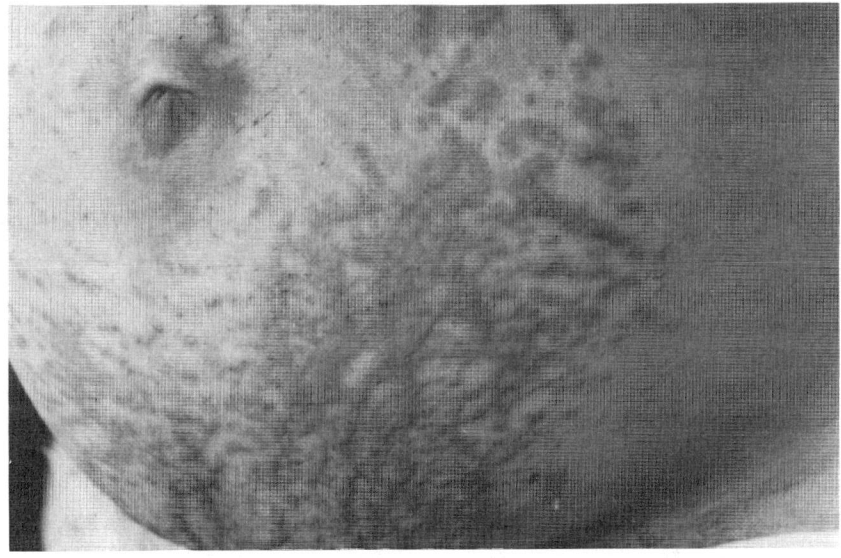

Figure 10 Erythematous urticarial plaques involving the striae atrophicae (distansae) in pruritic urticarial papules and plaques of pregnancy.

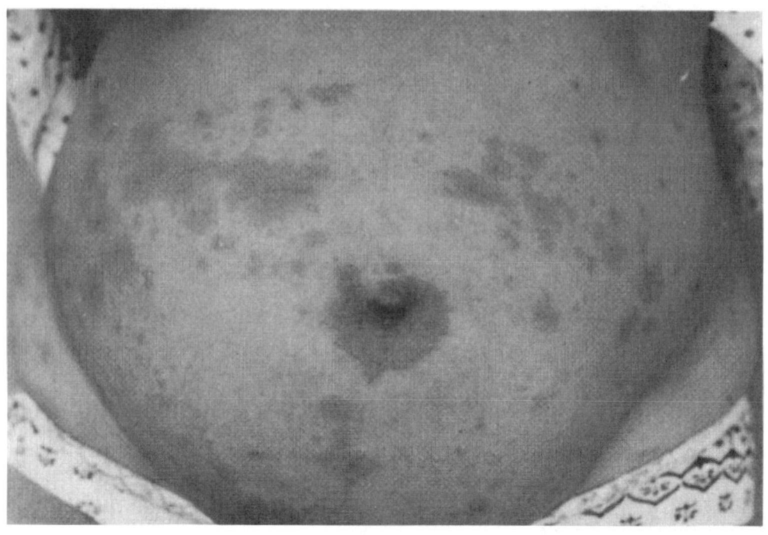

Figure 11 Pemphigoid gestationis: involvement of the umbilical area with typical urticarial plaques.

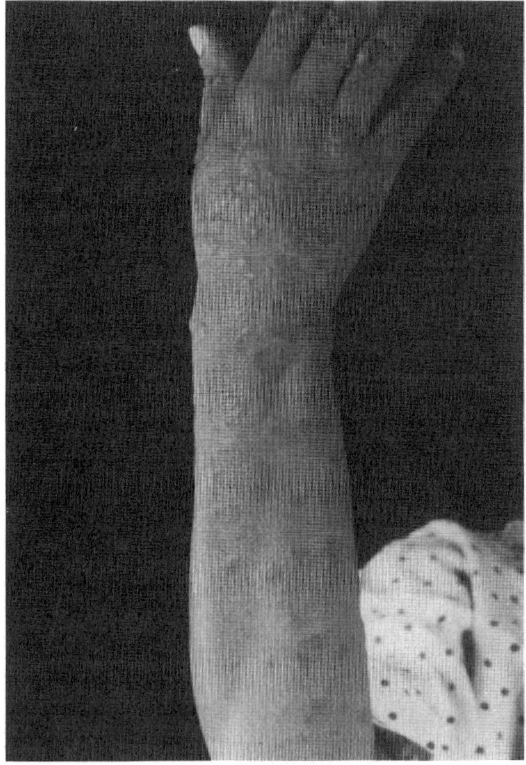

Figure 12 Pemphigoid gestationis: edematous papules and plaques.

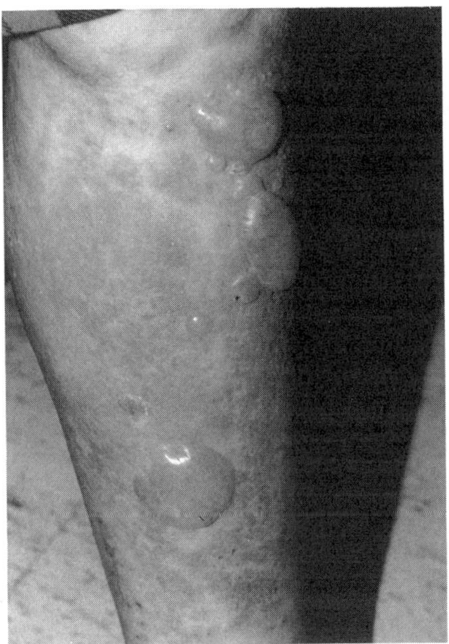

Figure 13 Pemphigoid gestationis. Tense blisters among urticarial plaques on the leg.

their undetermined safety during pregnancy and their ineffectiveness to induce somnolence. If eczematous changes are present, a low- to medium-potency topical steroid (e.g., hydrocortisone or 0.1% triamcinolone ointment) may be applied sparingly to selected areas BID (3).

IV. Pregnancy-Related Dermatoses (Table 2)

A. Pruritic Urticarial Papules and Plaques of Pregnancy

PUPPP occurs principally in primigravidas in the third trimester. It should be noted that some use the term "polymorphic eruption of pregnancy" in this condition (4). Urticarial, papular, and polycyclic lesions classically begin in the abdominal stria but then may spread to the trunk, arms, thighs, and buttocks (Figs. 9 and 10). Involvement above the breasts is uncommon. The lesions are usually very pruritic. PUPPP does not routinely flare postpartum, as does pemphigoid gestationis (PG). PUPPP has no tendency to recur in subsequent pregnancies. Maternal-fetal weight gain and the incidence of twins appears to be increased (5), but there is no increased fetal

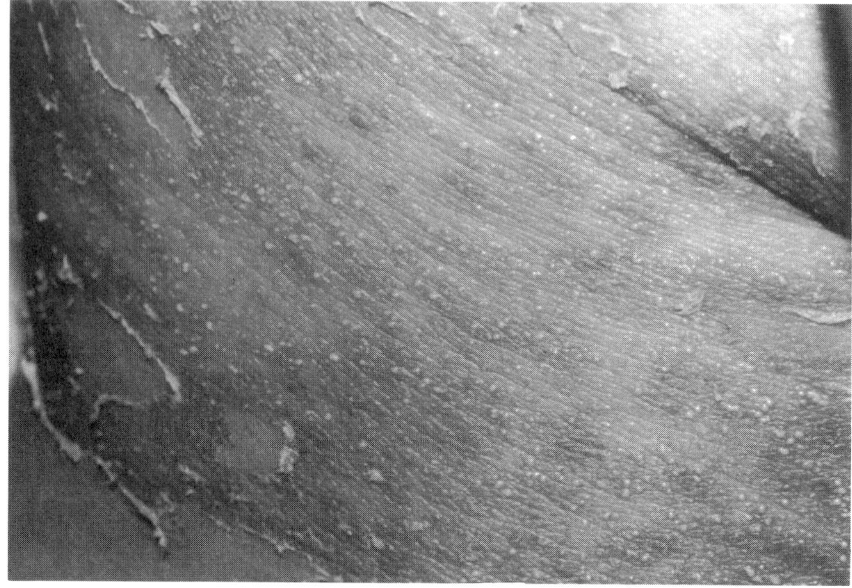

Figure 14 Impetigo herpetiformis. Sterile pustules on an erythematous background.

morbidity or mortality. In cases where pemphigoid gestationis is a consideration, direct immunofluorescence (DIF) of a skin biopsy should be performed. DIF is positive in PG but negative in PUPPP.

With regard to treatment, a medium- to high-potency topical steroid should be tried, and antihistamines appropriate for pregnancy may provide some relief. Systemic steroids may be needed (6). Therapeutic caesarian section has been reported on rare occasions near term in an attempt to relieve the severe intractable pruritus of PUPPP (7).

B. Pemphigoid Gestationis

Pemphigoid gestationis (PG), also known as herpes gestationis, is an uncommon, autoimmune, pregnancy-related, bullous eruption that is unrelated to any viral infection. It has its onset most commonly in the second and third trimester but may occur in the first or immediately postpartum (8). The skin lesions of PG often begin on the abdomen and include urticarial plaques, vesicles, and frank bulla (Figs. 10–13). Constitutional symptoms, e.g., fever, nausea, and malaise, may accompany the skin changes. The lesions may then extend to the upper thighs, arms, and legs, and finally to the palms and soles. Facial and oral mucosal involvement are uncommon. Pruritus may be significant. If there is any suggestion of pemphigoid gestationis, a skin biopsy with immunofluorescence is in order.

Histological examination of a vesicle or bulla shows subepidermal separation accompanied by a superficial and deep perivascular lymphohistiocytic infiltrate with eosinophils. DIF, a necessary diagnostic test to confirm PG, is positive in PG and reveals C3 along the basement membrane zone. IgG may or may not be present.

Flares have been noted after delivery, with the resumption of menses, ovulation, or beginning oral contraceptives (9). PG tends to recur in subsequent pregnancies but may not. Some studies have shown a tendency toward low-birth-weight and "small for dates" infants (10), with the presumed increased risk of fetal morbidity and mortality, although this conclusion is still controversial. The neonate presents with skin lesions of PG with a 5–10% occurrence rate. Of note, there is no evidence for a specific pregnancy-related entity characterized by circulating anti-BMZ IgM antibodies (11), as previously suggested.

With regard to pathophysiology, PG is an autoimmune disorder in which the body attacks the basement membrane zone (BMZ)—the junction between the epidermis and the dermis. Destruction of this area leads to subepidermal blistering. This initial attack on the BMZ is by a complement-fixing autoantibody (previously known as the herpes gestationis factor). Western blot analysis has demonstrated circulating IgG antibodies, mainly of the IgG1 subclass (12), which react primarily with an antigen of 180-kDa molecular weight, although a few patients' sera bind to a 220-kDa protein (13), and one patient's, a 200-kDa antigen (14). The 180-kDa antigen is a transmembrane protein associated with the hemidesmosomal plaque. The 220-kDa protein is the major antigen in bullous pemphigoid (BP) and represents a noncollagenous intracellular glycoprotein also associated with the hemidesmosomal plaque. The 200-kDa antigen is not as well characterized but has previously been described in BP and lichen planus pemphigoides. A recent study has shown that some PG and BP autoantibodies recognize a common antigenic site on the BP 180-kDa ectodomain (15). Why does PG arise in pregnancy? It appears that a placental antigen which cross-reacts with the skin triggers the immune response. Ortonne et al., for example, were able to demonstrate that the herpes gestationis factor was bound to the BMZ of the amnion (16).

With regard to treatment, antihistamines and potent topical steroids (beginning, for example, with 0.1% triamcinalone ointment BID and increasing as needed) should be tried initially. Systemic steroids are usually needed in the majority, however—e.g., prednisone, 40 mg/day initially, then tapered. Reports suggest that many patients can control their disease with 10–20 mg/day. The dose may be increased in anticipation of a post-partum flare (17). Plasmapheresis has been performed in severe cases (18).

C. Impetigo Herpetiformis

Impetigo herpetiformis (IH) has been called pustular psoriasis of pregnancy because of its resemblance clinically and histologically to pustular psoriasis (of von Zumbusch), although no personal or family history of psoriasis is usually found. The patient experiences the onset of innumerable superficial pustules studded on the periphery of erythematous plaques (Fig. 14). Lesions enlarge through peripheral extension. Nearly the entire cutaneous surface may become involved, as well as the oral and esophogeal mucosa. Fever, nausea, and diarrhea may accompany the skin changes. The pustules are initially sterile but may become secondarily infected. They may rupture, leading to limited or widespread erosions. Onset is typically in the third trimester, and it may recur with subsequent pregnancies. Histological examination shows intraepidermal pustule formation with a neutrophilic infiltrate.

Hypocalcemia has been reported to accompany IH and may be a precipitating factor (1). Tetany, delirium, and convulsions may occur. Stillbirths, placental insufficiency, and perinatal death are associated fetal complications. A flare of this disease precipitated by oral contraceptives has been reported (19).

With regard to treatment, the pustules should be cultured to rule out other diseases or secondary infection. Fetal status and maternal serum calcium levels should both be closely followed. Fluid replacement may be needed. A systemic corticosteroid (e.g., prednisone, 1 mg/kg/day) is usually begun, although UVB phototherapy is an alternative. In severe cases, therapeutic abortion, induction of labor and delivery (20), or caesaeran section (19) has been necessary. The disease usually remits after delivery.

D. Cholestasis of Pregnancy

Also known as pruritus gravidarum, cholestasis of pregnancy is characterized by generalized pruritus in the second half of pregnancy in the absence of any primary skin lesion. The disease is particularly common among Chileans (21). Transaminases and serum bile acids (postprandial measurement may be more sensitive) are elevated, and jaundice may develop (22). Associated complications include fetal distress, premature delivery, and perinatal mortality. The incidence of twins is significantly elevated (4). The disease may recur with subsequent pregnancies.

Because the cholestasis remits soon after delivery, interventions which ease the pruritus, such as antihistamines and emollients, may be all the treatment that is needed. If these fail, cholestyramine (e.g., 4 g, 2–3/ day), which binds bile salts in the gut lumen, has been used. Preliminary studies on the use of ursodeoxycholic acid (23) as well as dexamethasone (24) have been quite favorable. Close fetal monitoring is important.

E. Miscellaneous Eruptions of Pregnancy

Several other pruritic skin rashes under various names have been reported to occur during pregnancy. They include polymorphic eruption of pregnancy, prurigo of pregnancy, papular dermatitis of pregnancy, and pruritic folliculitis of pregnancy. The specific diagnostic criteria for these diseases is unclear. As stated above, this author favors using the term *polymorphic eruption of pregnancy* as a broad and all-encompassing term for this poorly defined category. As also noted above, some use the term *polymorphic eruption of pregnancy* to denote PUPPP (4).

V. Urticaria and Angioedema

Urticaria represents a common dermatological response to diverse physical, allergic, chemical, infectious, and emotional triggers, manifesting as circumscribed elevated pruritic and erythematous lesions. Edema of the superficial dermis characterizes the lesion. *Angioedema* results from extension of this edema to deeper areas of the dermis, subcutaneous tissue, and/or submucosa (25). For both urticaria and angioedema, convention defines acute disease as persistence of symptoms for less than 6 weeks and chronic as that persisting longer.

A. Incidence, Etiology, and Pathophysiology

Although at least one episode of urticaria is common in up to 20% of persons, chronic or recurrent symptoms are uncommon, occurring with a cumulative prevalence of less than 2% (25). For chronic urticaria/angioedema, causation remains unknown in over 90% of cases, leading to the classification of idiopathic urticaria/angioedema. During pregnancy, urticaria/angioedema can occur from any of the causes, agents, and mechanisms responsible during the nonpregnant state (Table 3). On the other hand, urticaria/angioedema may be limited to pregnancy and reoccur with subsequent pregnancies. This chronic urticaria/angioedema syndrome of pregnancy which occurred in 3 or 438 (0.5% incidence) consecutive pregnancies, possibly may be caused by allergic sensitization to endogenous hormones, particularly progesterone (26). As described above, sensitivity to progesterone during pregnancy has been termed *autoimmune progester-*

Table 3 Common Causes of Urticaria/Angioedema

IgE-mediated mechanisms
  Antibiotics (particularly penicillins and sulfonanides)
  Foreign proteins (heterologous sera, ACTH, hormones, enzymes, and venom)
  Therapeutic agents (allergen extracts, vaccines, muscle relaxants, ethylene ox-
    ide, latex, thiopental)
  Foods (peanuts, nuts, seeds, fish, shellfish, celery, fresh fruits, legumes, egg,
    milk)
Immune complex or complement-mediated mechanisms
  Blood products (whole blood, plasma, cyroprecipitate, immunoglobulin)
  Methotrexate
  Infections (bacterial, fungal, viral, helminthic)
Arachidonic acid metabolism-modulating agents
  Aspirin
  Nonsteroidal antiinflammatory drugs (NSAIDs)
Direct mediator-releasing agents
  Drugs (opiates. curare, contrast media, dextran, mannitol, pentamidine, poly-
    myxin B, and thiamine)
  Exercise
  Physical forces (cholinergic, trauma, pressure, stroking, water, heat, cold, and
    sun)
IgG-anti FcεRI antibodies
Hereditary conditions
  Hereditary angioedema (HAE)
  Familial cold urticaria
  Hereditary vibratory angioedema
  C3b inactivator deficiency
  Deafness, limb pain and urticaria with amyloidosis
Urticaria pigmentosa
  Cutaneous mastocytosis
  Systemic mastocytosis

---

one dermatitis of pregnancy since 1971, appearing as a papulopustular
eruption associated with transient arthritis, peripheral and tissue eosinophilia, miscarriage, and delayed intradermal sensitivity to aqueous progesterone (27). Moreover, administration of progesterone intramuscularly in
affected patients reproduces symptoms within 1 hr; in contrast, cyclically
administered conjugated estrogen appears to control the urticaria (27). As
noted above, progesterone injection has also been implicated in anaphylaxis during pregnancy (27).

B. Diagnosis

The cause of urticaria/angioedema, if one is to be found, can be elicited by a thorough history and careful physical examination. Should a cause not be readily identified, laboratory evaluation of chronic urticaria/angioedema should be limited to screening with a CBC, urinary analysis, and ESR. Diagnostic tests reserved for confirmation of diagnostic suspicions are noted in Table 4. Latex hypersensitivity reactions have recently been described after both natural delivery and caesarean section (28).

One must differentiate gestational urticaria/angioedema from such dermatological entities as (a) autoimmune progesterone dermatitis of pregnancy, (b) polymorphic eruptions of pregnancy, (c) other pruritic dermatoses of pregnancy, and (d) laryngopathia gravidarum. The first three disorders are discussed above and summarized in Table 2.

Laryngopathia gravidarum (LG) appears as an acute or chronic, noninfectious, somewhat inflammatory disorder of laryngeal tissue seen in the multigravida (29). Although the acute form presents prior to parturition, the chronic entity occurs throughout pregnancy, recurring with subsequent pregnancies. Spontaneous resolution occurs postpartum with both forms.

Table 4 Diagnostic Tests for Urticaria/Angioedema During Pregnancy

Suspected disorder	Procedure
Food, drug, inhalant allergy	Diary, avoidance trial, RAST/CAP test
Dermographism	Stroke skin with tongue blade
Cold urticaria	Ice cube on forearm for 5 min Cryoglobulin/cryofibrinogen
Solar urticaria	Expose skin to light wavelengths Porphyrins
Vibratory urticaria	Vortex skin for 4 min
Pressure urticaria	Weights to extremity for 10 min
Aquagenic urticaria	Expose hand to tap water at varying temperatures
Exercise	History
Infectious	Appropriate cultures/titers, stool for ova/parasites
Cutaneous vasculitis	Sed rate, antimicrosomal antibody, CH_{50}, skin/tissue biopsy with immunofluorescence, immunoglobulins
Hereditary angioedema (HAE)	Screening C_4 level, diagnostic C1-INH functional level

Typical symptoms of LG include (a) progressive dyspnea, sporadically requiring artificial ventilation, (b) hoarseness, (c) nonfebrile sore throat and odynophagia without fever, (d) malaise, (e) lymphadenopathy, (f) cough, and (g) elevated erythrocyte sedimentation rate (40–60 mm/hr) and mild leukocytosis. Patchy localized edema and congestion are noted in the larynx and frequently the epiglottis, but not the aryepiglottic folds, arytenoids, vestibular region, or true vocal cords. Microscopic abnormalities are limited to the submucosa, which appears edematous due to infiltration with lymphocytes and plasma cells. The pathogenesis of LG remains speculative, but owing to its resolution postpartum, pregnancy hormones have been implicated in its causation (29).

C. Prevention and Treatment

Identification and avoidance of triggering agents or causes (Table 3) remain the hallmark of treatment in order to prevent symptoms and obviate pharmacological intervention. Oral antihistamines should be used at the lowest effective dosage if clinically indicated. Based on the available data (29a), chlorpheniramine (4 mg up to every 4 hours or 8–12 mg slow-release up to twice a day) would be considered first followed by tripelennamine (25–50 mg every 6 hours or 100 mg sustained-release twice a day). If these are not effective, hydroxyzine (10–50 mg at the hour of sleep) could be considered, ideally after the first trimester. If sedation is a problem, second generation antihistamines (cetirizine, loratadine or terfenadine) could be considered after the first trimester (29a). Systemic corticosteroids occasionally are required for severe recalcitrant urticaria or angioedema. Acute, severe urticaria/angioedema requires aggressive therapy modeled after that used for anaphylaxis and starting with epinephrine (Chapter 12).

VI. Hereditary Angioedema

A. Incidence, Etiology, and Etiology

Hereditary angioedema (HAE) is a rare (estimated prevalence of 1:50,000 in the general population) (30), autosomal-dominantly transmitted systemic disorder caused by mutations within the C1-INH (inhibitor) gene leading to plasma deficiency of C1-INH (30–32). Two phenotypic variants exist in HAE: (a) type I (85% prevalence) has both low antigenic and functional levels of a normal C1-INH and (b) type II (15% prevalence) possesses normal or elevated antigenic levels of a dysfunctional mutant protein and lower levels of functional protein (30,31). C1-INH deficiency leads to unregulated proteolytic activation in the complement and kallikrein systems. In the complement system, the first component of complement (C1) activation is not controlled, leading to consumption of C4 and C2. Recent data suggest that the resulting formation of kininlike fragments and other pharmacologically active mediators trigger the myriad of clinical signs and symptoms of HAE. These include attacks of nonpruritic and nonurticarial angioedema of the subcutaneous tissue and submucosa of the extremities, abdomen, lips and face, and larynx, the frequency of which ranges from every few days to once a year (30,31). Severe abdominal colic, vomiting, and guarding without fever, leukocytosis, elevated sedimentation rate, or rigidity typically occur due to edematous involvement of the bowel wall. Differentiation of HAE-induced abdominal crises from a surgical or obstetric abdominal emergency is crucial to prevent needless exploratory surgery. HAE-induced laryngeal edema causes hoarseness, dysphagia, and occasionally life-threatening upper airway obstruction. While episodes are often sporadic, they may be often triggered by trauma (minor or major dental, surgical, and accidental), stress, infections, and wide fluctuations in temperature. A familial pattern is typical but not invariable.

During pregnancy, 23 of 25 pregnant women with HAE reported markedly fewer or an absence of attacks from the 4th to 9th months. Moreover, 10 women with a total of 25 pregnancies did not experience angioedema during vaginal delivery despite its traumatic potential (31). This favorable experience must be tempered by observations which report that (a) 4 of 7 deaths occurring in 21 families with HAE totaling 92 involved individuals happened during childbirth (33); (b) recurrent worsening occurred during multiple pregnancies (34); (c) postpartum exacerbations occur (34); (d) symptoms may diminish or intensify during pregnancy (31); and (e) protein S deficiency secondary to HAE and pregnancy may cause severe cutaneous necrosis (35). In addition, tragically, HAE has triggered localized perineal swelling after delivery, resulting in secondary irreversible shock and death (36). Moreover, a primary attack of HAE on the third postpartum day, precipitated by a spontaneous vaginal delivery, has been described recently, illustrating the importance of maintaining a high level of suspicion for emergence of this condition when evaluating labial swelling in the puerperium (37). HAE and selective IgA deficiency have been described to coexist during pregnancy, raising the potential for complications from either condition (38).

B. Genetics

HAE may be a recent disorder, since informative genealogical trees have generally found fewer than three generations involved. Moreover, up to 20% of affected kindreds may be new mutations, since parental analyses have frequently found both parents unaffected (30). HAE results from many mutations of a single gene of 1.7×10^4 base pairs on chromosome 11, consisting of 8 exons and 7 introns, which encodes for C1-INH, a SERPIN (serum protease inhibitor) protein (39). The C1-INH gene expression is enhanced and regulated by many elements, including androgens, interferon-γ, tumor necrosis factor-α, interleukin-6, and monocyte colony-stimulating factor (39). The isolation and cloning of the C1-INH gene has heralded a better understanding of the molecular biology of HAE, reviewed extensively recently (40–42). Type I HAE appears to be caused by gross deletions or insertions (or both) into exon IV and VII and its flanking introns, regions that are high in content of a family of sequences known as Alu repeats repeated in tandem, due to susceptibility of cleavage of the restriction enzyme isolated from *Arthrobacter luteus*. Type II HAE mutations generally involve point mutations in the codon from the reactive center in exon VIII of the C1-INH gene, which encodes for the arginine residue 444 at the reactive center of the protein (40–42). At this time almost 30 distinct mutations have been identified that cause type I HAE and about 10 responsible for type II HAE; more mutations are expected.

C. Diagnosis

Clinical Evaluation

HAE can be diagnosed based on clinical, demographic, and laboratory features. Clinically affected individuals present with a personal and/or family history of recurrent noninflammatory and nonurticarial edema of three predominant areas: (a) subcutaneous tissue (typically face, hand, arms, legs, genitalia, and buttocks) (Fig. 15); (b) abdominal viscera (stomach, gut, and bladder); and (c) the upper airway (mouth, tongue, and larynx) (30,31). These subcutaneous attacks generally persist for 2–5 days. Typical manifestations of allergic angioedema, as noted above, such as periorbital edema, are uncommon in HAE. The abdominal attacks, characterized by recalcitrant and continuous pain and vomiting without diarrhea, typically are particularly common in HAE (~75% incidence), and help to differentiate HAE from other forms of angioedema in which abdominal symptoms are absent. Laryngeal edema, which responds poorly to antianaphylaxis measures, indicates HAE until proven otherwise.

A recent syndrome experienced by two sisters who experience severe attacks of angioedema and some urticaria only with oral contraceptive ingestion and during pregnancy must be distinguished from HAE. Although several features of this syndrome resemble HAE, such as laryngeal edema, associated abdominal colic and nausea, exacerbation by trauma, and resistance to antihistamine and corticosteroid therapy, C1-INH levels and other complement components are consistently normal. The syndrome was re-

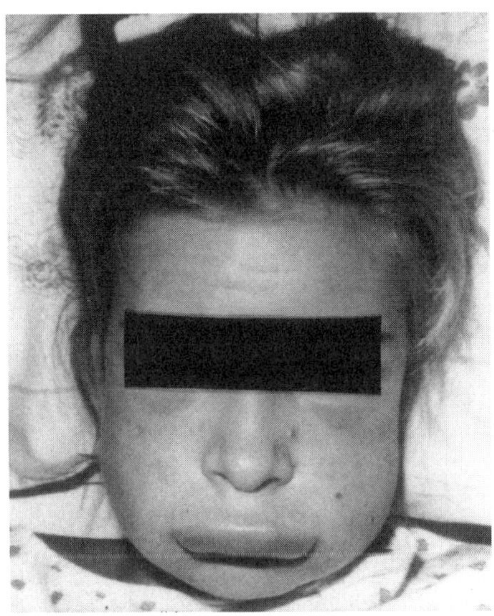

Figure 15 Hereditary angioedema. Typical facial and lip subcutaneous swelling during an acute attack. (Courtesy of Bruce Zuraw, MD.)

produced in one patient by challenge with estrogen but not with progesterone. In addition to supportive treatment of episodes, aminocaproic acid may have been beneficial in one sister, while epinephrine inhalation improved the oral swelling of the other sister (34).

Laboratory Evaluation

Initial laboratory screening includes determination of C4 levels, which are characteristically diminished between attacks (<2 SD from normal) and near absent during active episodes in both types I and II HAE. Definitive diagnosis of HAE rests with determination of C1-INH level functionally, which is <2 SD or below 40% of normal in both types of HAE. Type II HAE is distinguished from type I HAE by possessing normal or higher-than-normal levels of antigenic C1-INH on immunochemical measurement (30,31). Pregnancy has been associated with lower C1-INH levels in 3 of 23 patients (43), which returned to normal levels postpartum (34,44). These mild reductions of C1-INH levels in normal pregnancy are further lowered in patients experiencing eclampsia and preeclampsia during the third trimester (45). These reductions in C1-INH levels which occur during pregnancy (also after estrogen administration), due in part to hemodilution as well as hormonal effects, should preclude the making of a definitive initial diagnosis of HAE during pregnancy unless it is confirmed by further sophisticated tests such as complement or plasma contact system activation (cleaved) products, DNA analyses, or confirmatory C1-INH levels postpartum. Recently, investigation of a woman with pregnancy-associated HAE attacks noted activation of her plasma contact system which led to near-absent serum levels of high-molecular-weight kininogen (HMWK) and replacement by a lower-molecular-weight cleaved product (46). Determination of normal levels of HMWK help to confirm the absence of HAE in 20 normal pregnancies unaffected by HAE, but in which ~50% evidenced low C1-INH levels (45). Further confirmation of the sensitivity and specificity of HMWK in ruling out HAE during pregnancy is needed. Research laboratories can further characterize the genetic defect in individuals, if necessary.

D. Prevention and Treatment

Prevention of HAE Attacks

The prevention of HAE rests with avoiding its typical reported triggers, including trauma, surgery, dental procedures, and stress. Angiotensin-converting enzyme inhibitors are contraindicated in HAE patients, since such agents may potentiate the increased kininlike activity noted in HAE (47). Preventive pharmacotherapy of HAE must be individualized during pregnancy, as in the nonpregnant women. Attenuated androgen prophylaxis (based on dose titration of danazol or stanozolol to the minimum level necessary to prevent HAE attacks), through stimulation of C1-INH synthesis by the one normal gene, represents the treatment of choice in the *nonpregnant* women experiencing life-threatening HAE attacks. Androgen prophylaxis is generally not required nor warranted for the treatment of HAE during pregnancy, since the potential for drug-related fetal damage (48), including female masculination and pseudohermaphroditism and spontaneous abortion, are common (49). Effective contraception during androgen therapy is mandatory for women of child-bearing potential with HAE, to prevent these adverse fetal effects from occurring during early pregnancy, prior to confirmation of pregnancy. Women with HAE generally tolerate oral contraceptives, although estrogens may adversely affect some (50). Progestational agents are the hormonal contraceptives of choice in women with HAE, since these agents may help raise C1-INH levels. Optimally, conception should be attempted only after successful discontinuation of androgen prophylaxis.

Potential for HAE attacks following elective surgeries during pregnancy can be prevented by pretreatment with (a) C1-INH concentrate, if available (see below), (b) attenuated androgens (danazol 600 mg daily or stanozolol 6 mg daily for 6 days prior to and 3 days postsurgery), or (c) 2 units of fresh frozen plasma 24 hr prior to the procedure. Vaginal deliveries appear safe for HAE patients (31), while epidural anesthesia has been effective and is not likely to induce HAE (51). Caesarean section, on the other hand, requires preoperative transfusion of two units of fresh frozen plasma or C1-INH concentrate, if available (see below) to prevent attacks. Regional is preferred to general anesthesia in order to avoid endotracheal intubation, which could trigger laryngeal edema.

Treatment of Acute Attacks

HAE-induced abdominal pain during pregnancy must be carefully differentiated from a surgical or obstetrical abdominal emergency. It must be clearly understood that surgical exploration may precipitate HAE and should require prophylactic 2 units of fresh frozen plasma (48) or C1-INH concentrate (52–54). HAE-induced life-threatening laryngeal edema during pregnancy requires rapid and aggressive therapy. Standard emergent airway management, including intubation or tracheostomy, may be necessary and life-preserving. Generous intravenous fluid replacement may be needed to reverse hypovolemia induced by abdominal crises. Narcotics for severe pain should be considered.

The best acute pharmacotherapy for HAE and the future drug of choice in pregnant women with HAE rests with purified C1-INH (or recombinant human C1-INH, in the future), but this presently is an investigational drug. C1-INH is available in the United States through compassionate use (Immuno Clinical Research Corp, 750 Lexington Ave, New York, NY, 10022, 800–621–9824) or research centers. Administration of 1000 to 1500 units of C1-INH concentrate with 1 unit corresponding to the amount of C1-INH found in 1 ml of normal human plasma has been effective in reversing severe laryngeal edema and abdominal attacks in from 30 to 60 min and 60 to 120 min, respectively, in 82 of 83 infusions of HAE patients (30). Prior to 1986, non-A, non-B hepatitis occurred in some patients receiving C1-INH concentrate, but improved preparation of the concentrate, including vapor heating and PCR for HIV and hepatitis B and C, have prevented these infections (30). Fresh frozen plasma infusion should be avoided, since it may provide proportionally greater amounts of substrate (which could potentiate the attack) than C1-INH. The antifibrinolytic agent, epsilon aminocaproic acid (Amicar), due to its potential thrombogenic properties, should generally be avoided during pregnancy. The usual therapies for angioedema (epinephrine, antihistamines, and corticosteorids) typically are ineffective in HAE attacks; although epinephrine may be beneficial in an unusual HAE patient. Postpartum episodes of HAE must be recognized rapidly and aggressive therapy instituted, including large-volume fluid replacement of third-space losses and reinstitution of androgenic therapy, if indicated.

VII. Atopic Dermatitis

A. Incidence, Etiology, and Pathophysiology

Of 117 women with mild to severe atopic dermatitis, pregnancy was associated with clearing or definite improvement in 3% and definite exacerbation in 1% (55). In contrast, in a recent questionnaire-based study, atopic dermatitis was reported to worsen in 52%, improve in 24%, and remain unchanged in 24% of 50 women during 88 full-term pregnancies. Moreover, worsening of atopic dermatitis occurred by 20 weeks in 80% of those women reporting worsening of atopic dermatitis during pregnancy (56). Prospective natural history studies with clinical scoring are necessary to ascertain the real effect of pregnancy on atopic dermatitis.

The characteristic features of atopic dermatitis (Fig. 16), an eczematous disorder which occurs in about 1–2% of adults, include (a) pruritus, (b) chronicity, (c) typical morphology and distribution, and (d) a genetic predilection to develop allergic rhinitis, asthma, and food allergy. The spectrum of symptoms may extend from a mild, isolated, small, circumscribed patch (nummular eczema) to severe, generalized, exfoliative erythroderma. The acute condition evidences erythema, dermal edema, excoriations, and weeping, while the chronic stage reveals scaling, thickening, hyperpigmentation, and fissuring. The antecubital and popliteal fossae, neck, upper trunk, perioral and periorbital areas, and hands represent areas of predilection in adults (57).

Up to 70–80% of subjects with atopic dermatitis evidence elevated serum IgE levels, peripheral eosinophilia, and often specific IgE to foods (the majority during infancy) and inhalants, which historically may trigger the cutaneous symptoms. Alterations in cell-mediated immunity, reduced T lymphocytes, loss of circulating suppressor-cytotoxic T cells, increased numbers of circulating FcεRII mononuclear cells, depressed neutrophilic and mononuclear cell chemotactic activity, and elevated mononuclear cell phosphodiesterase activity have been observed to varying degrees in patients with atopic dermatitis (58). Abnormal cutaneous findings frequently include white dermographism (a white line rather than a wheal in response to skin stroking), a greater dermal constrictor response to cold, reduced whealing to histamine, reduced delayed hypersensitivity reactions upon

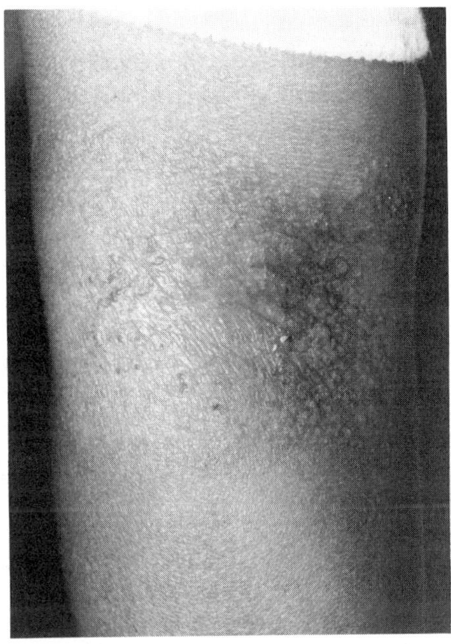

Figure 16 Atopic dermatitis. Erythematous, scaly lesions with predilection to the flexor surface.

patch testing, exaggerated response to methacholine, pallor instead of erythema to nicotinic acid, diminished reactions to beta-adrenergic stimulation, and increased dermal mast cells. These findings may also be observed, though less frequently, in patients with other chronic dermatoses. The pathogenesis of atopic dermatitis is thought to involve an abnormal immunological mechanism in atopics, which leads to the cutaneous release from mast cells of such mediators as histamine, eosinophilic chemotactic factors, leukotrienes, and others (58). Eczematous lesions evidence, depending on the severity of involvement, varying degrees of irregular parakeratosis and hyperkeratosis with irregular acanthosis and spongiosis. Recently, increased numbers of dendritic Langerhans' cells were found in chronic lesions; an elevated proportion of T-helper to T-suppressor lymphocytes was seen in dermal infiltrates; greater numbers of mast cells but not basophils were observed in lesions; and large quantities of eosinophil basic protein, a potentially toxic product of eosinophil leukocytes, were observed to permeate abnormal skin (59).

B. Diagnosis

To aid in the diagnosis of atopic dermatitis, specific diagnostic criteria have been formulated and are summarized in Table 5 (60). Typical-appearing atopic dermatitis is easily differentiated from such cutaneous disorders as (1) seborrheic dermatitis, which appears as greasy scaling areas on a yellow-red base over the scalp, forehead, and flexor areas; (b) allergic contact dermatitis, which manifests acute, patchy, and streaky lesions correlating with exposure to contactants; (c) other immunological disorders. These immunological conditions include (a) the hyper-IgE syndrome, which demonstrates recurrent cold abscesses, severe local and systemic infections to *Candida* and *Staphylococcus*, coarse facies and skeletal abnormalities, and markedly elevated serum IgE levels; (b) dermatitis herpetiformis, which has severe refractory pruritus, blistering, and excoriations frequently associated with sprue and wheat sensitivity; (c) the Wiskott-Aldrich syndrome, which presents with purpura from thrombocytopenia and systemic infections from immunological abnormalities; (d) chronic granulomatous disease, which manifests recurrent skin abscesses, fistulas, pneumonia, hepatosplenomegaly, and abnormal nitroblue tetrazolium test and generation of oxygen radicals; and (e) cutaneous lymphomas such as mycosis fun-

Table 5 Diagnostic Criteria for Atopic Dermatitis During Pregnancy

---

A. Absolute features
   1. Pruritus
   2. Flexural lichenification
   3. Chronic or recurrent tendency plus
B. Two or more of the following features
   1. Personal or family atopic history
   2. Specific IgE
   3. White dermographism (a white line instead of wheal with skin stroking)
   4. Anterior subscapsular cataracts or
C. Four of more of the following features
   1. Xerosis/ichthyosis/hyperlinear palms
   2. Pityriasis alba
   3. Keratosis pilaris
   4. Facial pallor/infraorbital darkening
   5. Dennie-Morgan infraorbital fold
   6. Elevated serum IgE level
   7. Keratoconus
   8. Tendency toward nonspecific hand dermatitis
   9. Tendency toward recurrent dermal infections

---

goides, Sezary's syndrome, and Hodgkin's disease, which may present early with pruritic dermatitic lesions involving linear thickening of flexural surfaces (57,58).

C. Prevention and Treatment

The treatment of atopic dermatitis during pregnancy must focus on avoidance of triggering factors, such as known (a) food and inhalant allergens, (b) irritating agents such as wools and chemicals, (c) excessive perspiration and heat, (d) unwarranted stress, (e) occlusive clothing, and (f) other known exacerbants. Topical therapies that have proven efficacious for atopic dermatitis include (a) moisturizes and lubricants to alleviate dryness (Neutrogena hand cream, Aveeno lotion, Eucerin cream), and (b) cleansers such as Cetophil lotion instead of soaps, and aluminum acetate (Burow's solution) or baking soda soaks to reduce inflammation, weeping, and pruritis. When clinically indicated, oral antihistamines should be administered at the lowest effective dose, initiating therapy with chlorpheniramine in doses similar to those given for urticaria/angioedema (page 350). Hydroxyzine may be necessary for recalcitrant pruritis. A similar conservative approach should be followed for topical corticosteroid usage. Corticosteroid treatment should be initiated, when clinically indicated, with the least potentially adrenal suppressive preparations, such as hydrocortisone (0.5–2.5%). Use of the more potent topical corticosteroid preparations should be reserved for the more recalcitrant areas or patients. Administration of corticosteroids by intralesional or systemic injections should be avoided. Infectious exacerbations, generally secondary to *Staphylococcus aureus* colonization, should be treated with penicillinase-resistant synthetic penicillins or erythromycin in those allergic to penicillin (see Chapter 14) (61).

VIII. Miscellaneous Cutaneous Immunological Disorders

A. Cutaneous Mastocytosis

Mast cell disorders characterized by mast cell infiltration of various tissues and organs, including mastocytoma, urticaria pigmentoisa, and diffuse and systemic mastocytosis, are rare conditions of humans. Release of potent mediators of inflammation, including histamine, leukotrienes, tryptase, proteases, heparin, and prostaglandins, causes the clinical manifestations associated with these disorders. The present discussion will involve only cutaneous mast cell disease; the reader is referred to a recent review for a more extensive treatise on mast cell disease (62). In addition to such myriad symptoms as urticaria/angioedema, bronchospasm, pruritus, headache, colic, diarrhea, anaphylaxis, and bone pain, the pregnant woman with mast cell disease is at particular risk for increase uterine irritability and preterm labor resulting mainly from histamine. Anaphylaxis may be provoked by alcohol, aspirin, or infections (see Chapter 12).

Clinical Manifestations

Urticaria pigmentosa, the most frequent manifestation of cutaneous mastocytosis, is characterized by small, yellow-tan to red-brown macules to slightly raised papules appearing on any skin surface but the palms, soles, face, and scalp. Clinical diagnosis is made by eliciting the Darier sign: urtication and erythema about a stroked or rubbed macule. Diagnosis should be confirmed by skin histopathology which reveals significantly increased numbers of mast cells in the dermis (63).

Telangiectasia macularis eruptiva perstans (TMEP) is a rare manifestation of mast cell disease, occurring in less than 1% of cases. TMEP characteristically shows tan-to-brown macules and patchy erythema with telangiectasia (Fig. 17). The first report of cutaneous mastocytosis complicating pregnancy revealed a 26-year-old woman gravida 4, para 1-0-2-

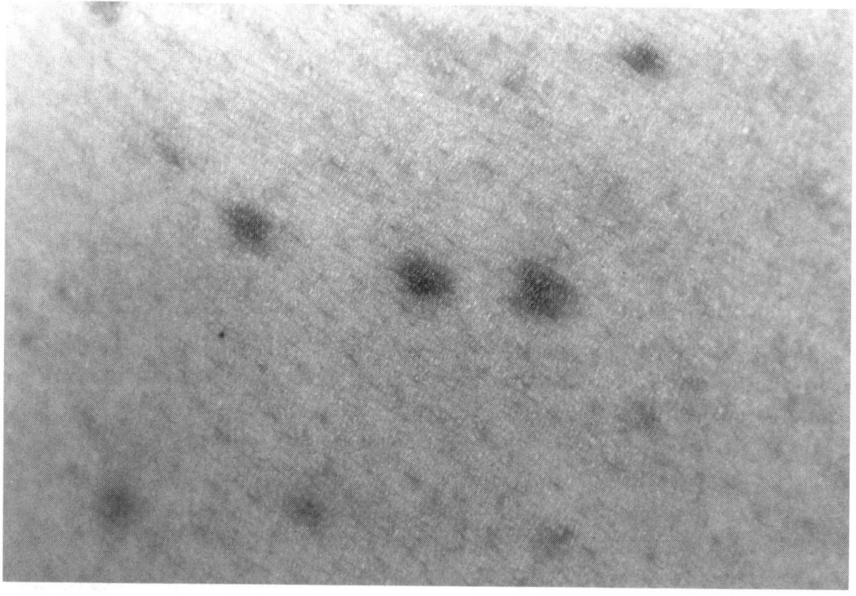

Figure 17 Telangietasia macularis eruptiva perstans. Macules with patchy erythema and telangiectasia on the trunk.

1, presenting at 19 weeks with a maculopapular rash occupying her trunk and upper extremities, bronchospasm, dyspnea, uterine contractions and fundal tenderness, vaginal bleeding, and a skin biopsy with increased numbers of perivascular mast cells diagnostic for TMEP. Treatment with hydroxyzine and imipramine initially relieved the dyspnea and uterine cramping, but preterm labor occurred frequently, which failed oral and required systemic tocolytics (magnesium sulfate) until 36 weeks gestation, when a repeat caesarean section delivered a healthy low-birth-weight infant. Urinary histamine excretion was 10 times normal levels (584 versus 5–24 μg/24 hr) and was hypothesized as being responsible for causing the uterine symptoms and preterm labor (64).

Prevention and Treatment

The hallmark of treatment is prevention of mast cell release by known triggers such as alcohol, aspirin, NSAIDs, infections, and other mediator-releasing agents (Table 3). Pharmacological therapy must be tailored to the pregnant patient, determined by the severity and troublesomeness of the symptoms, which may include pruritus, flushing, cramping, dyspepsia, diarrhea, and anaphylaxis. H_1-receptor antagonist antihistamines represent the first line of pharmacotherapy when medication is needed and have been discussed earlier (see urticaria/angioedema treatment above). H_2-receptor antagonists such as cimetidine may be needed to relieve gastric symptoms that are not controlled by antacids, but must be avoided during the first and possibly second trimesters due to the association with the potential for fetal antiandrogenic effects (Chapter 8). Cromolyn sodium (Gastrocrom) in dosages of 200 mg QID 30 minutes before meals and at bedtime is used to treat persistent GI symptoms in *nonpregnant* patients. Its role during pregnancy has not been determined, since it is not recommended for premature and term infants (65). The treatment of anaphylaxis in patients with mast cell disease is identical to that discussed for all types of anaphylaxis (Chapter 12).

B. Linear IgA Dermatosis

Linear IgA dermatosis (LAD) in adults is a rare, typically persistent (60%), autoimmune disorder characterized by bullous lesions and subepidermal blister formation with deposition of a linear band of IgA. LAD typically requires therapy with agents such as dapsone, sulfamethoxypyridazine, and sulfapyridine (64). The antigen in LAD is expressed in the amnion basement membrane, which shows deposited IgA in fetuses of affected women (65). A recent retrospective study of 12 patients with LAD who underwent 19 pregnancies revealed favorable maternal and fetal outcomes. LAD improved during pregnancy, with improvement first noted by 10 weeks' gestation. Three of 9 women with active disease prior to pregnancy remitted during pregnancy, allowing discontinuation of dapsone. Generally, dosages of prednisone and dapsone could be reduced in most of the women during pregnancy. Labor was uneventful, with only 1 episode each of fetal distress needing caesarean section and preterm birth at 38 weeks' gestation. Relapse occurred from 2 hr to 4 months postpartum in 14 of the 17 pregnancies in 10 of the 12 patients. Fetal outcomes were favorable, with only one newborn exhibiting a single transient blister remitting by 1 week. The improvement in LAD during pregnancy, the favorable fetal outcomes, and the relapse of LAD postpartum suggest that (a) pregnancy should not be discouraged in LAD, (b) medication should be tapered or discontinued when disease improvement/remission allows, and (c) patients should be counseled about relapse probabilities after birth (64).

References

1. Ellis DL. Pregnancy and sex steroid hormone effects on nevi of patients with the dysplastic nevus syndrome. J Am Acad Dermatol 1991; 25:467–482.
2. Holmes RC, Black MM. The specific dermatoses of pregnancy: a reappraisal with special emphasis on a proposed simplified clinical classification. Clin Exp Dermatol 1982; 7:65–73.
3. The Drugs and Pregnancy Study Group. Strategy of treatment of pruritus during pregnancy. Ann Pharmacother 1994; 28:17–20.
4. Roger D, Vaillant L, Fignon A, Pierre F, Bacq Y, Brechot JF, Grangepont MC, Lorette G. Specific pruritic diseases of pregnancy. A prospective study of 3192 pregnant women. Arch Dermatol 1994; 130:734–739.
5. Pauwels C, Bucaille-Fleury L, Recanati G. Pruritic urticarial papules and plaques of pregnancy: relationship to maternal weight gain and twin or triplet pregnancies. Arch Dermatol 1994; 130:801–802.
6. Bunker CB, Erskine K, Rustin MHA, Gilkes JJH. Severe polymorphic eruption of pregnancy occurring in twin pregnancies. Clin Exp Dermatol 1990; 15:228–231.
7. Beltrani VP, Beltrani VS. Pruritic urticarial papules and plaques of pregnancy: a severe case requiring early delivery for relief of symptoms. J Am Acad Dermatol 1992; 26:266–267.
8. Lawley TJ, Stingl G, Katz SI. Fetal and maternal risk factors in herpes gestationis. Arch Dermatol 1978; 114:552–555.
9. Holmes RC, Black MM, Jurecka W, Dann J, James DCO, Timlin D, Bhogal B. Clues to the aetiology and pathogenesis of herpes gestationis. Br J Dermatol 1983; 109:131–139.
10. Holmes RC, Black MM. The fetal prognosis in pemphigoid gestationis (herpes gestationis) Br J Dermatol 1984; 110:67–72.

11. Borradori L, Didierjean L, Bernard P, Tamm K, Gaucherand M, Zurn A, Saurat JH. IgM autoantibodies to 180- and 230- to 240-kd human epidermal proteins in pregnancy. Arch Dermatol 1995; 131:43–47.
12. Kelly SE, Cerio R, Bhogal BS, Black MM. The distribution of IgG subclasses in pemphigoid gestationis: PG is an IgG1 autoantibody. J Invest Dermatol 1989; 92:695–698.
13. Kelly SE, Bhogal BS, Wojnarowska F, Whitehead P, Leigh IM, Black MM. Western blot analysis of the antigen in pemphigoid gestationis. Br J Dermatol 1990; 122:445–449.
14. Kirtschig G, Collier PM, Emmerson RW, Wojnarowska F. Severe case of pemphigoid gestationis with unusual target antigen. Br J Dermatol 1994; 131: 108–111.
15. Giudice GJ, Emery DR, Zelickson BK. Bullous pemphigoid and herpes gestationis autoantibodies recognize a common non-collagenous site on the BP180 ectodomain. J Immunol 1993; 151:5742–5750.
16. Ortonne JP, Hsi BL, Verrando P, Bernerd F, Pautrat G, Pisani A, Yeh CJG. Herpes gestationis factor reacts with amniotic epithelial basement membrane. Br J Dermatol 1987; 117:147–154.
17. Shornick JR. Herpes gestationis. J Am Acad Dermatol 1987; 17:539–556.
18. Wiel AVD, Hart HC, Flinterman J, Kerckhaert JAM, Boeuff JAD, Imhof JW. Plasma exchange in herpes gestationis. Br Med J 1981; 281:1041–1042.
19. Oumeish OY, Farraj SE, Bataineh AS. Some aspects of impetigo herpetiformis. Arch Dermatol 1982; 118:103–105.
20. Wolf Y, Groutz A, Walman I, Luxman D, David MP. Impetigo herpetiformis during pregnancy: case report and review of the literature. Acta Obstet Gynecol Scand 1995; 74:229–232.
21. Reyes H, Gonzalez MC, Ribalta J, Aburto H, Matus C, Schramm G, Katz R, Medina E. Prevalence of intrahepatic cholestasis of pregnancy in Chile. Ann Intern Med 1978; 88:487–493.
22. Holzbach RT. Jaundice in pregnancy—1976. Am J Med 1976; 61:367–376.
23. Palma J, Reyes H, Ribalta J, Iglesias J, Gonzalez MC, Hernandez I, Alvarez C, Molina C, Danitz AM. Effects of urodeoxycholic acid in patients with intrahepatic cholestatsis of pregnancy. Hepatology 1992; 15:1043–1047.
24. Hirvioja ML, Tiumola R, Vuori J. The treatment of intrahepatic cholestatis of pregnancy by dexamethasone. Br J Obstet Gynaecol 1992; 99:109–111.
25. Soter NA, Wasserman SI. Clinical manifestations, pathogenesis, and therapeutic approaches in urticaria/angioedema. Dermatol Digest 1979; 18:17–32.
26. Champion RH, Roberts SOB, Carpenter RG, Roger JH. Urticaria and angioedema. Br J Dermatol 1969; 81:588–597.
27. Meggs WJ, Pescowitz OH, Metcalfe D, Loriaux DL, Cutler G Jr, Kaliner M. Progesterone sensitivity as a cause of recurrent anaphylaxis. N Engl J Med 1984; 311:1236–1238.
28. Laurent J, Malet R, Smiejan JM, Madelenat P, Herman D. Latex hypersensitivity after natural delivery. J Allergy Clin Immunol 1992; 89:779–780.
29. Bhatia PL, Singh M, Jha, BK. Laryngopathia gravidarum. ENT 1980; 60: 408 412.

29a. Schatz M, Petitti D. Antihistamines and pregnancy. Annals Allergy 1997; 78: 157–159.

30. Agostoni A, Cicardi M. Hereditary and acquired C1-Inhibitor deficiency: biological and clinical characteristics in 235 patients. Medicine 1992; 71: 206–215.

31. Frank MM, Gelfand JA, Atkinson JP. Hereditary angioedema: the clinical syndrome and its management. Ann Intern Med 1976; 4:580–593.

32. Chappatte O, De Swiet M. Hereditary angioneurotic oedema and pregnancy. Case reports and review of the literature. Br J Obst Gynaecol 1988; 95: 938–942.

33. Fontana L, Perricone R, DeCarolis C, Pizzolo JG, Casciani CU. Hereditary angioneurotic edema. Res Clin Lab 1989; 19:51–58.

34. Warin RD, Cunliffer WT, Greaves MW, Wallingtion TB. Recurrent angioedema: familial and estrogen induced. Br J Dermatol 1986; 115:731–734.

35. Perkins W, Downie I, Keefe M, Chisholm M. Cutaneous necrosis in pregnancy secondary to activated protein C. Resistance in hereditary angioedema. J R Soc Med 1995; 88:229–230.

36. Postnikoff IM, Pritzker KP. Hereditary angioneurotic edema: an unusual case of maternal mortality. J Forsensic Sci 1979; 24:473–478.

37. Cunningham DS, Jensen JT. Hereditary angioneurotic edema in the puerperium. A case report. J Reprod Med 1991; 36:312–313.

38. Peters M, Ryley D, Lockwood C. Hereditary angioedema and immunoglobulin A deficiency in pregnancy. Obst Gynecol 1988; 72(part 2):454–455.

39. Zahedi K, Prada AE, Davis AE 3rd. Structure and regulation of the C1 inhibitor gene. Behring Inst Mitt 1993; 93:115–119.

40. Donaldson VH, Bissler JJ. C1 inhibitors and their genes: an update. J Lab Clin Med 1992; 119:330–333.

41. Davis AE 3rd, Bissler JJ, Cicardi M. Mutations in the C1 inhibitor gene that result in hereditary angioneurotic edema. Behring Inst Mitt 1993; 93:313–320.

42. Donaldson VH. C1-inhibitor and its genetic alterations in hereditary angioneurotic edema. Int Rev Immunol 1993; 10:1–16.

43. Cohen AJ, Laskin C, Tarlo S. C1 esterase inhibitor in pregnancy. J Allergy Clin Immunol 1992; 90:412–413.

44. Ogston D, Warker J, Campbell DM. C1 inactivator level in pregnancy. Thromb Res 1981; 23:454–455.

45. Halbmayer WM, Hopmeier P, Mannhalter C, Heuss F, Leodolter S, Rudi K, Fischer M. C1-esterase inhibitor in complicated pregnancy and mild and moderate preeclampsia. Thromb Haemost 1991; 65:134–138.

46. Chhibber G, Cohen A, Lane S, Farber A, Meloni F, Schmaier AH. Immunoblotting of plasma in a pregnancy patient with hereditary angioedema. J Lab Clin Med 1990; 115:112–121.

47. Agostoni A, Cicardi M. Contraindications to the use of angiotensin converting enzyme inhibitors in patients deficient in C1 esterase inhibitor. Am J Med 1991; 90:278.

48. Stiller RJ, Kaplan BM, Andreoli JW. Hereditary angioedema and pregnancy. Obstet Gynecol 1984; 64:133–135.

49. Adverse effects of danazol in pregnancy (editorial). Ann Intern Med 1982; 96:672–673.

50. Borradori L, Marie O, Rybojad M, Vexiav P, Morel P. Hereditary angioedema and oral contraception. Dermatologica 1990; 181:78–79.

51. Wingtin LN, Hardy F. Epidural block during labour in hereditary angioneurotic oedema. Can J Anaesth 1990; 36:366.

52. Cox M, Holdcroft A. Hereditary angioneurotic oedema: current management in pregnancy. Anaesthesia 1995; 50:547–549.

53. Sim TC, Grant JA. Hereditary angioedema: its diagnostic and management perspectives. Am J Med 1990; 88:656–664.

54. Gadek JE, Hosea SW, Gelfand JA, Santaella M, Wickerhauser M, Triantaphyllopoulos DC, Frank MM. Replacement therapy in hereditary angioedema: successful treatment of acute episodes of angioedema with partly purified C1 inhibitor. N Engl J Med 1980; 302:542–546.

55. Roth HL, Kierland RR. The natural history of atopic dermatitis. Arch Dermatol 1964; 89:209–214.

56. Kemmett D, Tidman MJ. The influence of the menstrual cycle and pregnancy on atopic dermatitis. Br J Dermatol 1991; 125:59–61.

57. Zeiger RS. Atopic dermatitis of childhood: current concepts and management. Immunol Allergy Practice 1981; 3:198–210.

58. Hanifin JM. Atopic dermatitis. In Middleton E Jr, Reed EC, Ellis EF, Adkinson NF Jr, Yunginger JW, Busse WW, eds. Allergy: Principles and Practice, 4th ed. St. Louis: Mosby, 1993:1581–1604.

59. Sampson H. Pathogenesis of eczema. Clin Exp Allergy 1990; 20:459–467.

60. Schatz M, Zeiger RS. Allergic disease in pregnancy. In: Gleicher N, ed. Principles and Practice of Medical Therapy in Pregnancy. 2d ed. East Norwalk, CT: Appleton-Lange, 1992:435–454.

61. Schatz M, Hoffman CP, Zeiger RS, Falkoff R, Macy E, Mellon M. The course and management of asthma and allergic diseases during pregnancy. In Middleton E Jr, Reed EC, Ellis EF, Adkinson NF Jr, Yunginger JW, Busse WW, eds. Allergy: Principles and Practice. 4th ed. St. Louis Mosby, 1993:1301–1342.

62. Metcalfe DD. Mastocytosis syndromes. In Middleton E Jr, Reed EC, Ellis EF, Adkinson NF Jr, Yunginger JW, Busse WW, eds. Allergy: Principles and Practice. 4th ed. St. Louis: Mosby, 1993:1537–1551.

63. Donahue JG, Lupton JB, Golichowski AM. Cutaneous mastocytosis complicating pregnancy. Obstet Gynecol 1995; 85:813–815.

64. Collier PM, Kelly SE, Wojnarowska F. Linear IgA disease and pregnancy. J Am Acad Dermatol 1994; 30:407–411.

65. Kelly SE, Fleming S, Bhogal, Wojnarowska F, Black MM. Immunopathology of the placenta in pemphigoid gestationis and linear IgA disease. Br J Dermatol 1989; 120:733–743.

14

Immunologically Mediated Adverse Drug Reactions in Pregnancy

GILLIAN M. SHEPHERD

The New York Hospital–Cornell University Medical Center
New York, New York

I. Introduction

There are many types of adverse drug reactions. Only a small percentage, however, are immunologically mediated. In these cases, components of the immune system specifically recognize a drug and react with it. The resultant signs and symptoms vary depending on which part of the immune system is involved. The various immunologically mediated adverse drug reactions are noted in Table 1. The responsible immune mechanism is clearly defined for some, such as anaphylaxis and immune complex reactions. In other cases, such as the most frequent reaction, morbilliform rashes, the specific mechanism is less clear.

The spectrum of these reactions is not significantly different during pregnancy, although treatment should be modified in some cases. Serum albumin is decreased, so the concentration of protein-bound drug is generally lower and the concentration of free drug greater than in the non-pregnant patient. Gastrointestinal motility is slower during pregnancy, so peak drug levels occur later and are generally lower (e.g., 40% lower after 500 mg p.o. of ampicillin (1). The plasma volume and total body water are increased, but this does not change the volume of distribution of the

Table 1 Immunologically Mediated Adverse Drug Reactions

Reactions	Responsible immune mechanism, where known
Anaphylaxis	IgE antibody
Urticaria and angioedema	IgE antibody
Rash morbilliform	? T-cell mediated
Erythema multiforme minor	
Erythema multiforme major	
(Stevens-Johnson syndrome)	
Fixed drug eruption	
Erythema nodosum	T-cell mediated
Contact dermatitis	T-cell mediated
Fever	Release of pyrogenic cytokines, e.g., tumor necrosis factor, interleukin-1
Immune complex reactions (rash, fever, arthralgias, myalgias, lymphadenopathy, nephritis, vasculitis)	IgG and IgM antibody
Cytopenias	IgG and IgM antibody
Target organ-specific reactions	
Pulmonary	
Hepatic	
Renal	

Source: Adapted from Shepherd GM. Allergic reaction to drugs. In: Rakel RE, ed. Conn's Current Therapy. Philadelphia: Saunders, 1995:695–702.

drug as long as the weight of the patient is considered (2). Metabolism and excretion of drugs are variable; each drug must be evaluated separately. These changes, however, do not appear to significantly alter the frequency or clinical presentation of immunologically mediated drug reactions.

In general, most drugs administered to a pregnant patient after the fifth week will cross the placenta, except for very large or highly charged drugs (3). IgG is the only antibody that crosses the placenta. Other antibodies and immune cells have no specific receptors or are too large. Maternal IgG passes by binding to specific Fc gamma type III receptors (CD16) on trophoblasts, and is then internalized for active transport through the cell to the fetal side (4). The receptors have highest affinity for IgG1, and IgG3, followed by IgG4, and last for IgG2 (4).

Most neonatal IgG is acquired transplacentally, primarily during the third trimester. Small amounts are made by the fetus. IgM production is also low but can be initially detected in the mid-second trimester. Fetal lymphocytes can recognize foreign cells and respond, but much less efficiently than adults. Although there are data regarding immunosuppression in pregnancy (see Chapter 4), there are no significant data to answer whether this results in a decreased frequency of immunological drug reactions.

II. Diagnosis

There are two aspects to diagnosis. The first is prospective: identifying the patient at risk of an immune reaction *before* the physician administers the drug. This entails taking a detailed history of any possible immune reaction to the drug (or to a relative). If there is any suggestive history, ideally an alternative drug should be given. Although there is a tendency for a repeat immune reaction to mimic the first (e.g., repeat morbilliform rash), this is not reliable, as a more severe reaction may develop. If there is no suggestive history, the risk is theoretically no greater than for the general population and the desired drug can be given. There are no tests currently available that can prospectively identify patients at risk of an immunologically mediated drug reaction, except skin testing for penicillin. Skin testing can be done with other drugs and may provide some information, but the positive and negative predictive values are unknown. In all cases, however, skin testing only detects the presence of *IgE antibody* specific for the drug. It does not predict reactions caused by other immune mechanisms or the development of later reactions beyond the first day of drug administration. The IgE which is detected is preformed from past exposure to the drug. If the drug is given again, it can interact with the IgE, leading to reactions ranging from explosive anaphylaxis (85% of reactions within 1 hr) to urticaria within 1–2 days.

In other drug reactions the immune system starts to respond once it sees the drug, sometimes days later. The corresponding clinical symptoms usually develop over days. As stated, there is currently no way to predict who is going to develop a later reaction.

The other aspect of diagnosis is retrospective: Are the clinical signs and symptoms compatible with an immune reaction to a drug, or could they be due to other pathology? If drug allergy is possible, how can the culprit drug be identified? In most cases patients are on multiple drugs, thus complicating this task. The first question to ask is the nature of the reaction. Is it compatible with an immune-mediated reaction as listed on Table 1? If so, the next question is timing. What medication(s) was given prior to or concurrent with the reaction? In most cases a drug started within days to weeks is the most likely suspect, especially if the patient had a previous course within the year. Drugs given steadily for months rarely cause later allergic reactions. Occasionally rashes may develop within days after a drug has been discontinued, presumably in response to residual drug. The third question is the tendency of a particular drug to cause an immune-mediated reaction. This has to do with the chemical reactivity of the native drug or its metabolic products. Antibiotics followed by antiarrhythmics, anticonvulsants, and allopurinol frequently cause reactions. Within these groups there is a differential tendency to cause reactions—e.g., a rash is more likely to be due to penicillin than to erythromycin if both were started at similar times.

III. Treatment of Specific Reactions

A. Anaphylaxis

Anaphylaxis is due to specific IgE antibody bound primarily to mast cells. Upon exposure to specific drugs or drug metabolites, IgE becomes cross-linked, which results in a discharge of chemicals from the cells, the most notable being histamine. This causes the varied signs and symptoms of anaphylaxis, which can include any of the following: flushing, impending "sense of doom," lightheadedness from hypotension, shock, laryngeal edema, bronchoconstriction, and abdominal cramping (which may be from the uterus). A small percentage of women have intense vaginal itching as the initial symptom. If there is any question of a reaction to a drug, it should be stopped immediately. The treatment of anaphylaxis is described in Chapter 12. There is concern that the alpha- adrenergic effects of epinephrine might result in uterine vasoconstriction (4). However, the consensus of the 1993 National Heart, Lung, and Blood Institute (NHLBI) panel on management of asthma during pregnancy (2) was that subcutaneous epinephrine is still the treatment of choice for anaphylaxis, because it is mandatory for the fetus that adequate maternal blood pressure and oxygen saturation greater than 95% are maintained (5).

B. Urticaria and Angioedema

Like anaphylaxis, urticaria results from the interaction of specific IgE with a drug, which triggers a release of histamine and other mediators from skin mast cells. Angioedema is essentially the same reaction occurring deeper in the skin, with more diffuse edema. Typical locations of angioedema are the eyes, lips, tongue, palms, and soles. Urticaria and angioedema can occur immediately with the initial drug dose, as the only sign of anaphylaxis or as part of the constellation of signs and symptoms described above. It is unclear why some patients only have skin symptoms and others have systemic symptoms. Urticaria and angioedema can develop at any time during a course of treatment, although it is most common in the first week. In patients previously exposed to the drug, the reaction may occur more rapidly. In these cases the immune system presumably becomes stimulated once it encounters the drug. As the plasma cells consequently produce IgE, the patient gradually develops urticaria. This will not progress to an anaphylactic reaction unless the drug is discontinued and restarted after more than one day. As IgE antibody is produced, it is constantly binding to drug; therefore, in most cases, sufficient IgE necessary to cause anaphylaxis cannot collect if the drug is constantly present.

Other potential causes of urticaria and angioedema also need to be evaluated by a careful history. These include food allergy (if acute hives develop) and thyroid autoimmunity (6). Anecdotally, some cases of urticaria and angioedema are preceded by a viral infection, suggesting that this may be a trigger factor. Chronic urticaria (loosely defined as urticaria persisting beyond 6–8 weeks) unrelated to drug allergy can also occur during pregnancy (see Chapter 13). In nonpregnant patients, some of these cases appear to be an autoimmune reactions due to IgG antibody specific for the high-affinity IgE receptor on mast cells resulting in cross-linking and histamine release (7). Other cases may be due to excessive production of histamine-releasing factors (8). Some cases may be associated with stress or hormonal changes; it is a common observation that chronic urticaria may flare in women during the week before and the week of menses.

Treatment primarily involves stopping the drug. If the patient is on multiple drugs, the suspect one can usually be identified by looking at the timing of administration in relation to symptoms and at the propensity of the drug to cause urticaria, as discussed in the Diagnosis section. In most cases, urticaria and angioedema from drug allergy is a self-limited problem, usually peaking within 24 hr after stopping the drug and declining thereafter. If it persists beyond several days, other causes of urticaria should be explored, as discussed above.

Angioedema happens rapidly; the extravasated fluid then takes 2–3 days to become reabsorbed. The reaction appears confined to the skin; neither urticaria nor angioedema should affect the fetus. Treatment therefore is symptomatic but is often necessary to suppress the pruritus. H_1 antihistamines are the most effective. Those preferred for use during pregnancy are chlorpheniramine, 4 mg up to qid or 8–12 mg sustained-release bid, or tripelennamine (PBZ) 25–50 mg orally up to qid or 100 mg sustained-release bid (2). Use of specific antihistamines during pregnancy is discussed in detail in Chapters 8 and 11. Breast milk concentrations of antihistamines are very low, so they can usually be taken by nursing mothers. There are no data supporting a significant inhibition of lactation.

In some cases corticosteroids, in doses ranging from 20–50 mg of prednisone usually split bid, may be temporarily necessary to treat severe cases of urticaria. Although long-term corticosteroid use during pregnancy has been possibly associated with preeclampsia, intrauterine growth retardation, and preterm births, this is no evidence that short courses are associated with adverse outcomes (see Chapters 8 and 18). The effect on a child via breast milk is negligible, as only a very small amount of corticosteroids passes to the milk (9). One study found that breast milk concentration of prednisolone was 5–25% that of maternal serum. If the mother took 80 mg of prednisolone per day, the infant could ingest less than 0.1%, which represented less than 10% of the infant's daily cortisol production (9). Maternal serum and breast milk concentrations of prednisolone are in equilibrium, so it is preferable to breast-feed a baby as late as possible after maternal dosing (9).

C. Nonurticarial Rashes

A variety of nonurticarial rashes can result from drug reactions. The most common is referred to as *morbilliform* (resembling measles) or *maculopapular* (elevated discolored spots), a generally benign, self-limited problem. Another spectrum of potentially severe rashes ranging from erythema multiforme to severe bullous exfoliative dermatitis (Stevens-Johnson syndrome and toxic epidermal necrolysis) appear to be distinct from the morbilliform rash. Fixed drug eruptions and erythema nodosum from a drug reaction happen infrequently. Contact dermatitis from drugs can occur but is also rare.

Morbilliform rashes typically occur 4–10 days after the drug has been started but may occur earlier in sensitized patients or occasionally after the drug has been stopped. The responsible pathological mechanism is not clear but may be T-cell mediated. A morbilliform rash developing rapidly in 24–48 hr after semisynthetic penicillin has been associated with an infiltrate of CD_4-positive T cells (10). Morbilliform rashes are usually associated with pruritus but not urticaria. Unlike erythema multiforme rashes, they are usually not associated with significant constitutional symptoms.

In almost all cases this rash is self-limited and involves only the skin. A detailed physical exam of mucus membranes including the conjunctiva and oral cavity is mandatory to rule out an exfoliative dermatitis. The rash tends to appear centrally and proceed over days to the distal extremities, sometimes sparing the face. Moderate to severe rashes often result in a mild exfoliation of the epidermis, similar to peeling from a sunburn. Many physicians are concerned that a severe morbilliform/maculopapular rash will progress to an exfoliative dermatitis. In most cases, however, the exfoliative dermatitis reactions appear to be distinct from the morbilliform rashes. If there are no associated constitutional symptoms and no bullae are present after several days, progression is very unlikely.

As IgE antibody does not appear to be involved in the pathogenesis, skin testing with the drug(s) in question is not helpful. Common drugs that may cause morbilliform rashes include ampicillin, amoxicillin, sulfonamides, allopurinol, phenytoin, chlorpromazine, and barbiturates.

In contrast to the common morbilliform rashes, bullous exfoliative rashes are rare. However, approximately 50% of cases of Stevens Johnson syndrome and 80% or more of cases of toxic epidermal necrolysis are due to drugs, with mortality rates approaching 5% and 30%, respectively (11). Drug rashes with the potential to progress to severe exfoliation may present as erythema multiforme (EM) (raised erythematous circles with whiter centers resembling a target). This can run a spectrum from EM minor to major (usually considered synonymous with Stevens-Johnson syndrome, although some disagree) (11). EM minor is characterized by crops of target lesions occurring every 1–2 weeks and usually clearing by 4 weeks. The rash is most frequent on extensor surfaces, palms, and soles. EM major is more severe, with the development of vesicles and bullae on the underlying rash. It is often associated with a prodrome of systemic symptoms for 1–2 weeks. These include fever, malaise, myalgias, arthralgias, sore throat, cough, vomiting, and diarrhea. This is followed by an explosive onset of bullae on the skin and mucus membranes, especially the bulbar conjunctiva, oral mucosa, and lips.

Some physicians consider toxic epidermal necrolysis (Lyell's syndrome) to be a severe form of erythema multiforme major, while others consider it a separate entity (11). Patients presenting with toxic epidermal necrolysis have the above prodrome but also frequently have tenderness of the skin and a burning sensation of the conjunctiva. The onset of a bullous eruption occurs within hours to 2 days after the rash is noted in most cases.

Biopsies of EM rashes show mononuclear cells, which are predominantly CD8 and cytotoxic cells, similar to a graft-versus-host reaction. Granular IgM, complement, and fibrin are seen around dermal vessels. The antibody, however, does not appear to be antigen-specific, and the typical neutrophilic infiltrate seen with vasculitis is not present.

Fixed drug eruptions, by contrast, are generally mild reactions. They are red, round or ovoid lesions occurring in the same location (which can be any part of the body) each time the patient is exposed to the putative drug. Occasionally the lesions itch or burn, and they generally heal with hyperpigmentation. Potentially the hyperpigmentation may be enhanced with pregnancy; otherwise the reaction is fairly benign. Although ideally an alternative drug should be given, a history of a fixed drug eruption does not necessarily preclude future administration of the same drug.

Erythema nodosum is considered to be a delayed hypersensitivity reaction, most commonly to an infectious agent, but it has been noted in association with drugs, especially sulfonamides and rarely with birth control pills. Patients may have a prodrome of constitutional symptoms, primarily fever and malaise, followed by the appearance of recurrent crops of tender, deep red nodules on the extensor surfaces of the lower extremities. This generally resolves spontaneously in 3–6 weeks. Potassium iodide has been reported to help, but iodides are contraindicated in pregnancy.

As with all immune-mediated drug reactions, treatment of these rashes consists of stopping the drug as soon as the reaction is recognized. In the case of a nonpregnant patient it is sometimes possible to treat through mild morbilliform rashes. Usually no specific treatment of these rashes is necessary beyond emollients and antihistamines for relief of pruritus. If the morbilliform rash is severe, prednisone, 30–40 mg/day, may help. Comparable to morbilliform rashes, erythema multiforme minor is usually self-limited and does not require specific treatment. Use of steroids to treat erythema multiforme major (Stevens-Johnson syndrome) or toxic epidermal necrolysis is controversial (11), but more recent series suggest it may be beneficial, particularly in adults, if started as soon as possible at 1 mg/kg/day (12,13). Other immunosuppressant drugs have been used for bullous exfoliative drug reactions, including levamisole, azathioprine, dapsone, thalidomide, cyclosporin, and intravenous immunoglobulin (IVIG) (13). Of these only IVIG, possibly dapsone, and azathioprine can be used during pregnancy. All patients with vesicular-bullous disease should be observed very closely. If there is significant skin involvement they should be treated in a specialized burn unit for fluid and infection control. Most cases of erythema multiforme major recover fully; the mortality of toxic epidemeral mecrolysis, however, is very high.

D. Fever

Immune-mediated reactions to drugs can present as fever alone or in association with other signs and symptoms. The mechanism appears to be release of tumor necrosis factor, interleukin-1, and other pyrogens from active immune cells.

There is no obvious pattern to drug fever. Maximum temperature can be 40°C or higher. Likewise there are no associated signs or symptoms that suggest the fever is due to a drug. Eosinophilia is associated in only 20% of cases. Generally, patients appear somewhat better clinically than one would predict from the height of their fever. In one series the drugs responsible for 50% of cases of drug fever were penicillin derivatives, methyldopa, quinidine, phenytoin, procainamide, and cephalothin in respective order of frequency. There appears to be substantial variability in the time between initiation of the drug and start of the fever. That due to antineoplastics usually happens in several days, antimicrobials in 7–10 days, and generally longer, up to several weeks, for cardiac drugs (14).

The most important diagnostic point about drug fever is the recognition that in the overwhelming majority of patients the fever will resolve within 1–2 days after stopping the drug (14). If the patient is still febrile 2 days after discontinuing the drug, drug fever is very unlikely. In cases where the diagnosis is still questionable, studies have suggested that the drug can generally be readministered safely, with a return of fever but no other allergic reactions.

E. Immune Complex Reactions

Immune complex reactions typically result in clinical symptoms 7–10 days after starting a drug. They are a result of IgG or IgM antibody binding to the drug or a metabolite and forming complexes which are capable of passing through basement membranes. Complement binds to the complexes, leading to the recruitment of inflammatory cells to the area, which results in the typical pathology of vasculitis. Early in the course of drug administration the amount of IgG or IgM is low, so the complexes have excess antigen. These tend to be small and pass through the basement membranes without being trapped on the extravascular side. Later in the course, more antibody is made, resulting in "antibody excess" complexes which are large, generally cannot pass through basement membranes, and are cleared by the spleen and lymph nodes. Symptomatic immune complex disease occurs when the complexes contain slightly more drug than antibody. As time passes, more antibody is made and therefore this is usually a self-limited disease.

The complexes can pass through any basement membrane, so symptoms can range from cutaneous with palpable purpuric lesions to renal with glomerulonephritis. Most patients have fever, myalgia, arthralgia or arthritis, inflammation of serosal surfaces, and lymphadenopathy. Theoretically this may affect the fetus. Complexes are too large to pass through the placenta, but unbound IgG will, especially during the third trimester (4). If the relevant drug passes the placenta, theoretically complexes may form on the fetal side. There is, however, no documentation that this actually occurs.

The clinical picture may mimic other problems, such as a viral infection, or other causes of vasculitis such as lupus. Drug allergy should always be suspected, particularly if a new drug was started 7–10 days previously. Erythrocyte sedimentation rates are often elevated and a C4 level may be low as a result of utilization of complement. A skin or other biopsy will show vasculitis with deposition of IgG and complement in the vessel walls in a patchy distribution.

Immune complex reactions are most common with administration of heterologous antisera (e.g., horse anti-thymocyte globulin). In general, the higher the administered dose, the greater is the chance of a reaction.

Treatment consists of stopping the suspect drug. The reaction is self-limited over several days and may not need treatment if signs and symptoms are mild and the mother has normal pulmonary and renal function. If symptoms are moderate and any physiological function is compromised, prednisone should be given in doses from 30 to 60 mg, ideally split bid. As local histamine release may enhance extravasation of complexes from the vasculature, antihistamines, such as tripelennamine, 100 mg sustained-release bid, should be given as well.

F. Drug-Induced Cytopenias

Immune reactions to drugs can result in anemia, leukopenia, or thrombocytopenia (15). The mechanism is commonly IgG bound to drug attached to the cell surface. Complement then binds, which tags the cell for removal by the phagocytic system, or the cell is recognized by cytotoxic cells. If cytopenia is detected, a drug reaction should be suspected, particularly for those drugs started within 2 weeks.

Treatment is to discontinue the drug. If the reaction is severe, particularly if there is any risk of decreased fetal oxygenation or potential bleeding, then prednisone should be administered in doses ranging from 30 to 60 mg daily to bid.

G. Other Target-Organ Specific Reactions

Immune-mediated drug reactions can result in organ-specific pathology including pneumonitis, hepatitis and cholestasis, and interstitial nephritis. Pneumonitis from a drug is usually interstitial or alveolar. Associated eosinophilia, rash, or fever may occur. This has most commonly been associated with nitrofurantoin and sulfasalazine. Detailed information is available in a recent review (16).

Many hepatic reactions from drugs may be toxic, but some are probably immune-mediated, although specific mechanisms are generally not known. Sulfonamides, phenothiazines, anticonvulsants, and isoniazid may induce reactions. Drug-induced liver disease is discussed in detail in a recent review (17).

Renal manifestations of drug allergy are less common. Interstitial nephritis may occur with high doses of penicillin and is usually associated with eosinophilia, fever, and rash.

IV. Special Problems

A. Penicillin Allergy

Patient Requires Penicillin or Derivative but Has a History of Past Allergy

Ideally, any pregnant patient with a past history of an allergic reaction to penicillin should receive an alternative antimicrobial drug. If there is no suitable alternative, then penicillin skin testing should be done to determine the current status of the patient's allergy. When patients with any past history of a possible reaction to penicillin are skin tested, approximately 15% are found to be positive (18); if the history was anaphylaxis, up to 25% of patients may be positive (personal observation).

Skin testing requires use of specific reagents and expertise in the technique and analysis; therefore it should ideally be done by a specialist in allergy or specifically trained personnel. The details of testing are described elsewhere (18). Use of the major determinant benzyl penicilloyl (commercially available as PrePen, Bayer Corp.) and a mix of minor determinants (not commercially available) has a 99% negative predictive value: If negative, there is a 1% chance the patient will develop an immediate allergic reaction if given penicillin or any derivative (19). Use of penicillin G (most important minor determinant) as a substitute for the mix of minor determinants may be 98% predictive (18). In all of the reports of skin testing to date, the few reactions which have occurred in patients with negative skin tests have been mild.

If the skin test is clearly negative, the patient should receive a small test dose of the drug, approximately 1/1000th to 1/100th of the therapeutic dose. If no reaction occurs in 1 hr, the full therapeutic dose can be administered.

If the skin test is positive, there is a 50% chance the patient will react if given penicillin (18); therefore an alternative antimicrobial should be given. The only clear exception to this is the pregnant patient who requires treatment for syphilis. At present there is no acceptable alternative to penicillin. In this case the patient needs to undergo desensitization. This is a potentially dangerous procedure and should be supervised by an allergy specialist and performed in a monitored setting. It has been accomplished successfully in pregnant patients (20,21). Both oral and intravenous routes have been used, with initial low doses being doubled every 15–30 min until the therapeutic dose is reached. Most physicians prefer not to pretreat the patient with antihistamines, as early warning signs of a reaction may be blocked.

B. Cephalosporin Allergy

Patient Has a History of Allergy to Penicillin and Now Requires a Cephalosporin Antibiotic

Ideally, any pregnant patient with a history of penicillin allergy and the need for a cephalosporin antibiotic should use an alternative antimicrobial drug. The extent, if any, of clinically significant cross-reactivity between penicillin and cephalosporins is still not clear but is probably overestimated. Most patients lose allergy to penicillin over time. If a patient with a past history of allergy to penicillin, but a negative skin test to penicillin, is given a cephalosporin, the risk of an immediate reaction is no greater than in the general population (18). The predictive value of a positive skin test, however, to identify patients who may react to a cephalosporin is not clear; a recent review has suggested it may be of no value (22). As a result, the following recommendations have evolved as a guide to this problem.

1. It may not be worthwhile performing penicillin skin testing on these patients, as the positive predictive value may be limited or nonexistent.
2. If the patient's history of penicillin allergy is not anaphylaxis, a cephalosporin may be given, with the first dose under medical observation for 1 hr.
3. If the patient has a history of anaphylaxis to penicillin, she should receive incremental doses of the cephalosporin under medical observation.
4. Most early reports of reactions to cephalosporins in patients with a history of allergy to penicillin involved cephalothin and cephaloridine, which have side chains similar to benzyl penicillin (22). Other cephalosporins should be given to these patients.

Patient Has a History of Allergy to a Cephalosporin and Requires Penicillin

Ideally, an alternative drug should be given. If penicillin is required, penicillin skin testing can be done to determine the current status of the patient's allergy. If negative, the patient can receive penicillin; if positive, she needs to undergo desensitization.

Patient Has a History of Allergy to One Cephalosporin and Requires Another

The pregnant patient should ideally receive an alternative antibiotic. Skin testing with cephalosporins has not been validated, and the negative predictive value is unknown. If a different cephalosporin is required in a patient with a history of an adverse reaction, incremental dosing under observation is recommended.

Patients who are allergic to cephalosporins may have an immune reaction to a side chain of the drug rather than the central beta-lactam ring structure. If so, there is potential for a cross-reaction if another cephalosporin has the same side chain.

C. Immune-Mediated Reactions to Non-Beta-Lactam Antibiotics

Tetracycline and *quinolone* antibiotics should not be given during pregnancy. Tetracycline discolors permanent teeth as they develop, and quinolones may cause impaired cartilage development. *Sulfonamides* should be avoided in the third trimester near delivery, because of the possibility that their action as a folate antagonist will result in fetal/newborn jaundice, hemolytic anemia, or remotely kernicterus (3).

Vancomycin commonly causes immediate reactions; later rashes are uncommon. Intravenous administration over 1 hr can result in serum histamine release and potentially hypotension (23). Some patients may develop the nonimmunologically mediated "red man's syndrome," characterized by erythema usually from the trunk up, occasional severe pruritus, and hypotension. It is critical to avoid hypotension in the pregnant patient; therefore it may be advisable to give vancomycin more slowly (e.g., over 2 hr) to these patients. The addition of antihistamine prophylaxis (e.g., chlorpheniramine maleate, 8 mg) may help block the clinical symptoms.

Macrolides rarely cause immune-mediated drug reactions (24). If a specific reaction occurs, it should be approached as outlined in the treatment section. *Clindamycin* may result in maculopapular rashes in 1–2% of courses. Other reactions are unusual. Like clindamycin, maculopapular rashes may occur with *gentamycin,* but they rare, as are other immune reactions.

D. Immune-Mediated Reactions to Other Drugs

Protamine

Protamine is used primarily to reverse heparin anticoagulation during cardiac procedures and therefore is used rarely in pregnant patients unless there is an urgent problem. Like vancomycin, rapid infusion can result in hypotension. Major anaphylactic reactions with significant cardiovascular and respiratory symptoms have been reported. These are more frequent in diabetic patients exposed to protamine by NPH insulin, suggesting an IgE mechanism, yet a positive skin test or IgE ELISA assay specific for protamine does not seem to predict the patient at risk of a reaction (25).

Muscle Relaxants and Induction Agents

Muscle relaxants and induction agents may be responsible for anaphylactic reactions during general anesthesia. In one study the incidence was 0.67%; 7.5% of these reactions were fatal (26). Specific IgE antibody to muscle relaxants has been documented. These drugs, however, are known histamine liberators, and many reactions may result from this mechanism. All muscle relaxants have a common quaternary ammonium structure and should be considered cross-reactive (26). Reactions are more common in females and may occur on the initial contact, possibly from exposure to quaternary ammonium compounds in commercial materials. Reactions are also more common in patients with a history of atopy.

Intradermal skin tests and in-vitro tests for specific IgE to muscle relaxants are often positive after an anaphylactic reaction. The predictive value of these tests, however, is not established.

If a pregnant patient with a past history of a reaction to a muscle relaxant requires surgery, great caution must be exerted. There is no effective protocol available. A suggested approach is the following.

1. Try to avoid use of the suspect drug. If a muscle relaxant must be given, a different one should be selected from that suspected of causing the original reaction. Cross-reactivity is documented for these drugs, but it is not 100%, and successful administration of an alternative one has been noted (26). Atacurium may be a less potent histamine releaser than some of the other drugs in this group. It has been shown, however, to be potentially teratogenic in rabbits given one-half the human dose. The significant of this in humans is not known.

2. Consider pretreating the patient with prednisone and antihistamines (which will blunt a non-IgE-mediated anaphylactoid reaction but may not block a true allergic reaction).

3. Perform intradermal skin testing with the alternative drug as described elsewhere (28). Although the predictive value of this has not been precisely documented, a positive reaction, especially at a weak strength, suggests sensitivity.
4. Use a small initial test dose and administer it slowly. Rapid infusion rates are associated with hypotension. Dosing should be based on ideal body weight, not actual weight.

Immune-mediated reactions to induction agents are unusual. Rapid injection of thiopental, a barbiturate, is associated with marked hypotension and respiratory symptoms, but it is unlikely that this is immunologically mediated. If a patient has a suggestive history of a past reaction, the approach should be similar to that suggested above for muscle relaxants except that skin testing should not be done.

Insulin

Women may require insulin during pregnancy for control of gestational or ongoing diabetes, in part because oral agents are contraindicated (27). Immune reactions to insulin are infrequent but can result in local or systemic symptoms. Reactions are most common when insulin is used intermittently, e.g., with gestational diabetes during repeat pregnancies.

Skin testing can be performed with various insulin preparations. In general, human insulin is the least immunogenic and should be used preferentially during pregnancy. If the patient has persistent reactions to human insulin, desensitization to insulin can be done, as described elsewhere (28), and is usually successful.

Oxytocin

Anaphylactoid reactions to oxytocin are rare, but case reports exist, including one death attributed to a reaction to oxytocin (29). Although this is an unusual problem, obstetricians need to be aware of the possibility of such a reaction.

E. Nonimmunological Drug Reactions Which Simulate Immune Reactions

Aspirin and Nonsteroidal Anti-Inflammatory Drugs

Aspirin and nonsteroidal anti-inflammatory drugs (NSAIDS) can cause anaphylaxis, asthma, rhinitis, urticaria, and angioedema in sensitive patients. This results most likely from the effect of these drugs on the cyclooxygenase pathway with a subsequent shift in the production of prostaglandins and possibly leukotrienes.

A pregnant patient who has a history of reaction to aspirin or a NSAID in the past, and *absolutely* requires it again while pregnant, can undergo an extremely cautious, graded challenge, e.g., starting with 1/1000th of a 325-mg table and doubling every 30 min in a facility equipped to treat anaphylaxis. If a reaction occurs and aspirin is essential, aspirin desensitization may be considered, as described elsewhere (30).

Local Anesthetics

Local anesthetics are commonly perceived to cause frequent allergic reactions. Actual true immune-mediated reactions to these drugs are extremely rare, if they exist. Patients with a history of reaction to one local anesthetic should be incrementally challenged with an alternative one. Suggested protocols start with a full-strength prick test and progress through one to four incremental s.c. or i.d. doses, culminating in a final test dose of 1.0–3.0 cc (31). This should be donee using local anesthetic without epinephrine, as the latter may cause skin blanching and therefore confound reading of the test doses.

Angiotensin-Converting Enzyme Inhibitors

Within hours to approximately 1 week after starting an angiotensin-converting enzyme (ACE) inhibitor, angioedema may develop in 0.1% of patients. This has occurred more frequently in patients with a history of idiopathic angioedema. Life-threatening laryngeal edema has not occurred (32).

In 1.5–10% of treated patients, cough may develop, usually in 1–2 months (range 1–12 months) (32). The mechanism is not known. Although the cough has cleared in some patients despite continuation of the drug, it is preferable to discontinue ACE inhibitors in any patient with a cough who is pregnant. The cough usually clears within 4–6 days after discontinuing the drug.

Radiocontrast Media

Reactions to radiocontrast media (RCM) appear to be related to the hyperosmolality of the material. Use of newer, low-osmolar (nonionic) media is associated with a lower reaction rate. The signs and symptoms are those of an IgE-mediated reaction, although no IgE antibody is involved.

There is currently no way to predict who is at risk of a reaction if the patient has no prior history. If a pregnant patient has a history of a past reaction and absolutely needs administration of contrast media, then she should be pretreated with steroids and antihistamines (33) and receive low-osmolar contrast media. The patient should be off any beta-blockers because, if epinephrine is require for treatment, hypertension may occur from unopposed alpha-stimulation. There is no association between reactions to contrast media and iodine or shellfish allergy.

References

1. Philipson A. Pharmacokinetics of ampicillin during pregnancy. J Infect Dis 1977; 136:370–376.
2. NAEP Expert Panel Report. Management of asthma during pregnancy. U.S. Dept. of Health and Human Services, NIH publication 93-3279, 1993.
3. Briggs GG, Freeman RK, Yaffe SJ. Drugs in pregnancy and lactation. 3d ed. Baltimore: Williams & Wilkins, 1990:237–238, 520–521.
4. Landor M. Maternal-fetal transfer of immunoglobulins. Ann. Allergy Asthma Immunol 1995; 74:279–284.
5. Clark SL. Shock in the pregnant patient. Semin Perinatol 1990; 14:52–58.
6. Greaves MW. Current concepts: chronic urticaria. N Engl J Med 1995; 332: 1767–1772.
7. Hide M, Francis DM, Grattan VCEH, Hakim J, Kochan JP, Greaves MW. Autoantibodies against the high affinity IgE receptor as a cause of histamine release in chronic urticaria. N Engl J Med 1993; 328:1599–1604.
8. Claveau J, Lavoie A, Brunet C, Beclard PM, Hebert J. Chronic idiopathic urticaria: possible contribution of histamine-releasing factor to pathogenesis. J Allergy Clin Immunol 1993; 92:132–137.
9. Ost L, Wettrell G, Bjorkhem I, Ranc A. Prednisone excretion in human milk. J Pediatr 1985; 106:1008–1011.
10. Warrington RJ, Silviu-Dan F, Magro C. Accelerated cell mediated immune reactions in penicillin allergy. J Allergy Clin Immunol 1993; 92:626–628.
11. Roujeau JC, Stern RS. Severe adverse cutaneous reactions to drugs. N Engl J Med 1994; 331:1272–1285.
12. Patterson R, Miller M, Kaplan M, Doan T, Brown J, Detjen P, Grammer L, Greenberger PA, Hogan B, Latall J, Lowenthal M, Pongracic J, Sonenthal K, Zeiss CR. Effectiveness of early therapy with corticosteroids in Stevens-Johnson syndrome: experience with 41 cases and a hypothesis regarding pathogenesis. Ann Allergy 1994; 73:27–34.
13. Fine J-D. Management of acquired bullous skin disease. N Engl J Med 1995; 333:1475–1484.
14. Mackowiak PA, Lemaistre CF. Drug fever: a critical appraisal of conventional concepts. Ann Intern Med 1987; 106:728–733.
15. Gilliland BC. Drug induced autoimmune and hematologic disorders. In: Van Arsdel PP, ed. Immunology and Allergy Clinics of North America. Philadelphia: Saunders, 1991:525–554.

16. Obermiller T, Lakshminarayan S. Drug induced hypersensitivity reactions in the lung. In: Van Arsdel PP, ed. Immunology and Allergy Clinics of North America. Philadelphia: Saunders, 1991:575–594.

17. Willson RA. The liver: its role in drug biotransformation and as a target of immunologic injury. In: Van Arsdel PP, ed. Immunology and Allergy Clinics of North America. Philadelphia: Saunders, 1991:555–574.

18. Shepherd GM. Allergy to beta-lactam antibiotics. In: Van Arsdel PP, ed. Immunology and Allergy Clinics of North America. Philadelphia: Saunders, 1991:611–633.

19. Sogn DD, Evans R, Shepherd GM, Casale TB, Condemi J, Greenberger PA, Kohler PF, Saxon A, Summers RJ, Van Arsdel PP, Massicot JG, Blackwelder WC, Levine BB. Results of the National Institute of Allergy and Infectious Diseases collaborative clinical trial to test the predictive value of skin testing with major and minor penicillin derivatives in hospitalized adults. Arch Intern Med 1992; 152:1025–1032.

20. Wendel GD, Stark BJ, Jamison RB, Molina RD, Sullivan TJ. Penicillin allergy and desensitization in serious infections during pregnancy. N Engl J Med 1985; 312:1229–1232.

21. Ziaya PR, Hankins GDV, Gilstrap LC, Halsey AB. Intravenous penicillin desensitization and treatment during pregnancy. JAMA 1986; 256:2561–2562.

22. Anne S, Reisman RE. Risk of administering cephalosporin antibiotics to patients with histories of penicillin allergy. Ann Allergy Asthma Immunol 1995; 74:167–170.

23. Healy DP, Sahai JV, Fuller SH, Polk RE. Vancomycin induced histamine release and "RedMan syndrome": comparison of 1 and 2 hour infusions. Antimicrob Agents Chemother 1990; 34:550–554.

24. Slater JE. Hypersensitivity to macrolide antibiotics. Ann Allergy 1991; 66: 193–195.

25. Weiler JM, Gelhaus MA, Carter JG, Meng RL, Benson PM, Hotlel RA, Schillic KB, Vegh AB,, Clarke WR. A prospective study of the risk of an immediate adverse reaction to protamine sulfate during cardiopulmonary bypass surgery. J Allergy Clin Immunol 1990; 85:713–719.

26. Moneret-Vautrin DA, Gueant JL, Kamel L, Laxenaire MC, El Kholty S, Nicolas JP. Anaphylaxis to muscle relaxants: cross-sensitivity studied by radioimmunoassay compared to intradermal tests in 34 cases. J Allergy Clin Immunol 1988; 82:745–752.

27. Adam PAJ, Schwartz R. Diagnosis and treatment: should oral hypoglycemic agents be used in pediatric and pregnant patients? Pediatrics 1968; 42:812.

28. Mellon MH, Schatz M, Patterson R. Drug allergy. In Lawlor GJ, Fisher RJ, eds. Manual of Allergy and Immunology, 3rd ed. Boston: Little, Brown, 1995: 262.

29. Slater RM, Bowles BJM, Pumphrey RSH. Anaphylactoid reactions to oxytocin in pregnancy. Anesthesia 1985; 40:655.

30. Stevenson D, Simon R. Sensitivity to aspirin and non-steroidal antiinflammatory drugs. In: Middleton E, Reed CE, Ellis EF, Adkinson NF, Yuninger

JW, Busse WW, eds. Allergy Practice and Principles. St. Louis: Mosby, 1993: 1755–1756.
31. Schatz M. Skin testing and incremental challenge in the evaluation of adverse reactions to local anesthetics. J Allergy Clin Immunol 1984; 74:606–616.
32. Israili ZH, Hall WD. Cough and angioneurotic edema associated with angiotensin converting enzyme inhibitor therapy. Ann Intern Med 1992; 117: 234–242.
33. Greenberger PA, Patterson R. The prevention of immediate generalized reaction to radiocontrast media in high-risk patients. J Allergy Clin Immunol 1991; 87:867–872.

Part Four

ASTHMA

15

Effects of Asthma on Pregnancy and Labor

DONNA S. DIZON-TOWNSON

University of Utah School of Medicine
Salt Lake City, Utah

STEVEN L. CLARK

University of Utah School of Medicine
and Intermountain Health Care
  Perinatal Centers
Salt Lake City, Utah

I. Introduction

In the United States, asthma is responsible for 28 million office visits, 1 million emergency room visits, and over 130,000 hospitalizations per year (1,2). Asthma affects about 3–4% of the general population (3), and according to the Centers for Disease Control the prevalence of asthma increased during the years 1980–1987 (4). Asthma causes approximately 4000 deaths annually in the United States, and the mortality rate ranges from 1% to 3% (2,5). Unfortunately, despite advances in therapy and aggressive management of acute asthma, deaths from asthma have either remained steady or increased since the mid-1970s (6).

Asthma complicates from 0.4% to 1.5% of pregnancies (7,8), and is the most common obstructive pulmonary disease seen in pregnancy. Thus the obstetrician will frequently encounter a pregnant patient with acute airway hyperreactivity with reversible airflow obstruction.

Patients with asthma who are pregnant need treatment to ensure both their health and the health of their fetuses. Adequate control of asthma during pregnancy appears to be the best way to minimize any untoward effect of asthma on the mother or her fetus. (See Chapters 18 and 19.)

In order to consolidate the many clinical definitions of asthma, the American Thoracic Society's Joint Committee on Pulmonary Nomenclature has defined asthma as "a disease characterized by an increased responsiveness of the airways to various stimuli, manifested by slowing of forced expiration, which changes in severity either spontaneously or as a result of therapy (9). The definition may be modified by including words indicating triggering factors such as cold, exercise, or allergen-induced asthma. In comparison, status asthmaticus denotes severe asthma of any type not responding after a 30- to 60-min period of intensive therapeutic measures (1,10).

II. Clinical Course of Pregnancy Complicated by Asthma

Decades ago, an analysis of pregnancy complicated by asthma concluded: "The pregnant woman can be reassured that her asthma will have no bearing on her pregnancy or on the outcome of her delivery" (11). However, there now exists an overwhelming abundance of evidence supporting the contrary. Several large epidemiological studies have clearly defined the potential adverse effects of maternal asthma on pregnancy and the infant. Maternal complications in pregnancies complicated with asthma include pregnancy-induced hypertension, preeclampsia, gestational and insulin-dependent diabetes mellitus, preterm labor, hyperemesis gravidarum, vaginal hemorrhage, and induced and complicated labor. Fetal complications include an increased risk of perinatal mortality, intrauterine growth restriction, preterm birth, low birth weight, and neonatal hypoxia (12).

A. Maternal Considerations

Maternal Mortality

Severe asthma may be associated with maternal mortality. Nineteen maternal deaths due to bronchial asthma during pregnancy between 1950 and 1962 in England and Wales were described (13). Schaefer and Silverman describe with great detail 1 maternal death due to asthma among 293 pregnant asthmatic patients (11). In another cohort of 277 pregnant asthmatic patients, 2 maternal deaths due to asthma were described (14). In the same study, 2 other maternal deaths occurred within 1 year of delivery, and it was concluded that asthma is associated with a considerable risk to life, either during or proximate to pregnancy. Uncontrollable status asthmaticus in the third trimester may be an indication for termination of pregnancy by caesarean section in order to prevent maternal mortality; 3 case reports describe a dramatic improvement of maternal oxygenation occurring after delivery of the fetus (15,16).

Pregnancy-Induced Hypertension/Preeclampsia

In one of the earliest and largest retrospective analysis of pregnancy complicated by asthma, hyperemesis, hemorrhage, and toxemia were found to be significantly more frequent in asthmatics than in women without disease prior to pregnancy (17). They compared 381 women reporting bronchial asthma that had its onset either before or during the pregnancy with a control group of 125,423 pregnancies in women reporting no disease before or during the pregnancy. Of the 381 total pregnancies of women with a diagnosis of bronchial asthma, 40 (10.5%) also had a diagnosis of toxemia of pregnancy, as compared to 5856 (4.7%) of the 125,423 control subjects ($p < .001$). Hyperemesis gravidarum was documented in 8 (2.1%) of preg nant asthmatic patients, compared to 1041 (0.8%) of controls ($p < .01$). Vaginal hemorrhage was reported in 18 (4.7%) gravid asthmatics, compared to 2775 (2.2%) controls ($p < .001$). However, the authors discuss a number of limitations in this study, including the inherent bias of a retrospective analysis, lack of a classification of severity of asthma or criteria for toxemia, and no documentation of the medication used by the patients.

In a more recent retrospective evaluation of asthma and perinatal outcome, a stratification of the severity of asthma within the population studied and extensive detail of the medications used by the asthmatics were recorded (18). This case-controlled study looked at a total 183 deliveries which were coded for a diagnosis of asthma. Eighty-one required the chronic use of medications to control their disease process. Of the 81, 31 were steroid dependent and 50 were non-steroid-dependent. The outcome variables were compared among three groups: steroid-dependent asthmatics, non-steroid-dependent asthmatics, and controls. There were no statistically significant differences in the frequencies of chronic hypertension and preeclampsia among asthma and control groups.

Two prospective analyses have evaluated the outcome of pregnancy in women with severe steroid-dependent asthma in whom medication usage and degree of severity were well documented. Such study design allowed an attempt to distinguish the perinatal effects of uncontrolled asthma from those of medication (19,20). These two studies examined a total of 80 pregnancies in 73 gravidas with severe asthma who required inhaled and/ or systemic corticosteroids. The study population was divided into two groups: asthmatics not requiring emergency therapy (group 1a) and asthmatics requiring emergency therapy or having an episode of status asthmaticus (group 1b). There were no differences in the frequency of chronic hypertensive disorders or preeclampsia between these groups.

However, another prospective analysis designed to investigate whether carefully managed asthma is associated with an increased risk of pregnancy complications found an increased incidence of preeclampsia (21). One hundred and eighty-one asthmatic women were monitored during 198 pregnancies. Medication use was documented. A control group of 198 nonasthmatic pregnant women were matched in age and parity. Preeclampsia was observed significantly more often in the asthmatic group (especially those with severe asthma) than in the control population (14.6% versus 4.5% $p < .001$).

Lehrer also described an association between pregnancy-induced hypertension and asthma during pregnancy (22). This study retrospectively evaluated a study population of 24,115 women without a history of chronic hypertension. Asthma during pregnancy was defined as asthma that necessitated treatment. Medication profiles for the patients were not noted. Pregnancy-induced hypertension was defined as blood pressure of at least 140/90 mmHg or an increase of ≥ 30 mmHg in systolic pressure or ≥ 15 mmHg in diastolic pressure (22). Of the 24,115 women, 1307 had moderate pregnancy-induced hypertension (systolic blood pressure 140–160 mmHg and diastolic blood pressure 90–110), and 92 had severe pregnancy-induced hypertension (systolic blood pressure 160 mmHg or diastolic blood pressure >110 mmHg). In all, 1435 patients had a history of asthma and 136 had asthma during pregnancy. A significant association between pregnancy-induced hypertension and asthma during pregnancy was found ($p < .001$). There was a significant upward trend in the incidence of asthma during pregnancy in women with no pregnancy-induced hypertension, moderate pregnancy-induced hypertension, and severe pregnancy-induced hypertension ($p = .001$). In addition, an association between pregnancy-induced hypertension and a history of asthma was found ($p = .001$). The authors conclude that plausible explanations for this association may be: medications used to treat asthma may cause pregnancy-induced hypertension; the stress of hypertension may precipitate an asthma exacerbation; and finally, a circulating factor exists which affects smooth muscle reactivity which is important in the pathophysiology of both disease processes.

Medications that asthmatic patients require may alter the disease process of pregnancy-induced hypertension or preeclampsia. The incidence of preeclampsia among asthmatic patients has been reported to be affected by the use of theophylline during pregnancy (23,24). However the studies are conflicting, as Dombroski et al. (23) found a decrease in the incidence of preeclampsia associated with theophylline usage, while Stenius-Aarniala et al. (24) found an increase of the disease in patients receiving theophylline.

Gestational and Insulin-Dependent Diabetes Mellitus

There is less evidence that asthma influences the incidence of gestational and insulin-dependent diabetes mellitus. It seems likely that the presence of diabetes mellitus is the result of the steroid medications taken by the pregnant asthmatic and not a direct result of the disease process itself. In a retrospective analysis comparing steroid-dependent, non-steroid-medication-dependent asthmatics, and controls, steroid-dependent asthmatics were at significantly ($p = .01$) increased risk for gestational (12.9% versus 1.5%) and insulin-requiring diabetes (9.7% versus 0%) than were controls (18). Non-steroid-medication-dependent asthmatics, however, did not show a significantly increased occurrence of these complications compared to controls ($p = .6$) (18).

When steroid-dependent asthmatics not requiring emergency therapy were compared with steroid-dependent asthmatics requiring emergency therapy or status asthmaticus, there were no differences in the prevalence of gestational diabetes mellitus (19,20).

Even though steroid medications may influence the presence of diabetes during pregnancy, there is overwhelming evidence supporting the precis that steroids do not cause an increase of congenital malformations, and pregnancy should not preclude the use of these medications (18–21,25,26). The risk of hypoxemia to both the mother and fetus in a poorly controlled asthmatic far outweighs the risk of any potential dangers of corticosteroid administration.

B. Fetal Considerations

Miscarriage

Little is known concerning the risk of miscarrying a fetus when the new pregnancy is complicated by maternal asthma. In one series, spontaneous abortions occurred in 11.0% of patients with asthma, compared with 9.4% of all clinic patients who had abortions. The event of spontaneous abortion appeared to be unrelated to severe asthmatic attacks (11). In another study, spontaneous abortions occurred in 3 of 33 steroid-dependent, severe asthmatic patients. In all three pregnancies associated with abortion, the patient's asthma was considered to be under good control and not the etiology of the miscarriage (26). An additional reported case of life-threatening status asthmaticus at 12.5 weeks' gestation resulted in a normal pregnancy outcome (27).

Perinatal Mortality

In a large retrospective study comparing the outcome of pregnancy in 277 asthmatic women to that in a cohort of 30,861 gravidas, Gordon et al. observed a rate of perinatal mortality nearly double in asthmatic versus control women (5.9% versus 3.2%, $p < .05$) (14). While the risk of prematurity was not significantly increased, there were 16 perinatal deaths. All of the fetal deaths occurred antepartum and were generally associated with more significant asthmatic disease and complicating maternal illness. Four of the mothers were classified as having severe asthma. In addition, these investigators evaluated the condition of the infant at birth by reviewing Apgar scores at 1 and 5 min of age in infants of similar birth weight. No significant difference in the incidence of low scores (0–6) in the infants of the asthmatic patients were seen. In 16 women classified as having "severe asthma," there was a 28% perinatal death rate, 35% of these pregnancies resulted in low-birth-weight infants, and 12.5% of these infants manifested neurological abnormalities at 1 year of age. The authors concluded that the severity of maternal asthma was integral to the increase in perinatal mortality observed. Bahna et al. also demonstrated an increase in perinatal death rate among the infants of asthmatics (17). However, other studies have not confirmed an increase of perinatal mortality in the pregnancies of asthmatic compared to nonasthmatic women (19–21).

Intrauterine Growth

Several studies suggest that maternal asthma is responsible for impaired intrauterine growth resulting in an increase number of low-birth-weight infants and infants manifesting signs of intrauterine growth restriction. In reviewing these studies, it is important to distinguish preterm infants (≤ 37 weeks' gestation), low-birth-weight infants (< 2500 g), and infants with intrauterine growth restriction (< 10th percentile for gestational age).

Bahna et al. noted 7.1% of asthma patients and 3.7% of control patients ($p < .001$) as having infants of low birth weight (17). The mean gestation period in weeks for the asthma group (39.5) and for the control group (39.9) were similar. However, the mean birth weight in grams for the asthma group (3399.9) was significantly lower than in the control group (3496.7) ($p < .001$).

In the two series of steroid-treated asthmatics, a statistically significant increase in low-birth-weight infants was observed. When infants of gravidas who experienced at least one episode of status asthmaticus and infants of steroid-dependent asthmatics who had not required emergency therapy were compared, the mean birth weight of the infants of gravidas who had suffered an episode of status asthmaticus was decreased significantly ($p = .026$), and the frequency of intrauterine growth restriction was greater ($p = .056$) (19,20).

When steroid-dependent, non-steroid-dependent, and control groups were retrospectively compared, Perlow et al. (18) found that both asthmatic groups had a higher incidence of low-birth-weight infants when compared to their control population ($p < .05$). In addition, when steroid-dependent asthmatics were compared to non-steroid-dependent patients, there was a statistically significant increase in the number of low-birth-weight infants ($p = .004$) of steroid-dependent mothers (18).

An early prospective analysis of pulmonary function in bronchial asthma during and after pregnancy showed that patients with active disease tended to have smaller babies than patients with asthma in remission (28). These investigators were unable to demonstrate any significant longitudinal changes in FEV_1/FVC or FVC in the asthma or control groups during pregnancy.

Another well-designed study relating intrauterine growth to gestational pulmonary function prospectively surveyed 360 pregnancies in women with documented asthma who delivered singleton births beyond 20 weeks' gestation (29). Spirometry was obtained on each regularly scheduled monthly office visit as well as on extra visits required for the evaluation of increased symptoms. A significant ($p < .04$) correlation was demonstrated between individual mean percent predicted FEV_1 and birth weight in asthmatic individuals. In addition, lower maternal FEV_1 during pregnancy was associated with an increased likelihood of birth weight in the lower quartile of the population ($p < .002$) and ponderal indices <2.2 ($p < .05$). After calculating odds ratios and p values, an FEV_1 of 90% of predicted normal proved to be the most discriminating: Women with a mean $FEV_1 < 90\%$ of predicted normal were 2.5 times more likely to deliver an infant with low ponderal indices. No significant relationships were observed between lower FEV_1 and the incidences of preterm or low-birth-weight infants, chronic or gestational hypertension, or preeclampsia. The authors conclude that the findings from this study suggest that the goals for caring for the gravid asthmatic should include optimization of pulmonary function in addition to achievement of symptomatic control.

Preterm Birth

The issues of preterm birth and low birth weight in pregnancies complicated by maternal asthma are closely intertwined. The results of the two largest retrospective analyses are conflicting. Bahna et al. reported a significant increase of preterm delivery (<37 weeks' gestation). Also, 7.4% of patients with asthma delivered prematurely, compared to 5.0% of control patients ($p < .01$) (17). In contrast, Gordon et al. did not find an increase risk of prematurity in their patients (14). Another prospective study confirmed the results of Gordon (21). In this series, the mean gestational age for asthmatic patients was similar to that in controls.

In an evaluation of steroid-dependent asthmatics, the overall incidence of premature infants and low-birth-weight infants was slightly higher than in the general population (19,20). In patients requiring emergency therapy, 18.7% had premature births, compared to 9.6% of the general population.

Perlow et al. reported that both preterm delivery and preterm premature rupture of membranes occurred more frequently in both steroid-dependent and non-steroid-dependent asthmatics than in control patients (18). Both asthmatic groups were more likely to be admitted for preterm labor, to be delivered before 37 weeks, and to have their pregnancies complicated by preterm premature rupture of membranes ($p < .05$ for all three outcome variables).

Doucette recently demonstrated asthma as a risk factor in preterm labor and delivery (30). These investigators prospectively assessed the relation between maternal respiratory problems and preterm labor and delivery in a cohort of 3891 women who delivered a singleton livebirth. Women who reported a history of asthma had a higher risk of preterm labor [relative risk (RR) estimate = 2.33, 95% confidence interval (CI) = 1.03–5.26]. Although the results were not statistically significant, asthmatic women were reported to have an increased risk of preterm delivery (RR = 1.77, 95% CI = 0.60–5.24). However, gravidas reporting respiratory difficulty within the past year, while pregnant, were noted to have a statistically significant increased risk of preterm delivery (RR = 2.03, 95% CI = 1.08–3.82).

The mechanisms of potential adverse effects of asthma on pregnancy and the infant have not been fully defined. However, available information does suggest that poor asthma control may be the most important factor, and that adequate control of asthma during pregnancy is important in improving maternal and fetal outcomes (12).

C. Considerations for Labor and Delivery

The gravida with a recent history of severe asthma deserves considerable attention during labor and delivery. About 10% of pregnant asthmatics will have an exacerbation during labor and delivery (31). The risk of peripartum exacerbation is reported to be increased 18-fold following caesarean as compared with vaginal delivery (32). Bahna et al. (17) reported the percentage of induced labor to be statistically higher in asthmatic women (14.2%) than in controls (9.1%). "Complicated labor" was also more frequent among the asthmatics (14.4% versus 9.6%). "Interventions" during labor were slightly more frequent in asthmatic women (9.9%) than in controls (7.7%). Although the frequency of intervention was not statistically different between the two groups, the types of interventions mentioned included: artificial rupture of membranes (2.6% versus 1.4%), forceps or vacuum extraction (2.9% versus 2.4%), and caesarean section (1.8% versus 1.1%).

Other studies have confirmed these findings of an increased caesarean section and instrumental delivery rate in pregnant asthmatic women (21,33). The increased caesarean section rate may be related to a slightly higher rate of induction in asthmatic mothers. Lao et al. (33) reported that the labor of 24.1% of 87 asthmatic mothers was *induced*, compared to 19.5% of 87 control mothers. These authors also reported that the frequency distribution of indications for labor induction differed in the asthmatic versus control women. The indications for induction in asthmatic gravidas were: unstable asthma 5/21 (23.8%), postmaturity 5/21 (23.8%), prolonged leaking of amniotic fluid 5/21 (23.8%), other medical indications 3/21 (14.3%), suspected intrauterine growth retardation 2/21 (9.5%), and fetal abnormality 1/21 (4.8%). For controls the indications for induction of labor were: postdated pregnancy 13/17 (76.4%), prolonged rupture of membranes 3/17 (17.6%), and decreased fetal movement 1/17 (5.8%). The increased rate of instrumental deliveries in asthmatic women in this series may have been related to the use of epidural anesthesia, since (a) epidural analgesia was used in 40.2% of asthmatic women but only 3.4% of controls, and (b) asthmatic women receiving epidural analgesia had a lower incidence of spontaneous delivery (38.7%) than asthmatic women not receiving epidural analgesia (67.3%) ($p < .02$) (33).

During labor and delivery, precautions for prevention of an Addisonian-like adrenal crisis secondary to adrenal suppression from long-term corticosteroid use should be taken. Patients who have required chronic systemic corticosteroids during pregnancy should be given 100 mg of hydrocortisone every 8 hr until 24 hr postpartum to treat for possible adrenal suppression (12). The pediatrician should also be informed regarding chronic material steroid use, as transient neonatal adrenal suppression has occasionally been reported in such women.

In consultation with the anesthesiologist, the choice of a sedative for labor should include one of the non-histamine-releasing narcotics, such as fentanyl, as opposed to morphine (34). Furthermore, as endotracheal intubation has been associated with severe bronchospasm, consideration should be given to establishment of regional anesthesia and early placement of an epidural catheter (35). Finally, in the event of postpartum hemorrhage due to atony, PGE_2 and other uterotonics should be used in lieu of 15-methyl $PGF_{2\alpha}$. Clinically diminished pulmonary function associated with the administration of 15-methyl $PGF_{2\alpha}$ and significant bronchospasm in asthmatics receiving $PGF_{2\alpha}$ for mid-trimester abortion have been reported (36), as well as dangerous oxygen desaturation following 15-methyl $PGF_{2\alpha}$ given for postpartum hemorrhage (37).

III. Conclusions

In summary, the findings from these various studies suggest that the pregnancy complicated by maternal asthma is indeed a high-risk pregnancy and should be managed as such (see Chapter 20). Severe acute asthma in pregnancy poses a serious threat to both maternal and fetal well-being. Physiological alterations in pulmonary function render the pregnant woman susceptible to acute derangements in ventilation (see Chapter 3). In addition, fetal health may be in danger even in the early stages of asthma (see Chapter 2). Most recently, a study which controlled for potentially confounding variables and included the largest asthmatic population to date was reported (38). This prospective analysis compared 486 pregnant (<28 weeks) women with documented asthma to 486 pregnant nonasthmatic controls with normal pulmonary function. Active management of asthma in these gravidas was not associated with increased incidences of preeclampsia, perinatal mortality, preterm or low-birth-weight infants, intrauterine growth retardation, or congenital malformations. However, trends toward relationships between more severe asthma requiring emergency therapy or corticosteroids and increased incidences of preeclampsia and low-birth-weight infants were noted. For these reasons, the obstetrician should render aggressive therapy for the gravida suffering from asthma (see Chapters 18 and 19).

References

1. Summer WR. Status asthmaticus. Chest 1985; 87:87s–94s.
2. Corre KA, Rothstein RJ. Assessing severity of adult asthma and need for hospitalization. Ann Emerg Med 1985; 14:45–52.
3. Smith JM. Epidemiology and natural history of asthma, allergic rhinitis, and atopic dermatitis. In: Middleton E Jr, Reed CF, Ellis E, eds. Allergy: Principles and Practice. 3d ed. St. Louis: Mosby, 1988:899.

4. Centers for Disease Control. Asthma–United States, 1980–1987. Morbid Mortal Weekly Rep 1990; 39:493.
5. Franklin W. Treatment of severe asthma. N Engl J Med 1974; 290:1469–1472.
6. Woolcock AJ. Asthma. In: Murray JF, Nadel JA, eds. Textbook of Respiratory Medicine. Philadelphia: Saunders, 1988:1030–1068.
7. Mintz S. Pregnancy and asthma. In: Weiss EB, Segal MS, eds. Bronchial Asthma: Mechanisms and Therapeutics. Boston: Little, Brown, 1976:971–982.
8. de Swiet M. Diseases of the respiratory system. Clin Obstet Gynaecol 1977; 4:287–296.
9. Burrows B, Huang N, Hughes R, Johnston R, Kilburn K, Kuhn C, Miller W, Mitchell M, Snider G. Pulmonary terms and symbols: a report of the ACCP-ATS Joint Committee on Pulmonary Nomenclature. Chest 1975; 67:583–593.
10. Koch-Weser J, Webb-Johnson DC, Andrews JL. Bronchodilator therapy (second of two parts). N Engl J Med 1977; 297:758–764.
11. Schaefer G, Silverman F. Pregnancy complicated by asthma. Am J Obstet Gynecol 1961; 82:182–191.
12. Report of the Working Group on Asthma and Pregnancy. Management of Asthma During Pregnancy. National Asthma Education Program, National Heart, Lung, and Blood Institute, National Institutes of Health. NIH Publication 93-3279A, March 1993.
13. Williams DA. Asthma and pregnancy. Allergy 1967; 22:311.
14. Gordon M, Niswander KR, Berendes H, Kantor AG. Fetal morbidity following potentially anoxigenic obstetric conditions. Am J Obstet Gynecol 1970; 106:421–429.
15. Topilsky M, Levo Y, Spitzer SA, Lewinski U, Atsmon A. Status asthmaticus in pregnancy: a case report. Ann Allergy 1974; 32:151–153.
16. Gelber M, Sidi Y, Gassner S, Ovadia Y, Spitzer S, Weinberger A, Pinkhas J. Uncontrollable life-threatening status asthmaticus—an indicator for termination of pregnancy by cesarean section. Respiration 1984; 46:320–322.
17. Bahna SL, Bjerkedal T. The course and outcome of pregnancy in women with bronchial asthma. Acta Allergologica 1972; 27:397–406.
18. Perlow JH, Montgomery D, Morgan MA, Towers CV, Porto M. Severity of asthma and perinatal outcome. Am J Obstet Gynecol 1992; 167:963–967.
19. Fitzsimons R, Greenberger PA, Patterson R. Outcome of pregnancy in women requiring corticosteroids for severe asthma. J Allergy Clin Immunol 1986; 78:349–353.
20. Greenberger PA, Patterson R. The outcome of pregnancy complicated by severe asthma. Allergy Proc 1988; 9:539–543.
21. Stenius-Aarniala B, Piirila P, Teramo K. Asthma and pregnancy: a prospective study of 198 pregnancies. Thorax 1988; 43:12–18.
22. Lehrer S, Stone J, Lapinski R, Lockwood CJ, Schachter BS, Berkowitz R, Berkowitz G. Association between pregnancy-induced hypertension and asthma during pregnancy. Am J Obstet Gynecol 1993; 168:1463–1466.

23. Dombroski MP, Bottoms SF, Boike GM, Wald J. Incidence of preeclampsia among asthmatic patients lower with theophylline. Am J Obstet Gynecol 1986; 155:265–267.

24. Stenius-Aarniala B, Riikonen S. Slow-release theophyllline in pregnant asthmatics. Chest 1995; 107:642–647.

25. Snyder RD, Snyder D. Corticosteroids for asthma during pregnancy. Ann Allergy 1978; 41:340–341.

26. Greenberger PA, Patterson R. Beclomethasone diproprionate for severe asthma during pregnancy. Ann Intern Med 1983; 98:478–480.

27. Gilchrist DM, Friedman JM, Werker D. Life-threatening status asthmaticus at 12.5 weeks gestation. Report of a normal pregnancy outcome. Chest 1991; 100:285–286.

28. Sims CD, Chamberlain GVP, De Swiet M. Long function test in bronchial asthma during and after pregnancy. Br J Obstet Gynaecol 1976; 83:434–437.

29. Schatz M, Zeiger RS, Hoffman CP, Kaiser-Permanente Asthma and Pregnancy Study Group. Intrauterine growth is related to gestational pulmonary function in pregnant asthmatic women. Chest 1990; 98:389–392.

30. Doucette JT, Bracken MB. Possible role of asthma in the risk of preterm labor delivery. Epidemiology 1993; 4:143–150.

31. Schatz M, Harden K, Forsythe A, Chilingar L, Hoffman C, Sperling W, Zeiger RS. The course of asthma during pregnancy, post partum, and with successive pregnancies: a prospective analysis. J Allergy Clin Immunol 1988; 81: 509–517.

32. Mabie WC, Barton JR, Wasserstrum N, Sibai BM. Clinical observations on asthma in pregnancy. J Maternal-Fetal Med 1992; 1:45–50.

33. Lao TT, Huengsburg M. Labour and delivery in mothers with asthma. Eur J Obst Gynecol Reprod Biol 1990; 35:183–190.

34. Hermens JM, Ebertz JM, Hannifin JM, Hirshman CA. Comparison of histamine release in human skin mast cells induced by morphine, fentanyl, and oxymorphone. Anesthesiology 1985; 62:124–129.

35. Kingston HGG, Hirsham CA. Perioperative management of the patient with asthma. Anesth Analg 1984; 63:844–855.

36. Kreisman H, deWrel WV, Mitchell CA. Respiratory function during prostaglandin-induced labor. Am Rev Respir Dis 1975; 111:564–566.

37. Hankins GDV, Berryman GK, Scott RT Jr, Hood D. Maternal arterial desaturation with 15-methyl prostaglandin F2 alpha for uterine atony. Obstet Gynecol 1988; 72:367–370.

38. Schatz M, Zeiger RS, Hoffman CP, Harden K, Forsythe A, Chilingar L, Saunders B, Porreco R, Sperling W, Kagnoff M, Benenson AS. Perinatal outcomes in the pregnancies of asthmatic women: a prospective controlled analysis. Am J Respir Crit Care Med 1995; 151:1170–1174.

16

Effect of Pregnancy on Asthma: A Systematic Review and Meta-Analysis

ELIZABETH F. JUNIPER

McMaster University Medical Centre
Hamilton, Ontario, Canada

MICHAEL T. NEWHOUSE

McMaster University and St. Joseph's
   Hospital
Hamilton, Ontario, Canada

I. Introduction

The earliest reports of the effect of pregnancy on asthma started appearing in the 1930s. Since then there have been numerous case reports, case series, retrospective and prospective cohort studies, and reviews on the topic. Enormous variance in the results of the original research studies has led to confusion and diversity of opinion. Major contributors to these discrepancies have been inadequate study designs, methodological flaws, the use of different outcomes to measure asthma severity, and the selection of subjects from very different populations. As a result, the conclusions drawn by some investigators are at best questionable and sometimes invalid.

For this review, we have endeavored to locate all published reports on the effect of pregnancy on asthma. We conducted searches through *Medline, Citation Index,* and *Current Contents.* We also searched the references of papers on the topic and solicited the knowledge of experts in the field. Of the reports we identified, only original studies with more than 10 patients have been included. We have excluded individual case reports and case series with 10 patients or less.

Since 1953, 14 original studies have evaluated the effect of pregnancy on asthma with the results published in accessible journals (1–14). In this review, we critically appraise each of these studies for strength of evidence based on study design, subject sampling methods, outcome measures, whether other factors affecting asthma were considered, and statistical methods. We discuss the methodological strengths and weaknesses of the studies and consider how differences in conclusions may have arisen. In an attempt to determine whether any overall pattern arises from the results of these studies, we have pooled the results using meta-analytical techniques (Table 1).

II. Evaluation of an Intervention

To determine the effect of an intervention, usually a drug, on a specific condition, most investigators agree that the optimum study design is a double-blind, randomized, controlled trial (RCT). The strengths of such a design have been well documented, and RCTs have become the cornerstone of clinical drug evaluation. In fact, the results from any less rigorous design are usually viewed with extreme caution and awareness of potential biases.

However, in investigating the effect of an intervention, the study architecture alone is insufficient to exclude biases, and it is important that other factors are carefully controlled to ensure both the internal and the external validity of the conclusions. These include random or consecutive subject selection from a well-defined population, minimal loss to follow-up, validated objective and subjective measures of outcome, control of contaminants and cointerventions, and appropriate statistical analysis.

Pregnancy can be considered an intervention, and the evaluation of the effect of pregnancy on asthma is analogous to determining the effect of a drug on asthma. While a randomized controlled trial is clearly not possible, the most valid results can be obtained only through use of rigorous study design, with all factors that can affect outcome carefully controlled.

III. Study Design

If the effect of pregnancy on asthma could be evaluated with one or two well-designed, randomized controlled trials, much of the current confusion could be resolved very quickly. However, pregnancy cannot be randomized and therefore we are left with weaker study designs ranging in strength of

Table 1 Summary of Studies

First author (yr) country	Study design	Source of subjects	Asthma inclusion criteria	Time of enrollment	Number of subjects	Number of pregnancies	Outcomes	Other factors affecting outcomes considered
Jensen (1953) Denmark	Case series	Allergy consultation clinic	Married women with bronchial asthma	0–6 yr postdelivery	61	1–6 per subject	Patient recall	Eosinophils, allergy skin test, vital capacity
Gandev.a (1953) Australia	Case control	Allergy clinic	Women with asthma	Unknown	18	25	Patient recall	NIL
Turiaf (1958) France	Case series	General hospital	Women with asthma	Unknown	198	Unknown	Case records	NIL
Schaefe: (1961) USA	Case series	Obstetric–pulmonary clinic	Women with asthma	Unknown	271	Unknown	Patient recall	Seasonal allergens, climate, emotions, respiratory infection
Gammal (1963) Egypt	Case series	Chest service	Women with bronchial asthma	Unknown	112	1–6 per subject	Patient and physician recall, asthma attacks, therapy	Corticosteroids, season, duration of asthma
Wulfsohn (1964) S. Africa	Case series	Unknown	Bantu women with asthma	Postdelivery	18	Unknown	Patient recall	NIL

Table 1 Continued

First author (yr) country	Study design	Source of subjects	Asthma inclusion criteria	Time of enrollment	Number of subjects	Number of pregnancies	Outcomes	Other factors affecting outcomes considered
Hiddlestone (1964) New Zealand	Case series retrospective and prospective	Asthma clinic	Pregnant women with asthma	? During pregnancy	44	83	Case records, asthma assessment each trimester	Atopy, sex of foetus, menstrual asthma, puberty asthma
Williams (1967) UK	Case series	Asthma clinic	Women with asthma	Unknown	100	210 1–6 per patient	Case records, asthma attacks, therapy, hospitalizations	Menstrual asthma, season of delivery, respiratory infection, asthma severity
Sims (1976) UK	During cohort	Maternity hospital	Pregnant women with reversible bronchospasm in previous 3 yr	Pre-20-wk gestation	27	27	Spirometry (FEV, FVC), exercise induced ↓ in spirometry	FEV/VC, <70%
Gluck (1976) USA	During cohort	Prenatal clinic O and G emergency room	All pregnant asthmatics	During pregnancy	47	47	Observer record of asthma severity and therapy (change defined)	Asthma severity, IgE

Schatz (1988) USA	During–after cohort	Medical care program–prenatal clinic	All women with asthma history and reversible obstructive airway disease	During pregnancy	330	366	Patient recall, physician interpreted symptom and medication diary cards	NIL
Stenius-Aarniala (1988) Finland	During–after cohort	Maternity centers, outpatient practice	ATS and ACCP criteria of asthma	20% 1st trimester, 54% 2nd trimester, 26% 3rd trimester	181	198	Maintenance medication, (spirometry and daily PEFR not reported)	NIL
White (1989) UK	During–after cohort	Antenatal clinic	"Do you have asthma?"	During pregnancy	31	31	Patient recall, symptom and medication diary, daily PEFR	Asthma severity duration of asthma, menstrual asthma, season, smoking
Juniper (1989) Canada	Before–during–after cohort with controls	Asthma clinic, general practice, media	Airway hyperresponsiveness and current asthma symptoms	Preconception	16	16	Airway responsiveness, maintenance medications, asthma severity score, spirometry	Allergens, respiratory infection, reflux, inhaled steroids

evidence from the prospective cohort (with controls) to the case series (15). As one progresses from the prospective cohort to the case series, there is the potential for more and more of the well-described biases (16) to invalidate the conclusions. We start our critical appraisal of the 14 studies by examining the strengths and weaknesses of the various study designs, moving from the strongest study architecture, a before–during–after prospective cohort with controls, to the weakest, the case series.

A. Before–During–After Prospective Cohort with Controls

There is only one report that has used this design (14). This is mainly because it is very difficult to enroll women in a pregnancy study before they conceive. This study enrolled asthmatic women who had the potential to conceive and were trying to become pregnant (14). They were assessed regularly before conception, throughout their pregnancy, and 3 months thereafter. Data collected preconception and from the women who failed to conceive within 1 year were used as control data. The design provided strong before, during, and after data in the pregnant women, and the magnitude of change seen during pregnancy could be compared with the natural fluctuations of asthma in women who were not pregnant. A weakness of this design is that if women develop asthma for the very first time as a result of pregnancy, they would not be included.

B. During–After Prospective Cohort with No Controls

If one uses the drug intervention analogy, the during–after study design is equivalent to enrolling patients into a study after starting the drug and making the assumption that recovery after withdrawal returns the patient to the preintervention state. In our study, we showed that this is not always a valid assumption, because the patients who required regular inhaled steroids showed a significant improvement in airway responsiveness between preconception and postdelivery and this systematic change, which was independent of pregnancy, did not occur in the non-steroid-dependent patients (17). Late enrollment into a during–after study may also produce a series selection bias. Asthmatic patients who become symptom free during the first months of pregnancy, as a result of the pregnancy, are unlikely to meet the inclusion criteria, thus biasing the results in favor of patients who remain stable or deteriorate during pregnancy.

Several of the more recent studies have used the "during–after" study design (9–13). Asthmatic women were enrolled after conception and then followed during pregnancy and for various time periods thereafter. This allowed objective and subjective measurements to be made and permitted estimation of within-subject changes between pregnancy and postdelivery. None of these studies had matched nonpregnant asthmatic controls, which would have strengthened the inference that the observed changes could be attributed to pregnancy.

Two studies included a control cohort of pregnant nonasthmatic women (9,12). For Stenius-Aarniala et al. (12), these were ideal for addressing the primary question of the effect of asthma on pregnancy but not suitable for the secondary question of the effects of pregnancy on asthma. Sims et al. (9) had a similar control group with the same limitations.

IV. Loss to Follow-Up and Withdrawals

In drug intervention studies, one of the factors most profoundly affecting the validity of the results is the number of subjects who withdraw or are lost to follow-up. Patients may leave a study because they get much better or because they get much worse, and it is rarely possible to determine how their leaving affects the results. There is usually no way of knowing whether those who withdraw are different from those who remain in the study, and no amount of statistical gymnastics can alleviate the uncertainty. If there are more than 80% withdrawals from a clinical trial, most methodologists would challenge the validity of the conclusions. Loss to follow-up and withdrawals from pregnancy studies have exactly the same effect: They reduce the validity of the conclusions. Therefore an important component of reporting should be the number of withdrawals and, if possible, the reasons. Unfortunately, this is rarely done, and one is often forced to make the assumption that the investigators were not aware of this important source of error and that the number of withdrawals may have affected the results.

Schatz et al. (11) identified 573 potential subjects, of whom 463 entered the study. Three hundred and thirty were included in the final documentation. Reasons for leaving the study were identified as inconvenience, leaving the area, abortion, and not fulfilling the documentation criteria.

In our study (14), 26 women met the inclusion/exclusion criteria, but 6 dropped out after one clinic visit and before conception. The reasons were dislike of the breathing tests ($n = 3$), recommendation of a family doctor ($n = 1$), moving from the area ($n = 1$), and decision not to conceive ($n = 1$). The remaining 20 patients all completed the study.

The other 12 studies do not report how many of their enrolled subjects were not included in the final analysis. In terms of study validity, this is a serious omission.

V. Subjects

A. Sampling Strategies

Some of the differences in results between studies may be attributed both to sampling techniques and to the populations from which the study samples were drawn. A random sample of all women with asthma who are planning a pregnancy, entered consecutively, and with no refusals would provide the best estimate of outcome in a particular catchment area. However, such sampling would still miss women who develop asthma for the first time during pregnancy. In addition, the actual enrollment site may influence the results. For instance, women enrolled from a tertiary-care asthma clinic may have asthma that is more difficult to control and may respond differently to pregnancy compared with those enrolled from an obstetric clinic.

Sims et al. (9), White et al. (13), and Schatz et al. (11) appear to have achieved good generalizable samples by enrolling from obstetric populations. Sims et al. (9) included consecutive maternity hospital patients who had experienced as asthma attack in the previous 3 years, and White et al. (13) enrolled from an antenatal clinic by asking the question: "Do you have asthma?" Schatz et al. (11) asked all women from a medical care program who registered for prenatal care whether they had asthma or asthma symptoms. The limitation of this latter approach is that it is dependent on the patients' knowledge.

We (14) enrolled preconception and therefore could not use the unbiased obstetrical source. In an attempt to minimize the enrollment of patients with difficult asthma, only 30% came from an allergy clinic; the rest came from local family physicians and through advertising in the local media.

Patients studied by Jensen (1), Gandevia (2), Schaefer and Silverman (4), Gammal and Warraki (5), Hiddlestone (7), and Williams (8) all came from asthma or allergy clinics. These may have been biased toward women with more severe or difficult-to-control asthma. Stenius-Aarniala et al. (12) acknowledge that, because asthma patients were referred to their study, they may have tended to capture more severe cases. Jensen (1) actually excluded 22 of his 106 potential subjects because they did not have allergic disease during pregnancy. The generalizability of Wulfsohn and Politzer's (6) sample of Bantu women to other cultures is uncertain.

B. Inclusion Criteria

The inclusion/exclusion criteria are an essential part of a study protocol. Unless one knows the characteristics of the patients, both enrolled and excluded, it is very difficult to know whether the results are applicable to other patients. In addition, in studies examining the effect of pregnancy on asthma, one would at least like to have evidence that the women enrolled actually did have asthma. Ideally, investigators should use diagnostic criteria such as those specified in the American Thoracic Society Guidelines. History alone can be inadequate, because there is a risk of including patients who do not have the condition. The point was made by Yernault that dyspnoea, wheezing, and respiratory insufficiency during pregnancy may be cardiac rather than respiratory in origin (18). Evidence that this may be important is suggested in the study by Schaefer and Silverman (4), who noted that some of their patients did not manifest the classical symptoms of asthma.

Only three studies used objective, defined, and recognized entry criteria. Schatz et al. (11) required subjects to demonstrate variable airflow limitation, and the subjects of Stenius-Aarniala et al. (12) had to satisfy the diagnostic criteria for asthma set by the American Thoracic Society and the American College of Chest Physicians. We (14) required subjects to have current symptoms of asthma and airway hyperresponsiveness to methacholine.

In the remaining studies, inclusion appears to have been based on history alone. This runs the risk of not only including patients who might have been incorrectly diagnosed as having asthma, but also those currently in remission. Sims et al. (9) acknowledge that they may have included some of the latter in their sample when they set their entry criterion as having had an attack of reversible bronchospasm in the last 3 years.

C. Single Versus Multiple Enrollment

It is very tempting to enroll an eligible subject into a study twice or more. This may be ideal if one is examining the within-subject reproducibility of a response to an intervention. However, it is unacceptable when the primary question concerns the overall effect of an intervention. Hiddlestone (7) actually included one woman 10 times, for each of her 10 pregnancies. If a multigravid subject was consistently different from the true population mean, she would produce a series bias. Mixing within- and between-subject variance for examining the overall effect of pregnancy on asthma should be avoided.

VI. Measures of Outcome

A. Clinical Asthma Severity

Like study design and subject follow-up, the methods used to measure the primary outcome are crucial for ensuring the validity of the conclusions. In determining whether asthma "changes" as a result of pregnancy, it is essential to define exactly which measurement is being used to assess asthma severity (spirometry, medications, symptoms, airway responsiveness, etc.) and what magnitude of change actually constitutes an improvement or a deterioration. One of the major problems with trying to provide an overall review of the effect of pregnancy on asthma is that all the investigators who used objective measures used different ones, and the remainder used subjective judgment!

Clinical asthma severity can be estimated objectively from the combination of (a) severity of airflow limitation (symptoms and spirometry) and (b) medication requirements. If one is held constant, the other may be used to estimate the change in severity. When both change, estimation of severity becomes very complicated and the data difficult to interpret.

With objective outcome measures, magnitude of change can certainly be measured, but even here the magnitude of what constitutes a clinically important difference will vary between clinicians. In addition, for both objective and subjective outcomes, the magnitude of improvement necessary to be called an improvement may not be equivalent to the magnitude of deterioration interpreted as a deterioration. For instance, an exacerbation requiring additional medication may be more blatant and more readily interpreted as a deterioration than an equivalent improvement where change in medication is less dramatic. Therefore the bias in ordinal outcomes is likely to be underreporting of improvements. Applying the same reasoning, care should be taken in interpreting the studies by Williams (8) and Gluck and Gluck (10), who reported that women with more severe asthma prior to pregnancy were more likely to experience worsening of their asthma during pregnancy than women with milder prepregnancy asthma.

Sims et al. (9) were the first investigators to report objective data for all subjects from a prospective study. They measured spirometry but were unable to detect any changes due to pregnancy. However, they acknowledge that medications were altered as necessary, and this might have masked potential changes in spirometry.

Patients in our study (14) were instructed to keep their asthma symptoms well controlled on a minimum of medication, and they were given a definition of "well controlled." They were instructed to increase medications when symptoms deteriorated and to decrease medications when symptoms ameliorated. The estimate of asthma severity was therefore the amount of medication taken to maintain control. We also measured spirometry and asthma symptom scores to ensure that patients were compliant with the instructions.

Stenius-Aarniala et al. (12) also used medication requirements during pregnancy to estimate clinical severity and carefully defined criteria for increasing medications. However, they do not indicate what criteria were used for reducing medications, nor have they reported whether there were any changes in airflow limitation or symptoms during pregnancy, even though these were recorded. Assessments were made on enrollment, during the last month of pregnancy, and more frequently if symptoms were troublesome. This approach may have tended to overestimate deteriorations, since patients who improved or stayed the same would not have had these additional evaluations.

Complete objective data from the other prospective studies could have been more useful. White et al. (13) collected alternate-day peak flow measurements from all their patients and asked them to score the severity of asthma symptoms and bronchodilator use in a diary. They plotted the data, looked for patterns, and then unfortunately presented only the results from 10 subjects who reported a subjective improvement during the third trimester and 11 patients in whom there was a subjective deterioration postpartum.

The patients of Schatz et al. (11) kept daily symptom and medication diaries, but the results of only 75 of the 330 subjects who entered the study were presented. They were selected on the basis of the patient's own subjective assessment of how their asthma had been during their pregnancy and included 25 who reported an improvement, 25 a deterioration, and 25 who remained the same.

In the majority of the case series studies (1,4–6) and in two prospective ones (11,13), the patients' own recall of how their asthma behaved during pregnancy has been used as the primary outcome measure. There is no need to belabor the limitations of such assessments. Not only are physicians and asthmatics very unreliable at assessing the severity of asthma by symptoms alone (19,20), but pregnancy itself can alter many factors (e.g., mood, general health state, exercise) that may confound the perception of the asthma. Even back in 1953, Gandevia (2) recognized that "any retrospective investigation based on subjective phenomena is open to error . . . the patient's opinion regarding the state of her asthma while under treatment may be misleading." This is especially important if there is a delay between the pregnancy and the investigation. For instance, Jensen (1) interviewed patients several years after pregnancy.

In other studies (5,8,10), the investigators determined whether asthma had improved, deteriorated, or stayed the same using clinical outcomes such as wheeze, medication change, hospital admissions, exacerbations, etc. These are certainly more objective than the patient's own estimation but are still uncalibrated. What one investigator may consider a clinically important change might be interpreted by another as natural fluctuation in the disease. This may be one of the reasons that the results from these studies appear very contradictory. For instance, in Hiddlestone's study (7), 5% were reported as staying the same, whereas in the study by Gluck and Gluck (10), 43% fell in this category.

A further complication may be introduced by subacute or chronic bronchitis due to gastroesophageal reflux disease, with or without micro-aspiration, with clinical features that are indistinguishable from asthma exacerbations (see below).

B. Airway Responsiveness

There is an association between airway responsiveness to methacholine and clinical asthma severity (21), and therefore changes in responsiveness during pregnancy might be expected to be associated with the severity of the disease. We (14) measured airway responsiveness to methacholine before, during, and after pregnancy.

VII. Other Factors Affecting Asthma Severity During Pregnancy

Clinical research would be much simpler if the intervention of interest could be the only factor affecting the target disease. Unfortunately, this can rarely be the case, and in asthma we have a condition that is often affected by a number of external factors. These include allergen exposure, viral respiratory infections, the actual medications used to treat the condition, and, particularly during pregnancy, gastroesophageal reflux. Ideally, one would like to hold the effect of all of these constant, but the best that can be done is to minimize the effect, document exposure, and take exposure into account in the analysis. Very few studies have considered these sources of contamination and cointervention, and this omission may also have contributed to the discrepancies in results.

A. Asthma Medications

Studies have shown that the regular use of inhaled steroids can improve clinical asthma severity and airway responsiveness (22), while the regular use of high-dose inhaled beta-agonists alone may cause a worsening (23). In our study (14), all subjects used beta-agonists less than four times per day, but 8 of the 16 who conceived used inhaled steroids regularly throughout the study. In these 8 patients, the mean improvement in airway responsiveness between preconception and postdelivery was greater than a doubling concentration of methacholine, which was significantly different from the very stable airway responsiveness observed in the non-steroid-dependent patients. This inhaled-steroid effect accounts fully for the fact that the mean airway responsiveness for the entire group did not return completely to the preconception value after delivery and it occurred totally independent of the effect of the pregnancy on asthma. Similar medication effects do not appear to have been considered in other studies. However, systematic changes over time, independent of pregnancy, are difficult to detect unless one has preconception data.

B. Gastroesophageal Reflux

As serum progesterone rises during pregnancy, there is an associated relaxation of the smooth muscle of the lower esophageal sphincter (24), with the result that one-third of all women experience reflux, heartburn, and indigestion during pregnancy (25,26). In nonpregnant asthmatics, reflux is strongly associated with asthma (27), and surgical (28) and medical treatment (29) of the reflux has resulted in improvement in asthma symptoms. Although we (14) instituted a conservative treatment regimen for patients who developed reflux, there was a significant worsening of heartburn and flatulence during pregnancy. Both were also significant within-subject covariates for the primary outcomes, but adjusting for them did not affect the overall interpretation of the study. In some studies, where reflux was not treated during pregnancy, the increased asthma symptoms associated with the reflux may have been erroneously interpreted as being caused directly by the pregnancy.

C. Allergens

The inhalation of airborne allergens such as pollens, animal danders, and house dust will not only produce immediate bronchoconstriction in sensitized asthmatics but will often lead to increased airway responsiveness to methacholine and histamine as well as a deterioration in clinical asthma severity (30,31). Although it is often impossible to avoid these exposures, documentation of such events allows them to be taken into account in the analysis. Four studies considered the possible importance of allergen exposure and atopy. Williams (8) observed no relationship between the season of the year of delivery and the condition of asthma during pregnancy. Both Hiddlestone (7) and Stenius-Aarniala et al. (12) found that results in atopic and nonatopic subjects were similar, although Hiddlestone (7) did observe a trend toward greater improvement in extrinsic patients during pregnancy. In our study (14), patients were asked at each clinic assessment whether they were currently or had recently been in contact with an allergen to which they were sensitive. Exposures were scored and included as covariates in the statistical analysis. Although the effects of allergens appear to have made little difference to the results of studies where they have been taken into consideration, they should not be ignored. For instance, if by chance in a study a large number of pollen-sensitive women were pregnant during the late summer, this might erroneously be interpreted as a deterioration in asthma due to pregnancy rather than the allergen.

D. Upper Respiratory Tract Infections

Viral respiratory tract infections that produce acute bronchitis often result in an increase in asthma symptoms and a deterioration in airway responsiveness (32). There is some evidence that there is a decrease in cell-mediated immunity during pregnancy (33,34), which could make the patient more susceptible to viral infections, and it has been reported that viral infections are the most common precipitants of severe asthma during pregnancy (8). We (14) treated infections with antibiotics and, where necessary, increased asthma medications. Infections occurring within a month of any clinic assessment were scored similarly to allergen exposure, and these scores were included as covariates in the analysis. In our study (14), they did not make any difference to the conclusions, but in studies where infections are treated less vigorously, they might affect the outcome.

VIII. Results

A. Asthma Severity

The summary results of the 14 studies are presented in Table 2, showing the percentage of patients (with 95% confidence intervals) in each of three categories: (a) asthma improved during pregnancy; (b) asthma remained unchanged during pregnancy; and (c) asthma deteriorated during pregnancy.

Meta-analytical techniques are usually used to combine the results of high-quality, randomized controlled trials. Before an RCT can be included in such an analysis, it usually has to reach a high methodological standard, such as clearly defined intervention, clearly defined study population, minimal subject withdrawals, clearly defined and consistent outcomes, etc. In examining the effect of pregnancy on asthma, we have no RCTs, and only the intervention (pregnancy) was consistent between studies! Although we are very aware of the limitations in combining poor-quality study results,

Table 2 Study Results

First author (ref.)	Sample size	Improved % [95% C.I.]	Unchanged % [95% C.I.]	Deteriorated % [95% C.I.]
Jensen (1)	61	41 [29–53]	15 [5–25]	44 [41–57]
Gandevia (2)	25	48 [28–68]	28 [10–46]	24 [7–41]
Turiaf (3)	198	40 [33–47]	21 [15–27]	39 [32–46]
Schaefer (4)	271	3 [1–5]	93 [90–96]	4 [2–6]
Gammal (5)	112	35 [26–44]	25 [17–33]	40 [31–49]
Wulfsohn (6)	18	61 [38–84]	6 [0–17]	33 [11–55]
Hiddlestone (7)	83	39 [24–54]	35 [25–45]	26 [17–35]
Williams (8)	210	42 [35–49]	34 [28–40]	24 [18–30]
Sims[a] (9)	27	0	100	0
Gluck (10)	47	14 [4–24]	43 [29–57]	43 [29–57]
Schatz (11)	366	28 [23–33]	33 [28–38]	35 [30–40]
Stenius-Aarniala (12)	198	18 [12–24]	40 [33–47]	42 [35–49]
White (13)	31	69 [53–85]	22 [7–37]	6 [0–14]
Juniper (14)	11	73 [47–99]	12 [0–31]	18 [0–41]

All studies, except Sims, reported the percentage (number) of patients who experienced a change in asthma severity during pregnancy.

[a]Sims et al. reported the percentage of patients who experienced a change in spirometry.

nevertheless, clinicians still want to know whether pregnancy has an effect on asthma. Therefore we have combined the results of these studies using recognized meta-analytical techniques, but the results must be interpreted with extreme caution. They are probably more reliable than casting one's eye over the individual results and making a "guesstimate" of the overall effect in one's own mind, but they are definitely not robust!

We have performed the analysis in three stages, starting with the six most methodologically sound studies: the five prospective studies (10–14) and the one case-control study (2). We next added the three case series studies in which outcomes were determined from data extracted from case records. Finally, we included all the remaining case series studies. In the overall analyses, studies with stronger methodology were not given any additional weighting. We have not included the study by Sims et al. (9) in the meta-analysis because patients were allowed to alter medication use to control symptoms and the only outcome reported was spirometry. Not surprisingly, this did not change. From our own study (14), we have used the amount of medication needed to control asthma symptoms as the outcome for the meta-analysis.

The results of all three meta-analyses are presented in Table 3 and summarized in Fig. 1. In all three analyses, the test of homogeneity was

Table 3 Summary of Results Using Meta-Analytical Techniques

Subgroups	Test of homogeneity[a]	Improved % [95% C.I.]	Unchanged % [95% C.I.]	Deteriorated % [95% C.I.]
1. Gandevia (2), Gluck (10), Schatz (11), Stenius-Aarniala (12), White (13), Juniper (14)	$p < .0001$	28 [25–32]	36 [32–39]	36 [33–40]
2. Gandevia (2), Turiaf (3), Hiddlestone (7), Williams (8), Gluck (10), Schatz (11), Stenius-Aarniala (12), White (13), Juniper (14)	$p < .0001$	33 [31–36]	33 [30–35]	34 [31–37]
3. Jensen (1), Gandevia (2), Turiaf (3), Schaefer (4), Gammal (5), Wulfsohn (6), Hiddlestone (7), Williams (8), Gluck (10), Schatz (11), Stenius-Aarniala (12), White (13), Juniper (14)	$p < .0001$	29 [27–31]	41 [39–44]	30 [28–32]

[a]Based on Pearson chi-square test of independence of studies and outcome categories.

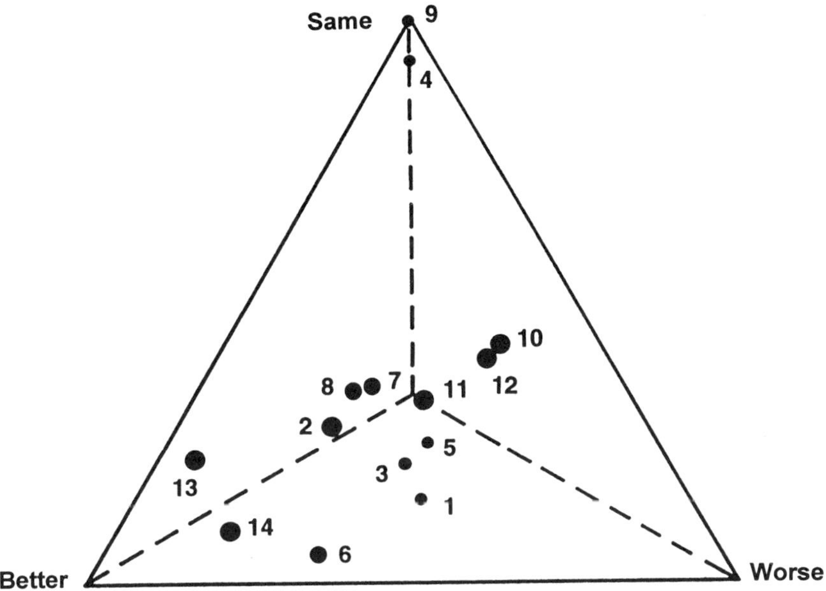

Figure 1 Effect of pregnancy on asthma. Summary of results from the studies in the meta-analysis: ● = better-quality studies (2,9–13); ● = moderate-quality studies (3,7,8); • = poor-quality studies (1,4–6). For interpretation of the figure, see text.

highly statistically significant ($p < .0001$), showing that the results of the studies are very inconsistent. All three analyses show that approximately one-third of women improved, one-third stayed the same, and one-third deteriorated during pregnancy.

Figure 1 presents the results pictorially. Each point represents a summary of the three outcomes (improved, the same, deteriorated) for one study. Let us take as an example the study by Schaefer (4). The point representing this study is near the apex of the triangle (#4), indicating that most of the patients stayed the same (93%) and the remainder were equally divided between "improved" and "deteriorated." In contrast, near the base of the triangle is a point representing the study by Wulfsohn (#6). In this study, very few patients were reported as having stayed the same (6%), whereas 61% improved and 33% deteriorated—hence the reason the point is closer to the left-hand corner of the triangle (better) than the right (worse).

Some studies provide us with additional information. Schatz and colleagues (11) found, based on the analysis of physician-interpreted diary cards, that (a) asthma symptoms seemed to improve in the last 4 weeks of pregnancy compared to weeks 17–36 (Fig. 2), (b) asthma symptoms in women reporting an improvement in asthma during pregnancy progressively decrease during pregnancy (Fig. 3), and (c) asthma symptoms in women reporting a worsening in asthma during pregnancy are particularly increased during weeks 29–36 (Fig. 3). However, since these 75 patients were not a random sample and there is no indication of the generalizability of these patients to the remaining 255, these patterns can only be interpreted with caution.

Data from our study (14) showed that the significant decrease in medication requirements during pregnancy (Table 4) was not at the expense of good control (Fig. 4). In fact, the FEV1 and FEV1/FVC ratios also tended to improve during pregnancy, but these differences did not reach statistical significance.

B. Airway Responsiveness

We (14) showed a twofold improvement in the mean PC20 between preconception and the second trimester, which deteriorated slightly but not significantly during the third trimester (Fig. 5). One month after delivery, the mean PC20 was not significantly different from that preconception. The overall effect of pregnancy on airway responsiveness was significant ($p = .033$), and the magnitude of this change was significantly greater than the natural fluctuations observed in the nonpregnant control data. There was a linear relationship between preconception PC20 and the magnitude of change during pregnancy, showing that the subjects with the most hyperresponsive airways initially showed the greatest improvement during pregnancy (Fig. 6). Of the 11 subjects who improved, 9 showed greater than twofold improvement in responsiveness, whereas in the 5 who deteriorated, the change was less than twofold.

C. Multiple Pregnancies

Jensen (1), Gammal and Warraki (5), Williams (8), Schatz et al. (11), and Stenius-Aarniala et al. (12) followed women during two or more pregnancies in order to evaluate whether the course of asthma during successive pregnancies is consistent. Once again, it is important when reviewing the results to take into consideration the biases associated with uncontrolled subjective recall, the method used in the majority of these studies. Nevertheless, the results are fairly consistent. Schatz et al. (11), looking at two consecutive pregnancies, demonstrated 58.8% concordance ($p = .019$) when patients were asked to rank asthma during each pregnancy as being better, the same, or worse than when they were not pregnant. Other data

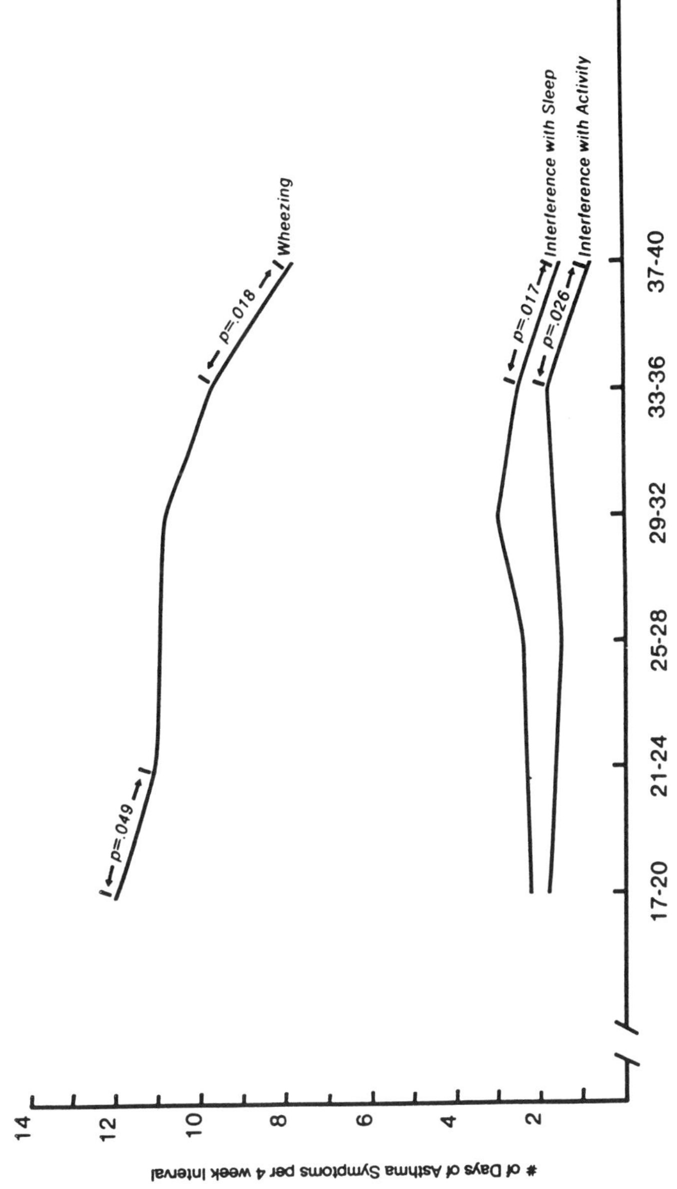

Figure 2 Mean number of symptomatic days (total days of wheezing, days of interference with sleep caused by asthma, days of interference with normal daily activity caused by asthma) versus 4-week gestational intervals in 75 selected women. (From Ref. 11.)

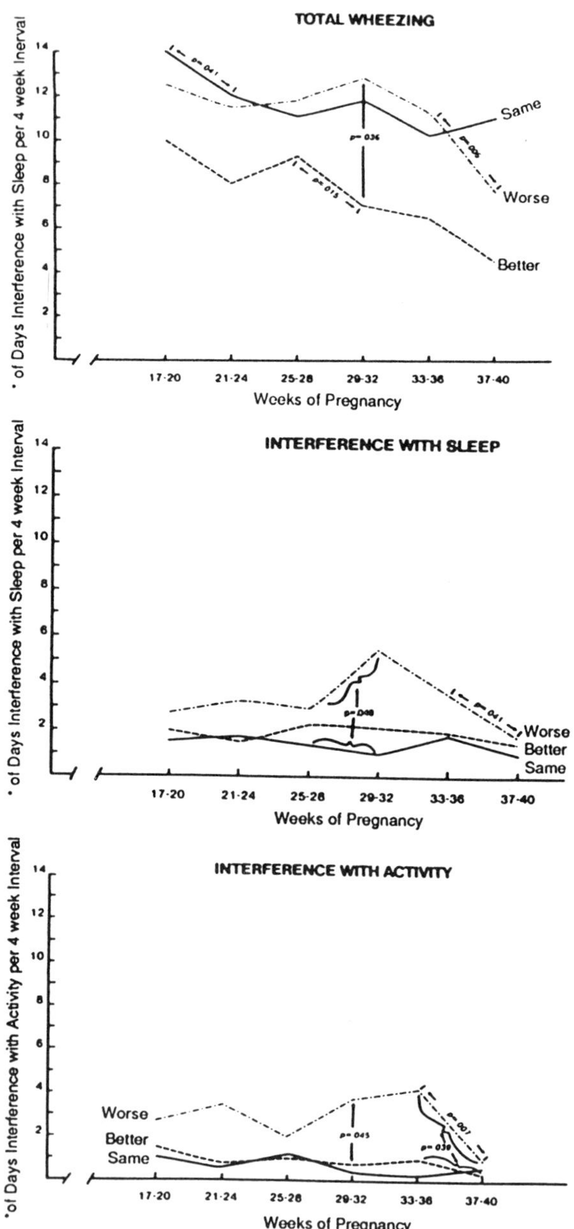

Figure 3 Mean number of symptomatic days versus 4-week intervals from 17 weeks of pregnancy to 12 weeks postpartum in each of 25 women who reported their asthma as getting better, getting worse, or staying the same during pregnancy. (From Ref. 11.)

Table 4 Medication Scores for the 11 Subjects Who Required Medications During Pregnancy

Subject	Preconception	Second trimester	Third trimester	Postdelivery
1	3	1	2	4
2	1.5	1.5	3	4
3	3	2	1	4
4	3.5	3.5	1.5	1.5
5	4	2.5	1	2.5
6	3.5	1	3.5	2
7	3	4	2	1
8	4	1	2.5	2.5
9	4	1.5	1.5	3
10	2	3.5	1	3.5
11	3.5	3.5	2	1
Mean	3.18	2.27	1.91	2.64

The effect of pregnancy on medication requirements was significant ($p = .0032$).

Scores were obtained by within-subject ranking of the minimum amount of medication required during each time period to keep symptoms controlled; 1 = least and 4 = largest amount of medication required.

Source: From Ref. 14.

support this observation. Gammal and Warraki (5) reported consistency in asthma deterioration in 29 or 33 patients and consistency of improvement in 23 of 28 patients. Williams (8) reported consistency in 63% of his subjects, but 21% of the subjects showed marked variation. Jensen (1) noted that each multipara stated that she responded in exactly the same manner during all her pregnancies. Although Stenius-Aarniala et al. (12) followed 13 women during more than one pregnancy, they report that medication was checked and adjusted at an earlier stage during the second pregnancy and, as a result, asthma may have been better controlled.

D. Symptoms During Labor and Delivery

There have been no controlled studies looking formally at the effect of labor and delivery on asthma severity, but two groups of investigators have reported their observations. Schatz et al. (11) reported the frequency of patient-reported asthma symptoms during labor and delivery. Ninety percent of their 366 subjects reported no symptoms of asthma at all during labor and delivery. Of the 37 patients who did have symptoms, 20 patients (54%) required no acute treatment, 15 patients (41%) used inhaled bronchodilators, and 2 patients (5%) received intravenous aminophylline. Sim-

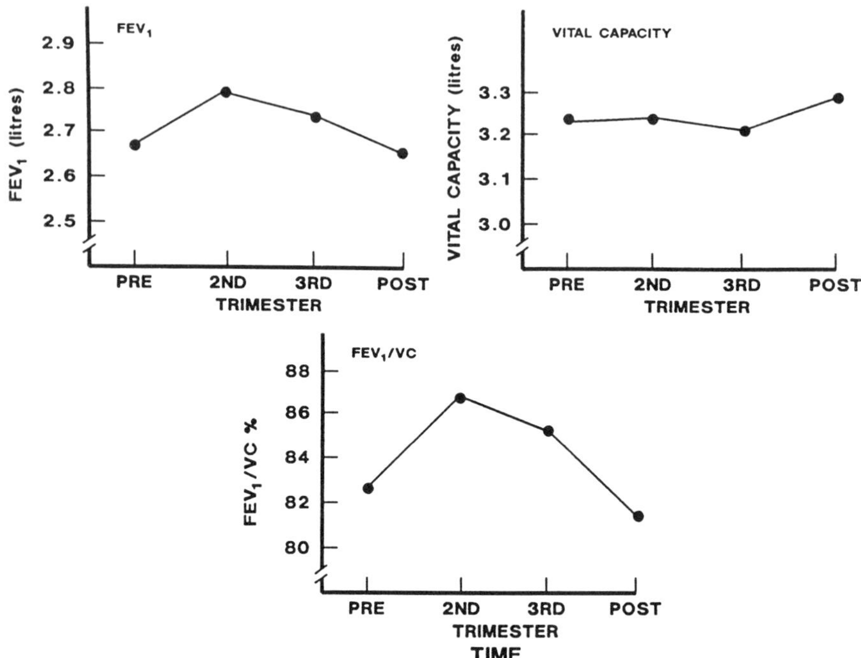

Figure 4 Spirometry measured before, during, and after pregnancy, showing that the significant reduction in medication use during pregnancy ($p = .032$) was not at the expense of good asthma control. (From Ref. 14.)

ilarly, Stenius-Aarniala et al. (12) reported that symptoms were mild during labor and easily controlled with an inhaled beta-agonist, and that no patients required intensive asthma treatment.

IX. Mechanisms

Our study (14) and the data of Gandevia (2), both of which included control data on nonpregnant women, suggest that the changes in asthma observed during pregnancy are more than just the random fluctuations in the natural course of the disease. This is supported by the observations of the majority of the uncontrolled during–after prospective cohort studies (10,11,13) and by the case series study by Jensen (1), all of which reported that asthma changes which occurred during pregnancy generally reverted to the prepregnancy state within 3 months postpartum. Although the mech-

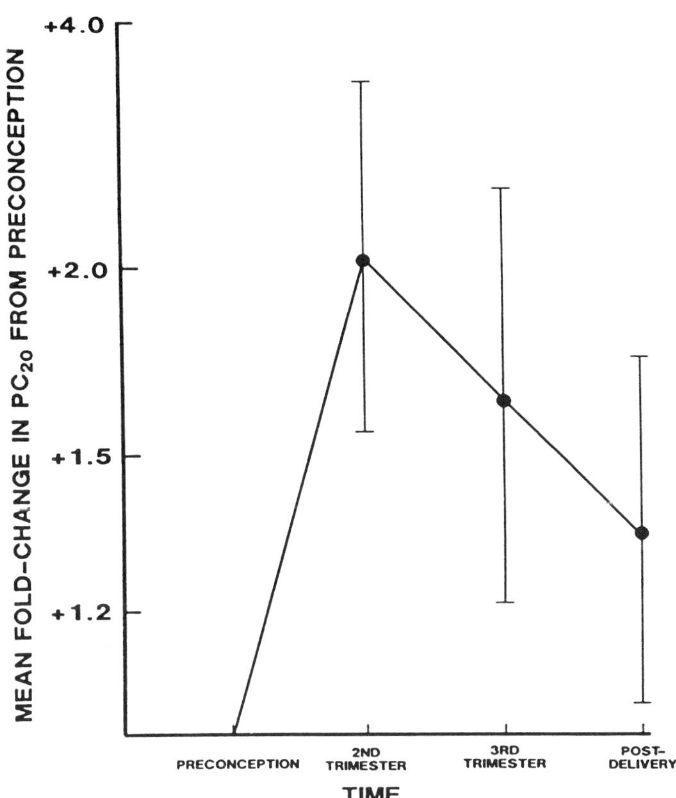

Figure 5 Within-subject mean change in airway responsiveness to methacholine from preconception expressed as a fold change in PC20. The overall effect of pregnancy was significant (p = .033). The difference between preconception and postdelivery is accounted for by subjects who required regular inhaled steroids through the study. (From Ref. 14.)

anisms involved in the changes in asthma during pregnancy have not been defined, there are a number of gestational physiological changes that have the potential to improve or worsen asthma, either directly or indirectly. Some of these have been proposed by Schatz and Zeiger (Table 5). Other possible mechanisms include the direct effect of progesterone and estrogen on airway smooth muscle and the suppressed proliferation of interleukin-2-dependent cells (14). Quite possibly some of the between-subject variance observed in the studies of the effect of pregnancy on asthma can be attributed to different mechanisms varying in impact between patients.

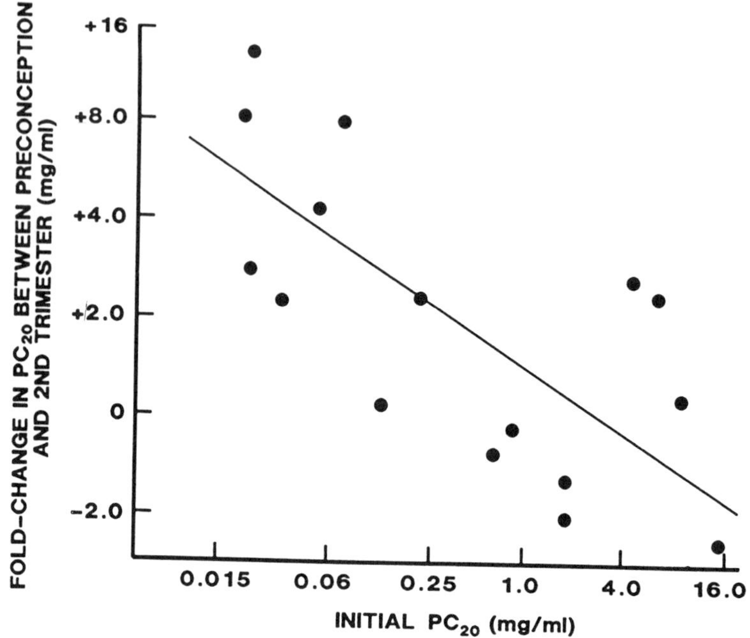

Figure 6 The relationship between the initial level of airway responsiveness and change in responsiveness between preconception and the second trimester, showing that subjects with the greatest improvements were most hyperresponsive initially ($p = .014$). (From Ref. 14.)

X. Conclusions

Although 14 reported studies have examined the effect of pregnancy on asthma, it is still not possible to draw any definite conclusions. In this review we have examined the practical difficulties associated with addressing this question and have considered some of the methodological problems and the pitfalls into which some studies have tumbled. We have looked at the importance of taking into consideration all the other factors that can affect asthma, such as medications, infections, reflux, and allergens. Although some studies have yielded results in which we can place far more confidence than others, there is still a need for further prospective work. Ideally, future studies should enroll consecutive patients, preconception, from a broad population base, and all patients should be accounted for at the end of the study. There should be matched, nonpregnant asthmatic controls. All data should be included in the analysis and reported,

Table 5 Physiological Changes During Pregnancy That May Affect the Course of Asthma

Factors that may improve asthma:

Progesterone-mediated bronchodilation

Estrogen or progesterone-mediated potentiation of beta-adrenergic stimulation

Decreased plasma histamine-mediated bronchoconstriction (due to increased circulating histaminase)

Pulmonary effects of increased serum free cortisol

Glucocorticoid-mediated increased beta-adrenergic responsiveness

Prostaglandin E-mediated bronchodilation

Prostaglandin I_2-mediated bronchial stabilization

Atrial natriuretic factor-induced bronchodilation

Increased half-life or decreased protein binding of endogenous or exogenous bronchodilators

Factors that may worsen asthma:

Pulmonary refractoriness to cortisol due to competitive binding to glucocorticoid receptors by elevated progesterone, aldosterone, and/or deoxycorticosterone

Prostaglandin $F_{2\alpha}$-mediated bronchoconstriction

Decreased functional residual capacity with resultant airway closure during tidal breathing and altered ventilation/perfusion ratios

Increased placental major basic protein reaching the lung

Increased viral or bacterial respiratory infection-triggered asthma

Increased gastroesophageal reflux-induced asthma

Increased stress

Source: From Schatz M. Asthma during pregnancy: interrelationships and management. Ann Allergy 1992; 68:123–133.

and the primary outcomes should be validated objective and subjective measurements of asthma severity. Until we have several methodologically sound studies showing consistent results, there will be uncertainty about the effect of pregnancy on asthma, and the search for possible mechanisms will be frustrated.

References

1. Jensen K. Pregnancy and allergic disease. Acta Allergol 1953; 6:44–53.
2. Gandevia B. Note on course of bronchial asthma and vasomotor rhinitis during pregnancy. Royal Melbourne Hosp Clin Rep 1953; 23:72–74.

3.   Turiaf J. L'asthme et ses rapports avec les secretions hormono-genitales. Donnees statistiques, physio-pathologiques et therpeutiques. J Francais de Medicine et Chirurgie Thoraciques 1958; 12:597–622.

4.   Schaefer G, Silverman F. Pregnancy complicated by asthma. Am J Obstet Gynecol 1961; 82:182–191.

5.   Gammal MT, Warraki S. Pregnancy and asthma. J Egypt Med Assoc 1963; 46:903–910.

6.   Wulfsohn NL, Politzer WM. Bronchial asthma during menses and pregnancy. S Afr Med J 1964; 38:173.

7.   Hiddlestone HJH. Bronchial asthma and pregnancy. N Z Med J 1964; 63: 521–523.

8.   Williams DA. Asthma and pregnancy. Acta Allergol 1967; 22:311–323.

9.   Sims CD, Chamberlain GVP, de Swiet M. Lung function tests in bronchial asthma during and after pregnancy. Br J Obstet Gynaecol 1976; 83:434–437.

10. Gluck JC, Gluck PA. The effects of pregnancy on asthma: a prospective study. Ann Allergy 1976; 37:164–168.

11. Schatz M, Harden K, Forsythe A, Chilingar L, Hoffman C, Sperling W, Zeiger RS. The course of asthma during pregnancy, post partum, and with successive pregnancies: a prospective analysis. J Allergy Clin Immunol 1988; 81: 509–517.

12. Stenius-Aarniala B, Piirila P, Teramo K. Asthma and pregnancy: a prospective study of 198 pregnancies. Thorax 1988; 43:12–18.

13. White RJ, Coutts II, Gibbs CJ, MacIntyre C. A prospective study of asthma during pregnancy and the puerperium. Respir Med 1989; 83:103–106.

14. Juniper EF, Daniel EE, Roberts RS, Kline PA, Hargreave FE, Newhouse MT. Improvement in airway responsiveness and asthma severity during pregnancy. Am Rev Respir Dis 1989; 140:924–931.

15. Department of Clinical Epidemiology and biostatistics, McMaster University Health Sciences Centre. How to read clinical journals: IV. To determine etiology or causation. Can Med Assoc J 1981; 124:985–990.

16. Sackett DL. Bias in analytic research. J Chronic Dis 1979; 32:51–63.

17. Juniper EF. The effect of pregnancy and the menstrual cycle on airway responsiveness and asthma severity. MSc. thesis, 1988, McMaster University, Hamilton, Ont., Canada.

18. Yernault JC. Dyspnoea, wheezing and respiratory insufficiency in pregnancy: was it bronchial or cardiac asthma? Eur Respir J 1990; 3:247–248.

19. Adelroth E, Hargreave FE, Ramsdale EH. Do physicians need objective measurements to diagnose asthma? Am Rev Respir Dis 1986; 134:704–707.

20. Burdon JGW, Juniper EF, Killian KJ, Hargreave FE, Campbell EJM. The perception of breathlessness in asthma. Am Rev Respir Dis 1982; 126: 825–828.

21. Hargreave FE, Ryan G, Thomson NC, O'Byrne PM, Latimer K, Juniper EF, Dolovich J. Bronchial responsiveness to histamine and methacholine in asthma: measurement and clinical significance. J Allergy Clin Immunol 1981; 68:347–355.

22. Juniper EF, Kline PA, Vanzieleghem MA, Ramsdale EH, O'Byrne PM, Hargreave FE. Effects of long-term treatment with an inhaled corticosteroid (budesonide) on airway hyperresponsiveness and clinical asthma severity in nonsteroid-dependent asthmatics. Am Rev Respir Dis 1990; 142:832–836.

23. Sears MR, Taylor DR, Print CG, Lake DC, Li Q, Flannery EM, Yates DM. Lucas MK, Herbison GP. Regular inhaled beta-agonist treatment in bronchial asthma. Lancet 1990; 336:1391–1396.

24. Bortoff A. Progesterone reduces slow wave propagation velocity and decreases electrical coupling between intestinal muscle cells. In: Weinbeck M, ed. Motility of the Digestive Tract. New York: Raven Press, 1982:445–450.

25. Fisher RS, Roberts, Grabowski CJ, Cohen S. Altered lower esophageal sphincter function during early pregnancy. Gastroenterology 1978; 74:1233–1237.

26. Ostrick DG, Cowley DJ, Sharp DS, Skinner L, Ganguli PC. A study of gastroesophageal reflux in late pregnancy. In: Vantrappen G, ed. Proceedings of the Fifth International Symposium of Gastrointestinal Motility. Belgium: Typoff Press, 1975: 358–362.

27. Kjellen G, Brundin A, Tibbling L, Wranne B. Oesophageal function in asthmatics. Eur J Respir Dis 1981; 62:87–94.

28. Perrin-Foyalle M, Bel A, Braillon G, Lombard-Platet R, Kofman J, Harf R, Montagnon B, Pacheco Y, Perpoint B. Asthme et reflux gastro-oesophagien. Resultats de la cure chirurgicale chez 50 malades. Poumon Coeur 1980; 36: 231–237.

29. Kjellen G, Tibbling L, Wranne B. Effect of conservative treatment of oesophageal dysfunction on bronchial asthma. Eur J Respir Dis 1981; 62:190–197.

30. Cockcroft DW, Ruffin RE, Dolovich J, Hargreave FE. Allergen-induced increases in non-allergic bronchial reactivity. Clin Allergy 1977; 7:503–513.

31. Boulet L-P, Cartier A, Thomson NC, Roberts RS, Dolovich J, Hargreave FE. Asthma and increases in nonallergic bronchial responsiveness from seasonal pollen exposure. J Allergy Clin Immunol 1983; 71:399–406.

32. Empey DW, Laitinen LA, Jacobs L, Gold WM, Nadel JA. Mechanisms of bronchial hyperreactivity in normal subjects after upper respiratory tract infection. Am Rev Respir Dis 1976; 113:131–139.

33. Finn R, St. Hill CA, Govan AJ. Immunological responses in pregnancy and survival of foetal homograft. Br Med J 1972; 3:150–152.

34. Jones E, Curzen P, Gaugas JM. Suppressed activity of pregnancy plasma on mixed lymphocyte reaction. J Obstet Gynaecol 1973; 80:603–607.

17

Diagnosis and Differential Diagnosis of Bronchial Asthma in Pregnancy

ALLAN T. LUSKIN

Rush Medical Center
Chicago, Illinois

I. Introduction

The clinical syndrome of cough, wheezing, and dyspnea associated with episodes of worsening and spontaneous or medication-induced improvement characterizes bronchial asthma. The diagnosis of this disorder usually is made without difficulty. However, the symptoms typical of bronchial asthma are not diagnostic of this disorder and are found in many cardiopulmonary disorders. Additionally, physiological changes associated with pregnancy may produce symptoms which mimic those of cardiopulmonary disease and offer the opportunity for diagnostic confusion. The course of asthma may vary in pregnancy, providing further diagnostic difficulties. Asthma previously undiagnosed and mild may worsen in pregnancy; or asthma occurring initially in infancy or childhood and which was in clinical remission for many years may reemerge; or asthma may become clinically evident for the first time during pregnancy (1–3). These factors complicate a differential diagnosis that is applicable to nonpregnant individuals as well.

II. Definition of Asthma

Although a universally accepted definition of asthma is not yet agreed upon, a widely utilized definition defines asthma as a lung disease with the following characteristics: (a) airway obstruction that is partially or completely reversible either spontaneously or with treatment; (b) airway inflammation; and (c) increased airway responsiveness to a variety of stimuli (4). A more recent definition in wide use expands on the previous definition: Asthma is a chronic inflammatory disorder of the airways in which many cells and cellular elements play a role, in particular mast cells, eosinophils, T lymphocytes, neutrophils, and epithelial cells. In susceptible individuals, this inflammation causes recurrent episodes of wheezing, breathlessness, chest tightness, and coughing, particularly at night or in the early morning. These episodes are usually associated with widespread but variable airflow obstruction that is often reversible either spontaneously or with treatment. The inflammation also causes bronchial hyperresponsiveness to a variety of stimuli (5). Recent evidence indicates that subbasement membrane fibrosis occurs in many affected individuals, and chronic asthma may be associated with long-lasting, perhaps permanent, airway abnormalities associated with airway remodeling which lead to persistent and irreversible changes in lung function (6). It is likely that this reflects chronic inflammation and will be incorporated into future definitions of this disorder.

III. Pathology and Pathophysiology

Studies of patients with asthma by postmortem examinations, biopsies, and bronchoalveolar lavage note (a) mucus hypersecretion and mucus plugs; (b) inflammatory cells with a predominance of eosinophils; (c) vasodilatation with exudation of serum proteins associated with microvascular leakage; and (d) shedding of epithelial cells and epithelial disruption. Airway smooth muscle is variably hypertrophied, and subepithelial and basement membrane hypertrophy is often noted. Many, but not all, of these changes may be modified by antiinflammatory pharmacotherapy (7–12).

The airway inflammation appears most often to involve mast cells and T lymphocytes, which secrete mediators acting directly on the airway, by recruitment of other inflammatory cells, or via neurally derived mediators (13). Lymphocyte, macrophage, and epithelial cell-derived mediators and cytokines may maintain chronic airway inflammation and may be associated with chronic cell damage and ongoing airway repair (14). There also appears to be a role for bronchial, lung, and vascular-derived adhesion molecules in facilitating the recruitment and access of the inflammatory cells to the airway; these may act to amplify and perpetuate the cycle of inflammation (15). This occurs in addition to the action of mediators, principally mast cell and neuronally derived, on airway vasculature, mucous-producing cells, and smooth muscle. These mediators include cysteinyl leukotrienes, and many of these mediators have dual effects, acting both directly on structural components of the airway and recruiting other inflammatory cells (16).

The airway changes described are associated with physiological abnormalities which characterize the disease. Bronchial hyperresponsiveness is a characteristic finding and is present in virtually all patients with asthma. Airway hyperreactivity reflects an exaggerated bronchoconstrictor response to a variety of clinical and pharmacological stimuli. The airways react in an exaggerated fashion, with both excessive and poorly modulated responses, as well as reacting to lower levels of stimuli than are necessary to cause a bronchoconstrictive response in normals. The degree of airway responsiveness is typically associated with the severity of the asthma clinically; marked hyperresponsiveness is seen most commonly in patients with severe asthma. Airway hyperresponsiveness may be seen in other conditions, although the degree of bronchial hyperreactivity is generally less.

The hyperresponsiveness may be seen clinically with symptoms and physiological changes of airflow obstruction in response to exercise, cold air, irritants, pollutants, and allergens. Airway hyperreactivity may be detected in the laboratory by response to a variety of pharmacological and nonpharmacological mediators, including cold air, hypertonic aerosols, exercise, or by inhalation challenge with pharmacological mediators (most commonly histamine and methacholine). Bronchial hyperreactivity is also associated with an exaggerated circadian variability in airway tone. The increase in airflow in midafternoon compared to early morning is approximately 5% in normals and may approach 50% in patients with marked bronchial hyperreactivity and severe asthma. Measurements of morning and afternoon peak flows may evidence this variability and are indicative of bronchial hyperresponsiveness.

Bronchial hyperresponsiveness is responsible for many of the characteristics of asthma, including the relationship between symptoms and environmental factors and reversibility. Airflow obstruction and resultant hyperinflation account for the characteristic symptoms of cough, chest tightness, dyspnea, and wheezing. The airflow obstruction is associated with four major factors affecting airway caliber: bronchoconstriction, airway edema, mucus hypersecretion, and airway remodeling.

Bronchoconstriction is seen in response to both allergic and nonallergic stimuli. Allergic stimuli cause bronchoconstriction via release of mediators from sensitized mast cells, including leukotrienes and other lipid-derived mediators as well as histamine (17). Nonallergic stimuli causing bronchoconstriction in patients with airway hyperreactivity are also characteristic of asthma and include cold air, irritant exposure, and exercise.

Airway edema impairs airflow and is associated with mediator-induced microvascular permeability. Mast cell and neurally derived mediators appear to be of prime importance.

Many mediators are secretegogues, including leukotrienes, platelet-activating factor, and neurally-derived mediators. The increased *mucus* and mucus plugging contribute to airflow limitation and appear to be a major factor in patients with severe chronic asthma.

Airway remodeling is associated with chronic airway inflammation and results in persistent and irreversible airflow obstruction. Basement membrane hypertrophy and deposition of collagen and subepithelial fibrosis characterize chronic bronchial asthma, and changes of airway remodeling may be seen relatively early in the disease process (18).

Atopy is a major risk factor for the presence of bronchial asthma and is present in most asthmatic children and young adults. Atopy is defined as the genetic susceptibility to produce IgE directed at common environmental allergens (19). Atopy may exist without evidence of bronchial asthma, but up to 40% of patients with atopy, particularly in association with symptomatic allergic rhinitis, have evidence of bronchial hyperreactivity, which is a hallmark of asthma. While nonatopic asthma occurs, it is far more common for asthma to be associated with atopy, particularly in the child-bearing years. It is likely that atopy represents a significant risk factor for the development of asthma and plays a role in the perpetuation and worsening of the disease (20,21). Adult-onset asthma is more often nonatopic than asthma which begins in childhood, but the inflammatory process appears similar (22). Nonetheless, a family history of atopy, a personal history of other atopic disorders including allergic rhinitis and atopic eczema, and/or biological evidence of IgE sensitivity are present in most young adults with asthma and represent important diagnostic considerations.

IV. Diagnosis of Asthma

In order to establish a diagnosis of asthma, the following criteria should be met: (a) There is evidence of airflow obstruction which is, at least in part, episodic and most typically related to exposure to identifiable factors; (b) airflow obstruction is at least partially reversible, either spontaneously or in response to therapy; and (c) alternative diagnoses are excluded. A directed medical history, appropriate physical examination, pulmonary function tests, and occasional additional tests typically will provide sufficient information to ensure an accurate diagnosis of bronchial asthma. Asthma remains a heterogeneous disorder, and symptoms often vary from patient to patient and may vary based on the situation in a particular patient over time.

A. History

Asthma should be considered in any patient with a history of wheezing, shortness of breath, cough, or chest tightness. Wheezing, particularly during exhalation, is a common symptom of asthma but is by no means diagnostic. While the presence of wheezing is a strong indicator of asthma, its absence does not exclude the diagnosis; in fact, many younger persons have asthma characterized only by cough (cough asthma) or recurrent dyspnea or chest tightness. A history of cough, recurrent wheezing, recurrent shortness of breath, or recurrent chest tightness each are sufficient to suggest asthma. Likely because of circadian variability in airway tone, symptoms typically worsen or occur only at night. Because of coexisting bronchial hyperreactivity, symptoms associated with airflow obstruction may worsen with exposure to irritant airborne chemicals, dust, exercise, viral infections, cigarette smoke, and laughing or crying. Because most women of child-bearing age with asthma are atopic, it is common to note onset or worsening of symptoms with exposure to allergens, including changes with the season associated with pollen or mold exposure or with exposure to dust mites or animals. Included in the history should be a family history of atopy and asthma. Thus, the medical history can identify symptoms and patterns of symptoms likely to be due to asthma, a family history of asthma and allergy, and possible precipitating factors. In addition, the history can assess the severity of asthma based in its frequency and its propensity to interfere with sleep and normal activity.

Any patient who manifests any of the following should be evaluated for asthma: (a) episodic or recurrent coughing, wheezing, or shortness of breath; (b) recurrent "chest colds"; (c) upper respiratory infections associated with lower respiratory symptoms; (d) coughing, wheezing or shortness of breath related to seasons or particular places or with specific exposures such as animals, tobacco smoke, or irritants; or (e) typical respiratory symptoms occurring at night, first thing in the morning, or with physical activity. The asthma history should include questions about specific symptoms including cough, wheezing, shortness of breath, chest tightness, and sputum production. The asthma history should ascertain the pattern of symptoms with particular attention to season, allergen or irritant exposures, frequency and severity of symptoms, potential aggravating factors, and response to therapy, if any. Particular attention should be placed on any lower respiratory complaints that occurred in childhood, even if the diagnosis of asthma was not made at that time. Childhood asthma is frequently misdiagnosed as recurrent croup, recurrent bronchiolitis, wheezy bronchitis, or chronic bronchitis. The majority of asthma in adulthood can be traced back with a careful history to onset prior to the age of 6. The presence of lower respiratory symptoms in childhood strongly suggests that current lower respiratory symptoms are asthmatic in origin. Family history, with particularly attention to upper and lower respiratory disease suggesting asthma or allergy, is important. Social and environmental history suggesting occupational or other allergen exposure is important, and particular attention should be directed toward current and childhood environmental tobacco smoke exposure.

B. Physical Examination

Physical examation should be performed with particular attention to the upper and lower respiratory tract and skin. Certain physical findings increase the probability of asthma. Hyperexpansion of the chest and use of accessory muscles of respiration suggesting more severe air flow obstruction should be noted. Wheezing during normal breathing or a prolonged expiratory phase suggests air flow obstruction. The presence of nasal polyps should be noted—they may be associated with asthma, cystic fibrosis, or aspirin sensitivity. Atopic dermatitis (eczema) correlates strongly with allergy and is a risk factor for asthma. Absence of clubbing and a cardiac examination assists in ruling out other causes for the respiratory symptoms noted (23) (see below).

C. Pulmonary Function Testing

Pulmonary function testing should be performed in all patients in whom the diagnosis of asthma is being considered. Spirometry with measurement of forced vital capacity, FEV_1, and FEV_1/FVC ratio before and after the administration of bronchodilators is appropriate. Air flow obstruction denoted by a decreased FEV_1 and FEV_1/FVC ratio with reversibility (24) helps confirm the diagnosis of bronchial asthma. Significant reversibility is defined as an improvement of greater than or equal to 12% and at least 200 mL in FEV_1 after administration of a short-acting bronchodilator. Absence of reversibility in the face of moderate or severe air flow obstruction may indicate the presence of fixed air flow obstruction due to long-standing asthma, an alternative diagnosis, or indicate the presence of marked in-flammation, edema, and mucous plugging. A 2- to 3-week course of corticosteroids may be necessary in order to establish reversibility (25,26). However, asthma which is mild may be associated with normal spirometry, and further testing may be necessary.

On occasion, additional pulmonary function studies may be indicated to rule out an alternative or coexisting disease, particularly when there is a historical suggestion of an alternative cause for chronic lung injury, such as heavy cigarette smoking. The diffusing capacity of the lung for carbon monoxide may be decreased in patients with chronic obstructive pulmonary disease due to smoking but is usually normal in patients with asthma. The presence of a restrictive defect (decreased FVC and FEV_1 with normal FEV_1/FVC ratio) on initial spirometric testing suggests that body plethysmography to obtain a measure of total lung capacity may be indicated. Morning and afternoon peak flow measures over a 2- to 3-week period may be helpful in establishing diurnal variations of 20% or greater, which strongly suggests asthma (27,28). This may be particularly helpful in patients with symptoms suggestive of asthma but in whom initial spirometric measures are normal. This same clinical situation may make bronchoprovocation with methacholine, histamine, exercise, or cold air helpful. Presence of bronchial hyperreactivity defined by these challenge studies helps confirm the diagnosis of asthma. In pregnancy, these studies should be carried out with great caution and only if absolutely necessary to establish a diagnosis which cannot otherwise be made. A negative bronchoprovocation test is strong evidence against bronchial asthma.

D. Additional Tests

A chest x-ray may be necessary to exclude other diagnoses. On occasion, allergy skin testing may be helpful, but because of the possibility, albeit remote, of systemic reactions, allergy skin testing is usually deferred during pregnancy. When necessary to guide environmental control, somewhat less sensitive in vitro tests may be helpful if allergy skin testing is deemed unwise. On occasion, other studies may give further evidence supporting a diagnosis of asthma or allergic nasal disease. The presence of eosinophils in sputum strongly suggests the diagnosis of asthma and in nasal secretions suggests an allergic origin for nasal symptoms. Neutrophilic nasal discharge is characteristic of infectious sinusitis. Rhinoscopy and sinus x-rays may be helpful in establishing an upper-airway cause for isolated cough, and evaluation for gastroesophageal reflux disorder may be helpful if cough is the primary symptom.

V. Differential Diagnosis

Alternative diagnoses should be considered in all patients who have asthma, whether pregnant or not (Table 1). Physiological *dyspnea of pregnancy* probably represents the most frequent alternative diagnosis to asthma. This is because dyspnea of pregnancy is commonly accepted as normal and expected. Thus, dyspnea during pregnancy may be underreported by patients to their caregiver because they consider it normal. In addition, respiratory symptoms may be mistakenly attributed to physiological dyspnea of pregnancy by caregivers for similar reasons.

Dyspnea of pregnancy often has its onset in early pregnancy, which obviously cannot be attributed either to the mechanical effects of the uterus decreasing venous return or altering respiratory or diaphragmatic function. It is estimated that, by midterm, half of patients notice dyspnea. The dyspnea of pregnancy, however, differs symptomatically from that of asthma and is often described as air hunger (29). In contrast, the dyspnea associated with asthma is typically described as associated with increased work or effort of breathing or with chest tightness. Symptoms of air hunger suggests dyspnea of pregnancy, whereas dyspnea associated with chest tightness suggests asthma. Likewise, dyspnea of pregnancy is not associated with cough or wheezing, and these symptoms should strongly suggest that dyspnea of pregnancy is not the explanation for shortness of breath. Symptoms associated with specific triggers, such as allergens or irritants, also strongly suggest asthma in contrast to dyspnea of pregnancy.

The etiology of dyspnea of pregnancy has been related to both changes in confirmation of the thorax and to hyperventilation associated with progesterone. Thoracic shape is altered in pregnancy (30), and the changes in subcostal angle occur prior to noting marked uterine enlargement. It is speculated that the changes in the shape of the thorax might affect respiratory muscle relationships and that the resulting mechanical disadvantage of respiratory musculature is associated with the presence of dyspnea (31).

Alternatively, it is suggested that the hyperventilation of pregnancy is a cause of dyspnea. Tidal volume increases in association with the increase in progesterone. This occurs in conjunction with increased respiratory muscle activity and increased work of breathing, since respiratory rate does not change (3,32). It has also been suggested that dyspnea may be due to an increased sensitivity to CO_2 and excessive ventilation out of proportion to metabolic demand (33).

The most conclusive data allowing one to differentiate dyspnea of pregnancy from asthma can be obtained from spirometry. Despite a variety of physiological changes which occur in cardiorespiratory status during

Table 1 Differential Diagnosis of Asthma During Pregnancy

Condition	Distinguishing features		
	History/physical	Pulmonary function	Laboratory
Dyspnea of pregnancy	No associated wheezing or cough	Normal	—
Mechanical obstruction (larynx, trachea, main bronchi)	History of injury, aspiration, hemoptysis Wheezing over the trachea	Inspiratory and expiratory obstruction on flow volume loop No response to bronchodilators Normal maximum mid-expiratory flow rate	Endoscopy diagnostic
Laryngeal dysfunction	Wheezing over the trachea	Same as above	Endoscopy reveals adduction of vocal cords during symptomatic episodes
Chronic bronchitis/ emphysema	Smoking Daily productive cough Family history of emphysema	Irreversible airway obstruction	α_1-antitrypsin deficiency
Pulmonary edema	Nocturnal dyspnea Wheezing may occur Cardiomegaly Gallop rhythm Valvular disease Tocolytic therapy	Decreased forced vital capacity	Chest x-ray: cardiomegaly, pulmonary venous hypertension; interstitial edema Echocardiography: mitral or aortic valve disease, left ventricular dilation or hypertrophy, hypocontractile left ventricle in peripartum cardiomyopathy

Table 1 Continued

| | Distinguishing features | | |
Condition	History/physical	Pulmonary function	Laboratory
Pulmonary embolism	Sudden onset of dyspnea/wheezing		Arterial hypoxemia Abnormal perfusion on ventilation/perfusion scan Pulmonary angiography diagnostic
Carcinoid syndrome	Episodes of flushing	—	Urinary 5-HIAA increased
Hyperventilation syndrome	Dyspnea without wheezing Perioral and peripheral paresthesias	Normal	Respiratory alkalosis (blood gases)
Amniotic fluid embolism	Acute respiratory distress during labor or delivery Cyanosis, shock, bleeding Wheezing may occur	—	Disseminated intravascular coagulation Demonstration of fetal elements in the maternal circulation
Upper airway cough	Medication use Sinusitis Reflux	Normal Normal Normal	— Abnormal sinus x-rays Demonstration of reflux on x-ray or esophageal pH monitoring

Source: Modified from Ref. 41.

pregnancy, the function of large airways does not change appreciably. FEV_1, FEV_1/FVC ratios, and conductance do not change during pregnancy. Flow volume loops are not altered. There is no change in respiratory muscle function during pregnancy (34–37). The total lung capacity is maintained, although the functional residual capacity (FRC) decreases in association with the enlarging uterus. However, despite the decreased FRC and the increased inspiratory capacity and decreased expiratory reserve volume, the flow rates do not change. Thus, spirometric measurements remain as accurate in assessing air flow obstruction during pregnancy as they are in the nonpregnant state. Similarly, abnormalities in FEV_1, FEV_1/FVC ratios, and peak flow rates cannot be ascribed to pregnancy and must be considered abnormal. Any diagnostic confusion suggested by dyspnea in pregnancy can be evaluated accurately by spirometric measurements. Abnormal spirometric measurements are inconsistent with the diagnosis of physiological dyspnea of pregnancy, and evidence of reversible air flow obstruction is strongly suggestive of asthma.

Mechanical obstruction of the airways by either benign or malignant growths either within or compressing the lumen of airways may mimic asthma. *Laryngeal dysfunction syndrome* may also mimic some of the symptoms of asthma, and patients may present with recurrent severe shortness of breath and wheezing. The correct diagnosis is suggested by stridorous sounds and typically an inspiratory "wheeze" heard maximally over the trachea. Flow-volume loops on pulmonary function testing may be helpful in defining intra- versus extrathoracic obstruction. Direct visualization of the upper airway may be necessary, and in laryngeal function is typically normal except during symptomatic episodes (38,39).

Chronic obstructive pulmonary disease may occur in highly susceptible individuals even at a young age with tobacco smoke exposure or antibody deficiency syndromes. Emphysema may occur at a young age in association with a familial deficiency in $alpha_1$ antitrypsin. Patients with chronic obstructive pulmonary disease typically have a history of daily sputum production and marked tobacco smoke exposure. There is often a family history of obstructive lung disease, suggesting a genetic susceptibility to the effects of tobacco smoke. Patients with cystic fibrosis or antibody deficiency syndromes associated with obstructive lung disease also typically have a history of chronic and/or recurrent sinusitis. While this may occasionally be confused with perennial allergic rhinitis associated with allergy in patients with asthma, the purulent nature of both upper and lower respiratory secretions are clues to the diagnosis. A chest x-ray is often helpful in detecting chronic changes, and complete pulmonary function tests (including diffusing capacity and body plethysmography) may be helpful as well. Some patients with chronic bronchitis, antibody deficiency syndromes, or cystic fibrosis may have some degree of reversibility after administration of bronchodilators; but this commonly does not approach the degree of reversibility seen in asthma, and bronchial hyperreactivity tends not to be as marked. Absence of reversibility on spirometry in the face of air flow obstruction and the presence of purulent secretions should suggest a diagnosis other than asthma. Emphysema occurring during the child-bearing ages is rare and typically associated with familial alpha$_1$ antitrypsin deficiency. The absence of a family history is strong evidence against this. Serum alpha$_1$ antitrypsin measurements and phenotyping can help confirm this diagnosis if necessary. The presence of clubbing on physical exam also strongly suggests an alternative diagnosis such as chronic bronchitis, emphysema, or cyanotic heart disease.

Pulmonary edema associated with congestive heart failure may cause symptoms which mimic asthma. Preexisting heart disease may be worsened in pregnancy, further confusing the diagnosis. The increase in blood volume and cardiac output during pregnancy may exacerbate symptoms associated with heart disease. Physical exam often provides clues to the diagnosis. The presence of heart murmur, arrhythmia, S3 or S4, cardiomegaly, rales, or signs of right-sided failure should indicate the need for a more complete cardiac evaluation to include electrocardiogram, chest x-ray, and often studies to evaluate cardiac output.

Pulmonary embolus may be associated with both dyspnea and cough as well as other symptoms, including chest pain, syncope, hemoptysis or cardiovascular collapse. Occasiopnally, wheezing may occur. Pregnancy represents a risk factor for pulmonary embolus. Tachycardia, tachypnea, cyanosis, hypotension, and cardiac abnormalities suggestive of pulmonary hypertension such as a loud P2 suggest pulmonary embolus. The chest x-ray may be normal but often shows atelectasis or pleural effusion. The electrocardiogram may show signs of right heart strain. None of these signs or symptoms is definitive for the diagnosis of pulmonary embolus, and many may be seen in severe asthma. This is also true of the typical arterial blood gas findings of hypoxemia and hypercapnia. The acute onset of symptoms in the absence of a previous history of respiratory disease and in the presence of chest pain, EKG abnormalities, chest x-ray abnormalities, and often signs of peripheral venous thrombosis make diagnostic confusion less likely.

Carcinoid syndrome is a rare cause of intermittent wheezing associated with flushing. *Hyperventilation syndrome* may be associated with dyspnea, but it is not associated with cough or wheezing. The presence of other symptoms, such as chest pain, dizziness, lightheadedness, and other central nervous system manifestations along with anxiety-related symptoms or symptoms associated with metabolic changes are usually sufficient to confirm this diagnosis. Typically, spirometric measures are normal in hyperventilation syndrome, and changes in spirometry associated with air flow obstruction should strongly mitigate against the diagnosis of hyperventilation. *Amniotic fluid embolism* usually presents with acute respiratory distress during labor and delivery associated with cyanosis, shock, and bleeding, but the presentation may include bronchospasm (40).

Isolated *cough* without shortness of breath or wheezing may be seen in asthma. However, cough may also occur due to drugs, particularly angiotensin-converting enzyme (ACE) inhibitors, although these drugs are rarely prescribed in individuals who are pregnant or attempting to become pregnant. Sinusitis may also cause cough and diagnostic confusion, since sinusitis may also be an exacerbating factor for bronchial asthma (23). Vigorous treatment of sinusitis usually results in resolution of the cough. Occasionally mild air flow obstruction can be seen, which resolves upon successful treatment of the sinusitis. This likely represents mild asthma worsened by sinusitis. Gastroesophageal reflux disorder may be a cause for isolated cough or may worsen bronchial asthma, and reflux occurs more commonly during pregnancy. Occasionally, sophisticated studies to assist in the diagnosis may be necessary, but these would not generally be performed during pregnancy. Simple treatment measures, such as antacids and elevation of the head of the bed, may be helpful in reducing heartburn due to reflux. More vigorous therapy may be necessary in order to effect improvement in asthma or cough.

VI. Conclusion

A correct diagnosis of asthma can usually be made on the basis of a carefully taken history, limited physical examination, and spirometry. Although the differential diagnosis of gestational asthma includes a number of entities unique to pregnancy as well as conditions that may be seen in nonpregnant women, the correct diagnosis can usually be made based on differential clinical and laboratory findings. Making a correct diagnosis of asthma is necessary to facilitate appropriate therapeutic intervention.

References

1. Gluck, JC, Gluck P. The effects of pregnancy on asthma, a prospective study. Ann Allergy 1976; 37:164–168.
2. Juniper EF, Daniel EE, Roberts RS, Kline PA, Hargreave FE, Newhouse MT. Improvement in airway responsive and asthma severity during pregnancy; a prospective study. Am Rev Respir Dis 1989; 140:924–931.

3. Schatz M, et al. The course of asthma during pregnancy, postpartum, and with successive pregnancies: a prospective analysis. J Allergy Clin Immunol 1988; 83:509–517.

4. American Thoracic Society. Standards for the diagnosis and care of patients with chronic pulmonary disease (COPD) and asthma. Am Rev Respir Dis 1987; 136:225–243.

5. National Heart, Lung, and Blood Institute. Global initiative for asthma. National Institutes of Health Pub 95-3659, 1995.

6. Roache WR Fibroblasts in asthma. Clin Exp Allergy 1991; 21:545–548.

7. Laitinen LA, Heino M, Laitinen A, Kava T, Haahtela T. Damage of the airway epithelium and bronchial reactivity in patients with asthma. Am Rev Respir Dis 1985; 131:599–606.

8. Beasley R, Roche WR, Roberts JA, Holgate, ST. Cellular events in the bronchi and mild asthma in bronchial provocation. Am Rev Respir Dis 1989; 139: 806–817.

9. Jeffrey PK, Godfrey RW, Adelroth E. Bronchial biopsies in asthma: an ultrastructural, qualitative study and correlation with hyperactivity. Am Rev Respir Dis 1989; 140:1745–1753.

10. Widdicombe JG, ed. Supplement: airway hyperreactivity from the International Symposium on Airway Hyper-reactivity October 1988, Sendai, Japan. Am Rev Respir Dis 1991; 1943:Sl–S82.

11. Djukanovic R, Roche WR, Wilson JW, et al. Mucosal inflammation in asthma. Am Rev Respir Dis 1990; 142:434–457.

12. Djukanovic R, Wilson JW, Britten KM. Effect of an inhaled corticosteroid on airway inflammation and symptoms of asthma. Am Rev Respir Dis 1992; 145:669–674.

13. Emmanuel MB, Howarth PH. Asthma and anaphylaxis: relevant model for chronic disease? An historical analysis of directions in asthma research. Clin Exp Allergy 1995; 25:15–26.

14. Robinson DS, Durham SR, Kay AB. Cytokines in asthma. Thorax 1993; 48: 845–853.

15. Albelda SM. Endothelial and epithelial cell adhesion molecules. Am J Respir Cell Mole Biol 1991; 4:195–203.

16. Horwitz RJ, Busse WW. Inflammation in asthma. Clin Chest Med 1995; 16: 583–602.

17. Marshall JS, Bienenstock J. The role of mast cell in inflammatory reactions of the airways, skin, and intestine. Curr Opin Immunol 1994; 6:853–859.

18. Laitinen A, Laitinen LA. Airway morphology: endothelium/basement membrane. Am J Respir Crit Care Med 1994; 150:Sl4–Sl7.

19. Larson GL Asthma in children. N Engl J Med 1992; 326:1540–1545.

20. Sporik R, Ingram JM, Price W, Sussman JH, Honsinger RW, Platts-Mills TAE. Exposure to house dust mite allergen (Der p I) and the development of asthma in childhood: a prospective study. N Engl J Med 1990; 323:502–507.

21. Martinez FD, Wright AL, Taussig LM, et al. Group Health Medical Associates. Asthma and wheezing in the first six years of life. N Engl J Med 1995; 332:133–138.
22. Walker C, Bode E, Boer L, Hausel TJ, Blaser K, Virchow JC. Allergic and nonallergic asthmatics have distinct patterns of T cell activation and cytokine production in peripheral blood and bronchoalveolar lavage. Am Rev Respir Dis 1992; 146:109–115.
23. Expert Panel Report II: Guidelines for the Diagnosis and Management of Asthma. U.S. Department of Health and Human Services. Public Health Service. National Institutes of Health. February 1997.
24. American Thoracic Society. Lung function testing: selection of reference values and interpretive strategies. Am Rev Respir Dis 1991; 144:1202–1218.
25. Bye MR, Kerstein D, Barsh E. The importance of spirometry in the assessment of childhood asthma. Am J Dis Child 1992; 146:977–978.
26. Li JT, O'Connell EJ. Clinical evaluation of asthma. Ann Allergy Asthma Immunol 1996; 76:1–13.
27. Enright PL, Lebowitz MD, Cockroft DW. Physiologic measures: pulmonary function tests. Asthma outcome. Am J Respir Crit Care Med 1994; 149: S9–S18.
28. Quackenboss JJ, Lebowitz MD, Krzyzanowski M. The normal range of diurnal changes in peak expiratory flow rates. Relationship to symptoms in respiratory disease. Am Rev Respir Dis 1991; 143:323–330.
29. Simon PM, et al. Distinguishable types of dyspnea in patients with shortness of breath. Am Rev Respir Dis 1990; 142:1009–1014.
30. Thomson KJ, Cohen ME. Studies on the circulation in pregnancy. II. Vital capacity observation in normal pregnancy women. Surg. Gynecol. Obstet 1938; 66:591–603.
31. Gilbert R, Epifano L, Auchincloss JH, Jr. Dyspnea of pregnancy: the syndrome of altered respiratory control. JAMA 1962; 182:1073–1077.
32. Field SK, Bell SG, Censiko DF. Relationship between inspiratory effort and breathlessness in pregnancy. J Appl Physiol 1991; 71:1897–1902.
33. Garcia-Rio F, et al. Regulation of breathing and perception of dyspnea in healthy pregnant women. Chest 1996; 110:446–453.
34. Contreras G, et al. Ventilatory drive and respiratory muscle function in pregnancy. Am Rev Respir Dis 1991; 144:837–841.
35. Cugell DW, Frank NR, Gaensler EA, Budger TL. Pulmonary function in pregnancy. Serial observations in normal women. Am Rev Tuberc 1953; 67: 568–597.
36. Craig DB, Toole MA. Airway closure in pregnancy. Can Anaesth Soc J 1975; 22:665–672.
37. Milne JA, Mills RJ, Howie AD, Pack AI. Large airway function during normal pregnancy. Br J Obstet Gynaecol 1977; 84:448–551.
38. Christopher KL, Wood RPII, Eckert RC, Blager FB, Raney RA, Souhrada JF. Vocal cord dysfunction presenting as asthma. N Engl J Med 1983; 308: 1566–1570.

39. Bucca C, Rolla G, Brussinol L, DeRose V, Bugiani M. Are asthma-like symptoms due to bronchial or extrathoracic airway dysfunction? Lancet 1995; 146: 791–795.
40. Scoggin CH. Pulmonary disorders. In: Abrams RS, Wexler P, eds. Medical Care of the Pregnant Patient. Boston: Little Brown, 1983:249.
41. Schatz M. The management of asthma during pregnancy. In: Schatz M, Zeiger RS, eds. Asthma and Allergy in Pregnancy and Early Infancy. New York: Marcel Dekker, 1993:270–271.

18

The Medical Management of Asthma During Pregnancy

MICHAEL SCHATZ

Kaiser Permanente Medical Center, San Diego
and University of California, San Diego, School of Medicine
La Jolla, California

I. Introduction

The management of asthma during pregnancy is important for both quantitative and qualitative reasons. Quantitatively, asthma is one of the most common potentially serious medical problems to complicate pregnancy. Retrospective data suggest that asthma complicates 1% of pregnancies (1), although it is currently estimated that the prevalence of asthma during pregnancy is 4% (2). Qualitatively, experiencing and managing asthma during pregnancy is different for the patient and her physician, because the effect of both the illness and the treatment on the developing fetus as well as the patient must be considered. This chapter reviews general concepts of asthma pathogenesis and therapy, specific goals of gestational therapy, and the nonpharmacological and pharmacological management of asthma during pregnancy. The obstetric management of the pregnant asthmatic patient is described in Chapter 20, and additional management guidelines for pregnant women with severe asthma are presented in Chapter 19.

II. Asthma: General Concepts

A. Definition

Symptomatic asthma may be defined as fluctuating degrees of chest wheezing, cough, and/or tightness associated with reversible obstructive airways disease and/or bronchial hyperreactivity. Although most patients with asthma report the symptom of wheezing and most patients who describe chest wheezing can be shown to have asthma, each may occur independently of the other. For example, in some patients cough or dyspnea without wheezing may represent the sole symptom of asthma (3,4). Conversely, wheezing may occasionally be caused by processes other than asthma (see Chapter 17).

B. Etiology and Pathogenesis

The cause of asthma is unknown. However, certain pathophysiological mechanisms are currently considered important. First, there appears to be a genetic predisposition to asthma, although the exact mode of inheritance and the specific inherited defect(s) remain to be defined (see Chapter 27). Second, the airway hyperreactivity of asthma may be related to airway wall thickening, epithelial injury, abnormalities of smooth muscle, and/or abnormalities of bronchoconstricting and bronchodilatory neurogenic reflexes (5,6). Third, eosinophil-rich airway mucosal inflammation, triggered by IgE-mediated reactions, viral infections, and possibly other mechanisms, is currently recognized as being important in both the clinical manifestations and bronchial hyperreactivity of asthma (7). Finally, abnormalities in production of mucus and in mucociliary function are documented in patients with asthma (8).

C. Triggering Factors

A number of exposures are known to trigger symptoms in patients with asthma (9). *Allergies* to pollen, mite, mold spores, and animal dander may trigger symptoms in allergic subjects. *Respiratory infections*, particularly viral infections and bacterial sinusitis, are probably the most important triggers of severe asthma, and may apparently induce long-lasting clinical asthma in previously asymptomatic subjects. *Exercise*, if it is vigorous enough, will trigger asthma in most patients, and some patients wheeze only with exercise. *Aspirin* and other nonsteroidal anti-inflammatory drugs may trigger wheezing in approximately 10% of adult asthmatics, especially steroid-dependent patients and those with nasal polyps. *Irritants, aeropollutants, emotional stimuli,* and *meteorological changes* may all trigger asthma, apparently nonspecifically. Finally, approximately one-third of women report exacerbation of their asthma several days *premenstrually* (10,11). Although premenstrual asthma occurs more frequently in women with more severe asthma, no clear relation has been documented between the occurrence of premenstrual asthma and the subsequent course of asthma during pregnancy.

D. Diagnosis

The diagnosis and differential diagnosis of asthma during pregnancy is discussed in Chapter 17. Most patients who complain of intermittent wheezing associated with chest tightness and/or cough can be shown to have asthma. Although the demonstration of auscultatory wheezing is more objective than subjective wheezing alone, the objective diagnosis of asthma depends on the demonstration of reversible obstructive airways disease on pulmonary function tests (12). It may be more difficult to demonstrate airway obstruction in patients with infrequent asthma episodes or those with cough-variant asthma. In these circumstances, the diagnosis may be confirmed by methacholine testing (13). However, since methacholine testing is not generally recommended during pregnancy (14), pregnant patients whose history is consistent with asthma but who lack pulmonary function confirmation thereof should be considered for therapeutic trials of antiasthma medication after other causes of symptoms (see Chapter 17) are excluded. A positive response to asthma therapy would support the diagnosis of asthma in such patients, which could then be confirmed by methacholine challenge postpartum, if indicated.

A number of conditions are particularly important in the differential diagnosis of asthma during pregnancy. *Dyspnea of pregnancy* generally presents in early or late pregnancy as dyspnea without wheezing or cough and with normal pulmonary function tests. Patients with asthma can usually differentiate this dyspnea from chest symptoms due to asthma. *Pulmonary embolism* may occur during pregnancy and usually presents with the sudden onset of chest pain, hemoptysis, and dyspnea, sometimes associated with wheezing. *Pulmonary edema* may cause wheezing ("cardiac asthma"), but the presence of cardiomegaly, left ventricular dysfunction, gallop rhythm, valvular disease, and interstitial pulmonary edema on physical examination, chest radiographs, and/or echocardiograms suggest the correct diagnosis. Two causes of pulmonary edema unique to pregnancy are tocolytic therapy (15) and peripartum cardiomyopathy (16). Finally, *amniotic fluid embolism* usually presents with acute respiratory distress during labor or delivery associated with cyanosis, shock, and bleeding, but the presentation may include bronchospasm (17).

III. Gestational Asthma Management

A. Goals of Therapy

Clinical data demonstrating the potential effects of asthma on pregnancy have been reviewed in Chapter 15. It is reassuring to know that asthma which is actively managed during pregnancy by specialists is not associated with increased incidences of perinatal mortality, low-birth-weight or pre-term infants, or congenital malformations compared to simultaneously followed nonasthmatic pregnant women (18,19). The results of two additional studies relate specifically to the goals of asthma therapy during pregnancy. First, data from Greenberger and Patterson (20) suggest that prevention of acute asthmatic episodes will improve perinatal outcome. These authors reported a significantly lower birth weight (2920 g) in the infants of mothers hospitalized for asthma during pregnancy compared to infants of mothers not requiring emergency therapy for gestational asthma (3,354 g) (20). Prevention of acute episodes potentially involves (a) avoiding triggering factors (see following discussion), (b) appropriate self-management behavior and early contact with the physician for increasing symptoms, and (c) optimizing pulmonary function.

Recent data further support optimizing pulmonary function as an important therapeutic goal during pregnancy. The Kaiser-Permanente Prospective Study of Asthma During Pregnancy has demonstrated a direct relationship between individual mean 1-sec forced expiratory volume (FEV_1) in asthmatic mothers during pregnancy and subsequent infant birth weight (21). Moreover, an inverse relationship between mean FEV_1 and the occurrence of asymmetric intrauterine growth retardation was demonstrated which was independent of the effects of maternal smoking or medication use (21). In addition to prevention of acute episodes and optimization of pulmonary function, other goals of gestational asthma management include controlling symptoms (including nocturnal symptoms), maintenance of normal activity levels (including exercise), avoidance of adverse effects from asthma medications, and, of course, giving birth to a healthy baby (2).

B. Monitoring the Asthmatic Patient

Careful follow-up by physicians experienced in managing asthma is an essential aspect of optimal gestational asthma management. In addition, all pregnant patients with asthma should have facilitated access to their asthma physician for increased symptoms (22). It is also important that effective three-way communication exists among the physician managing the asthma, the patient, and the obstetrician.

Asthmatic patients requiring regular medication should be routinely evaluated, at least monthly. These visits should evaluate the prior month's course in terms of frequency of day and nighttime symptoms, occurrence of acute episodes, and medication use. In patients using inhaled beta-agonists on an as-needed basis, the frequency of beta-agonist use is a particularly useful parameter to follow. Compliance with prophylactic medication also needs to be reinforced at each visit. In addition to symptomatic and auscultatory assessment, objective measures of respiratory status [optimally spirometry, minimally with peak expiratory flow rates (PEFR)] should be obtained at every clinic visit.

All patients with moderate or severe asthma should have a peak flow meter at home. Although home PEFR monitoring routinely twice daily may be optimal, many patients do not comply, particularly when experiencing few symptoms (23). At a minimum, a personal best PEFR should be established and exacerbations treated based on the decrease compared to their personal best (see later discussion). It is important to note that a personal best PEFR may not be determined immediately if the patient is initially inadequately controlled; several days or weeks of appropriate therapy may be required before a true personal best is established.

C. Nonpharmacological Aspects of Management

The identification and *avoidance* of potentially avoidable triggering factors is an important aspect of nonpharmacological asthma management which may improve clinical well-being and decrease the need for pharmacological intervention.

Identification of allergic and nonallergic triggering factors and allergen environmental control measures is discussed in Chapter 10. It is particularly important for the pregnant asthmatic woman to discontinue smoking during pregnancy. First, smoking may predispose to increased asthma, complicating bronchitis or sinusitis, leading to an increased need for medication. Second, the increased perinatal morbidity attributed to smoking may be additive to that conferred by maternal asthma (21).

Psychological changes during pregnancy and their implications for medical management are reviewed in Chapter 6. *Patient education* is particularly important for pregnant women with asthma. Appropriate education should improve patient compliance and reduce patient anxiety. Optimal patient education would include an understanding of asthma in general, the rationale for the patient's treatment regimen, appropriate self-management behavior for increased symptoms, the potential effects of asthma on pregnancy and pregnancy on asthma, and benefit–risk considerations regarding the use of asthma medications during pregnancy. One must attempt to prevent the discontinuation or reduction of necessary medication by pregnant asthmatic women out of fear of drug-induced fetal malformations; pregnant patients need to understand that such medication reduction may put the fetus at greater risk from uncontrolled asthma than would occur from the medication. Several examples of educational material for pregnant asthmatic patients have been published (22,24,25).

Immunotherapy may be indicated for some asthmatic women of child-bearing age. Immunotherapy during pregnancy is discussed in detail in Chapter 10. In general, it may be *continued* in patients who appear to be deriving benefit therefrom and who are not experiencing systemic reactions, but benefit–risk considerations do not favor *beginning* immunotherapy during pregnancy for most women.

D. Use of Specific Asthma Medications During Pregnancy

Safety data on the use of specific medications during pregnancy are discussed in Chapter 8. This section highlights certain benefit–risk considerations in the use of specific asthma medications during pregnancy. The National Asthma Education Program Working Group on Asthma and Pregnancy (2) evaluated the information available regarding the use of asthma medication during pregnancy. Based on the published animal and human data as well as on considerations such as efficacy, route of administration, and duration of experience with the drug, the Working Group recommended the drugs in Table 1 as "preferred" during pregnancy. The Working Group recommended avoidance during pregnancy of alpha-adrenergic compounds (other than pseudoephedrine), epinephrine (other than for anaphylaxis), iodides, sulfonamides (in late pregnancy), tetracyclines, and quinolones (2).

Inhaled beta-agonists provide rapid belief of bronchospasm via smooth muscle relaxation. Recent data in subjects using short-acting *inhaled beta-agonist bronchodilators* during pregnancy (18,26) support their gestational use. Their use is also supported by their efficacy with minimal associated side effects (27). Current data are insufficient to determine the safest specific inhaled beta-agonist bronchodilator to use during pregnancy, and the Working Group made no specific recommendation. Inhaled beta-agonists used in recent studies of gestational asthma have included albuteral (18), metaproterenol (26), and terbutaline (19). *Oral beta-agonists* are not generally recommended for use during pregnancy because of (a) lack of human data during early pregnancy, (b) potential inhibition of labor

Table 1 Preferred Drugs for Asthma and Associated Conditions During Pregnancy[a]

Drug class	Specific drug	Rationale
Anti-inflammatory	Cromolyn sodium	Topical; reassuring animal and human data
	Beclomethasone	Topical; reassuring human data, longer duration of experience than alternatives; efficacy
	Prednisone	Reassuring human data; benefits outweigh risks
Bronchodilator	Inhaled beta$_2$-agonist	Topical; reassuring human data
	Theophylline	Reassuring human data; long duration of experience
Antihistamine	Chlorpheniramine	Reassuring animal and human data; long duration of experience
	Tripelennamine	Reassuring animal and human data; long duration of experience
Decongestant	Pseudoephedrine	Reassuring animal and human data
	Oxymetazoline	Topical; reassuring human data

[a]Based on the recommendations of the National Asthma Education Program Report of the Working Group on Asthma and Pregnancy (2), and reprinted from Schatz and Zeiger (91).

during later pregnancy (28), and (c) increased side effects with little increased benefit in most subjects properly using inhaled beta-agonists. However, if a *systemic beta-agonist* is required, terbutaline is recommended due to the reassuring animal studies (29) and lack of adverse effect on uterine blood flow (30)

Theophylline is a longer-acting bronchodilator which has been a time-honored drug for use during pregnancy. However, its "first-line" use during pregnancy is being reevaluated due to (a) frequent gastrointestinal and central nervous system side effects, (b) occurrence of neonatal theophylline toxicity in some infants of mothers requiring theophylline at term (31), and (c) the availability of inhaled anti-inflammatory medications (*cromolyn, beclomethasone*), which appear to be safe during pregnancy (32,33), cause fewer maternal side effects, and which may have advantages over theophylline in their anti-inflammatory/prophylactic effects (34).

Cromolyn blocks both the early and late-phase pulmonary response to allergen challenge and prevents the development of airway hyperresponsiveness (35). Although the precise mechanism of action is unknown, cromolyn may stabilize mast cells as well as produce other anti-inflammatory effects (36). Chronic cromolyn treatment improves symptoms, pulmonary function, and bronchial hyperreactivity (36), but cromolyn is less effective than inhaled corticosteroids in reducing subjective and objective manifestations of moderate–severe asthma (37,38).

Glucocorticoids represent the most potent antiinflammatory agents available for the treatment of asthma. Inhaled corticosteroids have been shown to improve asthma symptoms, pulmonary function, and bronchial hyperreactivity (34,39), as well as to reduce hospitalizations (39) and possibly deaths (40) from asthma. Although inhaled corticosteroids may be associated with some demonstrable systemic effects at recommended doses, these changes are rarely clinically significant in adults (41). Beclomethasone is generally recommended when an inhaled corticosteroid is indicated during pregnancy, since it has been available longer and some reassuring data on its use have been published (33).

The overall role of *anticholinergic* bronchodilators in the treatment of asthma remains undefined. No human data exist on the use of inhaled atropine or ipratropium for asthma during pregnancy, although animal data for ipratropium are reassuring (29). Several studies do suggest that the effects of nebulized anticholinergics may be additive to the effects of inhaled beta-agonists in the treatment of acute asthma (42–45).

Although animal data have suggested adverse effects of the use of *systemic corticosteroids* during pregnancy (46), most of the human data have been reassuring (28). For example, there was no increase compared to the general population in the incidences of toxemia, perinatal mortality, preterm births, or congenital malformations in a series of case reports describing 261 pregnancies in women treated with corticosteroids for asthma (47). This difference may relate in part to the typical use of cortisone in animals as opposed to prednisone or methylprednisolone in humans, where the drugs have relatively poor fetal penetration (48,49). Although recent studies have reported increased incidences of preterm births, low-birth-weight infants, or preeclampsia in asthmatics requiring corticosteroids during pregnancy compared to non-steroid-treated patients (18,50), one cannot differentiate a medication effect from the effect of severe asthma in these studies. Several studies have evaluated the effects of oral corticosteroids during pregnancy in *nonasthmatic* women. Reinisch et al. (51) reported that the mean birth weight of 119 infants from mothers with prior pregnancy losses who received 10 mg of prednisone daily throughout gestation for pregnancy maintenance was significantly lower than that of 67 control infants from the same clinic. However, subsequent data did not reveal such an effect when prednisone was utilized at doses of 5–10 mg/day and discontinued within 3–24 weeks of conception (52,53), suggesting that the effect of prednisone on growth was a duration-dependent and/or dose-dependent effect. Although one study reported an increased incidence of preterm births and preeclampsia in pregnant women treated with corticosteroids for antiphospholipid antibodies in comparison to similar women treated with heparin (54), a subsequent larger study could not confirm this finding (55). In summary, the available literature neither excludes nor confirms an adverse effect of oral corticosteroids on the incidences of preeclampsia, preterm, or low-birth-weight infants. However, even if any or all of these are risks of oral corticosteroids, review of data on the adverse effects of severe asthma on pregnancy (Chapter 15), which may include maternal or fetal mortality, suggests that patients who require regular prednisone for control of their asthma would still be at greater risk from their uncontrolled disease than from the lowest effective dose of prednisone.

Two inhaled medications, salmeterol and nedocromil, have become available in this country since the Working Group completed its report. Nedocromil is an inhaled prophylactic medication which exerts a number of antiinflammatory effects in vivo and in vitro (56). Salmeterol is a long-acting (12-hr) inhaled beta-agonist bronchodilator (57). Animal studies with nedocromil have been reassuring (FDA class B), while those with salmeterol have not (FDA class C), but there are no published data in humans with either drug (29). Although these drugs would not generally be recommended for use during pregnancy instead of older beta$_2$-agonists, cromolyn, or beclomethasone, benefit–risk considerations may favor their continuation during pregnancy in patients who have demonstrated a good therapeutic response to either of these medications prior to becoming pregnant.

Two anti-leukotriene drugs have recently become available in this country, zafirlukast and zileuton. Animal studies with zafirlukast have been reassuring (FDA class B) while those with zileuton have not (FDA class C) (29). There are no human data for either drug, and they are both oral-medications. They cannot be recommended for use during pregnancy at this time.

Provider reluctance to prescribe asthma medications—especially corticosteroids—during pregnancy has been partially attributed to the fear of litigation if anomalies or fetal complications occur (58). However, the overall data reviewed in this chapter and in Chapters 8 and 15 suggest that the risk of uncontrolled asthma is greater than the risk of appropriate use of asthma medication; therefore, "a decision to avoid use of effective pharmacologic agents in a symptomatic pregnant asthmatic" may be viewed as "a willful act of neglect" (58).

E. Prophylactic Management of Chronic Asthma

Medications suggested by the Working Group on Asthma and Pregnancy (2) for the prophylactic management of mild, moderate, and severe chronic asthma are shown in Table 2. The reliance on the use of inhalational therapy seems quite appropriate during pregnancy, but respiratory tract penetration of the drugs must be optimized by appropriate inhaler technique and the use of spacer devices (27). Medications should generally be added one by one until adequate control is achieved. As has been pointed out previously, "inter-patient variability in asthma severity, compliance, and medication tolerance will lead to a variety of dosages and combinations of these medications which will ultimately be required to achieve acceptable asthma control in the individual patient" (59).

Mild Asthma

Inhaled beta-agonists by themselves are usually sufficient therapy for mild, intermittent asthma. If symptoms resolve and pulmonary function normal-

Table 2 Pharmacological Step Therapy of Chronic Asthma During Pregnancy[a]

Category	Frequency/severity of symptoms	Pulmonary function[b] (untreated)	Step therapy
Mild	<3 times per week Nocturnal symptoms <2 times per month	>80%	Inhaled beta$_2$-agonists as needed
Moderate	≥3 times per week Exacerbations affect sleep or activity	60–80%	Inhaled cromolyn Substitute inhaled beclomethasone Add oral theophylline
Severe	Daily Limited activity Frequent nocturnal symptoms Frequent acute exacerbations	<60%	Above + oral corticosteroids (burst for active symptoms, alternate day or daily if necessary)

[a]Based on the recommendations of the National Asthma Education Program Report of the Working Group on Asthma During Pregnancy (2), and reprinted from Schatz and Zeiger (91).
[b]FEV_1 or PEFR based on the norm for the patient, which may be standardized norms or personal best.

izes with inhaled beta-agonists, they can be used indefinitely on an as-needed basis. However, their use more often than three times a week usually indicates a need for inhaled anti-inflammatory therapy (see "Moderate Asthma").

Moderate Asthma

Patients with moderate asthma are those who have symptoms that are not controlled or are poorly regulated by episodic administration of a beta-agonist. Some patients have frequent (more than three times a week) asthmatic symptoms. Other patients with moderate asthma do not have acute exacerbations and can regulate symptoms by moderating their lifestyles, but their pulmonary function (FEV_1 or PEFR 60–80% of predicted) indicates potential compromise in airway function or maternal-fetal oxygenation.

Patients with moderate asthma should be considered for a trial with cromolyn, although a 4 to 6-week trial may be necessary to determine benefit for individual patients. The efficacy of cromolyn is less predictable than that of inhaled corticosteroids. Patients not adequately controlled by cromolyn should be switched to inhaled corticosteroids. Generally, beclomethasone would be recommended unless another specific inhaled corticosteroid appears to be uniquely beneficial for that individual patient. The usual dose would be 8–16 puffs per 24 hr in two to four divided doses, although up to 24 puffs per 24 hr may be considered for recalcitrant patients. For patients not adequately controlled on inhaled corticosteroids, sustained-release oral theophylline should be considered, with a recommended therapeutic range during pregnancy of 8–12 μg/mL (2).

Severe Asthma

Patients whose asthma is not controlled with maximal doses of bronchodilators and inhaled anti-inflammatory agents may need systemic corticosteroids on a routine basis. In this case, the lowest possible dose (alternate-day or single daily dose) should be used and administered under the supervision of an asthma specialist. Patients must be monitored closely for the potential adverse effects of corticosteroids, especially gestational diabetes, preeclampsia, and intrauterine growth retardation. The evaluation of these possibilities may be most appropriately managed in consultation with an obstetrician specializing in high-risk pregnancy case.

F. Management of Asthma Exacerbations

Exacerbations of asthma are acute or subacute episodes of progressively worsening wheezing, cough, chest tightness, and/or shortness of breath.

Exacerbations are characterized by decreases in expiratory air flow that can be documented and quantified by measurement of PEFR or spirometry. When asthma exacerbations occur during pregnancy, one must maintain a high index of suspicion for complicating bacterial respiratory infections, particularly for bacterial sinusitis, which has been estimated to be six times more common during pregnancy than in nonpregnant patients (60).

Home Management

Written action plans, prepared in advance with the asthma physician, help the patient to manage asthma exacerbations at home. Optimal home management involves (a) recognition of early indicators of an exacerbation, including symptoms and PEFR, (b) appropriate intensification of anti-asthma medications, including in many cases systemic corticosteroids, (c) removal of or withdrawal from a relevant environmental trigger, if possible, and (d) prompt communication between patient and health care provider about any serious deterioration and its appropriate treatment.

The home management of asthma exacerbations during pregnancy is summarized in Fig. 1. Patients receiving inhaled corticosteroids should also be advised to increase their dose routinely to at least 4 puffs four times daily when asthma exacerbations occur. Home PEFR determinations are an integral part of home management strategies. PEFR greater than 70–80% predicted suggest the exacerbation is being successfully managed, while PEFR <50% predicted in spite of therapy suggest that oral corticosteroids are indicated and/or that the patient should seek emergency therapy. Oral corticosteroids should also be generally used if the patient requires 12 or more puffs of inhaled beta agonist in 24 hr. Oral corticosteroids are usually prescribed as prednisone, 40–60 mg daily (in 1–3 doses) for 3–5 days, and then tapered over the next 5–10 days.

Emergency Assessment

The management of acute gestational asthma begins with a proper assessment (61–65). A brief history should attempt to ascertain the duration of the attack, the apparent precipitating event, the presence of upper respiratory infection (especially with fever and purulent mucus), current medication (especially theophylline and corticosteroids), and any prior history of respiratory failure or intubation. The physical examination should particularly attempt to identify features suggestive of severe asthma, including use of accessory muscles, diaphoresis, pulse paradoxicus >12, inability to lay down comfortably, pulse >120, or respiratory rate >30.

The first objective laboratory measurement to be obtained should be a PEFR or an FEV_1. Nowak et al. (66) have shown that patients with an

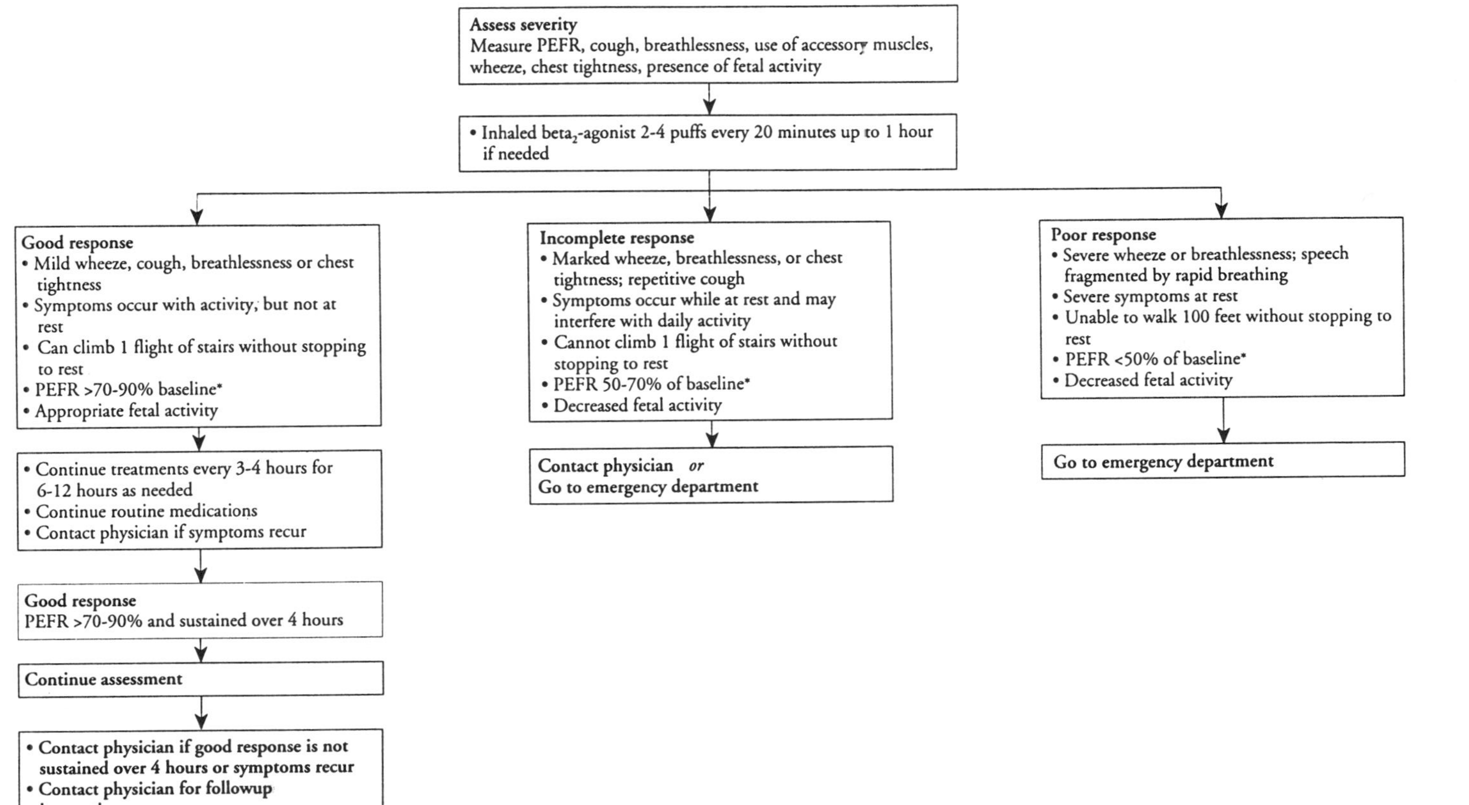

Figure 1 Home management of acute exacerbations of asthma during pregnancy. (From Ref. 2.)

457

initial FEV_1 >1 L or PEFR >200 L/min will have pO_2 >60 and a pCO_2 <42, and initial blood gases may be deferred in such patients. However, blood gases should be obtained in patients presenting with values less than the above or in those not responding to therapy. In interpreting blood gases in women with acute asthma during pregnancy, it must be remembered that blood gas analysis in the normal pregnant woman reveals a higher pO_2 (102–116 mmHg) and a lower pCO_2 (28–30 mmHg) than in the nonpregnant state (see Chapter 3). Thus, a pCO_2 ≥35 mmHg or a pO_2 <70 mmHg associated with acute asthma will represent more severe respiratory compromise during pregnancy than will similar blood gases in the nongravid state.

Pulse oximetry may be considered as a noninvasive alternative to blood gases when CO_2 retention appears unlikely. However, studies of the accuracy of oximetry and consideration of the oxyhemoglobin disassociation curve suggest that only an oximetry-determined O_2 saturation ≥95% can be considered sufficient evidence of adequate oxygenation (67).

A chest x-ray should not be obtained routinely, consistent with the recommended practice in nonpregnant patients presenting with acute asthma (68). However, a chest x-ray with a shielded abdomen is felt to constitute no increased risk during pregnancy (69) and should be obtained in patients in whom pneumonia, pneumothorax, or pneumomediastinum is suspected; in those not responding to therapy; and in those admitted to the hospital (61). A baseline serum potassium level should be obtained, since beta-agonists and corticosteroids may lower serum potassium, and a baseline serum glucose concentration should be obtained to evaluate possible hypoglycemia [to which pregnant patients may be unusually susceptible (70), particularly if not eating properly] or hyperglycemia (due to corticosteroids and/or pregnancy).

Emergency Therapy

Supplemental oxygen (initially 3–4 L/min by nasal cannula) should be administered, adjusting FiO_2 to maintain a pO_2 ≥70 mmHg and/or O_2 saturation by pulse oximetry ≥95% (2,63). Intravenous fluids (containing glucose if patient is not hyperglycemic) should be administered, initially at a rate of at least 100 cc/hr.

The recommended pharmacological management of acute gestational asthma is summarized in Table 3. Most authors suggest nebulized beta-agonists rather than epinephrine as the initial bronchodilator of choice for acute asthma in nonpregnant patients (61,62,65), and information on the use of inhaled beta-agonists during pregnancy (discussed above), as well as the apparent equal efficacy of epinephrine and inhaled beta-agonists in

Table 3 Pharmacological Management of Acute Asthma During Pregnancy[a]

1. Nebulized beta$_2$-agonist bronchodilator
   Up to 3 doses in first 60–90 min
   Every 1–2/hr thereafter until adequate response
2. Intravenous methylprednisolone (with initial therapy in patients on regular corticosteroids and for those with poor response during the first hour of treatment)
   1 mg/kg every 6–8 hr
   Taper as patient improves
3. Consider intravenous aminophylline (generally only if patient requires hospitalization). If it is to be used,
   6-mg/kg loading dose
   0.5-mg/kg/hr initial maintenance dose
   Adjust rate to keep theophylline level between 8 and 12 μg/mL
4. Consider subcutaneous terbutaline 0.25 mg if patient not responding to the above therapy

[a]Based on the recommendations of the National Asthma Education Program Report of the Working Group on Asthma During Pregnancy (2), and reprinted from Schatz and Zeiger (91).

the treatment of acute asthma (71–73), suggests that this recommendation does not need to be altered during pregnancy. In addition, recent studies suggest that beta-agonists administered by metered-dose inhaler (e.g., 4 puffs with a spacer device, waiting 1 min between puffs) may be as effective and safe as nebulized bronchodilators (74).

Three doses of inhaled beta-agonists spaced every 20–30 min can be safely given as initial therapy to patients without coexistent cardiovascular disease. Thereafter, the frequency of administration varies according to the severity of the patient's symptoms and occurrence of adverse side effects. In patients without cardiovascular disease, administration as frequently as every 1–2 hr is safe during periods of severe airflow obstruction (2,65).

Parenteral corticosteroids should be administered along with initial therapy to patients on regular corticosteroids. In addition, intravenous corticosteroids should be utilized in patients with severe airflow obstruction (PEFR <200 L/min or FEV$_1$ ≤40% predicted) after 1 hr of intensive beta-agonist therapy (2,62). There are no data on the pharmacokinetics of exogenous corticosteroids administered during pregnancy, and dosages of corticosteroids recommended for pregnancy are generally not different than those recommended for nonpregnant patients. Although there are insufficient data to determine the optimal dose of parenteral corticosteroids to be used in patients with acute asthma (65), 1 mg/kg methylprednisolone every 6–8 hr is recommended (2).

Intravenous aminophylline is not generally recommended in the emergency room management of acute gestational asthma because it has been demonstrated that aminophylline provides no additional benefit to optimal inhaled beta-agonist therapy in the first 4 hr of treatment (2). Moreover, when used in combination with intensive inhaled beta-agonist therapy, intravenous aminophylline causes increased adverse side effects without providing additional bronchodilation. (2)

Hospitalization

Up to 10–15% of non-pregnant patients presenting to the emergency room will require hospital admission (64). The following pulmonary function criteria for admission have been recommended: posttherapy FEV_1 <60% predicted (66), <2.0 L (75,76) or <400 cc greater than pretherapy (77) or posttherapy PEFR <300 L/min (76). Other criteria for admission include initial respiratory failure (even with improvement), the presence of complications such as pneumonia, pneumothorax, or cardiac arrhythmias, and repeat emergency room visit within 72 hr (64,78). Certainly, criteria for admission of the pregnant asthmatic should be no less liberal, and the coexistence of uterine contractions or fetal distress with acute asthma would also necessitate admission. When the pregnant asthmatic is hospitalized, both medical and obstetrical supervision is required. Patients in frank or impending respiratory failure (pCO_2 ≥35 mmHg) should be hospitalized in an intensive care unit.

In the hospital, oxygen, inhaled beta-agonists, and intravenous corticosteroids should be continued. Inhaled beta-agonists should be administered continuously to every 4 hr, depending on the severity and response. Nebulized ipratropium every 6 hr may be considered, since some data suggest that its bronchodilatory effect may be additive to that of inhaled beta-agonists (42–45). Since recent studies suggest that intravenous magnesium sulfate (1.0–2.0 g) may be beneficial in acute severe asthma as an adjunct to inhaled beta-agonists and intravenous corticosteroids (79,80), magnesium sulfate could also be considered, especially in patients with coexistent hypertension or preterm uterine contractions. In addition, intravenous aminophylline may be considered. When intravenous aminophylline is utilized, pharmacokinetic studies during pregnancy (81–83) suggest that the loading dose recommendation for theophylline requires no modification during pregnancy (6 mg/kg over 20–30 min), but the initial maintenance-dose guidelines should be more conservative (0.5 mg/kg/hr). In addition, studies have suggested that protein binding of theophylline decreases during pregnancy such that there is an approximately 15% increase in free drug for any total drug concentration (81,84). This suggests that a lower therapeutic range (8–12 μg/mL) than is usually recommended is appropriate during pregnancy (2).

Antibiotics should be utilized for hospitalized patients with purulent sputum or pneumonia documented on chest x-ray. In addition, a high index of suspicion for sinusitis must be maintained, and sinus films should be considered in hospitalized asthmatic subjects with substantial nasal congestion or postnasal drainage in the absence of purulent discharge. Based on the American Thoracic Society guidelines for the initial management of adults with community-acquired pneumonia (85) and on the organisms likely to cause sinusitis (see Chapter 11), intravenous cefuroxime is recommended initially for hospitalized pregnant asthmatic patients with suspected bacterial respiratory infections. Erythromycin should be included as part of initial therapy if *Mycoplasma pneumoniae*, *Chlamydia pneumoniae*, or *Legionella* infection is suspected. After the first 24–72 hr, oral therapy with amoxicillin-clavulanate or cefuroxime may be substituted for intravenous cephalosporin therapy in most hospitalized asthmatic patients with pneumonia or sinusitis.

Intubation was required in 2.3% of 811 consecutive hospitalized, nonpregnant patients (86) and in 8.0% of nonpregnant patients presenting with acute asthma and hypercapnia (mean pCO_2 = 54 mmHg) (87). Two cases during pregnancy have been recently reported (88). The criteria for intubation in nonpregnant patients are as follows (63–65,78): (1) pO_2 <60–65 mmHg on maximum supplemental O_2, (b) uncompensated respiratory acidosis (pCO_1 >55 mmHg, pH <7.2) in spite of intensive therapy, and (e) inability to clear secretions and the need to protect the airway due to altered mental status. Although these criteria may also be applied to pregnant patients, it has been suggested that pregnant patients should be intubated earlier in the stage of respiratory acidosis (pCO_2 $\geq$45 mmHg) (89).

Because of airway narrowing due to hyperemia, nasotracheal intubation should be avoided during pregnancy (63). When sedation and muscle paralysis are indicated, morphine sulfate and pancuronium bromide are recommended (63). Mechanical ventilation of the pregnant patient follows the same general principles as in nongravid patients (63). In general, the minute ventilation should be adjusted to aim for a pCO_2 of 30–32 mmHg, the normal level in pregnancy, and it is reasonable to aim for the usual gestational pO_2 of greater than 95 mmHg (63). Weaning parameters should also be the same as for nongravid patients, although it is recommended that pregnant patients maintain the lateral ducubitus position during weaning near term to minimize the inferior vena caval compression caused by the gravid uterus (63).

G. Asthma Management During Labor and Delivery

Fortunately, substantial asthma symptoms during labor in women whose asthma has been controlled during pregnancy are unusual. In one study (90), 90% of asthmatic women experienced no asthma symptoms during labor, and, of those who did, only half required treatment (4.1% inhaled bronchodilators, 0.5% intravenous aminophylline). Nonetheless, it is suggested that daily prophylactic medication (cromolyn, beclomethasone, or theophylline) be continued during labor. Asthma symptoms during labor requiring therapy should be treated initially with inhaled beta-agonists (Table 3). If the patient's asthma responds poorly to inhaled beta-agonists, intravenous methylprednisolone should be administered. For patients on regular corticosteroids or who have received frequent courses during pregnancy, supplemental parenteral corticosteroids for the stress of labor and delivery are recommended: 100 mg of hydrocortisone intravenously at admission, followed by 100 mg intravenously every 8 hr for 24 hr or until the absence of complications is established (2).

References

1. Gordon M, Niswander KR, Berendes H, Kantor AG. Fetal morbidity following potentially anoxigenic obstetric conditions. VII. Bronchial asthma. Am J Obstet Gynecol 1970; 106:421–429.
2. National Asthma Education Program Report of the Working Group on Asthma and Pregnancy: management of asthma during pregnancy. NIH Publication 93-3279A, September 1993.
3. Corrao WH, Brenner SS, Irwin RS. Chronic cough as the sole presenting manifestation of bronchial asthma. N Engl J Med 1979; 300:633–637.
4. DePaso WJ, Winterbauer RH, Lusk JA, Dreis DF, Springmeyer SC. Chronic dyspnea unexplained by history, physical examination, chest roentgenogram and spirometry. Chest 1991; 100:1293–1299.
5. O'Byrne PM. Airway hyperresponsiveness. In: Middleton E, Reed CE, Ellis EF, Adkinson NF, Yunginger, JW, Busse WW, eds. Allergy: Principles and Practices. 4th ed. St Louis: Mosby, 1993:1203–1213.
6. Barnes PJ. Neural mechanisms in asthma. In Holgate ST, Austen KF, Lichtenstein LM, Kay AB, eds Asthma: Physiology, Immunopharmacology, and Treatment. London: Academic Press, 1993:259–273.
7. Busse WW, Reed CE. Asthma: definition and pathogenesis. In: Middleton E, Reed CE, Ellis EF, Adkinson NF, Yunginger JW, Busse WW, eds. Allergy: Principles and Practices. 4th ed. St Louis: Mosby, 1993:1173–1201.
8. Chediak Ad, Wanner A. Airway mucus and the mucociliary system. In: Middleton E, Reed CE, Ellis EF, Adkinson NF, Yunginger JW, Busse WW, eds. Allergy: Principles and Practice. 4th ed. St. Louis: Mosby, 1993:694–711.

9. Mathison DA. Asthma in adults: diagnosis and treatment. In: Middleton E, Reed CE, Ellis EF, Adkinson NF, Yunginger JW, Busse WW, eds. Allergy: Principles and Practices. 4th ed. St. Louis: Mosby, 1993:1263–1299.

10. Gibbs, CJ, Coutts II, Lock R, Finnegan OC, White RJ. Premenstrual exacerbation of asthma. Thorax 1984; 39:833–836.

11. Eliasson O, Scherzer HH, DeGraff AC. Morbidity in asthma in relation to the menstrual cycle. J Allergy Clin Immunol 1986; 77:87–97.

12. Pennock BE, Rogers RM, McCaffree DR. Changes in measured spirometric index. What is significant. Chest 1981; 80:97–99.

13. Chai H, Farr RS, Froehlich LA, Mathison DA, McLean JA, Rosenthal RR, Sheffer AL, Spector SL, Townley RG. Standardization of bronchial inhalation challenge procedures. J Allergy Clin Immunol 1975; 56:323–327.

14. Physicians' Desk Reference. Oradell, NJ: Medical Economics, 1995:2050.

15. Hawker F. Pulmonary edema associated with beta$_2$ sympathomimetic treatment of premature labor. Anesth Intensive Care 1984; 12:143–151.

16. Adler AF, Davis MR. Peripartum cardiomyopathy: two case reports and a review. Obstet Gynecol Surv 1986; 41:675–682.

17. Elkayam U, Ostizega EL, Shoten A. Peripartum cardiomyopathy. In: Gleicher N, ed. Principles and Practice of medical Therapy in Pregnancy. 2d ed. Norwalk, CT: Appleton and Lange, 1992: 812–814.

18. Stenius-Aarniala R, Piirila P, Teramo K. Asthma and pregnancy: a prospective study of 198 pregnancies. Thorax 1988; 43:12–18.

19. Schatz M, Zeiger RS, Hoffman CP. Perinatal outcomes in the pregnancies of asthmatic women: a prospective controlled analysis. Am J Respir Crit Care Med 1995; 151:1170–1174.

20. Greenberger PA, Patterson R. The outcome of pregnancy complicated by severe asthma. Allergy Proc 1988; 9:539–543.

21. Schatz M, Zeiger RS, Hoffman CP, and the Kaiser-Permanente Asthma and Pregnancy Study Group. Intrauterine growth is related to gestational pulmonary function in pregnant asthmatic women. Chest 1990; 98:389–392.

22. Patterson R, Greenberger PA, Frederiksen MC. Asthma and pregnancy: responsibility of physicians and patients. Ann Allergy 1990; 65:469–472.

23. Garrett J, Fenwick JM, Taylor G, Mitchell E, Rea H. Peak expiratory flow meters (PEFMs)—who uses them and how and does education affect the pattern of utilisation? Austral NZ J Med 1994; 24:521–529.

24. Schatz M. Asthma and pregnancy: questions and answers. Asthma and Allergy Foundation of America N Engl Chap Bull 1989; 5(2).

25. Ziment I. Taking care of asthma when you're pregnant. J Respir Dis 1989; 10:91–92.

26. Schatz M, Zeiger RS, Harden K, Hoffman CP, Forsythe AB, Chilingar LM, Porreco RP, Benenson AS, Sperling WL, Saunders BS, Kagnoff MC. The safety of inhaled beta-agonist bronchodilators during pregnancy. J Allergy Clin Immunol 1988; 82:686–695.

27. Newhouse MT, Dolovich MG. Control of asthma by aerosols. N Engl J Med 1986; 315:870–874.

28. Schatz M, Hoffman CP, Zeiger RS, Falkoff R, Macy E, Mellon M. The course and management of asthma and allergic disease during pregnancy. In: Middleton E, Reed CE, Ellis EF, Adkinson NF, Yunginger JW, Busse WW, eds. Allergy: Principles and Practice. 4th ed St Louis: Mosby, 1993:1301–1342.

29. Physicians' Desk Reference. Oradell, NJ: Medical Economics, 1997.

30. Akerlund M, Andersson KE. Effects of terbutaline on human myometrial activity and endometrial blood flow. Obstet Gynecol 1976; 47:529–535.

31. Labovitz E, Spector S. Placental theophylline transfer in pregnant asthmatics. JAMA 1982; 247:786–788.

32. Wilson J. Utilization de cromoglycate de sodium a cours de la grossessa. Acta Ther 1982; 8(suppl):45–51.

33. Greenberger PA, Patterson R. Beclomethasone diproprionate for severe asthma during pregnancy. Ann Intern Med 1983; 98:478–480.

34. Du Toit JI, Salome CM, Woolcock AJ. Inhaled corticosteroids reduce the severity of bronchial hyperresponsiveness in asthma but oral theophylline does not. Am Rev Respir Dis 1987; 136:1174–1178.

35. Cockroft DW, Murdock KY. Comparative effects of inhaled salbutamol, sodium cromoglycate, and beclomethasone diproprionate on allergen-induced early asthmatic responses, and increased bronchial responsiveness to histamine. J Allergy Clin Immunol 1987; 79:734–740.

36. Shapiro GG, Konig P. Cromolyn sodium: a review. Pharmacotherapy 1985; 5:156–170.

37. Svendsen UG, Frolund L, Madsen F, Nielson NH, Holstein-Rathlou NH, Weeke B. A comparison of the effects of sodium cromoglycate and beclomethasone diproprionate on pulmonary function and bronchial hyperreactivity in subjects with asthma. J Allergy Clin Immunol 1987; 80:68–74.

38. Konig P. The risks and benefits of inhaled corticosteroids. Eur Respir Rev 1993; 3:15501–15510.

39. Salmeron S, Guerin JC, Godard P, Renon D, Henry-Amar M, Duroux P, Taytard A. High doses of inhaled corticosteroids in unstable chronic asthma: a multicenter, double-bind, placebo-controlled study. Am Rev Respir Dis 1989; 140:167–171.

40. Ernst P, Spitzer WO, Suissa S, Cockroft D, Habbick B, Horwitz RI, Boivin J-F, McNutt M, Buist AS. Risk of fatal and near-fatal asthma in relation to inhaled corticosteroid use. JAMA 1992; 268:3462–3464.

41. Barnes PJ. Inhaled glucocorticosteroids for asthma. N Engl J Med 1995; 332: 868–875.

42. Beck E, Robertson C, Galdes-Sebaldt M, Levison H. Combined salbutamol and ipratropium bromide by inhalation in the treatment of severe asthma. J Pediatr 1985; 107:605.

43. Ward MJ, MacFarlane JT, Davies D. A place for ipratropium bromide in the treatment of severe acute asthma. Br J Dis Chest 1985; 79:374–378.

44. Rebuck AS, Chapman KR, Abboud R, Pare PD, Kreisman H, Wolkove N, Vickerson F. Nebulized anticholinergic and sympathomimetic treatment of

asthma and chronic obstructive airways disease in the emergency room. Am J Med 1987; 82:59–64.

45. O'Driscoll BR, Taylor RJ, Horsley MG. Nebulized salbutamol with and without ipratropium bromide in acute airflow obstruction. Lancet 1989(June 24); 1418–1420.

46. Fainstat T. Cortisone-induced congenital cleft palate in rabbits. Endocrinology 1954; 55:502–508.

47. Schatz M, Hoffman CP, Zeiger RS, Falkoff R, Mellon M. The course and management of asthma and allergic diseases during pregnancy. In: Middleton E, Reed CE, Ellis EF, Adkinson NF, Yunginger JW, eds. Allergy: Principles and Practice. 3d ed. St. Louis: Mosby, 1988:1093–1155.

48. Beitins IZ, Bayard F, Ances IG, Kowarski A, Mieon CJ. The transplacental passage of prednisone and prednisolone in pregnancy near term. J Pediatr 1972; 81:936–945.

49. Levitz M, Jansen V, Dancis J. The transfer and metabolism of corticosteroids in the perfused human placenta. Am J Obstet Gynecol 1978; 32:363–366.

50. Perlow JH, Montgomery D, Morgan MA, Towers CV, Porto M. Severity of asthma and perinatal outcome. Am J Obstet Gynecol 1992; 167:963–967.

51. Reinisch JM, Simon NG, Karow WG, Gandelman R. Prenatal exposure to prednisone in humans and animals retards intrauterine growth. Science 1978; 202:436–438.

52. Smith KD, Steinberger E, Rodriguez-Rigan LJ. Prednisone therapy and birth weight. Science 1979; 206:96.

53. Lee F, Nelson N, Faiman C, Choi N-W, Reyes FL. Low-dose corticoid therapy for anovulation: effect on fetal weight. Obstet Gynecol 1982; 60:314–317.

54. Cowchock FS, Reece EA, Balaban D, Branch DW, Plouffe L. Repeated fetal losses associated with antiphospholpid antibodies: a collaborative randomized trial comparing prednisone with low-dose heparin treatment. Am J Obstet Gynecol 1992; 166:1318–1323.

55. Branch DW, Silver RM, Blackwell JL, Reading JC, Scott JR. Outcome of treated pregnancies in women with antiphospholipid syndrome. An update of the Utah experience. Obstet Gynecol 1992; 80:614–620.

56. Brogden RN, Sorkin EM. Nedocromil sodium: an updated review of its pharmacological properties and therapeutic efficacy in asthma. Drugs 1993; 45: 693–715.

57. Weinberger M. Salmeterol for the treatment of asthma. Ann Allergy 1995; 75:209–211.

58. Barron WM, Leff AR. Asthma in pregnancy. Am Rev Respir Dis 1993; 147: 510–511.

59. Schatz M, Zeiger RS. Allergic disease. In: Gleicher N, ed. Principles and Practice of Medical Therapy in Pregnancy. 2d ed. East Norwalk, CT: Appleton and Lange, 1992:435–454.

60. Sorri M, Hartikainen-Sorri AL, Karja J. Rhinitis during pregnancy. Rhinology 1980; 18:83–86.

61. Fitzgerald JM, Hargreave FG. The assessment and management of acute life-threatening asthma. Chest 1989; 95:888–894.
62. McFadden ER. Therapy of acute asthma. J Allergy Clin Immunol 1989; 84:151–158.
63. Hollingsworth HM, Irwin RS. Acute respiratory failure in pregnancy. Clin Chest Med 1992; 13:723–740.
64. McDonald AJ. Asthma. Emerg Med Clin N Am 1989; 7:219–235.
65. Leatherman J. Life-threatening asthma. Clin Chest Med 1994; 15:453–479.
66. Nowak RM, Tomlanovich MC, Sarkar DD, Kuale PA, Anderson JA. Arterial blood gases and pulmonary function testing in acute bronchial asthma: predicting patient outcome JAMA 1983; 249:2043–2046.
67. Ries AL. Oximetry—know thy limits. Chest 1987; 91:316.
68. Findley LJ, Sahn S. The value of chest roentgenograms in acute asthma in adults. Chest 1988; 80:535–536.
69. Swartz WM, Reichling BA. Hazards of radiation exposure for pregnant women. JAMA 1978; 239:1907–1908.
70. Myers SA, Gleicher N. Physiologic changes in normal pregnancy. In: Gleicher N, ed. Principles and Practice of Medical Therapy in Pregnancy. 2d ed. Norwalk, CT: Appleton and Lange, 1992:46.
71. Uden DL, Goetz DR, Kohen DP, Fifield GC. Comparison of nebulized terbutaine and subcutaneous epinephrine in the treatment of acute asthma. Ann Emerg Med 1985; 4:229–232.
72. Pancorbo S, Fifield G, Davies S, Fraser G, Helmink R, Heisler J. Subcutaneous epinephrine versus nebulized terbutaline in the emergency treatment of asthma. Clin Pharm 1983; 2:45–48.
73. Elenbaas RM, Frost GL, Robinson WA, Collier RE, McNabney WK, Ryan JL, Singsank MJ. Subcutaneous epinephrine vs. nebulized metaproterenol in acute asthma. Drug Intell Clin Pharm 1985; 19:567–571.
74. Idris AH, McDermott MF, Raucci JC, Morrabel A, McGorray S, Hendeles L. Emergency department treatment of severe asthma: metered-dose inhaler plus holding chamber is equivalent in effectiveness to nebulizer. Chest 1993; 103:665–672.
75. Verbeek PR, Chapman KR. Asthma; who to send home, when to hospitalize. J Respir Dis 1986; 7:15–31.
76. Nowak RM, Pensler MI, Sarkar DD, Anderson JA, Kvale PA, Ortiz AE, Tomlanovich MC. Comparison of peak expiratory flow and FEV_1 admission criteria for acute bronchial asthma. Ann Emerg Med 1982; 11:64–69.
77. Kelsen SG, Kelsen DP, Fleegler BF, Jones RC, Rodman T. Emergency room assessment and treatment of patients with acute asthma. Adequacy of the conventional approach. Am J Med 1978; 64:622–628.
78. Brenner BE, Bronchial asthma in adults: presentation to the emergency department. Part II. Am J Emerg Med 1983; 3:306–333.
79. Skobeloff EM, Spivey WH, McNamara RM, Greenspon L. Intravenous magnesium sulfate for the treatment of acute asthma in the emergency department. JAMA 1989; 262:1210–1213.

80. Bloch H, Silverman R, Mancherje N, Grant S, Jagminas L, Scharf SM. Intravenous magnesium sulfate as an adjunct in the treatment of acute asthma. Chest 1995; 107:1576–1581.

81. Gardner MJ, Schatz M, Cousins L, Zeiger R, Middleton E, Jusko WJ. Longitudinal effects of pregnancy on the pharmacokinetics of theophylline. Eur J Clin Pharmacol 1987; 32:289–295.

82. Frederiksen MC, Ruo TI, Chow MJ, Atkinson AJ. Theophylline pharmacokinetics in pregnancy. Clin Pharmacol Ther 1986; 40:321–328.

83. Carter BL, Driscoll CE, Smith GD. Theophylline clearance during pregnancy. Obstet Gynecol 1986; 68:555–559.

84. Connelly TJ, Rhuo TI, Fredericksen MC, Atkinson AJ. Characterization of theophylline binding to serum proteins in pregnant and non-pregnant women. Clin Pharm Ther 1990; 47:68–72.

85. American Thoracic Society Statement: Guidelines for the initial management of adults with community-acquired pneumonia: diagnosis, assessment of severity, and initial antimicrobial therapy. Am Rev Respir Dis 1993; 148: 1418–1426.

86. Scoggin CH, Sahn SA, Petty THJ. Status asthmaticus: a nine-year experience. JAMA 1977; 238:1158–1162.

87. Mountain RD, Sahn SA. Clinical features and outcome in patients with acute asthma presenting with hypercapnia. Am Rev Respir Dis 1988; 138:535–539.

88. Schreier L, Cutler RM, Saigel V. Respiratory failure in asthma during the third trimester: report of two cases. Am J Obstet Gynecol 1989; 160:80–81.

89. Stauffer JL. Emergency treatment of pregnant asthmatic patients. J Respir Dis 1983; (Nov.) 37–42.

90. Schatz M, Harden K, Forsythe A, Chilingar L, Hoffman C, Sperling W, Zeiger RS. The course of asthma during pregnancy, postpartum and with successive pregnancies: A prospective analysis. J Allergy Clin Immunol 1988; 81: 509–517.

91. Schatz M, Zeiger RS. Asthma and allergy during pregnancy. In: Bierman CW, Pearlman DS, Shapiro GG, Busse WW, eds. Allergy, Clinical Immunology and Asthma Management in Infants, Children and Adults. 3d ed. Orlando, FL: Saunders, 1996:729–742.

19

Prevention and Treatment of Severe Asthma During Pregnancy

PAUL A. GREENBERGER and ROY PATTERSON

Northwestern University Medical School
Chicago, Illinois

I. Introduction

Asthma is a disease characterized by smooth muscle contraction of large
or smaller bronchi, or both, with hypersecretion of viscid mucus (1). The
mucus contains eosinophils and ciliated epithelial cells that have been shed
and then expectorated. The smooth muscle contraction reverses with therapy or spontaneously, and bronchi are hyperresponsive. In severe asthma,
it is recognized increasingly that inflammation of the airways is the major
factor in the disease, as presented in detail later. For the purpose of this
chapter, *severe asthma* will be defined as asthma of such severity that daily
medications are necessary to prevent episodes of wheezing dyspnea, nocturnal wheezing, emergency room visits, hospitalizations, and fatalities.
The Working Group on Asthma and Pregnancy organized by the National
Heart, Lung, and Blood Institute of the National Institutes of Health (2)
has proposed a definition of asthma as a disease composed of airflow obstruction, airway inflammation, and increased airway responsiveness. Patients with severe asthma were characterized by "continuous symptoms,
limited activity level, frequent exacerbations, frequent nocturnal symptoms
and occasional hospitalization and emergency treatment (2).

II. Recent Advances in Asthma

There has been greater appreciation of mast cell activation products in asthma, such as bronchoconstricting prostaglandins (PG) (e.g., $PGF_{2\alpha}$ and PGD_2), leukotrienes C_4 and D_4, and platelet-activating factor (3), and specific antagonists have been effective in inhibiting agonist-induced bronchoconstriction (4–6). In addition, some leukotriene D_4, or 5-lipoxygenase, or cyclooxygenase antagonists have produced positive effects in chronic asthma. For example, the 5-lipoxygenase inhibitor zileutin has been shown to increase the $FEV_{1.0}$ and reduce asthma symptoms in a multicenter study that did not include pregnant women (7). At one time, asthma was considered to be a condition of β-adrenergic agonist deficiency and, indeed, it might be appealing to propose that the profound bronchial hyperresponsiveness of asthma is a form of denervation supersensitivity of the bronchi. There are no convincing data to support either hypothesis, and β-adrenergic agonists are useful pharmacological agents in the management of acute and chronic asthma. New knowledge of a series of compounds called neuropeptides has been the focus of continued investigation (8–10). Substance P, which is located in sensory nerves near the bronchial epithelium, can activate mast cells, cause increases in capillary permeability and bronchial glandular secretion, and induce bronchoconstriction (3). The quantity of substance P detected in tracheal tissue obtained during autopsies of patients with asthma (who did not necessarily expire from asthma) was less than in tracheal tissue from nonasthmatic subjects (10). One interpretation of this finding is that substance P had been released and degraded in patients with asthma (10). In contrast, lung tissue vasoactive intestinal polypeptide, a neuropeptide bronchodilator, was similar in samples from patients with asthma and nonasthmatic subjects (10). Asthma is characterized histologically by patchy denudation of bronchial epithelium in addition to mucous obstruction of bronchi and smooth muscle hypertrophy. Experimental evidence suggests that a bronchial epithelium-derived relaxing factor may be lost in asthma, which could contribute to bronchoconstriction in asthma (11).

Cellular products from eosinophils, such as major basic protein, have been identified at sites of bronchial epithelium denudation in asthma (12). Platelet-activating factor (PAF), synthesized by eosinophils (13), is a potent eosinophil chemoattractant, in addition to being a bronchospastic agonist and aggregator of platelets. Thus, the eosinophil not only produces major basic protein which results in bronchial epithelium injury, but produces PAF, which attracts even more eosinophils. Leukotriene B_4, which is synthesized by mast cells, has neutrophil and eosinophil chemoattractant effects that may be relevant in the late (3–11 hr) bronchial response following allergen challenge. Alveolar macrophages synthesize leukotrienes (LT), primarily LTB_4 (14), PAF (15), and cytokines which cause lymphocyte proliferation and activation (8). The relative contributory effects of mast cells, activated eosinophils, macrophages, activated CD25+ and $CD4+T_{H2}+$ lymphocytes, and neutrophils remain to be clarified (16), but the potential multicellular involvement emphasizes the tremendous complexity of asthma and the challenges involved in understanding the control of bronchial tone.

Asthma is now considered an inflammatory condition, especially in patients with long-term medication requirements when compared with patients who have sporadic asthma promptly managed by avoidance or by temporary bronchodilator use. Even patients with newly diagnosed mild asthma have evidence for bronchial mucosal eosinophilia and lymphocyte activation (17). Following inhalation of an allergen, some patients experience both an immediate bronchial reaction and a late reaction (8). Initially, it was thought that the late bronchial reaction resulted in greater bronchial hyperresponsiveness to other stimuli, such as exercise or cold air. Some evidence now suggests that bronchial hyperresponsiveness occurs several hours after the early bronchial response when airway caliber 1-sec forced expiratory volume (FEV_1) and forced vital capacity (FVC) is normal, but before the late bronchial response (18).

Patients usually are aware of an immediate bronchial response to an allergen, such as a cat, if there are acute symptoms. However, a late bronchoconstrictive response, hours later, may be indolent and severe, but not considered by the patient to be related to the exposure to cat dander hours earlier. Long-term exposure to an animal in a sensitive patient often results in daily respiratory symptoms, poorly controlled with an increasing number of medications. Patients may be unaware of or deny temporal associations between exposure and symptoms. Removal of the animal from the environment can reduce the concentration of airborne allergen such that there is improvement in respiratory status and decreased need for medications. This principle of antigen avoidance when possible is especially relevant during pregnancy (see Chapter 10).

The many advances in knowledge about asthma suggest that asthma should be considered a chronic condition of unknown etiology and one for which current approaches to management can result in outcomes for the gravida and fetus that are the same or close to what occurs in the general population (19–26). However, severe asthma during pregnancy can result in a greater incidence of low-birth-weight infants, need for caesarian delivery, and preterm deliveries (27).

III. Pregnancy Outcomes

A. General Population

Information concerning the outcomes of pregnancy in the general population has been published (19,28). *Prematurity*, defined as gestation of fewer than 37 weeks, occurs in about 10% of pregnancies (19). Birth weights of less than 2500 g are present in approximately 7%, and major malformations occur in 2.5–3.0%. These malformation figures can reach 6–9% if reexamination of the infant occurs in the first 9–12 months of life. The incidence of stillbirths is 8:1000, neonatal deaths (within the first month) 7:1000, and maternal deaths 8:100,000. The mean birth weight from the National Center for Health Statistics is 3370 g (19). Alternative "general population" data have been derived from a survey of 4412 pregnancies in medical residents and 4236 pregnancies in wives of medical residents (28). Miscarriages occurred in 12–14%, stillbirths in 2:1000–5:1000, preterm deliveries in 6.0–6.5%, and birth weights less than 2500 g in 3.0–4.3%.

B. Pregnancies in Gravidas with Asthma

The adverse effects of inadequately controlled asthma during gestation can be devastating in terms of pregnancy outcomes. Maternal fatalities have been reported in women who experienced frequent serious episodes of wheezing (29). Neonatal deaths and stillbirths have occurred in the same setting (30). Some studies have noted increased rates of preterm births and intrauterine growth retardation in the infants of gravidas with asthma (27,30–32). Alternatively, low-birth-weight (<2500 g) infants as a complication of severe asthma but without concomitant excessive intrauterine growth retardation has been reported (27). This latter finding occurred in 45.2% of prednisone-dependent gravidas, in 14.0% of non-prednisone-dependent gravidas versus 4.6% of control pregnancies (27). Pregnancy termination has been performed in an attempt to stop life-threatening episodes of asthma in the gravida (33). Several studies have demonstrated pregnancy outcomes similar or close to that of the general population (19–26,32). Effective control of severe asthma during gestation often requires use of oral corticosteroids, such as prednisone and inhaled beclomethasone dipropionate (2,19,23–25,32). The currently available information suggests that the failure to use these drugs in the management of severe asthma during pregnancy is a greater danger than the potential adverse effects from their use (34,35).

IV. Physiological Changes During Gestation

A. General (see also Chapters 1–4)

Progesterone concentrations increase and cause hyperventilation during gestation. Increases in plasma concentrations of estrone, estradiol, and estriol occur, but it is not established what, if any, effects relating to asthma occur. Similarly, both bound and free cortisol are elevated during gestation. There is a modest decrease in delayed hypersensitivity reactions during gestation, perhaps from increased free cortisol, but the clinical relevance to asthma is doubtful.

Uterine blood flow increases 10-fold, from about 50 mL/min in the nongravid state to as high as 500 mL/min at term (36,37). Uterine blood flow during gestation can be compromised by hypotension and severe hyperventilation with marked hypocarbia, (35), such as can occur in early acute asthma. Decreased fetal oxygen tension can result not only from maternal hypoxia but also apparently from hypocarbia-associated uterine artery vasoconstriction, reduced maternal venous return from increased intrathoracic pressure during acute asthma, and the leftward shift of the maternal oxyhemoglobin dissociation curve attributable to respiratory alkalosis. Additional complicating factors may include maternal anemia or hemoglobinopathy. In gravidas with normal hemoglobin levels, pregnancy does not change the P_{50}, or oxygen pressure in maternal blood at which hemoglobin is 50% saturated with oxygen (26–28 mmHg).

Cardiac stroke volume is unchanged, but diastolic pressure falls as peripheral resistance is reduced. The resting heart rate increases 10–20 beats/min, and cardiac output increases by 30–50% by the second trimester. Total body water expands by 8.5 L, mostly in the extravascular space. The blood volume increases by as much as 40–60% by term, and because the increase is in intravascular fluid, but not red cell mass, the hemoglobin concentration declines. The expected mild anemia of pregnancy can be aggravated in the presence of preexisting iron deficiency in gravidas who have not had prenatal care. The expansion of total body water and intravascular volume have some clinical implications for intravenous fluid therapy. Although dehydration must be corrected, excessive fluid administration in gravidas whose peripheral resistance is low can cause noncardiac pulmonary edema.

B. Respiratory Changes (see also Chapter 3)

The maternal hyperventilation during gestation alters the usual arterial blood gases such that the pO_2 ranges from 90 to slightly over 100 mmHg, depending on data in different studies (35). The pCO_2 drops to 25–32 mmHg, and pH varies from 7.40 to 7.47. A gravida who presents with acute asthma and has a pCO_2 of 35 mmHg is suffering from some degree of alveolar hypoventilation. The diaphragm moves cephalad, and there is a reduction in the generated negative intrathoracic pressure (38). In that an adaptive response during acute asthma is increased negative intrathoracic pressure (to apply more radial bronchodilating traction on bronchi), the gravida may become susceptible to more serious attacks of asthma during gestation. This theoretical possibility needs to be confirmed.

The major pulmonary function changes are 15–25% reductions of functional residual capacity (the amount of air remaining in the lung at the end of a normal or tidal breath) and residual volume (trapped gas) (39,40). The vital capacity is unchanged, but the quantity of air moved during resting ventilation (tidal volume) is increased. As the frequency of respiration is unchanged, the increased tidal volume results in greater minute ventilation. Minute ventilation rises by 20–50% over nongravid values. Serial measurements of bronchial responsiveness in women before the onset of pregnancy and during gestation did not reveal any large changes in bronchial tone (41). Thus, primary factors other than bronchial hyperresponsiveness must contribute to worsening of asthma during gestation.

V. Classification of Asthma Severity During Gestation

In evaluating the gravida, it is useful to define the type and severity of asthma. Some types of asthma are listed in Table 1. In the assessment of the patient with asthma who is pregnant, it is necessary to consider the physiological "dyspnea of pregnancy" that occurs in the first two trimesters (42). No wheezing or rhonchi are present in such patients.

Table 1 Classification of Asthma During Gestation

Asthma classification	IgE-triggering factors of asthma
Allergic	Yes
Nonallergic	No
Mixed	Yes
Potentially fatal asthma	Some cases
Malignant potentially fatal asthma	Some cases
Aspirin-sensitive asthma	Usually not
Adolescent asthma	Some cases
Asthma and allergic bronchopulmonary aspergillosis	Yes

Specific questions to determine the severity of the gravida's asthma include (a) current medications for asthma and other medical conditions, with emphasis on whether there is overuse of β-adrenergic agonists; (b) exercise tolerance; (c) presence of nocturnal wheezing and bronchodilator use; (d) coughing during inspiration; (e) recent hospitalizations or emergency treatment for respiratory symptoms; (f) development of asthma symptoms in association with viral upper respiratory syndromes, purulent rhinitis, bronchitis, or sinusitis; and (g) rapidity of respiratory compromise and previous nearly fatal asthma episodes.

VI. Special Considerations in Asthma Management

A. Potentially Fatal Asthma

It is important to identify patients who meet the criteria for the diagnosis of potentially fatal asthma (43) or malignant potentially fatal asthma (44). The cumulative fatality rate in nonpregnant patients with potentially fatal asthma is over 7% despite our very best efforts. This fatality rate is 1000 times higher than the overall fatality rate from asthma. Specific criteria for potentially fatal asthma are listed in Table 2. These criteria refer to major asthma events from which patients survive. However, rare patients do exist who suffer a life-threatening or fatal respiratory arrest from asthma without prior warning. Thus, these criteria for identifying the high-risk patient with asthma will not predict all patients who die of asthma. Some patients with potentially fatal asthma are so noncompliant with medications, office visits, and almost all physician's advice that they are a threat to themselves in terms of survival. The term *malignant potentially fatal asthma* has been proposed for such patients who are almost impossible to manage (44). Even long-acting injectable corticosteroids (45), which are undesirable because of the risk of adverse effects, especially hyperglycemia during gestation, become impossible to administer in these patients who are unable or unwilling to keep ambulatory appointments. An asthma severity index has been utilized in some patients with potentially fatal asthma (46).

Table 2 Criteria for the Diagnosis of Potentially Fatal Asthma

1. History of respiratory arrest or intubation from asthma
2. History of respiratory failure without intubation
3. Two or more episodes of status asthmaticus despite oral corticosteroids
4. Two or more episodes of pneumothorax or pneumomediastinum from asthma

B. Peak Expiratory Flow Monitoring

There is increasing interest in personal peak expiratory flow monitoring at home as well as during ambulatory visits (2,47,48). However, because certain patients, especially adolescents, may be noncompliant and submit "expected" values to their physicians, the actual benefit in terms of prevention of emergency room visits, hospitalizations, and in identifying subclinical asthma exacerbations remains to be established. For example, if a gravida is stable according to the first six parameters of assessment mentioned under "classification" above, is asymptomatic or has minimal symptoms, and has no wheezing on examination, the benefit of requiring her to record daily peak expiratory flow rates is questionable.

In the gravida with severe asthma, the main emphasis should be on moderate to high doses of inhaled beclomethasone dipropionate and alternate-day prednisone if necessary. This approach has been successful in preventing repeated exacerbations of asthma and in achieving clinical stability (25,32). Some physicians believe that use of personal expiratory flow rate monitoring formalizes the process of medication use and improves care from that perspective. In this context, the recordings represent an index of compliance.

C. Pregnancy in Adolescents

Pregnancy in adolescents with severe asthma has been associated with a high frequency of hospitalizations and emergency room visits (23). During 28 pregnancies in 21 adolescents with severe asthma, there were 22 hospitalizations and 20 emergency room visits during 56 asthma exacerbations. Most asthma exacerbations were attributable to upper respiratory tract infections or noncompliance with medical advice. No maternal or fetal deaths occurred. One infant was found to have cerebral palsy at the age of 9 months. The mother had episodes of status asthmaticus during gestation and was noncompliant. In an effort to prevent continued hospitalizations from asthma with its associated hypoxemia and respiratory distress, we administered a long-acting corticosteroid, depot methyl prednisolone, to help prevent a fatality in the gravida.

In the absence of asthma, the child born from an adolescent pregnancy has increased likelihood of physical and developmental abnormalities (49). Preterm births, low-birth-weight infants (50), and gestational hypertension are more frequent during adolescent pregnancies. From a management perspective, many adolescents desire to be medication-free. Repeated exacerbations of asthma that may be life-threatening can occur when the gravida has asthma of such severity and rejects effective long-term therapy. Emphasis in these patients should include regular administration of inhaled beclomethasone dipropionate in doses up to 840 μg per day, alternate-day prednisone on a maintenance basis, or short courses of daily oral corticosteroids such as prednisone (23). The latter are effective in preventing emergency room visits in adolescent gravidas whose asthma deteriorates (23).

VII. Choice of Therapy

A. General Measures

Asthma therapy requires accurate diagnosis, classification of asthma (see Table 1), consideration of additional major medical diagnoses (cystic fibrosis, allergic bronchopulmonary aspergillosis, substance abuse), avoidance measures, appropriate pharmacotherapy, and in some patients allergen immunotherapy. Communication with the physician managing the obstetrical aspects of the pregnancy is necessary (51). Some important general measures during gestation include smoking cessation, effective prenatal care, avoidance of recreational drugs and alcohol abuse, physician availability, prompt treatment for asthma exacerbations, and a management regimen that is not excessively demanding for the gravida. For example, especially for the adolescent gravida with severe or potentially fatal asthma, pharmacotherapy should include inhaled beclomethasone dipropionate and, if necessary, alternate-day prednisone as the cornerstones of maintenance therapy (23). Some general recommendations, as they apply to management of severe asthma, are listed in Table 3.

B. Pharmacotherapy

The appropriateness of pharmacotherapy during gestation has been established reasonably well for the management of asthma. Most of the commonly used medications are considered appropriate for use during gestation (2,19,21,22,24,25,26,52). General aspects of the use of medication during pregnancy are described in detail in Chapter 7, but certain points will be emphasized here.

The best data to support the administration of medication during gestation are derived from experience in human pregnancies in whom therapeutic doses are used at conception or during the first trimester. Information can be gained from a lack of case reports reporting teratogenic effects and from birth-defect registries. The period of organogenesis in human gestations is during days 13–56. The rest of the gestation is a period for growth and development. In humans the fraction of gestation during which organogenesis occurs is small, whereas growth and functional development is long compared with animals, which often are utilized for studies of tera-

Table 3 Some General Recommendations During Management of
Severe Asthma

---

1. Discontinue smoking and recreational drugs.
2. Consider IgE-mediated triggers of asthma, such as animals in the home.
3. Exclude allergic bronchopulmonary aspergillosis.
4. Appreciate limitations in pharmacotherapy as bronchodilators help mild more than severe asthma.
5. After emergency therapy, discharge gravidas on prednisone therapy.
6. Start oral steroids promptly for anticipated problem patients whose course deteriorates.
7. Antibiotics can help resolve purulent rhinitis or bronchitis, but oral corticosteroids likely will be required to prevent status asthmaticus.
8. After hospitalizations for asthma, alter discharge medications to prevent recurrences of status asthmaticus.
9. Choose medications of established efficacy and safety.
10. It is better to treat the gravida intensively during an exacerbation, rather than to undertreat.

---

togenic effects of drugs. As a generalization, many drugs that are considered appropriate for use in human pregnancies induce teratogenic effects in animals. For example, the administration of high doses of cortisone acetate to pregnant rabbits can induce cleft palate formation. However, systemic or oral corticosteroids in doses necessary for management of asthma do not produce an excessive number of teratogenic effects of any kind (24,32).

Most congenital malformations are not caused by maternal use of medications. However, examples of known human teratogens include lithium, isotretinoin, ethanol (dose-related), thalidomide, diethylstilbestrol, inorganic iodides, carbamazepine, valproic acid, tetracycline, and streptomycin.

Drugs for asthma considered appropriate for administration at conception and during gestation are listed in Table 4. Published data and long experience support the use of such medications (see Chapter 8). For acute exacerbations, either subcutaneous epinephrine or terbutaline may be administered. An alternative approach is use of metered-dose inhalers or nebulized delivery systems (see Chapter 18). Severely dyspneic gravidas may be unable to inspire deeply enough to permit delivery of inhaled β-adrenergic agonists to lower airways. Terbutaline is appropriate to administer in early gestation, but specific human data are limited (51). Other β-adrenergic agonists may be suitable alternatives (2,21,22), but there are

Table 4 Appropriate Therapy for Management of Severe Asthma During Gestation

1. General measures to reduce bronchial hyperresponsiveness
   Allergen avoidance
   Cessation of smoking
2. Inhaled beclomethasone dipropionate (420–840 μg daily)
3. Inhaled epinephrine or terbutaline (≤ 8 inhalations/day)
4. Prednisone or methylprednisolone
   Brief courses
   Alternate-day or rarely daily
5. Theophylline with caution (selected cases only)
6. Depot methylprednisolone for malignant potentially fatal asthma or noncompliant gravidas
7. Cromolyn[a]
8. Antibiotics: penicillins, erythromycin, older cephalosporins
9. Allergen immunotherapy
10. Influenza immunization (after first trimester)

[a]Cromolyn is not routinely used for management of ambulatory patients with severe asthma.

even fewer human data to support their use. Preliminary experience in the first trimester with albuterol during 38 pregnancies was associated with decreased birth weight, likely from ineffectively controlled asthma (53). An increase in teratogenicity was not observed, but the number of exposures was small. Theophylline is an effective bronchodilator on a short- or long-term basis and can be administered during gestation. Some recent studies in nonpregnant patients with asthma have not demonstrated benefit of theophylline when added to β-adrenergic agonists (54), and there is a raging controversy regarding use of β-adrenergic agonists in asthma (55). However, it appears premature to discard theophylline from the management of the acutely ill gravida who may not be responding to epinephrine or terbutaline. Nevertheless, most gravidas in status asthmaticus can be managed with intravenous corticosteroids and inhaled or injected β-adrenergic agonists without need for theophylline. Similarly for ambulatory patients, the use of inhaled beclomethasone dipropionate (up to 840 μg per day) with inhaled terbutaline or epinephrine provides a useful and appropriate medication regimen. Albuterol may be appropriate, but we have withheld using it until published data on safety in the first trimester are available.

For ambulatory management of many gravidas with severe asthma, beclomethasone dipropionate (420–840 μg daily) and inhaled terbutaline or epinephrine provide effective asthma control. Some gravidas will require

Table 5 Patient Information Sheet: Drug Therapy for the Pregnant Patient with Allergic Rhinitis or Asthma

Definitions: A drug or therapy that we consider appropriate for use in pregnancy is one that normally has been reported or otherwise shown to have no risk for the fetus or mother in human studies. This information is recorded in published medical journals. There are various drugs or therapies that may not be unsafe, but have not been proved to be appropriate; we do not recommend use of such drugs or therapies. The following drugs or therapies have been proved appropriate in human studies:

Antiasthmatic medications
    Epinephrine or terbutaline by inhalation or by injection
    Beclomethasone dipropionate by inhalation
    Cromolyn
    Prednisone
    Methylprednisolone
    Theophylline (selected cases only)
Allergen immunotherapy (allergy shots)
Influenza immunization in second or third trimester
Antibiotics
    Erythromycin
    Penicillin derivatives
Antirhinitis medications
    Chlorpheniramine
    Diphenhydramine
    Tripelennamine
    Beclomethasone dipropionate by nasal spray
    Cromolyn

All allergic and asthmatic patients can be managed by these drugs singly or in combination.

We consider it of great importance to prevent the low oxygen levels that may occur in the mother during asthmatic episodes. Early treatment of asthma episodes is indicated, and you should call your physician for increasing symptoms as well as keep scheduled outpatient visits.

We would be happy to discuss any questions or comments that you may have about this information.

Other medication may be required for pregnancy as evaluated and prescribed by your obstetrician.

Source: Modified from Ref. 51.

Table 6 Patient Information Sheet: Use of Cortisone-Type Medications for Asthma During Pregnancy

We believe that cortisone-type medications, such as prednisone or inhaled drugs of this type (e.g., Vanceril, Beclovent), are required to help control your asthma.

Poorly controlled severe asthma (frequent wheezing, coughing, and shortness of breath) is a risk to your health and may be a risk for your baby. A study done at Northwestern University determined that mothers with poorly controlled asthma delivered babies with smaller birth weights than babies born to mothers with well-controlled asthma. Thus, every effort is made to keep your asthma well controlled during pregnancy.

There are a variety of complications from cortisone-type medications that are dose-independent. Cleft palates have been reported in offspring of rabbits exposed to very high doses of cortisone-type compounds in early pregnancy. This had led to a fear that their use in humans might similarly affect the baby. However, the amount of cortisone-type compounds used to produce these abnormalities in rabbits was much greater than that required to control human asthma. Several studies of the use of cortisone-type compounds in human pregnancy, including studies done at Northwestern University, showed no abnormalities that could be associated with the treatment. Thus, we believe that prednisone and beclomethasone dipropionate (Vanceril or Beclovent) should be used during pregnancy to help control severe asthma. The smallest dose of Vanceril or Beclovent and prednisone necessary to prevent severe asthma will be used.

It is most important that your asthma be managed properly at all times and especially now that you are pregnant. No medications should be taken unless your physician prescribes them. If you are prescribed prednisone, you must notify your obstetrician of this because prednisone may increase your blood sugar levels. You may be required to have your blood sugar measured during your pregnancy.

Source: Ref. 51.

alternate-day prednisone, daily prednisone, or rarely depot methylprednisolone in cases of malignant potentially fatal asthma. Essentially all patients with severe asthma during pregnancy can be managed with these medications. The gravida must be taught effective inhaler technique whether or not an extender device is used. When the gravida develops severe coughing, wheezing dyspnea, or purulent bronchitis, rhinitis, or sinusitis, an increase in medication is indicated. A short course of prednisone, 30–60 mg daily, for 5–7 days may be advised and an appropriate antibiotic administered. The blood glucose concentration may be increased during gestation when oral corticosteroids are administered. During an exacerbation of asthma in gravidas who already require daily medication, theophylline or additional β-adrenergic agonists often produce limited or no additional benefit in terms of asthma control. More effective anti-inflammatory therapy, such as from a short course of prednisone, will help prevent emergency room visits and status asthmaticus.

Patient information sheets may be used for the asthmatic gravida, and some examples have been published concerning asthma during pregnancy (Table 5) and corticosteroids during pregnancy (Table 6) (51). Patients should contact their physicians when there has been a significant increase in symptoms so that additional pharmacotherapy can be instituted. Similarly, should the gravida be treated in the emergency room or office for an exacerbation of asthma, a short course of prednisone (56) should be administered to prevent complications from asthma that can result in maternal hypoxemia and stress for the fetus.

At the time of labor, hydrocortisone, 100 mg intravenously, should be administered to gravidas with severe asthma requiring corticosteroids and repeated every 8 h. This therapy provides for sufficient corticosteroid coverage should a caesarean section be required. Once the gravida is able to take her oral and inhaled medications, parenteral corticosteroids can be discontinued.

Acknowledgment

This work was supported by the Ernest S. Bazley Grant to Northwestern Memorial Hospital and Northwestern University Medical School.

References

1. American College of Chest Physicians, American Thoracic Society. Pulmonary terms and symbols. Chest 1975; 67:583–593.
2. Working Group on Asthma and Pregnancy. Management of asthma during pregnancy. National Institutes of Health, National Heart, Lung, and Blood Institute, National Asthma Education Program, Public Health Service, U.S. Department of Health and Human Services, NIH publication 93-3279, September 1993.
3. Friedman MM, Kaliner MA. Human mast cells and asthma. Am Rev Respir Dis 1987; 135:1157–1164.
4. Hsie HK-H. Effects of PAF antagonist, BN 52021, on the PAF-, methacholine-, and allergen-induced bronchoconstriction in asthmatic children. Chest 1991; 99:877–882.
5. Manning PJ, Watson RM, Margolskee DJ, Williams VC, Schwartz JI, O'Byrne PM. Inhibition of exercise-induced bronchoconstriction by MK-571, a potent leukotriene D_4-receptor antagonist. N Engl J Med 1990; 323:1736–1739.

6. Israel E, Juniper EF, Callaghan JT, Mathur PN, Morris MM, Dowell AR, Enas GE, Hargreave FE, Drazen JM. Effect of a leukotriene antagonist, LY171883, on cold air-induced bronchoconstriction in asthmatics. Am Rev Respir Dis 1989; 140:1348–1353.

7. Israel E, Rubin P, Kemp JP, Grossman J, Pierson W, Siegel SC, Tinkelman D, Murray JJ, Busse W, Segal AT, Fish J, Kaiser KB, Ledford D, Wenzel S, Rosenthal R, Cohn J, Lanni C, Pearlman H, Karaholios P, Drazen JM. The effect of inhibition of 5-lipoxygenase by zileuton in mild-to-moderate asthma. Ann Intern Med 1993; 119:1059–1066.

8. Woolcock AJ. Asthma—what are the important experiments? Am Rev Respir Dis 1988; 138:730–744.

9. Barnes PJ. Neuropeptides in the lung: localization, function and pathophysiologic implications. J Allergy Clin Immunol 1987; 79:285–295.

10. Lilly CM, Bai TR, Shore SA, Hall AE, Drazen JM. Neuropeptide content of lungs from asthmatic and nonasthmatic patients. Am J Respir Crit Care Med 1995; 151:548–553.

11. Barnes PJ, Cuss FM, Palmer JB. The effect of airway epithelium on smooth muscle contractility in bovine trachea. Br J Pharmacol 1985; 86:685–691.

12. Filley WV, Holley KE, Kephart GM, Gleich GJ. Identification by immunofluorescence of eosinophil granule major basic protein in lung tissues of patients with bronchial asthma. Lancet 1982; 2:11–16.

13. Lee TC, Lenihan DJ, Malone B, Roddy LL, Wasserman SI. Increased biosynthesis of platelet-activating factor in activated human eosinophils. J Biol Chem 1984; 259:5526–5530.

14. Martin TR, Altman LC, Albert RK, Henderson WR. Leukotriene B_4 production by human alveolar macrophages: a potential mechanism for amplifying inflammation in the lung. Am Rev Respir Dis 1984; 129:106–111.

15. Arnoux B, Duval D, Beneviste J. Release of platelet activating factor (PAF-acether) from alveolar macrophages by calcium ionophore A23187 and phagocytosis. Eur J Clin Invest 1980; 10:437–441.

16. Azzawi M, Johnston PW, Majumdar S, Kay AB, and Jeffery PK. T lymphocytes and activated eosinophils in airway mucosa in fatal asthma and cystic fibrosis. Am Rev Respir Dis 1992; 145:1477–1482.

17. Laitinen LA, Laitinen A, Haahtela T. Airway mucosal inflammation even in patients with newly diagnosed asthma. Am Rev Respir Dis 1993; 147:697–704.

18. Durham SR, Craddock CR, Cookson WO, Benson MK. Increases in airway responsiveness to histamine precede allergen-induced late asthmatic responses. J Allergy Clin Immunol 1988; 82:764–770.

19. Greenberger PA, Patterson R. The outcome of pregnancy complicated by severe asthma. Allergy Proc 1988; 9:539–543.

20. Schatz M, Harden K, Forsythe A, Chilingar L, Hoffman C, Sperling W, Zeiger RS. The course of asthma during pregnancy, postpartum, and with successive pregnancies: a prospective analysis. J Allergy Clin Immunol 1988; 81:509–517.

21. Steinus-Aarniala B, Piirila P, Teramo K. Asthma and pregnancy: a prospective study of 198 pregnancies. Thorax 1988; 43:12–18.
22. Schatz M, Zeiger RS, Harden KM, Hoffman CP, Forsythe AB, Chilingar LM, Porreco RP, Benenson AS, Sperling WL, Saunders BS, Kagnoff MC. The safety of inhaled β-agonist bronchodilators during pregnancy. J Allergy Clin Immunol 1988; 82:686–695.
23. Apter AJ, Greenberger PA, Patterson R. Outcomes of pregnancy in adolescents with severe asthma. Arch Intern Med 1989; 149:2571–2575.
24. Schatz M, Patterson R, O'Rourke J, Zeitz S, Melam H. Corticosteroid therapy for the pregnant asthmatic patient. JAMA 1975; 23:804–807.
25. Greenberger PA, Patterson R. Beclomethasone dipropionate for severe asthma during pregnancy. Ann Intern Med 1983; 98:478–480.
26. Stenius-Aarniala B, Rükonen S, Teramo K. Slow-release theophylline in pregnant asthmatics. Chest 1995; 107:642–647.
27. Perlow JH, Montgomery D, Morgan MA, Towers CV, and Porto M. Severity of asthma and perinatal outcome. Am J Obstet Gynecol 1992; 167:963–967.
28. Klebanoff MA, Shiono PH, Rhoads GG. Outcomes of pregnancy in a national sample of resident physicians. N Engl J Med 1990; 323:1040–1045.
29. Bahna SL, Bjerkedal T. The course and outcome of pregnancy in women with bronchial asthma. Acta Allergol 1972; 27:397–406.
30. Gordon M, Niswander KR, Berendes H, Kantor AG. Fetal morbidity following potentially anoxigenic obstetric conditions. VII. Bronchial asthma. Am J Obstet Gynecol 1970; 106:421–429.
31. Schatz M, Zeiger RS, Hoffman CP. Intrauterine growth is related to gestational pulmonary function in pregnant asthmatic women. Chest 1990; 98:389–392.
32. Fitzsimons R, Greenberger PA, Patterson R. Outcome of pregnancy in women requiring corticosteroids for severe asthma. J Allergy Clin Immunol 1986; 78: 349–353.
33. Gelber M, Sidi Y, Gassner S, Ovadia Y, Spitzer S, Weinberger A, Pinkhas J. Uncontrollable life threatening status asthmaticus: an indication for termination of pregnancy by caesarean section. Respiration 1984; 46:320–322.
34. Barron WM, Leff AR. Asthma in pregnancy. Am Rev Respir Dis 1993; 147: 510–511.
35. Greenberger PA, Patterson R. Management of asthma during pregnancy. N Engl J Med 1985; 312:897–902.
36. Assali NS, Rauramo L, Peltonen T. Measurement of uterine blood flow and uterine metabolism. VIII. Uterine and fetal blood flow and oxygen consumption in early human pregnancy. Am J Obstet Gynecol 1960; 79:86–98.
37. Quilligan EJ. Maternal physiology. In: Danforth DN, ed. Obstetrics and Gynecology. Philadelphia: Harper & Row, 1982:326–341.
38. Prowse CM, Gaensler EA. Respiratory and acid-base changes during pregnancy. Anesthesiology 1965; 26:381–392.
39. Alaily AB, Carrol KB. Pulmonary ventilation in pregnancy. Br J Obstet Gynaecol 1978; 85:518–524.

40. Cugell DW, Frank NR, Gaensler EA, Badger TL. Pulmonary function in pregnancy. I. Serial observations in normal women. Am Rev Tuberc 1953; 67: 568–597.

41. Juniper EF, Daniel EE, Roberts RS, Kline PA, Hargreave FE, Newhouse MT. Improvement in airway responsiveness and asthma severity during pregnancy. Am Rev Respir Dis 1989; 140:924–931.

42. Tenholder MF, South-Paul JE. Dyspnea in pregnancy. Chest 1989; 96: 381–388.

43. Greenberger PA. Potentially fatal asthma. Chest 1992; 101:401S–402S.

44. Detjen PF, Greenberger PA, Grammer LC, Patterson R. Malignant potentially fatal asthma: a management strategy. Allergy Proc 102; 13:27–33.

45. Chandler MJ, Grammer LC, Patterson R. Noncompliance and prevarication in life-threatening asthma. NER Allergy Proc 1986; 7:367–370.

46. Lowenthal M, Patterson R, Greenberger PA, Grammer LC. The application of an asthma severity index in patients with potentially fatal asthma. Chest 1993; 104:1329–1331.

47. Cross D, Nelson HS. The role of the peak flow meter in the diagnosis and management of asthma. J Allergy Clin Immunol 1991; 87:120–128.

48. Grampian Asthma Study of Integrated Care (GRASSIC). Effectiveness of routine self monitoring of peak flow in patients with asthma. Br Med J 1994; 308:564–567.

49. Martimer EA. Adolescent pregnancy. In: Berhrman RE, Vaugh VC III, eds. Nelson Textbook of Pediatrics. 12th ed. Philadelphia: Saunders, 1983:188.

50. Fraser AM, Brockert JE, Ward RH. Association of young maternal age with adverse reproductive outcomes. N Engl J Med 1995; 332:1113–1117.

51. Patterson R, Greenberger PA, Frederiksen MC. Asthma and pregnancy: responsibility of physicians and patients. Ann Allergy 1990; 65:469–472.

52. Wilson J. Utilization du cromoglycate de sodium au cours de la grosse. Acta Ther (suppl) 1982; 8:45–51.

53. Latall J, Greenberger PA, Yarnold PR. Effects of asthma control and asthma medications on pregnancy outcomes in 105 women. J Allergy Clin Immunol 1994; 93(2):260 (abstr).

54. Self JH, Abou-Shala N, Burns R, Stewart CF, Ellis RF, Tsiu SJ, Kellerman AL. Inhaled albuterol and oral prednisone therapy in hospitalized adult asthmatics. Does aminophylline add any benefit? Chest 1990; 98:1317–1321.

55. Barrett TE, Strom BL. Inhaled beta-adrenergic receptor agonists in asthma: more harm than good. Am J Respir Crit Care Med 1995; 151:574–577.

56. Chapman KR, Verbeek PR, White JG, Rebuck AS. Effect of a short course of prednisone in the prevention of early relapse after the emergency room treatment of acute asthma. N Engl J Med 1991; 324:788–794.

20

The Obstetrical Management of Pregnant Asthmatics

MITCHELL P. DOMBROWSKI

Wayne State University/Hutzel Hospital
Detroit, Michigan

I. Introduction

Asthma is probably the most common potentially serious complication of pregnancy (1). Approximately 4% of all gravidas have a history of asthma, but up to 10% of the population appears to have nonspecific airway hyperresponsiveness (2). In general, the prevalence, morbidity, and morality from asthma are increasing. The prevalence of asthma increased by 29% from 1980 to 1987, while hospitalizations increased threefold and mortality increased 31% from 1980 to 1987 (3). The obstetrical management of asthma is complicated because maternal exacerbations can cause serious fetal sequelae, the efficacy of common medical therapies has not been well studied, and medications may have untoward fetal and maternal effects.

The impact of asthma on any individual is highly dependent on the control of the disease that can be achieved by elimination of precipitating factors and medical therapy. The effects of pregnancy on asthma are controversial, since previous studies have had conflicting results (see Chapter 16). However, asthma during pregnancy has been associated with considerable maternal morbidity. In an inner-city clinic, Mabie et al. (4) reported that 42.5% of their patients required hospitalization for exacerbations of asthma during pregnancy, and an additional 18% had one or more emergency room (ER) visits for asthma. Similarly, Perlow et al. (5) reported a 46% rate of hospital admissions for their gravid asthmatics. In contrast, in a managed-care setting with a higher socioeconomic population, Schatz reported an ER visit rate of 12.6%, but a hospitalization rate of only 1.1% for asthma during pregnancy (6).

A number of investigators have reported that asthma during pregnancy is associated with an increased incidence of perinatal mortality, prematurity, low birth weight, and neonatal hypoxia (7–9). Perlow et al. reported a study of 81 moderate and severe asthmatics and found a 7.7-fold increase of preterm delivery <37 weeks, and a 4.0-fold increase of deliveries <32 weeks, compared to controls (5). Pregnant women with asthma have also been shown to have an increased risk of preeclampsia and delivery by caesarean section (9,10). In contrast, several studies have failed to confirm some or all of these previous observations (4,9,10,11). In a large prospective study lasting 11 years, Schatz compared 486 pregnant asthmatics to controls matched for age, parity, smoking, and year of delivery (12). The incidence of preeclampsia, preterm birth, perinatal demise, and low birth weight were not increased among subjects with asthma.

Although birth weight has commonly been used as an outcome measure, few studies have controlled for factors known to affect birth weight, such as maternal race, height, weight, parity, nutrition, chronic hypertension, and cigarette smoking. Asthmatics have increased frequencies of chronic hypertension and maternal smoking, which may also complicate the effects of other influences (6,11,12). Race may be a particularly important confounding factor in assessing the relationship between asthma and pregnancy outcomes, since African Americans (ages 15–44) are five times more likely to die from asthma and are twice as likely to be hospitalized from asthma as European Americans (3).

The mechanisms by which asthma may have adverse perinatal effects are not well defined. Poor control of asthma leading to chronic or episodic fetal hypoxia is thought to be important. Medications used in asthma treatment may also play a role, although the limited available data suggest minimal or no effects. However, steroids may be associated with low birth weight and preeclampsia (2). Furthermore, it is possible that extrapulmonary vascular autonomic nervous system abnormalities reported in asthmatic subjects may contribute to adverse perinatal outcomes in asthmatic women, independent of asthma control or medication use (8,13,14).

Studies have shown that patients with more severe asthma may have the greatest risk for complications during pregnancy (5,15). Quantitating this risk is problematic, because most studies have not categorized the severity of the asthma of their subjects. This problem is further complicated by the fact that there is no universally accepted definition of asthma severity during pregnancy. In 1993, the National Asthma Education Program (NAEP) published the working group's report, "Management of Asthma During Pregnancy" (2). This publication includes an overview on the pathogenesis, diagnosis, and management of asthma during pregnancy. The NAEP working group also defined mild, moderate, and severe asthma according to symptomatic and objective criteria.

> Mild asthma was defined as having brief (<1 hr) symptomatic exacerbations (wheezing, cough, and/or dyspnea) up to two times weekly. The peak expiratory flow rate (PEFR) is $\geq80\%$ of personal best, and FEV1 is $\geq80\%$ of predicted when asymptomatic.

> Moderate asthma was defined as having symptomatic exacerbations more than twice a week. Exacerbations can affect activity levels and may last for days. Pulmonary functions are compromised, with PEFR and FEV_1 ranging from 60% to 80% of predicted. Although not addressed, it would seem prudent to consider pregnant patients who require regular medications including β-agonist, theophylline, or inhaled steroids to also have moderate asthma.

> Severe asthma was defined as having continuous symptoms with frequent exacerbations which limit activity levels. Pulmonary functions are $<60\%$ of expected, and are highly variable. The need for medications was not addressed. However, pregnant patients who require regular oral corticosteroids for control of their asthma represent a level of risk which arguably places them in the severe category.

II. Asthma Management

The NAEP working group's statement emphasizes that the prime target of therapy should be adequate oxygenation of the fetus by prevention of hypoxic episodes in the mother. The NAEP working group concluded that effective management of asthma during pregnancy relies on four integral components, including: (a) objective measurements of maternal lung function and fetal well being, (b) patient education, (c) avoiding or controlling asthma triggers, and (d) pharmacological therapy. These aspects of the management of gestational asthma are described in detail in Chapters 10, 18, and 19.

III. Antenatal Management

The obstetrical management of asthma is complicated because maternal exacerbations can cause serious fetal sequelae, and asthma medications may have untoward fetal and maternal effects. Therefore, therapy and pregnancy interventions must be balanced according to maternal and fetal risks. While gravida with mild, well-controlled asthma may not have increased risks of adverse pregnancy outcomes, patients with moderate and severe asthma should be considered to have high-risk pregnancies. Patients with asthma may be at increased risk for other medical complications including chronic hypertension (11). Coexistent medical complications increase the risk of pregnancy complications for patients with asthma. Adverse outcomes are increased by underestimation of asthma severity and undertreatment of asthma exacerbations. Consultations with a perinatologist, especially with uncontrolled asthma or other pregnancy complications, is recommended (NAEP).

A. Initial Prenatal Visit

In addition to routine demographic information, obstetrical and medical histories, the first prenatal visit should also include a detailed medical history with attention to medical conditions which could complicate the management of asthma. These include diabetes, hypertension, cardiac disease, adrenal disease, hyperthyroidism, HIV, hemoglobinopathies, hepatic disease, and other active pulmonary disease (cystic fibrosis, bronchiectasis, tuberculosis, sarcoidosis, recurrent sino-pulmonary infections, bronchitis). A detailed asthma history should include the presence and severity of symptoms, episodes of nocturnal asthma, the number of days of work missed due to asthma exacerbations, history of acute asthma emergency care visits, and smoking history. The type and amount of asthma medications including the number of puffs on supplemental β_2-agonists used each day should be recorded.

Asthma severity should be classified by historical criteria and pulmonary function tests or PEFR. As discussed previously, it is probably appropriate to consider patients requiring continuous medications to have moderate asthma, and those requiring regular oral steroids to have severe asthma, regardless of symptoms or pulmonary function testing.

Patients should be instructed on proper dosing and administration of their asthma medications. Patients with moderate or severe asthma should be instructed on proper peak flow meter technique; PEFR should be determined with peak flow meters prior to medications, in the morning and after dinner. At each of these times the patient should make the measurement while standing, take a maximum inspiration, and note the reading on the instrument. Personal best PEFR should be determined, and management of asthma exacerbations based on the degree of deviation from the personal best PEFR should be carefully explained to the patient (see Chapter 18).

B. Estimating Gestational Age

Because asthma has been associated with intrauterine growth retardation (IUGR) and preterm birth, it is critical to accurately establish pregnancy dating. Ultrasound can be invaluable for accurate pregnancy dating, and ultrasounds performed early in gestation have greater precision (Table 1). For this reason, obtaining a routine crown–rump length measurement in the first trimester is optimal for patients with moderate and severe asthma.

Clinical assignment of fetal gestational age should be based primarily on a "reliable" last menstrual period (LMP). Reliable LMP is defined as the occurrence of regular menstrual cycles (28 ± 7 days) in patients who have not taken oral contraceptives during the 3 months before conception and who have no irregular bleeding. Additional clinical estimators of gestational age include basal body temperature or artificial insemination, pelvic examination between 12 weeks confirming appropriate uterine size, positive urine pregnancy test within 6 weeks of LMP, fetal heart tones by DeLee stethoscope <20 weeks, and fetal movement <20 weeks gestation.

C. Follow-Up Prenatal Visits

Patients with mild, well-controlled asthma should receive routine prenatal care. Moderate and severe asthmatics should have scheduling of prenatal visits based on clinical judgment. Most will need prenatal visits at least every 2 weeks, then weekly at 36 weeks' gestation. Each antenatal visit should include an evaluation of:

1. Weight, blood pressure, edema, proteinuria, fundal height, and fetal heart tones
2. Asthma severity and symptom frequency, including nocturnal asthma
3. FEV_1 or PEFR
4. Medications (assess compliance and dosage)
5. Emergency visits and hospital admissions for asthma exacerbations

Special considerations should be made for maternal complications which may be increased with asthma or asthma medications. Patients with

Table 1 Ultrasound Assignment of Gestational Age

Parameter	Weeks	(2 SD) days
Crown-rump length	5–12	±5
Biparietal diameter	12–20	±8
	20–30	±14
	>30	±21
Femur length	12–20	±7
	20–36	±11
	>30	±16

Source: Adapted from ACOG Technical Bulletin 187; SD = standard deviation.

asthma, especially if they are receiving systemic corticosteroids, may be at increased risk for developing preeclampsia. Systemic steroids may also potentiate the risk for weight gain and the development of gestational diabetes mellitus. Inhaled corticosteroids can cause thrush and hoarseness. Theophylline may cause nervousness, tremor, heart burn, palpitations, and nausea, side effects which may be difficult to differentiate from normal pregnancy symptoms.

D. Fetal Surveillance

Moderate and severe asthmatics require additional fetal surveillance in the form of ultrasound examinations and antenatal fetal testing. Ultrasound examinations are needed to evaluate gestational dating, fetal viability, major anomalies, multiple gestations, amniotic fluid volume, placental location, and interval fetal growth. Most patients will require at least one ultrasound examination in the second trimester for confirmation of gestational dating, fetal anatomy, and growth. Repeat ultrasound examinations are recommended for patients with suboptimally controlled asthma, and following asthma exacerbations to evaluate fetal activity, growth, and amniotic fluid volume. A careful examination following a severe fetal hypoxic episode should be performed to rule out anomalies including subsequent development of cerebral porencephalic cysts.

The intensity of antenatal fetal surveillance should be based on the severity of the asthma. All patients should be instructed to be attentive to fetal activity and to keep a record of fetal kick counts. In most cases, moderate and severe asthmatics should have fetal testing starting at 28 to

32 weeks' gestation, occurring at weekly or twice-weekly intervals. Most commonly, antenatal testing will consist primarily of nonstress testing (NST), but may also include biophysical profile testing (BPP), contraction stress testing (CST), and Doppler studies of the umbilical arteries or other vessels (16). An NST is considered reactive (normal) if there are two or more fetal heart rate accelerations (at least 15 beats/min above baseline lasting at least 15 sec) in a 20-min period of electronic monitoring. A CST is negative (normal) if fewer than 50% of spontaneous or induced contractions are followed by late decelerations. There must be at least three contractions in a 10-min period for the CST to be considered adequate. The BPP consists of a NST and a 30-min ultrasonographic evaluation of four other parameters. Each of the five parameters is scored 2 points if it is normal; the overall BPP is considered normal if the compiled score is 8 or 10. The five components are each normal if: (a) the NST is reactive; (b) there is at least one episode of fetal breathing lasting over 30 sec; (c) there are three or more discrete fetal body or limb movements; (d) there is at least one episode of extension and flexion of a fetal hand or extremity; and (e) the amniotic fluid is not abnormally decreased (oligohydramnios). Doppler flow assessment most commonly includes assessment of velocimetry of the umbilical arteries.

IV. Labor and Delivery Management

The patient's regularly scheduled asthma medications should be continued during labor and delivery. Although asthma is typically quiescent during labor, consideration should be given to assessing PEFRs upon admission and at 12-hr intervals. The parturient should be kept hydrated and should receive adequate analgesia in order to decrease the risk of bronchospasm. If the patient has received systemic corticosteroids in the past 4 weeks, then hydrocortisone (100 mg q 8 hr, IV) should be administered during labor and for the 24-hr period following delivery to prevent adrenal crisis (2).

Term patients in labor with well-controlled, mild asthma can be followed with either intermittent auscultation or continuous electronic fetal monitoring. Laboring patients with moderate, severe, or poorly controlled asthma should have continuous electronic fetal monitoring. The fetus is sensitive to maternal hypoxia, and abnormalities on fetal heart rate monitoring may be the initial indication that the mother is experiencing an asthma exacerbation. Fetal hypoxia and acidemia will result in changes in fetal heart rate including decreased variability, absence of accelerations, and the occurrence of late decelerations. Such changes can alert the clinician to begin measures including maternal oxygen, hydration, positional changes, and expedited delivery if appropriate, i.e., the fetus is not considered previable (17). With few exceptions, delivery should follow spontaneous labor, or induction of labor should be for obstetric indications. It is rarely necessary to perform a caesarean section for an acute asthma exacerbation. In most cases, maternal and fetal distress can be managed by aggressive medical management. An exception may be for a patient with unstable asthma with a mature fetus; in such instances delivery may improve respiratory status.

For patients with an unripe cervix, either laminaria tents or prostaglandin (PG) E_2 gel, which is not a bronchoconstrictor, may be used for cervical ripening (9,18). Oxytocin is the drug of choice for labor induction or augmentation (2). Either oxytocin or PGE_2 are indicated for the management of spontaneous or induced abortions, or postpartum hemorrhage (2). 15-Methyl PGF_2-alpha and methylergonovine can cause bronchospasm, and should be avoided (2,19). Magnesium sulfate, which is a bronchodilator (20), is commonly used for treating preterm labor. Indomethacin is a potent tocolytic which may be effective in arresting preterm labor when magnesium sulfate and beta-mimetics have not been efficacious. Indomethacin can induce bronchospasm in aspirin-sensitive patients, and should be avoided in such patients (2). If the patient is on a systemic beta-mimetic for asthma control, a non-beta-mimetic tocolytic should be used (2). There are no reports of the use of calcium channel blockers for tocolysis among patients with asthma.

Lumbar anesthesia is an excellent choice, since it also reduces oxygen consumption and minute ventilation during labor (21). For analgesia during labor, consideration should be given to using fentanyl rather than meperidine, which causes histamine release. However, meperidine use during labor is rarely associated with the onset of bronchospasm. Regional anesthesia is most appropriate for nonemergent caesarean delivery, although a 2% incidence of bronchospasm has been reported (22).

When general anesthesia is necessary, ketamine is useful for induction of anesthesia because it can prevent bronchospasm (23). While mechanical ventilation reduces the work of breathing, it may paradoxically increase bronchospasm (24). The use of sedation of intubated patients can reduce bronchoconstriction. Droperidol, which has been recommended, may have bronchodilating properties because of alpha-adrenergic antagonistic effects (24). Halogenated anesthetics have bronchodilating effects. Halothane, enflurane, and isoflurane are equally effective at preventing and reversing bronchoconstriction (25).

Communication among the obstetric, anesthetic, and pediatric care givers is important for optimal care. An analysis of maternal and fetal

Table 2 Possible Neonatal Complications Related to
Asthma and Drug Effects

Prematurity
Growth retardation
Hyperbilirubinemia
Theophylline toxicity—tachycardia, jitteriness, vomiting
Infection
Hypoglycemia
Sepsis
Respiratory distress syndrome
Bronchopulmonary dysplasia
Transient tachypnea of the newborn
Premature rupture of membranes
Hypoadrenalism
Asphyxia
Porencephalic cysts

---

status and the potential complications due to either asthma per se or asthma
pharmacological therapy should be communicated. Potential neonatal complications, which may also be due to prematurity, are listed in Table 2.

V. Breast Feeding

In general, only small amounts of asthma medications enter breast milk.
Prednisone, theophylline, antihistamines, beclomethasone, β-agonists, and
cromolyn are not considered to be contraindications for breast feeding
(2,26). However, increased sensitivity to theophylline may cause toxic effects in the neonate, including vomiting, feeding difficulties, jitteriness, and
cardiac arrhythmias.

References

1. Shatz M. Asthma and pregnancy. J Asthma 1990; 27:335–339.
2. National Asthma Education Program. *Management of asthma during preg-
    nancy*, Report of the Working Group on Asthma and Pregnancy. NIH Publi-
    cation 93-3279, September 1993.
3. National Asthma Education Program. Guidelines for the diagnosis and man-
    agement of asthma, Expert Panel Report. NIH Publication 91-3042, August
    1991.

4. Mabie WC, Barton JR, Wasserstrum N, Sibai BM. Clinical observations an asthma in pregnancy. J Mat Fet Med 1992; 1:45–50.

5. Perlow JH, Montgomery D, Morgan MA, Towers CV, Porto M. Severity of asthma and perinatal outcome. Am J Obstet Gynecol 1992; 167:963–967.

6. Schatz M, Zeiger RS, Harden KM, Hoffman CP, Forsythe AB, Chilingar LM, Porreco RP, Benenson AS, Sperling WL, Saunders BS, Kagnoff MC. The safety of inhaled β-agonist bronchodilators during pregnancy. J Allergy Clin Immunol 1988; 82:686–695.

7. Gordon M, Niswander K, Berendes H, Kantor A. Fetal morbidity following potentially anoxigenic obstetric conditions. Am J Obstet Gynecol 1970; 106; 3:421–429.

8. Bahna SL, Bjerkedal T. The course and outcome of pregnancy in women with bronchial asthma. Acta Allergol 1972; 27:397–406.

9. Lao TT, Huengsburg M. Labour and delivery in mothers with asthma. Eur J Obstet Gynec Rep Biol 1990; 35:183–190.

10. Stenius-Aarniala BS, Teramo PK. Asthma and pregnancy: a prospective study of 198 pregnancies. Thorax 1988; 43:12–18.

11. Dombrowski MP, Bottoms SF, Boike GM, Wald J. Incidence of preeclampsia among asthmatic patients lower with theophylline. Am J Obstet Gynecol 1986; 155:265–267.

12. Schatz M, Zeiger RS, Hoffman CP, Harden K, Forsythe AB, Chilingar LM, Saunders BS, Porreco RP, Sperling WL, Kagnoff, Bensenson AS. Perinatal outcomes in the pregnancies of asthmatic women: a prospective controlled analysis. Am J Respir Crit Care Med 1995; 151:1170–1174.

13. Kaliner M, Shelhamer, JH, Davis PB, Smith LJ, Venter JC. Autonomic nervous system abnormalities and allergy. Ann Intern Med 1982; 96:329–357.

14. Schatz M, Hoffman C. Interrelationship between asthma and pregnancy: clinical and mechanistic considerations. Clin Rev Allergy 1987; 5:301–315.

15. Greenberger PA, Patterson R. The outcome of pregnancy complicated by severe asthma. Allergy Proc 1988; 9:539–543.

16. American College of Obstetricians and Gynecologists. Antepartum fetal surveillance. ACOG Tech Bull 188. Washington, DC: ACOG, 1995.

17. Hack M, Wright LL, Shankaran S, Tyson JE, Horbar JD, Bauer CR, Younes N. Very low birth weight outcomes of the National Institute of Child Health and Human Development Neonatal Network, November 1989 to October 1990. Am J Obstet Gynecol 1995; 172:457–464.

18. Rayburn WF. Prostaglandin E2 gel for cervical ripening and induction of labor: a critical analysis. Am J Obstet Gynecol 1989; 160:529–534.

19. Fishburne JI Jr, Brenner WE, Braaksma JT, Hendricks CH. Bronchospasm complicating intravenous prostaglandin $F_2\alpha$ for therapeutic abortion. Obstet Gynecol 1972; 39:892–896.

20. Skobeloff EM, Spivey WH, McNamara RM, Greenspon L. Intravenous magnesium sulfate for the treatment of acute asthma in the emergency department. JAMA 1989; 262:1210–1213.

21. Hagerdal M, Morgan CW, Sumner AE, Gutsche BB. Minute ventilation and oxygen consumption during labor with epidural analgesia. Anesthesiology 1983; 59:425–427.
22. Fung DL. Emergency anesthesia for asthma patients. Clin Rev Allergy 1985; 3:127–141.
23. Hirshman CA, Downes H, Farbood A, Bergman NA. Ketamine block of bronchospasm in experimental canine asthma. Br J Anaesth 1979; 51:713–718.
24. Prezant OJ, Aldrich TK. Intravenous droperidol for the treatment of status asthmaticus. Crit Care Med 1988; 16:96–97.
25. Kingston HGG, Hirshman CA. Perspective management of the patient with asthma. Anesth Analg 1984; 63:844–855.
26. American Academy of Pediatrics Committee on Drugs. Transfer of drugs and other chemicals into human milk. Pediatrics 1989; 84:924–936.

Part Five

IMMUNOLOGICAL DISEASES

21

Systemic Lupus Erythematosus and Pregnancy

MICHAEL D. LOCKSHIN

National Institutes of Health
Bethesda, Maryland

I. Definition of Systemic Lupus Erythematosus

There are clinical ways and epidemiological ways to define systemic lupus erythematosus (SLE). The *clinical* diagnosis of SLE applies to patients with typical symptoms such as rash, arthritis, and glomerulonephritis. Most but not all patients with a clinical diagnosis of SLE have abnormal serological tests. Biopsy-proven disease of skin, spleen, or kidney suffices for clinical diagnosis, as do one or more typical symptoms in a person with anti-double-stranded (ds) DNA or anti-Smith (Sm) antibodies. Asymptomatic persons who have the same autoantibodies do not have SLE. The *epidemiological* definition requires that a patient fulfill at least four of 11 criteria (Table 1) (1). This definition establishes uniformity among published series but is too narrow a definition for care of the pregnant patient because it excludes clinically diagnosed patients who meet fewer than four criteria and it also excludes patients with related or overlapping disease, such as Sjogren's syndrome or mixed connective tissue disease (2,3).

   Whether a woman can be clinically or epidemiologically diagnosed to have SLE is less important for pregnancy prognosis than is her serological and clinical status at conception. SLE-associated autoantibodies affect

Table 1 ACR Criteria for the Classification of Systemic Lupus Erythematosus

1. Malar rash (flat erythema, sparing nasolabial folds)
2. Discoid rash (raised patches with follicular plugging and scarring)
3. Photosensitivity (skin rash after sun exposure)
4. Oral ulcers (painless, oral or nasopharyngeal, observed by a physician)
5. Arthritis (nonerosive, involving two or more joints, observed by a physician)
6. Serositis (pleurisy or pericarditis, confirmed by a physician)
7. Renal disorder (proteinuria >0.5 g/day or cellular casts)
8. Neurological disorder (seizure, psychosis)
9. Hematological disorder (hemolytic anemia or leukopenia [<4.0 × 10^9/L on two or more occasions] or lymphopenia [<1.5 × 10^9/L on two or more occasions)
10. Immunological disorder (positive LE cell preparation, antibody to dsDNA, antibody to Sm antigen; false-positive VDRL for at least 6 months)
11. Antinuclear antibody in the absence of drugs known to induce SLE

pregnancy outcome independent of clinical illness (Table 2). Pregnancies undertaken by women with SLE-caused organ damage carry risk independent of serology.

In this chapter, statements about SLE refer to patients who meet clinical criteria for this diagnosis. Because pathophysiology and risks are similar for pregnant women with undifferentiated connective tissue disease, Sjögren's syndrome, antiphospholipid antibody syndrome, suspect connective tissue disease, and well women with high-titer autoantibodies, most statements apply to women with these diagnoses as well. Specific references in the text highlight points relevant to non-SLE diagnoses.

II. Effects of SLE on Pregnancy

A. Effects of Disease Severity and Organ Damage

Effects of Global Disease Severity

Severity of SLE is graded as disease *activity* (the quantity and tempo of the immunological/inflammatory insult) and disease-induced *damage* (the quantity and permanence of injury to specific organ systems) (4,5). A pregnant patient with fever, anemia, arthritis, and rash has disease activity; another patient with renal insufficiency and hypertension has severe damage. Activity and damage are independent variables. A patient may have severe disease activity without damage, severe damage without disease activity, or any combination of the two.

Table 2 SLE-Related Autoantibodies Relevant to Pregnancy

Antibody to	Synonym	Disease	Putative effect
Phospholipid (β_2-glyco-protein I)	Anticardiolipin, lupus anti-coagulant	SLE, PAPS, (infection)[a]	Placental insufficiency, fetal death
Ro	SSA	SLE, Sjögren's	Neonatal lupus syndrome
La	SSA	SLE, Sjögren's	Neonatal lupus syndrome
nDNA	—	SLE	Confirms SLE, no known effect on pregnancy
Sm	Smith	SLE	Confirms SLE, no known effect on pregnancy

[a]When due to infection, antiphospholipid antibody is not pathogenic and is not β_2-glycoprotein I-dependent.

Disease activity harms a pregnancy in the general senses that an ill woman does not tolerate the added stress of pregnancy and that high fever may harm a fetus. Mildly to moderately active systemic disease in the absence of criteria listed below neither induces abortion nor precludes normal term delivery. Disease-induced damage of renal and hematological systems and specific immunological abnormalities may have measurable effects on pregnancy outcome.

Effects of Renal/Hypertensive Disease

Approximately half of SLE patients suffer renal lupus (6). Although a woman with lupus nephritis usually has a normal urinalysis and serum creatinine level, she may have borderline hypertension, modestly reduced creatinine clearance rate, or both. As intravascular volume physiologically increases in late pregnancy, such a patient may not be able to compensate and may develop hypertension, fluid overload, and toxemia. Reported frequencies of toxemia (primary or secondary) in series of SLE pregnancies range from 0% (7) to 51% (8). Hypertensive disorders of pregnancy account for an important proportion of adverse fetal outcomes (fetal deaths, growth-restricted infants, and premature deliveries) (9,9a,9b,9c,9d).

Lupus nephritis predisposes a patient to develop hypertension and toxemia but does not otherwise affect fetal outcome (10). Newborns can be normal despite maternal nephrotic syndrome or renal failure requiring dialysis. However, severe lupus nephritis during pregnancy may force the patient to choose between continuing the pregnancy (risking renal failure) or, because cyclophosphamide is teratogenic, terminating the pregnancy in order to take cyclophosphamide.

Differential diagnosis between toxemia and active lupus nephritis is difficult. Clinically measured serum complement (C3, C4, and CH_{50}), urinary protein, and platelet count may be abnormal in both conditions (11–13). Alternative pathway complement indicators and complement activation products (C4a, C5a, Ba, Bb, and C1s-C1 inhibitor complex) are abnormal in active SLE but not in toxemia. Rising levels of anti-dsDNA antibody and concomitant symptoms typical of SLE [lymphadenopathy, rash (but not erythema alone), mucosal ulcers, cellular urinary casts] suggest active SLE. Increasing signs of hepatic injury are more consistent with toxemia, fatty liver of pregnancy, or HELLP (*H*emolysis, *E*levated *L*iver enzymes, *L*ow *P*latelets) syndrome (13a). If the diagnosis is SLE, vigorous treatment for SLE may allow the pregnancy to continue; if the diagnosis is toxemia, induced delivery usually occurs.

Effects of Hematological Abnormalities

Leukopenia, anemia, thrombocytopenia, and lupus anticoagulant commonly occur in SLE patients (14). Leukopenia seldom reaches nadirs that predispose to infection, it does not affect either the course of the pregnancy or the health of the fetus. Anemia in SLE most commonly is of the "chronic disease" type but may be of the autoimmune hemolytic type. In patients with "chronic disease" anemia who are not in renal failure, the anemia varies with disease activity; it often will correct with prednisone treatment. Autoimmune hemolytic anemia is usually not severe. It, too, responds to prednisone, but splenectomy is occasionally necessary.

Severe anemia of any cause threatens fetal growth and well-being (15). Hence it is often necessary to treat pregnant women at lesser degrees of anemia than could be tolerated in nonpregnant women, for instance, a hemoglobin concentration of 8.0 g/dL. Autoantibodies that cause hemolysis are transmissible through the placenta and may cause hemolytic disease in the fetus and newborn.

Thrombocytopenia in pregnant patients with SLE may be due to SLE itself, antiphospholipid antibody syndrome, pregnancy thrombocytopenia, preeclampsia, or HELLP syndrome (16). Deciding the cause in an individual patient is difficult. When due to SLE, thrombocytopenia more often results from consumption coagulopathy than from autoantibody-mediated (ITP-like) mechanisms. High-titer antiphospholipid antibody, clinical toxemia, platelet counts that vary with multisystem disease activity, or falling platelet counts in an asymptomatic woman in late pregnancy all suggest consumption coagulopathy. A history of severe thrombocytopenia antedating the clinical diagnosis of SLE, especially with episodes of severe thrombocytopenia independent of multisystem disease, suggests ITP-like thrombocytopenia. Tests for platelet-associated antibody are commonly positive in SLE patients. Positive tests do not distinguish among causes (17).

If not associated with fetal thrombocytopenia, maternal thrombocytopenia does not directly harm the fetus but is a clue for complicating toxemia, HELLP syndrome, or antiphospholipid antibody syndrome. It is a predictor of possible fetal thrombocytopenia when it is due to maternal autoantibody.

Effects of Disease of Other Organ Systems

Other organ system disease activity or damage affect pregnancy only as the mother's functional health is limited. Neurological SLE, for instance, may damage a fetus through maternal anoxia during a seizure or through maternal neglect from dementia. Lupus arthritis, by limiting movement and strength, may compromise delivery and postpartum child care. Lupus rash may make breast feeding painful.

B. Effects of Autoantibodies and Associated Clinical Syndromes

Antiphospholipid Antibody and Fetal Death

"Antiphospholipid antibody" is a collective term, but a misnomer, for abnormal autoantibodies identified by: an enzyme-linked immunosorbent assay (ELISA) using a phospholipid (commonly cardiolipin) as the antigen; a phospholipid-dependent coagulation test for lupus anticoagulant; or a phospholipid-dependent test for syphilis (18,18a,18b,18c). Only the former two are associated with the clinical events that constitute the antiphospholipid antibody syndrome (19). New research indicates that the antigen to which these antibodies are directed is β_2-glycoprotein-I, a phospholipid-binding protein, rather than a phospholipid (20,21,21a,21b). The IgG isotype and high titer confer greater risk for the pregnancy than do low-titer antibodies and antibodies of other isotypes (18). A few investigators have reported that antibody specificity for the noncardiolipin phospholipids phosphatidylserine and phosphatidylethanolamine increases risk, but other investigators believe these findings to be artefacts of the test systems employed (22,22a). Infections such as syphilis and Lyme disease induce a β_2-glycoprotein-I-*independent* antiphospholipid antibody. Infection-associated antiphospholipid antibody gives a positive test in the standard ELISA system but usually not in the lupus anticoagulant test (18). It does not cause the antiphospholipid antibody syndrome (23).

Criteria for the diagnosis of the antiphospholipid antibody syndrome are high-titer antiphospholipid antibody and recurrent pregnancy loss or thromboembolism. Thrombocytopenia and livedo reticularis are commonly present. Antiphospholipid antibody syndrome patients who do not have diagnosable SLE or other rheumatic illness have the primary antiphospholipid antibody syndrome (24,25). Although approximately one-third of patients with SLE have antiphospholipid antibody, only those with fetal losses or thromboses have the syndrome (secondary antiphospholipid antibody syndrome) (26,26a). However, secondary antiphospholipid antibody syndrome is rare in patients with rheumatoid arthritis, scleroderma, or other definable rheumatic illnesses (18,27).

Fetal death rate in antiphospholipid antibody-positive pregnancies is about 20%. Any individual woman's risk for losing a current or future pregnancy depends more on her prior pregnancy history (the more losses, the higher the risk) than on her current antiphospholipid antibody titer, but both factors contribute to the risk (9b,28). Fetal loss is uncommon in normal women with antiphospholipid antibody, but in women with SLE, high-titer IgG antibody, and prior fetal losses, fetal death rate approaches 80% (8,29,30). Even in series with the worst fetal survival rates, a minority of untreated women who have both high-titer antibody and prior fetal losses deliver successfully. Some investigators believe that women with antiphospholipid antibody have an unusually high frequency and severity of toxemia (31–34). Antiphospholipid antibody-associated fetal death risks are similar for women with the primary and those with the secondary forms of the antiphospholipid antibody syndrome. For women with SLE, SLE risks are added to those for antiphospholipid antibody alone.

Antiphospholipid antibody-associated pregnancy loss occurs in the second trimester more frequently than in the first (34a,34b,34c). Affected pregnancies appear normal in the first trimester but then show, in sequence, decreased fetal growth rate, decreased amniotic fluid volume, worse fetal health profiles, and, eventually, fetal death (35). Affected infants are severely growth restricted but otherwise normal. The mode of fetal death is placental insufficiency.

Placental pathology shows an unusual vasculopathy, with inflammation, interpreted as ischemic-hypoxic change, and infarction (36,37, 38,38a,38b,38c,38d). Antiphospholipid antibody binds to a variety of placental structures and in-vitro interferes with several measured placental functions (39,40,40a,40b,40c). It co-localizes with β_2-glycoprotein-I in the placenta and impedes the natural anticoagulant action of placental anticoagulant protein I (annexin V) (41,42). Anticoagulation successfully treats both animal experimental and human fetal loss (43–45,43a,45a,45b, 45c,45d). Thus evidence from many sources implicates abnormal in-situ placental coagulation in the pathogenesis of antiphospholipid antibody-induced pregnancy complication. It is not clear, however, whether endothelial injury precedes or follows the local coagulopathy (46,46a).

Anti-Ro/La (SSA/SSB) Antibodies and Neonatal Lupus

Defining characteristics of the neonatal lupus syndrome are a distinctive, transient, photosensitive rash in the newborn period, in-utero acquired complete congenital heart block (with no associated development cardiac deformity), and maternal anti-Ro/SSA and anti-La/SSB antibodies present in neonatal serum (47). Cytopenias, hepatitis, other rashes, and other arrhythmias also occur. Infants with congenital heart block are born almost exclusively of mothers who carry antibodies to both the Ro/SSA (52-kDa) and La/SSB (48-kDa) antigens (48–50). Skin and other neonatal lupus manifestations occur in children of mothers with antibodies to either or both of the above antigens or to the 60-kDa Ro/SSA antigen. The risk to an anti-Ro/SSA or anti-La/SSB antibody pregnant woman that her child will develop cutaneous neonatal lupus may be as high as 25% and for complete congenital heart block <3% (51,52). If there has been one affected child, the likelihood for a second affected child is also up to 25%. In both monozygotic and dizygotic twins, discordance between twins is more frequent than is concordance (47,51). Some authors report an increased risk for an affected child in patients with high-titer antibodies, but even in these studies correlation between risk and titer is weak, and exact prediction for a given pregnancy is not possible (52).

Between one-quarter and one-third of SLE patients have anti-Ro/SSA or anti-La/SSB antibodies and are at risk to deliver a child with neonatal lupus (53). However, a large proportion of children with neonatal lupus are born of mothers with Sjögren's syndrome, undifferentiated connective tissue disease, or no recognizable rheumatic disease (53a,53b). Except in patients with SLE or Sjögren's syndrome, neonatal lupus is sufficiently rare that the screening of all pregnancies is unwarranted.

Cutaneous neonatal lupus usually appears several days to weeks after birth, often after the neonate is first exposed to sunlight or ultraviolet light; it spontaneously disappears as the infant's (maternal) antibody diminishes. Animal studies indicate that the antibody does attach to skin, suggesting that the autoantibody directly mediates the skin rash (54). Cardiac neonatal lupus is first demonstrable in mid-pregnancy. Although fetal complete heart block is usually the first indication, first- and second-degree heart block may antedate third-degree heart block, and inflammatory myocarditis may precede both (55,56). Temporary in-utero remissions of arrhythmia rarely occur, perhaps as a result of treatment (56a). Anti-La/SSB antibody may preferentially adsorb to fetal heart tissue; an in-vitro model of cardiac conduction potentials and an in-vivo mouse model of acquired fetal heart block both suggest that the antibody has direct pathogenic potential (57–59,59a). Recent studies indicate no quantitative differences in antibody levels between affected and unaffected infants, however (47,56).

III. Effects of Pregnancy on SLE

A. Global Disease Flare

Animal models of rheumatic disease and pregnancy suggest that pregnancy induces disease flare (60,61), and anecdotes concerning women who suffered severe disease exacerbation during or immediately after pregnancy support this contention. Available controlled and uncontrolled observations, however, are ambiguous, with some clinics noting higher flare rates in pregnancy, others no difference, and still others lower flare rates (7,62–66,66a). Study design variables likely account for the contrasting conclusions. In all studies, flare leading to important change in treatment is relatively uncommon.

B. Renal Effects

Patients entering pregnancy with documented lupus nephritis may suffer functional renal deterioration during pregnancy (10). Whether the deterioration reflects the inability of compromised kidneys to handle the increased workload, the hypertensive damage of toxemia, or activated inflammatory lupus nephritis is unknown. Renal functional deterioration sustained during pregnancy may not reverse (9a,9c,67,68). This concern is not specific to SLE. There is no convincing documentation that pregnancy causes renal deterioration in most patients, but, in mouse models of lupus pregnancy reduces survival (61). When pregnant patients are compared to controls, anti-DNA antibody increases no more frequently in pregnancy than expected (69). Proteinuria often increases during pregnancy, but microscopic evidence of lupus nephritis, hematuria, and erythrocyte casts does not. Serial biopsies are rarely performed in pregnant women, and serum complement, a proxy for renal disease activity, may be an unreliable measure in pregnancy.

Toxemia of pregnancy occurs in up to 51% of lupus pregnancies—the frequency may be higher if antiphospholipid antibody is present (8). The risk of toxemia is markedly increased in patients with preexisting nephritis, but not all patients with impaired renal function suffer this complication. Authors who report low frequency of toxemia appear to see a higher incidence of pregnancy-associated exacerbation of lupus nephritis (7). This suggests that clinics differ in assignment of diagnosis to pregnant SLE patients who develop proteinuria.

C. Hematological Effects

Due to physiological hemodilution, hemoglobin levels normally fall in pregnancy. Thus modest anemia commonly present in SLE patients may appear to worsen. Slight increases in leukocyte counts frequently occur in normal pregnancy. Lupus-induced leukopenia may therefore appear to improve. Platelet counts may increase or decrease during normal pregnancy; late-pregnancy thrombocytopenia is common in otherwise healthy women. Although falling platelet counts occur in pregnant SLE patients, other explanations than SLE flare are usual (see above). Autoantibody levels do not significantly change in uncomplicated lupus pregnancies; an increase in anti-DNA or antiphospholipid antibody may be an indication of activated SLE.

D. Other Organ Systems

In normal pregnancy, skin blood flow increases, particularly in the hands and face, and erythema results (70). Co-existing lupus rashes in these areas may appear to intensify. In normal pregnancy ligament loosening may result in small knee effusions (71). In joints with pre-existing arthritis, effusions and pain may increase. Chorea may occur in pregnancy independent of SLE (chorea gravidarum); fluid overload and hypertension, occuring in pregnancy, may lower a seizure threshold in a woman with prior brain lupus. Postpartum hair loss is also normal; it may be confused with lupus-associated alopecia. Other than these phenomena which imitate active SLE but are attributable to pregnancy superimposed on SLE, there is no specific effect of pregnancy on these organ systems in patients with SLE.

IV. Potential Effects of Specific Treatments on Pregnancy

A. Treatment

Treatment of Active SLE

Treatment for active SLE in a pregnant patient is like that in a nonpregnant patient, with the following qualifications. First, if clinical worsening occurs differential diagnosis must always consider pregnancy complications as well as SLE, particularly if the worsening includes proteinuria, hypertension, or thrombocytopenia. Second, immunosuppressive agents such as cyclophosphamide and methotrexate, which are teratogenic and abortifacients, should not be used (72,73,73a,74). Other interventions may be dangerous to the fetus also (see below).

Prophylaxis

For most patients, prophylactic treatment against lupus flare is unnecessary; physicians should use the same criteria for deciding to treat a pregnant woman as they do a nonpregnant one. Of course, specific symptoms (such as severe anemia) that threaten the baby may require earlier intervention in a pregnant woman.

Treatment of Antiphospholipid Antibody Syndrome

Patients with prior thromboembolic events should be anticoagulated with heparin during pregnancy and postpartum, since risk for recurrent thromboembolism is high. Warfarin, which is teratogenic, should be discontinued and heparin substituted prior to conception.

For the indication of prior pregnancy loss, subcutaneous heparin (10–12,000 units twice daily), usually used with aspirin (81 mg daily), initiated after pregnancy is confirmed, yields the best fetal and maternal outcomes (44,45). There is an important risk for osteoporosis (75,77,77a). Recent studies suggest that heparin doses as low as 5000 units twice daily may be equally protective of fetal life (45a,45b,45c). In experimental models of pregnancy loss, aspirin, heparin, a thromboxane antagonist, and interleukin-3 are all effective (78,80,80a). A small number of patients, in uncontrolled trials, have carried pregnancies successfully when given intravenous immunoglobulin, 400 mg/kg, for 5 consecutive days each month, beginning in the late first trimester (81,81a).

Because the postpartum period carries a high risk for thromboembolism, anticoagulation should be continued for at least 3 months after delivery, then gradually discontinued.

It is not established that asymptomatic women (regardless of high titer of IgG antiphospholipid antibody) and no or one prior pregnancy loss need be treated. Their prognoses are not defined at this time (82,83).

Treatment for Neonatal Lupus

It is not possible to predict which child of an anti-Ro/SSA, anti-La/SSB-positive mother will have neonatal lupus; prophylactic treatment to prevent neonatal lupus is therefore inappropriate. Only a small number of children, identified by fetal echocardiography to have myocarditis or congenital heart block, have been treated in utero. Prednisone, betamethasone, dexamethasone, and plasmapheresis have been used; resolution of effusions and anasarca, but not of arrhythmia, result (56,56a,84). There is no consensus for treatment, but the most experienced investigators suggest the use of betamethasone or dexamethasone, both of which are available to the fetus in active forms.

B. Medications Generally Considered Safe

Prednisone, which is highly metabolized by the placenta, is considered safe for the baby in lupus pregnancy. Because pregnancy itself may induce diabetes in the mother, the combination of pregnancy and prednisone may increase this risk. Prednisone may be associated with an excess frequency of premature rupture of amniotic membranes, leading to premature delivery (44). Low-dose aspirin (for anticoagulation) is also safe. Less information is available about high-dose aspirin. Heparin is safe for the infant but may lead to osteoporosis with fracture in the mother; in the relatively low doses used in pregnancy, hemorrhage risk is low.

C. Medications Generally Considered Unsafe

Small series of pregnancies suggest that hydroxychloroquine and azathioprine cause no permanent harm to infants; however, information on these drugs is insufficient to consider them harmless (73). Similarly, nonsteroidal antiinflammatory drugs are for the most part unstudied in pregnant women. Bolus intravenous corticosteroid may impair immunological function in experimental animals and in humans (85,86).

Methotrexate, cyclosporin, and cyclophosphamide are abortifacient and teratogenic (73,73a). Occasional children exposed to them late in pregnancy have been apparently normal at birth and in early childhood. Warfarin is also teratogenic. Use of this drug in late pregnancy, however, may be acceptable.

V. Optimal Gestational Management

A. Disease Monitoring

Monitoring of the pregnant SLE patient differs from that of the nonpregnant in the following ways: At diagnosis of pregnancy, full evaluation of all organ systems, with particular attention to renal function, serology, and platelet count, is mandatory; systematic reevaluations throughout the pregnancy should occur, for all systems at least each trimester, for renal function and platelet count at least monthly, other checks more frequently if abnormalities appear. Anti-Ro/SSA and anti-La/SSB antibody tests should be determined at the beginning of the pregnancy and need not be repeated. The presence of antiphospholipid antibody should also be determined early; it need not be repeated if positive, but if negative in the first trimester should be reexamined in the second because occasional patients do have an increase in titer during the pregnancy. Very close attention to blood pressure, using obstetrical criteria (90 mmHg diastolic is very abnormal) is required. Finally, physician flexibility in interpreting abnormalities, particularly proteinuria or thrombocytopenia, is necessary, since the assumption that these abnormalities reflect lupus flare rather than pregnancy complications is frequently wrong.

B. Fetal Monitoring

It is generally wise to ask a high-risk obstetrical/perinatology team to manage all SLE pregnancies. Maternal clinical and serological status dictate the extent of fetal monitoring. Decisions are based on whether the mother is well or ill, whether she has anti-Ro/SSA and anti-La/SSB antibodies, and whether she has antiphospholipid antibodies.

In the well SLE patient with negative antibody tests there is no need for special fetal monitoring. In the ill patient, particularly is she is hypertensive, fetal monitoring is individualized as determined by the obstetrician.

If the patient has anti-Ro/SSA and/or anti-La/SSB antibodies, close attention to fetal cardiac status is required. This consists of assuring normality of fetal heart rate at all visits, performing fetal echocardiography at approximately 15, 20, and 25 weeks (to verify ventricular function and absence of pericardial effusion) (55,56). New occurrence of fetal myocarditis or heart block after 25 weeks is rare. Postpartum, monitoring of the infant's platelet count for the first few days and observation for occurrence of rash for the first 6 months are appropriate.

Patients with antiphospholipid antibody have the highest risk for fetal demise. In them, frequent sonographic determination of fetal growth rate and amniotic fluid volume are appropriate. Noninvasive monitoring of fetal well-being should begin as soon as the obstetrical team and parents are willing to accept the possibility of having to terminate the pregnancy to deliver a viable infant if fetal health deterioration occurs (35). (Twenty-five weeks is a time accepted by many experienced physicians.) At this time weekly antepartum fetal heart rate tests ("nonstress tests") and sonographically determined biophysical profiles of the infant can give 1–2 weeks warning of impending fetal death. Umbilical artery waveform determinations by Doppler and sonographic assessments of the placenta give supplemental information. Occurrence of spontaneous or induced fetal (sinus) bradycardia or reversal of umbilical artery blood flow indicate imminent fetal death. Immediate delivery is the only effective treatment.

C. Delivery

In most patients, obstetrical criteria determine the route and timing of delivery. Whether thrombocytopenic patients need be delivered operatively is still controversial, but assessing fetal platelet count, when feasible, may help in the decision. For patients recently on corticosteroid therapy, addition of "stress" corticosteroid coverage is appropriate. In clinically well patients there is no need to give postdelivery corticosteroid therapy as prophylaxis against flare.

VI. Long-Term Outcome

Perinatal outcome of infants of lupus pregnancies does not differ from that of equally growth-restricted or premature infants born of non-SLE mothers. Prognosis for children born with complete congenital heart block is not uniformly good. Many later require pacemakers, and approximately one-third die in the first year of extrauterine life (52). Data are very sketchy, but there does not appear to be an increased risk that the child will later develop SLE even if he or she has had neonatal lupus. Although overall intelligence quotients and other tests of intellectual development show normal to above-normal development as SLE children enter and progress in school, small, not definitive studies suggest that a specific reading disability occurs more frequently in children of SLE patients than in matched children from neonatal intensive-care units (87–89). The cause of this impairment is unknown.

VII. Summary

Lupus pregnancy is complex and often difficult to manage. Fetal outcome is more often related to maternal serology than to specific components of maternal health, but toxemia and prematurity or fetal death are common events. Neonatal lupus is rare. Most children are normal except for prematurity. Long-term outcomes are not yet fully known.

References

1. Tan EM, Cohen AS, Fries JF, Masi AT, McShane DJ, Rothfield NF, Schaller JG, Talal N, Winchester RJ. The 1982 revised criteria for the classification of systemic lupus erythematosus. Arthritis Rheum 1982; 25:1271–1277.
2. Julkunen H, Kaaja R, Kurki P, Palosuo T, Friman C. Fetal-outcome in women with primary Sjogren's-syndrome—a retrospective case-control study. Clin Exp Rheum, 1995; 13:65–71.
3. Kaufman RL, Kitridou RC. Pregnancy in mixed connective tissue disease: comparison with systemic lupus erythematosus. J. Rheumatol 1982; 9: 549–955.
4. Gladman DD, Goldsmith CH, Urowitz MB, Bacon P, Bombardier C, Isenberg D, Kalunian K, Liang MH, Maddison P, Nived O, Richter M, Snaith M, Symmons D, Zoma A. Sensitivity to change of 3 systemic lupus erythematosus disease activity indices: international validation. J Rheumatol 1994; 21: 1468–1471.
5. Liang MH, Socher SA, Larson MG, Schur PH. Reliability and validity of six systems for the clinical assessment of disease activity in systemic lupus erythematosus. Arthritis Rheum 1989; 32:1107–1118.
6. Schur PH. Clinical features of SLE. In: Kelley WN, Harris ED Jr, Ruddy S, Sledge CB, eds. Textbook of Rheumatology. 4th ed. Philadelphia: Saunders, 1993:1026–1030.
7. Petri M, Howard D, Repke J. Frequency of lupus flare in pregnancy. The Hopkins lupus pregnancy experience. Arthritis Rheum 1991; 34:1538–1545.
8. Branch DW, Silver RM, Blackwell JL, Reading JC, Scott JR. Outcome of treated pregnancies in women with antiphospholipid syndrome: an update of the Utah experience. Obstet Gynecol 1992; 80:614–620.
9. Barron WM. Hypertension. In: Barron WM, Lindheimer MD, eds. Medical Disorders During Pregnancy. 2d ed. St. Louis: Mosby, 1995:1–36.
9a. Jones DC, Hayslett JP. Outcome of pregnancy in women with moderate or severe renal insufficiency. N Engl J Med 1996; 335:226–232.
9b. Martínez-Rueda JO, Arce-Salinas CA, Kraus A, Alcocer-Varela J, Alarcón-Segovia D. Factors associated with fetal losses in severe systemic lupus erythematosus. Lupus 1996; 5:113–119.
9c. Epstein FH. Pregnancy and renal disease (editorial). N Engl J Med 1996; 335: 277–278.
9d. Lindheimer MD, Grunfeld J-P, Davison JM. Renal disorders. In: Barron WM, Lindheimer MD, eds. Medical Disorders During Pregnancy. 2d ed. St. Louis: Mosby, 1995:37–62.
10. Hayslett JP. The effect of systemic lupus erythematosus on pregnancy and pregnancy outcome. Am J Reprod Immunol 1992; 28:199–204.
11. Buyon JP, Cronstein BN, Morris M, Tanner M, Weissman G. Serum complement values (C3 and C4) to differentiate between systemic lupus activity and preeclampsia. Am J Med 1986; 81:194–200.

12. Buyon JP, Tamerius J, Ordorica S, Young B, Abramson SB. Activation of the alternative complement pathway accompanies disease flares in systemic lupus erythematosus during pregnancy. Arthritis Rheum 1992; 35:55–61.

13. Levy RA, Qamar T, Lockshin M. Alternative complement pathway in hypocomplementemic/normal C1s-C1 inhibitor complex patients with SLE. Clin Exper Rheumatol 1990; 8:11–15.

13a. Knox TA, Olans LB. Liver disease in pregnancy. N Engl J Med 1996; 335: 569–576.

14. Schur PH. Clinical features of SLE. In: Kelley WN, Harris ED Jr, Ruddy S, Sledge CB, eds. Textbook of Rheumatology. 4th ed. Philadelphia: Saunders, 1993:1025–1026.

15. Letsky E. Hematologic disorders. In: Barron WM, Lindheimer MD, eds. Medical Disorders During Pregnancy. 2d ed. St. Louis: Mosby, 1995:228–241.

16. Letsky E. Hematologic disorders. In: Barron WM, Lindheimer MD, eds. Medical Disorders During Pregnancy. 2d ed. St. Louis: Mosby, 1995:251–258.

17. Pujol M, Ribera A, Vilardell M, Ordi J, Feliu E. High prevalence of platelet autoantibodies in patients with systemic lupus erythematosus. Br J Haematol 1995; 89:137–141.

18. Sammaritano LR, Gharavi AE, Lockshin MD. Antiphospholipid antibody syndrome: immunologic and clinical aspects. Sem Arthritis Rheum 1990; 20: 81–96.

18a. Piette J-C. 1996 diagnostic and classification criteria for the antiphospholipid/cofactors syndrome: a "mission impossible"? Lupus 1996; 5:354–363.

18b. Asherson RA, Cervera R, Piette J-C, Shoenfeld Y. The antiphospholipid syndrome: history, definition, classification, and differential diagnosis. In: Asherson RA, Cervera R, Piette J-C, Shoenfeld Y, eds. The Antiphospholipid Syndrome, Boca Raton, FL: CRC Press, 1996:3–12.

18c. Rai RS, Cliffor K, Cohen H, Regan L. High prospective fetal loss rate in untreated pregnancies of women with recurrent miscarriage and antiphospholipid antibodies. Human Reprod 1995; 10:3301–3304.

19. Sammaritano LR, Lockshin MD. Pregnancy loss in autoimmune diseases. Immunol Allergy Clin N Am 1994; 14:803–819.

20. Kandiah DA, Krilis SA. Beta$_2$-glycoprotein I. Lupus 1994; 3:207–212.

21. Hunt J, Krilis S. The fifth domain of β_2-glycoprotein I contains a phospholipid binding site (cys281-cys288) and a region recognized by anticardiolipin antibodies. J Immunol 1994; 152:653–659.

21a. Koike T, Matsuura E. Anti-β_2-glycoprotein I antibody: specificity and clinical significance. Lupus 1996; 5:378–380.

21b. Kandiah DA, Sheng YH, Krilis SA. β_2-glycoprotein I: target antigen for autoantibodies in the "antiphospholipid syndrome." Lupus 1996; 5:381–385.

22. Rote NS, Dostal-Johnson D, Branch DW. Antiphospholipid antibodies and recurrent pregnancy loss: correlation between the activated partial thromboplastin time and antibodies against phosphatidylserine and cardiolipin. Am J Obstet Gynecol 1990; 163:575–584.

22a. Vogt E, Ng AK, Rote NS. A model for antiphospholipid antibody syndrome—monoclonal antiphosphotidylserine antibody induces intrauterine growth restriction in mice. Am J Obstet Gynecol 1996; 174:700–707.

23. Aoki K, Matsuura E, Sasa H, Yagami Y, Dudkiewicz AB, Gleicher N. β_2-glycoprotein I-dependent and β_2-glycoprotein I-independent anticardiolipin antibodies in healthy pregnant women. Human Reprod 1994; 9:1849–1851.

24. Alarcon-Segovia D, Sanchez-Guerrero J. Primary antiphospholipid syndrome. J Rheumatol 1989; 16:482–488.

25. Asherson RA, Khamashta MA, Ordi-Ros J, Derksen RH, Machin SJ, Barquinero J, Out HH, Harris EN, Vilardell-Torres M, Hughes GR, The "primary" antiphospholipid antibody syndrome: major clinical and serologic features. Medicine (Baltimore) 1989; 68:366–374.

26. Vianna JL, Khamashta MA, Orid-Ros J, Font J, Cerevera R, Lopez-Soto A, Tolosa C, Franz J, Selva A, Ingelmo M, Vilardell M, Hughes GRV. Comparison of the primary and secondary antiphospholipid syndrome. A European multicenter study of 114 patients. Am J Med 1994; 96:3–9.

26a. Levy RA. Clinical manifestations of the aPL syndrome. Lupus 1996; 5: 393–397.

27. Kaburaki J, Kuwana M, Yamamoto M, Kawai S, Matsuura E, Ikeda Y. Disease distribution of β_2-glycoprotein I-dependent anticardiolipin antibodies in rheumatic diseases. Lupus 1995; 4:s27–s33.

28. Ramsey-Goldman R, Kutzer JE, Kuller LH, Guzick D, Carpenter AB, Medsger TA Jr. Pregnancy outcome and anticardiolipin antibody in women with systemic lupus erythematosus. Am J Epidemiol 1993; 138:1057–1069.

29. Lynch A, Marlar R, Murphy J, Davila G, Santos M, Rutledge J, Emlen W. Antiphospholipid antibodies in predicting adverse pregnancy outcome. Ann Intern Med 1994; 120:470–475.

30. Lockshin MD, Druzin ML, Qamar T. Prednisone does not prevent recurrent fetal death in women with anti-phospholipid antibody. Am J Obstet Gynecol 1989; 160:439–443.

31. Branch DW, Andres R, Digre KB, Rote NS, Scott JR. The association of antiphospholipid antibodies with severe preeclampsia. Obstet Gynecol 1989; 73:541–545.

32. Moodley J, Bhoola V, Duursma J, Pudifin D, Byrne S, Kenoyer DG. The association of antiphospholipid antibodies with severe early-onset preeclampsia. S Afr Med J 1995; 85:105–107.

33. Minakami H, Idei S, Koike T, Tamada T, Yasuda Y, Hirota N. Active lupus and preeclampsia—a life-threatening combination. J Rheumatol 1994; 21: 1562–1563.

34. Ornstein MH, Rand JH. An association between refractory HELLP syndrome and antiphospholipid antibodies during pregnancy; a report of 2 cases. J Rheumatol 1994; 21:1360–1364.

34a. Oshiro BT, Silver RM, Scott JR, Yu HX, Branch DW. Antiphospholipid antibodies and fetal death. Obstet Gynecol 1996; 87:489–493.

34b. Branch DW, Silver RM. Criteria for antiphospholipid syndrome: early pregnancy loss, fetal loss, or recurrent pregnancy loss? Lupus 1996; 5:409–413.

34c. Branch DW. Thoughts on the mechanism of pregnancy loss associated with the antiphospholipid syndrome. Lupus 1994; 3:275–280.

35. Druzin ML, Lockshin M, Edersheim TG, Hutson JM, Krauss A. Second trimester fetal monitoring and preterm delivery in pregnancies with systemic lupus and/or circulating anticoagulant. Am J Obstet Gynecol 1987; 157: 1503–1510.

36. Hanly JG, Gladman DD, Rose TH, Laskin CA, Urowitz MB. Lupus pregnancy. A prospective study of placental changes. Arthritis Rheum 1988; 31: 358–366.

37. Out HJ, Kooijman CD, Bruinse HW, Derksen HWM. Histopathological findings in placentae from patients with intra-uterine fetal death and antiphospholipid antibodies. Eur J Obstet Gynecol Reprod Biol 1991; 41: 179–186.

38. Magid M, Kaplan C, Lockshin M. Placental pathology in systemic lupus erythematosus—a prospective study. Mod Pathol 1995; 8:5p (abstr).

38a. Sammaritano L, Magid M, Kaplan C, Peterson M, Lockshin M. A prospective study of clinical features and placental pathology in systemic lupus erythematosus (SLE) with and without antiphospholipid antibodies. Arthritis Rheum 1995; 38:s218 (abstr).

38b. Nayar R, Lage JM. Placental changes in a first-trimester missed abortion in maternal systemic lupus erythematosus with antiphospholipid syndrome—a case report and review of the literature. Human Pathol 1996; 27:201–206.

38c. Sammaritano LR, Gharavi AE, Soberano C, Levy R, Lockshin MD. Phospholipid binding of antiphospholipid antibodies and placental anticoagulant protein. J Clin Immunol 1992; 12:27–35.

38d. Salafia CM, Starzyk KA, López-Zeno J, Parke A. Fetal losses and other obstetric manifestations in the antiphospholipid syndrome. In: Asherson RA, Cervera R, Piette J-C, Shoenfeld Y, eds. The Antiphospholipid Syndrome, Boca Raton, FL: CRC Press, 1996:3–12.

39. Rand JH, Wu XX, Guller S, Gil J, Guha A, Scher J, Lockwood CJ. Reduction of annexin-V (placental anticoagulant protein I) on placental villi of women with antiphospholipid antibodies and recurrent spontaneous-abortion. Am J Obstet Gynecol 1994; 171:1566–1572.

40. DiSimone N, DeCarolis S, Lanzone A, Ronsisvalle E, Giannice R, Caruso A. In vitro effect of antiphospholipid antibody-containing sera on basa and gonadotropin-releasing hormone-dependent human chorionic gonadotropin release by cultured trophoblast cells. Placenta 1995; 16:75–83.

40a. Katano K, Aoki K, Ogasawara M, Sasa H, Hayashi Y, Kawamura M, Yagami Y. Specific antiphospholipid antibodies (aPL) eluted from placentae of pregnant women with aPL-positive sera. Lupus 1995; 4:304–308.

40b. Peaceman AM, Rehnberg KA. The effect of aspirin and indomethacin on prostacyclin and thromboxane production of placental tissue incubated with immunoglobulin G fractions from patients with lupus anticoagulants. Am J Obstet Gynecol 1995; 173:1391–1396.

40c. Oliveira JA, Jesus NR, Albuquerque EMN, Avvad E, Silva RS, Porto LCMS, Levy RA. Immunolocalization of laminin and type IV collagen in SLE placentas: relationship with autoantibodies and histopathology. Arthritis Rheum 1996; 39:s204 (abstr).

41. La Rosa L, Meroni PL, Tincani A, Balestrieri G, Faden D, Lojacano A, Morassi L, Brocchi E, Delpapa N, Gharavi A, Sammaritano L, Lockshin M. Beta (2)-glycoprotein I and placental anticoagulant protein-I in placentae from patients with antiphospholipid-syndrome. J Rheumatol 1994; 21:1684–1693.

42. Sammaritano LR, Gharavi AE. Antiphospholipid antibodies and placental anticoagulant protein-I. Lupus 1994; 3:263–265.

43. Inbar O, Blank M, Faden D, Tincani A, Lorber M, Shoenfeld Y. Prevention of fetal loss in experimental antiphospholipid syndrome by low molecular weight heparin. Am J Obstet Gynecol 1993; 169:423–426.

43a. Krause I, Blank M, Shoenfeld Y. Immunomodulation of experimental APS: lessons from murine models. Lupus 1996; 5:458–462.

44. Cowchock FS, Reese EA, Balaban D, Branch DW, Plouffe L. Repeated fetal losses associated with antiphospholipid antibodies: a collaborative randomized trial comparing prednisone to low dose heparin treatment. Am J Obstet Gynecol 1992; 166:1318–1323.

45. Silver RK, MacGregor SN, Sholl JS, Hobart JH, Neerhof MG, Ragin A. Comparative trial of prednisone plus aspirin versus aspirin alone in the treatment of anticardiolipin antibody-positive obstetric patients. Am J Obstet Gynecol 1993; 169:1411–1417.

45a. Kutteh WH. Antiphospholipid antibody-associated recurrent pregnancy loss: treatment with heparin and low-dose aspirin is superior to low-dose aspirin alone. Am J Obstet Gynecol 1996; 174:1584–1589.

45b. Rai RS, Regan L, Dave M, Cohen H. Randomised trial of aspirin versus aspirin plus heparin in pregnant women with the antiphospholipid syndrome. Lupus 1996; 5:518 (abstr).

45c. Kutteh WH, Ermel LD. A clinical trial for the treatment of antiphospholipid antibody-associated recurrent pregnancy loss with lower dose heparin and aspirin. Am J Reprod Immunol 1996; 35:402–407.

45d. Cowchock S. Prevention of fetal death in the antiphospholipid antibody syndrome. Lupus 1996; 5:467–472.

46. Meroni PL, Khamashta MA, Youinou P, Shoenfeld Y. Mosaic of anti-endothelial antibodies. Review of the first international workshop on anti-endothelial antibodies: Clinical and pathological significance, Milan, 9 November 1994. Lupus 1995; 4:95–99.

46a. Meroni PL, Del Papa N, Beltrami B, Tincani A, Balestrieri G, Krilis SA. Modulation of endothelial cell function by antiphospholipid antibodies. Lupus 1996; 5:448–450.

47. Buyon JP. Neonatal lupus syndromes. Curr Opin Rheumatol 1994; 6:523–529.

48. Buyon JP, Slade SG, Reveille JD, Hamel JC, Chan EKL. Autoantibody responses to the "native" 52-kDa SS-A/Ro protein in neonatal lupus syndromes, systemic lupus erythematosus, and Sjogren's syndrome. J Immunol 1994; 152:3675–3684.

49. Buyon JP, Waltuck J, Caldwell K, Crawford B, Slade SG, Copel J, Chan EKL. Relationship between maternal and neonatal levels of antibodies to 48 kDa SSB(La), 52 kDa SSA(Ro), and 60 kDa SSA(Ro) in pregnancies complicated by congenital heart block. J Rheumatol 1994; 21:1943–1950.

50. Buyon JP, Winchester RJ, Slade SG, Arnett F, Copel J, Friedman D, Lockshin MD. Maternal antibodies to the 48 kD SSB/La and 52 kD SSA/Ro antigens but not to the 60 kD SSA/Ro antigen are associated with neonatal lupus syndromes. Arthritis Rheum 1993; 36:1263–1267.

51. Lockshin MD, Bonfa E, Elkon K, Druzin ML. Neonatal lupus risk to newborns of mothers with systemic lupus erythematosus. Arthritis Rheum 1988; 31:697–701.

52. Waltuck J, Buyon JP. Autoantibody-associated congenital heart block: outcome in mothers and children. Ann Intern Med 1994; 120:554–551.

53. Craft J, Hardin J. Antinuclear antibodies. In: Kelley WN, Harris ED Jr, Ruddy S, Sledge CB, eds. Textbook of Rheumatology. 4th ed. Philadelphia: Saunders, 1993:164–187.

53a. Press J, Uziel Y, Laxer RM, Luy L, Hamilton RM, Silverman ED. Long-term outcome of mothers of children with complete congenital heart-block. Am J Med 1966; 100:328–332.

53b. Tseng C-E, Di Donato F, Buyon JP. Stability of immunoblot profile of anti-SA/Ro-SSB/La antibodies over time in mothers whose children have neonatal lupus. Lupus 1996; 5:212–215.

54. Lee LA, Gaither KK, Coulter SN, Norris DA, Harley JB. Pattern of cutaneous immunoglobulin G deposition in subacute cutaneous lupus erythematosus is reproduced by infusing purified anti-Ro (SSA) autoantibodies into human skin-grafted mice. J Clin Invest 1989; 83:1556–1562.

55. Friedman DM. Fetal echocardiography in the assessment of lupus pregnancies. Am J Reprod Immunol 1992; 28:164–167.

56. Buyon JP, Waltuck J, Kleinman C, Copel J. In utero identification and therapy of congenital heart block. Lupus 1995; 4:116–121.

56a. Copel JA, Buyon JP, Kleinman CS. Successful in utero therapy of fetal heart block. Am J Obstet Gynecol 1995; 173:1384–1390.

57. Kalush F, Rimon E, Keller A, Mozes E. Neonatal lupus-erythematosus with cardiac involvement in offspring of mothers with experimental systemic lupus-erythematosus. J Clin Immunol 1994; 14:314–322.

58. Alexander E, Buyon JP, Provost TT, Guarnieri T. Anti-Ro/SS-A antibodies in the pathophysiology of congenital heart block in neonatal lupus syndrome, and experimental model. Arthritis Rheum 1992; 35:176–189.

59. Li JM, Horsfall AC, Maini RN. Anti-La (SS-B) but not anti-Ro (52) (SS-A) antibodies cross-react with laminin—a role in the pathogenesis of congenital heart block. Clin Exp Immunol 1995; 99:316–324.

59a. Garcia S, Nascimento JH, Bonfa E, Levy R, Oliveira SF, Tavares AV, de Carvalho AC. Cellular mechanism of the conduction abnormalities induced by serum from anti-Ro/SSA positive patients in rabbit hearts. J Clin Invest 1994; 93:718–724.

60. Ratkay LG, Zhang D, Tonzetich J, Levy JG, Watefield JD. Evaluation of a model for postpartum arthritis and the role of estrogen in prevention of MRL-lpr associated rheumatic conditions. Clin Exp Immunol 1994; 98:52–59.

61. McMurray RW, Keisler D, Izui S, Walker SE. Effects of parturition, suckling and pseudopregnancy on variables of disease activity in the B/W mouse model of systemic lupus erythematosus. J Rheumatol 1993; 20:1143–1151.

62. Lockshin MD. Pregnancy does not cause systemic lupus erythematosus to worsen. Arthritis Rheum 1989; 32:665–670.

63. Lockshin MD: Does lupus flare during pregnancy? Lupus 1993; 2:1–2.

64. Urowitz MB, Gladman DD, Farewell VT, Stewart J, Mcdonald J. Lupus and pregnancy studies. Arthritis Rheum 1993; 36:1392–1397.

65. Huong DLT, Wechsler B, Piette JC, Bletry O, Godeau P. Pregnancy and its outcome in systemic lupus-erythematosus. Quart J Med 1994; 87:721–729.

66. Buchanan NMM, Khamashta MA, Morton KE, Kerslake S, Baguley EA, Hughes GRV. A study of 100 high-risk lupus pregnancies. Am J Reprod Immunol 1992; 28:192–194.

66a. Ruiz-Irastorza G, Lima F, Alves J, Khamashta MA, Simpson J, Hughes GRV, Buchanan NMM. Increased rate of lupus flare during pregnancy and the puerperium—prospective study of 78 pregnancies. Br J Rheumatol 1996; 35: 133–138.

67. Hou S. Pregnancy in women with chronic renal disease. N Engl J Med 1985; 312:836–839.

68. Packham DK, Lam SS, Nicholls K, Fairley KF, Kincaid-Smith PS. Lupus nephritis and pregnancy. Quart J Med 1992; 83:315–324.

69. Lockshin MD, Reinitz E, Druzin ML, Murrman M, Estes D. Lupus pregnancy: case-control prospective study demonstrating absence of lupus exacerbation during or after pregnancy. Am J Med 1984; 77:893–898.

70. Aronson IK, Halaska BN. Dermatologic diseases. In: Barron WM, Lindheimer MD, eds. Medical Disorders During Pregnancy. 2d ed. St. Louis: Mosby, 1995:452–453.

71. Lowery CL. Sudden joint and extremity pain in pregnancy. Obstet Gynecol Clin N Am 1995; 22:173–190.

72. Briggs GG, Freeman RK, Yaffer SJ. Drugs in Pregnancy and Lactation—a Reference Guide to Fetal and Neonatal Risk. 2d ed. Baltimore: Williams & Wilkins, 1986.

73. Ostensen M. Optimization of antirheumatic drug-treatment in pregnancy. Clin Pharm 1994:486–503.

73a. Bermas BL, Hill JA. Effects of immunosuppressive drugs during pregnancy. Arthritis Rheum 1995; 38:1722–1732.

74. Lockshin MD, Druzin ML, Rheumatic disease. In: Barron WM, Lindheimer MD, eds. Medical Disorders During Pregnancy. 2d ed. St. Louis: Mosby Year Book, 1995:331.

75. Wise PH, Hall AJ. Heparin induced osteopenia in pregnancy. Br Med J 1989; 47:110–111.

76. Barbour LA, Kick SD, Steiner JF, LoVerde ME, Heddleston LN Lear JL, Baron AE, Barton PL. A prospective study of heparin-induced osteoporosis in pregnancy using bone densitometry. Am J Obstet Gynecol 1994; 170: 862–869.

77. Dahlman TC. Osteoporotic fractures and the recurrence of thromboembolism during pregnancy and the puerperium in 184 women undergoing thromboprophylaxis with heparin. Am J Obstet Gynecol 1993; 168:1265–1270.

77a. Douketis JD, Ginsberg JS, Burrows RF, Duku EK, Webber CE, Brill-Edwards P. The effect of long-term heparin therapy during pregnancy on bone density. A prospective matched cohort study. Thromb Haemost 1996; 75:254–257.

78. Fishman P, Falach-Vaknine, Zigelman R, Bakimer R, Sredni B, Djaldetti M, Shoenfeld Y. Prevention of fetal loss in experimental anti-phospholipid syndrome by in vivo administration of recombinant interleukin-3. J Clin Invest 1993; 91:1834–1837.

79. Shoenfeld Y, Blank M. Effect of long-acting thromboxane receptor antagonist (BMS 180,291) on experimental antiphospholipid syndrome. Lupus 1994; 3: 397–400.

80. Krause I, Blank M, Gilbrut B, Shoenfeld Y. The effect of aspirin on recurrent fetal loss in experimental antiphospholipid syndrome. Am J Reprod Immunol 1993; 29:155–161.

80a. Tincani A, Shoenfeld Y. Animal models of the antiphospholipid syndrome. In: Asherson RA, Cervera R, Piette J-C, Shoenfeld Y, eds. The Antiphospholipid Syndrome, Boca Raton, FL: CRC Press, 1996:71–82.

81. Spinnato JA, Clark AL, Pierangeli SS, Harris EN. Intravenous immunoglobulin therapy for the antiphospholipid syndrome in pregnancy. Am J Obstet Gynecol 1995; 172:690–694.

81a. Pregnancy Loss Study Group. Randomized, placebo-controlled trial of intravenous immune globulin (IVIG) in antiphospholipid syndrome (APS) in pregnancy: a progress report. Lupus 1996; 5:201 (abstr).

82. Harris EN, Spinnato JA. Should anticardiolipin tests be performed in otherwise healthy pregnancy women? Am J Obstet Gynecol 1991; 165:1272–1277.

83. Lockshin MD. Answers to the antiphospholipid-antibody syndrome? N Engl J Med 1995; 332:1025–1027.

84. Rider LG, Buyon JP, Rutledge J, Sherry DD. Treatment of neonatal lupus: case report and review of the literature. J Rheumatol 1993; 20:1208–1211.

85. Eishi Y, Hirokawa K, Hatakeyama S. Long-lasting impairment of immune and endocrine systems of offspring induced by injection of dexamethasone into pregnant mice. Clin Immunol Immunopathol 1983; 26:335–349.

86. Hensleigh PA, Herzenberg LA, Lipman SH, Malvehy RM, Medearis AL, Moore MH, Sutherland KK, Waters VB. Transient immunologic effects of

betamethasone in human pregnancy after suppression of pre-term labor. Am J Reprod Immunol 1983; 4:83–87.

87. Ross G, Sammaritano LR, Nass R, Lockshin M. Learning disabilities in offspring of women with systemic lupus erythematosus. Arthritis Rheum 1993; 36:s87 (abstr).

88. Schur PH. Fingerprint analysis of patients with systemic lupus erythematosus and their relatives. J Rheumatol 1990; 17:482–484.

89. Lahita RG. Systemic lupus erythematosus: learning disability in the male offspring of female patients and relationship to laterality. Psychoneuroendocrinology 1988; 13:385–396.

22

Rheumatoid Arthritis and Other Arthropathies During Pregnancy

J. LEE NELSON

Fred Hutchinson Cancer Research Center
and The University of Washington School
  of Medicine
Seattle, Washington

MONIKA E. ØSTENSEN

University Hospital of Trondheim
Trondheim, Norway

I. Introduction

Considerations of practical significance for a woman with rheumatic disease are what effect pregnancy is expected to have on her disease and whether it might affect the infant. This chapter is organized with practical considerations for women with rheumatoid arthritis considered first, followed by a discussion of investigative studies. Thereafter, existing data are summarized for pregnancy in women with juvenile chronic arthritis, adult-onset Still's disease, and spondyloarthropathies.

II. Rheumatoid Arthritis

A. Clinical Characteristics of Rheumatoid Arthritis in Women

Rheumatoid arthritis (RA) is a systemic, chronic inflammatory disorder, the hallmark characteristic of which is symmetrical polyarthritis. Extra-articular manifestations include subcutaneous nodules, lung disease, pericarditis, neuropathy, and vasculitis. RA is an autoimmune disorder of unknown etiology. The autoantibody rheumatoid factor, although neither wholly sensitive nor wholly specific, is characteristic of RA and can be detected in 80–90% of patients. The disease spectrum is wide, with patients with minor, limited arthritis on one end and patients with severe progressive joint destruction and/or extra-articular disease on the other. In many patients the disease is self-limited, with spontaneous remission not uncommon.

RA is a relatively common disorder, occurring in 1–2% of the population. About three times more women are affected than men. It is sometimes said that the peak incidence of RA in women occurs in middle years; however, this is erroneous. A number of studies have demonstrated that the incidence of RA in women continues to increase with advancing age, including into the seventh or even eighth decade of a woman's life (1–3). Particular histocompatibility genes (HLA) have been shown to be associated with RA. In most populations, specific subtypes of HLA-DR4 are increased among RA patients, and certain subtypes of DR1 and DR14 are also enriched in some RA populations (4). Although the RA-associated HLA genes are found with increased frequency in both men and women, gender-related differences in HLA associations have been described (5–8).

B.   Effect of Pregnancy on the Mother's Disease

Amelioration of the symptoms and signs of RA during pregnancy was initially described in 1938 by Dr. P. S. Hench (9). Hench reported relief of arthritis symptoms in 90% of women, and 18 of his 22 study patients had RA. Improvement of arthritis and reduction of swelling was described as often striking and frequently complete.

Confirmation of Hench's observation was forthcoming in subsequent studies. In two early retrospective studies, arthritis improved in 83% of 19 pregnancies (10) and in 54% of 24 patients with RA (11). In a larger retrospective study of 114 pregnancies, improvement occurred in 78%(12). Results from more recent retrospective studies are similar, reporting improvement in 62% of 56 pregnancies (13) and in 75% of 37 pregnancies (14). The number of pregnancies studied prospectively has been small, but the results confirm findings in retrospective studies. A 1960 report included prospective evaluation of 7 patients with RA, of whom 6 experienced improvement (86%) (15). In two other prospective studies, RA improved in 10 of 12 pregnancies (83%) and 10 of 14 pregnancies (71%) (16,17). Thus retrospective and prospective studies indicate that improvement of RA occurs in about three-quarters of pregnancies. The effect of pregnancy on extra-articular manifestations of RA is not known.

The presence or absence of rheumatoid fever, functional class (degree of disability), and duration of disease have not been found to predict pregnancy experience (13,16). An early report suggesting that a patient's age might be predictive for whether arthritis would improve during pregnancy (18) was not confirmed in later studies (13,19). Most studies are in agreement that if a woman improves during one pregnancy, she is likely to experience improvement in subsequent pregnancies

C. Timing of Improvement of RA During Pregnancy

In Hench's original paper, amelioration of RA was described as occurring early in pregnancy in most patients (9). Other retrospective studies have generally confirmed this observation. All of 13 patients who experienced improvement had relief in the first trimester, described in a 1964 report (11). In a larger study that evaluated 70 pregnancies, improvement occurred for 80% in the first trimester, in the second trimester for 17%, and in the third trimester for 3% (12). A more recent retrospective review of 35 pregnancics found that 57% improved in the first trimester, 34% in the second trimester and 9% in the third trimester (13). Østensen et al. (14) compared activity during pregnancy with preconception disease activity using an assigned mean activity score and found that initial arthritis relief occurred most frequently in the first trimester, with further improvement also observed in the second and third trimester for some patients. Once improvement occurred, it persisted and often became more nearly complete as gestation progressed.

Two small prospective studies have examined the timing of arthritis improvement. A 1960 report described remission in the last trimester in 6 of 7 patients (15). In a more recent study, 9 of 10 patients who improved had some relief in the first trimester; the 10th patient did not improve until 4 weeks prior to delivery (16). As part of research investigations of the maternal–fetal HLA relationship in pregnancies of women with RA (see below), 18 pregnancies were identified prospectively, 17 of which were characterized by remission or improvement (19). Patients were asked to rank their arthritis activity using a scale from 0 to 3 on a monthly basis extending from the 6 months prior to conception, throughout pregnancy, and in the 3 months postpartum. The study rheumatologist's examination and assessment of disease activity (remission, improvement, or active) was concordant with the patient's assessments in all pregnancies, although patients were often referred to the study when already pregnant, so the rheumatologist's assessment did not cover all time points. The timing of remission or improvement for these 17 women is shown in Fig. 1 and indicates that more than three-quarters experienced at least some improvement by the end of the first trimester (76%). In 14 pregnancies, once improvement began, it was either sustained or improved further (82%). Within

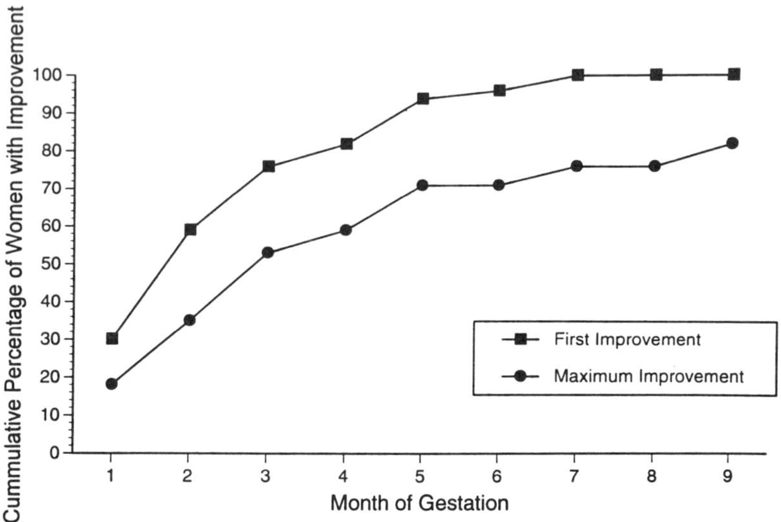

Figure 1 To examine the timing of arthritis amelioration during pregnancy, the experience of 17 women who had remission or improvement and were identified before or during pregnancy is summarized. Patients ranked arthritis activity each month on a scale of 0–3. Once improvement occurred, it was sustained or furthered in 14 pregnancies. However, 3 patients were better in the first and second trimesters than in the third (hence the percent with maximum improvement is not 100% in the third trimester). Of patients who experienced amelioration of arthritis, 53% had complete remission.

the category of improvement or remission, the percentage with complete remission was not indicated in earlier studies. Among the 17 pregnancies, 9 women had complete remission of all symptoms and signs of arthritis and took no medication, so that approximately half of patients who experienced disease amelioration had complete remission. If both retrospective and prospective pregnancies are included, 22 of 34 had complete remission (65%).

D. Pregnancy Complications, Preeclampsia, and Delivery

No study has specifically addressed the issue of pregnancy complications in RA patients. Mention of one patient with "mild" preeclampsia is made in a 1969 report (10). Because of the rarity of reported preeclampsia, the question has been asked as to whether the incidence might actually be reduced in RA patients. In a study of normal women, increased risk of preeclampsia was described both for women who had HLA-DR4 and also for mother–child pairs who shared HLA-DR4 (20). If this observation is confirmed, the absence of reports of preclampsia in women with RA becomes more striking, because an increase of DR4 is observed in women with RA and maternal–fetal sharing of DR4 would be expected more frequently.

No increase in premature labor has been observed in RA patients (10). With respect to delivery, in some cases vaginal delivery may be compromised by hip disease or prior total hip replacement, as has been reported for pregnancies of some women with juvenile chronic arthritis (21). However, hip disease and/or total hip replacement does not preclude the possibility of a normal vaginal delivery. In the patient requiring anesthesia and intubation, the usual precaution applies regarding possible involvement of the cervical spine by RA and instability.

E. Maternal Disease Activity Postpartum

Active arthritis characterizes the postpartum period, both for women who have experienced gestational remission and for those who have not. An early study described recurrence within 3 to 4 months after delivery in all 13 patients who had improvement during pregnancy (11). In an evaluation of 69 patients, recurrence was found in 36% within the first month postpartum, 69% by 2 months, 85% by 3 months, and 98% by the end of 4 months (12). Similar findings have been reported in more recent studies (13,14,16,22). Thus, almost all women have recurrent disease within 3 to 4 months of delivery. The return of arthritis has been found to be unrelated to resumption of menstration of lactation (14,16). Active arthritis following induced or spontaneous abortion has also been reported (18).

F. Drug Treatment During Pregnancy

Corticosteroids During Pregnancy and Lactation

The need for therapeutic intervention during pregnancy is often obviated, since patients with RA frequently show improvement or remission during pregnancy. For the patient who has active arthritis in one or a limited number of joints, intra-articular steroid injection(s) can be useful.

If medication is needed during pregnancy, prednisone is often prescribed. Corticosteroids may cross the placenta. With dexamethasone, fetal and maternal plasma levels are similar. In contrast to dexamethasone, when

prednisone is used, fetal plasma levels of the active metabolite, prednisolone, are 8–10 times lower than maternal levels (23). Therefore prednisone
is used when the purpose is to treat maternal disease and dexamethasone
is used when the purpose is to treat the fetus (e.g, for lung maturation).

Experimental studies from animals have shown an association of corticosteroids with neonatal malformations, particularly cleft palate (24–27).
There have been scattered reports of cleft palate, growth retardation, neonatal cataracts, and adrenal suppression in neonates of women exposed to
steroids during pregnancy (for review, see Ref. 28). However, substantial
clinical experience has accumulated in humans and does not indicate that
corticosteroid use results in a significant increased risk of fetal malformation, so patients with RA who have active disease can be reassured
regarding use of prednisone during pregnancy. For women who take corticosteroids during pregnancy, stress doses are given for labor and delivery.
Low-dose prednisone (<20 mg) is considered safe while breast feeding
(29). Studies have shown that following a 10-mg dose of prednisone, milk
concentrations of prednisone and prednisolone after 2 hr are 0.03 and 0.002
μg/mL, respectively (30).

Effect of Nonsteroidal Anti-Inflammatory Drugs (NSAIDs) on the Fetus and Newborn

Some patients may use NSAIDs to reduce signs and symptoms of arthritis.
NSAIDs inhibit cyclooxygenase, and may be expected to interfere with
pregnancy. A possible side effect of NSAIDs is inhibition of prostaglandin
synthesis in the fetus. Reduction of fetal renal output and a decrease in the
volume of amniotic fluid has been shown for indomethacin, ketoprofen,
and ibuprofen, and is likely to occur with other inhibitors of prostaglandin
synthesis (31,32). In premature infants exposed to standard doses of indomethacin, naproxen, and ketoprofen within 72 hr before delivery, impaired renal function has been reported (33–35). There is evidence that
renal function in the fetus recovers quickly after drug withdrawal (36).

In vitro studies have shown that acidic NSAIDs can constrict the
ductus arteriosus (37). Trials with indomethacin for inhibition of premature
labor have shown that constriction of the ductus occurs as early as the 27th
week of gestation. The effect was unrelated to fetal serum indomethacin
levels (38). NSAID-induced constriction of the ductus has been shown to
resolve within 24 hr after discontinuance of the drug, however (39). Østensen et al. (40) compared 49 patients with rheumatic disease using standard
doses of NSAID for an average of 15.3 weeks during gestation to 45
nonusers of NSAIDs. No adverse maternal or neonatal effects were ob-

served in users of NSAIDs, most probably due to the fact that NSAID were always discontinued 6 weeks before term.

Aspirin is prescribed by some physicians for symptoms of arthritis during pregnancy. In a study that included 14,864 women evaluated prospectively, no increase in the congenital malformation rate was found for almost 10,000 women who took moderate doses of aspirin during pregnancy (41). Aspirin is discontinued in the third trimester because of an increased risk of neonatal bleeding at delivery, including CNS hemorrhage, and because of the possibility of a constrictive effect of the ductus arteriosus (42,43).

Prophylactic Withdrawal Before Pregnancy, Use of DMARDs

Often patients with active arthritis will be taking NSAIDs alone or in combination with disease-modifying drugs (DMARDs) and will ask their doctors if they should stop all medication prior to becoming pregnant. Salicylates and NSAIDs such as indomethacin, fenoprofen, ibuprofen, ketoprofen, naproxen, diclofenac, mefenamic acid, and piroxicam are not known to be teratogenic in humans, so prophylactic cessation of therapy is not necessary (44,45) (Table 1).

There are no data that specifically address the issue of prophylactic withdrawal before pregnancy for DMARDs. Perhaps because of insufficient documentation in the literature, rheumatologists differ in their view of the advisability of DMARD during pregnancy. For antimalarial medications, among more than 200 reported human pregnancies exposed, only 58 occurred in patients treated for rheumatic disease. Experience with use of gold and penicillamine during pregnancy includes less than 100 pregnancies. Only sulfasalazine has a more extensive reported experience, with more than 2000 pregnancies exposed, but exclusively for the treatment of inflammatory bowel disease. The following is one suggested approach (Tables 1, 2). Patients on treatment with parenteral gold may receive their monthly injection on the first day of the menses so that gold can be withdrawn as soon as pregnancy is recognized. Transplacental passage of gold occurs, but there is no evidence of an increase in rate of neonatal malformations for women taking gold (46). Hydroxychloroquine has not been associated with reported fetal adverse effects and can be continued during pregnancy if strictly necessary (47,48). Whether penicillamine can act as a possible human teratogen has been debated. Some recommend prophylactic withdrawal before pregnancy (49), while others recommend slow tapering and withdrawal once pregnancy has been established (50,51). Sulfasalazine has been used in pregnant patients with inflammatory bowel

Table 1 Prophylactic Cessation of Treatment Prior to a Pregnancy

Drug	Risk of congential malformations	Prophylactic cessation recommended
NSAIDs		
Diclofenac	−[a]	No
Diflunisal	−	No
Ibuprofen	−	No
Indomethacin	−	No
Mefanamic acid	−	No
Naproxen	−	No
Piroxicam	−	No
Sulindac	−	No
Salicylates	−	No
DMARD		
Sulfasalazine	−	No
Chloroquine	?[b]	?
Hydroxychloroquine	0[c]	No
Gold	−	No
Penicillamine	?	No
Cyclosporine A	−	No
Cytotoxic drugs		
Azathioprine	−	No
Methotrexate	+[d]	3 months prior to conception
Cyclophosphamide	+	3 months prior to conception
Chlorambucil	+	3 months prior to conception
Glucocorticoids		
Prednisone	−	No

[a]Not proven.
[b]Possible.
[c]No congenital malformation reported.
[d]Increases risk of congenital malformations.

disease without harmful effects, and can be continued during pregnancy and breast feeding (52–54).

Cytostatic drugs including methotrexate, cyclophosphamide, and chlorambucil should always be withdrawn at least 3 months before trying to conceive. Methotrexate increases the risk of congenital malformations. The critical period is probably 6–8 weeks of gestation (for review, see Ref. 55), and the critical dose for the "aminopterin syndrome" is probably

Table 2 The Use of Antirheumatic Drugs During Pregnancy

Drug	Use during pregnancy
Disease-modifying drugs	
Salfasalazine	Can be given throughout
Chloroquine	Not to be started or continued
Hydroxychloroquine	Can be given if strictly indicated
Gold	Not to be started or continued
Penicillamine	Not to be started or continued
Cyclosporine A	Can be given if strictly indicated
Cytotoxic drugs	
Azathioprine	Azathioprine can be given during pregnancy if strictly indicated. All other cytotoxic drugs must be stopped before pregnancy.
Methotrexate	
Cyclophosphamide	
Chloramubucil	
Glucocortocoids	
Prednisone	Can be given during pregnancy

above 10 mg of methotrexate per week (55). Recovery from treatment with methotrexate may perhaps be enhanced by supplementation with folate (56). Azathioprine is not known to be teratogenic in humans. Almost 800 pregnancies with azathioprine use were summarized from renal transplant centers, and no increased risk of congenital malformation was found (57). The reader is referred to a recent review for more extensive information (46).

G. The Fetal Perspective—Pregnancy Outcome

Just as pregnancy in RA is beneficial from the maternal perspective, available data indicate that fetal outcome is good. A case report described an infant with intrauterine growth retardation (58) and another a newborn with congenital abnormalities and two stillborn infants (10). However, reports of series of RA patients have found no association between RA and any adverse pregnancy outcome (14,16). There is no indication that women with RA have an increase in spontaneous abortions, an increased frequency of premature infants, or a significant decrease in neonatal birth weight (10,14,16).

A report suggesting that the rate of spontaneous abortion is increased in RA patients prior to disease onset (59) was not confirmed in subsequent studies (60–62). Similarly, an earlier report suggesting an increase of stillbirths in women with RA prior to disease onset (60) was not confirmed in a later report from the same group (61) or in studies of other investigators (62). Thus there is also no indication that an adverse pregnancy outcome predisposes to the development of RA.

H. Prognosis According to Parity and According to Pregnancy Outcome

Because pregnancy most frequently results in improvement of RA but active disease predictably occurs postpartum, the question can be asked as to whether pregnancy positively or negatively affects the long-term outlook for women with RA. The answer to this question is not known. In fact, only one study has attempted to address it. In a retrospective analysis reported in 1966, a group of 100 consecutive patients with RA who had pregnancies was compared to an equal number without (63). No significant difference in functional capacity, disease activity, peripheral erosive arthritis, erythrocyte sedimentation rate, or hemoglobin was found. Fewer women who had been pregnant had a positive rheumatoid factor test (67%) than those who had not (83%). However, the analysis was not controlled for age, which has since been shown to influence rheumatoid factor positivity in women (6). In another study, no evidence was found to suggest that the prognosis of RA is better after an induced abortion than after a term pregnancy (18).

I. Fecundity and Fertility

In a population study of Cornwall England reported by Hargreaves in 1957, married women with RA were found to have smaller family sizes than control women (64). In 1965 Kay and Bach also reported decreased family size in women with RA (65). This result could be due to a decrease in the frequency of intercourse due to pain from RA (66). However, the latter authors included an analysis limited to events prior to RA onset and again found a decrease in family size. Results were interpreted as indicating that fertility (the ability to conceive a child) is diminished in women with RA (and predates disease onset). However, more recent studies have shown that nulliparous women are at increased risk for RA (see below). Therefore this conclusion may not be valid, since no attempt was made to exclude women who were nulliparous by choice.

We also did not find evidence for preexisting infertility in women who subsequently develop RA (67). Our study evaluated women with an opportunity for pregnancy and compared the pregnancy history prior to disease onset of 259 RA cases and 1258 matched controls. Of these women, 12% of cases and 11% of controls had attempted but never achieved pregnancy. Fertility is the ability to conceive a child and fecundity the probability of conception as a function of time. We did, however, find evidence of diminished fecundity of RA patients. Significantly, more RA patients reported a prolonged time to conception than control women (odds ratio 1.4, 95% CI 1.1, 1.9). Similar results were described by del Junco as part of a doctoral dissertation examining reproductive function in women with RA (68). del Junco's study included pregnancies prior to and after disease onset, both with significant reductions in time to conception (fecundity).

Numerous factors could potentially result in decreased fecundity without infertility, for example, ovulatory dysfunction, abnormalities of tubal transport or implantation, antibodies to spermatozoa, or insufficient progesterone secretion by the corpus luteum (luteal phase defect). Recent studies describing impairment of the hypothalamic-pituitary-adrenal axis in RA patients (69) suggest the additional possibility of a disturbance in the hypothalamic-pituitary-ovarian axis.

J. Pregnancy and Risk of Developing Rheumatoid Arthritis

In 1990 two separate studies reported that nulliparous women are at significantly more risk of developing RA than parous women. In a case-control study by Hazes et al. (70), the risk of RA was decreased by about half for women who had been pregnant compared to those who had not. Results of a study by Spectcor et al. (71) were similar but were described as a 1.8-fold increased risk in nulliparous compared to parous women. In a population-based prospective case-control study of newly diagnosed RA in women aged 18–64, we also found that nulliparous women were at greater risk of RA in comparison to parous women; however the difference was apparent only in the comparison of RA patients with onset aged 44 or younger with comparable controls (relative risk 1.9) (72). For reasons that are discussed further later on, the difference of risk in parous and nulliparous women may be best viewed as a protective effect of parity. Interestingly, when our analysis was carried out over an extended time period after pregnancy completion, parous women were at decreased risk of RA even many years after pregnancy completion. Comparing parous to nulliparous women, the odds ratios for developing RA 1–2 years after a term pregnancy was 0.4 (95% CI 0.1–1.1), for 2–3 years 0.3 (95% CI 0.2–0.7), and for 3–4 years 0.2 (95% CI 0.1–0.5).

K. Onset of RA During Pregnancy

Initial onset of RA can occur during pregnancy, as is evident from early reports (11,12,18). However, three case-control studies describe a reduced likelihood that a women will first develop RA during pregnancy. Silman et al. found an odds ratio of 0.3 for onset of RA during pregnancy (73). In our own study, the risk of developing RA during pregnancy was reduced to 0.2 (74); and in a report by Lansink et al. risk was reduced to 0.6 (75).

L. Onset of RA Postpartum

In 1953 Oka suggested that the initial onset of RA occurred with increased frequency in the postpartum period (12). RA can also begin after spontaneous or induced abortion (18). Recently, Silman et al. have demonstrated a statistically significant increased risk of RA onset in the first year postpartum (73). Similar findings have been reported in a study by Lansink et al. (75). Silman et al. found a greater than fivefold increased risk of RA in the first 3 months following delivery. A similar pattern is evident in the earlier report by Oka, who described 25, 21, 12, 8, and 8 cases of new RA in the first, second, third, fourth, and more than 4 months postpartum, respectively (12). Brennan et al. described a magnification of RA risk in the year after a first pregnancy for women who breast fed and postulated a proinflammatory role for increased levels of prolactin (76).

M. Treatment Trials of Pregnancy Products

Various treatment trials with pregnancy and placental products have been described in RA patients (Table 3). For the most part, treatment trials were not controlled and involved small numbers of patients. In 1947 Barsi described infusion of whole blood from pregnant women, with improvement in 64% of 28 patients (77). However, a subsequent study of 53 patients treated with pregnancy whole blood found no difference when compared to 49 patients given whole blood from nonpregnant donors (78). Subjective improvement was observed in 56% versus 44% and objective improvement in 19% versus 13% respectively. Trials in which postpartum plasma was administered were also conflicting. Eleven of 13 patients (85%) improved in one study that also described disappearance of rheumatoid nodules in 4 patients (79). However, no consistent improvement was found when separate observers ranked clinical findings and erythrocyte sedimentation rate was measured in a similar trial of 11 patients (80). Side effects included urticaria, temperature increase, and chilling.

Three reports described treatment with placental serum. The first study reported some improvement in 2 of 7 patients (81). A second study

Table 3 Some Treatment Trials of RA Patients with Pregnancy and Placental Products

Agent	No. of patients	Dose	Percent improved	Refs.
Pregnancy whole blood	28	300 mL IV "several times"	64%	77
Pregnancy whole blood	53	300 mL IV weekly	Similar to controls	78
Postpartum plasma	13	250 mL IV weekly	85%	79
Postpartum plasma	11	250–275 mL IV weekly	No improvement	80
Placental serum	7	10 mL IM twice weekly	29%	81
Placental serum	33	10 mL IM twice weekly	88%	82
Placental serum	15	30 mL IV a day	67%	83
Minced placenta tissue	35	25 g implanted subcutaneously	46%	84
Placenta eluted gamma-globulins	31	750–3500 mg IV daily, various daily/weekly/monthly protocols	60%	88,89

treated 33 patients and reported "slow" improvement in 88% (82). In a third study, subjective and objective improvement was reported in two-thirds of 15 patients (83); controls included administration of nonpregnant blood at some time during the treatment course. Minced placental tissue implanted subcutaneously has also been tried. Of 35 patients 46% experienced major improvement (and another 11% minor improvement) in arthritis as judged by subjective and objective measurements. Sustained improvement up to 3–4 years later was reported for some (84). In a case report, autologous postpartum plasma obtained 5 days postpartum was administered to a patient with RA, with transient benefit (85). In another case report of a patient with oligoarticular juvenile chronic arthritis, autologous pregnancy plasma was obtained by plasmaphereses in the third trimester and administered during a postpartum flare, with no benefit (86).

Administration of antibodies to HLA class II antigens has been shown to result in amelioration of arthritis in an experimental model of collagen-induced arthritis (87). Interestingly, controlled trials have shown benefit from the administration of gamma-globulins eluted from pooled human placentas (88,89). Antibody preparations were shown to contain alloantibodies to HLA class II antigens including HLA-DR and HLR-DQ (90). These studies included administration of retroplacental gamma-globulin as a control and follow-up extending for 10–22 months. Clinical assessments were made by an observer unaware as to treatment status, and a number of laboratory parameters were followed. Various daily, weekly, and monthly protocols were tried, with best results observed in patients receiving 1500 mg a day for 7 days each month. Sixty percent of patients experienced improvement in both subjective and objective parameters. Rheumatoid nodules disappeared in one patient. One patient developed proteinuria and another discontinued treatment because of development of nephrotic syndrome. Other side effects included headache, nausea, and lip edema. No significant overall change was observed in rheumatoid factor level as measured by Waaler-Rose and nephleometry. All patients treated with placenta-eluted gamma-globulins had demonstrated change in immunological tests including an increase in active E- and EA-rosette-forming cells and increased T-cell mitogen responsiveness. However, these changes occurred regardless of whether arthritis did or did not improve. Controls did not show improvement in clinical or laboratory parameters.

N. Proposed Reasons for Pregnancy-Induced Amelioration and Postpartum Exacerbation of RA (Table 4)

Early research by Hench into the cause of remission of RA during pregnancy contributed to the eventual discovery of cortisone, for which Hench shared a Nobel prize. Despite the tremendous importance of this discovery, subsequent studies showed that increased serum cortisol concentrations during pregnancy did not explain the amelioration of RA (15,91). Subsequent studies also failed to provide support for the possible explanation that elevated levels of sex hormones (at least estrogens) during pregnancy might be responsible for pregnancy-induced improvement of RA (92,93).

Table 4 Some Factors That Have Been Considered in the Modulation of Rheumatoid Arthritis Activity During Pregnancy and Postpartum

Changes in cortisol levels
Pregnancy associated α-2 globulin (PAG)
IgG immunoglobulins lacking the terminal galactose units (Gal[0])
Antibodies to HLA class II antigens
Sex hormone changes (?progesterone)
Fetal suppressor factors/fetal cells in maternal circulation
Hypothalamic-pituitary-adrenal axis dysregulation (corrected during pregnancy, reverting postpartum)
Prolactin (↑ postpartum associated with ↑ postpartum risk of new-onset RA)
Maternal-fetal disparity for HLA-Class II antigens (possibly mediated by T-cell receptor repertoire changes)
Change in cytokine production (T_H2 during pregnancy and T_H1 postpartum)

In the late 1970s a serum protein termed pregnancy-associated α-2-globulin (PAG) with immunosuppressive properties appeared promising (22). PAG levels increase markedly during most but not all pregnancies and return to normal within 6 weeks of delivery. Some studies have found a correlation of higher PAG levels with arthritis improvement during pregnancy (17,94), while others have not (95). In a recent report, significantly decreased levels of PAG correlated with the return of active arthritis postpartum, at which time IgM rheumatoid factor also increased significantly (96). With respect to rheumatoid factor, this study contrasts with earlier but smaller studies in which IgM rheumatoid factor did not correlate with changes of disease activity during pregnancy and postpartum (95,97).

Changes in the percentage of IgG immunoglobulins lacking the terminal galactose units in the oligosaccharide chains attached to CH2 regions have also been investigated as a possible explanation for amelioration of RA during pregnancy. The percentage of agalactosyl IgG (%Gal[0]) varies as a function of age in normal healthy individuals. However, in patients with RA, %Gal[0] exceeds age-related normal values, i.e., more IgG immunoglobulins lack terminal galactose units (98). Rook et al. (99) studied 8 pregnancies of women with RA and found that the %Gal[0] became normal during pregnancy in association with disease improvement and reverted in association with postpartum disease recurrence.

Pregnancy and postpartum neuroendocrine changes are likely to contribute to fluctuations in disease activity. An increasing body of literature strongly supports complex interactions between the neuroendocrine and immune systems (100,101). Chikanza et al. have shown that patients with RA have abnormalities of the hypothalamic-pituitary-adrenal axis response to immune stimuli (69) and also have dysregulated secretion of prolactin (102). The increased risk of developing RA postpartum associated with breast feeding suggests a role for prolactin (76). Consistent with this possibility, postpartum exacerbation of collagen-induced arthritis can be suppressed by treatment with bromocriptine, which inhibits prolactin (103).

We investigated maternal-fetal disparity for HLA antigens as a possible factor in the pregnancy-induced amelioration of RA. Pregnancy is an immunological experience of particular interest because of maternal exposure to fetal (paternal) HLA antigens. HLA molecules function in the distinction of self from other, in significant part determine transplantation compatibility, and are central to the generation of immune responses. With the exception of HLA-C, trophoblast cells have not been found to express classical HLA antigens (104,105). Nevertheless, by one or more mechanisms, exposure to fetal HLA does occur during pregnancy, as evidenced by antibodies to HLA antigens that are detected in the serum of many pregnant women (106). These observations, when considered together with the fact that RA is an autoimmune disease with an HLA class II association, caused us to ask whether a maternal response to fetal (paternal) HLA antigens might be related to the remission of RA during pregnancy. We studied maternal–child pairs for HLA antigens and compared pregnancies in which arthritis improved or remitted with those in which arthritis was active. This analysis examines the child's paternal HLA antigens from the maternal perspective; a disparity is present when, for example, the child's paternal HLA-DQ antigen differs from both of the mother's HLA DQ-antigens, and no disparity is present when the child's paternal HLA-DQ antigen is the same as either maternal HLA-DQ antigen. We found that maternal-fetal disparity in HLA class II antigens, HLA-DR, and DQ was significantly correlated with amelioration of arthritis during pregnancy (19).

The explanation for this observation is not known. Possible mechanisms that might account for the findings are considered. One possibility is that the maternal antibody response to paternal HLA antigens mediates a beneficial effect on the mother's arthritis. In support of this possibility, antibodies to class II antigens have been shown to abrogate or modulate diseases in animal models of autoimmune disease including collagen-induced arthritis (87) and, as mentioned above, a beneficial effect has been observed when placenta eluted gamma-globulins were administered to RA patients (88–90). A second possibility is that pregnancy induces regulatory T cells that suppress maternal autoimmune responses. A number of different studies have demonstrated DQ-restricted immune suppression (107–109). In this model a maternal deficiency in the ability to elicit DQ-restricted T suppressor cells to a self-peptide is remedied when DQ-restricted suppressor cells are successfully elicited by fetal HLA molecules or peptides.

A final hypothesis is that the beneficial effect of fetal (paternal) HLA disparity is mediated by an effect of fetal HLA peptides on the maternal T-cell repertoire. This hypothesis proposes that autoimmunity in RA patients results from a defect in the recognition (or presentation) of an HLA class II self-peptide. Recent studies have found that HLA molecules, in addition to presenting foreign antigens, also present self-peptides derived from other HLA molecules (110). Based on studies in collagen-induced arthritis, Zannelli et al. have proposed that HLA-DQ presents a peptide derived from the DR β1 chain (111). Immunological self-recognition could also include the presentation of more than one HLA peptide by other HLA molecules.

A second part of the above hypothesis addresses how fetal HLA class II disparity might translate into a correction of aberrant maternal autoimmunity. Concentrations of fetal HLA peptides high enough to result in effective direct competition at peripheral joints seems unlikely. HLA self-antigens are known to shape the T-cell repertoire, and introduction of non-self HLA has been shown to alter the T-cell receptor repertoire in experimental studies (112,113). A recent report of patients who received allogenic blood transfusions describes qualitative changes in the T-cell receptor repertoire temporally related to transfusion and dependent on the donor–recipient HLA relationship (114), lending support to this possibility. This could occur extrathymically, or possibly, as suggested in a recent paper, the thymus itself might be active during pregnancy (115). The foregoing possibilities are not necessarily exclusive. Certainly the explanation for disease remission is likely to be multifactorial. A facilitative role for sex hormones other than estrogens, especially progesterone, remains incompletely investigated (116). A shift in cytokine production during pregnancy from a T_H1 to T_H2 profile may also contribute to gestational disease amelioration (117, 118).

III. Juvenile Chronic Arthritis and Adult Still's Disease

A. Juvenile Chronic Arthritis

Juvenile chronic arthritis (JCA), by definition, starts before the age of 16. In addition to joints, JCA can affect extra-articular sites, notably the eye. Clinical features differ in subgroups of JCA. About 70% of patients experience spontaneous resolution of disease. History of JCA may affect pregnancy and motherhood even when the arthritis has subsided in the adult. Growth inhibition of the pelvis or hip joint prosthesis may preclude normal delivery. General anesthesia, if necessary, is potentially hazardous in patients who have had significant involvement of the cervical spine, temporomandibular joint, or cricoarytenoid joint. Therefore sequelae of JCA need to be considered when counseling pregnant women with a history of JCA.

Only one report has described a series of pregnancies in patients with JCA. Østensen et al. reported a retrospective study of 76 pregnancies in 51 women with JCA (21), which later was extended to include 61 patients and their 92 pregnancies (119). Overall the frequency of improvement in JCA was less than that observed in adult RA. When the effect of pregnancy on the mother's disease is broken down into subsets of JCA, improvement was most frequent in patients with that form of JCA most closely resembling adult RA, i.e., polyarticular JCA. In pregnancies of patients with polyarticular disease, 26 of 44 (59%) improved, whereas for patients with pauciarticular JCA, only 9 of 25 (36%) improved and of those with systemic disease, only 2 of 7 (29%) improved. In most patients, resolution of joint stiffness and tenderness or active synovitis took place in the second half of gestation. Four patients who had active anterior uveitis had continued active uveitis during pregnancy.

In 3 patients, renal symptoms developed during or shortly after pregnancy and were subsequently proven by renal biopsy to be caused by amyloidosis (119). Postpartum disease flares were common and usually occurred between 3 and 6 months. Moreover, a number of patients who had quiescent disease at the time of conception and throughout pregnancy, nevertheless had disease flares postpartum. In 20 pregnancies the patient's disease was quiescent at the time of conception. One patient with previously quiescent disease developed active disease during pregnancy, and another 11 developed active disease postpartum. However, in all patients for whom quiescent disease became active, the episode was transient. JCA was not permanently reactivated in any. Disease activity could vary in subsequent pregnancies for patients with multiple pregnancies (21). In 23 pregnancies the neonate was delivered by caesarean section, 17 of which were said to be related to JCA, 9 specifically because of hip prosthesis. No increase of adverse pregnancy outcome was found. Of the 92 pregnancies, there was 1 stillbirth, 1 infant with low birth weight, and 1 premature infant.

It appears from these data that pregnancy is not a risk factor for reactivating quiescent JCA and that it frequently improves symptoms of active polyarticular JCA. Bilateral hip involvement or hip prosthesis may sometimes preclude vaginal delivery. JCA has no adverse effect on the fetus or neonate. A risk of postpartum flare is present in about 60% of patients, and even in women with quiescent JCA.

B. Adult Still's Disease

Most of the literature describing Still's disease and pregnancy consists of case reports. The onset of Still's disease during pregnancy was described in five cases (120–122). Case reports also describe the initial onset of Still's disease postpartum; one patient had onset postpartum, subsequently resolved, and recurred postpartum in her next pregnancy (123), and another women with prior history of Still's had recurrence postpartum (124). Episodes of Still's during or after two pregnancies was described in another case (125). Improvement during a second pregnancy and relapse after a spontaneous abortion was described for another woman (126). Active disease during pregnancy was described in another case report (127). The only series was reported by LeLoet et al. who summarized the experience of 7 women with adult-onset Still's and their 9 pregnancies. No clear-cut effect of pregnancy on disease activity was found. Six pregnancies resulted in term infants, 2 in premature infants, and 1 in an induced abortion (122).

IV. Spondyloarthropathies

A case report described a patient with psoriatic arthritis (PA) who had temporary remissions in 3 pregnancies (128). In a prospective study of 10 patients with psoriatic arthritis, 8 improved in the first or second trimester. Two patients had a flare at mid-gestation but improved later. Several patients experienced complete remission. All patients had active disease postpartum (129). The timing of the onset of psoriatic arthritis was examined in a retrospective study of 33 women and onset in the postpartum period occurred in 18% (130).

One large retrospective study of 87 pregnancies in 50 patients by Østensen et al. (131) examined the effect of pregnancy on ankylosing spondylitis (AS). Remission was observed in just 18 (21%). Postpartum a flare of AS was reported in 45% but was of short duration. Fetal outcome was good. Østensen and Husby (16) also reported a smaller prospective study of patients with AS. In contrast to RA, only 5 of 13 (38%) improved. Moreover, in patients with active disease during pregnancy (62%), symptoms often worsened in the second and third trimesters. All but one patient had disease flare postpartum. Thus the pregnancy experience of women with AS contrasts to that of women with RA. Although the etiologies of both AS and of RA remain unknown, the contrast in pregnancy experience is perhaps not surprising given the differences observed in available knowledge of pathogenic mechanisms of these diseases. Whereas RA is clearly an autoimmune disorder, although AS is a rheumatic disease with some evidence for immunological aberration, both direct and indirect evidence of autoimmunity are lacking for AS (132).

V. Summary and Conclusions

Women with rheumatoid arthritis frequently experience amelioration of their arthritis during pregnancy. Improvement occurs in about three-quarters of pregnancies and is often noted in the first trimester. Once achieved, improvement is usually sustained or increases further with advancing gestation, but the disease recurs in the postpartum period. Analogous to the beneficial effect of pregnancy on women with preexisting RA, the chance of a women first developing RA during pregnancy is significantly reduced. There is no indication of adverse pregnancy outcome for women with RA. Juvenile chronic arthritis includes distinct subsets that are categorized by type of disease onset into polyarticular, pauciarticular, and systemic JCA. The experience of women with polyarticular JCA is most similar to adult RA and differs from pauciarticular JCA in that most of the former, compared to only one-third of the latter, experience improvement during pregnancy. Data for systemic-onset JCA are too infrequent for conclusions. Arthritis amelioration during pregnancy is uncommon for women with spondyloarthropathies. For all of these diseases, however, the postpartum period is a time when arthritis is likely to be active.

Because pregnancy often results in complete remission of RA, investigation into the possible reasons for improvement potentially might generate insight into disease pathogenesis. We questioned whether maternal immune response to fetal (paternal) HLA antigens might be related to the pregnancy-induced amelioration of arthritis. When the maternal–fetal HLA relationship was examined and pregnancies of women with improvement were compared to those with active disease, significantly greater disparity of HLA class II antigens was observed in the former group. This finding implicates the maternal immune response to fetal (paternal) HLA in the pregnancy-induced amelioration of RA. Future studies that elucidate the molecular mechanism(s) for this association may lead to a better understanding of the role that HLA molecules play in disease susceptibility, and possibly to novel treatment strategies for RA.

Table 5 Key Observations Regarding Rheumatoid Arthritis and Pregnancy

Remission or improvement RA occurs in three-quarters of pregnancies.

For women who improve, most experience initial relief in the first trimester.

Once achieved, improvement is usually sustained or increased with advancing gestation.

Analogous to the beneficial effect of pregnancy on women with preexisting RA, the chance of a woman first developing RA during pregnancy is significantly reduced.

With few exceptions, arthritis returns by the 3rd to 4th month after delivery.

Analogous to the postpartum flare of arthritis for women with preexisting RA, the chance of new onset of RA is increased in the first year after a pregnancy.

After the first year postpartum, risk of RA is reduced for parous women when compared with nulliparous women.

It is not known whether pregnancy affects the prognosis of RA.

There is some suggestion that women with RA may have a minimal reduction in fecundity.

There is no indication of adverse pregnancy outcome for women with RA.

Table 5 summarizes the key observations regarding rheumatoid arthritis and pregnancy.

References

1. Hochberg MC. Changes in the incidence and prevalence of rheumatoid arthritis in England and Wales, 1970–1982. Sem Arthritis Rheum 1990; 19: 294–302.
2. Linos A, Worthington JW, O'Fallon M, Curled LT. The epidemiology of rheumatoid arthritis in Rochester, Minnesota: a study of incidence, prevalence and mortality. Am J Epidemiol; 1980; 111:87–98.
3. Silman AJ. Hochberg MC. Rheumatoid Arthritis. In: Silman AJ, Hochberg MC, eds. Epidemiology of the Rheumatic Diseases. Oxford, New York, Tokyo: Oxford Medical Publications, 1993:7–68.
4. Winchester R. The molecular basis of susceptibility to rheumatoid arthritis. Adv Immunol 1994; 56:389–466.
5. Meyer JM, Han J, Singh R. Moxley G. Sex influences on the penetrance of HLA shared-epitope genotypes for rheumatoid arthritis. Am J Hum Genet 1996; 58:371–383.
6. Nelson JL, Dugowson CE, Koepsell TD, Voigt LF, Branchaud AM, Barrington RA, Wener MA, Hansen JA. Rheumatoid factor, HLA-DR4, and allelic DRB1 variants in recent onset rheumatoid arthritis in women. Arthritis Rheum 1994; 37:673–680.
7. Jaraquemada D, Ollier W, Awad J, Young A Silman A, Roitt IM, Corbett M, Hay F, Cosh JA, Maini RN, Venables PJ, Ansell B, Holborow I, Reeback J, Currey HLF, Festenstein H. HLA and rheumatoid arthritis: a combined analysis of 440 British patients. Ann Rheum Dis 1986; 45:627–636.
8. Young A, Jaraquemadda D, Awad J, Festenstein H, Corbett M, Hay F, Roitt I. Association of HLA-DR4/Dw4 and DR2/Dw2 with radiological changes in a prospective study of patients with rheumatoid arthritis. Arthritis Rheum 1984; 27:20–25.
9. Hench PS. The ameliorating effect of pregnancy on chronic atrophic (infectious rheumatoid) arthritis, fibrositis, and intermittent hydrathrosis. Proc Staff Meet Mayo Clinic 1938; 13:161–167.
10. Morris WIC. Pregnancy in rheumatoid arthritis and systemic lupus erythematosus. Austsal NZ J Obstet Gynaecol 1969; 9:136–144.
11. Betson JR, Dorn RV. Forty cases of arthritis and pregnancy. J Int Coll Surg 1964; 42:521–526.
12. Oka M. Effect of pregnancy on the onsent and course of rheumatoid arthritis. Ann Rheum Dis 1953; 12:227–229.
13. Neely NT. Persellin RH. Activity of rheumatoid arthritis during pregnancy. Texas Med 1977; 73:59–63.
14. Østensen M, Aune B, Husby G. Effect of pregnancy and hormonal changes on the activity of rheumatoid arthritis. Scand J Rheumatol 1983; 12:69 72.

15. Smith WD, West HF. Pregnancy and rheumatoid arthritis. Acta Rheum Scand 1960; 6:189–201.

16. Østensen M, Husby G. A prospective clinical study of the effect of pregnancy on rheumatoid arthritis and ankylosing spondylitis. Arthritis Rheum 1983; 26:1155–1159.

17. Unger A, Kay A, Griffin AJ, Panayi GS. Disease activity and pregnancy associated a2-glycoprotein in rheumatoid arthritis during pregnancy. B Med J 1983; 286:750–752.

18. Felbo M, Snorrason E. Pregnancy and the place of therapeutic abortion in rheumatoid arthritis. Acta Obst Gynecol Scand 1961; 40:116–127.

19. Nelson JL, Hughes KA, Smith AG, Nisperos BB, Branchaud AB, Hansen JA. Maternal-fetal disparity in HLA class II alloantigens and the pregnancy-induced amelioration of rheumatoid arthritis. N Engl J Med 1993; 329: 466–471.

20. Kilpatrick D, Gibson F, Livingston J, Liston W. Pre-eclampsia is associated with HLA-DR4 sharing between mother and fetus. Tissue Antigens 1990; 35:178–181.

21. Østensen M. Pregnancy in patients with a history of juvenile rheumatoid arthritis. Arthritis Rheum 1991; 34:881–887.

22. Persellin RH. The effect of pregnancy on rheumatoid arthritis. Bull Rheum Dis 1977; 27:922–928.

23. Beitins IZ, Bayard F, Ances IG, Kowarski A, Migeon CJ. The transplacental passage of prednisone and prednisolone in pregnancy near term. J Pediatr 1972; 81:936–945.

24. Walker B. Induction of cleft palate in rats with anti-inflammatory drugs. Teratology 1971; 4:39–42.

25. Walker B. Induction of cleft palate in rabbits by several glucocorticoids. Proc Soc Exp Biol Med 1967; 125:1281–1284.

26. Scott JR. Fetal growth retardation associated with maternal administration of immunosuppressive drugs. Am J Obstet Gynecol 1977; 128:668–676.

27. Bongiovanni A, McPaddan A. Steroids during pregnancy and possible fetal consequences. Fertil Steril 1960; 11:181–186.

28. Fraser FC, Sajoo A. Teratogenic potential of corticosteroids in humans. Teratology 1995; 51:45–46.

29. Committee on Drugs, American Academy of Pediatrics. The transfer of drugs and other chemicals into human breast milk. Pediatrics 1989; 84:924–936.

30. Katz F, Duncan B. Entry of prednisone into human milk. N Engl J. Med 1975; 293:1154–1158.

31. Hickok DE, Hollenbach KA, Reilly SF, et al. The association between decreased amniotic fluid volume and treatment with nonsteroidal anti-inflammatory agents for preterm labor. Am J Obstet Gynecol 1989; 160: 1525–1531.

32. Simeoni U, Messer J, Weisburd A, et al. Neonatal renal dysfunction and intrauterine exposure to prostaglandin synthesis inhibitors. Eur J Pediatr 1989; 148:371–373.

33. Briggs G, Freeman R, Yaffe S, eds. Indomethacin. Drugs in Pregnancy and Lactation. 3rd ed. Baltimore: Williams & Wilkins, 1990:313i–319i.

34. Wilkinson AR, Aynsley-Green A, Mitchell MD. Persistent pulmonary hypertension and abnormal prostaglandin E levels in preterm infants after maternal treatment with naproxen. Arch Dis Child 1979; 54:942–945.

35. Gouyon JB, Petion AM, Sandre D, et al. Renal insufficiency in a preterm infant aftre intrauterin exposure to ketoprofen. Arch Fr Pediatr 1991; 48: 347–348.

36. Wiggins DA, Elliott JP. Oligohydramnios in each sac of a triplet gestation caused by Motrin—fulfilling Kock's postulates. Am J Obstet Gynecol 1990; 162:460–461.

37. Momma K, Takeuchi H. Constriction of fetal ductus arteriosus by nonsteroidal anti-inflammatory drugs. Prostaglandins 1983; 26:631–643.

38. Veyver van den IB, Moise KJ, Ou CN, Carpenter RJ Jr. The effect of gestational age and fetal indomethacin levels on the incidence of constriction of the fetal ductus arteriosus. Obstet Gynecol 1993; 82:500–503.

39. Moise KJ Jr, Huhta JC, Sharif DS, Ou CN, Kirshon B, Wasserstrum N, Cano L. Indomethacin in the treatment of preterm labor. Effects on the fetal ductus arteriosus. N Engl J Med 1988; 319:327–331.

40. Østensen M, Østensen H. Safety of nonsteroidal anti-inflammatory drugs in pregnant patients with rheumatic disease. J Rheumatol 1996; 23:1045–1049.

41. Slone D, Siskind V. Heinonen OP, Monson RR, Kaufman DW, Shapiro. Aspirin and congential malformations. Lancet 1976; 1:1373–1375.

42. Stuart MJ, Gorss SJ, Elrad H, Graeber JE. Effects of acetylsalicylic-acid ingestion on material and neonatal hemostatis. N Engl J Med 1982; 307: 909–912.

43. Rumack CM, Guggenheim MA, Rumack BH, Peterson RG, Johnson ML, Braithwaite WR. Neonatal intracranial hemmorrhage and maternal use of aspirin. Obstet Gynecol 1981; 58(suppl 5):52S–56S.

44. Brooks PM, Needs CJ. The use of antirheumatic medication during pregnancy and in the puerperium. Rheum Dis Clin N Am 1989; 15:789–806.

45. Østensen M. Safety of nonsteroidal anti-inflammatory drugs during pregnancy and lactation. Immunopharmacology 1996; 4:31–41.

46. Østensen M. Optimization of anti-rheumatic drug treatment in pregnancy. Clin Pharmacokinet 1994; 27:486–503.

47. Parke AL. Antimalarial drugs, systemic lupus erythematosus and pregnancy. J. Rheumatol 1988; 15:607–610.

48. Lima F, Buchanan NMM, Kamashta MA, Kerslake S, Hughes GRV. Obstetric outcome in systemic lupus erythematosus. Sem Arthritis Rheum 1995; 25:184–192.

49. Roubenoff R, Hoyt J. Petri M, Hochberg MC, Hellman DB. Effects of anti-inflammatory and immunosuppressive drugs on pregnancy and fertiliy. Sem Arthritis Rheum 1988; 18:88–110.

50. Lyle WH. Penicillamine in pregnancy (letter). Lancet 1978; 1:606.

51. Jaffe I. Therapeutic stragegy in rheumatoid arthritis: a roundtable discussion. J Rheumatol 1981; S7:124–145.

52. Mogadam M, Dobbins WO, Korelitz BI, Ahmed SW. Pregnancy in inflammatory bowel disease: effect of sulfasalazine and corticosteroid on fetal outcome. Gastroenterology 1981; 80:72–76.

53. Järnerot G, Into-Malmberg M. Sulphasalazine treatment during breast feeding. Scand J Gastroenterol 1979; 14:869–871.

54. Esbjörner E. Järnerot G, Wranne L. Sulphasalazine and sulphapyridine serum levels in children to mothers treated with sulphasalazine during pregnancy and lactation. Acta Paediatr Scand 1987; 76:137–142.

55. Feldkamp M, Carey JC. Clinical teratology counseling and consultation case report: low dose methotrexate exposure in the early weeks of pregnancy. Teratology 1993; 47:533–539.

56. Kozlowski RD, Steinbrunner JV, MacKenzie AH, Clough JD, Wilke WS, Segal AM. Outcome of first trimester exposure to low-dose methotrexate in eight patients with rheumatic disease. Am J Med 1990; 88:589–592.

57. Rudolph J, Schweizer R, Bartus S. Pregnancy in renal transplant patients. Tranplantation 1979; 27:26–29.

58. Duhring JL. Pregnancy rheumatoid arthritis and intrauterine growth retardation. Am J Obstet Gynecol 1970; 108:325–326.

59. Kaplan J. Fetal wastage in patients with rheumatoid arthritis. J. Rheumatol 1986; 13:875–877.

60. Silman AJ, Roman E, Veral V, Brown A. Adverse reproductive outcomes in women who subsequently develop rheumatoid arthritis. Ann Rheum Dis 1988; 47:979–981.

61. Spector TD, Silman AJ. Is poor pregnancy outcome a risk factor in rheumatoid arthritis? Ann Rheum Dis 1990; 49:12–14.

62. Nelson JL, Voigt LF, Koepsell TD, Dugowson CE, Daling JR. Pregnancy outcome in women with rheumatoid arthritis before disease onsent. J Rheumatol 1992; 19:18–21.

63. Oka M, Vainio U. Effect of pregnancy on the prognosis and serology of rheumatoid arthritis. Acta Rheum Scand 1966; 12:47–52.

64. Hargreaves ER. A survey of rheumatoid arthritis in West Cornwall. A report to the empire rheumatism council. Ann Rheum Dis 1957; 16:61–75.

65. Kay A, Bach F. Subfertility before and after the development of rheumatoid arthritis in women. Ann Rheum Dis 1965; 24:169–173.

66. Yoshino S, Uchida S. Sexual problems of women with rheumatoid arthritis. Arch Phys Med Rehabil 1981; 62:122–123.

67. Nelson JL, Koepsell TD, Dugowson CE, Voigt LF, Daling JR, Hansen JA. Frequently before disease onset in women with rheumatoid arthritis. Arthritis Rheum 1993; 36:7–14.

68. del Junco DJ. The relationship between rheumatoid arthritis and reproductive function. Ph.D. thesis, University of Texas, Houston, TX, 1988.

69. Chikanza IC, Petrou P, Kingsley G, Chrousos G, Panayi S. Defective hypothalamic response to immune and inflammatory stimuli in patients with rheumatoid arthritis. Arthritis Rheum 1992; 35:1281–1288.

70. Hazes, JMW, Dijkmans BAC, Vandenbroucke JP, de Vries RRP, Cats A. Pregnancy and the risk of developing rheumatoid arthritis. Arthritis Rheum 1990; 33:1770–1775.

71. Spector TD, Roman E, Silman AJ. The pill, party, and rheumatoid arthritis. Arthritis Rheum 1990; 33:782–789.

72. Dugowson CE, Nelson JL, Koepsell TD, Voigt LF, Daling JR. Nulliparity as a risk factor for rheumatoid arthritis. Arthritis Rheum 1991; 34:S48 (abstr).

73. Silman A, Kay A, Brennan P. Timing of pregnancy in relation to the onset of rheumatoid arthritis. Arthritis Rheum 1992; 35:152–155.

74. Koepsell TD, Dugowson CE, Voigt LF, Nelson JL, Daling JR. Reduced incidence of rheumatoid arthritis during pregnancy. Arthritis Rheum 1990; 33: S29 (abstr).

75. Lansink M, de Boer A, Dijkmans B, Vandenbroucke J, Hazes J. The onset of rheumatoid arthritis in relation to pregnancy and childbirth. Clin Exp Rheumatol 1993; 11:171–174.

76. Brenna P, Silman A. Breast-feeding and the onset of rheumatoid arthritis. Arthritis Rheum 1994; 37:808–813.

77. Barsi I. A new treatment for rheumatoid arthritis. Br Med J 1947; 5:252–254.

78. Josephs C. Observations on the treatment of rheumatoid arthritis by transfusions of blood from pregnant women. Br Med J 1954; 2:134–135.

79. Granier LW. Clinical response of rheumatoid arthritis to postpartum plasma. JAMA 1951; 146:995–997.

80. Neustadt DH, Geiger J, Steinbrocker O. Effect of post-partum plasma in rheumatoid arthritis. Ann Rheum Dis 1954; 13:131–135.

81. Simson J, Bunim JJ. Effect of placental "serum" in rheumatoid arthritis. Am Rheum Dis 1952; 11:204–205.

82. Aronson W, Levy F, Besen LJ, Leff M. Placental serum therapy for rheumatoid arthritis. Am J Med Sci 1952; 223:144–150.

83. Spielberg M. Placental blood serum in the treatment of rheumatoid arthritis. Arch Intern Med 1953; 91:315–324.

84. Lintz RM. Placental tissue implantation for patients with rheumatoid arthritis. Geriatrics 1954; 9:106–110.

85. Scoville CD. Postpartum autologous plasma transfusion: effect on RA. Ann Rheum Dis 1992; 51:1342–1345.

86. Wallace DJ, Goldfinger D, Klineberg JR. Use of autologous pregnancy plasma to treat a flare of juvenile rheumatoid arthritis; case report and literature review. J Clin Apheresis 1987; 3:216–218.

87. Wooley PH, Luthra HS, Lafuse WP, Huse A, Stuart J, David CWS. Type II collagen-induced arthritis in mice III. Suppression of arthritis by using monoclonal and polyclonal anti-Ia antisera. J. Immunol 1985; 134:2366–2374.

88. Sany J, Clot J, Bonneau M, Andary M. Immunomodulating effect of human placenta-eluted gamma globulins in rheumatoid arthritis. Arthritis Rheum 1982; 25:17–24.

89. Combe B, Cosso B, Clot J, Bonneau M, Sany J. Human placenta-eluted gamma globulins in immunomodulating treatment of rheumatoid arthritis. Am J Med 1985; 78:920–928.

90. Moynier M, Cosso B, Brochier J, Clot J. Identification of class II HLA alloantibodies in placenta-eluted gamma globulins used for treating rheumatoid arthritis. Arthritis Rheum 1987; 30:375–381.

91. Wolfson WQ, Robinson WD, Duff IF. The probability that increased secretion of oxysteroids does not fully explain improvement in certain systemic diseases during pregnancy. J Mich State Med Soc 1951; 50:1019–1022.

92. Gilbert M, Rotstein J, Cunningham C, Estrin I, Davidson A. Norethynodrel with mestranol in treatment of rheumatoid arthritis. JAMA 1964: 190:235.

93. van den Brink H, van Everdingen A, van Wijk M, Jacobs J, Bijlsma J. Adjuvant oestrogen therapy does not improve disease activity in postmenopausal patients with rheumatoid arthritis. Ann Rheum Dis 1993; 52:862–865.

94. Persellin RH, Wiginton D, Rutstein J, Cohen M, Goehers H, Steele A, Philips V, Kradel P. Pregnancy alpha-glycoprotein (PAG) and rheumatoid arthritis (RA) activity: a prospective analysis during gestation. Arthritis Rheum 1982; 25(S): S6–S21.

95. Østensen M, vonSchoultz B, Husby G. Comparison between serum α2-pregnancy-associated globulin and activity of rheumatoid arthritis and ankylosing spondylitis during pregnancy. Scand J Rheumatoil 1983; 12: 315–318.

96. Quinn C, Mulpeter K, Casey E, Feighery C. Changes in levels of IgM RF and α-2 PAG correlate with increased disease activity in rheumatoid arthritis during the peurperium. Scand J Rheumatol 1993; 22:273–279.

97. Pope RM, Yoshinoya S, Rutstein J, Persellin RH. Effect of pregnancy on immune complexes and rheumatoid factors in patients with rheumatoid arthritis. Am J Med 1983; 74:973–979.

98. Rahman A, Isenberg D. Does it take sugar? Ann Rheum Dis 1995; 54: 689–691.

99. Rook G, Steele J, Brealey R, Whyte A, Isenberg D, Sumar N, Nelson JL, Bodman K, Young A, Willaims P, Scragg I, Edge C, Arkwright P, Ashford D, Wormald M, Rudd P, Redman C, Dwek R, Rademacher T. Changes in IgG glycoform levels may be relevant to remission of arthritis during pregnancy. J. Autoimmun 1991; 4:779–794.

100. Chowdrey H, Lightman H. Interaction between the neuroendocrine system and arthritis. Br J Rheumatol 1993; 32:441–444.

101. Breczi I. Prolactin, pregnancy and autoimmune disease. J. Rheumatol 1993; 20:1095–1100.

102. Chikanza IC, Petrou P, Chrousos G, Kingsley G, Panayi G. Excessive and dysregulated secretion of prolactin in rheumatoid arthritis: immunopathogenetic and therapeutic immplications. Br J. Rheumatol 1993; 32:445–448.

103. Whyte A, Williams RO. Bromocriptine suppresses postpartum exacerbation of collagen-induced arthritis. Arthritis Rheum 1988; 31:927–928.

104. King A, Boocock C, Charkey A, Gardner L. Beretta A, Siccardi A, Loke YW. Evidence for the expression of HLA-C Class I mRNA and protein by human first trimester trophblast. J. Immunol 1996; 156:2068–2076.

105. Hunt JS and Soares MJ. A novel major histocompatibility antigen, HLA-G. The placenta. In: Marsch JA, Kendall MD, eds. The Physiology of Immunity. Boca Raton, FL: CRC Press 1995.

106. Payne R. Leukocyte agglutinins in human sera. Arch Intern Med 1957; 99: 587–591.

107. Hirayama K, Matsushita S, Kikuchi I, Iuchi M, Ohta N, Sasazuki T. HLA-DQ is epistatic to HLA-DR in controlling the immune response to schistosomal antigen in humans. Nature 1987; 327:426–430.

108. Ottenhoff T, Walford C, Nishimura Y, Reddy N, Sasazuki T. HLA-DQ molecules and the control of *Mycobacterium leparae-specific* T cell nonresponsiveness in lepromatous leprosy patients. Eur J Immunol 1990; 20: 2347–2350.

109. Salgame P, Convit J, Bloom B. Immunological suppression by human CD8+ T-cells is receptor dependent and HLA-DQ restricted. Proc Natl Acad Sci USA 1991; 88:2598–2602.

110. Engelhard VH. Structure of peptides associated with class I and class II MHC molecules. Ann Rev Immunol 1994; 12:181–207.

111. Zanelli E, Gonzalezy-Gay MA, David CS. Could HLA-DRBI be the protective locus for rheumatoid arthritis? Immunol Today 1995; 16:274–278.

112. Zhou P, Anderson G, Savarirayan S, Inoko H, David C. Thymic deletion of Vβ11+, Vβ5+ T cell in H-2E negative, HLA-DQβ+ single transgenic mice. J Immunol 1991; 146:854–859.

113. Anderson GD, David CS. In vivo expression and function of hybrid Ia dimers (Eα Aβ) in recombinant and transgenic mice. J Exp Med 1989; 170: 1003–1008.

114. Munson JL, van Twuyver E, Mooijaart R, Roux E, ten Berge I J M, de Waal LP. Missing T-cell receptor Vβ families following blood transfusion. The role of HLA in development of immunization and tolerance. Hum Immunol 1995; 42:43–53.

115. Clarke A, Kendall M. The thymus in pregnancy: the interplay of neural, endocrine and immune influences. Immunol Today 1994; 15:545–551.

116. Masi AT, Feigenbaum SL, Chatterton RT. Hormonal and pregnancy relationships to rheumatoid arthritis: convergent effects with immunologic and microvascular systems. Sem Arthritis Rheum 1995; 25:1–27.

117. Wegmann TG, Lin H, Gilbert L, Mosmann TR. Bi-directional cytokine interactions in the material-fetal relationship: is successful pregnancy a TH2 phenomenon? Immunol Today 1993; 14:353–356.

118. Mosmann TR. Properties and functions of Interleukin-10. Adv Immunol 1994; 56:1–11.

119. Østensen M. The effect of pregnancy on ankylosing spondylitis, psoriatic arthritis, and juvenile rheumatoid arthritis. Am J Reprod Immunol 1992; 28: 235–237.

120. Green J, Kanter Y, Barzilai. Adult Still's disease associated with pregnancy. Isr J Med Sci 1982; 18:1037–1039.

121. Yebra Bango M, Garcia Paez JM, Solovera JJ, Merino MF, Giron Gonzalez JA. Adult-onset Still's disease: a case with onset during pregnancy. Arthritis Rheum 1985; 28:957.

122. Le Loet X, de Bandt M, Liote F, Daragon A, Kahn MF, Mejjad O. Adult-onset Still's disease and pregnancy. Rev Rheum 1993; 60:337–340.

123. Katz W, Starz T, Winkelstein A. Recurrence of adult Still's disease after pregnancy. J Rheumatol 1990; 17:373–374.

124. Leff RD. Recurrence of adult Still's after pregnancy. J Rheumatol 1990; 17: 1571–1572.

125. Elkon KB, Hughes GV, Bywaters EG, Ryan PF, Inman RD, Bowley NB, James MP, Eady RA. Adult-onset Still's disease: twenty-year followup and further studies of patients with active disease. Arthritis Rheum 1982; 25: 647–654.

126. Miguel de E, Cuesta M, Martin-Mola E, Gijon-Banos J. Adult Still's disease and pregnancy. J Rheumatol 1992; 19:498.

127. Stein GH, Cantor B, Panush RS. Adult Still's disease associated with pregnancy. Arthritis Rheum 1980; 23:248–250.

128. McNeill ME. Multiple pregnancy-induced remissions of psoriatic arthritis: case report. Am J. Obstet Gynecol 1988; 159:896–897.

129. Østensen M. Pregnancy in psoriatic arthritis. Scand J. Rheumatol 1988; 17: 67–70.

130. McHugh NJ, Laurent MR. The effect of pregnancy on the onset of psoriatic arthritis. Br J Rheumatol 1989; 28:50–52.

131. Østensen M, Romberg O, Husby G. Ankylosing spondylitis and motherhood. Arthritis Rheum 1982; 25:140–143.

132. Rose NR, Bona C. Defining criteria for autoimmune diseases. Immunol Today 1993; 14:426–430.

23

"Other" Autoimmune Diseases in Pregnancy

GEETA KHARE and HENRY N. CLAMAN

University of Colorado School of Medicine
Denver, Colorado

I. Introduction

Autoimmune diseases present a complex problem when they occur in the setting of pregnancy. The most common serious systemic autoimmune diseases Systemic Lupus erythematosus (SLE), rheumatoid arthritis, and the anticardiolipin syndrome) are covered in Chapters 21 and 22. The other autoimmune diseases are divided into systemic and organ-specific diseases. The systemic diseases include scleroderma, Sjogren's syndrome, Behcet's disease, and vasculitis. Under vasculitis, Wegener's granulomatosis and polyarteritis nodosa will be covered. The organ-specific diseases begin with those of hematological dysfunction, including autoimmune hemolytic anemia and autoimmune thrombocytopenia. Endocrine disorders include diabetes mellitus and thyroid disorders. The thyroid disorders include thyroid autoimmunity without overt disease, Graves' disease, and Hashimoto's thyroiditis. Neurological disorders include multiple sclerosis and myasthenia gravis. Dermatological diseases include pemphigoid gestationis and pemphigus vulgaris. And finally, dermatomyositis/polymyositis will be an example of a disease that involves more than one organ system.

Current affiliation: Consultant in Allergy and Clinical Immunology, Pueblo, Colorado

551

Each subject will be explored with regard to the effect of the disease on fertility as well as problems with spontaneous abortion. We will explore the effect of pregnancy on the disease as well as the effect of the disease on pregnancy, the fetus, the neonate, and the postpartum state.

II. Scleroderma

Scleroderma is a connective tissue disease with a wide spectrum of manifestations affecting the skin, gastrointestinal tract, kidneys, lungs, and other organ systems. There are two general categories of disease classification. In limited disease, usually the process is localized to the face as well as the hands with Raynaud's phenomenon. There is little or late organ involvement, and the prognosis is good in general. Diffuse scleroderma is also described as progressive systemic sclerosis. With generalized involvement, there is more widespread skin disease and it is a more aggressive illness. Raynaud's phenomenon is somewhat less common, though internal organ involvement is frequent.

Systemic sclerosis has a negative effect on fecundity. A history of infertility appears to precede the appearance of clinical disease (22,72). The risk of spontaneous abortion among women with scleroderma is controversial. Some investigators have reported a higher-than-expected incidence of spontaneous miscarriage (24,71). This may, however, reflect sampling error, as other reviews have reported no higher incidence of spontaneous abortion (22,39,71).

The effect of pregnancy on the disease is variable and depends on the type and severity of scleroderma. With the limited form, there is no effect. In diffuse cutaneous scleroderma, the effect of pregnancy depends on the severity of illness.

In general, the data regarding scleroderma in pregnancy are scant and the majority of serious complications are related to renal disease (71). Maymon et al. (49) studied 94 patients and found that 35 had worsening disease with pregnancy and 14 had pregnancy-related complications. However, one study investigated the histories of women with scleroderma who had had pregnancies versus those who were nulliparous. In these 48 patients, there was no difference in the incidence of hypertension, renal failure, or disease symptoms (78). In essence, the earlier information indicating a worsening of disease was gleaned from case reports and was, therefore, biased toward a more ominous prognosis. When approached in a case-controlled fashion, it appears that pregnancy probably does not worsen the disease.

Renal disease in scleroderma is of concern, as renal failure is the major cause of maternal death (8). In the past, renal disease with scleroderma was seen as a contraindication to pregnancy (8,45,49,50), but this is no longer the case. There are reports of women with scleroderma and renal disease in whom pregnancy was uneventful (4,76,88). These more recent observations are likely due to better management of pregnancy itself as well as of hypertensive renal crisis in general (4,71,76,88).

By contrast, scleroderma may lead to fetal problems, and the pathogenesis of these problems is probably vascular insufficiency (15,18). In 1974, Karlen (37) found that of 17 pregnancies, there were 5 perinatal deaths and 5 premature deliveries. In 1989, however, Steen et al., (78) found less frightening results. There was a slight increase in preterm births and low birth weight, but there was no difference in spontaneous abortions or perinatal deaths (78).

Specific obstetrical problems during labor and delivery include those regarding soft tissue/connective tissue. Intravenous access/venipuncture and sphygmomanometry may be difficult because of disease involvement of skin and blood vessels (91). Anaesthesia and intubation may be technically difficult (6). Cervical involvement has been reported to cause dystocia (84).

There have been no reported cases of neonatal scleroderma, suggesting that if there are IgG antoantibodies which cross the placenta, they may be either nonpathogenic or may have to be present for a significant period of time to cause neonatal disease. Depending on maternal serology, the neonate may have congenital complete heart block.

There appears to be no worsening of scleroderma in the postpartum period.

III. Sjögren's Syndrome

Sjögren's syndrome (SS) is a chronic inflammatory disorder with lymphocytic infiltration of lacrimal and salivary glands leading to xerostomia and keratoconjunctivitis sicca. It may be "primary" (in which case it seems to exist without other concomitant autoimmune syndromes), or "secondary," when it appears in the context of other autoimmune syndromes such as rheumatoid arthritis.

The effect of pregnancy on primary Sjögren's syndrome is unknown, but the probability is that the disease will be unaffected (66,73). Treatment is directed toward the specific maternal symptoms (e.g., dry eyes, dry mouth) (43). In secondary Sjögren's syndrome, the effect on pregnancy

Table 1 Summary[a]

	Effect of pregnancy on disease	Effect of disease on pregnancy	Effects of disease on fetus/newborn
Scleroderma	Probably no effect	Obstetric problems; soft tissue problems	Slight increase in pre-term births and low birth weight
Sjögren's syndrome	No effect	No	Congenital heart block if Ro Ab positive
Behcet's	Variable	No	No
Wegener's granulomatosis	Relapse frequent	No	IUGR
Polyarteritis nodosa	Onset before pregnancy— good; onset during pregnancy— poor prognosis	No	No
Organ-specific disorders: single organ			
Hematological			
Autoimmune thrombocyto-penic purpura	None	None	Fetal/neonatal thrombocytopenia
Autoimmune hemolytic anemia	None	None	Fetal/neonatal anemia
Endocrine			
Graves' disease	Improved	None	Neonatal thyrotoxicosis, IUGR, cardiac disease, and fetal goiter
Hashimoto's thyroiditis	Worse	Increased still birth and miscarriage	Neonatal hypothyroidism
Antithyroid anti-bodies with-out disease	None	Possible increased miscarriage	None
Neurological			
Multiple sclerosis	May improve	None	None
Myasthenia gravis	Variable	Increased fetal and neonatal wastage	IUGR, neonatal myas-thenia arthrogryposis
Dermatological			
Pemphigus gestationis	Occurs exclu-sively with pregnancy	None	None
Pemphigus vulgaris	None	Increased incidence of stillbirths	Neonatally transferred disease
Organ-specific disorders: multiorgan			
Dermatomyositis/ polymyositis	Variable	Variable	None

[a]See text for full discussion and references.

and the fetus depends on the associated autoimmune disease and the presence and titer of maternal autoantibodies. If the mother is SS-A (Ro) antibody positive, the fetus or neonate is at risk for complete congenital heart block (CHB) (43,46,66). The prevalence of CHB is about 5% and appears to be related to the presence of the antibody rather than whether the diagnosis is SLE or SS. Fetal monitoring to detect sustained bradycardia is essential.

IV. Behçet's Disease

Behçet's disease is an unusual, multisystem, seronegative disease manifested by iritis and recurrent oral and genital ulcerations. There appears to be a variable response of the disease to the pregnant state. Hamza et al., (29) studied 21 pregnancies in 8 patients. Disease expression varied from one patient to the next and from one pregnancy to the next. The ultimate outcome of pregnancy appears not to be affected by the disease, as there were 21 live births (29).

V. Wegener's Granulomatosis

Wegener's granulomatosis is a vasculitic syndrome with necrotizing granulomatous lesions affecting the upper respiratory tract (sinuses and especially the nasal septum), lungs, and kidneys (glomerulonephritis).

The effect of Wegener's granulomatosis on fertility is significant. The infertility rate is 50% of women of child-bearing age. These data, however, were based on patients who had received one year of cyclophosphamide therapy and had ovarian failure (33). Fortunately, oral contraceptives are thought to protect ovarian function in women receiving alkylating chemotherapy (17).

Pauzner et al., (55) reviewed 15 cases of Wegener's granulomatosis in pregnancy. The effects of the disease on the pregnancy and the fetus are considerable. Eight of 15 patients had known disease at the time of pregnancy. Five of these women suffered a relapse of disease, and one had an elective abortion. One of the 5 had her relapse postabortion and died. There were 7 cases diagnosed during pregnancy and postpartum. Of the 4 patients who had active disease during the pregnancy itself, there was one maternal death and one therapeutic abortion. One pregnancy was maintained to 28 weeks and one proceeded to term. Three patients had newly diagnosed disease postpartum, and in these patients the disease (with treatment) achieved either partial or complete remission.

If the fetus is viable, the disease, as well as treatment of the disease, affect it. Uncontrolled disease is more likely to result in intrauterine growth retardation. The usual treatment for Wegener's granulomatosis is cyclophosphamide and methylprednisolone, but cyclophosphamide is teratogenic (19,27,85). However, the necessity of aggressive treatment in Wegner's for maternal health is clear. Additionally, the teratogenic effects of cyclophosphamide may be markedly diminished later in pregnancy. Treatment decisions should be individualized. If cyclophosphamide may be avoided in early pregnancy without compromising maternal health, its use in late pregnancy appears to have leukopenia as its only fetal effect (23,82,87).

VI. Polyarteritis Nodosa

Polyarteritis nodosa is a systemic disease with multiorgan involvement. It is manifested by a segmental vasculitis of small and medium arteries. If polyarteritis nodosa (PAN) is diagnosed during pregnancy, there is a poor maternal outcome with high maternal mortality, usually in the postpartum period (53,57). There remains, however, a good fetal outcome (53,57). The treatment of PAN is cyclophosphamide and methylprednisolone, and the teratogenic issues are as described earlier.

Though fetal outcome is usually good, prematurity is frequent due to induced labor and caesarean section for maternal considerations. In general, the placenta is spared of vasculitis (40). There have been three reported cases of possible neonatal PAN. All of the mothers had disease limited to the skin. All three neonates also had cutaneous vasculitis only, and the illness was relatively short-lived (10,74,80). As PAN is usually believed to be caused by circulating antigen-antibody complexes, and these are not felt to be capable of passing the placenta, these three cases raise intriguing and as yet unanswered questions about the nature of this neonatal syndrome.

VII. Autoimmune Thrombocytopenic Purpura

Autoimmune thrombocytopenic purpura (AITP), also known as idiopathic thrombocytopenic purpura (ITP), may occur solely or with other autoimmune disorders. The disease involves an autoantibody of broad specificity against epitopes of platelet glycoproteins. It is usually treated with corticosteroids or intravenous immunoglobulin G (9,79).

Pregnancy appears not to affect the course of the disease. However, the disease does affect pregnancy outcome, because the autoantibody is of the IgG isotype and will therefore cross the placenta.

Fetal thrombocytopenia correlates with the mother's titer of anti-platelet antibodies but it does not correlate with maternal platelet count, which reflects both platelet destruction and compensation. The fetus, however, may not be able to compensate or may have a different conformation of platelet glycoprotein. In essence, the fetal and maternal milieu are different (14,21,64,67,83).

If the fetal platelet count becomes very low, there may be a risk of cerebral hemorrhage, especially peripartum (14). In general, however, this disease has a low fetal risk. Controversy does exist, however, about the management of labor and delivery. It is unclear if vaginal delivery or a cesarean section carry an equal risk of intracranial hemorrhage (14,21,64,67,83). Reports of perinatal mortality are variable, but more recent reviews and prospective data show no increased mortality (14,21,52,64,67,83).

Neonatal thrombocytopenia usually worsens in the first few days of life, reaching a nadir somewhere in days 1–10. It then spontaneously resolves without future relapse as maternal IgG is catabolized (44). Maternal treatment with steroids does not alter the disease course in the infant (3).

VIII. Autoimmune Hemolytic Anemia

Autoimmune hemolytic anemia (AIHA) has a wide spectrum of disease presentation and may occur with or without another autoimmune disorder. It may also be a manifestation of infectious mononucleosis. AIHA is defined by shortened in-vivo red cell survival, evidence of autoantibodies against red cells, and evidence of increased red cell production.

In AIHA, autoantibodies are directed against red blood cell antigens, causing hemolysis or opsonization and phagocytosis, all leading to anemia.

Autoimmune hemolytic anemia is not induced by the pregnant state, nor is it exacerbated by pregnancy. The effect of the disease on pregnancy and the fetus, however, may be significant. In most cases, the autoantibodies are of the IgG class (warm antibodies), which will cross the placenta. The fetus is then at risk for hemolysis, secondary to the maternal autoantibody. The degree of hemolysis in the fetus is usually mild; and, as with AITP, there is no correlation between the degree of maternal disease and the severity of fetal hemolysis (16). Diagnosis of the degree of fetal involvement is therefore more difficult, and fetal monitoring is of great importance. This includes serial ultrasounds to look for fetal hepatomegaly, ascites, or scalp edema. One may also look at amniotic fluid, antepartum heart rate, or perform biophysical testing.

However, the greatest threat to fetal survival is severe maternal anemia, especially at the level of hemoglobin <5 g/dL (16). The mother should therefore be treated with steroids and transfusion if she becomes severely anemic (54,75).

Autoimmune hemolytic anemia associated with pregnancy usually resolves with delivery, at which time blood should be available for exchange transfusion for the neonate. The neonate should also be serially monitored for hemolysis and persistence of antibodies (16).

IX. Graves' Disease

Graves' disease is a thyroid disorder of autoimmune etiology. It is caused by a family of thyroid-stimulating immunoglobulins (TSIs). These are antireceptor autoantibodies which bind to the TSH receptor and stimulate thyroid hormone production. Older studies noted a linkage between thyroid disease and pregnancy loss. However, this was usually later in pregnancy and associated with uncontrolled disease.

Graves' disease severity may change with the pregnant state. There may be a transient increase in serum thyroid hormone levels in the first trimester of pregnancy (2,30). This is usually without an associated change in the TSI level and is most likely secondary to an abnormal response of the Graves' thyroid gland to stimulation by placental HCG or chorionic thyrotropin.

In general, however, the disease severity in pregnancy decreases (13,63) due to a fall in TSI levels (28).

Congenital thyrotoxicosis has been traditionally ascribed to the crossing of TSIs across the placenta. Hollingsworth et al., (34) have questioned this assumption and have proposed that neonatal Graves is a primary disease found in families with a high incidence of thyroid autoimmunity (34).

Other fetal effects of maternal Graves' disease include intrauterine growth retardation (secondary to metabolic changes) (51), cardiac disease, and fetal goiter (32).

Therapy during pregnancy is directed toward maintenance of the euthyroid state. Interventions include thyroidectomy with thyroid hormone replacement, or medical therapy. In general, PTU is preferred over methimazole because there is less placental transfer of the drug (47).

As there may be decreased disease activity during pregnancy, the medication requirements are often decreased. Because of this fact (and of other poorly understood concepts), there may be a rebound, resulting in "postpartum thyrotoxicosis" (PPT) (28). This situation may be avoided by instituting a "block-and-replace" mode of therapy (31).

X. Hashimoto's Thyroiditis

Hashimoto's thyroiditis is an autoimmune disorder characterized by circulating antithyroid and antithyroglobulin autoantibodies. Cellular immune mechanisms may also be important. Patients usually have a transient hyperthyroidism followed by hypothyroidism. In general, there are higher rates of stillbirths and miscarriage in women with untreated hypothyroidism, and this fact applies to those with Hashimoto's thyroiditis (2,28). There is often a higher requirement for thyroid hormone replacement in hypothyroid pregnant women than in those who are not pregnant, and this should be considered in these patients (28).

The neonate, however, may experience hypothyroidism secondary to the placental transfer of antibody, though this is a transient phenomenon (48).

XI. Thyroid Autoimmunity Without Overt Disease

Thyroid autoimmunity without overt disease has become a subject of great interest. In this instance, organ-specific antibodies are directed against thyroglobulin or thyroid peroxidase (also known as antimicrosomal antibodies), or the TSH receptor. These antithyroid antibodies may be found in the serum of normal, healthy, euthyroid subjects. The prevalence can vary from 2% to 36%, with a higher prevalence in women and increased prevalence with age. Peak prevalence occurs during the reproductive years (11,12,59,86,90). It is not clear whether the presence of these autoantibodies is truly organ-specific or is a reflection of a more generalized immune perturbation.

Most of the investigation of thyroid autoimmunity without overt disease is with regard to the issue of recurrent miscarriage. This question was initially raised because of the association of systemic lupus erythematosus and recurrent spontaneous abortions. In 1990, Stagnaro-Green et al. (77) described in a prospective manner, pregnancy outcomes in women with and without thyroid autoimmunity. They found that 17% of patients with thyroid antibodies had spontaneous abortions, compared to 8.4% of those who did not have these antibodies. Pratt et al. (59) studied women who had three or more consecutive pregnancy losses and found there to be no increase in the frequency of thyroid autoantibodies. This study, however, was retrospective, and the control population was a random sample of blood donors. This group also included men, and there was no matching for age or determination of concurrent disease (81). In another study, however, Pratt et al. (60) found that in women who had habitual miscarriage, those with thyroid autoantibodies were more likely to have yet another miscarriage than were those who did not. Other investigators have also presented suggestive evidence to support the conclusion that women with thyroid autoantibodies have a higher incidence of spontaneous abortion (42).

In summary, though it appears that the presence of thyroid autoantibodies increases the risk of spontaneous miscarriage, this remains controversial. There is no evidence regarding the influence of pregnancy on the emergence of overt disease in these patients. Also, the fetus and neonate appear not to be affected if the pregnancy proceeds to term (25). At first, this sparing of the fetus and neonate from the effects of the mother's circulating autoantibodies seems to be at variance with the data on Hashimoto's thyroiditis presented above. It could be argued, however, that if the quality and quantity of the autoantibodies did not cause hypothyroidism in the mother, the offspring would be unaffected as well.

XII. Multiple Sclerosis

Multiple sclerosis is a chronic demyelinating central nervous system disease characterized by a variable course of neurological dysfunction. Its etiology is unknown. There is evidence that an autoimmune process may be triggered at a young age (20).

There appears to be no effect of multiple sclerosis on the ability of a women to get pregnant or stay pregnant (1). Multiple sclerosis appears to improve with pregnancy in some patients (7,20,62). There also appears to be a slightly higher relapse rate in the postpartum period (7,62,89), but there is an overall improvement in long-term relapse rate (7). Most investigators have ascribed these effects to the "immunosuppression of pregnancy," but (as discussed in Chapter 4) this phenomenon itself is probably nonexistent. It should be pointed out as well that these observations are not as firm as one would like, because of the variation of the course of the disease from patient to patient and its unpredictability even in a single woman. It is unclear why this is so.

There also appears to be no effect of the disease on the pregnancy, fetus, or neonate (20,89). This is consonant with the fact that, so far, transmission of the illness by cells or circulating factors has not been shown.

XIII. Myasthenia Gravis (MG)

Myasthenia gravis (MG) is a neurological disorder caused by antibodies affecting the acetylcholine receptor (AChR) at the neuromuscular junction. There does not appear to be any effect of the disease on the ability of a woman to get pregnant.

There is a variable effect of pregnancy on the course of the disease. Approximately 30% of women who become pregnant have no change in their disease activity, 40% get worse, and 30% get better (58). There are several possible reasons for this variable effect. These include the stress of pregnancy as an exacerbating factor as well as the difficulty in taking medication because of pregnancy-induced nausea (58). Furthermore, corticosteroids are frequently used to treat MG.

Myasthenia gravis may significantly affect pregnancy. In one series, there was significant fetal and neonatal wastage, including an abortion rate (some spontaneous, most therapeutic) of 12.2% and a perinatal mortality of 82/100,000 (58). There is also significant fetal disease, including intrauterine growth retardation, the transfer of the disease to the fetus, arthrogryposis, and polyhydramnios. Polyhydramnios and pulmonary hypoplasia are secondary to the decrease amplitude of fetal respirations and impaired fetal swallowing, if the fetus is affected.

Neonatal myasthenia gravis is a fascinating "experiment of nature" whose very existence demonstrates the pathogenicity of antibodies to AChR. It is certainly caused by the transfer of maternal IgG AChR to the fetus. [Some have suggested that the fetus may also synthesize these antibodies (41).] Neonatal MG is not a uniform occurrence. It appeared clinically in about 18% in one series (58). There is a rough correlation between the mother's titer of anti-AChR and the incidence and severity of neonatal MG, but this is far from being predictive.

It is not clear why clinical signs and symptoms do not appear until 12–48 hr after birth, nor why MG is rare in utero. It is clear that the waning of neonatal MG over a mean duration of 3 weeks reflects the newborn's metabolism of transferred antibody.

XIV. Pemphigoid Gestationis (PG)

Pemphigoid gestationis is a rare autoimmune disease of the skin which occurs exclusively with pregnancy. PG was previously called herpes gestationis, but this is a misonomer because it is not a herpetic nor even a viral illness. PG is characterized by a rash which may vary from intense pruritis to urticaria to a vesiculobillous eruption. It is related to bullous pemphigoid disorders. Typically, an urticarial, pruritic eruption will begin near the umbilicus and spread over the trunk and limbs. It usually persists until delivery. Pemphigoid gestationis may occur with another autoimmune disease (though this is unusual), and typically this is Graves' disease (69).

Pemphigoid gestationis may occur during any pregnancy, and it usually recurs with each subsequent pregnancy (35,38,68) and resolves in the postpartum period. There is a significant effect on the fetus and neonate. While there is no greater risk for miscarriage (35,68), there may be intrauterine growth retardation because of placental involvement (35,68,69). Pemphigoid gestationis is caused by a complement-binding IgG factor. There may be an increased representation of HLA DR3 and DR4 in those patients with this disease (38). Furthermore, anti-HLA antibodies are present in the serum of 85% of these patients (versus 15–25% in normal, multiparous women) (70). However, aberrant presentation of MHC class II antigens appear not to be occurring in the skin, but in the placenta (70). These facts suggest that an allogenic reaction is being initiated in the placenta, triggering an autoimmune response to placental and skin basement membrane antigens (38). The treatment for this condition is corticosteroids.

XV. Pemphigus Vulgaris

Pemphigus vulgaris is an autoimmune disease of the skin characterized by bullous changes. This is caused by IgG antibodies directed against intercellular connecting bridges between epidermal cells.

The condition is rare during pregnancy, and when it does occur in the gravid state, it is found disproportionately in those patients with myasthenia gravis who have a thymoma (26,65).

In reported cases of pemphigus vulgaris in pregnancy, there is a relatively high incidence of stillbirth (4/15) (26), all of whom have had autopsy evidence of placental transfer of disease-causing IgG antibody. Maternal therapy involves immunosuppression. The neonate may be treated with plasmapheresis to remove maternal antibody (26).

XVI. Dermatomyositis/Polymyositis

Dermatomyositis/polymyositis (DM/PM) is a diffuse inflammatory disease of striated muscle as well as characteristic skin involvement. It is characterized by variable degrees of diffuse and proximal muscle weakness and diffuse cutaneous eruptions.

There is no evidence that DM/PM affects fertility, though the disease is rare and few cases have coincided with the fertile years.

The outcomes of both fetus and mother varies with the temporal relationship of disease and the pregnancy. Of the reported cases (5,36,39,56,61), approximately half of the patients were first diagnosed in the first trimester. In these patients, the disease generally remained active throughout the pregnancy.

In patients with an established diagnosis at the time of pregnancy, a majority had inactive disease at the beginning of pregnancy (10/15 pregnancies) (56). Of these, two experienced an exacerbation, one leading to maternal death (36,56,61). [This death may have been secondary to noncompliance with medical therapy (56).] Of the patients who had active disease at the time of diagnosis (5/15 pregnancies), two improved, two had exacerbations during the third trimester, and one had an exacerbation during the second trimester (56).

Fetal outcome also appears to be worse when the disease first appears during pregnancy. Also, the incidence of fetal loss parallels the activity of maternal disease. Other than a high incidence of prematurity, no other effects on the newborn have been evident.

XVII. Summary

This chapter has reviewed a wide spectrum of autoimmune conditions and has assessed the effects of the illnesses on the mother and fetus, as well as the effects of pregnancy on the illness.

1. If the autoimmune condition is clearly related to IgG autoantibodies in the mother, then temporary "transmission" of the illness to the fetus or neonate may occur, although these situations are not frequent. Such phenomena are seen in Sjögren's syndrome (especially congenital heart block) and also occur in the form of neonatal myasthenia gravis, Graves' disease, autoimmune thrombocytopenia, and hemolytic anemia.
2. Other autoimmune illnesses are rarely if every transmitted to the fetus or newborn. In cases such as Wegener's granulomatosis and Behcet's syndrome, this is not unexpected, as we are not sure that circulating autoantibodies are pathogenic. In scleroderma, the failure to find the disease in newborns from affected mothers suggests (but does not prove) that antinuclear antibodies may *not* be pathogenic.
3. The effects of the autoimmune disease on pregnancy itself are variable. Only in rare instances is it so detrimental to the health of the mother or fetus that pregnancy needs to be terminated. Although good documentation is hard to find, we think that im-

proved prenatal care of the autoimmune condition has improved the prognosis for both mother and fetus.

References

1. Abramsky O. Pregnancy and multiple sclerosis. Ann Neurol 1994; 36: S38–S41.
2. ACOG Technical Bulletin. Thyroid disease in pregnancy. Int J Gynaecol Obstet 1993; 43:82–88.
3. al-Mofada SM, Osman ME, Kides E, al-Momen AK, al-Herbish AS, al-Mobaireek K. Risk of thrombocytopenia in the infants of mothers with idiopathic thrombocytopenia. Am J Perinatol 1994; 11:423–426.
4. Baethge BA, Wolf RE. Successful pregnancy with scleroderma renal disease and pulmonary hypertension in a patient using agiotensin converting enzyme inhibitors. Ann Rheum Dis 1989; 48:776–778.
5. Barnes AB, Link DA. Childhood dermatomyositis and pregnancy. Am J Obstet Gynecol 1983; 146:335–336.
6. Bellucci MJ, Coustan DR, Plotz RD. Cervical scleroderma: a case of soft tissue dystocia. Am J Obstet Gynecol 1984; 150:891–892.
7. Bernardi S, Grasso MG, Bertollini R, Orzi F, Fieschi C. The influence of pregnancy on relapses in multiple sclerosis: a cohort study. Acta Nuerol Scand 1991; 84:403–406.
8. Black CM, Stevens WM. Scleroderma. Rheum Dis Clin N Am 1989; 15: 193–212.
9. Blanchette VS, Kirby MA, Turner C. Role of intravenous immunoglobulin G in autoimmune hematologic disorders. Semin Hematol 1992; 29:72–82.
10. Boren JJ, Everett MA. Cutaneous vasculitis in mother and infant. Arch Dermatol 1965; 92:568–570.
11. Bouanani M, Piechaczyk M, Pau B, Bastide M. Significance of the recognition of certain antigenic regions on the human thyroglobulin molecule by natural autoantibodies from healthy subjects. J Immunol 1989; 143:1129–1132.
12. Boyden SV. The absorption of proteins on erythrocytes treated with taunic acid and subsequent hemagglutination by antiprotein sera. Proc R Soc Med 1957; 50:961.
13. Burrow GH. Thyroid status in normal pregnancy. J Clin Endocrinol Metab 1990; 71:274–275.
14. Burrows RF, Kelton JG. Pregnancy in patients with idiopathoc thrombocytopenic purpura: assessing the risks for the infant at delivery. Obstet Gynecol Surv 1993; 48:781–788.
15. Campbell PM, LeRoy EC. Pathogenesis of systemic sclerosis: a vascular hypothesis. Semin Arthritis Rheum 1975; 4:351–368.
16. Chaplin H Jr, Cohen R, Bloomberg G, Kaplan HJ, Moore JA, Dorner I. Pregnancy and idiopathic autoimmune hemolytic anemia: a prospective study during 6 months gestation and 3 months post-partum. Br J Haematol 1973; 24: 219–229.

17. Chapman RM, Sutcliffe SB. Protection of ovarian function by oral contraceptives in women receiving chemotherapy for Hodgkin's disease. Blood 1981; 58:849–851.

18. Claman HN. On scleroderma: mast cells, endothelial cells, and fibrosis. JAMA 1989; 262:1206–1209.

19. Coates A. Cyclophosphamide in pregnancy. Austral NZJ Obstet Gynaecol 1970; 10:33–34.

20. Davis RK, Maslow AS. Multiple sclerosis in pregnancy: a review. Obstet Gynecol Surv 1992; 47:290–296.

21. Druzin ML, Stier E. Maternal platelet count at delivery in patients with idiopathic thrombocytopenic purpura, not related to perioperative complications. J Am Coll Surg 1994; 179:264–266.

22. Englert H, Brennan P, McNeil D, Black C, Silman AJ. Reproductive function prior to disease onset in women with scleroderma. J Rheumatol 1992; 19: 1575–1579.

23. Gililland J, Weinstein L. The effects of cancer chemotherapeutic agents on the developing fetus. Obstet Gynecol Surv 1983; 38:6–13.

24. Giordano M, Valentini G, Lupoli S, Giordano A. Pregnancy and systemic sclerosis. Arthritis Rheum 1985; 28:237–238.

25. Glinoer D, Soto MF, Bordoux P, Lejeune B, Delange F, Lemone J, Kinthaert J, Robiyn C, Grun JP, de Nayer P. Pregnancy in patients with mild thyroid abnormalities maternal and neonatal repercussions. J Clin Endocrinol Metab 1991; 73:421–427.

26. Goldberg NS, DeFeo C, Kirshenbaum N. Pemphigus vulgaris and pregnancy: risk factors and recommendations. J Am Acad Dermatol 1993; 28:877–879.

27. Greenberg LH, Tanaka KR. Congenital anomalies probably induced by cyclophosphamide. JAMA 1964; 1988:423.

28. Hall R, Richards CJ, Lazarus JH. The thyroid and pregnancy. Br J Obstet Gynaecol 1993; 100:512–515.

29. Hamza M, Elleuch M, Zribi A. Behcet's disease and pregnancy. Ann Rheum Dis 1988; 47:350.

30. Hara T, Tamai H, Mukuta T, Fukata S, Kuma K. The role of thyroid stimulating antibody (TSAb) in the thyroid function of patients with post-partum hypothyroidism. Clin Endocrin (Oxf) 1992; 36:69–74.

31. Hashizume K, Ichikawa K, Nishii Y, Kobayashi M, Sakurai A, Miyamoto T, Suzuki S, Takeda T. Effect of administration of thyroxine of the risk of post-partum recurrence of hyperthyroid Graves' disease. J Clin Endocrinol Metab 1992; 75:6–10.

32. Hatjis CG. Diagnosis and successful treatment of fetal goitrous hyperthyroidism caused by maternal Graves disease. Obstet Gynecol 1993; 81:837–839.

33. Hoffman GS, Kerr GS, Leavitt RY, Hallahan CW, Lebovics RS, Travis WD, Rottem M, Fauci AS. Wegener granulomatosis: an analysis of 158 patients. Ann Intern Med 1992; 116:488–498.

34. Hollingsworth DR, Mabry CC. Congenital Grave's disease: four familial cases with long-term follow-up and perspective. Am J Dis Child 1976; 130: 148–155.

35. Holmes RC, Black MM. The fetal prognosis in pemphigoid gestationis (herpes gestationis). Br J Dermatol 1984; 110:67–72.

36. Ishii N, Ono H, Kawaguchi T, Nakajima H. Dermatomyosisis and pregnancy: case report and review of the literature. Dermatologica 1991; 183:146–149.

37. Karlen JR, Cook WA. Renal scleroderma and pregnancy. Obstet Gynecol 1974; 44:349–354.

38. Kelly SE, Fleming S, Bhogal BS, Wojnarowska F, Black MM. Immunopathology of the placenta in pemphigoid gestationis and linear IgA disease. Br J Dermatol 1989; 120:735–743.

39. Kitridou RC. Pregnancy in mixed connective tissue disease, poly/dermatomyositis and scleroderma (review). Clin Exp Rheumatol 1988; 6:173–178.

40. Klipple GL, Riordan KK. Rare inflammatory and hereditary connective tissue diseases. Rheum Dis Clin N Am 1989; 15:383–398.

41. Lefvert AK, Osterman PO. Newborn infants to myasthenic mothers: a clinical study and investigation of acetylcholine receptor antibodies in 17 children. Neurology 1983; 33:133–138.

42. Lejeune B, Grun JP, de Nayer P, Servais G, Glinoer D. Antithyroid antibodies underlying thyroid abnormalities and miscarriage or pregnancy induced hypertension. Br J Obstet Gynaecol 1993; 100:669–672.

43. Lockshin MD, Bonfa E, Elkon K, Druzin ML. Neonatal lupus risk to newborns of mothers with systemic lupus erythematosus. Arthritis Rheum 1988; 31:697–701.

44. Logsdon-Pokorny VK, Scott JR. Autoimmune-induced hematologic diseases in pregnancy. Immunol Allergy Clin N Am 1994.

45. Luiz DA, Moodley J, Naicher SN, Pudifin D. Pregnancy in scleroderma. S Afr Med J 1986; 69:642–643.

46. Manthorpe T, Manthorpe R. Congenital complete heart block in children of mothers with primary Sjogren's syndrome (letter). Lancet 1992; 340: 1359–1360.

47. Marchant B, Brownlie BE, Hart DM, Horton PW, Alexander WD. The placental transfer of propylthiouracil, methimazole and carbimazole. J Clin Endocrinol Metab 1977; 45:1187–1193.

48. Matsuura N, Yamada Y, Nohara Y, Konishi J, Kasagi K, Endo K, Kojima H, Wataya K. Familial neonatal transient hypothyroidism due to maternal TSH-binding inhibitor immunoglobulins. N Engl J Med 1980; 303:738–741.

49. Maymon R, Fejgin M. Scleroderma in pregnancy. Obstet Gynecol Surv 1989; 44:530–534.

50. Maymon R, Fejgin M, Ben-Aderet N, Bahary C. Scleroderma and pregnancy. Acta Obstet Gynecol Scand 1989; 68:469–470.

51. Mitsuda N, Tamaki H, Amino N, Hosono T, Miyai K, Tanizawa O. Risk factors for developmental disorders in infants born to women with Graves disease. Obstet Gynecol 1992; 80:359–364.

52. Moutet A, Fromont P, Farcet JP, Rotten D, Bettaieb A, Duedari N, Bierling P. Pregnancy in women with immune thrombocytopenic purpura. Arch Intern Med 1990; 150:2141–2145.

53. Nagey DA, Fortier KJ, Linder J. Pregnancy complicated by periarteritis nodosa: induced abortion as an alternative. Am J Obstet Gynecol 1983; 147:103–105.

54. Ng SC, Wong KK, Raman S, Bosco J. Autoimmune haemolytic anaemia in pregnancy: a case report. Eur J Obstet Gynecol Reprod Biol 1990; 37:83–85.

55. Pauzner R, Mayan H, Hershko E, Alcalay M, Farfel Z. Exacerbation of Wegener's granulomatosis during pregnancy: report of a case with tracheal stenosis and literature review. J Rheumatol 1994; 21:1153–1156.

56. Pinheiro G da R, Goldenberg J, Atra E, Pereira RB, Camano L, Schmidt B. Juvenile dermatomyosisis and pregnancy: report and literature review. J Rheumatol 1992; 19:1798–1801.

57. Pitkin RM. Polyarteritis nodosa. Clin Obstet Gynecol 1983; 26:579–586.

58. Plauche WC. Myasthenia gravis. Clin Obstet Gynecol 1983; 26:592–604.

59. Pratt D, Novotny M, Kaberlein G, Dudkiewicz A, Gleicher N. Antithyroid antibodies and the association with non-organ-specific antibodies in recurrent pregnancy loss. Am J Obstet Gynecol 1993; 168:837–841.

60. Pratt DE, Kaberlein G, Dudkiewicz A, Karande V, Gleicher N. The association of antithyroid antibodies in euthyroid nonpregnant women with recurrent first trimester abortions in the next pregnancy. Fertil Steril 1993; 60:1001–1005.

61. Rosenzweig BA, Rotmensch S, Binetti SP, Phillippe M. Primary idiopathic polymyositis and dermatomyositis complicating pregnancy: diagnosis and management. Obstet Gynecol Surv 1989; 44:162–170.

62. Runmarker B, Andersen O. Pregnancy is associated with a lower risk of onset and a better prognosis in multiple sclerosis. Brain 1995; 188:253–261.

63. Salvi M, How J. Pregnancy and autoimmune thyroid disease (review). Endocrin Metab Clin N Am 1987; 16:431–444.

64. Scott JR, Cruikshank DP, Kochenour NK, Pitkin RM, Warenski JC. Fetal platelet counts in the obstetric management of immunologic thrombocytopenic purpura. Am J Obstet Gynecol 1980; 136:495–499.

65. Scott JS. Single-system autoimmune diseases: lessons applicable to multisystem disease. In: Scott JS, Bird HA, eds. Pregnancy, Autoimmunity and Connective Tissue Disorders. Oxford: Oxford University Press, 1990.

66. Scott JS, Maddison PJ, Taylor PV, Esscher E, Scott O, Skinner RP. Connective tissue disease, antibodies to ribonucleoprotein, and congenital heart block. N Engl J Med 1983; 309:209–212.

67. Sharon R, Tatarsky I. Low fetal morbidity in pregnancy associated with acute and chronic idiopathic thrombocytopenic purpura. Am J Hematol 1994; 46:87–90.

68. Shornick JK. Herpes gestationis (review). Dermatol Clin 1993; 11:527–533.

69. Shornick JK, Black MM. Secondary autoimmune diseases in herpes gestationis (pemphigoid gestationis). J Am Acad Dermatol 1992; 26:563–566.

70. Shornick JK, Jenkins RE, Briggs DC, Welsh KI, Kelly SE, Garvey MP, Black MM. Anti-HLA antibodies in pemphigoid gestationis (pemphigoid gestationis). Br J Dermatol 1993; 129:257–259.

71. Silman AJ. Pregnancy and scleroderma. J Reprod Immunol 1992; 28:238–240.

72. Silman AJ, Black C. Increased incidence of spontaneous abortion and infertility in women with scleroderma before disease onset: a controlled study. Ann Rheum Dis 1988; 47:441–444.

73. Skopouli FN, Papanikolaou S, Malamou-Mitsi V, Papanikolaou N, Moutsopoulos HM. Obstetric and gynaecological profile in patients with primary Sjogren's syndrome. Ann Rheum Dis 1994; 53:569–573.

74. Smoller B. Cutaneous vasculitis in the newborn (letter, comment). J Am Acad Dermatol 1993; 29:665–666.

75. Sokol RJ, Hewitt S, Stamps BK. Autoimmune haemolysis: an 18-year study of 865 cases referred to a regional transfusion centre. Br Med J (Clin Res Ed) 1981; 282:2023–2037.

76. Spiera H, Krakoff L, Fishbane-Mayer J. Successful pregnancy after scleroderma hypertensive renal crisis. J Rheumatol 1989; 16:1597–1598.

77. Stagnaro-Green A, Roman SH, Cobin RH, el-Harazy E, Alvarez-Marfany M, Davies TF. Detection of at-risk pregnancy by means of highly sensitive assays for thyroid autoantibodies. JAMA 1990; 264:1422–1425.

78. Steen VD, Conte C, Day N, Ramsey-Goldman R, Medsger TA Jr. Pregnancy in women with systemic sclerosis. Arth Rheum 1989; 32:151–157.

79. Stiehm ER. Human gamma globulins as therapeutic agents. Adv Pediatr 1988; 35:1–72.

80. Stone MS, Olson RR, Weismann DN, Giller RH, Goeken JA. Cutaneous vasculaitis in the newborn of a mother with cutaneous polyarteritis nodosa. J Am Acad Dermatol 1993; 28:101–105.

81. Stricker RB. Antithyroid antibodies in recurrent pregnancy loss. Am J Obstet Gynecol 1994; 170:956–957.

82. Talbot SF, Main DM, Levinson AI. Wegener's granulomatosis: first report of a case with onset during pregnancy. Arth Rheum 1984; 27:109–112.

83. Tchernia G, Morel-Kopp MC, Yvart J, Kaplan C. Neonatal thrombocytopenia and hidden maternal autoimmunity. Br J Haematol 1993; 84:457–463.

84. Thompson J, Conklin KA. Anesthetic management of a pregnant patient with scleroderma. Anesthesiology 1983; 59:69–71.

85. Toledo TM, Harper RC, Moser RH. Fetal effects during cyclophosphamide and irradiation therapy. Ann Intern Med 1971; 74:87–91.

86. Tomer Y, Schoenfeld Y. Aging and autoantibodies. Autoimmunity 1988; 1: 141–149.

87. Wheeler GE. Cyclophosphamide-associated leukemia in Wegener's granulomatosis. Ann Intern Med 1981; 94:361–362.

88. Wilson AG, Kirby JD. Successful pregnancy in a woman with systemic sclerosis while taking nifedipine. Ann Rheum Dis 1990; 49:51–52.

89. Worthington J, Jones R, Crawford M, Forti A. Pregnancy and multiple sclerosis—a 3-year prospective study. J Neurol 1994; 241:228–233.

90.	Yadin O, Sarov B, Naggan L, Slor H, Shoenfeld Y. Natural autoantibodies in the serum of healthy women—a five-year follow-up. Clin Exp Immunol 1989; 75:402–406.
91.	Younker D, Harrison B. Scleroderma and pregnancy. Br J Anaesth 1985; 57: 1136–1139.

24

Human Immunodeficiency Virus Infection in Pregnancy

PAMELA STRATTON

National Institute of Child Health and
  Human Development
Bethesda, Maryland

**MARY JO O'SULLIVAN and
ADOLFO GONZALEZ-GARCIA**

University of Miami School of Medicine
Miami, Florida

I. Epidemiology and History

Heterosexual transmission is responsible for the majority of infections with the human immunodeficiency virus (HIV). The highest rates of infection in women occur in Africa, where 10–30% of pregnant women are HIV-infected (1). Recently, HIV infection has spread throughout parts of Southeast Asia. In the United States, an estimated 7000 HIV-infected women give birth annually (2).

In major cities in the Americas, Western Europe, and sub-Saharan Africa, HIV infection or the acquired immune deficiency syndrome (AIDS) has become the leading cause of death in reproductive-age men and women, and in children (1,3). The World Health Organization (WHO) estimates that 3 million women and children will die as a result of this epidemic by the year 2000 (4). AIDS causes secondary effects as well; some estimate that more than 9 million uninfected children in sub-Saharan Africa alone will be orphaned in the next 5 years (5).

Over half of the almost 60,000 U.S. women with AIDS have been reported to the United States Centers for Disease Control and Prevention (CDC) in the last 2 years (6). In 1994, 18% of the reported cases were

"

women, compared to 6% in 1986 (7). In the United States, a disproportionate number of black, Hispanic, and inner-city women are affected.

HIV infection is a chronic illness, often resulting in progression to the acquired immune deficiency syndrome (AIDS), and ultimately death. Initially, women appeared to have a shorter survival after the diagnosis of AIDS than men (8,9). In fact, this bias was due to several unrecognized factors. Women were diagnosed at a more advanced disease stage, were infected at a younger age, and had less access to health care including antiretroviral and other HIV-related therapies (10–13).

Worldwide, most pediatric HIV infection is perinatally transmitted. The risk of mother-to-child transmission ranges from 15% to 35% (14). The lowest rates are reported in Europe, the highest in Africa. Reanalysis of population-based data has shown that rates of vertical transmission are more consistent within geographic areas than was previously realized (15). This may reflect the occurrence of risk factors for mother-to-child transmission within a group of people. The nature of these factors is not known. It is possible that viral strains, obstetric practices, or population characteristics each play a role. Some factors could be altered over time, changing transmission rates.

A 67% reduction in perinatal transmission has demonstrated by ZDV administration during pregnancy, labor, and to the newborn (16). The U.S. Public Health Service, the American College of Obstetricians and Gynecologists, and the American Academy of Pediatrics strongly recommend routine prenatal counseling and screening for HIV and ZDV prophylaxis for HIV-infected women and their newborns (17,18).

II. Viral Biology

A retrovirus, by definition, has a reverse transcriptase enzyme which transcribes viral RNA into DNA which then becomes part of the infected cell's genome. The HIV, a retrovirus, has an inner core structure containing two strands of RNA surrounded by a host cell-derived trilaminar envelope (19). Its genome has three basic genes; *gag* (group-specific antigen/core), *pol* (polymerase), and *env* (envelope), which code for proteins that are vital for viral replication, as well as regulator genes *rev*, *tat*, and *nef*, which modulate infectivity by controlling the initiation or termination of transcription (20). The products of *gag*, *pol*, and *env* can be immunogenic, although antibody responses to any of the proteins may vary between individuals and over time within an individual.

The abbreviations "p" and "gp" are used to describe the protein and glycoprotein components of the HIV-1 virions and are followed by a number that corresponds to their molecular weight in kilodaltons. The HIV-1 *env* gene codes p92, which after glycosylation becomes gp160. Then gp160 is split intracellularly to form gp120, the major envelope glycoprotein, and gp41, the transmembrane protein. The *gag* gene encodes p55, which is cleaved into the core antigen p24. The *pol* gene encodes p150, which is then cleaved by a viral protease into reverse transcriptase. Antibodies to the viral products including gp160/120, gp41, and p24, are the basis for testing for infection (20).

In humans, HIV-1 may be transmitted by cell-free or cell-associated virus after mucosal or percutaneous exposure to infectious blood or secretions. Viral transmission may occur more readily with breaks in mucosal or other epithelial surfaces. HIV-1 preferentially infects cells expressing the CD4+ antigen on their surface, such as CD4+ T lymphocytes (helper/inducer) and cells of the monocyte lineage (macrophages, monocytes, and histiocytes) (21). Alternative receptors have recently been identified which account for heterogenicity of the virus in its ability to infect other cells such a capillary endothelium (22), neurons (22,23), epithelium (24,25), and placental tissue (26–31). Among these alternatives are the chemokine receptors CXCR4 and CCR5, which appear to facilitate fusion of the virus with the cell membrane (32,33). CXCR4 may be a primary receptor for some strains of the virus (34). More recently, the genetic absence of CCR5 has been linked with resistance to HIV infection and/or delayed progression (35–37). There may well be other yet-to-be-identified mechanisms by which virus gains entry into cells.

For many CD4+ T cells, the viral envelope glycoprotein, gp120, binds to the CD4+ antigen on the cell surface, and the envelope glycoprotein, gp41, facilitates fusion to the cell membrane. Fusion allows the viral core cell entry, where reverse transcriptase transcribed viral RNA to DNA. Most antiretroviral agents (nucleoside and non-nucleoside reverse transcriptase inhibitors) block transcription, the site of most viral mutations, with varying effectiveness (38,39). DNA is then transported into the nucleus and integrated into the genome by endonucleases (integrase) (40,41). Viral replication occurs when viral DNA is transcribed to RNA and translated into proteins by specific regulatory proteins, *tat* and *rev* (42,43). The protease enzymes render the virus infectious, and it is excreted form the infected cell by a process called budding (44). Other therapeutic interventions being developed to alter the viral life cycle include: inhibiting the endonucleases which cause viral transcription into the cell genome; blocking the transcription of RNA by *tat* and *rev*; inhibiting proteases preventing the intracellular production of infectious mature HIV particles; and developing specific gene therapy to control viral replication (45). Immunoregulatory therapeutic interventions are being developed and perhaps will offer more promise in terms of control/cure.

About 3–6 weeks after initial infection, 50–70% of patients have an acute mononucleosis-like syndrome associated with a significant viremia, during which HIV-1 is widely disseminated, particularly in lymphoid tissue (45,46). Within 1 week to 3 months, cellular and humoral responses to HIV-1 are detectable, usually associated with a dramatic decline in viremia to a set point between 10^2 and 10^6 HIV RNA copies/mL of plasma (47–49). Thereafter, the patient is usually asymptomatic for a long period (median 10 years) (46). Although cell-mediated and humoral immune responses may ultimately prove unsuccessful in containing the infection, they may contribute to the period of apparent latency (50).

Over time, immunosuppression (a significant decline in CD4 T lymphocytes), and increasing viremia (rising plasma HIV-RNA) develop. The latter as a measure of plasma viral load may be a better predictor of progression in asymptomatic patients than the CD4 lymphocyte count (51,52).

AIDS is the clinical manifestation of marked deterioration of the immune system. AIDS-defining illness include severe and persistent constitutional signs and symptoms, opportunistic and other infections, and neoplasms. Oral candidiasis, hairy leukoplakia, fever, and weight loss are more common in AIDS. Once a person has an AIDS-defining illness, he or she may die within 2 years, despite antiretroviral therapy (46). With the rapid advances in treatment of opportunistic infections, and recent advances in antiviral therapy, both progression to AIDS and prolongation of life with quality even after an AIDS diagnosis are realistic probabilities.

Progression to clinical AIDS is due to extremely high viral replication and mutation rates, which allow viral resistance to develop easily. In fact, within a few weeks, almost all wild-type virus can be replaced by drug-resistant variants in the presence of antiretroviral therapy (53). Multidrug therapy has demonstrated a decrease in the rate of progression to AIDS as compared to ZDV monotherapy (54,55). Approximately 5% of infected individuals remain clinically healthy and immunologically normal and are called long-term survivors or persons with long-term nonprogressive disease. They appear to have low levels of HIV-1 and multiple strong virus-specific immune responses (56). Although viral replication continues, the virus may be attenuated. Immune function and lymph node architecture remain intact (57). Long-term survivors have a defective *nef* gene; a normal *nef* gene may be required for the development of AIDS (58).

The U.S. AIDS case definition among adolescents and adults was expanded by the Centers for Disease Control and Prevention in 1993 to include all persons who have fewer than 200 CD4+ T lymphocytes/μL or a CD4+ T lymphocyte percentage less than 14% (59) (Table 1). Pulmonary tuberculosis, recurrent pneumonia, and invasive cervical cancer were added to the list of AIDS-defining illnesses. Those classified as AIDS based solely on CD4+ counts have a longer survival (60). Clinical status continues to play a major role in predicting survival for AIDS patients.

III. Laboratory Diagnosis

The enzyme immunoassay (EIA) for HIV-1 antibody was a high sensitivity and specificity and is the most common method of screening for HIV-1 infection in adults, and children over 15 months of age (61). The HIV-1 Western blot assay should be used to confirm HIV-1 infection on specimens that have a repeatedly reactive EIA. A Western blot is positive for HIV-1 if at least two of the following viral components are present: p24, gp41, or gp 120/gp160 (62).

HIV-1 specific IgG antibodies are passively transferred to the fetus during pregnancy, so their detection in the newborn reflects maternal rather than neonatal infection. Quantitative culture of either plasma or peripheral blood mononuclear cells (PBMC) had been the "gold standard" for both early diagnosis of HIV infection in infants and for viral load in adults. However, polymerase chain reaction (PCR) and/or plasma HIV-1 RNA are easier, more efficient, accurate, and cost-effective, and are rapidly replacing quantitative viral culture.

Detection of HIV-1 infection in neonates is done using PCR or plasma HIV-1 RNA levels. PCR is probably the most sensitive method for diagnosis of perinatally transmitted HIV infection (61). Like culture, PCR detects about 50% of infected newborn infants at birth and more than 90% by 3 months of age. In a reliable laboratory, PCR has high sensitivity and specificity. False-positive and false negative reactions may occur.

IV. Risk Factors for Transmission

A. Timing of Transmission

Today, more than 90% of pediatric AIDS is related to perinatal HIV-1 transmission during pregnancy, intrapartum, or postpartum. A limited understanding exists about the timing, mechanism, and route of transmission occurring before delivery. PCR helps delineate the timing of transmission (63).

Fetal infection has been confirmed by viral culture, immunohisto-chemistry, or in-situ hybridization in abortuses born to HIV-1-infected

Table 1 1993 Revised Classification System for HIV Infection and Expanded AIDS Surveillance Case Definition for Adolescents and Adults

	Clinical category		
CD4+ T-lymphocyte category	A*	B†	C‡
≥500/μL	A1	B1	C1
200–499/μL	A2	B2	C2
<200/μL[a]	A3[a]	B3[a]	C3

*Clinical category A: acute (primary) HIV infection; persistent generalized lymphadenopathy (PGL), and asymptomatic HIV-infected patients

†Clinical category B: symptomatic conditions occurring in an HIV-infected adolescent or adult, but not (A) or (C) conditions. Examples include:
Candidiasis, vulvovaginal; persistent, frequent or poorly responsive to therapy
Candidiasis, oropharyngeal (thrush)
Cervical dysplasia, moderate or severe/carcinoma in situ
Constitutional symptoms, e.g., fever (≥38.5°C) or diarrhea lasting >1 month
Hairy leukoplakis, oral
Herpes zoster (shingles), involving at least two distinct episodes or more than one dermatome
Idiopathic thrombocytopenic purpura
Listeriosis
Pelvic inflammatory disease; particularly if complicated by tubo-ovarian abscesses
Peripheral neuropathy

‡Clinical category C: AIDS-indicator conditions
Candidiasis of bronchi, trachea, or lungs
Candidiasis, esophageal
Cervical cancer, invasive[a]
Coccidioidomycosis, disseminated or extrapulmonary
Cryptococcosis, extrapulmonary
Cryptosporidiosis, chronic intestinal (>1 month's duration)
Cytomegalovirus disease (other than liver, spleen, or nodes)
Cytomegalovirus retinitis (with loss of vision)
Encephalopathy, HIV-related
Herpes simplex: chronic ulcer(s) (>1 month's duration) or bronchitis, pneumonitis, or esophagitis
Histoplasmosis, disseminated or extrapulmonary
Isosporiasis, chronic intestinal (>1 month's duration)
Kaposi's sarcoma
Lymphoma, Burkitt's (or equivalent term)
Lymphoma, immunoblastic (or equivalent term)
Lymphoma, primary, of brain

Table 1 Continued

Mycobacterium avium complex or *M. kansasii*, extrapulmonary
M. tuberculosis, any site (pulmonary[a] or extrapulmonary)
Mycobacterium, other or unidentified species, extrapulmonary
Pneumocystis carinii pneumonia
Pneumonia, recurrent[a]
Progressive multifocal leukoencephalopathy
Salmonella septicemia, recurrent
Toxoplasmosis of brain
Wasting syndrome due to HIV

[a]New AIDS-defining conditions added as of January 1, 1993.
Source: Centers for Disease Control and Prevention (53).

women (30,31,64,65). HIV has been detected in fetal and placental tissues of spontaneous fetal demises at a higher transmission rate than that observed in liveborn infants (31). If confirmed, either in-utero transmission of HIV infection increases the risk of pregnancy loss, or the disruption of the maternal placental barrier with spontaneous abortion may permit infection of the fetus and placenta.

Two patterns of HIV-1-related illness emerge in children, early onset within the first months of life, or later, after the first year. These two patterns may differentiate children infected in utero (early onset) from those infected intrapartum (symptomatic after the first year of life) (66–69). About 30–50% are PCR- or viral culture-positive either at or within days of birth, and are thought to be infected prior to labor (61,63,66). Fifty to seventy percent of infected infants who are initially PCR- or culture-negative become positive after 7 days, and are believed to have been infected late in pregnancy or around labor and delivery.

B. Viral Characteristics

HIV can be vertically transmitted from symptomatic or asymptomatic women and may be influenced by several factors (Table 2). An important determinant may be viral load, since an increased rate of perinatal transmission from women with a high viral load has been reported in a few small studies. In the AIDS Clinical Trials Group (ACTG) 076 study, viral load was not the only factor; there was no clear level below or above which virus was not transmitted (70) (see section E page 581). Viral load has been measured by quantitative culture (71–73), plasma RNA by the (PCR) (65), and RNA or DNA copy number (73). Other maternal immune or viral

Table 2 Potential Factors Influencing Perinatal HIV Transmission

Viral load/characteristics
CD4+ cell count
Neutralizing antibody
Placental pathology
Length of gestation
Cervical viral shedding
Duration of ruptured membranes
Duration of labor
Multiple births
Mode of delivery
Invasive procedures
Breast feeding

factors which has been associated with increased transmission reflecting viral load include: p24 antigenemia (71–75), low CD4 cell count (74,76–79), high CD8 cell count (76,79), high serum antibody to p24 (77), Western blot pattern (67), advanced clinical HIV disease (74,80), and increased neopterin or B_2 microglobulin (71,78). Women with primary HIV infection contracted during pregnancy or postpartum who have transmitted HIV infection to their infants may have had significant viremia (81,82).

Case series of mother–child pairs suggest that variation among HIV strains also influences transmission risk. Rapidly replicating viruses are more likely in mothers who transmit than in those who do not (83,84). Others have found that only select genetic variants are transmitted (85).

High maternal neutralizing antibody levels to the V3 loop of gp120 were thought to be associated with reduced transmission (83,86), but this finding has not been supported (84,87). Differences in laboratory methods, groups studied, and variations in the affinity between the V3 antibodies and the V3-loop peptide might account for the disparities. Protection against transmission may be conferred if high-affinity antibodies reacting against a wide range of epitopes are used. Studies of passive immunization to prevent HIV transmission may help answer these questions.

C. Pregnancy and Delivery

The role of placenta in HIV transmission or prevention is poorly understood. Placentas from normal term pregnancies are impervious to cell-free HIV in laboratory studies (88). In cell culture studies, both human trophoblast and Hofbauer cells at different gestational ages have successfully been infected (26–29), yet the rate of placental HIV infection detected in HIV-infected women has varied (30,89). Detection of HIV-1 in placental tissue has not correlated with transmission.

Chorioamnionitis and sexually transmitted diseases are also risk factors for mother-to-child transmission of HIV (76,90–93). Both are associated with preterm delivery and possibly with an increased viral load in the genital tract. Theoretically, chorioamnionitis could facilitate transmission either by fetal exposure to infected maternal cells or by disrupting the placental barrier. Advanced HIV disease and other sexually transmitted infections may increase the likelihood of viral shedding. Because it has been technically difficult to isolate virus from cervical and vaginal secretions, little is known about the amount of HIV in these fluids or whether infectious virus is predominately cell-free or cell-associated. HIV-1 is inactivated in the acid pH of the vagina, yet grows well in the neutral pH of blood, cervical mucus, amniotic fluid, and semen (94). During labor, cervical mucus, blood, and ruptured membranes raise the vaginal pH and may enhance the survival of HIV in the lower genital tract. In fact, an increased risk of transmission has been correlated with exposure to maternal blood in labor (75).

An international registry of 100 pairs of twins was used to infer that intrapartum transmission occurs as a result of exposure to infected secretions (95). In 22 pairs discordant for HIV infection, caesarean-delivered and/or second-born twins had a lower risk of HIV-1 infection. Conclusions from this study are hampered by the fact that the infection status of one-third of the twins in the registry was unknown, and little information about each pregnancy and intrapartum course was gathered.

A meta-analysis suggests that caesarean delivery offers some protection against mother-to-child HIV transmission (96–98). Infants delivered vaginally are more likely exposed to vaginal secretions and ruptured membranes than those born by elective caesarean delivery. The studies lack critical details about intrapartum events which increase the risk of comingling of maternal and fetal secretions, such as duration of ruptured membranes, use of fetal scalp electrodes, intrauterine pressure catheters, or fetal scalp sampling. The European Collaborative Study reported a 12% perinatal transmission rate associated with caesarean birth, contrasted to 18% for those delivered vaginally (96). Currently, the effectiveness of elective caesarean delivery for reduction of transmission is being studied prospectively in a randomized clinical trial in Europe.

It is difficult to limit fetal exposure to blood during caesarean delivery. A uterine stapling device does decrease blood loss and therefore blood exposure, but stapling a thickened lower uterine segment such as occurs prior to labor is technically difficult. The device, at present, is expensive, slightly cumbersome, and of limited availability. Although it has been used, no significant data are available (99).

Other obstacles to caesarean delivery include late entry into prenatal care, making it difficult to date fetal age accurately. Assuring fetal lung maturity requires an invasive procedure (amniocentesis) which itself may increase the risk of vertical transmission. Additionally, caesarean delivery increases the exposure of health care workers to infectious blood and secretions. A caesarean has a higher risk of morbidity and mortality compared to a vaginal delivery even in non-HIV-infected women, and may pose additional risks for HIV-infected women according to at least one study. Progression to AIDS appears to be associated with delivery method. In the 4 years following delivery, women who had emergency (30%) versus elective (20%) caesareans had more rapid progression to AIDS than those delivered vaginally (15%) (100). Whether this difference represents the heterogeneity of HIV infection, or is truly an effect of delivery method, must be confirmed in other studies. HIV-infected women, particularly those with CD4 counts below 200 cells/μL, have a higher risk of serious infections compared to other women (100). Surgery might further increase the risk of serious life-threatening morbidity for HIV-infected women.

Vaginal disinfection by cleansing with a nonspecific virucidal agent during labor and delivery did not decrease the mother-to-child transmission for women who had chlorhexidine vaginal swabbing during labor (101).

D. Breast Feeding

HIV has been cultured from both the cellular and cell-free components of breast milk (81). Transmission has been reported in breast-fed babies whose mothers acquired HIV after delivery (102) and, one case, when breast feeding was continued in the presence of a breast abscess (82). The transmission rate had been correlated with both the duration of breast feeding (103) and a lack of HIV-specific secretory antibodies (IgM) in breast milk (104). Two cohort studies show a doubling of transmission risk in breast-fed infants (105,106). The additional risk of transmission through breast feeding is approximately 14% (107). Whether maternal antiretroviral therapy would decrease this risk is unknown but is being studied in Africa and Haiti. Where adequate nutrition can be achieved safely through infant formulas, breast feeding by HIV-infected women should be discouraged.

E. Reduction of Perinatal Transmission with Zidovudine Treatment

For asymptomatic women without other medical or obstetric problems, initiation of zidovudine (ZDV) after the first trimester of pregnancy, through the intrapartum period, and in the newborn decreases the transmission rate of HIV (ACTG 076) (16). In a randomized controlled clinical trial, 8% (95% CI: 3.9–12.8) of infants in the zidovudine group were infected compared with 26% (95% CI: 18.4–32.5%) in the placebo group, a 67% reduction in transmission risk (p = .000056). The safety and effectiveness of this regimen in decreasing transmission from women who are symptomatic, have AIDS, other medical conditions, or received ZDV prior to pregnancy is not known. The U.S. Public Health Service recommends the use of ZDV to reduce perinatal HIV transmission (17) (Table 3).

V. Screening, Counselling, and Testing

Recommendations by the U.S. Public Health Service, the American College of Obstetrics and Gynecology, and the American Academy of Pediatrics state that *all* pregnant women should be routinely offered HIV counseling and antibody testing with informed consent (17,18). The risk of HIV infection may increase if a woman has high-risk behaviors such as substance abuse, prostitution, other sexually transmitted diseases, multiple sex partners, or a known HIV-infected sex partner. In these circumstances, it

Table 3 Initiation of Antiretroviral Therapy for Maternal Health

Status	Recommendation
Symptomatic	Therapy recommended for all; first choice ZDV + 3TC because of synergism.
Asymptomatic, CD4+ count < 500 cells/mm^3	Therapy recommended for all.
Asymptomatic, CD4+ count > 500 cells/mm^3	[a]Therapy recommended for all with HIV RNA > 30,000–50,000 copies/mL or a rapidly decreasing CD4+ count. Therapy should be considered with HIV RNA > 5,000–10,000 copies/mL.
CD4 < 200	ZDV, 3TC + protease inhibitor. Consider drug changes based on viral load as above.

[a]Applies to both pregnant and nonpregnant women.
Source: Ref. 111.

is appropriate to consider retesting later in pregnancy (108). However, risk-based screening has proved to be an insensitive predictor of HIV infection, missing as many as 50% of seropositive individuals (109).

The optimal time to screen for HIV infection is prior to or early in pregnancy. To make an informed decision about testing, a woman needs to know how HIV infection is acquired and its impact on her health and that of her infant. Counseling can help the uninfected assess their current or future risk of acquiring HIV infection and offers the opportunity to reinforce risk-reduction behaviors, such as not sharing needles, limiting the number of sexual partners, avoiding anal intercourse, and/or using condoms.

The risk of perinatal transmission should be discussed with HIV-infected women so they can make decisions about their current or future pregnancies. Whatever reproductive option they choose should be supported. Reducing the risk of vertical transmission by ZDV therapy and the avoidance of breast feeding should be discussed. Diagnosis of HIV infection would allow indicated maternal treatment of HIV infection, prophylaxis against *Pneumocystis carinii* pneumonia (PCP), and the early detection of HIV-related diseases as well as early diagnosis and early treatment of the infant. It is vital that clinicians understand the patient's dilemma and provide social supports to help her cope with the stress and possible discrimination she and her family might experience.

Treatment does not cure HIV infection. Initiation of zidovudine during the asymptomatic period has not been shown to increase longevity (110). Current recommendations suggest treating all symptomatic HIV-1-infected adults, those who are asymptomatic but have CD4+ T-lymphocyte counts below 500 cells/μL or whose CD4+ counts are rapidly dropping or whose HIV RNA viral load is greater than 30,000–50,000 copies/mL (111) (Table 4). Treatment is defined as follows: zidovudine (ZDV)/didanosine (ddI, Videx), ZDV/zalcitabine (ddC, HIVID), ZDV/lamivudine (3TC, Epivir), or ddI monotherapy. Whether protease inhibitors should be used as part of a triple therapy regimen early on or saved to be used later in the infection remains to be seen. It should not be assumed that these drugs will be effective against the virus long term.

VI. Treatment with Zidovudine to Prevent Mother-to-Child Transmission

For pregnant women, these recommendations differ such that all HIV-infected women and their newborns should be given antiretroviral prophylaxis because of the proven reduction in perinatal transmission. The pro-

Table 4 Zidovudine Prophylaxis Regimen to Prevent Mother-to-Child Transmission *(Modification of CDC Recommendations)*

Candidates:	HIV-infected, ≥14 wks, gestation
Prenatal	100 mg zidovudine orally 5 times daily every 4 hr while awake, or 200 mg 3 times a day[a]
Intrapartum	Intravenous loading dose: 2 mg/kg body weight over 30–60 min, followed by 1 mg/kg/hr until delivery in a separate intravenous access from other drugs
Neonate	Ideally, start zidovudine oral syrup within 12 hr of birth. Dose: 2 mg/kg body weight every 6 hr for 6 weeks

[a]ZDV, unless contraindicated, should be offered in labor and to the neonate even if patients did not receive prenatal drug.

phylaxis recommended is ZDV, because it has demonstrated effectiveness in two studies, ACTG 076 and ACTG 185 (17,111) (Table 4) (see Notes Added in Proof). Women already on antiretroviral treatment for their own health care should continue that therapy in pregnancy. In labor they should be offered intravenous ZDV if there is not contraindication, and their babies should receive ZDV syrup for the first 6 weeks of life. Those with an AIDS-defining condition, or who are severely immunocompromised and previously unidentified, may have additional benefits with the initiation of antiretroviral treatment and PCP prophylaxis during pregnancy. It is essential that, once delivered, the HIV-infected woman (and her infant) be enrolled in a care system to continue therapy as needed and/or ongoing HIV follow-up. This is the health care providers' responsibility.

Adverse effects of indicated ZDV therapy in nonpregnant adults include anemia in 20% at doses of 400 mg/day (compared to 34% taking 1200 mg/day) and neutropenia (112,113). Dose interruption or reduction is recommended for a hemoglobin less than 8.0 g/dL and granulocytopenia less than 750 cells/mm^3. Hematologic toxicity has been decreased using recombinant erythropoietin (114). Zidovudine is metabolized by the liver. Anecdotal cases of fatty liver sometimes resulting in death have been reported in women receiving ZDV (115,116). Nonmetastasizing vaginal tumors have been reported in long-term, high-dose ZDV studies in rodents (117); toxicology experts believe that it is unlikely that this observation predicts human carcinogenicity.

Zidovudine may reduce perinatal transmission by reducing maternal HIV burden in peripheral blood, placenta, or cervico-vaginal secretions; providing preexposure prophylaxis to the infant; or eliminating early infection in the placenta, fetus, or infant. Transplacental passage of ZDV has been confirmed (118). Zidovudine does not cause malformations in animals (117,119); however, it has been shown to be embryotoxic (120). The effect of first-trimester exposure in humans is unknown. No significant fetal malformations have been noted in two observational studies (121,122). Transient, reversible anemia was observed in newborns when zidovudine was given during pregnancy, labor, and to the newborn for 6 weeks (16).

VII. Other Therapies for HIV Infection

Four other nucleoside analogs are available as licensed alternatives to zidovudine for those who cannot tolerate or who experience disease progression on zidovudine. Little information is available about the safety or effectiveness of any of these during pregnancy. They are didanosine (ddI, dideoxyinosine, Videx), currently being studied in a Phase 1 pregnancy trial; stavudine (d4T, Zerit), for which a similar Phase I trial is being initiated; zalcitabine (dideoxycytidine, ddC, HIVID); and 3TC (Lamivudine), which is being incorporated into a combination perinatal prophylaxis study planned by the pediatric ACTG. Didanosine has less hematological toxicity than ZDV, but has been associated with pancreatitis and peripheral neuropathy (123). Zalcitabine may cause peripheral neuropathy and, less frequently, pancreatitis (124). Stavudine may also cause peripheral neuropathy (125). Lamivudine appears to cause less peripheral neuropathy or pancreatitis and has no apparent marrow suppressant effect (126).

Non-nucleoside analogs such as nevirapine and delavirdine rapidly decrease viral load (127). Since nevirapine is associated with rapid development of viral resistance, it may be most useful for short-term treatment or in combination with another therapy. Nevirapine is currently being studied in Phase I clinical trials in newborns and their mothers.

A new class of drugs, the protease inhibitors, has been approved by the FDA for treatment of HIV infection. Saquinavir (Inverase), the first, is highly effective (as are the others) in decreasing viral load by as much as threefold (128). It, indinavir, and ritonavir will be studied in Phase I protocols in pregnant women within a year.

VIII. Pregnancy Effects

Pregnancy does not appear to have an adverse effect on the course of HIV disease, at least as measured by decline in CD4 counts over time (129). However, early in the epidemic, women were identified as HIV infected sometime after they delivered a child diagnosed with AIDS. Since progression to death was noted with 2 years after delivery, it was thought that pregnancy affected disease progression (130,131). Prospective studies show pregnancy uncomplicated by injection drug use or symptoms of HIV infection despite mild to moderate immunosuppression does not strongly influence progression to AIDS (132–137).

Whether cell-mediated immunity is altered in pregnancy and whether this is accounted for by changes in circulating T-cell numbers or functions is debatable. There are reports of altered CMI (138–141) but, as discussed at length in Chapter 4 of this volume, these changes are small in magnitude and are probably of minor clinical significance. A decline of circulating CD4+ T cells in late pregnancy with a return to baseline postpartum was observed in a small series of HIV-1-infected and HIV-uninfected pregnant women (142) but has not been confirmed (143, 144). Comparing HIV-infected pregnant women to HIV-infected nonpregnant women, CD4+ lymphocyte counts decline at similar rates regardless of pregnancy or the number of pregnancies (129). A decrease in CD4+ T cells could increase the risk of opportunistic infection during pregnancy. In one study, 5 of 16 HIV-1-infected women with CD4 counts less than 300 cells/μL had serious or opportunistic infections during pregnancy (100). Zidovudine (or any retroviral) may increase or stabilize CD4 counts (11,110–114), and blunt any pregnancy- or HIV-induced changes in cell-mediated immunity or CD4+ T-lymphocyte counts.

Early in the epidemic, PCP was the most commonly reported cause of AIDS-related mortality during pregnancy or in the year following delivery (145). This risk has been minimized with routine PCP prophylaxis for those with CD4+ counts below 200 cells/μL. Tuberculosis could become the most common cause of AIDS-related mortality in women, as it has become in Africa (146). Nonetheless, most pregnant women with CD4+ T-cell counts below 200 cells/μL do not develop other opportunistic infections. Thus, although AIDS can occur during pregnancy, survival time may not be reduced compared with nonpregnant women (134).

There is no evidence that HIV-1-infected women are less fertile than uninfected women; in fact, there is a relatively high rate of second pregnancies (147–149). The spontaneous abortion rate may be higher in some populations of HIV-1-infected women than in uninfected women, perhaps related to STDs or HIV, rather than hormonal abnormalities (31,150). HIV-1 infection does not seem to be teratogenic. Although, initially an HIV-1-related craniofacial dysmorphism was described, a comparison group was lacking (151,152), and prospective studies have subsequently failed to demonstrate an HIV-1-related dysmorphism (153–155).

Early in the epidemic, there were concerns that HIV-1 infection increased preterm birth, low birth weight, premature rupture of membranes, and obstetric infectious morbidity (156,157). Prospective studies comparing asymptomatic HIV-1-infected women to uninfected women of similar race, socioeconomic status, and drug use show no significant differences in the rates of preterm birth, low birth weight, low Apgar scores, or premature rupture of membranes (136,137,158). HIV-infected infants are of similar birth weight and gestational age as those who serorevert (loss of maternal HIV-1 antibody in exposed, uninfected infants) (159–161). The effect of the timing of HIV-1 transmission on short-term pregnancy outcome remains unknown, but infection rarely seems to increase the obstetrical complications of pregnancy.

African studies report a higher rate of advanced HIV-1 disease in pregnant women than the European and American cohorts. Preterm birth, low birth weight, a decreased head circumference-to-height ratio, and chorioamnionitis are significantly more common in symptomatic HIV infection during pregnancy compared to asymptomatic seropositive or seronegative mothers (76,79,80,162–164). While this may be related to HIV-1 infection itself, it could also reflect poor nutrition, other maternal infections initiating preterm labor, or poor access to HIV-1 treatment and care.

IX. Neonatal/Infant Outcome

HIV-1-infected lymphocytes are sequestered in fetal tissues such as fetal thymus (31). However, the natural history of the infection in children differs from that in adults. Signs and symptoms are rarely present at birth and may develop over months or years (67–69,165). For about 25% of infected children, progression to AIDS occurs rapidly in the first year of life; presumably these infants were infected in utero. The mortality for children with HIV infection is high, approaching 28% by 5 years of age in several studies. The rapid progression and death in children compared with adults is possibly related to immaturity of the immune system at the time of infection, inability to mount an appropriate response over time, or factors unique to perinatal transmission of infection. Infants with HIV infection experience primary infection with opportunistic organisms, rather than reactivation of such infections as occurs in adults. Early identification and aggressive treatment has lead to a decrease in HIV-related pediatric mortality, but children generally remain persistently infected with HIV throughout their life. There have been reports of transiently positive cultures or PCR tests during the first 6 months of life which became negative and the children have remained culture-, PCR-, and antibody-negative. These children represent transient infection with clearing of the virus or, less likely, a false-positive diagnosis because of technical problems with the assays (166).

X. Principles of Prenatal Care

In general, obstetricians should coordinate comprehensive health care of women newly diagnosed with HIV infection or those women with symptoms, especially when first identified in pregnancy, during prepregnancy counseling, or as a result of routinely offered screening during annual gynecological visits. Nonspecific symptoms including fatigue, weight loss, and difficulty swallowing and breathing should be carefully evaluated, as they may be early signs of HIV-related disease. Unless the obstetrician has had significant experience with HIV infection in women, an infectious disease specialist should be consulted. Antepartum testing, including sonography, nonstress testing, and intrapartum fetal monitoring, should be done only if otherwise clinically indicated, not solely because the woman is HIV-infected.

ZDV therapy to prevent transmission requires monthly maternal monitoring for bone marrow suppression or liver damage (17). The drug should be interrupted or stopped if the hemoglobin is less than 8 g/dL, absolute neutrophil count is less than 750 cells/μL, or AST or ALT is greater than 5 times the normal value. A CD4+ T-cell lymphocyte count should be done initially and a viral load considered before initiating ZDV treatment. These tests should be repeated later in pregnancy, especially if the CD4+ count is initially low, i.e., between 200 and 500 cells/μL. PCP prophylaxis should be initiated when the maternal CD4+ count is <200 cells/μL. At birth, 6 weeks, and 12 weeks of age, the newborn should have a CBC and differential. Published recommendations for diagnosing HIV infection in infants, and for initiating PCP prophylaxis and antiretroviral therapy for those infected, should be followed.

HIV-1-infected women who do not have evidence of previous hepatitis B infection can be immunized; both pneumococcal and flu vaccines should be considered (167).

Since HIV infection affects mucosal immunity, genital tract infections, especially candida and human papilloma virus, occur commonly in both pregnant and nonpregnant HIV-infected women (168,169). Accordingly, care of the HIV-infected pregnant women should include screening and treatment of candida and sexually or vertically transmitted diseases known to influence pregnancy outcome. In particular, syphilis is more common in HIV-infected pregnant women and requires treatment to prevent congenital disease (170).

Screening for tuberculosis is an essential part of prenatal care for HIV-infected women. It includes a medical history, tuberculin skin test [Mantoux test of purified protein derivative (PPD)] with an anergy panel using candida, mumps, or tetanus skin test antigens. If indicated, a baseline chest radiograph should be obtained (171). If tuberculosis treatment is warranted, it should be monitored to decrease the likelihood of drug-resistant disease resulting from treatment noncompliance.

A common AIDS-defining infection, PCP, has a mortality rate of 5–20% after the first episode and a high recurrence rate for those not receiving prophylaxis (12,172). The U.S. Public Health Service recommends that patients at high risk for PCP receive primary and secondary prophylaxis to reduce the frequency of initial episodes and relapses (173). Lifetime prophylaxis is indicated for those with a history of PCP, or CD4+ count less than $200/\mu L$ or 20% of total circulating lymphocytes. Those with oropharyngeal candidiasis unrelated to medication therapy or with unexplained, persistent fever for more than 2 weeks should also receive antifungal prophylaxis. Preventive therapy for PCP and several other infections, including disseminated *Mycobacterium avium* complex, toxoplasma encephalitis, and cryptococcal meningitis, has been discussed elsewhere (108,174–178). Since the fetal safety of HIV-related therapies may not be known, the benefits of beginning treatment must be weighed against the potential adverse fetal effects and the risk of delaying treatment until after delivery (179).

Every attempt should be made to minimize fetal or newborn exposure to infectious maternal blood and secretions (Table 5). During labor and delivery, anti-infection precautions must be used to prevent the woman and health care workers from unnecessary exposure to HIV or other pathogens (180,181). Gloves, masks, eye shields, caps, and water-repellant gowns should be worn for every delivery. Meconium should be suctioned as indicated by mechanical suction.

Breast feeding should be avoided. Women should be informed about contraceptive and risk-reduction behaviors to decrease the risk of sexual transmission, e.g., abstinence, condoms, etc. The possibility of transmission through needle sharing should be discussed and, if appropriate, enrollment in a drug treatment program is indicated. The use of nonintravenous drugs such as crack cocaine is an indirect risk factor for HIV infection; women who are addicts may trade sex for drugs.

Table 5 Approaches to Reduce the Transmission of HIV from Mother to Child

Avoid breast feeding
Zidovudine prophylaxis during pregnancy, delivery, and to the neonate
Investigate other antiretroviral agents
Treat sexually transmitted diseases
Reduce exposure to maternal blood and secretions
   Avoid invasive procedures
      Amniocentesis, especially through an anterior placenta
      External cephalic version
      Chorion villus sampling
      Percutaneous umbilical blood sampling
      Fetal scalp sampling
      Fetal scalp monitoring
      Amnioinfusion
      Episiotomy
      Artificial amniotomy
      Caesarean section
      Investigate vaginal disinfection
Investigate immunotherapy for the mother or infant
   Passive therapy
   Active immunization

XI. Future Considerations

As the epidemic continues among women and children, with prophylaxis available to reduce perinatal transmission, screening for HIV infection during pregnancy is important for both maternal and child health. When obstetricians know a woman is HIV-infected, they can provide optimal health care, offer ZDV prophylaxis and/or other antiretroviral indicated therapy, treat HIV-related infections, limit invasive procedures that may increase risk of mother-to-child transmission, and be sure the women is in the health care system and referred for the proper social services for her and her child. Pediatricians can be aware of the potentially infected child, provide prophylaxis, determine infection status early, and potentially initiate aggressive early infant treatment as indicated.

HIV treatments are rapidly evolving, and women are receiving multiple therapies during pregnancy. Many newer drugs have unknown toxicities during pregnancy, so it is important to gather information about their benefits and side effects in both nonpregnant as well as pregnant adults, and to anticipate their potential benefits and toxicities for HIV-infected mothers and their children. Ideally this should be done in controlled trials. All women who are on antiretrovirals should be included in the Burroughs-Wellcome, Glaxo-Wellcome Registry, to gather information about the effects of these agents.

As a result of AIDS Clinical Trials Group Protocol 076, progress has been made in reducing perinatal transmission in a specific group of asymptomatic pregnant women given ZDV during pregnancy intrapartum and to the neonate for the first 6 weeks of life; whether ZDV will have a significant impact on a broader population is unknown. Several research questions remain. Why did transmission occur for some, despite ZDV? The reduction in viral load in the ZDV-exposed women does not entirely explain the decreased perinatal transmission. The relative efficacy of the three components of the ZDV regimen must be delineated. To simplify the ZDV regimen, the safety and pharmacokinetics of oral ZDV during labor is being studied. Whether perinatal transmission of maternal ZDV-resistant HIV occurs is being explored. The risk of minor and major congenital anomalies with first-trimester antiretroviral use must be determined, although to date there have been no reported abnormalities related at least to ZDV. The long-term risks of ZDV to the woman and/or her child are being assessed by two AIDS clinical trials, one for women and one for all children exposed during pregnancy.

Other interventions for reducing perinatal transmissions are being pursued with the goal of complete prevention of transmission. One study, a randomized, double-blind, controlled clinical trial of the use of HIV-IgG versus IV-IgG in pregnant women who were also receiving ZDV was stopped early. Their newborns received the standard ZDV regimen (ACTG 185). This was stopped because ZDV is effective and HIVIG did not work. (See Note Added in Proof.) A Phase III study using nevirapine is being planned for women who enter prenatal care late in pregnancy or who refuse ZDV. Phase I safety and pharmacokinetic studies are ongoing or planned to evaluate the use of several other antiretroviral agents during pregnancy or delivery. The drugs studied will include ddI, d4T, and the protease inhibitors. Once initial data are obtained, a triple-therapy trial will likely be the next step to attain a goal of nearly total elimination of perinatal HIV transmission. One vaccine trial has been completed; the data are being tabulated. Other immune therapy strategies are awaiting drug development and better understanding of viral heterogenecity and cell penetrance.

Tremendous progress has been made in understanding HIV and its characteristics. Unfortunately, the long-awaited cure has not arrived. The rapid spread of infection in women and their children significantly affects the family, and leaves orphaned HIV-infected and uninfected children. Certainly all pregnant women should be offered HIV counseling and testing with appropriate follow-up. All men and women should also be offered the same opportunity. Obstetrician-gynecologists and other primary-care providers have a unique opportunity to integrate this screening as part of preventive health care. The continued education of the public at large is essential.

Note Added in Proof

ACTG 185, a randomized, double-blind, controlled clinical trial of the use of HIV-IgG versus IV-IgG in pregnant women and infants who were receiving the standard doses of ZDV to prevent mother-to-child transmission was discontinued early. The transmission rates in the HIV-IgG and IV-IgG groups were 4.7% and 4.8%, demonstrating that 1) ZDV is effective in preventing transmission, even in those who are sicker with HIV infection and 2) HIV-IgG offers no added benefit in reducing transmission.

Acknowledgment

The opinions expressed in this article are those of the author and do not represent the official position of the U.S. Public Health Service

References

1. Nicoll A, Timaeus I, Kigadye RM, Walraven G, Killewo J. Impact of the human immunodeficiency virus epidemic on mortality in children under 5 years of age in sub-Saharan Africa: a demographic and epidemiologic analysis. AIDS 1994; 8:995–1005.
2. Gwinn M, Redus MA, Granade TC. HIV-1 serologic test results for one million newborn dried blood specimens: assay performance and implications for screening. J Acquir Immun Defic Syndr 1992; 5:505–512.
3. National Center for Health Statistics. Annual summary of births, marriages, divorces, and deaths: United States, 1993. Monthly Vital statistics Report. Vol. 42, No. 13. Hyattsville, MD: U.S. Public Health Service, 1994.
4. Chin J. Current and future dimensions of the HIV/AIDS pandemic in women and children. Lancet 1990; 336:221–224.
5. McCarthy M. World bank warns of AIDS economic threat. Lancet 1994; 344:1628.
6. Centers for Disease Control and Prevention. HIV/AIDS Surveillance Report 1994; 6(no. 2):1–39.
7. Ellerbrook TV, Bush TJ, Chamberland ME, Oxtoby MJ. Epidemiology of women with AIDS in the United States, 1981 through 1990: a comparison with heterosexual men with AIDS. JAMA 1991; 265:2971–2975.

8. Whyte BM, Swanson CE, Cooper DA. Survival of patients with the acquired immunodeficiency syndrome in Australia Med J Austral 1989; 150:358–362.

9. Moore RD, Hidalgo J, Sugland BW, Chaisson RE. Zidovudine and the natural history of the acquired immunodeficiency syndrome. N Engl J Med 1991; 324:1412–1416.

10. Lemp GF, Hirozawa AM, Cohen JB, Derish PA, McKinney KC, Hernandez SR. Survival for women and men with AIDS. J Infect Dis 1992; 166:74–79.

11. Lagakas S, Fischl MA, Stein DS, Lim L, Volberding P. Effects of zidovudine therapy in minority and other subpopulations with early HIV infection. JAMA 1991; 266:2709–2712.

12. Bastian L, Bennett CL, Adams J, Waskin H, Divine G, Edlin BR. Differences between men and women with HIV-related *Pneumocystis carinii* pneumonia: Experience from 3,070 cases in New York City in 1987. J Acquir Immun Defic Syndr 1993; 6:617–623.

13. Chaisson RE, Keruly JC, Moore RD. Race, sex, drug use, and progression of human immunodeficiency virus disease. N Engl J Med 1995; 333:751–756.

14. Newell ML, Peckham C. Risk factors for vertical transmission of HIV-1 and early markers of HIV-1 infection in children. AIDS 1993; 7(suppl):S91–S97.

15. The Working Group on Mother-to-Child Transmission of HIV. Rates of mother-to-child transmission of HIV in Africa, America, and Europe: results from 13 perinatal studies. J Acquir Immune Defic Syndr 1995; 8:1495–1497.

16. Connor E, Sperling RS, Gelber R, Kiselev P, Scott G, O'Sullivan MJ, VanDyke R, Bey M, Shearer W, Jacobson R, Jimenez E, O'Neill E, Bazin B, Delfraissy JF, Culnane M, Coombs, R, Maha-Elkins M, Moye J, Stratton P, Balsley J. Zidovudine decreases the rate of maternal-infant transmission of human immunodeficiency virus 1. N Engl J Med 1994; 331:1173–1180.

17. Centers for Disease Control and Prevention. Recommendations for the use of zidovudine to reduce perinatal transmission of human immunodeficiency virus. Morbid Mortal Weekly Rep 1994; 43(RR-11):1–20.

18. The American Academy of Pediatrics and The American College of Obstetricians and Gynecologists. Joint statement on human immunodeficiency virus screening, August 1995.

19. Haseltine WA. Molecular biology of the human immunodeficiency virus type 1. FASEB J 1991; 5:2349–2360.

20. Parslow TG, Hope TJ. Structure and expression of the HIV-1 genome. In: Cohen PT, Sande MA, Volberding PA, eds. The AIDS Knowledge Base. 2d ed. 1994; chap. 3.2:1–7.

21. Koyanagi Y, Miles S, Mitsuyasu R, Merrill JE, Vinters HV, Chen ISY. Dual infection of the central nervous system by AIDS viruses with distinct cellular tropisms. Science 1987; 236:819–822.

22. Wiley C, Schrier R, Nelson J, et al. Cellular localization of human immunodeficiency virus infection within the brains of acquired immune deficiency syndrome patients. Proc Natl Acad Sci USA 1986; 83:7089–7093.

23. Cheng-Meyer C, Tutka J, Rosenblum M, McHugh T, Sites DP, Levy JA. Human immunodeficiency virus can productively infect cultured human glial cells. Proc Natl Acad Sci USA 1987; 84:3526–3530.

24. Nelson JA, Reynolds-Kohler C, Margaretten W, Wiley CA, Reese CE, Levy JA. Human immunodeficiency virus detected in bowel epithelium from patients with gastrointestinal symptoms. Lancet 1988; i:259–262.

25. Phillips DM, Bourinbaiar AS. Mechanism of HIV spread from lymphocytes to epithelia Virology 1992; 186:261–273.

26. Maury W, Potts BJ, Rabson AB. HIV-1 infection of first-trimester and term human placental tissue: a possible mode of maternal-fetal transmission. J Infect Dis 1989; 160:583–588.

27. Phillips DM, Tan X. HIV-1 infection of the trophoblast cell line BeWo: a study of virus uptake. AIDS Res Hum Retro 1992; 8:1683–1691.

28. Zachar V, Norskov-Lauritsen N, Juhl C, Spire B, Chermann JC, Ebbesen P. Susceptibility of cultured human trophoblasts to infection with human immunodeficiency virus type 1. J Gen Virol 1991; 72:1253–1260.

29. Mano H, Chermann JC. Replication of human immunodeficiency virus type 1 in primary cultured placental cells. Res Virol 1991; 142:95–104.

30. Lewis SH, Reynolds-Kohler C, Fox HE, Nelson JA. HIV-1 in trophoblastic and villous Hofbauer cells, and hematologic precursors in eight-week fetuses. Lancet 1990; 335:565–568.

31. Langston C., Lewis DE, Hammill HA, Popek, EJ, Kozinitz CA, Kline MN, Hanson IC, Shearer WT. Excess intrauterine fetal demise associated with maternal fetal immunodeficiency virus infection. J Infect Dis 1995; 172:1451–1460.

32. Feng Y, Broder CC, Kennedy PE, Berger EA. HIV-1 entry cofactor functional cDNA cloning of a seven transmembrane G protein-coupled receptor. Science 1996; 272:872–877.

33. Berson JF, Long D, Doranz BJ, et al. A seven transmembrane domain receptor involved in fusion and entry of T-cell-tropic human immunodeficiency virus type 1 stains. J. Virol 1996; 70:6288–6295.

34. Levy JA. Infection by human immunodeficiency virus—CD4 is not enough. N Engl J Med 1996; 335:1528–1530.

35. Liu R, Paxon WA, Choe S, et al. Homozygous defect in HIV-1 co-receptor accounts for resistance for some multiple exposed individuals to HIV-1 infection. Cell 1996; 86:367–377.

36. Samson M, Libert F, Doranz BJ et al. Resistance to HIV-1 infection in caucasian individuals bearing mutant alleles of the CCR-5 chemokine receptor gene. Nature 1996; 382:722–725.

37. Dean M, Carrington M, Winkler C, et al. Genetic restriction of HIV-1 infection and progression to AIDS by a deletion allele of the CKR5 structural gene. Science 1996; 273:156–162.

38. Preston BD, Piesz BJ, Loeb LA. Fidelity of HIV-1 reverse transcriptase. Science 1988; 242:1168–1171.

39. Robert JD, Bebenek K, Kunkel TA. The accuracy of reverse transcriptase from HIV-1. Science 1988; 242:1171–1173.

40. Lewis P, Hensel M, Emerman M. Human immunodeficiency virus infection of cells arrested in the cell cycle. EMBO J 1992; 11:3053–3058.

41. Sakai H, Kawamura M, Sakuragi J, et al. Integration is essential for efficient gene expression of human immunodeficiency virus type 1. J Virol 1993; 67: 1169–1174.

42. Frankel AD. Activation of HIV transcription by Tat. Curr Opin Genet Devel 1992; 2:293–298.

43. Malim MK, Hauber J, Fenrick R, et al. Immunodeficiency virus rev trans-activator modulates the expression of the viral regulatory genes. Nature 1988; 335:181–183.

44. Kohl NE, Emini EA, Schleif WA. Active human immunodeficiency virus protease is required for viral infectivity. Proc Natl Acad Sci USA 1988; 85: 4686–4690.

45. Tindall B, Cooper DA. Primary HIV infection: host responses and intervention strategies. AIDS 1991; 5:1–14.

46. Pantaleo G, Graziosi C, Fauci AS. The immunopathogenesis of human immunodeficiency virus infection. N Engl J Med 1993; 328:327–335.

47. Mellors JW, Kinsley LA, Rinaldo CRJ, et al. Quantitation of HIV-1 RNA in plasma predicts outcome after seroconversion. Ann Intern Med 1995; 122: 575–579.

48. Daar ES, Moudgil T, Meyer RD, Ho DD. Transient high levels of viremia in patients with primary human immunodeficiency virus type 1 infection. N Engl J Med 1991; 324:961–964.

49. Clark SJ, Saag MS, Decker WD, Campbell-Hill S, Roberson JL, Veldkamp PJ, Kappes JC, Hahn BH, Shaw GM. High titers of cytopathic virus in plasma of patients with symptomatic primary HIV-1 infection. N Engl J Med 1991; 324:954–960.

50. Fauci AS. Immunopathogenesis of HIV infection, J Acquir Immun Defic Syndr 1993; 6:655–662.

51. Mellors JW, Rinaldo CR, Gupta G, et al. Prognosis in HIV-1 infection predicted by the quantity of virus in the plasma. Science 1996; 272:1167–1170.

52. O'Brien WA, Hartigan PM, Martin D, Eisenhart J. Changes in plasma HIV-1 RNA and CD4+ lymphocyte count relative to treatment and progression to AIDS. N Engl J Med 1996; 334:426–431.

53. Wei X, Ghosh SK, Taylor ME, et al. Viral dynamices in human immunodeficiency virus type 1 infection. Nature 1995; 73:117–122.

54. Hammer SM, Kagenstein DA, Hughes MD, et al. A trial comparing nucleociole monotherapy with combination therapy in HIV infected adults with CD4 cell counts from 200 to 500 per cubic millimeter. N Engl J Med 1996; 335:1081–1090.

55. Delta Coordinating Committee. A randomized double blind controlled trial comparing combinations of zidovudine plus didanosine or zalcitabine with zidovudine alone in HIV infected individuals. Lancet 1996; 348:283–291.

56. Cao Y, Qin L, Zhangl, Safrit J, Ho DD. Virologic and immunologic characterization of long-term survivors of human immunodeficiency virus type 1 infection. N Engl J Med 1995; 332:201–208.

57. Pantaleo G, Menzo S, Vaccarezza M, Graziosis C, Cohen OJ, Damarest JF, Montefiori D, Orenstein JM, Fox C, Schrager LK, Margolick JB, Buchbinder S, Giorgi JV, Fauci AS. Studies in subjects with long-term nonprogressive human immunodeficiency virus infection. N Engl J Med 1995; 332:209–216.

58. Kirchhoff F, Greenough TC, Brettler DB, Sullivan JL, Desrosiers. Brief report: absence of intact nef sequences in a long term survivor with nonprogressive HIV-1 infection. N Engl J Med 1995; 332:228–230.

59. Centers for Disease Control and Prevention. 1993 revised classification system for HIV infection and expanded surveillance case definition for AIDS among adolescents and adults. Morbid Mortal Weekly Rep 1992; 41(RR-17):1–19.

60. Vella S, Chiesi A, Volpi A, Giuliano M, Floridia M, Dally LG, Binkin N. Differential survival of patients with AIDS according to the 1987 and 1993 CDC case definitions. JAMA 1994; 271:1197–1199.

61. Report of a Consensus Workshop, Siena, Italy, January 17–18, 1992. Early diagnosis of HIV infection in infants. J Acquir Immun Defic Syndr 1992; 5: 1169–1175.

62. Centers for Disease Control. Interpretation and use of Western blot for serodiagnosis of human immunodeficiency virus type 1 infection. Morbid Mortal Weekly Rep 1989; 38(suppl):S1–S7.

63. Simonon A, Lepage P, Karita E, Hitimana DG, Dabis F, Msellati P, Van Geothem C, Nsengumuremyi F, Bazubagira A, Van de Perre P. An assessment of the timing of mother-to-child transmission of human immunodeficiency virus type 1 by means of polymerase chain reaction. J Acquir Immun Defic Syndr 1994; 7:952–957.

64. Jovaisis E, Koch MA, Schafer A, Stauber A, Stauber M, Lowenthal D. LAV/HTLV-III in a 20-week fetus. Lancet 1985; 2:1129.

65. Sprecher S, Soumenkoff G, Puissant F, Degueldre M. Vertical transmission of HIV in a 15-week fetus. Lancet 1986; 2:288–289.

66. Bryson YJ, Luzuriaga K, Sullivan JL, Wara DW. Proposed definition for in utero versus intrapartum transmission of HIV-1. N Engl J Med 1992; 327: 1246–1247.

67. Rouzioux C, Costagliola D, Burgard M, Blanche S, Mayaux MJ, Griscelli C, Valleron AJ, and the HIV Infection in Newborns French Collaborative Study Group. Timing of mother-to-child HIV-1 transmission depends on maternal status. AIDS 1993; 7(suppl 2):S49–S52.

68. The European Collaborative Study. Natural history of vertically acquired human immunodeficiency virus-1 infection. Pediatrics 1994; 94:815–819.

69. Italian Register for HIV Infection in Children. Features of children perinatally infected with HIV-1 surviving longer than 5 years. Lancet 1994; 343: 191–195.

70. Sperling RS, Shapiro DE, Coombs R, et al. Maternal viral load and the success of zidovudine for the reduction of maternal infant HIV-1 transmission. N Engl J Med 1996; 335:1621.

71. Borkowsky W, Krasinski K, Cao Y, et al. Correlation of perinatal transmission of human immunodeficiency virus type 1 with maternal viremia and lymphocyte phenotypes. J Pediatr 1994; 125:345–351.

72. Weiser B, Nachman S, Tropper P, Viscosi KH, Grimson R, Baxter G, Fang Guowei, Reyelt C, Hutcheon N, Burger H. Quantitation of human immunodeficiency virus type 1 during pregnancy: relationship of viral titer to mother-to-child transmission and stability of viral load. Proc Natl Acad Sci USA 1994; 91:8037–8041.

73. Roques P, Marce D, Courpotin C, et al. Correlation between HIV provirus burden and in utero transmission. AIDS 1993; 7(suppl 2):S39–S43.

74. Mayaux MJ, Blanche S, Rouzioux C, Chenadec JL, Chambrin V, Firtion G, Allemon MC, Vilmer E, Vigneron NC, Tricoire J, Guillot F, Courpotin C, and the French Pediatric HIV Infection Study Group. Maternal factors associated with perinatal HIV-1 transmission: the French Cohort Study: 7 years of follow-up observation. J Acquir Immun Defic Syndr Hum Retro 1996; 8:188–194.

75. Boyer PJ, Dillon M, Navaie M, Deveikis A, Keller M, O'Rourke S, Bryson YJ. Factors predictive of maternal-fetal transmission of HIV-1: preliminary analysis of zidovudine given during pregnancy and/or delivery. JAMA 1994; 271:1925–1930.

76. St. Louis ME, Kamenga M, Brown C, Nelson AM, Manzila T, Batter V, Behets F, Kabagabo U, Ryder RW, Oxtoby M, Quinn TC, Heyward WL. Risk for perinatal HIV-1 transmission according to maternal immunologic, virologic, and placental factors. JAMA 1993; 269:2853–2859.

77. Bredberg-Raden U, Urassa W, Urassa E, Lyamuya E, Msemo G, Kawo G, Kazimoto T, Massawe A, Grankvist O, Mbena E, Karlsson K, Mhalu F, Biberfeld G. Predictive markers for mother-to-child transmission of HIV-1 in Dar es Salaam, Tanzania. J Acquir Immun Defic Syndr Hum Retro 1995; 8:182–187.

78. Erb P, Krauchi S, Burgin D, Biedermann K, Camli C, Rudin C, and the Swiss HIV and Pregnancy Collaborative Study Group. Quantitative anti-p24 determinations can predict the risk of transmission. J Acquir Immun Defic Syndr 1994; 7:261–264.

79. Temmerman M, Nyong'o AO, Bwayo J, Fransen K, Coppens M, Piot P. Risk factors for mother-to-child transmission of human immunodeficiency virus-1 infection. Am J Obstet Gynecol 1995; 172:700–705.

80. Ryder RW, Nsa W, Hassig SE, et al. Perinatal transmission of the human immunodeficiency virus type 1 to infants of seropositive women in Zaire. N Engl J Med 1989; 320:1643–1648.

81. Palasanthiran P, Ziegler JB, Stewart GJ, et al. Breast-feeding during primary maternal human immunodeficiency virus infection and risk of transmission from mother to infant. J Infect Dis 1993; 167:441–444.

82. Van de Perre P, Simonon A, Msellati P, et al. Postnatal transmission of human immunodeficiency virus type 1 from mother to infant. N Engl J Med 1991; 325:593–598.

83. Scarlatti G, Albert J, Rossi P, Hodara V, Biraghi P, Muggiasca L, Fenyo EM. Mother-to-child transmission of human immunodeficiency virus type 1: correlation with neutralizing antibodies against primary isolates. J Infect Dis 1993; 167:207–210.

84. Klik SC, Wara DW, Landers DV, Levy JA. Features of HIV-1 that could influence maternal-child transmission. JAMA 1994; 272:467–474.

85. Wolinsky SM, Wike CM, Korber BTM, et al. Selective transmission of human immunodeficiency virus type-1: variants from mothers to infants. Science 1992; 255:1134–1137.

86. Rossi P, Moschese V, Broliden PA, et al. Presence of maternal antibodies to human immunodeficiency virus 1 envelope glycoprotein gp120 epitopes correlates with the noninfective status of children born to seropositive mothers. Proc Natl Acad Sci USA 1989; 86:8055–8058.

87. Parekh BS, Shaffer N, Pau C-P, et al. Lack of correlation between maternal antibodies to V3 loop peptides of gp120 and perinatal HIV-1 transmission: the NYC Perinatal HIV Transmission Collaborative Study. AIDS 1991; 5: 1179–1184.

88. Bawdon RE, Gravell M, Hamilton R, Sever J, Miller R. Gibbs CJ. Studies on the placental transfer of cell-free human immunodeficiency virus and p24 antigen in an ex vivo human placental model. J Soc Gynecol Invest 1994; 1:45–48.

89. Peuchmaur M, Delfaissy JF, Pons JC, et al. HIV proteins absent from placentas of 75 HIV-1 positive women studied by immunochemistry. AIDS 1991; 5:741–745.

90. Jauniaux E, Nessmann C, Imbert C, et al. Morphological aspects of the placenta in HIV pregnancies. Placenta 1988; 9:633–642.

91. Chandwani S, Greco MA, Mittal K, et al. Pathology and human immunodeficiency virus expression in placentas of seropositive women. J Infect Dis 1991; 163:1134–1138.

92. Nelson AM, Firpo A, Kamenga M, et al Pediatrics AIDS and perinatal HIV infection in Zaire: epidemiologic and pathologic findings. Prog AIDS Pathol 1992; 3:1–33.

93. Nair P, Alger L, Hines S, Seiden S, Hebel R, Johnson JP. Maternal and neonatal characteristics associated with HIV infection in infants of seropositive women. J Acquir Immun Defic Syndr 1993; 6:298–302.

94. Ongradi J, Ceccherini-Nelli L, Pistell M, et al. Acid sensitivity of cell-free and cell-associated HIV-1: clinical implications. AIDS Res Hum Retro 1990; 6:1433–1436.

95. Goedert JJ, Duliege AM, Amos CI, et al. High risk of HIV-1 infection for first-born twins. Lancet 1991; 338:147–1474.

96. The European Collaborative Study. Caesarean section and risk of vertical transmission on HIV infection. Lancet 1994; 343:1464–1467.

97. Dunn DT, Newell ML, Mayaux MJ, Kind C, Hutto C, Goedert JJ, Andiman W, and Perinatal AIDS Collaborative Transmission Studies. Mode of delivery and vertical transmission of HIV-1: a review of prospective studies. J Acquir Immun Defic Syndr 1994; 7:1064–1066.

98. Villari P, Spino C, Chalmers TC, Lau J, Sacks HS. Caesarean section to reduce perinatal transmission of human immunodeficiency virus. Online J Curr Clin Trials 1993; 2:July 8 (Doc. no. 74).

99. Burkett G, Jensen L, Lai A, O'Sullivan MJ Evaluation of surgical staples in caesarean section. Am J Obstet Gynecol 1990; 161:540–547.

100. Minkoff HL, Willoughby A, Mendez H, et al. Serious infections during pregnancy among women with advanced human immunodeficiency virus infection. Am J Obstet Gynecol 1990; 162:30–34.

101. Bigger RJ, Miotti PG, Taha TE, et al. Perinatal intervention trial in Africa: effect of a birth canal cleansing intervention to prevent HIV transmission. Lancet 1996; 347:1647–1650.

102. Ziegler JB, Johnson RO, Cooper DA, et al. Postnatal transmission of AIDS-associated retrovirus from mother to infant. Lancet 1985; 1:896–897.

103. De Martino M, Tove PA, Tozzi AE, et al. HIV-1 transmission through breastmilk: appraisal of risk according to duration of feeding. J Acquir Immun. Defic Syndr 1992; 6:991–999.

104. Van de Perre P, Simonon A, Hitimana DG, et al. Infective and anti-infective properties of breastmilk from HIV-1 infected women. Lancet 1993; 341: 914–918.

105. European Collaborative Study. Risk factors for mother-to-child transmission of HIV-1. Lancet 1992; 339:1007–1012.

106. The HIV Infection in Newborns French Collaborative Study Group. Comparison of vertical human immunodeficiency virus type 2 and human immunodeficiency virus type 1 transmission in the French prospective cohort. Pediatr Inf Dis J 1994; 13:502–506.

107. Dunn DT, Newell ML, Ades AE, Peckham CS. Risk of human immunodeficiency virus type 1 transmission through breast-feeding. Lancet 1992; 340: 585–588.

108. Stratton P. Treatment options and care of HIV-infected pregnant women. Ped AIDS HIV Inf 1996; 5:333–343.

109. Institute of Medicine. Prenatal screening for HIV infection. In: Hardy LM, ed. HIV Screening of Pregnant Women and Newborns. Washington, DC: National Academy Press, 1991:33.

110. Volberding PA, Lagakos SW, Grimes JM, Stein DS, Balfour HH, Reichman RC, Bartlett JA, Hirsch MS, Phair JP, Mitsuyasu RT, Fischl MA, Soeiro R, for the AIDS Clinical Trials Group of the National Institute of Allergy and Infectious Diseases. The duration of zidovudine benefit in persons with asymptomatic HIV infection: prolonged evaluation of protocol 019 of the AIDS Clincial Trials Group. JAMA 1994: 272:437–442.

111. Carpenter CC, Fischl MA, Hammer SM, et al. Antiretroviral therapy for HIV infection in 1996. Recommendations of an international panel. JAMA. 1996; 276: 146–154.

112. Fischl MA, Richman DD, Grieco MH, et al. The efficacy of azidothymidine (AZT) in the treatment of patients with AIDS and AIDS-related complex. A double-blind, placebo-controlled trial. N Engl J Med 1987; 317:185–191.

113. Volberding PA, Lagakos SW, Koch MA, et al. Zidovudine in asymptomatic human immunodeficiency virus infection: a controlled trial in persons with fewer than 500 CD4-positive cells per cubic millimeter. N Engl J Med 1990; 322:941–949.

114. Fischl M, Galpin JE, Levine JD, et al. Recombinant human erythropoietin for patients with AIDS treated with zidovudine. N Engl J Med 1990; 322:1488.

115. Freiman JP, Helfert KE, Hamrell MR, Stein D. Hepatomegaly with severe steatosis in HIV-seropositive patients. AIDS 1993; 7:379–385.

116. Shuman P, Kinzie J, Merlino N, et al. Fatty infiltration of the liver associated with lactic acidosis in 3 women with HIV infection. 32nd Interscience Conference on Antimicrobial Agents and Chemotherapy, 1992, abstr 1085.

117. Toltzis P. Rationales for treating the human immunodeficiency virus-infected woman during pregnancy. Clin Perinatal 1993; 20:47–60.

118. O'Sullivan MJ, Boyer PJ, Scott GB, Parks WP, Weller S, Blum MR, Bolsky J, Bryson Y, and the Zidovudine Collaborative Working Group. The pharmacokinetics and safety of zidovudine in the third trimester of pregnancy for women infected with human immunodeficiency virus and their infants. Phase I Acquire Immunodeficiency Syndrome Clinical Trials Group Study (protocol 082). Am J Obstet Gynecol 1993; 168:1510–1515.

119. Klug S, Lwandowski CL, Merker HJ, et al. In vitro and in vivo studies on the prenatal toxicity of five virustatic nucleoside analogues in comparison to acyclovir. Arch Toxicol 1991; 65:283–288.

120. Toltzis P, Marx CM, Kleinman N, et al. Zidovudine-associated embryonic toxicity in mice. J Infect Dis 1991; 163:1212–1215.

121. Sperling RS, Stratton P, O'Sullivan MJ, Boyer P, Watts DH, Lambert JS, Hamill H, Livingston EG, Gloeb DJ, Minkoff H, Fox HE. A survey of zidovudine use in pregnant women with human immunodeficiency virus infection. N Engl J Med 1992; 326:857–861.

122. Kumar RM, Hughes PF, Khurranna A. Zidovudine use in pregnancy: a report of 104 cases and the occurrence of birht defects. J Acquir Immun Defic Syndr 1994; 7:1034–1039.

123. Flexner C. New antiretroviral agents in clinical development. Curr Opin Infect Dis 1992; 5:798–805.

124. Abrams DI, Goldman AI, Launer C, Korvick JA, Neaton JD, Crane LR, Grodesky M, Wakefield S, Muth K, Kornegay S, Cohn DL, Harris A, Luskin-Hawk R, Markowitz N. Sampson JH, Thompson M, Deyton L, and the Terry Beirn Community Programs for Clinical Research on AIDS. A comparative trial of didanosine or zalcitabine after treatment with zidovudine in patients with human immunodeficiency virus infection. N Engl J Med 1994; 330:657–662.

125. Pavia AT, Gathe J, BMS-019 study group investigators. Clinical efficacy of stavudine (d4T, Zerit) compared to zidovudine (ZDV, Retrovir) in ZDV-pretreated HIV positive patients. In: Abstracts of the 35th Interscience Conference on Antimicrobial Agents and Chemotherapy, San Francisco, September 17–20, 1995. Washington, DC: American Society of Microbiology, 1995: 235 (abst).

126. Eron JJ, Benoit SL, Jemsek J, MacArthur RD, Santana J, Quinn JB, Kuritzkes DR, Fallon MA, Rubin M for the North American HIV Working Party. Treatment with lamivudine, zidovudine, or both in HIV-positive patients with 200 to 500 CD4+ cells per cubic millimeter. N Engl J Med 1995; 333: 1662–1669.

127. Havlir D, Cheeseman SH, McLaughlin M, et al. High-dose Nevirapine: safety pharmacokinetics, and antiviral effect in patients with human immunodeficiency virus infection. J Infect Dis 1995; 171:537–545.

128. Kitchen VS, Skinner C, Ariyoshi K, et al. Safety and activity of saquinavir in HIV infection. Lancet 1995; 345:952–955.

129. O'Sullivan M, Lai S, Yasin S, Helfgott A. The effect of pregnancy on lymphocyte counts in HIV infected. Oral presentation, HIV Infection in Women Conference, Washington, DC, Feb. 22–24, 1995.

130. Scott GB, Fischl M, Klimas N, et al. Mothers of infants with acquired immunodeficiency syndrome. JAMA 1985; 253:363–366.

131. Minkoff H, Nanda D, Mendez R. Pregnancies resulting in infants with acquired immunodeficiency syndrome or AID's related complex: follow-up of mothers and children and subsequently born siblings. Obstet Gynecol 1987; 69:288–291.

132. Hocke C, Morlat P, Chene G, et al. Prospective cohort study of the effect of pregnancy on the progression of human immunodeficiency virus infection. Obstet Gynecol 1995; 86:886–891.

133. Deschamps MM, Pape JW, Desvarieux M, Williams-Russo P, Madhavan S, Ho JL, Johnson WD Jr. A prospective Study of HIV-seropositive asymptomatic women of childbearing age in a developing country. J Acquir Immun Defic Syndr 1993; 6:446–451

134. Johnstone FD, Willcox L, Brettle RP. Survival time after AIDS in pregnancy. Br J Obstet Gynaecol 1992; 99:633–636.

135. Gloeb DJ, Lai S, Efantis J, O'Sullivan MJ. Survival and disease progression in human immunodeficiency virus-infected women after an index delivery. Am J Obstet Gynecol 1992; 167:152–157.

136. Selwyn PA, Schoenbaum EE, Davenny K, et al. Prospective study of human immunodeficiency virus infection and pregnancy outcomes in intravenous drug users. JAMA 1989; 261:1289–1294.

137. Alger LS, Farley JJ, Robinson BA, Hines SE, Berchin JM, Johnson JP. Interactions of human immunodeficiency virus infection and pregnancy. Obstet Gynecol 1993; 82:787–796.

138. Weinberg ED. Pregnancy-associated depression of cell-mediated immunity. Rev Infect Dis 1984; 6:814–831.

139. Sridama V, Pacini F, Yang LS, et al. Decreased levels of helper T-cells—a possible cause of immunodeficiency in pregnancy. N Engl J Med 1982; 307: 352–356.
140. Castilla JA, Rueda R, Vargas ML, et al. Decreased levels of circulating CD4+ T lymphocytes during normal human pregnancy. J Reprod Immunol 1989; 15:103–111.
141. Weinberg ED. Pregnancy associated immune suppression: risks and mechanisms. Microbiol Pathogen 1987; 3:747–749.
142. Biggar RJ, Pahwa S, Minkoff H, et al. Immunosuppression in pregnant women infected with human immunodeficiency virus. Am J Obstet Gynecol 1989; 161:1239–1244.
143. Johnstone FD, Thong KJ, Bird AG, Whitelaw J. Lymphocyte subpopulations in early human pregnancy. Obstet Gynecol 1994; 83:941–946.
144. Miotti PG, Liomba G, Dallabetta GA, Hoover DR, Chiphangwi JD, Saah AJ. T-lymphocyte subsets during and after pregnancy: analysis in human immunodeficiency virus type 1-infected and -uninfected Malawian mothers. J Infect Dis 1992; 165:146–149.
145. Koonin LK, Ellerbrock TV, Atrash HK, Rogers MF, Smith JC, Hogue CJ, Harris MA, Chavkin W, Parker AL, Halpin GG. Pregnancy associated deaths due to AIDS in the United States. JAMA 1989; 261;1306–1309.
146. Leroy V, Msellati P, Lepage P, Butungwanayo J, Hitimana DG, Taelman H, Bogaerts J, Boineau F, Van de Perre P, Simonon A, Salamon R, Dabis F. Four years of natural history of HIV-1 infection in African women: a prospective cohort study in Kigali (Rwanda), 1988–1993. J Acquir Immun Defic Synd Hum Retro 1995; 9:415–421.
147. Sunderland A, Minkoff HL, Handte J, Moroso G, Landesman S. The impact of human immunodeficiency serostatus on reproductive decisions of women. Obstet Gynecol 1992; 79:1027–1031.
148. Sheon AR, Fox HE, Rich KC, Tuomala R, Stratton P, Mendez H, Diaz C, Carrington J, Alexander G. The women and infants transmission study (WITS) of maternal-infant HIV transmission: study design, methods, and baseline data. J Women's Health 1996; 5:69–78.
149. Lindsay MK, Grant J, Peterson HB, Willis S, Nelson P, Klein L. The impact of knowledge of human immunodeficiency virus serostatus on contraceptive choice and repeat pregnancy. Obstet Gynecol 1995; 85:675–679.
150. Miotti PG, Dallabetta G, Ndovi e, et al. HIV-1 and pregnant women: associated factors, prevalence, estimate of incidence and role in fetal wastage in central Africa. AIDS 1990; 4:733–736.
151. Marion RW, Wiznia AA, Hutcheon RG, et al. Human T-cell lymphotropic virus type III (HTLV-III) embryopathy. A new dysmorphic syndrome associated with intrauterine HTLV-III infection. Am J Dis Child 1986; 140: 638–640.
152. Iosub S, Bamji M, Stone RK, et al. More on human immunodeficiency virus embryopathy. Pediatrics 1987; 80:512–516.

153. Embree JE, Braddick M, Datta P, et al. Lack of correlation of maternal human immunodeficiency virus infection with neonatal malformations. Pediatr Infect Dis J 1989; 8:700–704.
154. Carlin ME, Bauer M. Does the human immunodeficiency virus affect morphogenesis? Clin Res 1988; 36:58A.
155. Qazi QH, Sheikh TM, Fikrig S, et al. Lack of evidence for craniofacial dysmorphism in perinatal human immunodeficiency virus infection. J Pediatr 1988; 112:7–11.
156. Minkoff H, Nanda D, Mendez R, et al. Pregnancies resulting in infants with acquired immunodeficiency syndrome or AIDS-related complex. Obstet Gynecol 1987; 69:285–287.
157. Gloeb DJ, O'Sullivan MJ, Efantis J. Human immunodeficiency virus infection in women. The effects of human immunodeficiency virus on pregnancy. Am J Obstet Gynecol 1988; 159:756–761.
158. Minkoff HL, Henderson C, Mendez H, et al. Pregnancy outcomes among mothers infected with human immunodeficiency virus and uninfected control subjects. Am J Obstet Gynecol 1990; 163:1598–1604.
159. Lindgren S, Anzen B, Bohlin AB, Lidman K. HIV and child-bearing: clinical outcome and aspects of mother-to-child transmission. AIDS 1991; 5:1111–1116.
160. Hutto C, Parks WP, Lai S, et al. A hospital-based prospective study of perinatal infection with human immunodeficency virus type 1. J Pediatr 1991; 118:347–353.
161. Gabiano C, Tovo PA, DeMartino M, et al. Mother to child transmission of human immunodeficiency virus type 1: Risk of infection and correlates of transmission. Pediatrics 1992; 90:369–374.
162. Braddick MR, Kreiss JK, Embree JE, et al. Impact of maternal HIV infection on obstetrical and early neonatal outcome. J AIDS 1990; 4:1001–1004.
163. Temmerman M, Chomba EN, Ndinya-Achola J, et al. Maternal human immunodeficiency virus-1 infection and pregnancy outcome. Obstet Gynecol 1994; 83:495–501.
164. Lepage P, Dabis F, Hitimana DG, Msellati P, Van Goethem C, Stevens AM, Nsengumuremyi F, Bazubagira A, Serufilira A, De Clerq A, Van de Perre P. Perinatal transmission of HIV: lack of impact of materna HIV infection on characteristics of live births and on neonatal mortality in Kigali, Rwanda. AIDS 1991; 5:295–300.
165. Kind C, Brandle B, Wyler C-A, et al. Epidemiology of vertically transmitted HIV-1 infection in Switzerland; results of a nationwide prospective study. Eur J Pediatr 1992; 151:442–448.
166. Bryson YJ, Pang S, Wei LS, Dickover R, Diagne A, Chen ISY. Clearance of HIV infection in a perinatally infected infant. N Engl Med 1995; 332:833–838.
167. Centers for Disease Control and Prevention. Recommendations of the Advisory Committee on Immunization Practices (ACIP): use of vaccines and immunoglobulins in persons with altered immunocompetence. Morbid Mortal Weekly Rep 1993; 42(RR-5):1–18.

168. Carpenter CCJ, Mayer KH, Stein MD, et al. Human immundeficiency virus infection in North American women: experience with 200 cases and a review of the literature. Medicine (Baltimore) 1991; 70:307–325.

169. Clark RA, Brandon W, Dumestre J, Pindaro C. Clinical manifestations of infection with the human immunodeficiency virus in women in Louisiana. Clin Infect Dis 1993; 17:165–172.

170. O'Sullivan MJ, Helfgott A, Yasin S, LaVoie L. Incidence of syphilis/gonorrhoeae in HIV(+) compared to HIV(−) women. Poster presentation, HIV Infection in Women Conference, Washington, DC, 1995.

171. Centers for Disease Control. Purified protein derivative (PPD)-tuberculin anergy and HIV infection: guidelines for anergy testing and management of anergic persons at risk of tuberculosis. Morbid Mortal Weekly Rep 1991; 40:27.

172. Fleming PL, Ciesielski CA, Byers RH, Castro KG, Berkelman RL. Gender differences in reported AIDS-indicative diagnoses. J Infect Dis 1993; 168: 61–67.

173. Centers for Disease Control. Recommendations for prophylaxis against *Pneumocystis carinii* pneumonia for adults and adolescents infected with human immunodeficiency virus. Morbid Mortal Weekly Rep 1992; 41:1.

174. Masur H. Prevention and treatment of pneumocystis pneumonia. N Engl J Med 1992; 327:1853–1860.

175. Schneider MME, Hoepelman AIM, Karel J, et al. A controlled trial of aerosolized pentamidine or trimethoprim-sulfamethoxazole as primary prophylaxis against *Pneumocystis carinii* pneumonia in patients with human immunodeficiency virus. N Engl J Med 1992; 327:1836–1841.

176. Masur H. Public Heath Service Task Force on Prophylaxis and Therapy for *Mycobacterium avium* complex. Recommendations on prophylaxis and therapy for disseminated *Mycobacterium avium* complex disease in patients infected with the human immunodeficiency virus. N Engl J Med 1993; 329: 898–904.

177. Carr A, Tindall B, Bre BJ, et al. Low dose trimethoprim-sulfamethoxazole prophylaxis for toxoplasmic encephalities in patients with AIDS. Ann Intern Med 1992; 117:106–111.

178. Quagliarello VJ, Viscoli C, Horwitz RI. Primary prevention of cryptococcal meningitis by flucconazole in HIV-infected patients. Lancet 1995; 345: 548–552.

179. Minkoff HL, Moreno JD, Drug prophylaxis for human immunodeficiency virus infected pregnant women: ethical considerations. Am J Obstet Gynecol 1990; 163:1111–1114.

180. Centers for Disease Control. Recommendations for prevention of HIV transmission in health care settings. Morbid Mortal Weekly Rep 1987; 36: 189–202.

181. Centers for Disease Control. Guidelines for prevention of transmission of human immunodeficiency virus and hepatitis b virus to health-care and public-safety workers. Morbid Mortal Weekly Rep 1989; 38:1–37.

25

Immune Deficiency During Pregnancy

FREDERICK M. SCHAFFER

Mississippi State University
Starkville, Mississippi

I. Introduction

This chapter reviews several primary and acquired immunodeficiency disorders that affect the mother and fetus. The discussion is restricted to the most common disorders and their infectious and obstetrical complications that could compromise pregnancy and/or fetal viability. The major T-lymphocyte disorder affecting women during their reproductive years is AIDS, which is discussed in Chapter 24. Most primary T-lymphocyte or combined T- and B-cell disorders (e.g., severe combined immunodeficiency) are rare and require vigorous intervention early in life. Therefore, these disorders will not be reviewed. The section on granulocyte disorders concentrates on neutropenia, since the primary granulocyte disorders (e.g., chronic granulomatous disease) are usually identified and treatment initiated during the first 5 or 6 years of life.

II. Prevalence of Primary Immunodeficiency Disorders

Studies in Europe, the United States, and Japan demonstrate that the antibody deficiency disorders are the most common forms of primary immunodeficiency (Table 1). These B-lymphocyte disorders include selective IgA deficiency, the most common primary immunodeficiency disease, and common variable immunodeficiency. Less frequently encountered are the granulocyte and complement deficiencies which can adversely affect pregnancy.

III. Clinical B-Lymphocyte Disorders

A. IgA Deficiency

Incidence and Definition

IgA deficiency (IgA-D) is the most common primary immunodeficiency disorder, with a prevalence of 1 in 700 individuals of European ancestry (1). IgA-D was first recognized in 1961 as part of the spectrum of ataxia-telangiectasia (2). It was evident that the degree of humoral and cellular immune defects was variable in affected individuals. In symptomatic individuals, IgA-D is associated with recurrent sinopulmonary infections, atopy, autoimmune disorders, gastrointestinal disorders, genetic disorders, and malignancy (3).

Selective IgA-D is defined by a serum IgA concentration of less than 5 mg/dL with normal serum concentrations of the other immunoglobulin classes (3). Approximately 20% of individuals with IgA-D have an associated IgG2 subclass deficiency (4). Most individuals with IgA-D are asymptomatic, whereas the majority of symptomatic individuals have an

Table 1 Prevalence of Specific Disorders Among Patients with Primary Immunodeficiencies

Disorder	Prevalence
Antibody deficiencies	50%
Combined T-cell and B-cell deficiencies	20%
Granulocyte deficiencies	18%
T-cell deficiencies	10%
Complement deficiencies	2%

Source: Ref. 39.

IgA and IgG subclass deficiency (5). These latter individuals have a propensity to develop anti-IgA antibodies after exposure to blood products (e.g., IV gamma-globulin). Thus, these individuals have an increased risk of developing anaphylactic reactions upon subsequent exposure to blood products (6).

Etiology

IgA-D is phenotypically characterized by an arrest in B-lymphocyte differentiation, the extent of which may determine clinical variability. This immunodeficiency disorder is associated with a normal number of IgA-bearing B lymphocytes. However, these B cells are relatively immature and fail to undergo terminal differentiation into IgA-secreting plasma cells (Fig. 1) (3). Peripheral blood IgA-bearing B cells, acquired from individuals with IgA-D, resemble their counterparts in neonatal blood (8). The expression of surface IgA antibodies by phenotypically immature B lymphocytes in IgA-D provides evidence for the integrity of the IgA antibody heavy- and light-chain gene segments. This concept is also supported by noting that the offspring of individuals with IgA-D demonstrate normal expression of the IgA genes. Furthermore, in a study of IgA-D patients, all had intact IgA antibody heavy-chain $C\alpha1$ and $C\alpha2$ gene segments (9). The majority of individuals with IgA deficiency do not secrete both IgA1 and IgA2. Therefore, one would have to envision an extensive gene deletion encompassing the $C\alpha1$ and $C\alpha2$ gene segments, with three other intervening heavy-chain gene segments, for IgA-D to be based on a structural defect of the constant-region gene segments (3,7). One would have to envision an even larger gene deletion to implicate a structural genetic defect in common variable immunodeficiency (discussed below). Since B cells in both disorders express all immunoglobulin isotypes, the genetic elements required for isotype switching are probably intact. These factors support the concept of an immunoregulatory gene defect as the underlying cause of IgA-D and common variable immunodeficiency, rather than defects in the immunoglobulin structural genes.

Some studies demonstrated that only one of identical twins had IgA deficiency (10). This information further supports the hypothesis of an immunoregulatory gene defect as the underlying cause of IgA-D. Furthermore, acquired forms of IgA-D have occurred following the use of certain medications (11). Acquired IgA-D has also been associated with specific neonatal infections (12). These results suggest a role for environmental factors, possibly influencing an immunoregulatory gene(s), in the pathogenesis of IgA-D.

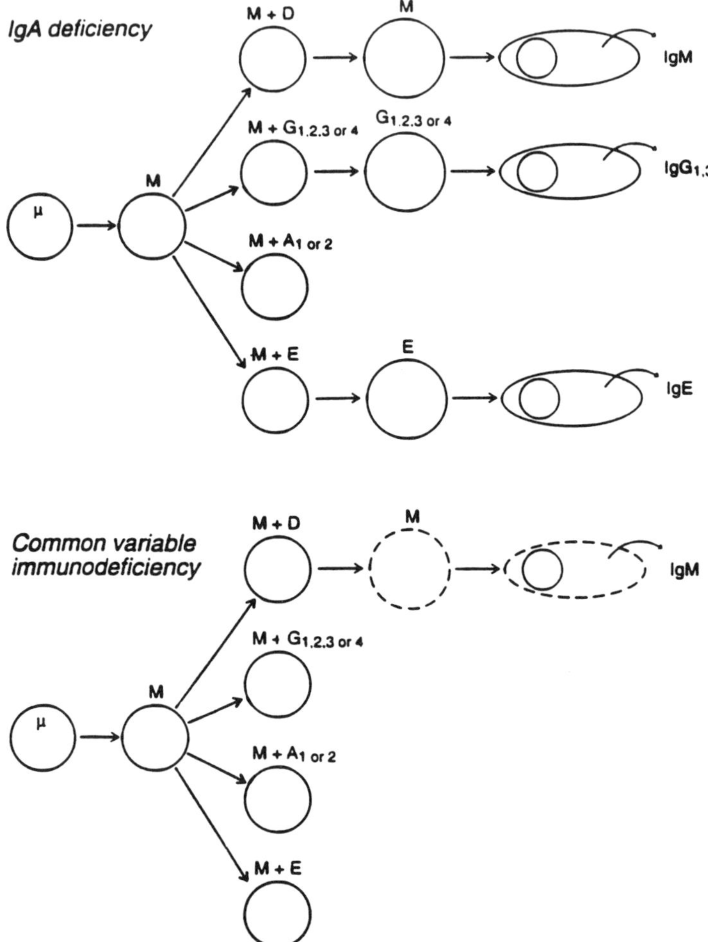

Figure 1 The B-cell differentiation arrest of Ig-D and CVID. Both disorders are associated with an arrest in B-cell differentiation, characterized by the presence of a normal number of immature B cells that express multiple immunoglobulin isotypes on the cell surface (capital letters; Arabic numbers represent IgG and IgA subclasses). In IgA-D, this results in a paucity of IgA and in 20% of cases, IgG2 (or 4)-secreting (curved arrows) plasma cells (oval cells). In CVID, this results in a lack of all antibody-secreting plasma cells for most patients; however, a few of these individuals do have IgM-secreting plasma cells (illustrated as cells with broken borders). (From Ref. 3.)

B. Common Variable Immunodeficiency

Incidence and Definition

Common variable immunodeficiency (CVID), defined by panhypoglobulinemia is a heterogeneous disorder with a variable degree of T-lymphocyte dysfunction (7,13). The reported prevalence of CVID varies from 1 in 50,000 to 1 in 200,000 individuals. This immunodeficiency disorder is usually diagnosed between the second and fourth decades of life. Thus, it is not uncommon to diagnose CVID in a woman during or shortly after pregnancy. Most forms of CVID are associated with a normal number of phenotypically immature peripheral blood B lymphocytes and an arrest in B-cell differentiation just prior to the plasma cell stage (3,7). This differentiation arrest is associated with minimal antibody secretion and the resultant panhypogammaglobulinemia (Fig. 1) (7). A minority of individuals diagnosed with CVID have normal concentrations of serum IgM, reflecting an incomplete arrest in B cell differentiation. In contrast a small number of individuals with CVID have a diminished number of peripheral blood B lymphocytes, which contributes to diminished antibody synthesis and secretion.

Recent studies have demonstrated defects in triggering of the T-cell receptor in CVID (reviewed in Ref. 7). Normal T- and B-lymphocyte interactions are required for B cells to differentiate into antibody-secreting plasma cells. It is intriguing to speculate that the characteristic arrest in B-cell differentiation associated with CVID is caused by aberrant T-cell signaling mechanisms.

Pathogenesis and Infections

A panhypogammaglobulinemic state (i.e., CVID) is associated with an increased susceptibility to recurrent and severe infections. Several pathogenic mechanisms have been suggested. Mucosal protection is impaired by a lack of secretory antibody synthesis that is associated with CVID and IgA-D (i.e., decreased IgA2 synthesis). Thus, pathogenic organisms, after mucosal attachment, develop a local infection which can result in respiratory and gastrointestinal infections often seen in individuals with antibody deficiency disorders (14). Dissemination of a focal mucosal infection to the CNS, joints, or lungs often occurs in the absence of neutralizing or cytotoxic antibody production. Also, deficient antibody-antigen complex formation may result in diminished complement activation. In turn, this results in diminished chemotaxis, opsonization, and phagocytosis (15). These processes are required for effective clearance and destruction of pathogenic organisms.

Sinopulmonary infections are the hallmark of antibody deficiency disorders. Recurrent upper respiratory tract infections are common to IgA-D and may persist throughout life (3). In contrast, individuals with CVID are more prone to recurrent upper and lower respiratory tract infections (13,14). Recurrent lower respiratory tract infections have been associated with the development of bronchiectasis in a significant percentage of CVID patients and in some individuals with IgA-D (14,16).

A recurrent or chronic gastrointestinal infection is the second most common infectious disorder seen in antibody deficiency disorders. Typically, chronic gastrointestinal infections occur more frequently in individuals with CVID (14). The following organisms have been associated with chronic enteritis in antibody deficiency disorders: giardia, salmonella, shigella, campylobacter, rotavirus, and less frequently cryptosporidium (14,17). A spruelike syndrome has been reported in individuals with either CVID or IgA-D (3). At times, an intestinal biopsy is required to differentiate this disorder from other causes of chronic enteritis.

Most individuals with IgA-D only experience infections of the mucosal surfaces; however, as is evident in CVID, systemic infections do occur. Susceptibility to these infections may be dependent on both the extent of the humoral and cellular immune deficiency. Examples of systemic infections reported in the past include meningoencephalitis, fatal viral hepatitis, disseminated CMV, and mycoplasma arthritis.

Vaccinations

Since cellular immune deficiency may contribute to the clinical spectrum of CVID and in some cases IgA-D (e.g., ataxia-telangiectasis), vaccination of individuals with live viral vaccines could result in viremia and death (3,18). Thus, individuals in whom a cellular immune deficiency exists, as evident in a significant proportion of those with CVID, should not be vaccinated. However, the majority of individuals with IgA-D have normal cellular immune function and can be vaccinated if no other contraindications (e.g., pregnancy) exists.

Autoimmune Disorders

A wide range of autoimmune disorders is associated with antibody deficiency syndromes. In selective IgA-D, rheumatoid arthritis and systemic lupus erythematosus (SLE) occur in up to 7% of individuals (19). Other disorders associated with CVID and IgA-D include idiopathic thrombocytopenic purpora, Henoch-Schonlein purpura, hemolytic anemia, autoimmune neutropenia, celiac disease, lupoid hepatitis, sarcoidosis, juvenile rheumatoid arthritis (JRA), Graves' disease, juvenile-onset diabetes, Sjogren's syndrome, dermatomyositis, and Addison's disease (3,18). The high incidence of autoimmune disease in antibody deficiency disorders may be related to autoantibody production (more common in IgA-D). Individuals with IgA-D and autoimmune disease synthesize autoantibodies against pancreatic cells, smooth muscle cells, adrenal gland cells, thyroglobulin, and nuclear proteins (3,20–22). This autoantibody production may be the initiation of an autoimmune disease characterized by subsequent immune-complex formation and deposition.

The antibody deficiency disorders appear to have minimal effect on the severity of the particular autoimmune disease in question except in a few specific cases. Individuals with IgA-D and pauci- or polyarticular JRA seem to have a more benign disease course than their counterparts with a normal immune status. Individuals with antibody deficiencies frequently have sinopulmonary (and/or other) infections. During the course of these infections, other disease activity (e.g., JRA, SLE, and diabetes) may increase.

Gastrointestinal Disorders

There is an association of a wide spectrum of gastrointestinal disorders with antibody deficiency disorders. Disorders of malabsorption such as celiac disease, inflammatory bowel disease, pancreatic insufficiency, and disaccharidase deficiency have been diagnosed in individuals with CVID or IgA-D (3,18,20). Pernicious anemia, as a result of gastric atrophy or secondary to autoantibody production to intrinsic factor, has occurred in CVID and less frequently in IgA-D (3). Nodular lymphoid hyperplasia has often been associated with CVID and less often with IgA-D (3,18,20.) Hepatic disorders such as cholelithiasis, primary biliary atresia, and chronic active hepatitis have also been associated with antibody deficiency disorders (22,23).

Malignancy

Individuals with CVID or IgA-D have an increased risk for the development of malignancies. Neoplastic disorders encountered by these patients are primarily gastric and colonic adenocarcinomas and lymphoreticular malignancies. Specifically, there is a 50-fold increase in gastric carcinoma in CVID. There is also an increased risk for the development of lymphoma. However, women with CVID have a much greater risk than do their male counterparts. Less frequently encountered malignancies in IgA-D include acute lymphoblastic leukemia, lymphosarcoma, ovarian cancer, hepatoma, malignant thymoma, melanoma, and multiple myeloma (3,7,18,20).

Etiological Association with the Major Histocompatibility Complex (MHC) Genes

We hypothesized that CVID and IgA-D have a common genetic basis (24,25). This concept is based on several lines of evidence: Both disorders occur in several members of the same family; an arrest in B-cell differentiation is a central cellular phenotype of both disorders; several individuals with IgA-D developed panhypogammaglobulinemia; IgA-D was previously associated with specific extended MHC haplotypes (26), and we have demonstrated that the same MHC haplotypes were associated with CVID (24,25). Based on our molecular studies, we suggested that susceptibility to CVID and IgA-D was associated with an MHC class III region immunoregulatory gene (or genes).

The prevalence of IgA-D and CVID is different in different population groups. For example, IgA-D is more than 25-fold less common in Japan than in northern Europe. This striking contrast suggests that genetic backgrounds, possibly differences in the expression of specific MHC susceptibility genes, are important parameters in disease pathogenesis.

Treatment

IgA-D

Antibody replacement therapy is not indicated in most cases of IgA-D. This is due to the short half-life of the IgA antibody, and the knowledge that serum IgA is a poor source for acquiring secretory IgA. Furthermore, since individuals with IgA-D have a high proclivity for anti-IgA antibody synthesis, the administration of exogenous IgA may result in anaphylactic reactions (6,27). The practitioner should address possible etiological factors such as the association of specific congenital infections (cytomegalovirus and *Toxoplasma gondii*) with IgA-D; some late-onset forms of CVID and IgA-D have been documented following Epstein-Barr viral infections; and the use of some antiseizure medications and specific medications for rheumatoid arthritis and inflammatory bowel disease have resulted in drug-induced reversible IgA-D (28–30).

In general, individuals with IgA-D and associated autoimmune, gastrointestinal, or allergic disorders should be treated in the same manner as those without antibody deficiency disorders. For those individuals with recurrent infections (e.g., IgA-D with an IgG subclass deficiency), aggressive antibiotic management may be needed. A small subset of such patients may also require antibody replacement therapy in the form of intravenous gamma-globulin (IVIG) therapy (3,18,20). The use of IVIG administration is recommended in the event that a functional antibody deficiency is demonstrated, and "breakthrough" infections occur despite the use of aggressive antibiotic management. In order to decrease the possibility of anaphylactic reactions, the patient should receive IVIG that has been depleted of IgA itself (31). To assess the risk of an anaphylactic reaction for a patient, anti-IgA antibody serum titers should be measured prior to and after the initiation of IVIG therapy (6). If a blood transfusion is required, only matched blood from an individual with IgA-D or double-washed, matched, packed red blood cells should be administered (3,18).

CVID

Most individuals with CVID have serum IgG concentrations of less than 200 mg/dL (normal >700 mg/dL) and minimal functional antibody titers (7,32). These individuals require antibody replacement therapy in the form of IVIG to avoid recurrent and life-threatening infections (16,33). The half-life of IgG is 23 days; therefore, appropriate administration should occur every 3–4 weeks. After IVIG therapy has started, plateau (steady-state) serum IgG concentrations are achieved after 3–6 months (33). Recent studies have demonstrated significant clinical improvement with the use of high-dose (600 mg/kg/dose) rather than low-dose (~200/mg/kg/dose) IVIG (16,33). This improvement in clinical status was reflected by a decreased number of sinopulmonary infections and hospitalizations, an improvement in pulmonary function studies, and (in some cases) a diminished extent of bronchiectasis. This improved clinical status was associated with a trough serum IgG concentration of greater than 500 mg/dL (33). In most cases, disorders associated with CVID should be treated in the same manner as individuals with normal serum antibody concentrations.

IV. Pregnancy and Clinical B-Lymphocyte Disorders

A. IgA Deficiency

The majority of individuals with IgA-D are asymptomatic and should be treated similar to pregnant women without this condition. For symptomatic individuals, specific precautions need to be considered. A subset of symptomatic individuals with IgA-D do well solely with the use of prophylactic antibiotic therapy (3,18,20). The practitioner should prescribe the use of antibiotics that will have no deleterious effects upon the fetus. For pregnant women with symptomatic IgA-D who are treated with IVIG, it is important to prevent potential anaphylactic reactions. This can be achieved by utilizing IVIG depleted of IgA and by following serum anti-IgA titers prior to and throughout pregnancy (6,31). As is true for CVID, the treatment of the associated disorders (e.g., autoimmune disease) should follow the treatment guidelines for affected pregnant women without IgA-D.

B. Common Variable Immunodeficiency

Pregnant women with CVID have a higher risk of antepartum infection than do their counterparts without hypogammaglobulinemia (34). Their offspring also have a high risk for the development of prenatal and neonatal infections (35–39). This is due to the minimal quantity of maternal IgG that is transported transplacentally during pregnancy in CVID (35–39). Serum IgG is the predominant antibody directed against bacteria, viruses, and fungi. Diminished serum levels are associated with an increased incidence of infections. Full-term neonates do not synthesize appreciable quantities of IgG until approximately 4–6 months of age. Normal newborn serum IgG concentrations range from ~425 to 1600 mg/dL and steadily decreases to as low as 200 mg/dL by 4 months of age. This decrease in (maternally acquired) serum IgG is a result of the 23-day half-life of IgG and minimal neonatal IgG synthesis during this time period (34). Thus, transplacentally acquired material IgG is the major component of humoral immunity for the neonatal prior to delivery and for several months after birth.

Transplacental transfer of maternal IgG1 occurs by an active transport process during the end of the second trimester and throughout the third trimester of pregnancy, while the other IgG subclasses are passively transported (34). IgG1 is the predominant subclass (~65–70% of normal adult total serum IgG), while the IgG3, and IgG4 subclasses account for smaller fractions of total serum IgG. Newborn IgG subclass ratio reflect the maternal values. These ratios soon change due to minimal newborn IgG2 synthesis until after 18 months of age. The offspring of untreated women with CVID have minimal IgG serum concentrations, since the maternal IgG pool size is quite small in comparison to pregnant women with normal IgG concentrations. The IgG pool size naturally falls as pregnancy progresses, due to the hemodilutional effect of the increasing maternal blood volume (40). Therefore, the CVID minimal IgG placental transport occurs as a result of a small initial serum IgG pool, which is further diminished by a hemodilutional effect. This is exemplified by reviewing the maternal serum (pretreatment) and cord blood IgG concentrations for patients 1 and 2 in Table 2.

To prevent significant antepartum infections for women with CVID, antibody replacement therapy should ideally begin prior to pregnancy or, at the latest, during the first trimester in order to achieve "protective" serum IgG concentrations (16,33,41). "Protective" steady-state serum IgG concentrations of greater than 500 mg/dL are associated with lower morbidity (16,33) and are achieved only after 3–6 months of monthly IVIG administration (33). Moreover, fetal protection occurs as in indirect by-

Table 2 Literature Survey of IVIG Administration During Pregnancy

Ref.	Patient no.	Mode and frequency of treatment	Onset of treatment	Maternal serum IgG concentration (mg/dL)		Cord blood IgG conc. (mg/dL)
				Pretreatment	Posttreatment	
35	1	None	None	11	Not reported	11
36	2	None	None	139	Not reported	194
42	3	IMIG 25 mg/kg/wk	Prepregnancy	6	Not reported	Not reported
	4	IMIG 25 mg/kg/wk	Prepregnancy			
	5	IMIG 25 mg/kg/wk	4 wk prior to delivery	80	520	144
	6	IVIG 200 mg/kg/5 wk	Prepregnancy	230	400	633
	7	None	After delivery	210	Not reported	80
45	8	Weekly IVIG	First trimester	226	240	240
46	9	20 ml daily of IMIG solution s.c.	First trimester	12	620	880
43	10	IVIG every 2 wk	Second trimester	120	300–700	940
44	11	IVIG 100 mg/kg	First trimester	123	442	217
		IVIG 200 mg/kg/2 wk	Second/third trimester			
	12	IVIG 200 mg/kg/2 wk	Third trimester	58	326	232
	13	IVIG 200 mg/kg/2 wk	Third trimester	109	333	304
41	14	IVIG 400 mg/kg/3 wk	First trimester	102	703	774

Source: Ref. 41.

product of the prevention of maternal infections (which may jeopardize fetal viability) and directly by the acquisition of a larger quantity of maternal IgG.

Several groups have reported the use of large doses of IVIG that were administered frequently during the third trimester of pregnancy (42–44). We (41) and a few others (45,46) have published protocols in which IVIG is administered throughout pregnancy. Table 2 summarizes the reports of gamma-globulin replacement therapy in pregnant women with CVID. Only four of these studies (patients 6, 9, 10, and 14) used treatment regimens that resulted in cord blood IgG concentrations greater than 425 mg/dL (normal range). In the majority of studies, frequent IVIG administration schedules (from daily to every 2 weeks) were reported (42–46). Ideally, as previously described, the frequency of IVIG administration should be every 3–4 weeks throughout pregnancy, which is associated with lower medical costs and placing fewer restraints on the patient's daily activities (47).

By administering IVIG throughout pregnancy rather than during the third trimester only, the following issues are addressed: the prevention of maternal infections prior to the third trimester; the 3- to 6-month time period needed to acquire "protective" steady-state serum IgG levels; or the avoidance of low fetal IgG levels resulting from fluctuating (nonsteady-state) maternal serum IgG concentrations during the third trimester (34,41).

Term infants will have serum IgG levels that are approximately 110% of the maternal serum IgG concentration (34). In contrast, premature neonates or those with intrauterine growth retardation never achieve these levels. Only four of the protocols listed in Table 2 (patients 6, 9, 10, and 14) reported normal cord blood IgG concentrations >100% of the maternal serum concentrations. The results of the other studies are consistent with the reported low IgG concentrations of prematurity.

In summary, the principles used for the treatment of CVID are generally applicable during pregnancy. The administration of IVIG prior to and throughout pregnancy is clinically beneficial to the mother and fetus. Furthermore, the treatment of the associated disorders (e.g., allergies, autoimmune disease, and gastrointestinal disorders) should follow the treatment guidelines for affected women without CVID.

Since CVID and IgA-D are immunogenetic disorders and several family members may be diagnosed with an antibody deficiency syndrome, newborns in these families should undergo periodic immunological evaluation during childhood (3,41,48).

V. Complement Deficiencies

A. The Classical and Alternative Complement Pathways

The complement system consists of over 20 plasma proteins that interact with antibodies and cell membranes. Upon activation, the complement system plays a crucial role in bacterial lysis, as well as phagocytosis and inflammatory reactions (15,49). There are two independent pathways that can trigger the activation of the terminal portion of the complement cascade. This terminal portion consists of the C5 through C9 complement components (50).

The classical pathway is activated by immune complexes consisting of IgG or IgM and antigen or antibody aggregates (51). The classical pathway can be activated by the binding of the C1 complement component to specific enzymes or cell membrane molecules. Activation of the classical pathway results in enzymatic reactions involving the C1, C4, and C2 complement molecules. Components of this pathway are responsible for enhancing antibody-dependent cellular cytotoxicity, phagocytosis, leukocytosis, prevent immune complex precipitation, and neutralizing of viruses (15,49). Also, animal studies have demonstrated that the complement components C2, C3, and C4 play a role in both antibody isotype switching and amnestic responses to a recall antigen (52–55). Of note, our molecular studies demonstrated that a significant number of individuals with IgA-D and CVID express either a C4A gene deletion and/or rare C2 alleles (24,25). Our results suggest that a gene(s) in close association with these complement genes may be a susceptibility gene(s) for IgA-D and CVID.

The alternative pathway is activated by venom, thrombin, polysaccharides, certain enzymes, and immunoglobulins (56,57). Activation of this pathway requires the presence of the C3b product of the enzymatically cleaved C3 complement component. The C3b product complexes with other proteins of this pathway and like the classical pathway, forms a C5 convertase which plays a role in the activation of the terminal complement components. Activation of either pathway can result in activation of the C5 through C9 molecules that form the membrane attack complex (50,56,57). After activation, the membrane attack complex attaches to and then disrupts the cell membrane surface, leading to cytolysis (50,58). Individual terminal complement components have other immunological functions. For example, C5a is a neutrophil chemotactic and activating factor in local immunological reactions. Furthermore, C7, C8, and C9 promote neutrophil intracellular bacteriacidal activity (15,50,58,59).

Etiology of Complement Deficiency

Complement deficiencies are commonly the result of acquired rather than hereditary disorders. Acquired disorders such as liver disease affect the synthesis of complement proteins, while disorders such as a protein-losing enteropathy or nephrotic syndrome are associated with an increased catabolic rate. An increased consumption of complement components, as occurs in immune-complex disorders, is another well-known cause of hypocomplementemia (15).

Hereditary complement deficiency states are uncommon, with a prevalence of 0.35% in the general population (60). The most common familial deficiency states are the complement component C2 and C4 deficiencies (61,62). Molecular studies have demonstrated that most C2-deficient individuals lack the C2 protein due to a 28-base-pair deletion in the C2 gene's sixth exon (63). The lack of expression of the C4A and C4B genes has been attributed to point mutations and gene deletions (64). Recently, Barba et al. (65) demonstrated that a collection of individuals failed to express the C4A protein due to a 2-base-pair insertion in exon 29 which resulted in the formation of a termination codon.

Complement Deficiencies and Susceptibility to Recurrent Infections

Approximately 20% of the individuals with either a C1, C2, or C4 complement component deficiency have systemic infections. In addition, about 45% of these individuals experience recurrent episodes of otitis and/or sinopulmonary infections (15). The most common organisms cultured are *S. pneumoniae*, *H. influenzae*, and *Neisseria* species (14,15). Individuals with such a classical pathway complement deficiency demonstrate impaired complement activation, which results in recurrent infections (due to diminished chemotaxis, phagocytosis, and a defective humoral immune response).

Seventy percent of those rare individuals with a C3 complement component deficiency experience systemic infections. The majority of these infections are due to pneumococcus and *Neisseria* species (15,49). These individuals demonstrate several immunological defects, including a defective humoral immune response, decreased chemotaxis, diminished phagocytosis, decreased complement dependent bactericidal activity, and diminished neutrophil activation.

The spectrum of infectious disease susceptibility for deficiencies of the alternative complement pathway varies. If the primary deficiency leads to a secondary C3 complement component deficiency, then the spectrum increases. Properdin is an important component of the alternative complement pathway. Recent studies identified three forms of properdin deficiency associated with recurrent meningococcal infections (66,67). Type I deficiency is characterized by very low levels of properdin and absent function. Types 2 and 3 deficiencies are associated with low levels of a dysfunctional glycoprotein, and a normal amount of properidin without detectable function (68–71). Properdin deficiency is an X-linked disorder and has been mapped to a structural gene location (DXS-255) on the short arm of the X chromosome (72,73). Other reported deficiencies of the alternative complement pathway directly affect consumption of C3, and therefore, infectious disease susceptibility is similar to that discussed for C3 deficiency.

Complement deficiencies of the late complement components (C5–C9) share an impaired bactericidal activity which results in a greater than 50% frequency of meningococcal disease. Because of a high frequency of complement deficiencies, it has been suggested that individuals with meningococcal infections from serotypes W135, X, Y, or nontypable strains be tested for a potential complement deficiency state (74). Recent studies demonstrate that individuals with complement deficiencies who receive a meningococcal vaccine fail to synthesize adequate titers of antibodies directed against particular capsular polysaccharides (15). Thus, diminished bactericidal activity and decreased antibody titers may contribute to the recurrent meningococcal disease experienced by individuals with C3 and C5–C9 complement component deficiencies.

Treatment

Since there are minimal side effects associated with the administration of the pneumococcal, *H influenzae* type B, and meningococcal vaccines, the use of these is recommended. Due to the high prevalence *of Neisseria* species infections, the meningococcal vaccine is recommended for all individuals with complement deficiencies. Individuals with a C1–C4 deficiency should receive the pneumococcal, *H influenzae* type B, and meningococcal vaccines.

Potter et al. (75) demonstrated the efficacy of antibiotic prophylaxis in decreasing the frequency of *Neisseria* species infections in individuals with complement deficiencies. We recommend the use of daily prophylaxis with oral antibodies for the subset of individuals with recurrent infections or during periods of meningococcal epidemics (15). The duration of antibiotic prophylaxis and the potential development of antibiotic-resistant organisms are issues that require further study.

The use of fresh-frozen plasma as a source of exogenous complement has been reported for individuals hospitalized for systemic infections with complement deficiencies (76,77). It use is controversial because the recipient may develop antibodies directed against the missing complement component. Further exposure to particular blood products may lead to anaphylaxis.

B. Hereditary Angioedema

Hereditary angioedema (HAE) was first described by Osler in 1888 (78). It is an autosomal dominant disorder with incomplete penetrance that is characterized clinically by recurrent episodes of edema unaccompanied by urticaria or pruritis. There is a deficiency or dysfunction of the C1 esterase inhibitor, an inhibitor of the activated complement component C1, factor XII, and plasma kallikrein. This state leads to an unchecked activation of the classical complement pathway, the kallikrein-kinin system, and the fibrinolytic system. In turn, the release of bradykinin and other mediators occurs. Release of these mediators can result in edema of subcutaneous tissues, abdominal viscera, the genitourinary system, mucous membranes, and at times, of the upper airway which can lead to airway obstruction and death.

Symptoms of classical HAE are usually present by 4 years of age, and recurrent attacks occur throughout life. Typical attacks last several hours and seldom persist longer than 4 days. Of note, patients have undergone needless laparotomy from a misdiagnosis of an acute abdomen during an abdominal crisis. This occurs because vomiting, colicky abdominal pain, and rarely diarrhea are also consequences of abdominal viscera edema. The correct diagnosis may require ultrasound studies for evidence of ascites and an edematous intestinal tract. However, the typical fever and leukocytosis of an acute abdomen are usually absent with an HAE abdominal attack (79–81,83). Also, women with HAE often experience urinary tract infections, probably as a result of partial urinary tract obstruction from edema (82). There are many triggers for HAE attacks. These include physical or emotional stress, infection, trauma, surgical or dental procedures, pregnancy, and from the use of oral estrogen preparations.

Diagnosis and Etiology

The clinical history, especially in view of a positive family history, is suggestive of the diagnosis. However, about 20% of cases occur from "spontaneous" mutations. In these cases, no evidence of other affected family members exist. The best screening test for HAE is the serum C4 level. If this is normal, the disease is effectively ruled out. If it is low, then direct measurement of the C1 esterase inhibitor protein (C1-E1) functional activity and concentration aid in differentiating the two most common forms of this disorder. C1-E1 functional activity is measured as a percentage of normal controls, while an antigenic assay is used to determine concentration. Most affected individuals have a C1-E1 functional activity of less than 35% of normal. This low functional percentage arises from the translated product of the one normal allele. About 85% of individuals with hereditary angioedema have a deficiency of the C1-E1 (HAE type 1); whereas, the remaining 15% of individuals have a dysfunctional C1-E1 (HAE type II). HAE type 1 is typically associated with minimal quantities of normally produced C1-E1, resulting in marked reduction of activity and serum level. In contrast, HAE type 2 is characterized by a normal or elevated (antigenically determined) level, while the activity assay reveals minimal function. A few forms of acquired angioedema have been reported which are associated with neoplastic disorders such as lymphoma, or with autoimmune disorders such as SLE. In the acquired forms of angioedema, an autoantibody is produced and directed against the C1-E1, which results in the same clinical picture at HAE (83).

To elucidate the molecular mechanism associated with a complete deficiency of the C1 esterase inhibitor protein (HAE type 1), two families exhibiting this disorder were recently studied. The study results demonstrated that point mutations in exons of genes coding for two of the three polypeptide chains of the inhibitor protein resulted in a termination codon and a single base exchange (84). In turn, the C1 esterase inhibitor protein was not formed or secreted. Other gene deletions and rearrangements (associated with either deletions or duplications) have also been associated with HAE (83).

The majority of individuals with the acquired form of angioedema have a normal amount of the C1 esterase inhibitor protein (83,85). One recent study has mapped two epitopes in the C1-E1 that bind specific autoantibodies. The binding of autoantibodies to these epitopes may mediate the process of the C1-E1 dysfunction (85).

Individuals with HAE have low serum C4 and C2 concentrations (83). However, other disorders, such as SLE, may exhibit similar biochemical results. Therefore, to confirm a suspected diagnosis of HAE, the C1-E1 plasma concentration and activity level should be measured.

Functional C1-E1 molecules bind to the C1 complement component and regulate the initial activation steps of the classical complement pathway. The C1 complement component is a trimolar complex containing one molecule of C1q and two molecules of C1r and C1s (15). Upon activation, a catalytic reaction releases the activated C1r and C1s subunits. The C4 and C2 complement proteins are the substrates of these activated proteases. In HAE, low C4 and C2 plasma levels are the result of unregulated activation of the C1 complex and the subsequent proteolytic cleaving of plasma C4 and C2 molecules (15,81).

Treatment

Prophylaxis

Classic prophylaxis involves one or more modes of therapy for HAE. The medications most often used to prevent HAE attacks are the anabolic steroids stanazolol or Danazol, and less frequently, the antifibrinolytic agent ϵ-aminocaproic acid, or the use of exogenous C1-E1 in the form of fresh-frozen plasma (FFP). The use of stanazolol (synthetic derivative of testosterone) or Danazol (synthetic steroid derived from ethisterone) increases serum concentrations of the C1-E1 and can prevent episodes of angioedema. Maintenance doses (stanazolol 1–4 mg; Danazol 50–300 mg) can be administered daily, every other day, or in some cases on every third day (80,86). The majority of patients are well controlled on this regimen (80–84). Liver functions studies should be evaluated regularly while using these agents. Typical side effects include irregular menses, virilization and hirsutism, weight gain, depression, and growth retardation in children due to the premature closing of long-bone epiphyses. Higher doses are required for prophylactic use in untreated patients about to have surgery. Specifically, an adult Danazol does of 600 mg daily or a 6 mg daily dose of stanazolol for 6 days preoperative and for 3 days postoperative has proven to be effective (80). Effective prophylaxis requires careful monitoring of the clinical response. The appropriate frequency of administration and dose of medication is dependent on the clinical response and the avoidance of medication side effects.

Oral administration of ϵ-aminocaproic acid also prevents episodes of angioedema by inhibiting the fibrinolytic-dependent generation of kininlike peptides. Its use has not been as effective as Danazol or stanazolol. In addition, treatment with ϵ-aminocaproic acid in cases complicated by hematuria or a bleeding diaphesis is contraindicated.

The intravenous administration of FFP has been used successfully to prevent episodes of edema associated with dental procedures. A series of such infusions results in an approximate 150% increase in the mean plasma C1-E1 concentration (79). Nevertheless, with the current availability of human C1-E1 concentrations, prophylaxis with FFP will probably become a treatment modality of the past.

Recently, the prophylactic intravenous administration of concentrates of human C1-E1 has proven (in Europe) to be very successful before surgical and anesthetic procedures (80,86). Case reports (80) demonstrated the efficacy of administering 1000–1500 units of human C1-E1 intravenously prior to intubation for surgical procedures. The administration of this does provided prophylaxis for 4–5 days. Double-blind crossover studies were conducted in the United States to determine the clinical efficacy of administering the C1-E1 concentrate to patients with HAE (79). Treatment with the C1-E1 concentrate significantly reduced the frequency of extremity, abdominal, genitourinary tract, and laryngeal edema. However, Stanazolol (or Danazol) is currently recommended for long-term prophylaxis in adult patients because of the current high cost and limited availability of the C1-E1 concentrate.

Hospitalization for Acute or Impending HAE Attacks

In the past, approximately 33% of individuals with HAE died of upper airway obstruction (78,87). Currently, more than 10% of patients have undergone intubation or tracheostomy during an attack of angioedema (88,89). In the event of upper airway edema, hospitalization and treatment are needed to prevent obstructive laryngeal edema. Moderately severe episodes of abdominal or extremity angioedema may also require hospitalization. Upper airway edema also arises from the process of intubation; therefore, medical prophylaxis and an anesthesiologist well versed in HAE are of utmost importance. Some patients requiring hospitalization, or those admitted for an anesthetic and/or surgical procedure, would benefit from short-term prophylaxis, and in the event of an acute HAE attack, treatment with the C1-E1 concentrates (79,80,86).

C. Complement Deficiencies and Pregnancy

Complement Deficiencies

Symptomatic individuals with an early complement component (C1–C4) deficiency usually exhibit systemic or recurrent sinopulmonary infections before 5 years of age (15). In contrast, individuals with a late complement component deficiency (C5–C9) may not exhibit a *Neisseria* species infection until after 16 years of age (14,15,49,74). In the former case, if diagnosed, these individuals will have been vaccinated and possibly given antibiotic prophylaxis; however, in the latter case, manifestations of infectious and/or collagen vascular disease may not be present until pregnancy occurs (90). Diagnosis and prevention of systemic maternal infections will also provide fetal protection. Aggressive antibiotic therapy is recommended in women with complement deficiencies with suspected infections, whether pregnant or not. It is recommended that these individuals be vaccinated preferably before pregnancy, but in any event, as soon as possible. Since the vaccines under discussion are not attenuated live viral vaccines, they are safe to administer during all phases of pregnancy.

Unlike IgG molecules, the complement proteins do not cross the placenta (91). Thus, neonatal deficiencies are (except for rare inherited disorders) the result of aberrant synthesis or catabolism of the complement components. This is exemplified by the well-documented C3 deficiency associated with premature neonates. This C3 deficiency is believed to be the result of decreased synthesis by the newborn (91,92).

Hereditary Angioedema

The majority of women with HAE do well throughout pregnancy, but a minority of these women have an increased risk of spontaneous abortions and premature labor (82). Several women with complications of HAE during pregnancy have successfully undergone normal deliveries and caesarian sections without adverse effects. Antifibrinolytic agents and fresh-frozen plasma were used with success in these cases. Nevertheless, these medications are not always effective in preventing laryngeal edema and death (93). Pregnant women with moderate complications of HAE, such as abdominal viscera edema, or cutaneous edema and necrosis, should be treated with intravenous C1-E1 concentrates (80,94). Prevention of attacks can be effectively mediated by the administration of Danazol (or stanazolol); however, it is a known teratogenic agent. In addition, ϵ-aminocaproic acid is classified as a pregnancy category C medication.

Abdominal pain during pregnancy can be a result of edematous viscera, an obstetrical problem, or a gastrointestinal disorder. The use of ultrasonography (as discussed above) can be helpful in delineating the correct etiology.

In some women with HAE, the anxiety and trauma associated with a spontaneous vaginal delivery can precipitate an attack. Local trauma in the uterogenital region may lead to local edema formation and complicate or possibly prevent what was expected to be a normal delivery. Thus, the prophylactic administration of C1-E1 concentrates should be considered prior to delivery (82). An effective regimen of C1-E1 concentrates treatment was reported by Cox et al. (80). In the event of a caesarian section, the C1-E1 regimen described above for surgical and anesthetic procedures should suffice.

A lyophilyzed vapor-treated C1-E1 concentrate has been used to prevent viral transmission (79,80). In the previously described U.S. study, over 100 infusions of C1-E1 concentrate were administered. Patients were followed for up to 4 years without evidence of HIV, hepatitis B, or C seroconversion. Furthermore, no evidence of anti-C1-E1 autoantibody synthesis was detected (79).

VI. Granulocyte Disorders

A. Neutropenia

The granulocyte compartment of the immune system is multifunctional. Two of the more prominent functions are phagocytosis and killing of pathogenic organisms. The most common form of a granulocyte disorder is one of quantity. Neutropenia in most cases is a consequence of either peripheral neutrophil destruction (e.g., autoimmune neutropenia) or decreased neutrophil synthesis (e.g., infiltrative disorder of the bone marrow). The normal adult neutrophil number is more than 2500 cells/mm^3, and neutropenia is defined as less than 1000 cells/mm^3. When significant neutropenia occurs (i.e., fewer than 500 cells/mm^3), an increased incidence of infections ensues. In particular, life-threatening infections caused by *S. aureus*, *P. aeruginosa*, *S. marscesens*, and less frequently *Aspergillus fumigatus* are complications of chronic neutropenic states (14). Thus, diagnosis and an early intervention with aggressive antibiotic therapy is required to diminish morbidity. Table 3 lists several causes of neutropenia.

Autoimmune Neutropenia

One of the most common acquired forms of neutropenia is autoimmune-mediated neutropenia. Autoimmune neutropenia can occur as part of the spectrum of an autoimmune disorder such as seen in Felty's syndrome (rheumatoid arthritis, splenomegaly, and neutropenia) or as an isolated transient disorder. Differentiation of autoimmune from other causes of neutropenia (see Table 3) requires the detection of antigranulocyte autoantibodies and an examination of the bone marrow. In most cases, autoimmune neutropenia is associated with peripheral granulocyte destruction. In such cases, a bone marrow aspiration demonstrates myeloid cell hyperplasia with a shift to the left. In contrast, there have been reported cases of autoantibodies directed against bone marrow myeloid precursor cells with bone marrow aspiration demonstrating a paucity of these cells. Common neutrophil antigens demonstrated to be the targets of autoantibodies are NA1, NA2, and NB1 (95,96).

Clinical Signs and Symptoms

Some of the associated findings with chronic or recurrent neutropenia include gingival hypertrophy, oral apthous ulcers, and hepatosplenomegaly. If these findings are evident upon physical examination, disorders associated with neutropenia should be considered. The skin, oropharynx, lungs, and genitourinary system are the common sites of infection in a neutropenic individual. Individuals with recurrent otitis should be vigorously

Table 3 Causes of Neutropenia

Bone marrow injury	Bone marrow infiltration	Maturation defects
Drugs	Malignancies (lung, breast, prostate, lymphoproliferative tumors)	Folic acid deficiency
Radiation		B_{12} deficiency
Chemicals	Fibrosis	Congenital neutropenia
Congential neutropenia	Agnogenic myeloid metaplasia	PNH[a]
Infectious: *viral* (hepatitis, parvovirus, AIDS)	Chronic mylogenous leukemia	Acute nonlymphocytic leukemia
	Radiation injury	Myelodisplastic syndrome
Infectious: *bacterial* (mycobacterium)	Chronic cytotoxic drug therapy	Polycythemia vera
	Acute megakaryocytic leukemia	

[a]Paroxysmal nocturnal hemaglobinuria.
Source: Ref. 79.

treated in order to prevent hearing loss. Also, careful attention to oral hygiene is recommended to avoid recurrent gingival and periodontal infections (97). Erythroderma and cellulitis are more frequently encountered initially than abscesses and furunculosis in individuals with neutropenia. Neutropenic patients with pneumonia may exhibit nonpurulent sputum and only minimal bilateral infiltrates; however, these individuals are quite ill. In a similar fashion, lab studies of neutropenic patients with pyelonephritis may not demonstrate evidence of pyuria. Neutropenic individuals with pharyngitis may manifest only mild erythrema and injection of the oropharynx without purulent exudates. Although these presentations may appear to be mild initially, a disseminated disease state can quickly occur (97–99). Individuals with these presentations, or neutropenic individuals with a fever or unknown origin, require a thorough workup including cultures, followed by the hospitalization and the administration of broad-spectrum antibiotics (at least until culture results are known).

Treatment

The treatment of autoimmune neutropenia initially involves observation. If the patient is experiencing a benign course, then no intervention is required. In contrast, if evidence of infectious complications exists, then the initial requirement is the acquisition of cultures and the administration of antibiotics. For those individuals with significant morbidity, therapy should also be directed to increasing the neutrophil count. This can be accomplished by the administration of steroids, with the use of IVIG, or by splenectomy. The use of steroids usually results in a significant but transient increase in the neutrophil count (96–98, 100). Similarly, the administration of IVIG also results in a rapid but transient increase in the neutrophil count (95,98,101). The use of steroids is associated with more significant side effects than IVIG (see treatment discussion in the alloimmune neonatal neutropenia section below). Finally, in some rare cases, splenectomy has resulted in improving neutrophil counts, but the potential infectious disease consequences need to be fully assessed prior to taking this step (97,101).

VII. Pregnancy and Granulocyte Disorders

A. Cyclical Neutropenia

Pregnancy is associated with a relative leukocytosis which becomes more pronounced during labor and the immediate postpartum period (102). This relative leukocytosis may contribute to the benign course experienced in some forms of neutropenia during pregnancy. Cyclical neutropenia is characterized by periodic episodes of neutropenia that at times precede local and systemic infections. A decreased entry of granulocytic precursor cells into the process of granulopoiesis is thought to be the basis of this disorder (103). Recent case reports have documented that women with cyclical neutropenia had benign courses during pregnancy with increased mean absolute neutrophil counts (104,105). Studies on a larger population of individuals are required to substantiate these preliminary observations.

B. Alloimmune Neonatal Neutropenia

Definition and Pathogenesis

Alloimmune neonatal neutropenia is a rare disorder that usually affects the offspring of multiparous women or those who have received numerous blood transfusions (102,106–108). This is a neonatal acquired form of autoimmune neutropenia. Severe neutropenia can be documented at birth and is shortly followed by infection (102,106–108). Neutropenia is a result of the transplacentally acquired maternal IgG antibodies directed against the neutrophil NA1, NA2, and other neutrophil-specific antigens (95,96). Several reports have demonstrated that the anti-neutrophil antibody is usually targeted against a paternal neutrophil antigen that is expressed by the offspring but not the mother (106–108). Apparently, exposure to fetal cells expressing the paternal antigen in previous pregnancies, or exposure during previous blood transfusions, precipitated the anti-neutrophil antibody production by the mother.

Treatment

Neonates with alloimmune neonatal neutropenia are at risk for infection. Vigorous antibiotic therapy is required when sepsis is suspected. In some cases, neutropenia may persist for 4–5 months, and close observation may be required (106). We shall briefly discuss a treatment modality for autoimmune neutropenia of infancy and relate it to the treatment of alloimune neonatal neutropenia. Autoimmune neutropenia of infancy is characterized by severe neutropenia associated with recurrent infections. As is evident in alloimmune neonatal neutropenia, antineutrophil antibodies directed against the neutrophils NA1, NA2, and other antigens appear to be the cause of this disorder. However, in contrast to alloimmune neonatal neutropenia, these are autoantibodies that are not maternally acquired. The time period required for exposure to the putative antigen and to produce IgG autoantibodies may be the reason that the mean age of presentation is at 8 months (98). Several studies have demonstrated the efficacy of administering IVIG to infants with autoimmune neutropenia (95,98). In the majority of cases, there is a quick (approximately 3 days) increase in the absolute neutrophil count (98). Only in one case report has the administration of IVIG proven to diminish the neutrophil count. In this particular report, a neonate received IVIG which contained antineutrophil antibodies. Others have successfully treated autoimmune neutropenia with oral steroids (96–98, 100). However, some individuals treated with steroids developed fungal infections (96). Furthermore, the risk of severe viral infections or overwhelming sepsis is a risk that must be considered if the chronic use of steroids is contemplated. Therefore, for neonates with alloimmune neonatal neutrophil and infectious complications, antibiotics and the administration of IVIG should be considered. Treatment protocols vary from 500 mg/kg/day for 4 days to 1/kg/day until the absolute neutrophil count (ANC) is greater than 1000 cells/mm^3 (95,98). With the latter protocol, the mean time period required to raise the ANC above 1000 cells/mm^3 was 3 days. In addition, the ANC remained above 1000 cells/mm^3 for approximately 9–14 days (95,98). A few patients needed repeated infusions of IVIG, depending on their ANC and the recurrence of infections (98).

Prior to the initiation of treatment, the diagnosis of autoimmune neutropenia should be confirmed. Some other disorders to be considered include the acute-phase reversible neutropenia of neonatal sepsis, drug-induced leukopenia, Kostmann's syndrome (severe congenital neutropenia), the neutropenia associated with autoimmune hemolytic anemia and thrombocytopenia, and congenital dysgranulopoietic neutropenia.

C. Preeclampsia and Neonatal Neutropenia

Infants born to mothers with preeclampsia often develop neutropenia. In a recent review of 301 cases of low-birth weight infants of mothers with preeclampsia, 48% of these neonates were found to be neutropenic prior to 12 hr of age (109). Neonates with neutropenia were found to be premature, products of pregnancies with severe preeclampsia, and small for gestational age. Statistical analysis demonstrated that a low ANC was the prominent factor associated with early-onset sepsis. Similar results were also reported by Koenig and Christensen (110). They studied 72 infants whose mothers were hypertensive during pregnancy. Forty-nine percent of these infants were neutropenic, some for up to 30 days. Noscomical infections occurred in 8 infants (23%) compared to only 1 non-neutropenic newborn (3%).

Until recently, few options were available to effectively treat this form of neutropenia, which has been suspected to result from an arrest in progenitor cell differentiation (110). In several forms of neutropenia, with a similar arrest in granulopoieses, treatment with recombinant granulocyte colony stimulating factor (G-CSF) has been quite effective. G-CSF treatment enhanced neutrophil recovery, decreased the duration of neutropenia, and diminished the frequency of life-threatening infections experienced by these individuals (111–115).

Makhlouf et al. (115) demonstrated that the administration of G-CSF significantly increased the ANC in 8 or 9 neutropenic infants studied who were born to women with preeclampsia. The rise in ANC occurred within 6 hr and lasted at least 72 hr. Other preliminary studies have demonstrated similar results for G-CSF treatment of neutropenic neonates born to mothers with preeclampsia (114). These preliminary studies show promise. Nevertheless, in a recent report, two neutropenic patients (with Kostmann's syndrome) developed acute myeloid leukemia while undergoing G-CSF treatment (112). Further studies are required to determine the efficacy, safety, and best clinical settings for the administration of G-CSF.

References

1. Bachman R. Studies on the serum γA-globulin level. III. The frequency of a-γA-globulinemia. Scand J Clin Lab Invest 1965; 17:316–320.
2. Thieffry S, Arthuis M, Aicardi J, Lyon G. L'ataxie-telangiectasie (7 observations personelles). Rev Neurol 1961; 105:390–405.
3. Schaffer FM, Monteiro RC, Volanakis JE, Cooper MD. IgA deficiency. Immunodef Rev 1991; 3:15–45.
4. Oxelius VA, Laurell AB, Lindquist B, Golebiowska H, Axelsson U, Biorkander J, Hanson LA. IgG subclasses in selective IgA deficiency: Importance of IgG2-IgA deficiency. N Engl J Med 1981; 304:1476–1477.
5. Preud'homme JL, Hanson LA. IgA subclass deficiency. Immunodef Rev 1990; 2:129–149.
6. Burks AW, Sampson HA, Buckley RH. Anaphylactic reactions after gammaglobulin administration in patients with hypogammaglobulinemia. Detection of IgE antibodies to IgA. N Engl J Med 1986; 314:560–563.
7. Rosen FS, Cooper MD, Wedgwood RJP. The primary immunodeficiencies. N Engl J Med 1995; 333:431–440.
8. Conley MA, Cooper MD. Immature IgA B cells in IgA-deficient patients. N Engl J Med 1981; 305:495–497.
9. Hammarstrom L, Carlsson B, Smith CIE, Wallin J, Wieslander L. Detection of IgA constant region genes in IgA deficient donors: evidence against gene deletions. Clin Exp Immunol 1985; 60:661–664.
10. Lewkoma RM, Gardner D, Doe WF. IgA deficiency in one of identical twins. Br Med J 1976; 1:311–313.
11. Aarli JA. Drug-induced IgA deficiency in epileptic patients. Arch Neurol 1976; 33:296–299.

12. Soothill, JF, Hayes K, Dudgeon JA. The immunoglobulins in congenital rubella. Lancet 1966; 1:1385–1388.

13. Good R, Zak S, Condie R, Bridges R. Clinical investigation of patients with agammaglobulinemia and hypogammaglobulinemia. Pediatr Clin N Am 1960; 7:397–414.

14. Stiehm ER, Chin TW, Haas A, Peerless AG. Infectious complications of the primary immunodeficiencies. Clin Immunol Immunopathol 1986; 40:69–86.

15. Figueroa JE, Denson P. Infectious diseases associated with complement deficiencies. Clin Microbiol Rev 1991; 4:359–395.

16. Roifman CM, Levison H, Gelfand EW. High-dose versus low-dose intravenous immunoglobulin in hypogammaglobulinemia with chronic lung disease. Lancet 1986; 1:1075–1077.

17. Cunningham-Rundles C. Disorders of the IgA system. In: Stiehm ER, ed. Immunologic Disorders of Infants and Children. Philadelphia: Saunders, 1996:423–442.

18. Burks AW Jr, Steele RW. Selective IgA deficiency. Ann Allergy 1986; 57: 3–8.

19. Cassidy JT, Burt A, Petty R, Sullivan D. Selective IgA deficiency in connective tissue diseases. N Engl J Med 1969; 280:275.

20. Klemola T. Deficiency of immunoglobulin A. Ann Clin Res 1987; 19: 248–257.

21. Buckley RH, Dees SC. Correlation of milk precipitins with IgA deficiency. N Engl J Med 1969; 281:465–469.

22. James SP, Jones EA, Schafer DF, Hoofnagle JH, et al. Selective immunoglobulin A deficiency associated with primary biliary cirrhosis in a family with liver disease. Gastroenterol 1986; 90:283–288.

23. Donan YL, Dinari G, Garty BZ, Horodruceau C, et al. Cholelithiasis in children with immunoglobulin A deficiency: a new gastroenterologic syndrome. J Pediat Gastroenterol Nutr 1983; 2:663–666.

24. Schaffer FM, Palermos J, Zhu Z, Barger B, et al. Individuals with IgA deficiency and common variable immunodeficiency share polymorphisisms of major histocompatibility complex class III genes. Proc Natl Acad Sci USA 1989; 86:8015–8019.

25. Volanakis JE, Zhu ZB, Schaffer FM, Macon KJ, et al. MHC class III genes and susceptibility to IgA deficiency and common variable immunodeficiency. J Clin Invest 1992; 89:1914–1922.

26. Wilton AN, Cobain TJ, Dawkins RL. Family studies of IgA deficiency. Immunogenet 1985; 21:333–342.

27. Vyas GN, Perkins HA, Fudenberg HH. Anaphylactoid transfusion reactions associated with anti-IgA. Lancet 1968; 2:312–315.

28. Saulsbury FT. Selective IgA deficiency temporarily associated with Epstein-Barr virus infection. J Pediatr 1989; 115:268–270.

29. van Riel PLCM, van de Putte LBA, Gribnau FWJ, et al. IgA deficiency during aurothioglucose treatment. Scand J Rheum 1984; 13:334–336.

30. Delamere JP, Fart M, Grindulis KA. sulphasalazine induced selective IgA deficiency in rheumatoid arthritis. Br Med J 1983; 286:1547–1548.

31. Cunningham-Rundles C, Wong S, Bjorkander J, Hanson LA. Use of an IgA depleted intravenous immunoglobulin in a patient with an anti-IgA antibody. Clin Immunol Immunopathol 1986; 35:141–143.

32. Rosen FS, Janeway CA. The gamma globulins. 3. The antibody deficiency syndromes. N Engl J Med 19866; 10:117–121.

33. Ochs HD, Fischer SH, Wedgwood RJ, et al. Comparison of high-dose and low-dose intravenous immunoglobulin therapy in patients with primary immunodeficiency diseases. Am J Med 1984; 76:78–82.

34. Sacher RA, King JC. Intravenous gamma-globulin in pregnancy: a review. OB GYN Surv 1988; 44:25–34.

35. Bridges RA, Condie RM, Zak SJ, Good RJ. The morphological basis of antibody formation development during the neonatal period. J Lab Clin Med 1959; 53:331–337.

36. Holland NH, Holland P. Immunologic maturation in an infant of an agammaglobulinaemic mother. Lancet 1966; 1:1152–1155.

37. Kobayashi RH, Hyman CJ, Stiehm ER. Immunologic maturation in an infant born to a mother with agammaglobulinemia. Am J Dis Child 1980; 134:942.

38. Gitilin D, Janeway CA. Agammaglobulinemia: congenital acquired and transient forms. Prog Hematol 1956; 1:318–329.

39. Conley ME, Stiehm ER. Immunodeficiency disorders: general considerations In: Stiehm ER, ed. Immunologic Disorders in Infants and Children. Philadelphia: Saunders, 1996:201–252.

40. Pritchard JA. Changes in blood volume during pregnancy and delivery. Anesthesiology 1965; 26:393–399.

41. Schaffer FM, Newton JA. Intravenous gamma globulin administration to common variable immunodeficient women during pregnancy: case report and review of the literature. J Perinatol 1994; 14:114–117.

42. Williams PE, Leen CLS, Heppleston AD, Yap PL. IgG replacement therapy for primary hypogammaglobulinaemia during pregnancy: report of 9 pregnancies in 4 patients. Blut 1990; 60:198–201.

43. Smith CIE, Hammarstrom L. Intravenous immunoglobulin in pregnancy. OB GYN 1985; 66:39S–40S.

44. Sorenson RU, Tomford JW, Gyves MT, Judge NE, Polman SE. Use of intravenous immune globulin in pregnant women with common variable hypogammaglobulinemia. Am J Med 1984; 76:73–77.

45. Hausser C, Buriot D. Gamma globulin therapy during pregnancy in mother with hypogammaglobulinemia. Am J Obstet Gynecol 1982; 144:112.

46. Berger M, Cupps TR, Fauci AS. High-dose immunoglobulin replacement therapy by slow subcutaneous infusion during pregnancy. JAMA 1982; 247:2824–2825.

47. Morell A, Schnoz M, Barandun S. Build-up and maintenance of IgG serum concentrations with intravenous immunoglobulin in patients with primary humoral immunodeficiency. Vox San 1982; 43:212–219.

48. Wollheim FA, Williams RC Jr. Immunoglobulin studies in six kindreds of patients with adult hypogammaglobulinemia. J Lab Clin Med 1965; 66: 433–445.

49. Primary immunodeficiency diseases. Report of a WHO scientific group. Clin Exp Immunol 1995; 99:S2–S25.

50. Muller-Eberhard HJ. The membrane attack complex of complement. Annu Rev Immunol 1986; 4:503–528.

51. Cooper NR. The classical complement pathway: activation and regulation of the first complement component. Adv Immunol 1985; 37:151–216.

52. Bottger EC, Bitter-Suermann D. Complement and the regulation of humoral human immune responses. Immunol Today 1987; 8:261–264.

53. Ochs HD, Wedgwood RJ, Frank MM, Heller SR, Hosea SW. The role of complement in the induction antibody responses. Clin Exp Immunol 1983; 53:208–216.

54. Ochs, Wedgwood RJ, Heller SR, Beatty PG. Complement membrane glycoproteins, and complement receptors: their role in regulation of the immune system. Clin Immunol Immunopathol 1986; 40:94–104.

55. O'Neil KM, Ochs HD, Heller SR, Cork LC, Morris JM, Winkelstein JA. Role of C3 in humoral immunity. Defective antibody production in C3-deficient dogs. J Immunol 1988; 140:1939–1945.

56. Pangburn MK. The alternative pathway. In: Ross GD, ed. Immunobiology of the Complement System. Orlando, FL, Academic Press, 1986:45–62.

57. Pangburn MK, Muller-Eberhard HJ. The alternative pathway of complement. Springer Semin Immunopathol 1984; 7:163–192.

58. Harriman GR, Podack ER, Braude AI, Corbeil C, et al. Activation of complement by serum-resistant *Neisseria gonorrhoeae.* Assembly of the membrane attack complex without subsequent cell death. J Exp Med 1982; 156:1235–1249.

59. Harriman GR, Esser AF, Podack ER, Wunderlich AC, et al The role of C9 in complement mediated-killing of *Neisseria.* J Immunol 1981; 127: 2386–2390.

60. Hassig AJ, Borel JF, Ammann P. Essentialle hypokomplementamie. Pathol Microbiol 1964; 27:542–547.

61. Alper CA, Awdeh Z, Yunis EJ. Frequency of the C2 deficiency gene among normal caucasians. Complement 1987; 4:125.

62. Hauptmann G, Goetz J, Uring-Lambert B, Grosshans E. Component deficiencies. 2. The fourth component. Prog Allergy 1986; 39:232–249.

63. Sullivan KE, Winkelstein JA. Prenatal diagnosis of heterozygous deficiency of the second component of complement. Clin Diag Lab Immunol 1994; 1: 606–607.

64. Carroll MC, Palsdottir A, Belt KT, Porter RR. Deletion of complement C4 and steroid 21-hydroxylase genes in the HLA class III region. EMBO J 1985; 4:2547–2552.

65. Barbara G, Rittner C, Schneider PM. Genetic basis of human complement C4A deficiency. Detection of a point mutation leading to nonexpression. J Clin Invest 1993; 91:1681–1686.

66. Sjoholm AG. Absence and dysfunction of properdin as a basis for susceptibility to meningococcal disease. Immunol Immunopathol Immunother Forum 198; 4:3–12.

67. Sjoholm AG. Inherited complement deficiency states: implications for immunity and immunologic disease. Acta Pathol Microbiol Immunol Scan Sect C 1990; 98:861–874.

68. Densen P, Weiler M, Griffiss JM, Hoffman JL. Familial properdin deficiency and fatal meningococcemia: correction of the bactericidal defect by vaccination. N Engl J Med 1987: 316:922–926.

69. Sjoholm AG. Braconier JH, Sodestrom C. Properdin deficiency in a family with fulminant meningococcal infections. Clin Exp Immunol 1982; 50: 291–297.

70. Sjoholm AG, Soderstrom C, Nilsson LA. A second variant of properdin deficiency: the detection of properdin at low concentrations in affected males. Complement 1988; 5:130–140.

71. Sjoholm AG, Kuijper EJ, Tijsen CC, Jansz A, Bol P, Spanjaard L, Zanen HC. Dysfunctional properdin in a Dutch family with meningococcal disease. N Engl J Med 1988; 318:33–37.

72. Goonewardena P, Sjoholm AG, Nilsson LA, Pettersson U. Linkage analysis of the properdin deficiency gene: suggestion of a locus in the proximal part of the short arm of the X chromosome. Genomics 1988; 2:115–118.

73. Goundis, D, Holt SM, Boyd Y, Reid KB. Localization of the properdin structural locus to Xp11.23-Xp21.1. Genomics 1989; 5:56–60.

74. Swart AG, Fijen CA, Bulte MT, Daha MR, et al. Complement deficiencies and meningococcal disease in the Netherlands. Ned Tijdschr Geneeskd 1993; 137:1147–1152.

75. Potter PC, Frasch CE, van der Sande WJ, Cooper RC, et al. Prophylaxis against *Neisseria meningitidis* infections and antibodyresponses in patients with deficiency of the sixth component of complement. J Infect Dis 1990; 161:932–937.

76. Barrett DJ, Boyle MD. Restoration of complement function in vivo by plasma infusion in factor I (C3b inactivator) deficiency. J Pediatr 1984; 104: 76–84.

77. Rao CP, Minta JO, Laski B, Alper CA, Gelfand EW. Inherited C8 beta subunit deficiency in a patient with recurrent meningococcal infections: in vivo functional kinetic analysis of C8. Clin Exp Immunol 1985; 60:183–190.

78. Osler W. Hereditary angioneurotic oedema. Am J Med Sci 1888; 95: 362–367.

79. Waters AT, Rosen FS, Frank MM. Treatment of hereditary angioedema with a vapor-heated C1 inhibitor concentrate. N Engl J Med 1996; 334: 1630–1634.

80. Cox MB, Holdcroft A. Hereditary angioneurotic edema: current management in pregnancy. Anaesthia 1995; 50:547–549.
81. Cicardi M, Agostoni A. Hereditary angioedema. N Engl J Med 1996; 334: 1666–1667.
82. Nielson EW, Gran JT, Straume B, Mellbye OJ, et al. Hereditary angio-oedema: new clinical observations and autoimmune screening, complement and kallikrein-kinin analyses. J Intern Med 1996; 239:119–130.
83. Horan RF, Schneider LC, Sheffer AL. Allergic skin disorders and mastocytosis. JAMA 1992; 268:2858–2868.
84. Petry F, Le DT, Kirschfink M, Loos M. Non-sense and missense mutations in the structural genes of complement component C1q A and C chains are linked with two different types of complete selective C1q deficiencies. J Immunol 1995; 155:4734–4738.
85. He S, Tsang S, North J, Chohan N, et al. Epitope mapping of C1 inhibitor deficiency. J Immunol 1996; 156:2009–2013.
86. de Wazieres B, Dupond JL, Hory B, Humbert P, et al. Hereditary angioneurotic edema: an underestimated medical emergency. Apropos of 33 cases. Ann Dermatol Venereol 1995; 122:11–15.
87. Donaldson VH, Rosen FS. Hereditary angioneurotic edema: a clinical survey. Pediatr 1966; 37:1017–10127.
88. Agostini A, Cicardi M. Hereditary and acquired C1-inhibitor deficiency: biological and clinical characteristics in 253 patients. Medicine 1992; 71: 206–215.
89. Pruet CW, Kornblut AD, Brickman C, Kalimer MA, et al. Management of the airway in patients with angioedema. Laryngoscope 1983; 93:749–754.
90. Hironaka K, Makino H. Amano T, Ota Z. Immune complex glomerulonephritis in a pregnant woman with congential C9 deficiency. Intern Med 1993; 32:806–809.
91. Sawyers MK, Ferguson ML, Lanier SR, Stiehm ER. Developmental aspects of the human complement system. Biol Neonate 1974; 19:142–162.
92. Winkelstein JA, Kurlandsky LE, Swift AJ. Defective activation of the third component of complement in the sera of newqborn infants. Pediatr Res 1979; 13:1093–1096.
93. Nielsen EW, Kjernlie DF, Aaseth J. A fatal case of hereditary angioedema. Tdsskr Nor Laegeforen 1995; 115:43–44.
94. Perkins W, Downie I, Keefe M, Chisholm M. Cutaneous necrosis in pregnancy secondary to activated protein C resistance in hereditary angioedema. J R Soc Med 1995; 88:229P–230P.
95. Lalezari P. Monoochehr K, Petrosova M. Autoimmune neutropenia of infancy. J Pediatr 1985; 109:764–769.
96. Lalezari P, Jiang AF, Yegen L, Santorineou M. Chronic autoimmune neutropenia due to anti-NA2 antibody. N Engl J Med 1975; 293:744–747.
97. Bagby GC Jr. Leukopenia. In: Wyngaarden JB, Smith LH Jr, eds. Cecil Textbook of Medicine. Philadelphia: Saunders, 1988:661–667.

98. Bussel J, Lalezari P, Fikrig Senih. Intravenous treatment with γ-globulin of autoimmune neutropenia of infancy. J Pediatr 1988; 112:298–301.

99. Turgeon PL, Laverdiere M, Perron L. Successful treatment of *Pseudomonas meningitis* and septicemia in a leukemic neutropenic adult. Am J Clin Pathol 1975; 63:135–141.

100. Boxer LA, Greenberg Ms, Boxer GJ, Stossel TP. Autoimmune neutropenia. N Engl J Med 1975; 293:748–753.

101. Wordell CJ. Immunotherapy of ideopathic thrombocytopenia purpora and autoimmune neutropenia. Pharmacotherapy 1987; 7:S41–S47.

102. Ledger WJ. Immunity. In: Infection in the female. Philadelphia: Lea & Febiger, 1986:73–76.

103. Greenberg PL, Bax J, Levin J. Andrews TM. Alteration of colony-stimulating factor output, endotoxemia, and granulopoiesis in cyclic neutropenia. Am J Hematol 1976; 1:375–385.

104. Polcz TE, Stiller RJ, Whetham JC. Pregnancy in patients with cyclic neutropenia. Am J Obstet Gynecol 1993; 169:393–394.

105. Pajor A, Szakacs Z. Pregnancy in cyclic neutropenia. Gynecol Obstet Invest 1991; 32:189–190.

106. Puig N, Montoro JA, Villalaba JL, Gimeno M, et al. Alloimmune neonatal neutropenia: flow cytometry study of the first patient described in Spain with identification of an anti-NA1. Sangre 1993; 38:235–238.

107. Rios E, Heresi G, Arevalo M. Familial alloimmune neutropenia of NA-2 specificity. Am J Pediatr Hematol Oncol 1991; 13:296–299.

108. Skacel PO, Stacey TE, Tidmarsh CE, Contreras M. Maternal alloimmunization to HLA, platelet and granulocyte-specific antigens during pregnancy: its influence on cord blood granulocyte and platelet counts. Br J Haematol 1989; 71:119–123.

109. Doron MW, Makhlouf RA, Katz VL, Lawson EE, Stiles AD. Increased incidence of sepsis at birth in neutropenic infants of mothers with preeclampsia. J Pediatr 1994; 125:452–458.

110. Koenig JM, Christensen RD. Incidence, neutrophil kinetics, and natural history of neonatal neutropenia associated with maternal hypertension. N Engl J Med 1989; 321:557–562.

111. Naparstek E. Granulocyte colony-stimulating factor, congenital neutropenia, and acute myeloid leukemia. N Engl J Med 1995; 333:516–518.

112. Dong F, Byrnes RK, Tidow N, Welte K, et al. Mutations in the gene for the of granulocyte colony-stimulating-factor receptor in patients with acute myeloid leukemia preceded by severe congenital neutropenia. N Engl J Med 1995; 333:487–493.

113. La Gamma EF, Alpan O, Kocherlakota P. Effect of granulocyte colony-stimulating factor on preeclampsia-associated neonatal neutropenia. J Pediatr 1995; 126:457–459.

114. Russell AR, Davies EG, Ball SE, Gordon-Smith E. Granulocyte colony stimulating factor treatment for neonatal neutropenia. Arch Dis Child Fetal Neonatal Ed 1995; 72:F53–F54.

115. Makhlouf RA, Doron MW, Bose CL, Price WA, Stiles AD. Administration of granulocyte colony-stimulating factor to neutropenic low birth weight infants of mothers with preeclampsia. J Pediatr 1995; 126:454–456.

26

Immunological Causes of Fetal Loss

HENRY N. CLAMAN

University of Colorado School of Medicine
Denver, Colorado

I. Introduction

A successful pregnancy is the felicitous result of a very large number of processes which operate over a long period of time. It is expected, therefore, that a wide variety of factors may be important in causing the pregnancy to terminate prior to the point of extrauterine viability. The reasons for such spontaneous miscarriages or abortions can be grouped in several general categories:

Genetic
Anatomic
Infectious
Hormonal
Autoimmune
"Idiopathic" (not clearly any of the above)

This book is not concerned with the first four categories, and autoimmune reasons for pregnancy loss have been covered in Chapters 21, 22, and 23. This chapter will cover the subject of *recurrent pregnancy loss* and its possible immune basis.

II. Frequency of Spontaneous Pregnancy Loss

The frequency of pregnancy loss is a subject in which definitions and new methods of diagnosis are forcing changes in medical thinking. It is necessary to state clearly the criteria for the presence of a pregnancy in order to be clear about the frequency of pregnancy loss. For clinically recognized pregnancies, it is often stated that 15% terminate spontaneously as a miscarriage (1). Now, however, "early" (preclinical) pregnancies can be diagnosed using hormonal methods, and even "very early" pregnancies (fertilized ova present before uterine implantation) can be detected (2,3). When these newer methods of detection are used, the results support the thinking of many observers, i.e., that far more than 15% of pregnancies end in spontaneous abortion. One study noted that 15% of very early pregnancies were lost, another 22% of early pregnancies failed, and only 9% of clinically apparent pregnancies failed. This is an overall loss rate of 46%, with 80% of the losses occurring before a clinical pregnancy was defined (3).

If these results are applied to the general population of women who are able to become pregnant, it is quite certain that many women who are considered nulliparous or primigravidas will have had previous unrecognized spontaneous miscarriages. Nevertheless, the detection of early and very early pregnancy losses is not yet routine, and most studies are confined to those instances of *clinically apparent pregnancies.*

III. Definitions of Recurrent Spontaneous Abortion

It is important to recognize right at the outset that there is no agreement about the definition of recurrent spontaneous abortion (RSAb). Criteria vary from one study to another, and understanding this variability may be crucial for the proper analysis of the results of surveys, as well as therapeutic trials. The most frequently used criterion for the designation of RSAb is the occurrence of three or more spontaneous miscarriages of clinical pregnancies. (It is usually assumed but not always stated that the woman's partner is the same for at least three losses.) Nevertheless, at least one study proposes that two losses are sufficient to make a diagnosis of RSAb (4). It is also generally considered that a designation of RSAb will allow no more than one pregnancy of 28 weeks or more (5). Some workers believe that women with RSAb and one successful pregnancy ("secondary aborters") should be considered separately from women with RSAb who have never had a successful pregnancy ("primary aborters"). This item is controversial.

The point in pregnancy at which the fetus is lost is an additional important variable. It is customary to distinguish first-trimester from second-trimester losses. Since, however, it is possible to establish the existence of a pregnancy before it is "clinical" (see above), it would be optimal to categorize losses as very early, early, and clinical. As yet, these distinctions have not been widely made in the analysis of RSAb. One can reasonably ask whether, with regard to *any* cause of fetal loss, the responsible factors are likely to be the same for very early versus early pregnancies or as compared with clinically apparent pregnancies. One suspects that the responsible factors will be found to be different in these three categories.

IV. Causes of Recurrent Spontaneous Abortion

It is generally agreed that about 50% of RSAbs can be accounted for by genetic, anatomic, hormonal, infectious, and autoimmune problems.

Idiopathic or *unexplained* are terms used to designate the other 50% of cases, in which an etiology cannot be found. It is in these situations that the question has arisen: *Are there immunological reasons for RSAb that are not accounted for by overt autoimmune disorders?* That is the subject of the remainder of this chapter. It is important to recognize two facts. First, the subject is very controversial. There are strongly held opinions on several "sides" of the question. Second, the literature on this subject is large, often redundant, and of variable quality.

V. Immunological Causes of Recurrent Fetal Loss

A. Immunological Considerations in RSAb

At least four areas of inquiry lead one to consider whether some of the idiopathic cases of RSAb have important immunological components. First, as was discussed in Chapters 21, 22, and 23, overt (or perhaps subclinical) autoimmune disease may lead to pregnancy loss. Second, there is an interesting mouse model of RSAb in which both genetic and immunological components are important (see below). Third, the beneficial effects of outbreeding in animal husbandry (larger litters, healthier pups) may have an immunological component. Fourth, some clinical anecdotes, while not rigorously collated, are intriguing and suggest immunological (and also genetic) factors. Consider the following generic scenario. Mary marries Bob and they have three children. Mary gets divorced, marries John, and they have three miscarriages. It is obvious that Mary can get pregnant and go to term, but only if Bob is the father. Are there immunological factors that lead to pregnancy success with Bob but fail with John? (If advancing maternal age seems to be a possible explanation, the order of delivery and miscarriage can be reversed.)

However, three types of data indicate that immunological considerations may not be important in pregnancy nor in RSAb. On the humoral side, women with common variable immunodeficiency (CVID) have severe hypogammaglobulinemia. They make little if any antibody to conventional antigens or to paternal HLA antigens. Nonetheless, they can go to term, and CVID is not known to be associated with RSAb. On the cellular side, mice with SCID (severe combined immunodeficiency) lack effective T (and B) cell systems, yet can reproduce. Finally, although inbreeding of genetically identical animals does lead to smaller litters and more runts, still, these couples reproduce fairly well. After all, the spectacular success of modern immunobiology has depended to a large extent on the ready availability of genetically identical strains of mice which are themselves the progeny of MHC-identical brother–sister matings.

In view of the above three considerations, it would be safe to say that, in general, if immunological factors are important in RSAb, they are likely to be operating in an auxiliary rather than in a definitive way.

B. An Animal Model for RSAb

A mouse model for RSAb exists. In this model, DBA/2 males mated to CBA females have normal pregnancy rates but high rates of embryo loss. (Mice have bicornuate uteri, in which the embryos—sometimes as many as 10—are arranged much like peas in a pod. Embryo loss in mice is not usually associated with loss of the entire litter but rather by death and resorption of individual fetuses.) This phenomenon is associated with several immunological abnormalities, including infiltration and activation of suppressor T cells and their products (6). Recently, experiments have shown that NK function is not normal in these pregnancies and that NK cells may be responsible for fetal loss (7,8). Of great interest to people who treat RSAb with immunotherapy (see below) are experiments showing that the embryo failure rate can be diminished by leukocyte immunization. It is important to recognize, however, the immunological specificity of this immunization. A previous pregnancy by a BALB/c male (which carries the same MHC as the DBA/2 male) will protect the CBA female from aborting fetuses in a subsequent pregnancy by a DBA/2 male. Furthermore, immunologically nonspecific procedures such as treatment with complete Freund's adjuvant, injections of poly I-C, reduction of TNF-α levels in vivo, or injections of GM-CSF will all decrease the miscarriage rate. Conversely, other nonspecific measures such as giving anti-GM-CSF or anti-CD8 will increase the abortion rate (8).

While it is not always possible to apply the results of animal studies directly to humans, the existence of animal models facilitates progress in understanding complex biological phenomena. In the case of immunology, it is important to recognize that most phenomena identified in mice have been shown to be significant in humans.

VI. Maternal Immune Responses and RSAb

Are there data to support the idea that maternal immune responses might be abnormal in women with RSAb?

A. Blocking Factors in Serum

In 1976, Rocklin and colleagues reported provocative experiments (9). They investigated the production of "migration inhibitory factor" (MIF) in mixed leukocyte reactions (MLRs). This was perhaps the first T-cell cytokine, and it was believed to be an important mediator in DTH, but the readout was a cumbersome in-vitro bioassay. Their findings were that:

1. MIF was produced during MLRs of PBL from either successful or RSAb couples.
2. The serum of successful multiparous women had an IgG factor that was able to block the MLR, but
3. The serum of women with RSAb was not able to block the MLRs.

The paradigm which emerged was that most couples, successful or with RSAb, had maternal antipaternal reactivity of a DTH type (as shown by the MLR) but successful women had a serum factor which thwarted this potentially harmful mechanism. The investigators thought that the IgG was probably directed to class II paternal antigens.

Similar experiments were reported by others (10). Still a third group showed that the serum-blocked factors in RSAb women could be increased by leukocyte transfusions (11,12).

These experiments are difficult to do, and have not been pursued by many groups. However, it is interesting to note that the concept that normal pregnancy may be associated with an antibody which downregulates a DTH response is very much in consonance with the most recent generalization that a normal pregnancy is associated with a "tilt" from TH_1 to TH_2 responses (13).

Natural killer (NK) cells are non-T, non-B mononuclear cells which are operationally defined by their ability to kill certain tumor targets in vitro. This killing shows no clonal specificity, nor is there immunological memory in the NK system. These characteristics have suggested that NK cells might be important in "immune surveillance" against mutant clones of malignant cells. Might they also be important in maternal surveillance of "foreign" paternal antigens on the fetus?

Although many NK cells carry the CD3-TcR complex, target lysis does not appear to involve this complex, and many NK cells lack this complex. Many cells with NK activity bear markers such as NK1.1, CD16, and CD56. While NK cells appear in peripheral blood at a modest level, it has been intriguing that rodent and mammalian decidua are considerably enriched in cells with NK markers. In the uterus, these cells have the morphology of large granular leukocytes (LGL) and are frequently designated U-LGL. The predominant human phenotype for such cells is $CD2^+3^-16^-45^+56^+57^+$ (reviewed in Ref. 14, chap. 2).

Whether NK cells are important in pregnancy remains an unsettled question. NK-deficient mice have normal pregnancies (15). In humans, NK cells are more frequent in the decidua than in the peripheral blood, but NK *activity* is decreased in decidua (16).

Studies have also tried to tie abnormal NK numbers or function with failed pregnancies. Several years ago, a report appeared in which NK cells were counted immunohistochemically in the mouse model of RSAb described above (7). There was a clear increase in decidual NK cells in those embryos which were being resorbed. Comparable changes in T or B cells were not seen. These results suggest that increased NK cell numbers (lytic activity was not measured) accompanied fetal loss, although it was not possible to invoke a cause-and-effect relationship. A recent paper studied NK cells in human pregnancies which ended in delivery, in blighted ova, or in RSAb. The numbers of decidual NK cells did not differ in these three situations, but decidual NK *activity* was higher in the two failed pregnancy categories than in the successful women (17). Thus, the role of NK cells in pregnancy continues to unfold.

B. Embryotoxic Factors

Recent work has suggested that women with RSAb have leukocytes which respond in culture with trophoblastic antigens to produce soluble factors which are toxic to cultured mouse embryos (18). The nature of these factors is as yet unknown. Furthermore, the production of embryotoxic factors is associated with an increase in T-cell proliferation against trophoblast antigens, a phenomenon found in 53% of RSAb women and 0% of controls

(19). These observations indicate that many RSAb women have abnormal T-cell reactivity to trophoblastic antigens. Whether this is causally related to RSAb remains to be seen.

VII. RSAb and Sharing of MHC Antigens

The concept that genetic similarities, i.e., sharing of MHC alleles, may promote RBSb is currently a subject of great interest. It is likely that this idea developed as a result of a number of considerations, and it has been in the medical literature at least since 1977 (20). From the Darwinian standpoint, extensive HLA sharing between partners would promote MHC homozygosity in the offspring. This, in turn, might favor the expression of certain lethal genes which are MHC-linked (21,22). In fact, homozygosity in general, considered as a form of inbreeding, is felt to be unfavorable for the population as a whole. Finally, the reason that Mary and Bob had children while Mary and John had miscarriages might mean that there was more HLA sharing in the latter situation. (This has not been rigorously shown in more than occasional cases.)

There is already an extensive literature which has investigated the question of whether couples with RSAb share more HLA antigens than do successful couples. Unfortunately, there is no agreement on the answer to this question.

A number of reports have indicated that there is more HLA sharing between couples with RSAb than there is in couples with successful pregnancies. With regard to HLA class I loci, there are reports that RSAb is associated with increased sharing at the A but not B locus (23) or increased sharing at both A and B loci (24–26). Some reports show an increase in homozygosity at the B locus in RSAb women and a weak association with HLA-B sharing (27). There are data showing increased sharing at class II (DR) loci (28). Some reports also looked at mixed leukocyte culture reactivity in RSAb couples as compared with successful couples. Decreased MLR reactivity did not correlate well with HLA-DR sharing (25,26). However, it is important to note that all of these studies used only serological typing methods for class II locus assignment. Had DNA-based methods been used, serological HLA-DR sharing and significant MLR activity might be discovered to be actually instances of DR disparity at the peptide level.

At the same time, concomitant studies from different investigators did not show that RSAb couples had more HLA sharing (29–34).

Finally, more recent studies have used DNA-based typing methods. Unfortunately, this technological and conceptual advance has also not produced a consensus on this subject. For instance, one group has found that RSAb is correlated with HLA sharing at the DQα locus (a gene in the class II region) (35), but a different report has not confirmed this (36).

HLA *sharing* may, perhaps, not be the best way to analyze the problem. In terms of maternal allorecognition of MHC-antigens on the fetus, it is the antigens which are *not shared* which are important. Consider the following couple:

	Woman	Man
HLA-A	1,2	2,2
HLA-B	8,8	5,8
HLA-DR	1,2	3,4

This couple can be considered to share two antigens HLA-A2 and -B8. However, since she is homozygous for B8, it turns out that rather than the man having 4 antigens which she does not have (i.e., 6 total minus 2 shared), he has only 3 (namely, B5, and DR-3 and -4). Similarly, one can think of homozygosity in terms of possible inheritance of MHC-linked recessive genes, or, in terms of homozygosity in the male, as one more reason for there to be a decrease in unshared HLA antigens.

In summary, the literature is conflicting concerning the question of whether RSAb is associated with more HLA sharing (or fewer HLA disparities) than is found in successful couples.

A. Immunotherapy for RSAb

Based partly on concepts derived from studies of HLA sharing (and other studies), immunotherapeutic maneuvers have been tried in the treatment of RSAb. This section reviews this topic. It is safe to say at the outset, however, that no sector in the difficult area of RSAb has been the scene of so much heat and disagreement as that of immunotherapy.

The rationale for using immunotherapy in RSAb today seems to rest on one or more of several concepts. First, immunological processes may be responsible for a significant proportion of otherwise unexplained RSAbs. Such processes might include the failure of desirable immunological events (e.g., failure to make some blocking cell or factor) or the intrusion of an undesirable influence such as autoantibodies or embryotoxic factors. The second concept is the experiences of animal and human transplantation teams in which pretransplant treatment with donor-specific or nonspecific leukocytes increased graft acceptance (37). Third is the concept that RSAb couples shared more MHC antigens than expected and thus represented a form of unwanted but inadvertent "inbreeding." These three concepts are not mutually exclusive.

B. Leukocyte Immunotherapy

Immunotherapy with leukocytes appears to have been reported first in 1981 (38). That report and a subsequent one (although both uncontrolled) looked promising (39). These reports were followed by a number of other papers, most prominent being one by Mowbray (40). This trial was prospectively controlled, and women who received husband's blood as immunogen had a far better rate of delivery in the next pregnancy (77%) than did women who received their own white cells as a placebo (33%). This study has been criticized, as have all controlled studies of leukocyte immunization for RSAb (reviewed in (14), chap. 6).

The criticisms of these trials are based on a number of items, including (a) selection of patients particularly with regard to whether two- or three-or-more miscarriages are needed for inclusion, (b) ethnic or racial heterogeneity of patient populations (which would influence the incidence of HLA sharing), (c) randomization of controls, (d) decisions to use (or not use) secondary aborters, (e) cell dose and route of administration, (f) presence or absence of other concomitant therapeutic maneuvers, such as hormonal supplements, and so on.

Implicit in all the discussions of these variables is the question: "What is the chance that a woman who has had three SAbs with the same partner will have a delivery on the next pregnancy if immunotherapy is not used?" This, of course, represents the control group. The answer to this question turns out to be most interesting, at least partly because the expectation that a fourth pregnancy (after 3 Sabs) will be successful seems to have risen over the past 20 years. A review of earlier studies suggested that after three Sabs, a successful delivery occurred in the next pregnancy in 25–46% (41). More recent reports indicate that success on the fourth pregnancy is to be expected 50% of the time (34,42). (It is generally agreed that the success rate will fall as the number of prior Sabs rises beyond three.) If this rising delivery rate represents a real increase in pregnancy success in women with RSAb, it most likely represents better prenatal care (perhaps including hormonal supplements), and thus makes it imperative to use concomitant randomized controls in any therapeutic trials. As the next paragraph will discuss, the rate appears to continue to rise.

The most recent comprehensive report on this controversial subject comes from a collaborative observational study and meta-analysis of 15 clinical centers that used controlled trials of allogeneic leukocytes in the treatment of RSAb (43). There were nine randomized trials and six nonrandomized trials. Somewhat surprisingly, the results were very similar when the two types of trials were compared. The results showed that pregnancy success was more frequent in the alloimmunized women than in the controls—but the differences were small. Taking the two types of trials together, treated women had an 8–10% better chance of achieving a delivery than did untreated women (p = .02–.03). There were differences in success rates between centers. One interesting feature is that control women (with three, four, or five previous Sabs) had a delivery rate of 60.8%—higher than that seen in many studies to date. Immunized women had a delivery rate (live births) of 68.4%.

In summary, one would need to immunize 11 women with RSAb to get one additional live birth.

The result is better than the skeptics expected but not nearly as good as the enthusiasts had hoped. Whether such a treatment will survive cost–benefit analyses remains to be seen.

C. Intravenous Immunoglobulin (IVIG)

IVIG is known to be an immunomodulating reagent (in addition to its recognized ability to provide passive antimicrobial immunity). It is used for Kawasaki's disease and for the treatment of autoimmune thrombocytopenia (AITP). Its immunomodulatory properties may be related to its content of anti-idiotypic antibodies, and its use in AITP is associated with its ability to produce RES blockade. It has also been used in the treatment of RSAb, and the results are controversial. Recently, however, a prospective controlled trial has been reported. Women with two or more consecutive Sabs were given either pooled IVIG (500 mg/kg) or albumin starting at the follicular phase of the cycle when pregnancy was desired and, when pregnant, monthly until 28–32 weeks of gestation or until delivery. Of 29 women receiving IVIG, 18 (62%) delivered and 11 had an SAb. Of 32 women receiving placebo, 11 (38%) delivered and 21 had an SAb. The difference is statistically significant (p = .04) (44).

This report has a problem, and it is the same problem as was seen in the Mowbray study of leukocyte immunotherapy (40). In both studies, while more treated women than controls delivered, the difference appears to be due not to the high degree of success in the treated women, but to the low percentage of delivery in the controls (33% in the Mowbray study and 38% in the IVIG study by Coulam et al. (44). In fact, the success rate for *treated* women in the IVIG study (62%) is almost exactly the same as the delivery rate in the *control* women reported in the meta-analysis of leukocyte immunotherapy (43). The reasons for such discrepancies are not known.

Table 1 Immunological Mechanisms Possibly Accounting for Recurrent Fetal Loss

Autoimmune disease—overt
SLE, anticardiolipin syndrome, etc.
—cryptic
Failure of maternal recognition of paternal antigens
Excessive HLA sharing in parents
Failure to develop "blocking factors"
Increased NK cell activity
Embryotoxic factors

Therefore, although both leukocyte immunotherapy and IVIG infusions seem to hold some promise in the treatment of RSAb, their efficacy has not been established beyond cavil.

VIII. Summary

There are a number of known immunological reasons for recurrent pregnancy loss (RSAb) (Table 1). Autoimmune problems were discussed in Chapters 21–23. This chapter reviewed the question as to whether there may be immunological reasons for RSAb in women who do not have overt autoimmune disease or any chromosomal, endocrinological, anatomical, or infectious factors in place. Several areas of evidence favor the concept that pregnancy is more successful if there is little genetic similarity between the partners. Some data show that spontaneously aborting couples share more HLA antigens than do successful couples. Other data suggest that women with RSAb fail to make blocking factors able to interfere with potentially harmful maternal–antipaternal immunological reactions. However, the field of inquiry is not settled and continues to be controversial.

For these and other reasons, there are several immunological approaches to the treatment of RSAb. The most widely used are paternal leukocyte immunization and IVIG. A meta-analysis of controlled trials of leukocyte immunization showed that immunized women had a significantly better delivery rate than controls, but the difference was not great. Some trials with IVIG showed promise, but not enough have been completed to make a convincing case for the success of this modality.

References

1. Lauritsen JG. Genetic aspects of spontaneous abortion. Dan Med Bull 1977; 24:169–188.
2. Little AB. There's many a slip 'twixt implantation and the crib. N Engl J Med 1988; 319:241–242.
3. Wilcox AJ, Weinbert GR, O'Connor JF, Baird DD, Schlatterer JP, Canfield RE, Armstrong EG, Nisula BC. Incidence of early loss of pregnancy. N Engl J Med 1988; 319:189–194.
4. McIntyre JA, Coulam CB, Faulk WP. Recurrent spontaneous abortion. Am J Reprod Immunol 1989; 21:100–104.
5. Johnson PM. Reproductive immunopathology. In: Lachmann PJ, Peters SK, Rosen FS, Walport MJ, eds. Clinical Aspects of Immunology. 5th ed. Boston: Blackwell 1993:2137–2152.
6. Clark DA, Chaout G. What do we know about spontaneous abortion mechanisms? Am J Reprod Immunol Microbiol 1989; 19:28–38.
7. Gendron RL, Baines MG. Infiltrating decidual natural killer cells are associated with spontaneous abortion in mice. Cell Immunol 1988; 113:261–267.
8. Clark DA, Chaouat G, Mogil R, Wegmann TG. Prevention of spontaneous abortion in DAB/2-mated CBA/J mice by GM-CSF involves CD8$^+$ T cell-dependent suppression of natural effector cell cytotoxicity against trophoblast target cells. Cell Immunol 1994; 154:143–152.
9. Rocklin RE, Kitzmiller JL, Carpenter CB, Garovoy MR, David JR. Maternal-factor relation: absence of an immunologic blocking factor from the serum of women with chronic abortions. N Engl J Med 1976; 295:1209–1213.
10. Stimson WH, Strachan AF, Shepherd A. Studies on the maternal immune response to placental antigens: absence of a blocking factor from the blood of abortion-prone women. Br J Obstet Gynecol 1979; 86:41–45.
11. Unander AM, Cindholm A. Transfusions of leukocyte rich erythrocyte concentrates: a successful treatment in selected cases of habitual abortion. Am J Obstet Gynecol 1984; 154:516–520.
12. Unander AM, Lindholm A, Olding LB. Blood transfusions generate/increase previously absent/weak blocking antibody in women with habitual abortion. Fertil Steril 1985; 44:766–771.
13. Wegmann TG, Lin H, Guilbert L, Mosmann TR. Bidirectional cytokine interactions in the maternal-fetal relationship: is successful pregnancy a T_H2 phenomenon? Immunol Today 1993; 14:353–356.
14. Claman HN. The Immunology of Human Pregnancy. Totowa, NJ: Humana Press, 1993:
15. Croy BA, Gambel P, Rossant J, Wegmann TG. Characterization of murine decidual natural killer (NK) cells and their relevance to the success of pregnancy. Cell Immunol 1985; 93:315–326.
16. Hunt JS, Andrews GK, Wood GW. Normal trophoblasts resist induction of class I HLA. J Immunol 1987; 138:2481–2487.

17. Chao K-H, Yang Y-S, Ho H-N, Chen S-U, Chen HF, Dai HJ, Huang SC, Gill TJ. Decidual natural killer cytotoxicity decreased in normal pregnancy but not in anembryonic pregnancy and recurrent spontaneous abortion. Am J Reprod Immunol 1995; 34:274–280.

18. Ecker JL, Laufer MR, Hill JA. Measurement of embryotoxic factors is predictive of pregnancy outcome in women with a history of recurruent abortion. Obstet Gynecol 1993; 81:84–87.

19. Yamada H, Polgar K, Hill JA. Cell-mediated immunity to trophoblast antigens in women with recurrent spontaneous abortion. Am J Obstet Gynecol 1994; 170:1339–1344.

20. Komlos L, Samir R, Joshua H, Halbrecht I. Common HLA antigens in couples with repeated abortions. Clin Immunol Immunopathol 1977; 7:330–335.

21. Gill TJ, III. Immunogenetics of spontaneous abortions in humans. Transplantation 1983; 35:1–6.

22. Awdeh ZL, Raum D, Yunis EJ, Alper CA. Extended HLA/complement allelic haplotypes: evidence for a T/t-like complex in man. Proc Natl Acad Sci USA 1983; 80:259–263.

23. Gerencer M, Kastelan A, Drazancic A, Kerhin-Brkjacic V, Madjaric M. The HLA antigens in women with recurrent abnormal pregnancies of unknown etiology. Tissue Antigens 1978; 12:223–227.

24. Beer AE, Quebbeman JF, Ayers JWT, Haynes RF. Major histocompatibility complex antigens, maternal and paternal immune responses and chronic habitual abortions in humans. Am J Obstet Gynecol 1981; 141:987–999.

25. McIntyre JA, Faulk WP. Recurrent spontaneous abortion in human pregnancy: results of immunogenetical, cellular, and humoral studies. Am J Reprod Immunol 1983; 4:165–170.

26. Thomas ML, Harger JH, Wagener DK, Rabin BS, Gill TJ, III. HLA sharing and spontaneous abortion in humans. Am J Obstet Gynecol 1985; 151: 1053–1057.

27. Johnson PM, Chia KV, Risk JM, Barnes RMR, Woodrow JC. Immunological and immunogenetic investigation of recurrent spontaneous abortion. Disease Markers 1988; 6:163–171.

28. Takakuwa K, Kanazawa K, Takeuchi S. Production of blocking antibodies by vaccination with husband's lymphocytes in unexplained recurrent aborters: the role in successful pregnancy. Am J Reprod Immunol Microbiol 1986; 10:1–9.

29. Sargent IL, Wilkins T, Redman CWG. Maternal immune responses to the fetus in early pregnancy and recurrent miscarriage. Lancet 1988; 2:1099–1104.

30. Cauchi MN, Tait B, Wilshire MI, Koh SH, Mraz G, Kloss M, Pepperell R. Histocompatibility antigens and habitual abortion. Am J Reprod Immunol Microbiol 1988; 18:28–31.

31. Caudle MR, Rote NS, Scott JR, DeWitt C, Barney MF. Histocompatibility in couples with recurrent spontaneous abortion and normal fertility. Fertil Steril 1983; 39:793–798.

32. Lauritsen JG, Kristensen T, Grunnet N. Depressed mixed lymphocyte culture reactivity in mothers with recurrent spontaneous abortion. Am J Obstet Gynecol 1976; 125:35–39.

33. Oksenberg JR, Pesitz E, Amar A, Schenker J, Segal S, Nelken D, Brautbar C. Mixed lymphocyte reactivity non-responsiveness in couples with multiple spontaneous abortions. Fertil Steril 1983; 39:525–529.

34. Houwert-de Jong MH, Termijtelen A, Eskes TKAB, Mantingh A, Bruinse HW. The natural course of habitual abortion. Eur J Ob Gyn Reprod Biol 1989; 33:221–228.

35. Ober C, Steck T, van der Ven K, Billstrand C, Messer L, Kwak J, Beaman K, Beer A. MHC class II compatibility in aborted fetuses and term infants of couples with recurrent spontaneous abortion. J Reprod Immunol 1993; 25: 195–207.

36. Dizon-Townson D, Nelson L, Scott JR, Branch DW, Ward K. Human leukocyte antigen DQ a sharing is not increased in couples with recurrent miscarriage. Am J Reprod Immunol 1995; 34:209–212.

37. van Rood JJ. Pretransplant blood transfusion: sure! But how and why? Transplant Proc 1983; 15:915–916.

38. Taylor C, Faulk WP. Prevention of recurrent abortion with leukocyte transfusion. Lancet 1981; ii:68–70.

39. Taylor C, Faulk WP, McIntyre JA. Prevention of recurrent spontaneous abortions by leukocyte transfusion. J R Soc Med 1985; 78:623–627.

40. Mowbray JF, Gibbings C, Liddell H, Reginald PW, Underwood JL, Beard RW. Controlled trial of treatment of recurrent spontaneous abortion by immunisation with paternal cells. Lancet 1985; 4/27/85 issue:941–943.

41. Roman E. Fetal loss rates and their relation to pregnancy order. J Epidemiol Community Health 1984; 38:29–35.

42. Knudsen UB, Hansen V, Juul S, Secher NJ. Prognosis of a new pregnancy following previous spontaneous abortions. Eur J Ob Gyn Reprod Biol 1991; 39:31–36.

43. Coulam CB, Clark DA, Collins J, Scott JR, Schlesselman JS. Worldwide collaborative observational study and meta-analysis on allogenic leukocyte immunotherapy for recurrent spontaneous abortion. Am J Reprod Immunol 1994; 32:55–72.

44. Coulam CB, Krysa L, Stern JJ, Bustillo M. Intravenous immunoglobulin for treatment of recurrent pregnancy loss. Am J Reprod Immunol 1995; 34: 333–337.

Part Six

DEVELOPMENT/PREVENTION OF ALLERGIC DISEASES IN INFANCY

27

The Genetic Basis of Asthma and Allergic Disease

WILLIAM O. C. M. COOKSON

John Radcliffe Hospital
Oxford, England

I. Introduction

Asthma is almost certainly not one disease but many. In children, 95% of asthma is allergic, also known as atopic. The term atopy, meaning "strange disease," was invented by Coca and Cooke in 1926 to describe a familial syndrome of asthma, seasonal rhinitis (hay fever), and infantile eczema.

The familial nature of atopy and asthma implies that they are due at least in part to inherited genetic factors. Study of their genetics will increase understanding of the etiology and pathophysiology of these diseases. It may be hoped that the early identification of children at genetic risk of asthma may open new approaches to the prevention of illness. The involvement of particular genes may identify a particular clinical course and response to therapy. Eventually, and perhaps most distantly, genetics may lead to new pharmacological treatment for asthma.

Asthma is a complex disease that is likely to be due to the interaction of several genes with important environmental factors. In contrast to single-gene disorders, such as cystic fibrosis or muscular dystrophy, genes predisposing to asthma will not contain mutations. Rather, as in the genes influencing lipid metabolism, they will be variants of normal genes, whose evolutionary advantage has been lost in the current Western environment.

Of the various types of asthma, atopic asthma is clinically most easily recognized and defined, and has the most obvious familial clustering. For this reason, most effort toward elucidating the genetic causes of asthma have been directed at asthma in children and in young adults, and at the underlying condition of atopy.

The identification of genes causing disease is through two processes: the study of candidate genes, or by genetic linkage and positional cloning. These two approaches, which will be described in more detail below, both begin with a definition of phenotype, which may be the disease itself or the choice of disease-related parameter (known as an intermediate phenotype). The choice of phenotype may be critical in the eventual ability to identify the genotype, the genetic lesions, or variations that predispose to disease.

II. Asthma and Atopy Phenotypes

Asthma may be recognized by questionnaire, physical examination, and the demonstration of variable reduction of air flow. In the absence of an attack of asthma, air flow limitation can be demonstrated by challenge tests. Challenges in common use include exercise, cold air, and inhaled bronchial spasmogens such as histamine or methacholine. Of these challenges, spasmogen inhalation gives the most reliable measure of underlying airway lability. Challenge tests have been widely used in the investigation of asthma, both in the clinical setting and in large epidemiological surveys.

Atopy is distinguished by Immunoglobulin E (IgE) responses to inhaled proteins, known as allergens. Typical allergen sources include house dust mite (HDM), grass pollens, and animal danders (sheddings from skin and fur). The total annual exposure to allergens is small, often of the order of micrograms. IgE binds by its high-affinity receptor (FcϵRI), most notably to mast cells in the skin and in mucosal surfaces of the lung and intestines. Mast cells possess dense granules, which contain histamine and other inflammatory mediators, in addition to proinflammatory cytokines. In sensitized individuals, exposure to allergen produces cross-linking of IgE, triggering of high-affinity receptors, and release of mast cell granules. The subsequent inflammation is in two waves, the first immediate and the second some hours later. Inflammation produces airway narrowing, with wheeze when occurring in the lung or sneezing and obstruction when in the nose. The regulation of IgE and of some components of early and late inflammation are under the control of antigen-specific T cells.

The atopic state is detected most easily by skin-prick tests. In these, allergen in dilute solution is placed on the skin, and a superficial prick is made to introduce minute amounts of allergen below the dermis. Sensitization and mast cell degranulation is detected by a wheal which is maximal after 10–15 min. A significant wheal is judged to be between 2 and 4 mm greater than a negative control.

Atopy may also be detected by elevation of the total serum IgE, or by elevation of serum IgE titres against common allergens. Elevation of antigen-specific IgE is detected by RAST or ELISA techniques. In the affluent populations of the West, there is a close correlation between prick skin tests, specific IgE titers (RASTs), the total serum IgE, and symptoms of wheeze or rhinitis. Despite these close correlations, the relationship among the variables is complex.

Atopy, defined by skin tests, is very common, and has been shown in several large Western population samples to affect between 40% and 50% of young adults (2 4). The prevalence of asthma has risen steadily through this century (1). The prevalence of seasonal rhinitis also appears to have risen, although the evidence for this is less clear. The reasons for this increase, which cannot be due to changes in the gene pool, must be environmental (see below).

Any trait as common as atopy cannot be considered abnormal, and it is obvious that the atopic state gives some advantage to those who carry it. The most likely evolutionary reason for atopy to exist is that IgE is particularly important in handling parasite infestations (5,6). In our society, we are now largely free of parasite infection, the implications of which are also discussed in the section on environment below.

III. Factors Confounding Genetic Studies of Atopy

The high population prevalence of atopy may seriously confound genetic studies (7). If atopy is present in 40–50% of the population, then a fifth of marriages may be between two atopics. Any large pedigree is therefore likely to contain several atopy genes introduced through different individuals, rather than a single abnormal gene introduced through one progenitor. If atopy was due to a single gene disorder, then many of the population would be homozygous. If, as is likely, more than one gene predisposes to the syndrome, then many individuals will carry two or more of these genes.

The substantial prevalence of atopy means that great care has to be taken in the recruitment of families for genetic studies. Ascertainment by public appeals for families with asthma (8) or with eczema (9) produced samples in which 70% and 80%, respectively, were atopic, with considerable loss of power to detect linkage (8). For this reason, in Oxford we now recruit families either from population samples (i.e., complete ascertainment), or through a defined proband with atopic disease.

For the purposes of genetic investigations, it is necessary to decide which measures of the atopy or asthma phenotype should be studied. The total serum IgE is an attractive parameter for genetic study, as it has well-established normal values, and in large population surveys correlates well with the presence of asthma. However, about 45% of the variation in the total serum IgE is attributable to the specific IgE (RAST) to HDM or grass pollen (10). When multiple regressions are carried out on population data, asthma and bronchial hyperresponsiveness are found to relate to variation in the specific IgE, most notably to HDM (10,11). Once specific IgE is taken into account, the residual total IgE does not correlate with the presence of asthma. The specific IgE, either detected indirectly by skin tests or directly in the serum by RAST or ELISA techniques, may therefore be suitable for genetic analysis. Bronchial hyperresponsiveness is a further intermediate phenotype which is currently being investigated.

It is also possible to study asthma as the principal phenotype. If this is done, care needs to be taken that the asthma being investigated is as clinically homogeneous as possible, which will usually mean the asthma of children and young adults. As there is no clear-cut division between normal and abnormal individuals, studies of asthma should exclude marginal phenotypes, and concentrate on "barn door" affected and unaffected subjects.

Selection will affect the type of genetic effects found in particular samples of subjects or families. Even if total or specific IgE is used as phenotype, the factors influencing the IgE in asthmatics may be different from those affecting the IgE in children with eczema, or in subjects selected for the presence of positive skin tests rather than for symptoms.

The behavior of atopy with age presents a particular problem for geneticists. While many diseases have increasing penetrance throughout life, atopy has a low penetrance in infancy, which rises to a maximum from 15 to 25 years of age. Thereafter the serum IgE and skin-prick test responses decline steadily, until at the age of 45 the serum IgE may be half of its value at the age of 15 (2).

IV. The Inheritance of Atopy

Geneticists have traditionally carried out segregation analysis as a first step in the study of a genetic disorder. Segregation analysis is intended to detect the presence of major genes predisposing to the disease, or to suggest that the illness is polygenetic or environmental, or a mixture of environmental and genetic factors. Segregation analysis may be used to estimate the values of parameters, related to the mode of inheritance of a trait, its penetrance, and its prevalence. Taken together, the estimates from segregation analysis make up a model which can be used to test for genetic linkage of a trait to particular chromosomal regions.

The pattern of inheritance of atopy has been the subject of much debate. In 1916 Cooke and Van der Veer (12), in a study of 1000 patients, found that if one parent was allergic, then 50% of the children were similarly affected, and that if both parents were allergic, then so too were 75% of their children. This neat Mendelian finding was disputed by Schwartz, who found families in which atopic children has only normal parents, so that he proposed a dominant model of inheritance tempered with incomplete penetrance (13). Weiner et al. observed a similar pattern in 1936 (14).

These early authors studied the inheritance of the whole syndrome, without reducing it to its component parts. Later studies concentrated on the inheritance of specific illnesses such as asthma or hay fever. In these circumstances a pattern of inheritance was much harder to define. Sibbald and Turner-Warwick (15) studied the first-degree relatives of atopic and nonatopic asthmatics, mostly by questionnaire, and found some evidence of familial aggregation of atopy without any clear-cut pattern of inheritance. Edfors-Lubs studied 7000 twin pairs for asthma and atopy, relying primarily on responses to a questionnaire. She concluded that asthma was polygenic (16).

After atopy was shown to be mediated by IgE, workers then concentrated on the genetics of this parameter, as it was quantifiable in a way not possible with symptoms alone. Bazaral et al. (17) studied IgE levels in infants and mothers, concluding that there was simple Mendelian inheritance of basal IgE levels. A subsequent study by the same investigators (18) showed identical twins to be highly concordant for total serum IgE, and that this effect was not linked to HLA haplotypes. The result indicated an important genetic component to the control of the total serum IgE. Hanson et al. (19) studied pulmonary function, total serum IgE, and specific IgE responses (RAST) in mono- dizygotic twins reared together and apart. He too found that monozygotic twins reared apart or together were concordant for the total IgE but differed in their specific IgE responses.

Marsh and his colleagues (20) studied many families for the inheritance of total IgE. They found that there was no simple pattern of Mendelian inheritance of the high-IgE trait, but that a model in which high IgE was recessive best fitted the data. Gerrard et al. (21) also studied many families with complex segregation analysis, concluding that a major locus controlled IgE levels, with a recessive allele determining high IgE levels, but that other genes influenced the trait. Blumenthal et al. (22), however, considered that a dominant allele coded for high IgE levels in some families and a recessive in others.

Borecki et al. studied a Canadian population for the inheritance of atopy. They found that if the total serum IgE was the only measure of atopy, then an autosomal recessive pattern of inheritance best fitted the data. When they included symptoms in their definition, they then found that a dominant pattern of inheritance best explained their findings (23).

Using a definition of atopy which included the responses to skin-prick tests and serum specific IgE estimation in addition to the total IgE (which they termed IgE responsiveness), Cookson and Hopkin examined the genetics of atopy in a limited number of nuclear and extended families (24). Their findings suggested that there was a major genetic component to atopy. As with the kindreds studied by Marsh, at least 10% of atopic subjects did not have atopic parents, which the authors attributed to dominant inheritance with incomplete penetrance (24).

Thus, diverse models have been proposed for the inheritance of atopy at different times, with varying definitions of atopy and different methods of analysis. It is perhaps as a result of the diversity of approaches that dominant, dominant with incomplete penetrance, recessive, and polygenic modes of inheritance have all been suggested. None of these hypotheses explains the results of many studies which have shown that the risk of atopy is much higher in the children of atopic mothers than in the children of atopic fathers. That asthmatic mothers had more asthmatic children than asthmatic fathers was reported 60 years ago (25), and large studies have shown a similar maternal pattern to the inheritance of elevations of cord blood IgE (26,27), atopic symptoms (28,29), and skin-prick test responses to common allergens (30). This finding may be due to interactions between the mother and her child in utero through the placenta or postpartum through the breast milk. Genomic imprinting, in which a paternal "atopy gene" may be suppressed during spermatogenesis, is also possible (31).

One new approach to the problem of a complex phenotype has been the application of regressive models to segregation analysis. Despite the close correlations among symptoms, total serum IgE, and specific IgE, genetic effects independently modifying these different variables can be dissected out with these models. This type of segregation analysis has been applied to the total serum IgE. The results demonstrate that, at least in the population studied, the total IgE is influenced by at least one gene which is independent of genes affecting skin tests or positive RAST tests (32).

The failure to show a simple consistent model of inheritance is most simply explained by accepting that the most likely possibility is that of several genes interacting with a strong environmental component. For the purpose of identifying genes causing atopy, an eclectic approach to phenotype definition is necessary, allowing for potential differences in the genes influencing skin tests and RASTs, the total serum IgE, or disease states such as asthma.

V. Finding Genes

As with other complex diseases, genes contributing to atopy may be found either by examining candidate genes or by genetic linkage. The most obvious candidate genes for atopy include *IL4*, *γ-interferon*, *IL10*, *G-CSF*, and the genes making up the high- and low-affinity receptors for IgE. Also included in this list should be the corresponding ligands or receptors. The enormous increase in understanding of the complex cytokine networks that influence atopy, however, has meant that a plausible case could be put for as many as 20 different candidates. The role of candidate genes may be assessed by defining polymorphisms within the receptor genes and testing for associations with disease. At the moment, a systematic search through the various candidates has not yet been carried out. Two candidates, *IL-4*, and the beta chain of the high-affinity receptor for IgE (*FcεRIβ*) have been implicated by genetic linkage studies.

Genetic linkage relies on the demonstration of co-inheritance of disease and genetic markers of known chromosomal localization. This approach has the advantage of not requiring any preexisting knowledge of the pathophysiology of the disease. However, the power to detect linkage in multigenic diseases is very limited (Table 1), so several hundred families may be necessary to detect linkage to a gene affecting a third of subjects with disease. A further problem with complex diseases is that of replication of linkage (33). Linkage to a heterogeneous trait will normally only be found fortuitously, in samples which contain an exceptional proportion of individuals or families influenced by that particular gene. Simulation experiments have shown that, in these circumstances, many studies may be necessary before replication occurs.

VI. Genes Influencing Asthma and Atopy

Many different kinds of genes may be involved in atopy and asthma. These can be divided into four classes: (a) genes predisposing in general to IgE-mediated inflammation, (b) genes influencing the specific IgE response, (c) genes influencing bronchial hyperresponsiveness independently of atopy, and (d) genes influencing non-IgE-mediated inflammation (Table 2).

Table 1 The Power to Detect Linkage

Fraction linked	Recessive inheritance	Dominant inheritance	Imprinted inheritance
0.80	22	69	29
0.50	62	181	87
0.30	181	508	253
0.20	412	1152	571
0.10	1662	4637	2310

The table shows the number of affected sibling pairs required to detect loci at p = .05 with 90% power at ϕ = 0.005, with different proportions of families linked to the putative locus. The required number of sibpairs is estimated for three modes of inheritance. The table assumes 70% marker informativeness.
Source: Table courtesy of Dr. Alan Young, Statistical Genetics Group, Wellcome Centre for Human Genetic Disease, Oxford, UK.

A. Class 1 Asthma Genes: Genes Influencing Generalized IgE Responses

Genes predisposing to generalized atopy have been identified on chromosome 11 and chromosome 5, by a combination of genetic linkage and candidate-gene approaches.

Chromosome 11q12-13

The first suggested linkage of atopy was to the marker d11s97 on chromosome 11q13 (34,35). Following some controversy (36), this linkage has been replicated by two further groups (37,38). This linkage was confounded by the high prevalence of atopy and because the linkage was seen predominantly in maternal meioses (37,39). In the largest study described,

Table 2 Classes of Genes Influencing Asthma

I	Genes predisposing in general to IgE-mediated inflammation	FcɛRI-β IL-4
II	Genes influencing the specific IgE response	HLA TCR-α
III	Genes influencing bronchial responsiveness independent of atopy	β-Adrenergic receptor
IV	Genes influencing non-IgE-mediated inflammation	TNF

linkage was exclusively maternal (39). The reasons for the maternal linkage are not known, and it is not clear that this maternal phenomenon corresponds to the phenotypic maternal inheritance of atopy which has been previously noted.

Recognition of the maternal linkage allowed better localization of the atopy locus, to within a cM 1-lod unit support interval (40,41). This interval was centromeric to and excluded the original d11s97 marker to which linkage was first observed. A lymphocyte surface marker, *CD20*, was noted to be within the interval. *CD20* shows sequence homology to the beta chain of the high-affinity receptor for IgE (*Fc∈RIβ*), and has been localized close to that gene on mouse chromosome 19 (42). The human *Fc∈RIβ* was subsequently found to be on chromosome 11q13, in close genetic linkage to atopy (40). Two coding polymorphisms have now been identified within the gene, *Fc∈RIβ Leu181* and *Fc∈RIβ Leu181/Leu183* (43). These both show strong associations with atopy when maternally inherited. The population prevalence of *Fc∈RIβ Leu181/Leu183* is about 4% (44), and *Fc∈RIβ Leu181* has been reported in 15% of asthmatics (43).

These results with *Fc∈RIβ* variants have not been replicated outside the Oxford group, and a reliable assay system for the variants has not yet been established. *Fc∈RIβ Leu181* does not show functional differences from the wild-type receptor (J. P. Kinet, personal communication). A further complication is the detection of a third homologous gene, *Htm4*, in close proximity to *Fc∈RIβ* and *CD20* (45), so that it is not clear how many members of the gene family are present. As it stands, it is therefore not yet established if the chromosome 11q atopy gene is *Fc∈RIβ*, or if it is some other gene in linkage disequilibrium with the *Fc∈RIβ* variants.

Chromosome 5

Linkage of the total serum IgE to markers near the cytokine cluster on chromosome 5q31-33 has been demonstrated by Marsh et al. (46). Marsh and his colleagues studied Amish pedigrees, selected to contain members with positive skin-prick tests. Linkage was strongest, however, in families with the lowest serum IgE. The result was replicated by Myers et al. (47) in Dutch asthmatic families. Linkage has not been found in other studies of extended families (S. Rich, personal communication). My group has tested 1500 individuals from 300 nuclear families, and find no evidence for linkage either by sib-pair or by lod score methods. However, in order to test the claim that linkage is seen predominantly with the low-IgE phenotype, we have used class D regressive models to account for the specific IgE response. The residual IgE shows evidence of linkage to a microsatellite repeat found in IL4, but not to the other polymorphic markers studied by Marsh or Myers (Dizier et al., in preparation). We find no linkage to asthma or bronchial responsiveness at this locus.

The region contains a number of cytokines, the most important of which from the point of view of atopy are *IL-4*, *IL-13*, the p40 subunit of *IL-12*, and *IL-5*. Other cytokines include *IL-9* and granulocyte-colony stimulating factor (*G-CSF*). A substantial amount of work is now required to establish which of these various candidates accounts for the linkage.

B. Class 2 Asthma Genes: Genes Influencing Specific IgE Responses to Particular Allergens

Atopic individuals differ in the particular allergens to which they react. This difference is of clinical significance, as asthma and bronchial hyper-responsiveness are associated with allergy to house dust mite (HDM) but not grass pollens (10,11). It is therefore of interest to examine whether particular genes influence the IgE response to specific allergens. In addition, study of these genes may give an insight into the inheritance of normal variation within the immune system, and the functional consequences of such variation.

Two classes of genes are likely candidates for constraining specific IgE reactions. These are the genes encoding the human leukocyte antigen (HLA) proteins and the genes for the T-cell receptor (TCR). These molecules are central to the handling and recognition of foreign antigen.

Inhaled allergen sources such as HDM are complex mixtures of many proteins. A number of "major allergens," to which the IgE responses are consistently found in most individuals, have been identified from each allergen source. It is likely that genetic associations will be better detected with reactions to purified major allergens rather than with complex allergen sources. Major allergens include *Der p* I (25.4 kDa) and *Der p* II (14.1 kDa) from the house dust mite *Dermatophagoides pteronyssinus*, Alt a I (28 kDa) from the mould *Alternaria alternata*, *Can f* I (25 kD) from the dog *Canis familiaris*, *Fel d* I (18 KDa) from the cat *Felis domesticus*, and *Phl p* V (30 kDa) from Timothy grass, *Phleum pratense*.

HLA

The human major histocompatibility complex (MHC) includes genes coding for HLA class II molecules (HLA-DR, DQ, and DP), which are involved in the recognition and presentation of exogenous peptides.

An HLA influence on the IgE response was first noted by Levine et al. (48), who found an association between HLA class I haplotypes and IgE responses to antigen E derived from ragweed allergen (*Ambrosia artemisifolia*). This association has been subsequently found to be due to restriction of the response to a minor component of ragweed antigen (*Amb a* V) by HLA-DR2 (49). To date the association of *Amb a* V (molecular weight 5000) and HLA-DR2 is the only HLA association to have been consistently confirmed (48–50). Other suggested associations are of the rye grass antigens *Lol p* I, *Lol p* II, and *Lol p* III with HLA-DR3 (in the same 53 allergic subjects) (51,52), American feverfew (*Parthenium hysterophorus*) and HLA-DR3 in 22 subjects from the Indian subcontinent (53), the IgE response to *Bet v* I, the major allergen of birch pollen, and HLA-DR3 in 37 European subjects (54), and an HLA-DR5 association with another ragweed antigen, *Amb a* VI, in 38 subjects (55).

Other authors have reported negative associations with particular allergens. These include HLA-DR4 and IgE responses to mountain cedar pollen (37 subjects) (56) and HLA-DR4 and melit (from bee venom) (22 subjects) (57). Nonresponsiveness to Japanese cedar pollen may be associated with HLA-DQw8 (58).

There is to date no confirmation of many of these results, and the number of subjects has generally not approached that required to establish an unequivocal HLA association. In addition, there has not been recognition of the problems of reactivity to multiple allergens: significant relationships between HLA-DR alleles and five antigens (*Amb a* V, *Lol p* I, *Lol p* II, *Lol p* III, and *Amb a* 6) have been claimed from the same pool of approximately 200 subjects (49,51,52,55).

In order to test more definitively if HLA class II gene products have a general influence on the ability to react to common allergens, we have genotyped for HLA-DR and HLA-DP in a large sample of atopic subjects from the British population (59). The subjects were tested for IgE responses to the most common British major allergens.

Four hundred and thirty-one subjects from 83 families were genotyped at the HLA-DR and HLA-DP loci and serotyped for IgE responses to six major allergens from common aeroallergen sources. Three hundred subjects were used as controls. The subjects and the controls came from the same relatively homogenous population. In the United Kingdom and Europe, allergens other than *Bet v* I and those tested for in our study are uncommon causes of sensitization and IgE-mediated allergy.

The results showed only weak associations between HLA-DR allele frequencies and IgE responses to common allergens. A possible excess of HLA-DR1 was found in subjects who were responsive to *Fel d* I compared to those who were not [odds ratio (OR) = 2, *p* = 002], and a possible excess of HLA-DR4 was found in subjects responsive to *Alt a* I (OR = 1.9, *p* = .006). Increased sharing of HLA-DR/DP haplotypes was seen in sibling pairs responding to both allergens. *Der p* I, *Der p* II, *Phl p* V, and *Can f* I were not associated with any definite excess of HLA-DR alleles.

No significant correlations were seen with HLA-DP genotype and reactivity to any of the allergens.

Of the possible associations, that of *Alt a* I with HLA-DR4 and of *Fel d* I with HLA-DR1 were supported by a finding of excess sharing of a HLA haplotype in affected sibling pairs. Regression analysis shows that the apparent association of *Phl p* V with HLA-DR4 is due to the presence of many individuals who have reacted with an IgE response both to *Alt a* I and *Phl p* V. The association of HLA-DR1 and *Fel d* I is the strongest statistically, and is significant even taking the multiple comparisons into account.

The study was the first to investigate HLA-DP alleles and reactivity to common allergens. As no definite correlation was found between any antigen response and HLA-DP genotypes with substantial numbers of subjects, HLA-DP genes are unlikely to have a major role in restricting IgE responses to these allergens.

The results suggest that HLA-DR alleles do modify the ability to mount an IgE response to particular antigens. However, the odds ratio for the association of *Alt a* I with HLA-DR4 was only 1.9, and that of *Fel d* I with HLA-DR1 was 2.0. Thus class II HLA restriction seems insufficient to account for individual differences in reactivity to common allergens. It is therefore likely that environmental factors or other loci such as T-cell receptor genes may be of greater relevance in determining an individual's susceptibility to specific allergens.

The T-Cell Receptor

The T-cell receptor (TCR) is usually made up of α and β chains, although 5% of receptors consist of γ and δ chains. The β-chain locus is on chromosome 7, and the α-chain locus is on chromosome 14. The δ-chain genes are found within the α-chain locus.

An enormous potential for TCR variety follows from the presence of many variable (V) and junctional (J) segments within the TCR loci. However, the usage of the TCR Vα and Vβ segments by lymphocytes is not random and may be under genetic control (60–63).

In order to examine whether the TCR genes influence susceptibility to particular allergens, we have tested for genetic linkage between IgE responses and microsatellites from the TCR-α/δ and TCR-β regions (64). Two independent sets of families, one British and one Australian, were investigated. Because the mode of inheritance was unknown, and because of interactions from the environment and other loci, affected sibling pair methods were used to test for linkage.

No linkage of IgE serotypes to TCR-β was detected, but significant linkage of IgE responses to the house dust mite allergens *Der p* I and *Der p* II, the cat allergen *Fel d* I, and the total serum IgE to TCR-α was seen in both family groups. The results show that a locus in the TCR α/δ region is modulating IgE responses. The close correlation between total and specific IgE makes is difficult to determine if the locus controls specific IgE reactions to particular allergens or confers generalized IgE responsiveness. Nevertheless, linkage was strongest with highly purified allergens, suggesting that the locus primarily influences specific purposes. The pattern of allele sharing seen with some serotypes suggests a recessive genetic effect, making it possible that this linkage corresponds to the recessive atopy locus implied by previous segregation analyses (32,65).

Replication of positive results of linkage in a second set of subjects is important in interpreting this study. Differences between the populations for the serotypes showing TCR-α allele sharing may be due to different allergen exposures, as grass pollen responses were much more common in Australian subjects. In addition, British subjects were recruited through clinics, whereas Australian subjects were not selected by symptoms.

No association was seen between particular IgE responses and specific TCR-α microsatellite alleles, implying that the microsatellite is not in immediate proximity to the IgE-modulating elements. The degree of linkage disequilibrium across the TCR-α/δ locus seems low (66), and the microsatellite has only been localized within a 900-kb yeast artificial chromosome (67). The observed linkage may therefore be with any elements of TCR-α or TCR-δ, or with other genes in the locality.

Several Vα genes have been recognized to be polymorphic (68), and limitation of the response to an allergen may correspond to these polymorphisms. Particular TCR-Vα usage may induce IL-4 dominant (Th2) helper T cells which enhance IgE production (69). A reported nonrandom usage of Vα13 usage in *Lol p* I specific T-cell clones supports independently the possibility of Vα genes controlling IgE responses (70).

The TCR-δ locus is also a candidate for this linkage. The function of TCR-γ/δ cells is not known, but their location on mucosal surfaces, where allergens initiate IgE responses, could suggest a role in IgE regulation (71).

This study has therefore identified a further genetic locus affecting atopy. The genetic restriction of specific IgE responses may be of clinical significance and may be of general interest in understanding the control of humeral immunity. Further localization of this genetic effect requires the identification of TCR α/δ elements showing allelic associations with specific IgE responses. Studies are also needed to investigate the interactions between this chromosome 14 linkage and the HLA class II genes.

C. Class 3 Asthma Genes: Genes Influencing Bronchial Responsiveness

No genes have yet been identified which predispose to bronchial hyper-responsiveness independent of atopy. Variants in the beta-adrenergic receptor have been identified, and it has been suggested that these may be associated with nocturnal asthma or other subdivisions of the asthma phenotype (72).

D. Class 4 Asthma Genes: Genes Influencing Non-IgE-Mediated Inflammation

Airway inflammation is a characteristic of asthma which may be independent of mechanisms controlling atopy. Tumor necrosis factor-alpha (TNF-α) is a potent proinflammatory cytokine, that shows constitutional variations in the level of secretion which are linked to polymorphisms in the TNF gene complex (73–75). We have therefore investigated TNF polymorphisms for association with asthma in 800 normal and abnormal subjects from general population and asthma clinic samples. We found that asthma was significantly increased in subjects with alleles associated with increased secretion of TNF-α, most notably the TNF-α promoter polymorphism TNFα-308. Considering unrelated subjects only (the parents) from both populations, the odds ratio for asthma in individuals homozygous for the high-secretor allele was 3.9 compared to homozygotes for the low-secretor alleles (95%CI: 1.4–11.0, $p = .007$) (76).

VII. Whole-Genome Screens for Atopy and Asthma

The four loci described above do not account for all atopy. The chromosome 11 and 5 genes do not seem to have major effects on the population as a whole, and HLA and TCR-α loci modify the specific response rather than endowing any general predisposition to atopy. Segregation analysis is unable to predict with any accuracy the number and nature of genes contributing to atopy and asthma. In order to discover if atopy is a genuine polygenic disorder, my group has carried out a complete genome screen in 80 nuclear families, with 300 markers spaced at approximately 10% recombination. Using sib-pair analysis we have discovered nine potential new linkages ($p < .001$) to the serum IgE or other asthma-associated phenotypes. These results are currently being evaluated for their significance in further sets of subjects. Similar large-scale genome scans are to be carried out in the United States and Canada, so it is likely that general agreement will soon be reached on the number and nature of the most important loci causing atopy.

VIII. Genes and Environment

No description of the genetics of asthma would be complete without some consideration of the effects of environment. It is self-evident that, in the absence of environmental precipitants, allergic asthma and hay fever would not exist. Such conditions are found on mountains, where there is little pollen, and where the low humidity prevents house dust mite growth. Schoolchildren raised at high altitude develop less allergy than those raised at sea level (77). Similarly, children living in the dry interior of Australia develop less allergy than those living in more humid conditions near the coast (4).

Data from a number of sources indicate that events in early infancy are critical in determining the subsequent course of allergic disease. In the Scandinavian countries a short, intense spring flowering of birch trees is accompanied by symptoms in many individuals. Children born in the 3 months around the pollen season carry an increased risk of allergy to birch pollen for the rest of their life (78). In English children the level of house dust mite in infants' bedding during the first year of life correlates with the subsequent risk of childhood asthma (79).

The enormous increase in the prevalence of asthma in the past two decades cannot be attributed to changes in gene frequencies in the affected populations and must be due to an environmental factor or factors. Air pollution has been suggested as a cause of this increase, although atmospheric pollution has declined steadily since the 1950s in England and Western Europe, and ozone levels remain stable despite an increase in the number of cars. Comparative studies of the prevalence of asthma have been carried out between East and West Germany, two regions with genetically similar populations, and with far higher levels of atmospheric pollution in the East (80). Surprisingly, the prevalence of asthma is lower in the East than in the West. This decrease is matched by a lower prevalence of atopy, as detected by skin tests to common allergens (81). Similar results are seen when the prevalence of asthma in the Baltic states is compared to that of Sweden (82). This difference may be attributable to childhood respiratory infections, as pollution and overcrowding, both of which are more common in the East, predispose to infantile infection. Support for this hypothesis is given by the finding that the youngest children in large sibships have significantly less asthma than their older siblings (83). At the cellular level it is suggested that early infections program the immature immune system toward a Th2 rather than a Th1 helder-cell profile, thereafter favoring a cellular rather than humeral immune response.

Thus, even in genetically similar people, the dose and timing of allergen exposure will have important effects on subsequent manifestations of the atopy phenotype. This places an additional requirement for careful study design and interpretation in attempts to unravel the genetics of atopic disease.

Another environmental factor to consider is parasitism. Slumdwelling Venezuelan children have higher levels of serum IgE and lower levels of asthma that their more affluent compatriots (84). In endemically parasitized Australian Aborigines, the presence of a positive RAST to HDM correlates poorly both with skin-test responses to the same allergen and the presence of asthma (85). Multiple regression shows that the discrepancy between RAST and skin tests can be accounted for by the elevation of total serum IgE. The results fit the hypothesis that parasitism, by causing an increase in polyclonal IgE, is protective against atopy.

IX. Screening

The increase in prevalence of asthma in recent decades has an important corollary: Asthma is preventable. Recognition of children or infants genetically predisposed to asthma is likely to be the first step in strategies for prevention by environmental manipulation or vaccination in the first year of life. It is likely that many genetic variants which predispose to asthma will be identified in the near future, and that a comprehensive estimation of genetic risk to a particular infant will be feasible by the end of the decade.

References

1. Strachan DP, Anderson HR, Limb ES, O'Neill A, Wells N. A national survey of asthma prevalance, severity, and treatment in Great Britain. Arch Dis Child 1994; 70:174–178.
2. Cline MG, Burrows BB. Distribution of allergy in a population sample residing in Tuscon, Arizona. Thorax 1989; 44:425–432.
3. Holford-Strevens V, Warren P, Wong C, Manfreda J. Serum total immunoglobulin E levels in Canadian Adults. J Allergy Clin Immunol 1984; 73: 516–522.
4. Peat JK, Britton WJ, Salome CM, Woolcock AJ. Bronchial hyperresponsiveness in two populations of Australian school children III. Effect of exposure to environmental allergens. Clin Allergy 1987; 17:271–281.
5. Ogilvie BM, Jones VE. Protective immunity in helminth diseases. Proc R Soc Med 1969; 62:298–301.
6. Capron M, Capron A. Immunoglobulin E and effector cells in schistosomiasis. Science 1994; 264:1876–1877.

7. Cookson WOCM. Atopy: a complex genetic disease. Ann Med 1994; 26: 351–353.

8. Moffatt MF, Sharp PA, Faux JA, Young RP, Cookson WOCM, Hopkin JM. Factors confounding genetic linkage between atopy and chromosome 11q. Clin Exp Allergy 1992; 22:1046–1051.

9. Coleman, R, Trembah RC, Harper JI. Chromosome 11q13 and atopy underlying atopic eczema. Lancet 1993; 341:1121–1122.

10. Cookson WOCM, De Klerk NH, Ryan GR, James AL, Musk AW. Relative risks of bronchial hyper-responsiveness associated with skin-prick test responses to common antigens in young adults. Clin Exp Allergy 1991; 21: 473–479.

11. Sears MR, Herbison GP, Holdaway MD, Hewitt CJ, Flannery EM, Silva PA. The relative risks of sensitivity to grass pollen, house dust mite and cat dander in the development of childhood asthma. Clin Allergy 1989; 18:419.

12. Cooke RA, van der Veer A. Human sensitisation. J. Immunol 1916; 1: 201–305.

13. Schwartz M. Heredity in bronchial asthma. Acta Allergol 1952; 5(suppl 2): 3–288.

14. Weiner A, Zieve I, Fries J. The inheritance of allergic diseases. Ann Eugen 1936; 7:141–162.

15. Sibbald B, Turner-Warwick M. Factors influencing the prevalence of asthma in first degree relatives of extrinsic and intrinsic asthmatics. Thorax 1979; 34: 332–337.

16. Edfors-Lubs ML. Allergy in 7000 twin pairs. Acta Allergol 1971; 26:249–285.

17. Bazaral M, Orgel HA, Hamburger RN. IgE levels in normal infants and mothers and an inheritance hypothesis. J Immunol 1971; 107:794–801.

18. Bazaral M, Orgel HA, Hamburger RN. Genetics of IgE and allergy: serum IgE levels in twins. J Allergy Clin Immunol 1974; 54:288–304.

19. Hanson B, McGue M, Roitman-Johnson B, Segal NL, Bouchard TJ Jr, Blumenthal MN. Atopic disease and immunoglobulin E in twins reared apart and together. Am J Hum Genet 1991; 48:873–879.

20. Marsh DG, Meyers DA, Bias WB. The epidemiology and genetics of atopic allergy. N Engl J Med 1981; 305:1551–1559.

21. Gerrard JW, Horne S, Vickers P, MacKenzie JWA, Goluboff N, Garson JZ, Maningas CS. Serum IgE levels in parents and children. J Pediatr 1974; 85: 660–663.

22. Blumenthal MN, Namborrdiri K, Mendell N, Gleich C, Elston RC. Genetic transmission of serum IgE levels. Am J Med Genet 1981; 10:219–228.

23. Borecki I, Rao DC, Lalouel JM, McGue L, Gerrard JW. Demonstration of a common major gene with pleiotrophic effects on immunoglobulin E and allergy. Genet Epidemiol 1985; 2:327–338.

24. Cookson WOCM, Hopkin JM. Dominant inheritance of atopic immunoglobulin-E responsiveness. Lancet 1988; i:86–88.

25. Bray GW. The hereditary factor in hypersensitivity anaphylaxis and allergy. J Allergy 1931; II:205–224.

26. Magnusson CG. Cord serum IgE in relation to family history and as predictor of atopic disease in early infancy. Allergy 1988; 43:241–251.

27. Halonen M, Stern D, Taussig LM, Wright A, Ray CG, Martinez FD. The predictive relationship between serum IgE levels at birth and subsequent incidences of lower respiratory illnesses and eczema in infants. Am Rev Respir Dis 1992; 146:866–870.

28. Arshad SH, Matthews S, Grant C, Hide DW. Effect of allergen avoidance on development of allergic disorders in infancy. Lancet 1992; 339:1493–1497.

29. Åberg N. Familial occurrence of atopic disease: genetic versus environmental factors. Clin Exp Allergy 1994; 23:829–834.

30. Kuehr J, Karmaus W, Forster J, Frischer T, Hendel-Kramer A, Moseler M, Stephan V, Urbanek R, Weiss K. Sensitisation to four common inhalant allergens within 302 nuclear families. Clin Exp Allergy 1993; 23:600–605.

31. Hall JG. Genomic imprinting. Arch Dis Child 1990; 65:1013–1016.

32. Dizier MH, Hill M, James A, Faux J, Ryan G, le Souef P, Musk AW, Lathrop M, Demenais F, Cookson W. Genetic control of IgE level after accounting for specific atopy. Genet Epidemiol 1993; 10:333–334.

33. Suarez BK, Hampe CL, Van Eerdewegh P. Problems of replicating linkage claims in psychiatry. In: Gershon ES, Cloninger CR, eds. Genetic Approaches to Mental Disorders. American Psychiatric Press, Washington, DC: 1994: 23–46.

34. Cookson WOCM, Sharp PA, Faux JA, Hopkin JM. Linkage between immunoglobulin E responses underlying asthma and rhinitis and chromosome 11q. Lancet 1989; i:1292–1295.

35. Young RP, Lynch J, Sharp PA, Faux JA, Cookson WOCM, Hopkin JM. Confirmation of genetic linkage between atopic IgE responses and chromosome 11q13. J Med Genet 1992; 29:236–238.

36. Marsh DG, Myers DA. A major gene for allergy—fact or fancy? Nature Genet 1992; 2:252–254.

37. Shirakawa T, Morimoto K, Hashimoto T, Furuyama J, Yamamoto M, Takai S. Linkage between severe atopy and chromosome 11q in Japanese families. Clin Genet 1994; 46:125–129.

38. Collée JM, ten Kate LP, de Vries HG, Kliphuis JW, Bouman K, Scheffer H, Gerritsen J. Allele sharing on chromosome 11q13 in sibs with asthma and atopy. Lancet 1993; 342:936.

39. Cookson WOCM, Young RP, Sandford AJ, Moffatt MF, Shirakawa T, Sharp PA, Faux JA, Julier C, Nakumuura Y. Maternal Inheritance of atopic IgE responsiveness on chromosome 11q. Lancet 1992; 340:381–384.

40. Sandford AJ, Shirakawa T, Moffatt MF, Daniels SE, Ra C, Faux JA, Young RP, Nakamura Y, Lathrop GM, Cookson WOCM, Hopkin JM. Localisation of atopy and the β subunit of the high affinity IgE receptor (FcεRI) on chromosome 11q. Lancet 1993; 341:332–334.

41. Sandford AJ, Moffat MF, Daniels SE, Nakamura Y, Lathrop GM, Hopkin JM, Cookson WOCM. A genetic map of chromosome 11q, including the atopy locus. Eur J Hum Genet 1995; 3:188–194.

42. Hupp K, Siwarski D, Mock BA, Kinet JP. Gene mapping of the three subunits of the high affinity FcR for IgE to mouse chromosomes 1 and 19. J Immunol 1989; 143:3787–3791.

43. Shirakawa TS, Li A, Dubowitz M, Dekker JW, Shaw AE, Faux JA, Ra C, Cookson WOCM, Hopkin JM. Association between atopy and variants of the β subunit of the high-affinity immunoglobulin E receptor. Nature Genet 1994; 7:125–129.

44. Hill MR, James AL, Faux JA, Ryan G, Hopkin JM, le Souef P, Musk AW, Cookson WOCM. FcεRI-β polymorphism and risk of atopy in a general population sample. Br Med J 1995; 311:776–779.

45. Adra CN, Lelias J-M, Kobayashi H, Kaghad M, Morrison P, Rowley JD, Lim B. Cloning of the cDNA for a haemopoietic cell-specific protein related to CD20 and the beta subunit of the high-affinity of IgE receptor: Evidence for a family of proteins with four membrane spanning regions. Proc Natl Acad Sci USA 1994; 91:10718–10182.

46. Marsh DG, Neely JD, Breazeale DR, Ghosh B, Friedhoff LR, Erlich-Kautzky E, Schou C, Krishnaswamy G, Beaty TH. Linkage analysis of IL4 and other chromosome 5q31.1 markers and total serum IgE concentrations. Science 1994; 264:1152–1155.

47. Myers DA, Postma DS, Panhuysen CIM, Xu J, Amelung PJ, Levitt RC, Bleeker ER. Evidence for a locus regulating total serum IgE levels mapping to chromosome 5. Genomics 1994; 23:464–470.

48. Levine BB, Stember RH, Fontino M. Ragweed hayfever: genetic control and linkage to HL-A haplotypes. Science 1972; 178:1201–1203.

49. Marsh DG, Meyers DA, Bias WB. The epidemiology and genetics of atopic allergy. N Engl J Med 1981; 305:1551–1559.

50. Blumenthal MN, Awdeh Z, Alper C, Yunis E. Ra5 immune responses, HLA antigens and complotypes. J Allergy Clin Immunol 1985; 75:155 (abstr.).

51. Freidhoff LR, Ehrlich-Kautzky E, Meyers DA, Ansari AA, Bias WB, Marsh DG. Association of HLA-DR3 with human immune reponse to Lol p I and Lol p II allergens in allergic subjects. Tissue Antigens 1988; 31:211–219.

52. Ansari AA, Freidhoff LR, Meyers DA, Bias WB, Marsh DG. Human immune responsiveness to Lolium perenne pollen allergen Lol p III (rye III) is associated with HLA-DR3 and DR5 [published erratum appears in Hum Immunol 1989; 26:149]. Hum Immunol 1989; 25:59–71.

53. Sriramarao P, Selvakumer B, Damodaran C, Rao BS, Prakash O, Rao PV. Immediate hypersensitivity to *Parthenium hysterophorus*. I. Association of HLA antigens and *Parthenium* rhinitis. Clin Exp Allergy 1990; 20:555–560.

54. Fischer GF, Pickl WF, Fae I, Ebner C, Ferreira F, Breiteneder H, Vikoukal E, Scheiner O, Kraft D. Association between IgE response against Bet v I, the major allergen of birch pollen, and HLA-DRB alleles. Hum Immunol 1992; 33:259–265.

55. Marsh DG, Freidhoff LR, Ehrlich-Kautzky E, Bias WB, Roebber M. Immune responsiveness to *Ambrosia artemisiifolia* (short ragweed) pollen allergen

Amb a VI (Ra6) is associated with HLA-DR5 in allergic humans. Immunogenetics 1987; 26(4–5):230–236.

56. Reid MJ, Nish WA, Whisman BA, Goetz DW, Hylander RD, Parker WA Jr, Freeman TM. HLA-DR4-associated nonresponsiveness to mountain cedar allergen. J. Allergy Clin Immunol 1992; 89:593–598.

57. Lympany P, Kemeny DM, Welsh KI, Lee TH. An HLA-associated nonresponsiveness to mellitin: a component of bee venom. J Allergy Clin Immunol 1990; 86:160–170.

58. Sasazuki T, Nishimura Y, Muto M, Ohta N. HLA-linked genes controlling immune response and disease susceptibility. Immunol Rev 1983; 70:51–75.

59. Young RP, Dekker JW, Wordsworth BP, Schou C, Pile KD, Matthiesen F, Rosenberg WMC, Bell JI, Hopkin JM, Cookson WOCM. HLA-DR and HLA-DP genotypes and immunoglobulin E responses to common major allergens. Clin Exp Allergy 1994:24:431–439.

60. Loveridge JA, Rosenberg WMC, Kirkwood TBL, Bell JI. The genetic contribution to human T-cell receptor repertoire. Immunology 1991; 74:246–250.

61. Moss PAH, Rosenberg WMC, Zintzaras E, Bell JI. Characterization of the human T cell receptor α-chain repertoire and demonstration of a genetic influence on Vα usage. Eur J Immunol 1993; 23:1153–1159.

62. Gulwani-Akolar B, Posnett DN, Janson CH, Grunewald J, Wigzell H, Akolkar P, Gregersen PK, Silver J. T cell receptor V-segment frequencies in peripheral blood T cells correlate with human leukocyte antigen type. J Exp Med 1991; 174:1139–1146.

63. Robinson MA. Usage of human T-cell receptor V beta, J beta C beta and V alpha gene segments is not proportional to gene number. Hum Immunol 1992; 35:60–67.

64. Moffatt MF, Hill MR, Cornélis F, Schou C, Faux JA, Young RP, James AL, Ryan G, le Souef P, Musk AW, Hopkin JM, Cookson WOCM. Genetic linkage of the TCR-α/δ region to specific immunoglobulin E responses. Lancet 1994; 343:1597–1600.

65. Gerrard JW, Rao DC, Morton NE. A genetic study of immunoglobulin E. Am J Hum Genet 1978; 30:46–58.

66. Robinson MA, Kindt TJ. Genetic recombination within the human T-cell receptor alpha-chain complex. Proc Natl Acad Sci USA 1987; 84:9089–9093.

67. Cornélis F, Hashimoto L, Loveridge J, MacCarthy A, Buckle V, Julier C, Bell J. Identification of a CA repeat at the TCRA locus using yeast artificial chromosomes: a general method for generating highly polymorphic markers at chosen loci. Genomics 1992; 13:820–825.

68. Cornélis F, Pile K, Loveridge J, Moss P, Harding C, Julier C, Bell JI. Systematic study of human αβ T-cell receptor V segments shows allelic variations resulting in a large number of distinct TCR haplotypes. Eur J Immunol 1993; 23:1277–1283.

69. Heinzel FP, Sadick MD, Mutha SS, Locksley RM. Production of interferon gamma, interleukin 2, interleukin 4, and interleukin 10 by CD4+ lymphocytes

in vivo during healing and progressive murine leishmaniasis. Proc Natl Acad Sci USA 1991; 88:7011–7075.

70. Mohapatra SS, Mohapatra S, Yang M, Ansari AS, Parronchi P, Maggi E, Romagnani S. Molecular basis of cross-reactivity among allergen-specific human T cells. T-cell receptor Vα gene usage and epitope structure. Immunology 1994; 81:15–20.

71. Holt PG, McMenamin C. IgE and mucosal immunity: studies on the role of intraepithelial Ia+ dendritic cells and α/γ T-lympocytes in regulation of T-cell activation in the lung. Clin Exp Allergy 1991; 21(suppl): 148–152.

72. Turki J, Pak J, Green SA, Martin RJ, Liggett SB. Genetic polymophisms of the beta-2 adrenergic receptor in nocturnal and non-nocturnal asthma. J Clin Invest 1995; 95:1635–1641.

73. Jacob CO, Fronek Z, Lewis GD, Koo M, Hansen JA, McDevitt HO. Heritable major histocompatibility complex class II-associated differences in production of tumor necrosis factor α: relevance to genetic predisposition to systemic lupus erythematosis. Proc Natl Acad Sci USA. 1990; 87:1233–1237.

74. Messer G, Spengler U, Jung MC, Honold G, Blömer K, Pape GR, Riethmüller G, Weiss EH. Polymorphic structure of the tumor necrosis factor (TNF) locus: an NcoI polymorphism in the first intron of the human TNF-β gene correlates with a variant amino acid in position 26 and a reduced level of TNF-β production. J Exp Med 1991; 173:209–219.

75. Wilson AG, Symons JA, McDowell TL, di Giovine FS, Duff GW. Effects of a tumour necrosis factor (TNF-α) promotor base transition on transcriptional activity. Br J Rheumatol 1994; 33:89 (abstr.).

76. Moffatt MF, Cookson WOCM. TNF-α promoter polymorphism and asthma. Submitted.

77. Charpin D, Birnbaum J, Haddi E, Genard G, Lanteaume A, Toumi M, Faraj F, Van der Brempt X, Vervolet D. Altitude and allergy to house dust mites. A paradigm of the influence of environmental exposure on allergic sensitisation. Am Rev Respir Dis 1991; 143:983–986.

78. Holt PG, McMenamin C, Nelson D. Primary sensitisation to inhalant allergens during infancy. Pediatr Allergy Immunol 1990; 1:3–15.

79. Sporik R, Holgate S, Platts-Mills TAE, Cogswells JJ. Exposure to house dust mite allergen Der P1 and the development of asthma in children. N Engl J Med 1990; 323:502–507.

80. von Mutius E, Fritzsch C, Weiland SK, Roell G, Magnussen H. Prevalence of asthma and allergic disorders among children in united Germany: a descriptive comparison. Br Med J 1992; 305:1395–1399.

81. von Mutius E, Martinez FD, Fritzsch C, Nicolai T, Roell G. Thiemann HH. Prevalence of asthma and atopy in two areas of West and East Germany. Am J Respir Crit Care Med. 1994; 149:358–364.

82. Bråbäck L, Breborowicz A, Dreborg S, Knutsson A, Pieklik H, Björkstén B. Atopic sensitization and respiratory symptoms among Polish and Swedish school children. Clin Exp Allergy 1994; 24:826–835.

83. von Mutius E, Martinez FD, Fritzsch C, Nicolai T, Reitmer P, Thiemann HH. Skin test reactivity and number of siblings. Br Med J. 1994; 308:692–695.
84. Lynch NR, Hagel I, Perez M, Di Prisco MC, Lopez R, Alvarez N. Effect of antihelmintic treatment on the allergic reactivity of children in a tropical slum. J Allergy Clin Immunol 1993; 92:404–411.
85. Paré PD, Faux JA, Hill MR, Kan R, Bremmer P, Musk M, Murray C, le Souef PN, Musk AW, Cookson WOCM. Skin test responses and specific IgE levels to common aeroallergens in Australian aborigines. Am J Respir Crit Care Med 1995; 151:A214.

28

Risk Factors in the Development of Allergy

BENGT BJÖRKSTÉN and N-I MAX KJELLMAN

University Hospital
Linköping, Sweden

I. Introduction

Sensitization, as proven by the demonstration of low levels of IgE anti-bodies directed against environmental allergens, appears to be part of the normal immune response (1). In most instances, at least in children, these antibodies are only temporary, as the continuing IgE antibody formation is rapidly suppressed (2). But when genetically predisposed individuals are exposed to an allergen at a time when the regulation of the immune system is immature, then higher levels of IgE antibodies, lasting for a long time, may appear (3). The more susceptible to sensitization that the individual is, the lower is the allegen dose needed for this to occur. The fact that an individual is sensitized does not, however, necessarily mean that clinical symptoms, i.e., allergic disease, will develop. It is not known which factors decide what allergic manifestations will appear in an atopic individual, e.g., whether he or she will suffer from atopic dermatitis, asthma, hay fever, gastrointestinal allergy or several of them. It is likely, however, that the selection of target organ is also at least partially under genetic control.

Sensitivity to allergens and manifest disease are thus the end results of an interaction between genetically determined susceptibility to atopy, exposure to allergen, and exposure to adjuvant factors. In this chapter, environmental factors that may either enhance or reduce the likelihood of sensitization and trigger clinical disease in sensitized individuals will be discussed (Table 1), emphasizing particularly their significance in individuals with a genetically determined susceptibility to allergic manifestations and variations in the susceptibility.

II. Epidemiology

Recent epidemiological studies show that there are large regional differences in the prevalence of asthma and allergies both in children and in adults (4–6). With the exception of a few isolated groups of people, the reported differences between populations are not genetically determined. Rather, they seem to be explained by differences in living conditions. Factors associated with "Western lifestyle" appear to have resulted in a large increase in the prevalence of allergic disorders over the past few decades (7–9). The increase is particularly obvious in children and young adults. It is likely that environmental factors that are encountered in early childhood are of particular significance and that the increasing prevalence seen in young adults is a result of a cohort effect.

These suggestions are supported by the results from studies in genetically similar populations living under different conditions in the same country and studies comparing migrants with those who remained in their community of origin. Thus, the prevalence of allergic disease in developing countries seems to be higher in people living under privileged conditions

Table 1 Risk Factors in the Development of Allergy

Genetic susceptibility:
    Family history of allergy
    Presence of predictive marker, e.g., elevated serum-IgE, IgE antibodies to allergens, eosinophilia, various immunological findings
Prenatal:
    Maternal medication
    Maternal tobacco smoking
Infancy and early childhood:
    Exposure to tobacco smoke
    Early formula feeding
    High-level exposure to allergens
    Certain infections, e.g., RSV
Few infections during the first years of life?

than among the poor. More than 20 years ago Morrison Smith observed that the prevalence of asthma was low in children migrating to Britain from the West Indies with their parents (10). Interestingly, the prevalence of asthma in the younger children in these families, who were born in Britain, was similar to that of the native British children. A South African study yielded similar results, in that children of the Xhosa tribe who were born in a rural area had much less asthma and other allergies than Xhosa children raised in Cape Town (11). The influence of living conditions on childhood asthma has also been noted among Tokelauans living in their home environment in the Pacific and in New Zealand, with a much more lower prevalence of disease among the former (12).

Environmental differences in the prevalence of allergy are also recorded between urban and rural areas in industrialized countries. As an example, two recent Swedish studies showed that the relative risk for a positive skin-prick test is 70% higher among 11-year-old children living in a moderately polluted town in Northern Sweden than among children living in the neighboring countryside (13,14).

The understanding of the role of environmental factors has become complicated however by some recent observations. Air pollution is a major problem in many formerly socialist countries in Central and Eastern Europe, yet the prevalence of atopy among children there is much lower than in Western Europe. As an example, the prevalence of positive skin-prick tests in Leipzig in eastern Germany is less than half of that among children of the same age living in Munich in western Germany (15,16). Similarly, atopic sensitization is much lower in Konin in central Poland and in Estonia than it is in northern Sweden, despite generally less environmental pollution in the latter region (Table 2) (14,17,18). The low prevalence of atopy was not associated with less respiratory disease in Estonia and Poland, however. Thus, the responses to questionnaires given to 2600 11-year-old children revealed that symptoms of bronchial hyperreactivity and wheezing were similar or higher than in Sweden, although the diagnosis "asthma" was much more common in Sweden. The relative influence of known risk factors, such as exposure to tobacco smoke, living in a town with air pollution, and a family history of allergy, was similar, however, in the three countries.

These very recent studies in formerly socialistic countries of Eastern and Central Europe strongly indicate the other factors connected with "Western lifestyle" are important for the development of allergy.

Table 2 Prevalence of Positive Skin-Prick Tests and Respiratory Symptoms Among 11–12-Year-Old School Children in Five Locations in the Baltic Sea Region and the Levels of Some Air Pollutants

	Sweden		Poland	Estonia	
	Rural	Urban	Konin	Tallinn	Tartu
≥1 pos SPT (%)	24.2	35.3	13.7	14.3	8.1
Crude OR	1	1.71	0.49	0.46[a]	0.28[a]
Cough >2 weeks during common cold (%)	5.7	12.0	15.1	18.8	13.8
Resp. inf. > 6 time/yr (%)	6.3	8.0	14.0	10.4	10.5
Wheezing (%)	9.3	11.6	10.4	9.4	5.8
Asthma diagnosis (%)	6.7	9.5	2.9	3.2	2.5

[a]Odds ratio for a positive skin-prick test in Tallinn (coastal, industrialized town), as compared to Tartu (university town) was 1.81.
n.d. = not determined.
Source: Data from Refs. 14 and 18.

III. Immunological Aspects

There are two major types of T-helper cells, TH-1 and TH-2 (19). The former are associated with a lymphokine profile that stimulates, e.g., IgM and IgG antibody formation, while suppressing IgE antibody synthesis. In contrast, the TH-2 cells are associated with IgE antibody formation and the appearance of mast cells and eosinophils. Recent development on basic and clinical immunology and the results of several epidemiological studies have given rise to a model for IgE immunoregulation, viz., that the magnitude of the IgE component of the antigen-specific immune responses to persistent allergens is ultimately determined by the relative balance between antigen-specific TH-1 and TH-2 cells that become established in relevant T-memory populations (20).

Animal experiments show that repeated inhalation of an allergen by immunologically naive rat pups usually results in a transient low-level IgE antibody response. Susceptibility to this form of tolerance induction is genetically determined (20), but can be markedly influenced by a range of environmental factors, including chemical air pollutants and also infection. The T-cell responses in rat pups of A strain with the normal low propensity to IgE antibody formation, "low responders," were mostly of the TH-1 type, while the TH-2 phenotype dominated in pups of an IgE high-responder strain, indicating that the propensity for a certain type of immune response was genetically determined (Fig. 1). The ultimate expression of TH profiles however, was influenced by environmental factors. Thus, the TH-2 responses in the high-responder rat pups could be suppressed by exposure to infections and microbial adjuvants concomitantly with the allergen and by high antigen doses. A switch toward a TH-2 response could be induced in pups of the low-responder strain by simultaneously exposing them to allergen and air pollutants, e.g., tobacco smoke.

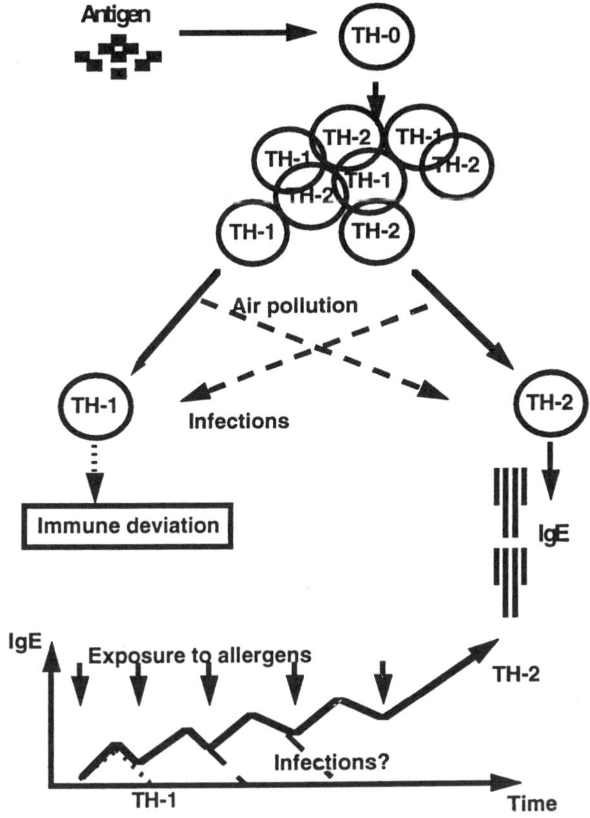

Figure 1 Primary immune responses to inhaled allergens in rat pups with a low (normal) and high propensity for IgE antibody formation. A low-grade IgE antibody formation is seen in both rat strains. In the low-responder rats, the IgE response is suppressed upon repeated allergen exposures while in the high responders it is gradually boosted. An immune deviation toward a TH-1-type response is enhanced by infections and other microbial stimulation, while an "allergic" TH-2-type response is enhanced by air pollutants, e.g., exposure to tobacco smoke and NO_2.

It is important to note that it was only possible to induce tolerance in animals via inhalation or ingestion against antigens to which the animals were immunologically naive; i.e., once stable immunological memory is established in the TH-2 population; and persistent IgE responses develop, further exposure to the relevant antigens only further boosts the ongoing responses. Additionally, this form of tolerance is preferentially directed against IgE, as the animals typically manifest IgG responses against the same allergens (21).

The data accumulating on cytokine regulation of IgE synthesis in humans are broadly consistent with the major predictions from the animal models. The human immune system appears to begin responding to ubiquitous inhalant allergens in early infancy. There are also indications that blood mononuclear cells from infants with a family history of allergy have less capacity to produce IFN-γ which would support a less efficient induction of TH-1 type response in them (22–24). Furthermore, infants who develop allergic disease during their first 18 months of life have elevated serum levels of IL-4, which is the major cytokine from TH-2 cells (25).

The clinical relevance of the data generated in animal studies is further supported by some data from epidemiological studies that are discussed in more detail in Section VII.D. These studies lend some support to the notion that recurrent infections in infancy could protect against sensitization to inhalant allergens.

The kinetics of humoral antibody responses to food antigens and inhalant allergens in infants and young children lend further support to the relevance of the animal model. Thus, IgG antibodies to ubiquitous environmental antigens appear very early in life and remain detectable in serum from the majority of both atopic and normals throughout life (26). The picture for IgE antibodies is markedly different, however. Prospective analysis of serum IgE levels to environmental allergens in individual children indicates that antibodies to foods are commonly detected both in atopic and nonatopic infants during the first year of life, although the magnitude of the responses is higher and of longer duration in the former (2,27). In virtually all children, however, these initial IgE responses to foods are terminated spontaneously by age 2–4 years, leaving intact IgG responses to the same antigens which persist into adulthood. In support of these findings, transient skin-test reactivity to food allergens is also common during this period (28).

The pattern for IgE responses to ingested and inhaled allergens differs in at least two significant aspects. First, the latter responses rarely appear until after 1 year of age, i.e., at a higher age than the IgE responses to foods. Secondly, whereas IgE responses against foods do not usually persist beyond early childhood, a much larger proportion of children continue to produce IgE antibodies against one or more inhalant allergens into adulthood. The induction of antibody responses to both groups of allergens appear to be induced very early in life, however.

IV. Prenatal Factors

A. Intrauterine Sensitization

Maternal IgE is not supposed to pass through the human placenta (29). The human fetus seems capable of producing IgE antibodies, as such antibodies have been demonstrated in in-vitro studies of fetal lung and liver tissues and they have also been isolated in amniotic fluid (29,30). Under normal circumstances this production is limited, as the IgE levels in cord blood are usually very low, often even below the detection level of a sensitive assay. However, elevated levels of cord blood IgE, i.e., above about 0.8 kU/L, do occur in some newborns. Such elevated levels are associated with an increased risk for development of allergic disease during infancy and childhood (summarized in Ref. 31). In some cases these antibodies may indicate intrauterine sensitization, since low levels of IgE antibodies against cow's milk can be detected in some cord blood samples (32–36). Furthermore, positive skin-prick tests have been elicited in newborns to penicillin, helminths, cow's milk, and grass pollen (34,37,38). It is possible that the fetus is not completely protected from allergenic material and may be sensitized in utero, although this is only rarely associated with allergic manifestations. This possibility is indicated by the observation that proteins eaten by pregnant rats can be isolated both in serum of their pups and in the amniotic fluid (39). In humans, food allergens are often present in the serum of adults after ingestion of milk and egg (40), but so far there is no documentation of food allergens in the fetal circulation.

An even more likely explanation for the presence of elevated serum-IgE levels in some atopic infants at birth, however, could be that they are the consequence of nonspecific spontaneous IgE synthesis, perhaps due to a lack of suppression. This notion would be supported by the negative outcome of prospective studies of manipulation of the maternal diet during pregnancy (41,42).

Transplacental transfer of maternal anti-idiotypic antibodies is yet another possible explanation for the occasional finding of IgE antibodies in cord blood. Such maternal IgG antibodies directed against the antigen specific parts of other antibodies have a structure similar to the antigen and can replace it as an immunological stimulus. As a consequence, anti-idiotypic antibodies would have the capacity to stimulate fetal antibody formation. This has been demonstrated as a possible mechanism for transfer of immunity to polio virus and certain strains of *Escherichia coli* from mother to baby (43). It has been suggested that the IgE synthesis in a newborn baby may be stimulated by a similar mechanism, but so far there is no convincing evidence of such prenatal sensitization.

Recent studies demonstrate that cord blood lymphocytes respond to stimulation in vitro to food and inhalant allergens (22,44). It is not known whether these responses indicate "sensitization" in the sense that they are the forerunners of allergy, or whether they are part of the normal maturation of the immune system.

B. Maternal Immunity

The fetus is protected from various external influences by the placental barrier. This barrier is selective and, e.g., maternal IgG antibodies pass through it (45). Immunity to various infectious agents is thus transferred to the fetus.

Less is known about the role of transplacental transfer of maternal immunity for the development of allergy in her infant. IgG antibodies to good antigens are present in cord blood at a higher concentration than in corresponding maternal blood (46).

There are several ways by which transplacentally transferred immunity by maternal IgG antibodies in theory could protect the baby, e.g., by protecting the newborn infant against infections. Such infections could otherwise possibly change mucosal barrier function and influence immune responses to antigens, including enhanced allergic sensitization. By increasing the maternal intake of milk and eggs during pregnancy, for example, it is possible to increase maternal antibody concentrations to these foods, and by decreasing the intake there is a corresponding decrease in antibody concentration (46,47). There are indications that maternal IgG antibodies against various foods may protect the infant from sensitization (48,49). The latter study, however, was presented only as an abstract and not as a full paper. Moreover, in two more recent and larger studies, there was no relationship between maternal IgG antibody levels to foods and protection of allergy (46,47,50).

Yet another interesting possibility was indicated by a recent study reporting that elevated levels of IgG anti-IgE antibodies in the cord blood were associated with less allergy during the first 18 months of life (51). This was particularly obvious in babies with a strong family history of allergy. This finding and the reported individual variations in the composition of human milk (Section V of this chapter) indicate that maternal immunity may be an important environmental factor influencing the risk for allergic manifestations in her child, even many years later. It is also possible that reports of a stronger influence of genetics when atopy is inherited from the maternal side rather than from the paternal (52) is not explained by genetic imprinting but by an early environmental influence exerted by the mother.

C. Maternal Diet During Pregnancy

The fact that foods are the dominating allergens in infants, as well as the possibility of prenatal induction of IgE antibody formation has prompted studies of maternal dietary restriction during pregnancy as a means to prevent the development of the IgE antibodies and allergy in the babies. Some of these studies are difficult to evaluate, however, as the maternal diet was not limited to pregnancy, but continued into the lactation period. This is discussed more in detail in Chapter 30.

Two prospective studies that were limited to studying the effects of dietary manipulation during pregnancy both failed to reveal any protective effect. In one of the studies, pregnant women with a family history of allergy were randomly assigned to an unrestricted diet or to an elimination diet during the last trimester of pregnancy (41,47). Allergenic foods such as cow's milk, egg, fish, and peanuts were excluded in the intervention group. In another prospective study of similarly selected mothers, the participants either had a diet low in these foods or had a diet with increased amounts of milk and eggs, i.e., at least 1 L of milk and 1 egg daily (50). In contrast to the effect of dietary manipulation of breast-feeding mothers (vide infra), none of the diets during pregnancy were associated with a reduced risk for food allergy, nor of other symptoms of atopic disease in their babies. Thus, neither avoidance of certain allergenic foods nor increased amounts of them in order to stimulate IgG antibody formation had any appreciable effects on clinical symptoms.

The studies indicate that dietary manipulation of the mothers during pregnancy is not associated with less allergy in their babies, unless continued into the lactation period. Consequently, no dietary restrictions should be imposed on pregnant women as a means for allergy prevention in her baby.

D. Other Pre- and Perinatal Factors

There is little doubt that maternal smoking during pregnancy is a health hazard for her baby, including growth retardation (53). Studies of the possible role of this habit for the development of allergy and asthma in her baby is more difficult to study, as very few mothers who smoke during pregnancy quit when the baby is born. It is therefore difficult to confirm whether the increased prevalence of allergy and asthma is a consequence of maternal smoking during pregnancy, smoke exposure of the infant, or both. As summarized in (53), however, there is some evidence that maternal tobacco smoking during pregnancy may increase the risk for childhood allergy and wheezing disorder.

There are also indications that certain medication to pregnant women may affect the rate of allergy in their children. Observations include a possible increase in neonatal IgE concentration in babies of mothers treated with the beta-blocking agent metoprolol (54). Intrauterine exposure to metoprolel tended to be associated with an increased incidence of atopic disease during the first years of life, as compared to children of placebo-treated mothers.

The influence of maternal disease during late pregnancy on the rate of allergic disease in their children has not been adequately assessed in prospective studies, although there are suggestions that the lack of well-being of pregnant asthmatics may add to the genetic risk for development of atopic disease in their babies (55).

Perinatal stress factors are associated with respiratory problems during the first years of life. It has also been suggested that they could increase the risk for sensitization to allergens. These studies (summarized in Ref. 56) were all retrospective, however, and they did not control for various other possibilities. In a recent Swedish study, prematurity was associated as a moderate risk factor for hospitalization in early childhood due to wheezing (57).

In conclusion, although much remains to be studied, it is reasonable to assume that maternal immunity, health, and medication, at least during the final part of pregnancy, all may have consequences for the incidence of respiratory disease and allergy in their babies, at least during early childhood. Whether prenatal factors may also affect the prevalence of allergy later in life remains to be studied.

V. Infant Feeding

As discussed in more detail in Chapter 30, early weaning to cow's milk formulas has been associated with an increased rate of allergic disease. The data are conflicting, however, as there are many studies in which prolonged breast feeding was not protective against allergy (summarized in Ref. 58). The explanation for the apparently conflicting results seems to lie in selection of patients for the studies, in the necessity for other dietary precautions, and how the outcome was assessed. Studies showing a protective effect of prolonged, exclusive breast feeding have included infants with a genetic propensity to allergy, rather than an unselected group of infants. Also, the breast feeding in these cases was associated with an avoidance of other foods, e.g., juices and solid foods. Thus, late introduction of foreign foods, i.e., after 6 months of life, appears to lower the frequency of infants producing IgE antibodies to cow's milk and to be associated with less allergic symptoms, as compared to introduction of cow's milk products before that age (59,60). It is also possible that any long-term effects, if real, are limited to respiratory disease rather than to allergy in itself (61).

As poor breast feeding is associated with early introduction of formula and solid foods, it is not fully understood to what extent development of allergy is a consequence of exposure to foreign allergenic foods and to what extent it is a consequence of not receiving breast milk, which contains many components that may modify the immune responses of the infant (reviewed in Ref. 62). There are therefore several possible explanations for a protective role of breast milk against allergy, including low content of allergens, protection against intestinal and respiratory infections, passive transfer of immunity from the mother by secretory IgA antibodies, and transfer of components that stimulate the maturation by secretory IgA antibodies, and transfer of components that stimulate the maturation of the infantile immune system. It is well established that human milk may contain food antigens such as cow's milk proteins and egg if these items are ingested by the mother (summarized in Refs. 62 and 63). This may sensitize the breast-fed baby. The small amounts of allergens that may be present in breast milk can thus be sufficient to cause a high grade of sensitization in a genetically predisposed infant—and to evoke allergic symptoms during lactation (20).

Passive transfer of immunity is another possibility by which human milk is protective, as in one study it was reported that high levels in breast milk of IgA antibodies against cow's milk protein were associated with less allergic symptoms in the babies (64). This observation, however, could not be confirmed in a larger, prospective study (47).

Several recent studies indicate that human milk may exert a regulatory role on infant immunity. Observations include an early stimulation of IgA antibody synthesis in breast-fed infants (65,66) and transfer of cell-mediated immunity (67,68) and cytokines (69,70). The precise relation between breast feeding and infant allergy is thus not fully understood. It is reasonable to assume that any allergy-protective effects of breast feeding may vary with the individual mothers, as both their diet and their immune status appear to play a role. Also, an allergy-preventing effect of human milk seems to be limited to babies with a genetically determined increased risk for allergic disease (58). This lends further support to the notion that environmental factors associated with an increased rate of allergic disease in children are operative mainly in individuals with a genetic propensity for allergic sensitization and disease.

The effect of various hypoallergenic diets to lactating mothers and infants as a means of primary prevention of allergy are discussed in Chapter 30.

VI. Exposure to Inhalant Allergens

Several clinical studies indicate that there is a period in early infancy during which exposure to inhalant allergens may result in the development of allergy several years later. In a large epidemiological study comprising 40,000 individuals, a Finnish team observed a significantly higher prevalence of allergy to birch and grass pollen in 10-year-old children who were born in the spring, as compared to children who were born at other times of the year (71). Subsequently the authors reported that the risk of pollen allergy, as diagnosed at 10 years of age, was affected not only by the month of birth, but also by the intensity of the pollen season the year they were born (72). The intensity of the first pollen season even had a stronger impact than the intensity of the pollen season when their symptoms first appeared.

Similar results have been reported for ragweed allergy in individuals born in the United States, before and during the peak ragweed pollen season (73). In a Swedish study, however, it was observed that the relationship between season of birth and allergy development was limited to children with elevated IgE levels in the cord blood, i.e., with a congenital propensity for allergy (74), again supporting the notion that manifestations of disease are the result of an interaction between environmental and genetic factors.

Similar to the apparent effects of early exposure to pollen, early contacts with animal epithelia and house dust appear to influence the incidence of allergy. Thus, children born in the autumn, i.e., before the main indoor season, seem to be more prone to sensitization to indoor allergens than babies born at other times of the year (75–77). These observations in pollen-, dander- and mite-sensitive individuals all indicate that early exposure to an allergen increases the risk for allergy. The association between exposure to allergens early in life and clinical symptoms to inhalant allergens appearing several years later could be explained by the development of immune responses during the first years of life, as discussed in Section III of this chapter.

In conclusion, although sensitization may occur at any age, the first years of life and the conditions under which the primary encounter with an allergen takes place seem to be particularly important, even if the consequences may not become apparent until many years later.

The fact that exposure to high levels of allergens early in life appears to be a risk factor for sensitization and allergic manifestations later in life has prompted studies of the possible effects of allergy prevention. The results of these studies are discussed in detail in Chapter 30, but in summary indicate a marginal protective effect against sensitivity to the particular allergens that were avoided. From current knowledge of the kinetics of the primary immune responses as discussed in Section III, it is not reasonable to expect a general allergy-preventive effect by the avoidance of certain allergens but merely a possible prevention or delayed sensitization to that particular allergen.

VII. Non-Specific Environmental Factors

It is well established that various environmental factors may enhance sensitization and also trigger an allergic reaction in a sensitized individual (Table 3). While allergy to most of the compounds listed in the table is rare, these compounds do play a role in both enhancing sensitization to allergens and in eliciting and aggravating clinical symptoms.

A. Air Pollution

Air pollution such as ozone, SO_2, and NO_2 may all enhance sensitization, at least in experimental animals (reviewed in Refs. 1 and 78). Data are less

Table 3 Adjuvant Factors Thought to Be Involved Either in Sensitization or Manifestations of Allergic Disease

Air pollution and sources:
   Tobacco smoke
   Industry and traffic; solid particles, SO_2, NO
   Combustion by-products; CO_2, CO, SO_2, NO_2, NO, formaldehyde, volatile
     vapors
   Photochemical reactions; ozone, NO_2
Building materials; formaldehyde, decoration, and paints; solvents, furnishings
Tight, poorly ventilated homes
Presicides and consumer products; organic substances, aerosols
Respiratory tract infections; viral, pertussis
Ongoing allergic reaction [facilitates sensitization to new allergens]

clear-cut in humans, but in an epidemiological survey of 5300 children in Sweden, bronchial hyperactivity and pollen allergy were both more common in children living near a moderately air polluting paper factory than among children living in a forested, unindustrialized area about 40 km away from the factory (79). If the parents smoked at home, then the prevalence of bronchial hyperactivity and allergy were further increased, indicating a synergistic effect between the two pollutants.

As mentioned in the previous section, the prevalence of allergic manifestations is lower in rural than it is in nearby urban areas in Western Europe. The most likely explanation for this is different levels of air pollution. A similar difference was also noted in the formerly Soviet-occupied Estonia (Table 2). Thus, the prevalence of at least one positive skin-prick test was significantly higher in Tallinn, an industrialized coastal city with considerable pollution, than in Tartu, which is an inland university town.

B. Exposure to Tobacco Smoke

Tobacco smoke is the major indoor air pollutant. Tobacco smoke is strongly associated with allergic sensitization, asthma, and other respiratory diseases. Increased serum IgE levels and an increased prevalence of positive skin tests toward occupational allergens have been shown in multiple studies (reviewed in Ref. 53). Thus, smokers are sensitized more easily to occupational allergens than are nonsmokers who are exposed to the allergens to a similar degree (80).

The effect of tobacco smoke is not limited to active smoking, however. Infants and young children are particularly susceptible to the adjuvant effects of tobacco smoke as trigger of sensitization and wheezing. Children of parents who smoke at home have a significantly earlier onset of allergy and wheezy bronchitis than children of nonsmoking parents (53).

The effect of tobacco smoke on sensitization to allergens may be explained by a local effect on the airways, or by a direct effect on the immune system. The former notion is supported by the finding that smoking rats exposed to antigen in aerosol develop higher IgE responses than subcutaneously immunized animals and nonsmoking aerosol-immunized controls (81).

In conclusion, passive smoking is by far the best-identified risk factor for the development of allergic disease, particularly in early childhood, and this is independent of how "allergy" is defined. There is little doubt that exposure to tobacco smoke is the most important environmental risk factor for childhood allergy and respiratory disease that has been identified so far. The long-term effects of childhood exposure to tobacco smoke are unknown.

C. Housing

Most children in Europe and North American spend at least 90%m of their time indoors. It is therefore likely that the indoor environment is even more important than geographic and other macroenvironmental factors. Modern, well-insulated buildings with poor ventilation represent a definite risk factor for allergic sensitization (summarized in Ref. 82). Many new compounds are used in modern buildings, e.g., plastic material, synthetic paints, and chemical substances with unknown effects on human health. Combined with efficient insulation and a reduced ventilation, this has created a new indoor climate. In temperate climates, energy crisis and increased interest in energy-conserving measures have resulted in changed building standards, particularly better insulation and reduced ventilation. This in turn has resulted in more "sick buildings," characterized by damage due to dampness, indoor mold growth, and presence of various symptoms among people dwelling in the houses. At least one well-documented consequence of this is a much increased prevalence of sensitivity to house dust mite allergens in regions with a temperate climate (83–85). Sensitivity to these allergens used to be rare in climates with cold and dry winters, but the creation of a warm and humid "subtropical" indoor climate has changed this.

In an epidemiological survey, it was found that homes with damage due to dampness were associated with both a higher incidence of atopic disease and/or bronchial hyperactivity in the children. In children living in houses with damage by dampness and whose parents in addition smoked at home, there was a marked increase in allergic asthma and bronchial hyperactivity, as compared with children exposed to only one of these factors. The effects of the living conditions were most marked for children with a family history of asthma. This supports the notion that environmental influences play a particular role in individuals with a genetic susceptibility to allergic disease.

Much more has to be learned about the role of the indoor climate for sensitization and triggering of allergic manifestations, e.g., the role of molds and other micro-organisms. It is, however, reasonable to conclude that a search for environmental factors influencing the development of asthma and allergy should be directed toward factors affecting the indoor climate.

D. Infections

The role of infections, notably in the respiratory tract, as risk factors for the development of childhood allergic disease is complex. An infection induces an inflammatory reaction in the respiratory mucosa, which in turn modifies the local immune response. They may also possibly alter the immune defence and act as adjuvants or as allergens. Furthermore, it is common knowledge that infections may trigger clinical symptoms in already-sensitized individuals and that infections increase bronchial hyperactivity. Earlier animal experiments support clinical observations showing enhanced IgE production after allergen exposure and concomitant viral infection (1,86).

Epidemiological studies of the relation between infections and manifestation of allergic disease are complicated, however, by the fact that symptoms such as a runny nose, wheezing, and cough may all be caused by either an infection or an allergic reaction and that the etiology of the symptoms is therefore not always easily identified by patients and researchers.

Certain infectious agents, e.g., respiratory syncytial virus (RSV), Epstein-Barr virus, and *Bordetella pertussis* seem to be of particular interest, as they appear to enhance sensitization. The mechanisms are probably different, however. Bronchiolitis caused by RSV in early infancy has been associated with the development of atopy and asthma. The mechanism may be that the G protein of RSV may directly stimulate TH2-like cells, thus enhancing IgE antibody formation and other components of the allergic inflammation.

The relationship between bronchiolitis caused by RSV during the first 6 months of life and the development of asthma was recently studied prospectively in 47 infants; (87). For each child, two matched controls were selected, making a study population of 140 participating in the follow-up at 3 years. Asthma, defined as three episodes of bronchial obstruction verified by a physician, was found in 11 of the 47 children with RSV bronchiolitis (23%) and in only one of 93 controls. A positive test for IgE antibodies against a mixture of allergens was recorded in 32% of the RSV children and 9% of the controls ($p = .02$). Of particular interest was the observation that among the former children, 6 of 11 children with a family history of allergy developed asthma, as compared to only 5 of 36 without this family history. Thus, the risk for asthma after RSV bronchiolitis was much higher in infants with a genetic propensity to allergy.

Among the infectious agents, *Bordetella pertussis* is of particular interest, as it is a well-established adjuvant for the induction of IgE antibody formation in experimental animals (88). Furthermore, whooping cough is associated with bronchial hyperactivity for several months (89). It has also been shown that IgE antibodies to pertussis toxin appear after an infection (90) and after immunization against pertussis (91). The latter observation raises a question about a possible role of vaccinations as a risk factor for allergic disease. This notion is further strengthened by the fact that aluminum, which is used as an adjuvant in many vaccines, is also one of the most potent adjuvants for IgE antibody synthesis in animals (92). Properly designed epidemiological studies are needed to clarify a possible relationship between routine immunizations of infants and the development of atopic disease.

Infection with Epstein-Barr virus is associated with atopic disease (93). This is possibly explained by the general stimulatory effects on B cells that is exerted by the virus.

The understanding of the interaction between infections and sensitization has become more complicated recently in the light of experimental studies and epidemiological observations. As discussed in Section III, rat pups who are protected against infections are more easily sensitized to inhaled allergens than are pups exposed to various microbial agents (20). Data from recent animal experiments are supported by the results of epidemiological studies. In a British study, an inverse relationship between many respiratory tract infections and atopy was observed (94). An inverse relationship between the number of siblings (16), particularly older siblings (95), and atopy has also been reported, indicating that many infections during the first year of life could protect against sensitization. Very recently it was observed that the prevalence of positive skin-prick tests may be lower in tuberculin-positive than in tuberculin-negative children, indicating that bacterial infections and vaccinations early in life may possibly enhance the downregulation of the IgE antibody formation to allergens encountered at the time of the infection. Reports of less atopy among school children in the formerly socialist countries of Eastern Europe (14,16,19,96) lend some support to the relevance of these findings.

Based on the experimental and clinical findings, Holt (20) suggested that improvements in public health and general living standards in the developed countries over the last two or three generations has progressively reduced the level of exposure of infants and young children to the natural microbial environment. According to this hypothesis, the lowered microbial stimulation has resulted in a delayed postnatal development of immune competence, resulting in a prolonged period during which the immune system is at risk of generating a TH-2-type immune response with IgE antibody formation and stimulation of mast cell and eosinophil proliferation.

E. Other

Animal studies and clinical observations have indicated that stress alters the immune response, as measured by various laboratory tests of inflammatory responses, immunoglobulin production, and cell-mediated immunity (97,98). Clinical studies also indicate that stress may cause reduced resistance to infections (99,100). It is clinically well established that psychological factors influence the severity of asthmatic symptoms and allergic reactions in affected patients. For example, dysfunctional patterns of interaction and relations are more common in the families of children with severe asthma than in families of children with another severe chronic disease, i.e., diabetes mellitus (101,102). Patterns of low flexibility ("rigidity") and too much closeness ("enmeshment") dominated among the dysfunctional families. Family therapy to such families reduced the severity of the asthma in the affected children.

A recent prospective study addressed the question of whether the disturbed family interaction is a primary finding or a consequence of disease. The study included the families of 100 infants with a strong family history of allergy (103). The entire family participated in a standardized family test when the children were 3 and 18 months old, assessing the ability to adjust to demands of the situation ("adaptability") and the balance between emotional closeness and distance ("cohesion"). An unbalanced family interplay was common at 3 months (37%), but it was not predictive for respiratory illness. At 18 months a dysfunctional interaction was significantly more common in families of children with eczema and obstructive symptoms, as compared to families of healthy children. The study indicates that a dysfunctional family interaction is the result, rather than a cause, of recurrent wheezing in infancy. Further studies are needed to clarify the role of psychological factors for variations in individual susceptibility to allergic manifestations over time.

As already discussed, the prevalence of allergy in the formerly socialist countries in Central and Eastern Europe is much lower than in Western Europe, despite the fact that air pollution is often higher in the former. The studies strongly indicate that other factors connected with Western lifestyle are more important than air pollution for the development of allergy, although the latter also plays an obvious role. The fact that the differences in the prevalence of sensitivity to inhaled allergens between eastern and western Germany are limited to populations who were born after 1960 indicates that they are explained largely by factors encountered early in life (96).

The living conditions in the formerly socialistic countries of Europe are in many respects similar to those that prevailed in Western Europe 30–40 years ago, including type of air pollution, panorama of childhood infections and immunizations, building standards, and food. The low prevalence of allergy in these countries supports the general feeling that the prevalence of allergy has increased substantially in the West over the past decades. The nature of the factors associated with the environment and/or changing living conditions are unknown. In all the studies however, there was an inverse relation between sensitization and manifestations of allergy on one hand and crowded dwellings and the number of respiratory infections among the children on the other hand. In currently ongoing studies, differences in the intestinal flora, dietary habits, and infections in early childhood, as well as other factors related to lifestyle, are being studied as possible explanations for the different outcome of exposure to ubiquitous inhalant allergens in Western industrialized countries and other parts of the world.

VIII. Concluding Remarks

A number of environmental factors may increase the risk for sensitization in early childhood and the subsequent development of allergic disease. Environmental factors may already operate during fetal life, e.g., maternal health and medication. After birth, the first months of life appear to be a period during which babies are particularly susceptible to sensitization, although the clinical manifestations of respiratory allergy may not appear until several years later. Infants with a genetic propensity to develop allergy and atopic disease seem particularly susceptible to the various environmental influences. There are distinct differences in the early immune responses to allergens in atopic and nonatopic infants. It is possible that the apparent increase in the prevalence of atopic disease in many countries over the past decades are caused by unknown changes in lifestyle operating in early life. Even if all the known factors that may influence the incidence of allergic disease are added, however, this can only explain a fraction of the regional differences and changes over time in the prevalence of allergy. In order to implement effective prevention of allergy, it is necessary to identify these environmental factors and the infants who are at risk in life, and then to support their families and encourage them to take allergy-preventive measures.

References

1. Björkstén B. Risk factors in early childhood for the development of atopic diseases. Allergy 1994; 49:400–407.
2. Hattevig G, Khellman B, Björkstén B. Appearance of IgE antibodies to ingested and inhaled allergens during first 12 years of life in atopic and nonatopic children. Pediatr Allergy Immunol 1993; 4:182–189.

3. Holt P. Postnatal maturation of immune competence during infancy and childhood. Pediatr Allergy Immunol 1995; 6:59–70.
4. Burney P. Epidemiology of asthma. Allergy 1993; 48:17–21.
5. Burney PG, Luczynska C, Chinn S, Jarvis D. The European Community Respiratory Health Survey. Eur Respir J 1994; 7:954–960.
6. Pearce N, Weiland S, Keil U, Langridge P, Anderson HR, Strachan D, Bauman A, Young L, Gluyas P, Ruffin D. Self-reported prevalence of asthma symptoms in children in Australia, England, Germany and New Zealand: an international comparison using the ISAAC protocol. Eur Respir J 1993; 6: 1455–1461.
7. Åberg N. Asthma and allergic rhinitis in Swedish conscripts. Clin Exp Allergy 1989; 19:59–63.
8. Burney P, Chinn S, Rona R. Has the prevalence of asthma increased in children? Evidence from the national study of health and growth 1973–86. Br Med J 1990; 300:1306–1310.
9. Burr M, Butland B, King S, Vaughan-Williams E. Changes in asthma prevalence: two surveys fifteen years apart. Arch Dis Child 1989; 64:1452–1456.
10. Morrison Smith J. Skin tests and atopic allergy in children. Clin Allergy 1973; 3:269–275.
11. van Niekerk C, Weinberg E, Shore S, de V Heese H, van Schalkwyk D. Prevalence of asthma: a comparative study of urban and rural Xhosa children. Clin Allergy 1979; 9:319–324.
12. Waite D, Eyles E, Tonkin S, O'Donnell T. Asthma prevalence in Tokelauan children in two environments. Clin Allergy 1980; 10:71–75.
13. Bråbäck L, Kälvesten L. Urban living as a risk factor for atopic sensitization in Swedism schoolchildren. Pediatr Allergy Immunol 1991; 2:14–19.
14. Bråbаčk L, Breborowicz A, Dreborg S, Knutsson A, Peiklik H, Björkstén B. Atopic sensitization and respiratory symptoms among Polish and Swedish schoolchildren. Clin Exp Allergy 1994; 24:826–835.
15. von Mutius E, Sherrill D, Fritzsch C, Martinez F, Lebowitz M. Air pollution and upper respiratory symptoms in children from East Germany. Eur Respir J 1995; 8:723–728.
16. von Mutuis E, Martinez FD, Fritzsch C, Nicolai T, Roell G, Thiemann HH. Prevalence of asthma and atopy in two areas of West and East Germany. Am Respir Crit Care Med 1994; 149(2 pt 1):358–364.
17. Bråbäck L, Breborowicz A, Julge K, Knutsson A, Riikjarv MA, Vasar M, Bjorksten B. Risk factors for respiratory symptoms and atopic sensitization in the Baltic area. Arch Dis Child 1995; 72:487–493.
18. Riikjïv M, Julge K, Vasar M, Bråbäck L, Knutsson A, Björkstén B. The prevalence of atopic sensitization and respiratory symptoms among Estonian school children. Clin Exp Allergy 1995; 25:1198–1204.
19. Romagnani S. Human TH1 and TH2 subsets: doubt no more. Immunology Today 1991; 12:256–257.

20. Holt P. Environmental factors and primary T-cell sensitization to inhalant allergens in infancy: reappraisal of the role of infections and air pollution. Pediatr Allergy Immunol 1995; 6:1–10.
21. McMenamin C, Holt PG. The natural immune response to inhaled soluble protein antigens involves major histocompatibility complex (MHC) class I-restricted CD8+ T cell-mediated but MHC class II-restricted CD4+ T cell-dependent immune deviation resulting in selective suppression of IgE production. J Exp Med 1993; 178(3):889–899.
22. Warner J, Miles E, Jones A, Warner J. Is deficiency of interferon gamma production by allergen triggered cord blood cells a predictor of atopic eczema? Clin Exper Allergy 1994; 24:423–430.
23. Tang MLK, Kemp AS, Thorburn J, Hill DJ. Reduced interferon-γ secretion in neonates and subsequent atopy. Lancet 1994; 344:983–985.
24. Rinas U, Horneff G, Wahn V. Interferon-gamma production by cord-blood mononuclear cells is reduced in newborns with a family history of atopic disease and is independent from cord blood IgE-levels. Pediatr Allergy Immunol 1993; 4:60–64.
25. Björkstén B, Borres M, Einarsson R. Interleukin-4, soluble CD23, and interferon-γ levels in serum during the first 18 months of life. Int Arch Allergy Immunol 1995; 107:34–36.
26. Kemeny DM, Urbanek R, Ewan P, HcHugh S, Richards D, Patel S, Lessof MH. The subclass of IgG antibody in allergic disease: II. The IgG subclass of antibodies produced following natural exposure to dust mite and grass pollen in atopic and non-atopic individuals. Clin Exp Allergy 1989; 19: 545–549.
27. Hattevig G, Kjellman B, Johansson SGO, Björkstén B. Clinical symptoms and IgE responses to common food proteins in atopic and healthy children. Clin Allergy 1984; 14:551–559.
28. Van Asperen P, Kemp A. The natural history of IgE sensitization and atopic disease in early childhood. Acta Padiatr Scand 1989; 78:239–245.
29. Madani G, Heiner DC. Antibody transmission from mother to fetus. Curr Opin Immunol 1989; 1:1157–1164.
30. Miller DL, Hirvonen T, Gitlin D. Synthesis of IgE by human conceptus. J Allergy Clin Immunol 1973; 52:182–188.
31. Kjellman N-IM. IgE determinations in neonates is not suitable for general screening. Ped Allergy Immunol 1994; 5:1–4.
32. Businco L, Marchetti F, Pellegrini G, Perlini R. Predictive value of cord blood IgE levels in "at-risk" newborn babies and influence of type of feeding. Clin Allergy 1983; 13:503–508.
33. Delespesse G, Sarfati M, Lang G, Sehon A. Prenatal and neonatal synthesis of IgE. Monogr Allergy 1983; 18:83–95.
34. Kimpen J, Callaert H, Embrechts P, Bosmans E. Influence of sex and gestational age on cord blood IgE. Acta Paediatr Scand 1989; 78:233–238.
35. Høst A, Halken S. A prospective study of cow milk allergy in Danish infants during the first 3 years of life. Allergy 1990; 45:587–596.

36. Høst A, Husby S, Gjesing B, Larsen J, Løwenstein H. Prospective estimation of IgG, IgG subclass and IgE antibodies to dietary proteins in infants with cow milk allergy. Allergy 1992; 47:218–229.

37. Levin S, Altman Y, Sela M. Penicillin and dinitrophenyl antibodies in newborn and mothers detected with chemically modified bacteriophage. Pediatr Res 1971; 5:87–88.

38. Weil G, Hussain R, Kumareaswami V, Tripathy S, Phillips K, Oliessen E. Prenatal allergic sensitization to heminth antigen in offspring of parasite-infected mothers. J Clin Invest 1983; 71:1124–1129.

39. Dahl GMK, Telemo E, Wesström BR, Jacobsson I, Lindberg T, Karlsson BW. The passage of orally fed protein from mother to foetus in the rat. Comp Biochem Physiol 1984; 74:199–201.

40. Husby S, Schultz Larsen F, Petersen PH. Genetic influence on the serum levels of naturally occurring human IgG antibodies to dietary antigens. Quantitative assessment from a twin study. J Immunogenet 1987; 14:131–142.

41. Fälth-Magnusson K, Kjellman N-IM. Allergy prevention by maternal elimination diet during late pregnancy—a 5-year follow-up of a randomized study. J Allergy Clin Immunol 1992; 89:709–713.

42. Zeiger R, Heller S, Mellon M, Helsey J, Hamburger R, Sampson H. Genetic and environmental factors affecting the development of atopy through age 4 in children of atopic parents: a prospective randomized study of food allergen avoidance. Pediatr Allergy Immunol 1992; 3:110–127.

43. Mellander L, Carlsson B, Hansson L-Å. Secretory IgA and IgM antibodies to *E. coli* and poliovirus type I antigens occur in amniotic fluid, meconium and saliva from newborns. A neonatal immune response without antigenic exposure: a result of anti-idiotype induction? Clin Exp Immunol 1986; 63: 555–561.

44. Piccinni MP, Mecacci F, Sampognaro S, Manetti R, Parronchi P, Maggi E, Romagnani S. Aeroallergen sensitization can occur during fetal life. Int Arch Allergy Immunol 1993; 102:301–330.

45. Bramwell F. The transmission of antibodies. In: Bramwell F, ed. The Transmission of Immunity from the Mother to the Young. Amsterdam: North-Holland, 1970: 242–250.

46. Lilja G, Dannaeus A, Fälth-Magnusson K, Graff-Lonnevig V, Johansson SG, Kjellman NI, Oman H. Immune response of the atopic woman and foetus: effects of high- and low-dose food allergen intake during late pregnancy. Clin Allergy 1988; 18:113–142.

47. Fälth-Magnusson K, Öman H, Kjellman N-IM. Maternal abstention from cow milk and egg in allergy risk pregnancies. Effect on antibody production in the mother and the newborn. Allergy 1987; 42:64–73.

48. Dannaeus A, Johansson S, Foucard T. Clinical and immunological aspects of food allergy in childhood. II. Development of allergic symptoms and humoral immune responses to foods in infants of atopic mothers during the first 24 months of life. Acta Paediatr Scand 1978; 67:497–504.

49. Casimir G, Gossart B, Vis H, Duchateau J. Antibody against betalactoglobulin (IgG) and cow's milk allergy. J Allergy Climinal Immunol 1985; 75: 206.

50. Lilja G, Dannaeus A, Foucard T, Graff-Lonnevig V, Johansson S, Öman H. Effects of maternal diet during late pregnancy and lactation on the development of atopic diseases in infants up to eighteen months of age—in vivo results. Clin Exp Allergy 1989; 19:473–479.

51. Vassella C, Odelram H, Kjellman N-I, Borres M, Vanto T, Björkstén B. High anti-IgE levels at birth are associated with a reduced allergy incidence in early childhood. Clin Exp Allergy 1994; 24:771–777.

52. Cookson W, Young R, Sandford AJ, Moffatt MF, Shirakawa T, Sharp PA, Faux JA, Julier C, Nakumuura Y. Maternal inheritance of atopic IgE resonsiveness on chromosome 11q. Lancet 1992; 340:381–384.

53. Halken S, Høst A, Nilsson L, Taudorf E. Passive smoking as a risk factor for development of obstructive respiratory disease and allergic sensitization. Allergy 1995; 50:97–105.

54. Björkstén B, Finnström O, Wichman K. Intrauterine exposure to the beta-adrenergic receptor-blocking agent metoprolol and allergy. Int Arch Allergy Appl Immunol 1988; 87:59–62.

55. Nelson H. Pregnancy and allergic diseases. In: Bierman C, Pearlman D, eds. Allergic Diseases of Infancy, Childhood and Adolescence. Philadelphia: Saunders, 1980: 675–680.

56. Björkstén B, Kjellman N-I. Perinatal environmental factors influencing the development of allergy. Clin Exp Allergy 1990; 20(suppl 3):3–8.

57. Rylander E, Pershagen G, Eriksson M, Nordvall L. Parental smoking and other risk factors for wheezing bronchitis in children. Eur Epidemiol 1993; 9:517–526.

58. Björkstén B. Does breast feeding prevent the development of allergy? Immunol Today 1983; 4:215–217.

59. Fergusson D, Horwood L, Shannon F. Early solid feeding and recurrent childhood eczema, a 10-year longitudinal study. Pediatrics 1990; 86: 541–546.

60. Kajosaari M, Saarinen UM. Prophylaxis of atopic disease by six months total solid food elimination. Acta Paediatr Scand 1983; 72:411–414.

61. Saarinen U. Breastfeeding as prophylaxis against atopic disease: prospective follow-up study until 17 years old. Lancet 1995; 346:1065–1069.

62. Duchén K, Björkstén B. Sensitization via the breast milk. In: Mestecky J, ed. Immunology of Milk and the Neonate. New York: Plenum Press, 1991: 427–436.

63. Goldman A. Immunologic system in human milk. Pediatr Gastroenterol Nut 1986; 5:343–345.

64. Machtinger S, Moss R. Cow's milk allergy in breast-fed infants: the role of allergen and maternal secretory IgA antibody. J Allergy Clin Immunol 1986; 77:341–347.

65. Robinson G. Identification of a secretory IgA receptor on breast-milk macrophages: evidence for specific activation via these receptors. Pediat Res 1991; 29:429–434.

66. Prentice A. Breast feeding increases concentrations of IgA in infatns' urine. Arch Dis Child 1987; 62:792–795.

67. Pittard W, Bill K. Immunoregulation by breast milk cells. Cell Immunol 1979; 42:437–441.

68. Schlesinger J. Evidence for transmission of lymphocyte responses to tuberculin by breast-feeding. Lancet 1977; 1:529–532.

69. Delespesse G. Presence of IgE suppressive factors in human colostrum. Eur J Immunol 1986; 16:1005–1008.

70. Chiba, Minagawa T, Mito K, Nakane A, Suga K, Honjo T, Nakao T. Effect of breast feeding on responses of systemic inferferon and virus-specific lymphocyte transformation in infants with respiratory syncytial virus infection. J Med Virol 1987; 21:7–14.

71. Björkstén F, Suoniemi I, Koski V. Neonatal birch-pollen contact and subsequent allergy to birch pollen. Clin Allergy 1980; 10:585–591.

72. Björkstén F, Suoniemi I. Time and intensity of first pollen contacts and risk of subsequent pollen allergies. Acta Med Scand 1981; 209:229–303.

73. Settipane R, Hagy G. Effect of atmospheric pollen on the newborn. Rhode Island Med J 1979; 62:477–482.

74. Croner S, Kjellman N-IM. Predictors of atopic disease: cord blood IgE and month of birth. Allergy 1986; 41:68–70.

75. Rowntree S, Cogswell J. Platts-Mills T, Mitchell E. Development of IgE and IgG antibodies to food and inhalant allergens in children at risk of allergic disease. Arch Dis Child 1985; 60: 727–735.

76. Sporik R, Holgate S, Platts-Mklls T, Cogswell J. Exposure to house-dust mite allergen (*Der p I*) and the development of asthma in childhood. N Engl J Med 1990; 323:502–507.

77. Suoniemi I, Björkstén F, Haahtela T. Dependence of immediate hypersentivity in the adolescent period on factors encountered in infancy. Allergy 1981; 36:263–268.

78. Holt P, McMenamin C, Nelson D. Primary sensitization to inhalant allergens during infancy. Pediatr Allergy Immunol 1990; 1:3–13.

79. Andrae S, Axelson O, Björkstén B, Fredriksson M, Kjellman N-IM. Symptoms of bronchial hyperractivity and asthma in relation to environmental factors. Arch Dis Child 1988; 63:473–478.

80. Zetterström O, Osterman K, Machado L, Johansson S. Another smoking hazard: raised serum IgE concentration and increased risk of occupational allergy. Br Med J 1981; 282:1215–1217.

81. Zetterström O, Nordvall SL, Björkstén B, Ahlstedt S, Stelander M. Increased IgE antibody responses in rats exposed to tobacco smoke. J Allergy Clin Immunol 1985; 75:594–598.

82. Munir A, Björkstén B. Indoor air pollution and allergic sensitization. In: Knöppel H, Wolkoff P, ed. Chemical Microbiological Health and Comfort. Brussels: ECSC, EEC, 1992: 181–199.
83. Wickman M. Residential characteristics and allergic sensitization in children especially to mites [Medical Dissertation]. Stockholm, 1993.
84. Wickman M, Nordvall SL, Pershagen G. Risk factors in early childhood for sensitization to airborne allergens. Pediatr Allergy Immunol 1992; 3: 128–133.
85. Munir AKM, Björkstén B, Einarsson R, Ekstrand-Tobin A, Moller C, Warner A, Kjellman NI. Mite allergens in relation to home conditions of asthmatic children from three climatic regions. Allergy 1995; 50:55–64.
86. Frick OL, Brooks DL. Immunoglobulin E antibodies to pollens augmented in dogs by virus vaccines. Am J Vet Res 1983; 44:440–445.
87. Sigurs N, Bjarnason R, Sigurbergsson F, Kjellman B, Björkstén B. Asthma and IgE antibodies after respiratory syncytial virus bronchiolitis: a prospective cohort study with matched controls. Pediatrics 1995; 95:500–505.
88. Pauwels R, van der Straeten M, Platteu B, Bazin H. The non-specific en hancement of allergy. In vitro effects of *Bordetella pertussis* vaccine on IgE synthesis. Allergy 1983; 38:239–246.
89. Sen D, Arora S, Gupta S, Sanyal R. Studies of adrenergic mechanisms in relation to histamine sensitivity in children immunized with Bordetella pertussis vaccine. J Allergy Clin Immunol 1974; 54:25–31.
90. Hedenskog S, Björkstén B, Blennow M, Granström G, Granström M. Immunoglobulin E response to pertussis toxin in whooping cough and after immunization with a whole-cell and an acellular pertussis vaccine. Int Arch Allergy Appl Immunol 1989; 89:156–161.
91. Blennow M, Granstöm M, Björkstén B. Immunoglobulin E response to pertussis toxin after vaccination with accellular pertussis vaccine. In: Manclark CR, ed. Proceedings of the Sixth International Symposium on Pertussis. Bethesda, MD: Department of Health and Human Services, U.S. Public Health Service, 1990:184–188.
92. Björkstén B, Turner K. Regulation of IgE antibody formation in the airways. In: Mygind N, Pipkorn U, Dahl R, ed. Rhinitis and Asthma. Copenhagen: Munksgaard, 1990:100–122.
93. Strannegård I-L, Strannegård Ö. Epstein-Barr virus antibody in children with atopic disease. Int Arch Allergy Appl Immunol 1981; 64:314–319.
94. Strachan D. Hay fever, hygiene and household size. Br Med J 1989; 289: 1259–1260.
95. Strachan D. Epidemiology of hay fever: towards a community diagnosis. Clin Exp Allergy 1995; 25:296–303.
96. Wichman H. Environment, life-style and allergy: the German answer. Allergy J 1995; 4:315–316.
97. Husband A, King M, Brown R. Behaviorly conditioned modification of T cell subset ratios in rats. Immunol Lett 1987; 14:91–94.

98. King M, Husband A, Kusnecov. Behavioral conditioning of the immune system: from laboratory to clinical application. In: Sheppard J, ed. Advances in Behavioral Medicine. Vol. 4, Sydney: Cumberland College of Health Sciences, 1987:110–117.
99. Jemmott JI, Borysenko J, Borysenko M, McClelland DC, Chapman R, Meyer D, Benson H. Academic stress, power motivation, and decrease in secretion rate of salivary secretory immunoglobulin A. Lancet 1983; 1:1400–1402.
100. Anonymous. Depression, stress and immunity. Lancet 1987; 1:1467–1488.
101. Gustafsson PA, Kjellman N-IM, Cederblad M. Family therapy in the treatment of severe childhood asthma. J Psychosomat Res 1986; 30:369–374.
102. Gustafsson PA, Kjellman N-IM, Ludvigsson J, Cederblad M. Asthma and family interaction. Arch Dis Child 1987; 62:258–263.
103. Gustafsson PA, Björkstén B, Kjellman N-IM. Family dysfunction in asthma—A prospective study of illness development. J Pediat 1994; 125: 493–498.

29

The Natural History of Allergic Disease and Asthma in Childhood

STEVEN W. RUBINSTEIN

Lucille Packard Children's Hospital at Stanford
Stanford, California

I. Introduction

The duration of any illness of condition is paramount to both the physician and the patient. Knowledge of any precautionary measures that can be taken to ameliorate the severity or shorten the duration of the condition is instrumental in patient care. Longitudinal data can enable physicians, regardless of specialty, to responsibly counsel individuals and parents of those with allergic and asthmatic conditions. This counseling can outline reasonable expectations for the duration of the condition, as well as any interventions that can be taken to minimize its severity. Numerous long-term studies have been undertaken, both retrospectively and prospectively, to evaluate the duration of atopic conditions, particularly asthma, and the risk factors for their persistence.

Unfortunately, most studies assessing the natural history of allergic disease are wrought with inherent methodological difficulties. Comparing these studies is even more arduous. Nevertheless, analysis of these studies reveals surprisingly consistent findings. This chapter should help the practitioner more confidently and honestly convey predictions of disease outcome to their patients.

                                    Rubinstein

This review assesses both the outcomes and the risk factors determining these outcomes for the most common allergic conditions of childhood. Some epidemiological factors, such as the prevalence or incidence of these conditions, are discussed only in terms of early childhood. Other epidemiological patterns, particularly in later childhood and adulthood, are beyond the scope of this chapter and are reviewed elsewhere (1).

II. The Natural History of Atopy and Asthma in Early Childhood

The presence of atopic conditions in infancy and early childhood is influenced by numerous factors. The most significant of these is a familial tendency toward atopy (3–6). There is increasing evidence, however, that environmental exposures in infancy may affect an individual's symptomatic expression of atopy, not only through childhood, but well into adulthood (7–9). Similarly, infectious episodes of the lower respiratory tract in infancy may result in life-long bronchial hyperreactivity (2,5,10,11).

Two general types of studies have evaluated the epidemiology of atopy: longitudinal studies of atopic subjects or those at higher risk for atopy (i.e., infants of atopic parents), and general population cohort studies in which all subjects are evaluated for the presence and persistence of atopic conditions. Many of these studies are reviewed later in this chapter when the specific atopic condition is discussed.

Prospective studies by Van Asperen and Kemp (12) in Australia, Cogswell et al. (13) in Great Britain, and Zeiger et al. (14–16) and the Tuscon Children's Respiratory Study (17,18) in the United States delineate the early natural history of atopy and skin-test reactivity from infancy through early childhood. Their findings are consistent with similar earlier studies (19). Van Asperen and Kemp prospectively studied 79 infants with a family history of atopy every 4 months from birth to 20 months, and again at age 5 (12). Each infant was evaluated clinically and by skin testing to milk, egg, wheat, and dust mite. Cogswell and his group followed 73 children who had at least one atopic parent prospectively from birth to age 5 (13). Each study patient had a physical examination with skin testing every 3 months from birth through 12 months, and then yearly through age 5. Skin testing was performed for reactions to egg, milk, rye grass, dust mite, dog, and cat. Zeiger et al. have prospectively followed 288 children of atopic parents (~50% bilaterally atopic) from birth with evaluations at 4, 12, 24 months (14), again at 36 and 48 months (15), and most recently at 7 years (16). Evaluations included physical examinations, skin testing, food challenges, nasal cytologies, and IgE determinations. The Tuscon Children's

Respiratory Study prospectively evaluated children from infancy through age 6 with IgE determination, pulmonary function studies (including selected subjects during infancy), and skin testing (17). The results of these studies are discussed later.

A. Atopic Dermatitis

The cumulative prevalence of atopic dermatitis (AD) in the first 12 months of life in these prospective studies ranged from a low of 11% (14) to a high approaching almost 50% (12) in Van Asperen's study of children with one or two atopic parents. Most cases start by 4–8 months of age, with few new cases developing after 1–2 years. Van Asperen found that the cumulative prevalence of AD by age 5 increased only to 58% in the high-risk groups (12). Most children improve significantly or remit by age 5. In fact, Cogswell et al. found that 90% had symptomatically resolved by 1 year of age (13). Zeiger at al. noticed only a 6% period and 20% cumulative prevalence at 4 years of age (15).

The presence of adverse reactions to foods, as well as possible skin tests to foods, is much higher in infants with AD than with other atopic conditions. Cogswell et al. found that 58% of subjects under age 2 with AD had skin-test positivity (13); 86% of those with positive tests reacted to foods. Zeiger et al. noted that 67% of infants with atopic dermatitis evidence positive food skin tests (14). Those with AD had statistically higher serum IgE levels, and egg was the only antigen statistically correlated with the presence of AD (13). Those who had skin-test positivity were significantly more likely to have persistence of their skin symptoms through age 5 and to have other associated atopic conditions. By age 5, however, the nature of the skin test reactivity in those with persistent AD appears to change. As the frequency of positive reactions to foods declines, positive reactivity to inhalants increases.

B. Rhinitis

Few studies have investigated the incidence of persistent, noninfectious rhinitis in the first several years of life. About 50% of children of atopic children of atopic parent(s) in Van Asperen's study had prolonged (over 4 weeks) continuous rhinitis by 1 year of age. Two-thirds developed rhinitis by age 5 (12). Most children with rhinitis had episodic symptoms, although about 14% were observed to have continuous symptoms from infancy through age 5. This rhinitis started by 4 months of age in most children. In contrast, Zeiger et al., employing symptoms, nasal eosinophilia, and positive skin tests to diagnose allergic rhinitis, could not identify allergic rhinitis in any of their 4-month-old infants, but found that the frequency of allergic rhinitis increases steadily from a cumulative prevalence of 4% at 1 year to 28% by 4 years to 40% at age 7 (14–16). At each time interval, the period and cumulative prevalences for allergic rhinitis were similar, indicating that by 4 years of age allergic rhinitis tends to persist, rather than improve/remit as in the case of atopic dermatitis (14,15). Zeiger also found that those with a history of food allergy before age 4 were nearly twice as likely to have rhinitis at age 7 (16).

Healthy newborns followed in a health maintenance organization in Tuscon, Arizona, were studied prospectively by questionnaire from birth through age 6 (18). A diagnosis of allergic rhinitis was made by physician diagnosis with or without positive skin-prick tests at ages 1, 2, 3, and 6. One-half of those with allergic rhinitis at age 6 had the onset of persistent rhinitis symptoms before the age of 1. In addition, significantly more infants with the onset of persistent rhinitis in the first year of life had allergic rhinitis at age 6 versus those with onset after the first year of life. Interestingly, these children were also more likely to have persistent cough and/or asthma at age 6, but were not more likely to have positive skin tests. Those with rhinitis at age 6 had higher IgE levels at both 9 months and 6 years of age. At age 3, 79% of those with allergic rhinitis had already developed a seasonal pattern to their symptoms (primarily in the fall) (18).

C. Wheezing, Asthma

Children experiencing a single episode of wheezing (unrelated to bronchiolitis) in the first few years of life appear to be at no higher risk of developing asthma than a child never having a wheezing episode (12,13,17,20). Children of atopic parents, however, are about twice as likely to wheeze by age 5, with about one-half of children of atopic parents experiencing at least one episode of wheezing by that age. Approximately 20% of these children will wheeze at least once by 12 months of age. Two or more episodes of wheezing occur by 4 years in about 25% of children of atopic parents (15).

Cohort studies of general population groups have shown variable results in the percentage of children who experience one or more episodes of wheezing. In Britain and Australia, these studies show that about 20% of children by age 7, and 25% by age 16, will have at least one episode of wheezing (4,5). In the Tuscon study, where reporting was more closely monitored, 49.5% had at least one wheezing episode by age 6 (17). Sixty percent that had wheezed before age 3 had stopped for at least 1 year by age 6. At age 6, 28.7% of all children had experienced a wheezing episode in the prior year. This contrasts notably with Anderson's findings of more persistent asthma symptoms in only 8% of 8806 British children in the year prior to age 7 (21).

Ultimately, by the mid-teen years, there is a cumulative prevalence of recurrent wheezing of 10–15% (5,8). Anderson found the prevalence of asthma symptoms in the prior year to be 5% at age 11 and 3% at age 16 (21). In contrast, in those with a parental atopic history, asthma occurs in approximately one in three children by age 5 (12,13). Similarly, Zeiger found a significant increase in the period prevalence of asthma from age 4 (~20%) to age 7 (~30%) in genetically predisposed children (16).

About one-half of those with recurrent wheezing at age 5 started wheezing before 1 year of age (12). Recurrent wheezing was rarely found, however, before 4 months of age (19). In those with multiple atopic conditions, asthma generally follows the appearance of atopic dermatitis, persistent rhinitis, and possibly food allergy. The Tuscon Respiratory study found that children with late-onset wheezing (present at age 6, but not at age 3) were more likely to have persistent rhinitis in the first year of life (17). High-risk children who develop recurrent wheezing in childhood concurrently experience other atopic conditions, including an increased likelihood of having positive skin tests (13). Cogswell et al. found 89% of asthmatics at age 5 had at least one positive skin test to a battery of six antigens (13).

Those children younger than 2 years of age with atopic parent(s) are more likely to develop recurrent wheezing (asthma) should they have positive skin tests, elevated serum IgE levels, and/or nasal eosinophilia (9,13,15). Similarly, those with earlier symptoms of recurrent wheezing are significantly more likely to have positive skin tests (at any age) (8,9,13). Persistence of wheezing in early childhood is also related to the degree of bronchial hyperreactivity (20). Bronchial hyperreactivity is further discussed in the next section of this chapter, as are other risk factors for the development of asthma (see Table 1).

If airway obstruction is present in the mid-childhood years (age 5–9), it is likely to persist into later childhood and early adulthood (22). Once asthma and/or bronchial hyperreactivity is present in later childhood, the risk for its persistence into adulthood is high (23,24). Further work by Burrows and others, in a prospective evaluation of general population groups, confirmed that atopically predisposed individuals (as measured by serum IgE and skintesting) are much more likely to manifest asthma in childhood and adulthood (25–27). In addition, only persons with elevated serum IgE had or went on to develop asthma (25,26). These studies, as well as numerous studies cited later, suggest that environmental factors play a crucial role in allowing the atopic gene(s) to be expressed.

Table 1 Risk Factors for Presence of Asthma in Childhood

Definite[a]
    Family history of atopy/asthma
    Early lung disease/bronchiolitis
    Elevated IgE
    Positive skin tests/RAST
    Maternal smoking
    Concurrent allegic rhinitis, especially if onset <1 year of age
    Concurrent atopic dermatitis, especially if early onset
    Male sex
    House dust/dust mite allergy
    High dust mite levels in home (with positive family history of atopy)
Probable[b]
    Black race
    House dampness
    Immediate food reactivity/early food reactivity
    Presence of furred animal in home (with positive family history)
    Blood eosinophilia (adult > children)
    Maternal smoking while pregnant
    Low birth weight
Possible[c]
    Air pollution
    Nasal eosinophilia in early childhood
    Skin-test reactivity to milk, egg, peanut under 1 year of age
    Not breast-fed as an infant
    Season of birth
    Paternal smoking
    Cockroach allergy (with positive family history)
    Hispanic ethnicity
    Childhood obesity
    Young maternal age (<20)
    Day care attendance
    Central-city residence
    Low family income
    Presence of wood/charcoal burning stove in home
    Cord IgE levels
Unlikely[d]
    History of urticaria
    Delayed food reactions
    Lower respiratory infections after infancy
No association
    IgA, IgG levels
    Presence of gas stove in home
    Proportion of protein/fish in diet

---

[a]Multiple studies show strong statistical significance.
[b]Multiple studies show statistical significance; occasional studies do not.
[c]Some studies show statistical significance and a similar number do not, or a single study showed statistical significance and not evaluated in other studies.
[d]Most studies do not show statistical significance.

D. Skin Test Reactivity and Radioallergosorbent Testing

Infants and children with elevated serum IgE levels and positive skin tests or positive radioallergosorbent tests (RASTs) in early childhood are more likely to have positive skin tests and clinical atopy when prospectively studied into later childhood and adulthood (8,16,28). This positivity, however, does not necessarily predict persistent clinical symptomatology (discussed later).

Positive skin tests to inhalants in infancy tend to persist and are significantly associated with the early onset of respiratory symptoms (9,12,14). Positive skin tests to inhalants develop later than to foods (Fig. 1) (12–14). Those to foods tend to develop in infancy and are associated with the presence of atopic dermatitis (12–14) and food allergy (14), but not generally with recurrent wheezing. These positive tests to foods often remit (see Chapter 32), whereas inhalant sensitivity tends to persist in childhood (12–14) and often into adulthood (29).

The number of infants with positive skin tests or RAST tests under 1 year of age varies greatly among studies. Soothill et al. found a 48% prevalence of specific IgE reactivity in infants of atopic parent(s) (30), whereas Rowntree et al. showed that less than 10% had specific reactivity (19). The likelihood of skin test or RAST positivity is statistically higher

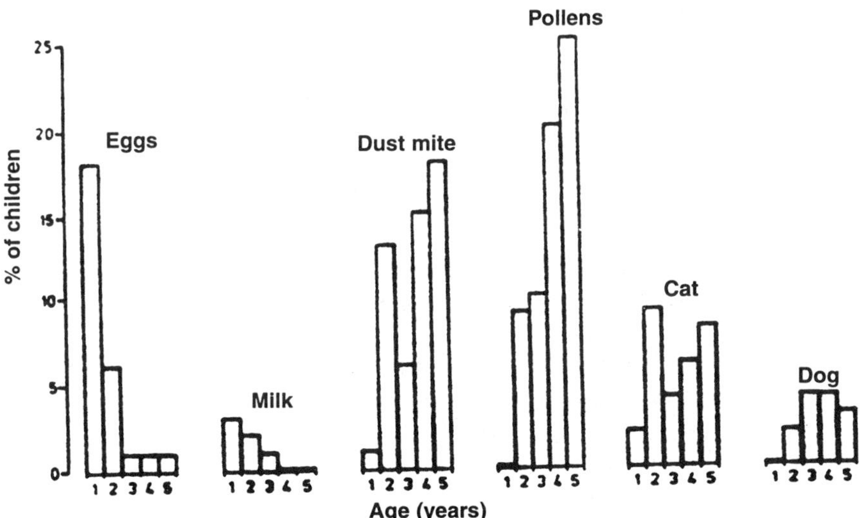

Figure 1 Percentage of children with positive results to skin tests for the six common allergens. (From Ref. 13.)

under age 1 (versus nonatopic controls) in children with atopic dermatitis, recurrent wheezing, and immediate food reactions (12,14,31). In infancy there is no correlation between positive skin tests and persistent rhinitis, a single episode of wheezing, gastrointestinal symptoms, or delayed food reactions. In older children, skin-test positivity occurs primarily to inhalants and is significantly associated with asthma and allergic rhinitis, but not other atopic conditions (5).

Infants and young children who have specific IgE reactivity to foods only, and not to inhalant allergens, are statistically more likely to develop atopic dermatitis by age 5 (12,13,15). In addition, their symptoms are more likely to persist. Those who react to inhalants with or without food reactivity are significantly more likely to develop ongoing or recurrent respiratory symptoms by age 5. They are also much less likely to lose their skin-test reactivity by this age; in fact, skin-test positivity to inhalants tends to persist for years, often into adulthood (8, 29).

In terms of reactivity to specific allergens, prospective studies of infants of atopic parent(s) have noted about a 15% cumulative prevalence of positive skin tests to egg at 1 year of age (12,14). Conversely, between 2% and 5% reacted to dust mites (12–14). Reactivity to animal proteins and pollens has been reported at this age, but is quite rare (32).

By age 4–5, between 50% and 70% of infants who had been skin-test-positive to foods become negative (12,13,15). Zeiger found that those skin-test-positive to foods at age 4, however, tend to have persistent positivity through age 7 (16). At age 7, skin test reactivity to peanut was higher than to other foods; reactivity to milk and egg at this age was quite rare.

Specific reactivity to dust mites increases dramatically by age 2 and continues to rise through at least age 5 (see Fig. 1). Between 15% and 20% of children with atopic parent(s) are skin-test-positive to dust mite by age 4 (13,15). This approaches 30% by age 7 (16). Animal reactivity, as manifested by positive skin tests to dog or cat, reaches a cumulative prevalence of 10% by age 4 in infants of atopic parents (15). Pollen reactivity begins later, generally by age 3, probably owing to the more intermittent exposure to pollen than to other aeroallergens. By age 5, however, 25% of Cogswell's subjects reacted to grass, more than any other antigen tested (13). Wright et al. also found grass to be the most commonly positive skin test in 6-year-olds with allergic rhinitis followed prospectively from birth in Arizona (18). In the prospective study by Zeiger et al. (15), 4-year cumulative prevalences for skin-test reactivity to grass was 12% and to mold (*Alternaria* or *Cladosporium*) was 21%. Skin reactivity to dust mite, grass, and other aeroallergens increased to a statistically significant degree between ages 4 and 7 in these genetically predisposed atopic children (16).

As childhood progresses into adulthood, the number of positive skin tests increases in individuals with atopic respiratory conditions, with some studies showing up to 88% skin reactivity to at least one inhalant (8,28). In older children and younger adults with clinically apparent allergic conditions and negative skin tests, skin-test reactivity nearly always develops over the next few years if the condition persists (28). Conversely, in adults with positive skin reactivity to both pollens and dust mite, but no clinical manifestations of allergy/asthma, symptoms are likely to develop over time in a significant number (33,34).

As in younger children, skin-test reactivity to inhalants in older children, once present, tends to persist (29). At 8 years follow-up, Gerritsen found 94% of children initially studied at age 9 to have persistence of skin reactivity to grass pollen, with 74% persistence of animal dander reactivity (8). All patients maintained reactivity to house dust mite at follow-up, as was also found in a study by Sporik et al. (9).

III. Risk Factors for the Development of Allergic Disease/Asthma

The primary risk factors for the development of atopy in childhood are detailed in Chapters 27 and 28. The risk factors for the persistence of asthma, once present, are discussed at length later in this chapter. A discussion of the risk factors for the development of bronchial hyperreactivity and/or asthma follows below, and a summation of the risk factors for the development of asthma itself are shown in Table 1. The risk factors most related to the *development* of an atopic condition, as opposed to its ongoing *persistence* over time, are the presence of an elevated IgE level, positive skin tests, or both. Although these are definite risk factors for the presence of asthma and other atopic conditions, they cannot predict the likelihood of their persistence in an individual patient.

A. Bronchial Hyperreactivity

A genetic predisposition toward allergy and excessive airway hyperreactivity is the most important determinant for the development of asthma. This has been shown in numerous general population cohort studies (3,6), and is beyond the scope of this chapter. Prospective studies of newborn infants have also shown that an inherent reduction of pulmonary function predisposes to subsequent lower respiratory infections with wheezing. Martinez et al. studied pulmonary function (respiratory conductance measured by force oscillometry) in newborn infants and found that those who developed wheezing with or without lower respiratory tract infections had significantly lower pulmonary function shortly after birth (35). Those infants who measured in the lowest third for certain pulmonary function parameters were 10–16 times more likely to have a wheezing illness. Those with recurrent wheezing episodes in the first year of life had a sixfold risk of a low respiratory conductance value (53).

This early wheezing and reduced pulmonary function do not necessarily lead to later asthma. In fact, it appears that a genetic predisposition to increased bronchial hyperreactivity beyond infancy, in conjunction with environmental influences, are much stronger contributors to the development of asthma. In a later study, Martinez found that those infants with reduced pulmonary function were at higher risk for transient wheezing episodes only, and at age 6 were no more likely to wheeze than those who had never wheezed (17). Conversely, those who had later onset and/or persistent wheezing between at age 6 had normal pulmonary function in infancy.

This observation that infantile bronchial hyperreactivity in itself may not be persistent unless certain environmental circumstances are present has been found in other studies. Van Asperen found that the presence of wheezing in infancy was in itself not a risk for the presence of bronchial hyperreactivity at age 7 (20). Only those with other atopic conditions or positive skin tests were at risk for later bronchial hyperreactivity. Zeiger recently confirmed such observations in 7-year-old children with asthma (16).

Infants have an inherent increase in bronchial reactivity as measured by bronchial responsiveness to methacholine and histamine when compared to older children and adults (36,37). Infants with a family history of asthma show increased histamine responsiveness as early as 1 month of age (37). This reactivity decreases linearly from about age 5 months through adulthood for a variety of proposed reasons (36,38,39). This decline is not seem, however, in atopic children (with or without a history of asthma) (40). Hence, the presence of atopy itself may predispose to prolonged airway hyperreactivity.

B. Inhalant Reactivity

Inhalant exposures, both allergic and nonallergic, in early childhood are definite risk factors for the development of asthma. Nonallergic inhalant exposures (i.e., tobacco smoke) are more likely to be risk factors in children with or without a genetic tendency toward atopy, whereas allergenic factors, particularly indoor allergens such as dust mite, generally play a role primarily in those with an allergic family history.

Skin-test positivity to house dust mites and high levels of exposure to these mites are definite risk factors for the development of asthma and allergic rhinitis in both children and adults (9,41–44). A negative atopic family history reduces, but does not eliminate, this risk.

Kuehr et al., in a study of a large general population cohort of children entering primary school, revealed that the prevalence of asthma in children was statistically higher in those skin-test-positive to not only mites, but to cats and dogs as well (44,45). Only sensitivity to mite, however, was associated with new onset asthma in these children between ages 7 and 10.

Van Asperen et al. found six children in his prospective study to be skin-test-positive to dust mites at 12 months of age (12). All of these children went on to develop asthma. In another study, every child (119 between ages 6 and 14) with asthma referred to a university allergy clinic in the Netherlands was skin-test positive to dust mite (8).

Sporik et al., in a follow-up of Cogswell's original study group, found that those wheezing in the prior year or actively taking asthma medications at age 11 were significantly more likely to be skin-test-positive to dust mites (9). Most of those taking regular bronchodilators were reactive to dust mites as early as age 2. Those who had wheezing before age 5, but had stopped wheezing by age 11, were significantly less likely to be mite-sensitive. The relative risk of having asthma at age 11 if one was skin-test-positive to mites approximated 20. Kuehr et al. likewise found that children not wheezing at age 7, but who had developed asthmatic symptoms by age 10, were much more likely to be mite-sensitive (45).

Similarly, Van Asperen et al. found that bronchial hyperreactivity (as measured by responsiveness to methacholine or histamine) was significantly higher in 5- and 7-year-olds who were skin-test-positive to dust mites and cats, but not to grass or selected foods (20).

Studies from France and China have correlated the degree of mite exposure with the presence of asthma and skin-test reactivity to mite (41,42). When mite-infested blankets were introduced into a "mite-free area" in New Guinea, the incidence of adult asthma increased from 0.15% to 7.3%. All of those who developed asthma were skin-test positive to mites. General population cohort studies have shown a significantly increased likelihood of wheezing children living in damp houses, an environment where mites (and molds) thrive (7,46).

Several studies have estimated the actual level of dust mite exposure needed to develop clinical sensitivity. Korsgaard (47) and Lau et al. (48) found that the critical level of exposure for the development of mite sensitization was above 2 μg of the major mite allergen (Der p 1) per gram of house dust (about 100 mites per gram). There was a statistically significant correlation between exposures above this level and RAST values to mite, as well as the presence of clinical symptomatology. Eight-six percent of those exposed to more than 10 μg/g showed positive histamine release from leukocytes, as opposed to 17% of those exposed to less than 0.4 μg/g (48).

Correlating the level of mite exposure in infancy (mite levels determined at 1–2 years of age in bedding and carpet) to the presence of asthma at age 11, Sporik et al. noted that all but 1 of 17 children with persistent wheezing at age 11 were exposed to levels of more than 10 μg/g of mite (9). In addition, there was a significant relation between the level of exposure at age 1 and the first episode of wheezing. No child exposed to less than 2 μg/g Der p 1 of dust had symptoms of asthma, and none was skin-test- or RAST-positive to mites at age 11.

Although not studied in such detail, early exposure to high levels of any inhalant antigen is likely to be a risk factor for the development of atopic respiratory conditions. This has been increasingly found in numerous studies of exposure to furry mammals, particularly cats, and to house dampness (molds and dust mites) in early childhood (7,12,44,46,49,50). Suoniemi et al. found that adolescents 15–17 years old were statistically more likely to have atopic illness if they had a cat (but not a dog) in the home in the first 6 months of life (50). The month of an individual's birth, implying increased pollen or other aeroallergen exposure, in conjunction with a familial tendency, also appears to be a risk factor for the development of allergic disease (51,52). Prospective likelihood similarly suggest that exposure to cats and cockroaches increases the likelihood of allergic rhinitis and asthma (53). All of the data signify the importance of early environmental intervention in those with allergic family histories in the ultimate prevention or minimization of allergic disease.

C. Food Allergens

The role of early exposure to food allergens in the development of respiratory allergic disease is unclear. Early retrospective studies (54,55) suggested a possible protective role of breast feeding and a possible contributory role of formula feeding to the development of respiratory allergy in infants with a strong family history of atopy. Recent prospective studies (12,15,16) have not shown such a correlation in later childhood, but there appears to be a correlation between early food hypersensitivity and allergy test positivity (especially to egg), and the later presence of allergic rhinitis and asthma (16). The role of food allergens in the development of atopy are discussed in detail in Chapter 32. The likelihood of food allergies persisting once present are discussed later in this chapter.

D. Irritants

In addition to the risk of early exposure to aeroallergens, early exposure to aerosolized irritants is a risk factor for the development of ongoing respiratory conditions. These irritants could (a) damage mucosal surfaces or lung tissue itself, or (b) facilitate penetration of foreign substances, predisposing an individual to allergic sensitization. Many studies have shown that children exposed to high levels of air pollution are more likely to have allergic rhinitis and asthma (7,56,57). Andrae et al. found an increased prevalence of both conditions in children living in close proximity to a pulp plant in Sweden (7). More specifically, high levels of early exposure to air pollutants (sulfur dioxide, ozone) has been shown to enhance allergic sensitization through respiratory mucosal tissue (58–60). On the other hand, the Harvard Six Cities Study, which correlated air-quality monitoring with childhood lower respiratory symptoms over a multiyear period, found no association between pollutant levels and the prevalence of childhood asthma (61). This study did not, however, follow children from birth.

E. Passive Smoke

Parental smoking is an obvious factor resulting in both upper and lower airway disease in children. Although some, mostly retrospective studies, show only a marginal relation between parental smoking and childhood wheezing or asthma (44,62–65), later well-controlled, prospective studies have undeniably shown a causative relation (16,17,57,66–69). This risk is higher when the mother smokes, indicating a probable dose-related risk of smoke, since children usually spend more time with their mothers than with their fathers (16,70–72). Weitzman et al., in studying data from the Child Health Supplement to the 1981 National Health Survey, found an odds ratio of 2.6 for the presence of asthma (recurrent wheezing episodes) in the first year of life if a mother smoked over one-half pack of cigarettes per day (73). The odds ratio was 2.1 for acquiring asthma by age 5 and 4.7 for the use of chronic asthma medications at age 5 if the mother smoked. Interestingly, Martinez found that maternal smoking was a risk factor for asthma only when mothers were less educated, indicating that increased recognition of the adverse effects of smoking could result in less exposure to the child (17).

This risk can appear as early as infancy. Young et al. found that as early as 1 month of age, infants of smoking mothers had an enhanced bronchial response to histamine (37). Early exposure to parental tobacco smoke may have more long-term adverse impact on lung function than later exposure. Frischer et al. showed increased bronchial hyperreactivity in 7-year-olds whose mothers smoked during the first year of life; there was no increased risk in this study if the mother smoked during pregnancy or she smoked currently (74).

Cogswell et al. found that the cumulative prevalence of wheezing by age 5 (independent of serum IgE levels) reached 62% with smoking parents versus 37% with nonsmoking parents (13). Neuspiel et al. further demonstrated that this statistical association persisted to at least age 10 in a prospective national cohort study in England (46). Britten et al., in a multidecade general population cohort study in Great Britain, suggested that this risk persists at least into the mid-30s age range (56).

Studies examining pulmonary function in children (independent of respiratory symptoms) have also shown a detrimental effect of parental smoking, which potentially may impinge on later respiratory function (65,66,69,70,76,77). Zeiger recently confirmed this by showing that increased home environmental tobacco smoke exposure, as reflected by urinary cotinine levels, were associated with a significantly reduced FEV1 and FEF25-75 in 7-year-old children (16). Interestingly, these children also showed significantly increased skin reactivity to aeroallergens.

Some studies have demonstrated that this increased risk of asthma from passive parental smoke may not be restricted to postnatal exposure. Collins et al. found that fetal rats showed lung hypoplasia with decreased number of alveoli when exposed to tobacco (78). Infants of smoking mothers with no personal or family history atopy have shown elevated levels of cord IgE and increased development of asthma and other atopic conditions (79). Martinez et al. found that maternal smoking while pregnant was statistically associated with bronchial hyperreactivity in 9-year-olds, while current smoking was not (80). Confirming studies are needed before these findings can be fully accepted.

F. Sex, Race

Male children are more likely to develop asthma. Black children (in the United States) appear to be at higher risk of becoming asthmatic than other race groups (16,81).

G. Prematurity, Birth Weight

Various types of studies have statistically correlated low birth weight to the development of asthma (44,81,82). Kuehr et al. found a higher incidence of skin-test reactivity and asthma in children entering school who had a history of low birth weight and low gestational age (44). Follow-up of low-birth-weight babies has revealed not only diminished lung function, but increased bronchial hyperreactivity as well (82,83).

H. Miscellaneous Risk Factors

Holberg et al. showed an increased risk of wheezing and lower respiratory infections in children up to 3 years of age attending day care with more than three children (84). This was found to be a risk factor independent of numerous other variables, including smoking exposure.

The Second National Health and Nutrition Examination Survey (NHANES II) evaluated 5672 children between the ages of 6 months and 11 years selected randomly in 64 U.S. locations between 1976 and 1980 (81). The risk of developing asthma and/or persistent wheezing was statistically correlated to a number of epidemiological factors. Increased risk factors for asthma development included black race, male sex, prematurity/low birth weight, lack of breast feeding, low family income, the presence of coal/wood stoves in the home, and several nutritional factors. The latter data included body mass index, tricep skinfold thickness, and total food energy intake, and suggested that heavier children were more likely to develop asthma. No association between persistent wheezing was found when correlated with other nutritional factors, including protein intake, calcium/vitamin C/zinc intake, fish in the diet, and transferrin saturation (81).

In this same study, young maternal age (under age 20) was found to be a significant risk factor for the development of asthma, even after controlling for other socioeconomical/racial variables (81). Central-city residence was also found to be a risk factor. This corroborates with the initial work of Gelber et al., in which increased antigen load by cockroach exposure resulted in higher rates of atopic disease in inner-city locations (53).

I. Multiple Risk Factors

Many of the risk factors listed in Table 1 are cumulative. Peat et al. found a sixfold risk of moderate or severe bronchial hyperreactivity if a subject had a history of respiratory infection in infancy, a parent with asthma, and positive skin tests (5). There was a twofold risk if the skin-test positivity occurred with either early respiratory infection or positive family history. Smoking also appears to by synergistic with other factors in increasing the risk for the development of asthma (62,85). The most notable of these appears to be concurrent atopy, particularly atopic dermatitis (86). Wright found that the early onset of rhinitis (prior to age 1), maternal smoking, and elevated IgE levels at age 6 were cumulative risk factors for the development of asthma by age 6 (but not for allergic rhinitis itself) (18).

IV. Asthma: Retrospective Studies

Numerous retrospective studies examined the outcome of childhood asthma over various time periods (1). Those studies published since 1960 with a minimum of 10-year follow-up are listed in Table 2 (87–93). These studies cannot be directly compared because of their differing definitions of asthma, its severity, and length of follow-up. Nevertheless, examinations of these studies generally reveal consistent patterns. Roughly one-half of those children with asthma had some degree of respiratory symptoms at follow-up, even after three decades. Approximately one-half of these patients had periodic, mild symptoms; the other half had more severe and persistent symptoms. Jonsson et al. studied a more severe population of asthmatics requiring hospitalization near the onset of their asthma (93). The results after 23–31 years of follow-up were similar, with 47% claiming to be symptom-free at follow-up. At 20-years follow-up, Buffum and Settipane found only a 5% persistence of severe symptoms in those presenting in childhood with "severe, debilitating" asthma (91). Hence, most of those patients with symptoms at follow-up did experience an overall improvement in their condition, as will be demonstrated again when the prospective studies are discussed.

Mosfeldt Laursen et al. recently found a much higher rate of symptomatic persistence in more severe asthmatics (those requiring at least one inpatient hospitalization) (94). Only 13% of those interviewed by telephone between ages 12 and 23 claimed to have no symptoms of asthma in the prior 2 years. In those who were asymptomatic, the median duration of symptoms before remission was 9 years.

Two of these retrospective studies have examined asthmatic children at both the 10- and 20-year intervals, with contradictory findings. Buffum found that the percentage of those with ongoing symptoms decreased from 57% at 10 years to 37% at 20 years (91). Blair looked at the same individuals at 10 years and again at 20 years after the onset of asthma and found more patients symptomatic at 20 years than at 10 years, indicating a marked number (27%) with recurrence of asthma after prolonged symptom-free intervals (92). The mean age of "remission" was 10 years, with the average age of recurrence of being 19. This finding of symptomatic recurrence has been demonstrated not only in the prospective studies of asthma, but also in long-term observations of most other atopic conditions.

Whether individuals "outgrow" their asthma symptomatically may be a separate issue than persistence of airway hyperreactivty. As some prospective studies have revealed, many patients with a history of asthma who have become symptom-free still maintain bronchial hyperreactivity.

Table 2 The Natural History of Asthma: Retrospective Studies

Author (Ref.)	No.	Age at onset (yr)	Follow-up (yr)	No symptoms at follow-up (%)	Ongoing symptoms at follow-up			(%) Total	Recur (%)
					Mild	Persistent	Severe		
Ryssing, Flensborg (87)	442	Under 15	NS	37	9	54		63	
Buffum (88)	51	NS	10–16	55				45	
Barr, Logan (89)	336	Under 14	17–27	50				48	
Whatley, Guerrant (90)	115	Under 16	15 (median)	53	25	21		46	
Buffum, Settipane (91)	518	"Child"	10	41			6	57	
	136	"Child"	20	55			5	37	
Blair (92)	244	Under 12	10	35	25	37		65	3
	244	Under 12	20	28	24	21		72	27
Jonsson et al. (93)	123	Under 15	22–32	55[a]	27	5	13	45	
Konlg (111)	175 (total)	6 (mean) Range 0.2–1.6	8.4	15[b]				85[b]	
	84 (mild)[c]			17[b]	69[b]	3[b]	11[b]	83[b]	
	57 (moderate)[c]			13[b]	36[b]	23[b]	28[b]	87[b]	
	34 (severe)[c]			11[b]	30[b]	5[b]	54[b]	89[b]	
Mosfeldt Laurence (94)	224	Under 5	4–20	13				87	

NS, not stated.

[a]These patients had been symptom-free for a mean of 17 years.

[b]Condition at onset of study. Mild group received only pro beta-agonists, moderate group inhaled cromolyn sodium, and severe group inhaled corticosteriods.

[c]All of these figures are approximations from graphs presented in reference. Overall, there was clinical improvement in 17% of the initially mild group, 49% of the moderate group, and 47% of the severe group.

Jonsson later studies asthmatics who had become symptom-free with pulmonary function studies and found 23% to have significant abnormalities (29). These individuals would certainly be more prone to symptomatic relapse over time.

V. Asthma: Prospective Studies

The prospective studies examining the long-term course of asthma have shorter follow-up periods than do the retrospective ones (Table 3) (4,8,95–101). On initial inspection, the results of the prospective studies appear to vary greatly. Once again, however, the populations studies, methods of evaluation, and definitions of asthma vary markedly among studies. Some studies followed selected symptomatic patients (31,100), others followed randomized cohorts (96,97,101), and others followed entire population cohorts (4,98). Although the percentage of asthmatics with symptoms at follow-up appears to vary greatly, there is general consistency between the type of study performed and the frequency of symptomatic persistence. The general population cohort studies usually include any individual with a personal or parental reporting of wheezing at any one time. Overreporting is likely common in younger age groups, when infectious upper bronchitis or even upper respiratory infections are mistaken as asthmatic episodes. In these studies, children at follow-up would be less likely to have symptoms than in those studies including only asthmatic children. In these general population studies, roughly one-fourth to one-third of individuals are symptomatic at follow-up evaluation.

Johnstone's study, in which all patients were asthmatics followed by an allergy specialist, found the highest percentage of symptomatic persistence at follow-up (78%) (100). Sixty-three asthmatic children under age 16 were followed up at 4 to 14 years. This preselection bias for increased disease severity as well as the shorter length of follow-up probably explains the higher percentage of patients with persistence compared with other studies.

Foucard and Sjoberg, on the other hand, studied a much younger population (mean age of onset 10 months) 12 years after presentation with wheezy bronchitis (31). Because of the young age, many of these patients were presenting for the first time when studied and likely had an infectious cause for their initial respiratory symptoms. The low percentage of persistent wheezing at follow-up probably reflects the likelihood that many of these individuals may not have had associated atopy and that their presentations may have been isolated infections.

Table 3 The Natural History of Asthma: Prospective Studies

Author (Ref.)	No.	Age first studied (yr)	Age at follow-up (yr)	Follow-up (yr)	No symptoms at follow-up (%)	Ongoing symptoms at follow-up (%)	Wheeze (%) at follow-up			Symptoms recur (%)
							Rare	Occa-sional	Fre-quent	
Gerritsen et al. (8)	119	6–14	22–31	14–20	57	43		75	25	
Friberg et al. (95)	20	10.6 (median)	24.9 (median)	14	0	100				
Anderson et al. (4)	1608									
Severe symptoms		7[a]	11	4	36	64 (17% severe)				
At age 7		7	16	9	64	36 (4% severe)				
All patients	7	11	4	72	28					
	7	16	9	84	16					
Strachan et al. (98)[b]	1608	7[a]	23	11	34	66				
Martin et al. (96)	331	7[a]	14; 21	7; 14	29	71	21	27	23	45[d]
Kelly et al. (97)[c]	293	7[a]	28	21	32	68[e]	20	22	26	27[f]
Foucarfd and Sjoborg (31)	81	10 mo (median)	12–17	12	72	28[a]				
Giles et al. (99)	218	7	13; 20	6; 13	78	22				
Johnstone (100)	63	NS	16	4–14	22	78	8	51	19	
Sherrill et al. (101)	696	7	15	8	64	36				

NS, not stated

[a]These patients has a history of wheezing at or before age 7.
[b]Continued study of Anderson's population.
[c]Continued study of Martin's population.
[d]Symptoms recurred between ages 14 and 21.
[e]Of these, 24% improved, 26% worsened, 50% did not change their condition between ages 21 and 28.
[f]Symptoms recurred between ages 21 and 28.
[g]All but one patient with ongoing symptoms improved clinically.

Two studies in the South Pacific have prospectively followed birth cohorts of children born in a single year, initially by health questionnaires, and later by interview and pulmonary function studies. Giles et al. followed all children born in Tasmania in 1961 (99), and Sherrill et al. followed all children born in a single hospital in New Zealand in 1972–1973 (101). In both studies, questionnaire surveys directed toward respiratory symptoms of wheezing and cough were sent to all families at regular intervals, starting at age 7 in Giles' study and at age 3 in Sherrill's study. Any child with a history of any wheezing episode was asked to be included in these surveys. Hence, numerous patients with single episodes of vague symptomatology and etiology were likely to be included. These subjects would be expected to be less likely to wheeze at follow-up, and this probably explains the low number of patients with persistent symptoms at age 15 in Sherrill's study (36%), and at age 20 in Giles' study (22%).

Anderson and Strachan similarly followed a much larger and randomized cohort of 10,557 individuals born in a single week in Britain in 1958 (4,98). Families were sent questionnaires asking if their child "ever had attacks of breathing with wheezing." Follow-up at ages 11, 16, and 23 was performed by questionnaire or interview, with numerous other health and social items also included in the survey. The low prevalence of symptoms at follow-up again probably reflects the liberal inclusiveness of the original survey. When children in this study with more frequent wheezing were evaluated, nearly two-thirds had wheezing at age 11, and approximately one-third had wheezing at age 16. Nevertheless, as most other studies show, nearly all patients demonstrated improvement in their condition, as gauged by frequency of symptoms. This was particularly apparent by age 23, when only 10% of those who had wheezed at or before age 7 had clinical symptoms in the prior year (98).

As noted, all prospective studies show that, even when asthma symptoms persist, they usually improve after prolonged follow-up intervals. This holds true even for those with more severe asthma. Friberg et al. studied 20 males in early adolescence and then again in their mid-20s (95). When initially studied, all had been persistently symptomatic from under 5 years of age, and 60% had been on a long-term systemic corticosteroid regimen. That this was a markedly more severe group than the other studies probably explains the 100% persistence after the 14-year follow-up interval. Despite this persistence, however, only 20% continued to use bronchodilators regularly, and no individual required regular systemic corticosteroids after the age of 12.

The most thorough and well performed of the prospective studies has taken place through Royal Children's Hospital in Melbourne (95,96). Randomly selected asthmatics from a single-aged cohort and controls were studied at age 7, 14, 21, and 28. Follow-up included questionnaires, interviews, physical examinations, and pulmonary function testing. At follow-up, the patients were classified into four general categories: (1) no episode of wheezing within the prior 3 years of review; (2) no episodes within 3 months, but within 3 years; (3) an episode within 3 months, but neither very frequent nor persistent symptoms; (4) very frequent or persistent symptoms over the prior year. The myriad of statistics at the three follow-up periods can be summarized numerous ways. Overall, approximately two-thirds of all patients who had wheezed at or before age 7 had some history of wheezing within 3 years of follow-up at ages 21 and 28. Twenty percent of these individuals with persistent symptoms fell into category 2, and approximately one-quarter fit into category 3. In other words, although these patients had persistent symptoms, they were either infrequent or generally mild. Another quarter of the patients had frequent symptoms (more than once per week). Further categorization of prognosis based on severity (frequency) of wheezing is discussed later under the risk factors for asthma persistence.

Of particular note in the Martin and Kelly group (95,96) is the high frequency of recurrence after prolonged symptom-free intervals, similar to the findings of Blair (92). Of those wheezing at age 7, but not at 14 or 21, 27% recurred by age 28. For those wheezing at 7 and 14, but not at 21, 31% recurred by age 28 (95,96).

Gerritsen et al., in a study of 119 children referred to a university allergy department in the Netherlands, found similar percentages of symptomatic persistence (8). After an average of 16 years follow-up, 43% of those clinically similar to Martin and Kelly's foregoing categories 3 and 4 had symptomatic asthma. An interesting side finding was that the average age of symptomatic disappearance occurred at age 15, somewhat later than age 10 found by Blair (92).

The only abnormal physical finding at any age in Martin's and Kelly's studies was an increased prevalence of barrel chest noted at age 14 in the most severe group (95,96). This was not seen at age 21 or 28. There was no alteration of growth in any group at any age. Friberg and associate's more severe, smaller population sample also had several individuals with barrel chest (and reduced height) when initially studied, but this had resolved by follow-up in their mid-20s (95).

A. Pulmonary Function Testing (PFT)

Selected patients and controls in Martin and Kelly's study received full pulmonary function testing at age 21 and spirometry at age 28 (97,102). Decrements in pulmonary function were proportional to the severity class at both ages. At age 21, those in categories 3 and 4, and at age 28, those in categories 2 through 4, showed significant abnormalities in most pulmonary function values compared with control groups. Those in category 2 showed evidence of small-airway obstruction with significantly diminished FEF25-75 (forced expiratory flow, mid expiratory phase). Although those in category 1 statistically had normal results of their PFTs, more than 10% still showed evidence of significant small-airway obstruction. Fifty-nine percent of this group (no wheezing for at least 3 years) still showed abnormal reactivity to histamine inhalation challenge, indicating exaggerated bronchial reactivity despite the absence of symptoms. This suggests that the potential for symptom recurrence is high, particularly under the proper environmental circumstances. Other retrospective studies in asymptomatic adolescents and young and middle-aged adults with a prior history of asthma similarly reveal mild abnormalities of pulmonary function (2,40,102,103). The ultimate clinical significance of these abnormalities is unknown.

Giles et al. (99) and Sherrill et al. (101) also prospectively examined pulmonary function tests, and similar to Martin and Kelly, found lower pulmonary function in those with persistent wheezing. In addition, both groups found that nonwheezers in the preteen years with abnormal pulmonary functions were significantly more likely to become symptomatic by age 13–15.

Other studies show that former asthmatics now symptom-free for some time have significantly reduced PFTs versus normal controls (29,94). Mosfeldt Laursen et al. found that 18-year-olds with a history of severe asthma who has no symptoms for more than 2 years were significantly lower in all flow parameters versus normal controls. In fact, their PFTs were virtually indistinguishable from those with mild asthma requiring regular medications (94). Friberg also showed that significant reductions in pulmonary flow rates (as compared to adult control populations) persisted into adulthood in those wheezers who became asymptomatic ($p < .001$) (95). Sherrill found that children with any degree of increased bronchial responsiveness (as measured by methacholine challenge test) had significantly diminished rates of lung growth versus controls (101). Hence, those children with a history of severe asthma who have become asymptomatic appear likely to maintain reduced PFTs indefinitely and hold a high risk for symptomatic recurrence. This recurrence is unlikely to become severe, however.

Conversely, symptomatic children with normal PFTs may be more likely to remit over time. Sherrill found that 9-year-old symptomatic asthmatics with normal methacholine challenges were more likely to remit by age 15, although diminished FEV1/VC did persist (101).

Watanabe did show that bronchial hyperreactivity could possibly be reversed with routine treatment of inhaled anti-inflammatory bronchodilators (105). Cromolyn sodium alone was administered to 34 Japanese asthmatic children in Japan continuously (20 mg tid) over a 3-year period. A significant reduction in bronchial responsiveness to histamine was demonstrated. The influence of therapy on symptomatic persistence is further explored below.

VI. Risk Factors for the Persistence of Asthma

The discussion that follows details the risk factors for the persistence of asthma once present. The risk factors for the development of asthma itself are discussed in Chapter 28.

A. Severity and Frequency

All studies examining the natural history of asthma have found persistence to correlate directly with the severity of the asthma. Most studies used frequency of symptoms as the indicator of severity, since it is an easy parameter to follow up by questionnaire or interview in large studies. Severity based on morbidity, as represented by frequency of asthma hospitalizations, is certainly a risk factor for the ongoing persistence of asthma (29,69,70,94). In addition, prospective studies that followed asthmatics referred to allergy/asthma centers (where asthma severity is more likely to be greater) show higher frequencies of asthma persistence than general population cohort studies. The risk of asthma persistence from childhood and adolescence into early adulthood is best summarized by collation of Martin and Kelly's data (Table 4) (96,97). In individuals with occasional wheezing at age 14, one-fourth will actually have more frequent symptoms at age 21 and one-third will have more at age 28. In individuals with frequent or persistent symptoms at age 14, two-thirds will still have frequent symptoms at age 28, and only 2% will be symptom-free. These numbers can give the clinician a good idea of the likelihood of asthma persistence in a patient based on the current severity (frequency) of asthma symptoms.

B. Other Atopy

With the exception of urticaria, the presence of other atopic disease, particularly if persistent or early in onset, has been shown by numerous authors to increase the likelihood of asthma persistence (Table 5) (4,18,31,85,87–90,94,95,98,104). Giles et al. estimated a fourfold risk of

Table 4 The Risk of Future Wheezing in All Patients Studied (A) and Based on Asthma Severity (B)

	Age 21(%)	Age 28(%)
A. If wheezing is present before age 14, will it be present at age 21? At 28?		
None	34	32
Rare	21	20
Occasional	27	22
Frequent	23	26
B. If wheezing is not or rarely present at age 14, will it be present at 21? At 28?		
None	55	54
Rare	25	19
Occasional	16	20
Frequent	3	7
If occasional wheezing is present at age 14, will it be present at 21? At 28?		
None	20	16
Rare	20	22
Occasional	35	30
Frequent	25	32
If frequent or persistent wheezing is present at age 14, will it be present at 21? At 28?		
None	4	2
Rare	14	19
Occasional	7	11
Frequent	55	68

Source: Collated from Refs. 96 and 97.

asthma persistence at age 20 if atopic dermatitis or allergic rhinitis was present (99). In the prospective cohort studies of Anderson et al., several statistical correlations predicting the risk of asthma from ages 7 to 16 were found (4,21). Most notable was the 15-fold greater likelihood of wheezing at age 16 in children with both allergic rhinitis and atopic dermatitis at age 7, as compared with those without these disorders (4). Johnstone found that all the asthmatics with concurrent allergic rhinitis had persistent asthma at follow-up (100).

The presence of atopic dermatitis with wheezing appears to be one of the most predictive of all risk factors for persistent asthma (100). Two studies (86,93) found a profound of risk of asthma persistence when an individual presented with asthma and atopic dermatitis, but not with other atopic conditions. In contrast with this data and the results of many addi-

Table 5 Persistent Asthma: Association with Other Atopic Disease

Author (Ref.)	Allergic rhinitis (AR)	Atopic dermatitis (AD)	AR and AD	Food allergy	Eosinophilia	Elevated IgE	Positive skin test
Anderson et al. (4)	+[a](5-7x)	+[a]	+[a] (15X)				
Barr, Logan (89)		+	+				
Blair (92)	+		+[a]	+			−
Buffum, Settipane (91)		+					Egg +, other −
Foucard, Sjoberg (31)	+	+				−[b]	Cat, pollen + other −
Geller-Bernstein et al. (106)						−[b]	
Gerritsen et al. (8)	−	−			−	−[b]	−[b]
Giles et al. (99)	+ (4x)	+ (4x)					
Johnstone (100)	+[c]	−					Grass +, other −
Jonsson et al. (93)	−	+					
Kelly et al. (97,107)	+	+[d]			+	+[e]	
Kjellman, Dalen (28)						−[a]	−[a]
Murray, Morrison (85)	+	+					
Ryssing, Flemsborg (87)	+						Mold +, other −
Sporik et al. (9)							Dust mite +
Whatley, Guerrant (90)							−
Sherrill et al. (101)							Dust mite, cat + other −

[+]Indicates statistically significant association of this condition or test with persistent asthma.
[−]Indicates no statistically significant association of this condition or test with persistent asthma.
[a]Significant only if condition present at follow-up.
[b]Indicates predictive of the presence of asthma, but not of asthma persistence.
[c]All subjects with asthma before or concurrent with AR had persistence.
[d]Only the most severe asthmatics had associated AD.
[e]These associations were made in young adult asthmatics followed into later adulthood.

tional studies (4,31,87,89–92,97,99,100,106,107), the presence of other atopic conditions was not related to asthma persistence in 119 asthmatic children originally studied at age 6–14 and then reevaluated 14–20 years later (when a 57% remission rate was observed) (8).

Wright et al. found that those infants with the onset of persistent rhinitis before age 1 were significantly more likely to have asthma at age 3 and at age 6 than those who developed rhinitis after 1 year of age (18).

C. Clinical Markers of Atopy

An elevated IgE and multiple positive skin tests are definite predictors of general allergic disease or the risk of developing asthma itself, but numerous studies in asthmatics and other atopic conditions have shown that these laboratory measurements are not statistically predictive of persistence in any one person over prolonged time intervals (8,20,31,92,94,106). This was recently reconfirmed in the study by Mosfeldt Lauren et al., in which no difference in skin reactivity was found between current asthmatics and former asthmatics at age 18 (94).

Recent studies over shorter periods of time have shown that an elevated IgE and positive skin tests to inhalants in children under 7 years of age with asthma may be predictive of persistence over short-term intervals (<4 years) (16,17,45). In addition, follow-up of Kelly and Martin's childhood asthmatic population into adulthood demonstrated that the number of positive skin tests, elevated IgE, and eosinophilia were predictive of asthma presence at age 28 (107). Specific skin test reactivity to dust mite does appear to be a risk factor for the persistence of asthma into later childhood, but the risk into adulthood is unclear. Specifically, infants and children under age 5 with wheezing were more likely to have persistent asthma at follow-up in later childhood if they were skin-test-reactive to dust or dust mite (20). In addition, children demonstrating skin-test reactivity to mite after an episode of bronchiolitis evidence a greater incidence of asthma symptoms at follow-up (108). However, Gerritsen et al. found that, although skin-test reactivity to dust mite almost invariably persisted from childhood to 30 years of age, most patients at that time no longer experienced asthma symptoms (8).

Skin-test reactivity to other antigens may also be predictive of future wheezing (45,101). Sherrill et al. showed that 9-year-olds with asthma and skin-test reactivity to cats (and dust mites) were statistically more symptomatic at age 15 than those who were skin-test-negative (101). These same individuals also showed a significantly lower growth in both FEV1/VC and FEV1, whereas other antigens (grass, dog, mold, horse) did not have these associations. As shown in Table 5, however, skin reactivity as a predictor of asthma persistence is generally inconsistent. Retrospectivity, although several studies have shown that those adults showing skin test positivity to inhalants were more likely to have had asthma as a child (8,107), others could not confirm these findings (25).

In Gerritsen's study of childhood asthmatics followed after 10 years, numerous statistical trends were found in relation to the presence of asthma and persistence of skin test positivity, but none of the clinical variables studied initially proved to be predictive of asthma prognosis (8). Those who had asthma symptoms at follow-up showed no significant specific IgE to antigens (animal dander, dust, pollen, mold), total IgE, or eosinophilia from those who were symptom-free. Kjellman, following 58 children admitted for asthma (average age 9) over 8 subsequent years (28), similarly found skin test reactivity increased with age, but its presence was not predictive of asthma symptoms at follow-up.

Overall, these conflicting data suggests that the presence of an elevated total IgE and positive skin tests must be used cautiously in prognosticating outcome in any single child with asthma.

D. Heredity

Several studies have shown that a history of atopy or asthma in family members, particularly first-degree relatives, places an individual at higher risk for asthma persistence (31,87,92). Ryssing found that 67% of those with a "familial predisposition" were symptomatic at follow-up, versus 58% without a family history (87). Blair found that 73% of those asthmatics having a first-degree relative with an atopic condition had chronic or recurrent asthma at follow-up (92). This compares with only 27% of those who were symptom-free at the end of the study.

E. Sex

Although the prevalence of asthma is higher in males, the rate of persistence into early adulthood appears to be higher in females. Sherrill found that asthmatic boys had a slower rate of FEV1 and vital capacity (VC) increase than asthmatic girls (101), whereas Weiss et al. showed the opposite trend (22). Follow-up into early adulthood, however, has shown that females tend to maintain symptoms more than males (4,96). Kelly's follow-up data at age 28, however, suggest that this trend may not continue into later adulthood (97).

F. Respiratory Infection

Retrospective studies in adults generally show an association of chronic obstructive pulmonary disease (COPD) with a history of childhood respiratory disease (2,109). These studies have numerous methodological flaws, however, particularly for recall bias or lack of control populations.

The role of bronchiolitis in infancy as a risk factor for the development of persistent wheezing is discussed in depth later in this chapter. Several studies have noted an association between recurrent upper respiratory illnesses or croup in childhood and wheezing persistence or abnormal pulmonary function studies later in childhood (2,4,110).

G. Age of Onset

Most studies show no correlation between age of onset of wheezing in childhood and the persistence of symptoms into later childhood and adulthood (4,89,91,92,94,100). Some studies have shown that children with the onset of symptoms later in childhood are at a higher risk for ongoing symptoms than those with onset in the first two years of life (24,31), whereas other have found the opposite (93). This correlates with the findings of Martinez (17) and Van Asperen (20) discussed earlier, in which lower respiratory symptomatology under the age of 6–12 months did not predict future asthma.

H. Asthma Therapy

Undertreatment of asthma appears to be a risk factor for the continuation of reactive airway disease into adulthood (24,87,111). In addition, undertreatment has been suggested to lead to various degrees of fixed airway obstruction. The influx of inflammatory cells, particularly in the late-phase reaction of an asthma attack, has been hypothesized to result, over time, in some irreversible damage to the airways. Burrows found that patients with a chronic history of undertreated bronchospasm had a greater decline of 1-sec forced expiratory volume (FEV1) with age than did asthmatics under good control (103).

Obviously, all studies of asthmatics over time by their nature assume ongoing therapy of the disease. However, the impact of specific anti-inflammatory therapy on the natural history of asthma in children over prolonged periods of time is just starting to be investigated. Watanabe did show a reduction in bronchial hyperreactivity (as measured by bronchial histamine challenge) in an open 3-year study of Japanese asthmatic children treated only with cromolyn sodium (105). Konig (111) retrospectively evaluated 175 asthmatics over a mean of 8 years and categorized the severity of their asthma based on the International Guidelines (112). Pulmonary function and a detailed clinical history was documented at the end of the study. Children with mild asthma received only beta-agonist therapy on an as-needed basis, while children with moderate disease received inhaled cromolyn sodium regularly and those with severe disease received ongoing inhaled corticosteroids. Those in the latter two groups were statistically more likely to remain unchanged or improve than the mild group, in which disease progression was more common. While symptoms, school absence, emergency room visits, and hospitalizations were initially higher in the moderate and severe groups, by the last year of the study there were no differences between groups. He concluded that therapy with these anti-inflammatory medications compared to bronchodilators produced significant improvement in both clinical severity and lung function, likely altering, at least in part, the natural history of asthma (personal communication).

Haahtela et al. prospectively showed significant, persistent improvement in symptoms and lung function in newly diagnosed, mild asthmatics over a 2-year time frame when treated with inhaled corticosteroids versus beta-agonists (113). This improvement was maintained in only one-third of the patients after they were taken off the inhaled corticosteroids, indicating that ongoing therapy is likely necessary for most chronic asthmatics. Interestingly, asthmatics treated earlier with inhaled corticosteroids seemed to maintain some degree of clinical improvement for longer than did those patients who started this form of therapy later (114). These studies suggest that earlier intervention with corticosteroids may favorably alter the natural course of asthma over time.

Immunotherapy appeared to have little effect on asthma persistence in the few studies in which it has been addressed. Only Johnstone's study found that immunotherapy improved asthma outcome (115). He found that over a 4- to 14-year duration, 72% of those asthmatic children receiving allergen immunotherapy were symptom-free by age 16, as opposed to only 22% of placebo-treated controls. This study had a 40% dropout rate, suggesting that a high proportion of individuals were likely to have had an improvement in their symptoms and did not require further therapy or follow-up. The very low rate of improvement or remission in the placebo group is inconsistent with nearly all of the studies discussed earlier. The 72% improvement in the treated group, however, corresponds to the trends in the other studies in which immunotherapy was not considered.

Other epidemiological studies evaluating immunotherapy have found no effect on asthma outcome. In Rackemann and Edwards' landmark 20-year follow-up study of 449 childhood asthmatics, no difference was found in the 19 patients who received allergen immunotherapy (116). Kraepelien followed 100 asthmatic children receiving immunotherapy for 8–10 years (117). Only 12% were symptom-free and 55% were considerably improved, consistent with the outcome of other follow-up studies in which immunotherapy was not evaluated.

More recently, Jonsson's prospective study of previously hospitalized asthmatic children over two to three decades found no difference in outcome between those who had received immunotherapy and those who did not (93). In fact, 68% (48/56) of those not receiving immunotherapy were symptom-free at follow-up, as compared with 43% (26/61) of those who had been treated in this manner. This difference was not statistically different, but does indicate a trend toward treatment with immunotherapy in those asthmatics with more severe disease.

Johnstone suggested from his studies that specific immunotherapy for allergic rhinitis may prevent the ultimate development of asthma (100,115). This was based on the eventual development of asthma in 50% of children with allergic rhinitis who were in the placebo group in an immunotherapy study. There were only 22 subjects in this group, however. Furthermore, this observation has never been confirmed and is strongly tempered by many of the studies cited earlier, in which the onset of asthma occurs before or coincident with rhinitis (12,14,93,116). Hence, based on the availability of current data, there is no indication for initiating immunotherapy to prevent the onset of asthma or to alter its natural history.

I. Allergen Exposure

Ongoing exposure to inhalant allergens in sensitized individuals increases the likelihood of asthma persistence. This was shown most clearly in Sporik et al.'s prospective study of children to age 11, in whom levels of mite exposure correlated with not only the presence of asthma, but also its persistence (9). Long-term studies on environmental control avoidance measures are required to determine whether such measures affect asthma persistence. Although Johnstone found that the degree of dust-proofing appeared not to affect asthma outcome (100), more recent studies confirm the real benefit of dust mite avoidance on reducing bronchial hyperreactivity (118). Retrospective data also suggest that ongoing small-mammal exposure, and possibly pollen exposure, similarly increase the likelihood of persistent symptoms (45,49,51,93).

J. Smoking

Although parental or patient smoking is a risk factor for the development of respiratory symptoms and childhood asthma and diminished pulmonary function status, no definitive study has implicated smoking as a risk factor for the persistence of wheezing (4,31). In fact, some studies show no increased rate of wheezing in those patients who take up smoking in late adolescence (4,99). On the other hand, retrospective studies in adults with

COPD (including asthma) have generally found a relation between smoking and asthma persistence or recurrence (2,103). As reviewed earlier, however, numerous studies have revealed a higher prevalence of respiratory illness as well as pulmonary function testing in children of smokers.

K. Air Pollution

The Harvard Six Cities Study correlated respiratory symptoms in general population cohorts of children with air pollution levels over a 20-year time frame (61). No association could be found between levels of pollutants and the incidence of asthma. A correlation was noted, however, between pollutant levels, symptomatic flares, and symptomatic persistence in those already with underlying asthma.

Children raised in northern England (an industrial area) were found to have a higher rate of asthma persistence than those in other locations (56). Those exposed to higher levels of air pollution were at higher risk for symptoms at age 15, but not at 20 or 25.

L. Breast Feeding

Studies conflict on the effect of breast feeding on asthma persistence. While Geller-Bernstein (106) and Blair (92) found that breast-fed infants were statistically less likely to wheeze in late childhood and adolescence, other studies failed to show this association (4).

M. Miscellaneous Risk and Associated Factors

A history of pneumonia or whooping cough before age 7 was a risk factor for wheezing at age 16, but not at 23 (4). Similar to the possible risk of parental smoking, these findings show that the risk of early childhood exposure to irritants or infectious agents may initially result in symptomatic persistence, but that by early adulthood these symptoms resolve. Any subclinical effect on pulmonary status, or the ultimate effect on possible respiratory status in later adulthood, however, has not been evaluated.

Young maternal age has repeatedly been found to a risk factor for ongoing symptoms (15,20,21), just as it is a risk factor for the presence of asthma itself. Further statistical evaluations of the British cohort study found that a history or recurrent abdominal symptoms and associated congenital disabilities were risk factors for ongoing symptoms (21,119).

A summary of the risk factors predictive of asthma persistence are listed in Table 6. In addition, factors that were and were not associated with (but not necessarily predictive of) persistent asthma are also listed.

Table 6 Factors Predictive of and Associated with Persistent Asthma

---

Definitely predictive[a]
  Severity/frequency of symptoms
  Concurrent allergic rhinitis
  Family history of asthma in first-degree relatives
  Lower respiratory of infection in infancy
  Maternal smoking
Probably predictive[b]
  Concurrent atopic dermatitis
  Overcrowded housing conditions in childhood
  History of pneumonia with asthma
  Dust mite allergy
  Cat allergy/cat exposure in the home
Possibly predictive[c]
  Air pollution exposure as a child
  Undertreatment of asthma
  Food allergy
  Young maternal age
  History of recurrent abdominal symptoms in childhood
  Coincident birth defect(s)
Erratically predictive[d]
  Female sex
  Smoking as adolescent/young adult
  Lower social class
  Absence of breast feeding
  Total IgE
  Skin test reactivity (except dust mite)
  Dog allergy
  Low birth weight
Not predictive
  Eosinophilia
  Onset age
  Pneumonia without asthma before age 7
  History of urticaria
No association with persistence
  Parental occupation
  Birth order
  History of measles
  Single parent in home

---

[a]Multiple studies show statistical significance.
[b]Multiple studies show statistical significance, occasional studies do not; or, a limited number of studies show statistical significance.
[c]A majority of studies show statistical significance; or a single study shows statistical significance.
[d]Some studies show statistical significance, but many others do not.

Britten found that the social class of an individual and the number of occupants of a child's bedroom were associated with ongoing symptoms, whereas Anderson did not (21,56).

N. Relation Between Bronchiolitis and Subsequent Wheezing or Asthma

Bronchiolitis is a viral infection of the lower respiratory tract occurring most commonly under 2 years of age. It is invariably associated with some degree of airway obstruction, although there is a wide spectrum of clinical severity. Numerous studies, both retrospective and prospective, have been performed evaluating the persistence of both clinical airway symptoms as well as the persistence of both clinical airway symptoms and the presence of functional airway abnormalities (Table 7) (106,108,120–126). However, difficulties are encountered in comparing these studies because of marked differences between them in (a) the time interval until follow-up evaluation, (b) the age of onset of the initial illness and its severity [(varying from those severely affected and hospitalized in early infancy (120), to those younger than 2 years of age treated as outpatients for wheezing with respiratory infection (125)], and (c) the criteria established to determine persistent symptomatology. Nevertheless, consistent patterns occur, providing the practitioner with data to assess the risk and risk factors for the development of asthma after lower respiratory tract infection early in life.

Table 7 lists these studies in order of duration of follow-up. In general, the longer the duration of follow-up, the more likely it is that clinical symptoms of airway obstruction (wheeze, cough) will improve (122,125,126). Pullan retrospectively found that 38% of young infants with bronchiolitis experienced wheezing in the subsequent 4 years, but that by 10 years after the index illness, only 22% had recent wheezing (126). Duiverman retrospectively showed that 62% of infants had some degree of wheezing at follow-up, but only 12% remained symptomatic after age 6 (125).

Most prospective studies show higher rates of symptomatic persistence than do retrospective ones, probably indicating a recall bias, particularly when follow-up was by parental interview only. Milder symptoms of wheezing during infancy generally led to a lower incidence of persistence (32%) at follow-up (106). In contrast, when the index bronchiolitis episodes were more severe (requiring hospitalization), generally higher incidences of symptomatic persistence occurred, indicating that those with a specific diagnosis of bronchiolitis were more likely to having ongoing symptoms (108,120). Moreover, a study which included only infants with documented respiratory syncytial virus (RSV) disease demonstrated higher

Table 7 Bronchlolitis/Lower Respiratory Tract Infection Follow-Up Studies

Author (Ref.)	Study type	No.	Onset age	Follow-up time	Symptomatic at follow-up	Abnormal PFTs
Stokes et al. (120)	Retro No cont	18	1.5–5 mo	12–15	67% (ongoing wheeze)	1. 40% increase thoracic gas volume 2. 75% abnormal airway resistance and/or conductance
Geller-Bernstein et al. (106)	Prosp No cont In+Outpt	80	6–24 mo (avg 13 mo)	4 yr (q6 mo)	32% (ongoing wheeze in prior year)	
Welliver et al. (121)	Prosp No cont	38	Under 6 mo	4 yr	1. 53% ever wheeze 2. 32% over 3 episodes	
Sly and Hibbert (122)	Prosp No cont	48	2 wk–10 mo (avg 3 mo)	5 yr (q1 yr)	1. 71% "asthmatic" 2. 17% on daily meds 3. 92% has further episodes	1. 3% FEV1<80% predicted 2. 30% FEV1/FVC<80% predicted 3. 60% (+) histamine challenge
Mok and Simpson (123)	Prosp Control Outpt	200	Infancy	7 yr	60% symptomatic (47% wheeze, 36% cough)	1. If sx present, all flow studies within 80% predicted, but still significantly reduced versus controls 2. If no symptoms, only FEV1/FVC reduced versus controls 3. 38% (+) exercise challenge
McConnochie and Roghman (124)	Retro Control In+Outpt	77	Under 25 mo	7.7 yr	1. 44% regularly wheeze in last 2 yr (13% control) 2. 55% wheeze with colds (25% control)	

Study	Design	N	Age at onset	F/U	Symptoms	PFTs
					3. 18% on routine meds for asthma (4% control)	
					4. 22% wheeze with exercise (7% control)	
Sims et al. (108)	Retro Control	26	Under 12 mo	8 yr	56% (ongoing wheeze)	
Duiverman et al. (125)	Retro Control	16	1–18 mo	2.5–12.8 yr (avg 8 yr)	62% recurrent resp sx; 12% after age 6	1. If no sx, airway caliber (by force oscillometry) and histamine challenge normal 2. If + sx, 70% abnormal smooth muscle tone, and + histamine challenge
Pullan and Hey (126)	Retro Control	130	Under 1 yr (avg 14 wk)	10 yr	1. 42% ever wheeze (19% control) 2. 38% in first 4 yr (15% control) 3. 22% in last 2 yr (13% control) 4. 5% on routine meds (Same as control)	1. 16% FEV1/FVC < 72% (1.8% control) 2. 10% FEV1/FVC < 72% with no further wheeze 3. 15% (+) exercise challenge (5% cont) 19% (+) histamine challenge (6% cont) 25% (+) exercise and/or histamine challenge (6% control) 4. All had normal nitrogen washout studies

F/U, follow-up; Retro, retrospective study; Prosp, prospective study; Inpt, inpatient study; Outpt, outpatient study; No cont, uncontrolled study; sx, symptoms; PFTs, pulmonary function studies; (+), positive.

rates of persistence than any other study (122). In this latter study, 92% of infants had subsequent wheezing episodes and 71% had "symptoms suggestive" of asthma (by parental questionnaire) at 5-year follow-up, 42% of which had physician-diagnosed asthma (122).

Studies that include general pediatric population control groups or control groups of pediatric asthmatic patients (123–126) have shown a significant increase in the likelihood of both clinical symptomatology and functional airway abnormalities in those children with bronchiolitis in infancy, when compared with age-matched controls. McConnochie et al. found that 44% of those infants who had bronchiolitis experienced wheezing in the 2 years before follow-up at 7.7 years, as opposed to 13.6% in a private-practice pediatric population ($p < .0001$) (124). Of these, 18.6% had "current asthma," versus 4% of the control group ($p < .001$). Other patterns of recurrent lower respiratory symptoms, such as wheezing with exercise, also showed strong statistical significance in index cases versus controls (see Table 7). Although most studies found similar trends for lower airway symptomatology, Pullan found no difference at 10-year follow-up between index cases and controls for those children who required regular bronchiolitis therapy (126).

A review of those studies evaluating pulmonary function shown approximately a threefold risk of abnormal pulmonary function tests (PFTs) or increased bronchial reactivity following bronchiolitis. Abnormalities in airway resistance or specific conductance were found in 75% of infants 15 months after bronchiolitis (120), whereas 30% evidence FEV1/forced vital capacity (FVC) less than 80% predicted 5 years post-bronchiolitis (122). Longer intervals of follow-up have found that pulmonary flow rates tend to normalize eventually to within normal limits (higher than 80% predicted) following bronchiolitis (123,125,126). Nevertheless, when compared with control groups, these values are still significantly reduced (127). Pullan found that 16% of the total index cases had FEV1/FVC of less than 72% predicted, as opposed to only 1.9% of controls ($p < .005$) (126). Ten percent of infants with bronchiolitis but no subsequent wheezing for 12 years after the initial illness had FEV1/FVC of less than 72% predicted, as opposed to none of the 84 control patients without a history of wheezing.

Bronchial hyperreactivity occurred more often in ex-bronchiolitis than in controls. At 5 years follow-up, 60% had a positive bronchial histamine challenge (122), compared with 19% after 10 years (126); however, even this lower incidence was six times more frequent than in controls (126). Duiverman found that 70% of those with symptoms at follow-up had abnormal smooth muscle tone as measured by forced oscillometry, whereas those without symptoms were normal (125). All patients studied by Pullan had normal nitrogen washout studies, indicating the absence of persisting ventilation abnormalities years after the bronchiolitis episode (126).

A summary of the associated risk factors for the persistence of wheezing following bronchiolitis is shown in Table 8. Those studies with younger index cases showed higher percentages of symptoms at follow-up (120,122,125). This finding is consistent with the persistent symptoms often seen after early lung damage from other types of lower respiratory tract infections of infancy, including pertussis and croup (83,128,129), as well as from other traumatic conditions such as respiratory distress syndrome (130), bronchopulmonary dysplasia (131), tracheo-esophageal fistula (132), and foreign body aspiration (133). Even seemingly benign newborn res-

Table 8 Risk Factors for Persistence of Wheezing Following Bronchiolitis

Definite[a]
  Documented RSV infection
  Presence of RSV IgE titers
  Younger age at initial illness
Probable[b]
  Associated atopy
  First-degree relative with atopy, particularly asthma
  Parental smoking
Possible[c]
  Elevated IgE
  Poor socioeconomic background
  Bottle feeding
  Eosinophilia
  Specific IgE reactivity to dust mite
  Initial unresponsiveness to bronchodilators
Doubtful
  Sex
  Other specific skin/RAST tests
Other factors not associated with risk of persistence in single studies

Race	Day care
Family size	Forced-air heat
Presence of dog/cat	Older sibling in preschool
Serum immunoglobulins	

[a]Multiple studies show statistical significance.
[b]Most studies show statistical significance, an occasional study does not.
[c]The majority of studies show statistical significance, but many do not; or a single study shows statistical significance; or studies show these to be risk factors for the development of bronchiolitis itself, but not necessarily for the persistence of wheezing after bronchiolitis.

piratory conditions, such as transient tachypnea of the newborn, have been associated with persistent pulmonary abnormalities (134). These findings suggest that respiratory insults in infancy have the potential to significantly damage the lower airways, sometimes indefinitely.

Children with confirmed RSV bronchiolitis are at higher risk for persistent symptoms (122). Welliver et al. found that those infants demonstrating the highest RSV IgE titers in nasopharyngeal secretions were much more likely to have subsequent wheezing (70%) than those who did not develop an RSV IgE response (20%) (120). This was recently confirmed in the Tuscon Children's Respiratory study (17).

Most studies show that the development of other atopic conditions (120,123,124), or a history or atopy in a first-degree relative (123,124,126,135), or both, are risk factors for persistent wheezing in infants with bronchiolitis. Other studies show that eosinophilia, an elevated serum IgE, and dust mite sensitivity during the initial illness are risk factors, although other specific allergic sensitivities (by skin test or RAST) are not (108,126). Even those studies that did not show these factors to be a risk for subsequent wheezing did show that they were still risk factors for the development of bronchiolitis itself (123,124).

Although Pullan found significantly more girls as index cases (126), other studies found boys to be at higher risk for symptomatic persistence (121,124). A single study found that infants of younger parents were at higher risk (123), but race, family size, and other socioeconomic variables have not been found to be significant risk factors (123,124,126). Likewise, many other environmental factors do not appear to be important. The primary exception is parental smoking, which in most studies has been shown to be a significant risk factor for both the acquisition of bronchiolitis and subsequent wheezing (106,108,122,124,126,136).

In studying the relative odds of future wheezing after bronchiolitis, McConnochie found that many of these factors have cumulative risk potential (Table 9) (124). The relative odds of wheezing at follow-up was 4 for those who had bronchiolitis without other atopy or without a smoking parent, 7 for those with bronchiolitis and a smoking parent, 15 for those with bronchiolitis and associated allergy, and 28 when all three factors were present. When these other risks variables were controlled, bronchiolitis was a more significant factor for future wheezing than the other two variables.

In summary, roughly two-thirds of infants experiencing bronchiolitis go on to have further recurrent wheezing episodes. Improvement does occur over time, particularly in terms of frequency of symptoms. Despite the symptomatic improvement, however, bronchial hyperreactivity persists. Even in those studies with the longest follow-up intervals, those index

Table 9 Occurrence of Risk Factor Groups, Relative Odds of Wheezing, and Attributable Risk for Wheezing

Upper respiratory tract allergy	Bronchiolitis	Passive smoking	Raw data	Occurrence	Relative odds	Population attributable risk
0	0	0	6/64	34.64	1.00	2.35
0	0	+	9/77	41.68	1.87	5.00
0	+	0	3/10	0.72	3.99	0.16
0	+	+	7/26	1.89	7.46	0.67
+	0	0	1/15	8.09	3.79	1.75
+	0	+	8/21	11.32	7.08	3.86
+	+	0	3/6	0.43	15.12	0.23
+	+	+	13/17	1.23	28.27	0.83
			50/236	100.00		14.85

Symbols used: 0, absent; +, present.
Definitions are as follows: "Raw data" are presented as a number of subjects wheezing/total number of subjects in each cell. "Occurrence" of risk-factors groups in the pediatric practice population was based on the observed frequencies in the control and index groups and on the bronchiolitis attack rate of 4.27/100 children in the first 2 years of life. Figures represent frequency with which children were observed in each risk-factor group per 100 children in the practice population. "Relative odds" are those obtained from multivariate analysis. They range from 1.00, for children exposed to none of the risk factors in the model, to 28.27, for children who experience all three risk factors. "Population attributable risk" is presented as the number of children in each of the cells who report wheezing out of every 100 children in the practice population. Calculations are based on occurrence and on rate of wheezing in each risk-factor group as predicted by logistic regression analysis. The total number of wheezing children per 100, 14.85, derived from predicted values, varies slightly from that deviated from the observed values, 14.87.
Source: Ref. 125.

cases without wheezing have more frequent coughing and episodes of bronchitis. Although pulmonary function studies are usually within normal limits in these infants at follow-up, they are statistically below control values, and evidence of bronchial abnormalities are unclear, but retrospective studies of adults do show a higher risk for increased symptoms and lower FEV1 in those with a history of childhood respiratory illness, especially when younger than age 2 (2,137).

These findings indicate that there appears to be a propensity for those with familial atopic tendencies to be not only at risk for the persistence of wheezing after bronchiolitis, but for bronchiolitis itself. On the other hand, there is strong evidence that the infection itself may be a catalyst toward early manifestations of atopy and bronchial hyperreactivity (10). Hence, the ultimate chicken-egg dilemma has been only partially solved: Bronchiolitis does predispose to ongoing lower airway abnormality, but does a genetic propensity for airway hyperreactivity predispose an infant to bronchiolitis?

VII. Persistence of Atopic Dermatitis

The natural history of atopic dermatitis under the age of 5 is discussed earlier in this chapter. Well over half of those with atopic dermatitis in childhood will evidence some persistent atopic dermatitis at follow-up at one to three decades (Table 10) (138–140). Rystedt et al. interviewed patients directly and performed physical examinations at frequent intervals for as long as 32 years in over 90% of patients (138). In 549 patients requiring hospitalizations for severe atopic dermatitis, 62% had continuing disease at a follow-up of 24–32 years (138). Forty percent of those with moderate atopic dermatitis who were evaluated as outpatients showed persistent disease at the same follow-up intervals (138). In a supportive 20-year follow-up study using retrospective questionnaires, patients with severe or moderate atopic dermatitis had 79% and 60% persistence, respectively (139).

Table 10 Atopic Dermatitis: Follow-Up Studies

Author (Ref.)	No.	Age of onset (yr)	Follow-up interval (yr)	Age at follow-up (yr)	Severity	Persistent symptoms (%)
Roth and Kierland (139)	271 221	Child	20	NS	Mild Severe	60 79
Musgrove and Morgan (140)	99	Under 5	15–17	NS	NS	57
Rystedt (138)	40 549	Under 14	24–32	24–44	Moderate Severe	40 62[a]

NS, not stated.
[a]Persistent hand eczema in 51% of severe, 35% of moderate cases.
Severe disease persisted in 13% of severe onset cases, 3% overall.

Despite the frequent chronicity of atopic dermatitis, the clinical severity generally diminishes over long periods of time. Only 13% of those initially presenting with severe eczema, and only 2–3% of the overall study population, continued to have severe disease at follow-up. The severity at initial presentation exists as the most significant risk factor for persistence of atopic dermatitis (138).

Other risk factors associated with disease continuation were (in decreasing order of significance): family history of atopic dermatitis, concurrent atopic disease, age of onset, and female sex (138). When these latter two factors were present, there was an 80% chance of persistence at follow-up. If none of the factors was present, persistence declined to 15% (138).

About one-third of patients with chronic atopic dermatitis have a history of asthma, whereas one-half have a history of allergic rhinitis (138). A higher risk for the persistence of atopic dermatitis occurred in those with chronic asthma or allergic rhinitis or with the onset of symptoms before age 3 (138).

Although a family history of atopic dermatitis was a significant risk factor for persistence, a family history of other skin conditions or atopic disease was not. The presence of a positive family history for atopy or other skin conditions did increase the risk of acquiring atopic dermatitis, but did not increase the risk for persistence (138).

Similar to several studies with asthma, Rystedt found that 25% of the population initially studied had recurrences after prolonged symptom-free intervals (138). Most of the patients with persistence or recurrence of atopic dermatitis experienced only hand involvement at follow-up. Fifty-one percent of those with severe symptoms at presentation, and 25% of those in the moderate group, had primarily hand eczema at follow-up. Approximately 10% of these cases were disabling (138).

Although those with severe and moderate atopic dermatitis exhibited 45% and 26% incidence of elevated serum IgE, respectively, total IgE and total eosinophil counts did not correlate with persistence of atopic dermatitis. This is consistent with the findings in the asthma studies, which indicate the lack of prognostic value of IgE and eosinophilia. Positive patch testing also did not correlate with persistence (138). No relation was found between personality type, academic achievement, recreational activities, or financial success with the persistence of atopic dermatitis (140).

VIII. Persistence of Chronic Urticaria

Acute urticaria is generally self-limited, and its cause is often identifiable. A certain proportion of these patients, however, will go on to develop chronic or recurrent urticaria. What time frame constitutes "chronic urticaria" is unclear. Nevertheless, several studies assessing the risk of urticaria persisting for at least 6 weeks have found that one-half to two-thirds of these patients have continuing symptoms at 1–3 years follow-up (Table 11) (141–145). Longer follow-up has shown that approximately two-thirds remain symptom-free for prolonged periods (143,144). In one study of 86 patients of all ages with urticaria, the duration of the urticaria exhibited a mean of 4 years and a median of 1.5 years, indicating that several cases had extremely long duration (141).

The prognosis of chronic urticaria with angioedema appears to be the same as chronic urticaria alone (141), although one study suggested a more prolonged course if both entities were present (146). Other generalizations can be made concerning the natural history of chronic urticaria. Age, sex, history of other atopic conditions, total serum IgE, eosinophil count, RAST analysis, and skin testing are of no value in predicting the natural course of urticaria. In general, those patients with an identifiable cause for their chronic urticaria have the same course of illness as those patients in whom no cause can be found, although exceptions exist (143).

The longer the urticaria persists, the worse is the prognosis. Those patients with urticaria persisting for longer than 24 months had an 81% chance of symptomatic persistence 5–14 years after onset (142). As seen with other atopic conditions, disease severity in those with persistent symptoms generally tends to decrease over time.

Several other observations from these urticaria studies are worthy of note. Kauppinen found that 30% of those with acute urticaria (under 2 months duration) developed chronic urticaria (142). Harris found a mean duration of 16 months for urticaria in 52 children younger than age 16 (145). Most studies show that fewer than 25% and frequently fewer than 10% of patients have an identifiable cause for their chronic urticaria (141,142,144–146).

IX. Persistence of Food Allergy and Intolerance

A. Reaction Types

Most adverse reactions to food begin in infancy, usually before the first birthday. Approximately one-fourth of those with a positive family history of allergy in a first-degree relative will have a parentally reported adverse

Table 11 Chronic Urticaria: Follow-Up Studies

Author (Ref.)	N	Age	Duration at onset	Follow-up interval	Asymptomatic at follow-up (%)	Symptomatic at follow-up (%)	Improved at follow-up (%)	Known etiology[a] (%)
Quaranta et al. (141)	86	33 yr (mean)	6 wk	3 yr	68	32	NS	10
Kauppinen et al. (142)	99	$\frac{1}{2}$–16 yr	2 mo	3.8 yr (mean)	47	53	36	25
Smith et al. (143)	100	NS	6–24 mo	6 mo–14 yr	52	48	NS	NS
	46		6 mo		67	33	22	
	38		6–24 mo		47	53	18	
	16		24 mo		19	81	NS	
Pecourd and Genton (144)	83	40 yr (mean)	6 mo	15–236 mo (mean 82)	65	35	6	26[b]
Harris et al. (145)	52	16 yr	6 wk	12 mo	58[c]	42	NS	12

NS, not stated.

[a]Those with food or food-additive triggered urticaria not included.

[b]13% of total group resolved with cessation of specific foods/additives/analgesics.

[c]37% had no symptoms for 12 months; 21% has no symptoms for 6 months.

reaction to a food in the first 2 years of life (12,13). The prevalence of food allergy in prospective studies does not increase after 1 year of age (16). The immediacy of the adverse reaction, the severity, the type of offending food, the organ site involved, and whether the reaction is IgE-mediated appear to affect the persistence of food allergy. In general, severe reactions that occur immediately and that are IgE-mediated persist for longer periods than do more vague, later-onset, and non-IgE-mediated reactions. Immediate reactions occur within 4 hr of ingestion and usually involve milk, eggs, peanut, soy, fish, or nuts. These reactions often affect multiorgan system, including the respiratory system. Delayed reactions often involve grains, meats, and fruits and affect the gastrointestinal and dermatological systems exclusively. These delayed reactions almost never involve the respiratory system or cause anaphylaxis. Regardless of these categorizations, however, the ultimate prognosis for food allergies is good (discussed later).

Those children experiencing immediate-onset reactions to foods often have other evidence of atopic disease, a family history of atopy, and elevated serum IgE (147). These patients are more likely to have a correlation between double-blind, placebo-controlled food challenges (DBPCFC) and a positive skin test or RAST to the food involved (148,149). Dermatitis is the most common symptom experienced, followed by gastrointestinal upset, urticaria, and respiratory symptoms.

The delayed-onset reactivities to food usually occur in the first 3 years of life. Positive delayed-type DBPCFC results are rare after 3 years of age (149). Delayed reactions occur 3–4 hr after ingestion and are almost always confined to the gastrointestinal tract or skin (150). Bock found that no isolated behavioral changes occurred in 1014 DBPCFC in 480 children referred for evaluation of food hypersensitivity. Similarly, no ear problems were found after challenge in children with a history of recurrent or persistent middle ear problems (149).

B. Prognosis

Double-blind, placebo-controlled food challenges are the gold standard for the diagnosis of true adverse reactivity to a food and are discussed in detail in Chapter 21.

As noted earlier (also see Chapter 21), most adverse reactions to food occurring in early childhood are mild and transient. Those with delayed-type reactions are more likely to develop partial or complete tolerance to their food sensitivities (148,150). Reactions are more likely to persist if they are generalized, urticarial, or respiratory. Those with higher RAST or skin-test reactivity also have an increased risk of persistent symptoms

(147,148). After 1 year follow-up in all of the studies cited, no patients worsened in their sensitivity or reactivity (147–153).

Those patients with chronic symptoms generally continue to have positive RAST or skin-test results to the offending food, although these reactions tend to diminish over time. Positive test results tend to lag behind clinical tolerance. Dannaeus found that RAST titers to milk parallel the clinical course (148). Overall, these titers tend to increase between 12 and 18 months of age and decline thereafter. Conversely, Sampson found no correlation between the clinical course and skin reactivity to egg in children with atopic dermatitis (151). As had been observed with other types of atopic disease, total serum IgE is not predictive of outcome (147,153).

Bock followed 480 children from birth to age 3 referred for possible food intolerance (150). Twenty-eight percent of these children had some suspected reactivity to food, but these could be confirmed by challenge in only 8%. The average time until the food was in the diet was 9 months. All but four patients were able to tolerate the offending food by age 3. He found an astonishingly high rate of reactivity to fruits and fruit juices. These reactions were generally dermatological or gastrointestinal, and they were not associated with any skin-test reactivity. Orange was the primary offender, followed by tomato, apple, and grape.

In terms of severe food reactions (anaphylactic, urticarial, asthmatic), Bock found that 80% occurred in the first year of life, with a mean age of onset at 6 months (152). Of nine children studied, all had milk reactions, one had soy reaction, and two had egg reactions. By age 3, three of nine were able to tolerate the offending foods in normal amounts, four were able to tolerate small quantities, and two remained reactive to even small quantities of the offending food.

Atopic dermatitis appears to be the most persistent of all food reactions (12,13,151). Sampson rechallenged 70 patients with challenge-proven food symptoms 1 year after presentation; two-thirds of these had persistent symptoms (152). Dannaeus followed 82 older children (mean age 4.5 years) for 2–5 years: reactions in two-thirds of those with eczema persisted, while half of those with an asthmatic reaction persisted (147).

C. Specific Foods

One-third of those developing milk allergy do so after the first few exposures (147). Of those infants reacting, 60% have an immediate and more severe type of reactivity, whereas 40% have a delayed generally less dramatic reaction. Danneaus followed 47 infants for 1–4 years after the development of milk sensitivity (147). At follow-up, 29% had developed complete tolerance, 32% were able to ingest small amounts without complete tolerance, 21% were improved but had continued significant symptoms, and 18% were unchanged. In the delayed group, 75% developed complete tolerance and only 5% remained unchanged.

Reactivity to egg persists for longer periods. The reactions to egg occur in 90% of reactors by the first several exposures (153). Ford and Taylor found the mean age of onset to be 17 months of age (153). They followed 25 patients with egg sensitivity for 2–2.5 years; at follow-up, 44% had developed complete tolerance.

Reactions to peanut, fish, and nuts have a higher tendency to persist, although the severity improves with time (147). There is a loose correlation between RAST reactivity to these foods and clinical course, although severe reactors are likely to have persistent symptoms.

X. Conclusion

Most allergic conditions are likely to persist, although they tend to improve over time. Even when these conditions appear to remit completely, they frequently recur, even after prolonged intervals. The clinical relevance of these observations are self-evident: Clinicians may be cautiously optimistic about eventual outcome, but blind reassurance that an individual will outgrow allergies or asthma can be quite misleading. Furthermore, the foregoing review leaves little doubt that early environmental intervention must be strongly considered in attempts to minimize the onset of respiratory allergic conditions, especially asthma, in individuals with a strong family history of atopy. In addition, these interventions will likely affect the persistence, recurrence, and possibly the severity of these respiratory allergic conditions once they present.

Roughly 50–60% of children with asthma have symptoms at follow-up, even through three decades (the length of the longest follow-up studies). Most cases, however, become mild and episodic. Children tend to improve into their early teenage years, but approximately 25% of those who have seemingly "outgrown" their asthma have recurrence of symptoms in their late teens or 20s.

Those with the most severe allergic conditions or those with the presence of multiple concurrent atopic conditions are significantly more likely to have continuation of their symptoms. A strong family history of general atopy, an elevated total IgE, and positive specific allergy tests can identify an individual likely to develop allergies, but cannot predict if that individual will have prolonged symptomatic illness. Nevertheless, ongoing exposure to provocative factors, such as passive tobacco smoke, infectious agents, and/or substantial house dust or other indoor allergens, appears to predispose to ongoing symptoms over the years. Empirically this should lead to aggressive environmental intervention, but this has not been specifically studied to ascertain if it affects ultimate outcome.

Any review of the natural history of an illness should attempt to answer two fundamental questions: (a) what are the ultimate implications of disease persistence? and (b) how does treatment or prevention alter disease outcome?

In nonasthmatic atopic conditions, the primary importance of persistence is in the realm of patient comfort. Ongoing problems with allergic rhinitis, atopic dermatitis, or urticaria may be disconcerting to a patient, but the inherent nature of these conditions and the myriad of safe treatment modalities available make prolonged or intractable morbidity unlikely. On the other hand, the implications of ongoing asthma on morbidity and mortality, although specifically unknown, are potentially quite severe. Adults with substantial pulmonary obstruction have repeatedly been shown to have accelerated declines in pulmonary flow studies (FEV1) with age (154). In addition, FEV1 appears to be the single most important predictor of morbidity and mortality in COPD (155). Retrospectively, adults with respiratory symptoms and diminished pulmonary function have stronger histories of childhood respiratory problems (2). Whether asthmatics have an accelerated rate of decline of FEV1 with age (as those with emphysema do) is unclear (103), but is hypothetically quite realistic with the ongoing inflammatory changes that occur in the airways of those with asthma (156). Minimizing this inflammation by preventing it, or attempting to reverse it once present with anti-inflammatory medications, would then be essential. We hope the continuation of many of the studies cited in this chapter will more definitely address the role of childhood asthma in the morbidity and mortality in COPD.

The major pathological role of inflammation in asthma has been recently stressed, as has the consequent universal recommendation of ongoing anti-inflammatory therapy, once again to minimize disease morbidity (157). Over short intervals, aggressive preventative measures and the extended use of anti-inflammatory inhaled medications, such as corticosteroids or cromolyn sodium/nedocromil, are likely to prevent asthma morbidity in children. Over various periods of time (up to 10 years), inhaled corticosteroids have been shown to significantly reduce airway inflammation in adults (158). Unfortunately, how these interventions ultimately influence disease outcome, particularly from childhood into late adulthood, when the complications of COPD arise, is unknown. Early studies, however, suggest that aggressive use of inhaled corticosteroids or cromolyn early in the course of asthma may have extended benefit on the overall natural history of this condition (111,114). This, in conjunction with the general observation that any perpetual adverse stimulation of a body organ is likely to be harmful, appears to more than justify aggressive intervention in the childhood asthmatic.

References

1. Evans R III. Epidemiology and natural history of asthma, allegic rhinitis, and atopic dermatitis. In: Middleton E, Reed CE, Ellis EP, Adkinson NF, Yunginger JW, Busse WW, eds. Allergy: Principles and Practice. Vol. 2. St. Louis: Mosby, 1993:1109–1136.
2. Burrows B, Knudson RJ, Lebowitz MD. The relationship of childhood respiratory illness to adult obstructive airway disease. Am Rev Respir Dis 1977; 115:761–760.
3. Cookson WOCM, Hopkin JM. Dominant inheritance of atopic immunoglobulin-E responsiveness. Lancet 1988; 1:86–88.
4. Anderson HR, Bland JM, Patel S, Packham C. The natural history of asthma in childhood. J Epidemiol Community Health 1986; 40:121–129.
5. Peat JK, Britton WJ, Salome CM, Woolcock AJ. Bronchial hyperresponsiveness in two populations of Australian schoolchildren. II. Relative importance of associated factors. Clin Allergy 1987; 17:283–290.
6. Huang SK, March DG. Immunogenetics of allergic disease. In: Middleton E, Reed CE, Ellis EP, Adkinson NF, Yunginger JW, Busse WW, eds. Allergy: Principles and Practice. Vol. 1. St. Louis: Mosby, 1993:60–72.
8. Gerritsen J, Koeter GH, de Monchy JGR, Knol D. Allergy in subject with asthma from childhood to adulthood. J Allergy Clin Immonol 1990; 85: 116–125.
9. Sporik R, Holgate ST, Platts-Mills TAE, Cogswell JJ. Exposure to house-dust mite allergen (Der p 1) and the development of asthma in childhood. N Engl J Med 1990; 323:502–507.
10. Frick OL, German DL, Mills J. Development of allergy in children. Association with virus infections. J Allergy Clin Immunol 1979; 63:228–241.
11. Busse WW. Respiratory infections: their role in airway responsiveness and the pathogenesis of asthma. J Allergy Clin Immunol 1990; 85:671–683.
12. Van Asperen PP, Kemp AS. The natural history of IgE sensitisation and atopic disease in early childhood. Acta Paediatr Scand 1989; 78:239–245.
13. Cogswell JJ, Mitchell EB, Alexander J. Parental smoking, breast feeding, and respiratory infection in development of allergic diseases. Arch Dis Child 1987; 62:34–38.
14. Zeiger RS, Heller S, Mellon MH, O'Connor R, Hanbunger RN, Schatz M. Effect of combined maternal and infant food allergen avoidance on development of atopy in early infancy: a randomized study. J Allergy Clin Immunol 1989; 84:72–74.
15. Zeiger RS, Heller S, Mellon MH, Halsey JF, Hamburger RN, Sampson HA. Genetic and environmental factors affecting the development of atopy

through age 4 in chldren of atopic parents: a prospective randomized study of food allergen avoidance. Pediatr Allergy Immunol 1992; 3:110–127.

16. Zeiger RS, Heller S. The development and prediction of atopy in high-risk children: follow-up at age seven years in a prospective randomized study of combined maternal and infant food allergen avoidance. J Allergy Clin Immunol 1995; 95:1179–1190.

17. Martinez FD, Wright AL, Taussig LM, Holberg CJ, Halonen M, Morgan WJ. Asthma and wheezing in the first six years of life. N Engl J Med 1995; 332:133–138.

18. Wright AL, Holberg CJ, Martinez FD, Halonen M, Morgan W, Taussig LM. Epidemiology of physician-diagnosed allergic rhinitis in childhood. Pediatrics 1994; 94:895–901.

19. Rowntree S, Cogswell JJ, Platts-Mills TAE, Mithcell EB. Development of IgE and IgG antibodies to food and inhalant allergens in children at risk of allergic disease. Arch Dis Child 1985; 60:727–735.

20. Van Asperen PP, Kemp AS, Mukjhi A. Atopy in infancy predicts the severity of bronchial hyperresponsiveness in later childhood. J Allergy Clin Immunol 1990; 85:790–795.

21. Anderson HR, Bland JM, Peckham CS. Risk factors for asthma up to 16 years of age. Chest 1987; 91:127S–130S.

22. Weiss ST, Tosteson TD, Segal MR, Tager IB, Redline S, Speizer FE. Effects of asthma on pulmonary function in children. Am Rev Respir Dis 1992; 145: 58–64.

23. Hopp RJ, Townley RG, Biven BE, Bewtra AD, Nair NM. The presence of airway reactivity before the development of asthma. Am Rev Respir Dis 1990; 141:2–6.

24. Lebowitz MD, Holberg CJ, Knudson RJ, Burrows B. Longitudinal study of pulmonary function as a predisposing factor for wheezing respiratory illness in infants. N Engl J Med 1988; 319:1112–1117.

25. Burrows B, Halonen M, Lebowitz MD, Knudson RJ, Barbee RA. The relationship of serum immunoglobulin E, allergy skin tests, and smoking to respiratory disorders. J Allergy Clin Immunol 1982; 70:199–204.

26. Burrows B. The natural history of asthma. J Allergy Clin Immunol 1987; 80:373–377.

27. Sunyer J, Anto JM, Sabria J, Roca J, Morell F, Rodriquez-Roison R, Rodrigo MJ. Relationship between serum IgE and airway responsiveness in adults with asthma. J Allergy Clin Immunol 1995:699–706.

28. Kjellman B, Dalen G. Long-term changes in inhalant allergy in asthmatic children. Allergy 1986; 41:351–356.

29. Johsson J, Boe J. Asthma as a child. Symptoms-free as a adult? Ann Allergy 1992; 69:300–301.

30. Soothill JF, Stokes CR, Turner MV, Norma AP, Taylor B. Predisposing factors and the development of reaginic allergy in infants. Clin Allergy 1976; 6:305–319.

31. Foucard T, Sojberg O. A prospective 12-year follow-up study of children with wheezy bronchiolitis. Acta Paediatr Scand 1984; 73:577–583.

32. Kaufman HS. Allergy in the newborn: skin test reactions confirmed by the Prausnitz-Kustner test at birth. Clin Allergy 1971; 1:363–367.

33. Hagy GW, Settipane GA. Prognosis of positive allergy skin tests in an asymptomatic population. J Allergy Clin Immunol 1971; 48:201–211.

34. Ohman JL, Sparrow D, MacDonald MR. New onset wheezing in an older male population: evidence of allergen sensitization in a longitudinal study. J Allergy Clin Immnol 1993; 91:752–757.

35. Martinex FD, Morgan WJ. Wright AL, Holbert CJ, Taussig LM. Diminished lung function as a predisposing factor for wheezing respiratory illness in infants. N Engl J Med 1988; 319:1112–1117.

36. Mongomery GL, Tepper RS. Changes in airway reactivity with age in normal infants and young children. Am Rev Respir Dis 1990; 142:1372–1376.

37. Young S, Le Souef PN, Geelhoed GC, Stick SM, Chir B, Turner KJ, Landau LI. The responsiveness in early infancy. N Engl J Med 1991; 324: 1168–1173.

38. Landau LI, Stick S, Turnbull S, LeSoeuf PN. Increased bronchial responsiveness in infants compared with children. Am Rev Respir Dis 1989; 139: A128–A133.

39. Moreno RH, Hogg JC, Pare PD. Mechanics of airway narrowing. Am Rev Respir Dis 1986; 133:1171–1180.

40. Dave NK, Hopp RJ, Biven RE, Degan J, Bewta AK, Townley RG. Persistence of nonspecific bronchial reactivity in allergic children and adolescents. J Allergy Clin Immunol 1990; 86:147–153.

41. Charpin D, Kleisbauer JP, Lanteaume A, Razzouk H, Vervolet D, Toumi M, Fadel F, Charpin J. Asthma and allergy to house dust mites in populations living at high altitude. Chest 1988; 93:758–761.

42. Wen T. Mites and mite allergy in the Shanghai region of China. In: de Weck AL, Todt A, eds. Mite Allergy. Brussels: UCB Institute, 1988:75–79.

43. Dowse GK, Turner KJ, Stewart GA, Aplers MP, Woolcock AJ. The association between *Dermatophagoides* mites and the increasing prevalence of asthma in village communities within the Papau New Guinea Highlands. J Allergy Clin Immunol 1985; 75:75–80.

44. Kuehr J, Frischer R, Karmaus W, Meinert R, Barth R, Herrman-Kuna E, Forster J, Urbanek R. Early childhood risk factors for sensitization at school age. J Allergy Clin Immunol 1992; 90:358–362.

45. Keuhr J, Frischer T, Meinert R, Barth R, Schraub S, Urbanek R, Karmaus W, Forster J. Sensitization to mite allergens is a risk factor for early and late onset of asthma and for persistence of asthmatic signs in children. J Allergy Clin Immunol 1995; 95:655–662.

46. Neuspiel DR, Rush D, Butler NR, Golding J, Bijur PE, Kurzon M. Parental smoking and post-infancy wheezing in children: a prospective cohort study. Am J Public Health 1989; 79:168–171.

47. Korsgaard J. Mite asthma and residency: a case-control study on the impact of exposure to house dust mites in dwellings. Am Rev Respir Dis 1983; 128: 231–235.

48. Lau S, Falkenhorst G, Weber A, Werthmann I, Lind P, Beuttner-Goetz P, Wahn U. High mite-allergen exposure increases the risk of sensitization in atopic children and young adults. J Allergy Clin Immunol 1989; 83:718–725.

49. Kjellman B, Petterson R. The problem of furred pets in childhood atopic disease. Allergy 1983; 38:65–73.

50. Suoniemi I, Björkstén F, Haahtela T. Dependence of immediate hypersensitivity in the adolescent period on factors encountered in infancy. Allergy 1981; 36:263–268.

51. Björkstén F, Suoniemi I, Koski V. Neonatal birch-pollen contact and subsequent allergy to birch pollen. Clin Allergy 1980; 10:585–591.

52. Peat JK, Britton WJ, Woolcock AJ. Bronchial hyperresponsiveness in two populations of Australian schoolchildren. III. Effect of exposure to environmental allergens. Clin Allergy 1987; 17:291–300.

53. Gelber L, Pollart SM, Chapman MD, Platts-Mills TAE. Serum IgE antibodies and allergen exposure as a risk factor for acute asthma (abstr). J Allergy Clin Immul 1190: 85:193.

54. Glaser J, Johnstone DE. Prophylaxis of allergic disease in the newborn. JAMA 1953; 153:620–624.

55. Gruskay FL. Comparison of breast, cow, and soy feedings in the prevention of onset of allergic disease. Clin Pediatri 1982; 21:487–491.

56. Britten N, Davies JMC, Colley JRT. Early respiratory experience and subsequent cough and peak expiratory flow rate in 36 year old men and women. Br Med J 1987; 294:1317–1320.

57. Dodge R. The effects of indoor pollution on Arizona children. Arch Environ Health 1982; 37:151–215.

58. Ware JH, Ferris JR. BG, Dockery DW, Spengler, JD, Stram DO, Speizer FE. Effect of ambient sulfur oxides and suspended particules on respiratory health in preadolescent children. Am Rev Respir Dis 1986; 133:834–842.

59. Osebold JW, Gerschwin LJ, Zee YC. Studies on the enhancement of allergic lung sensitization by inhalation of ozone and sulfuric acid aerosol. J Environ Pathol Toxicol 1980; 3:221–234.

60. Riedel F, Kramer M, Scheibenboge C, Reiger CHL. Effects of SO_2 exposure on allergic sensitization in the guinea pig. J Allergy Clin Immunol 1988; 82: 527–534.

61. Speizer FE. Asthma and persistent wheeze in the Harvard Six Cities Study. Chest 1990; 98:191S–195S.

62. Schilling RSF, Letai AD, Hui SL, Beck GJ, Schoenberg JB, Bouhuys AH. Lung function, respiratory disease, and smoking in families. Am J Epidemiol 1977; 106:274–283.

63. Ekwo EE, Weinberger MM, Lachenbruch PA, Huntley WH. Relationship of parental smoking and gas cooking to respiratory disease in children. Chest 1983; 64:662–668.

64. Colley JR, Holland WW, Corkhill RT. Influence of passive smoking and parental phlegm on pneumonia and bronchitis in early childhood. Lancet 1974; 1:529–532.

65. Lebowtiz MD, Burrows B. Respiratory symptoms related to smoking habits of family adults. Chest 1976; 69:42–50.

66. Weiss ST, Tager JB, Speizer FE, Rosner B. Persistent wheeze: its relation to respiratory illness, cigarette smoking, and level of pulmonary function in a population sample of children. Am Rev Respir Dis 1980; 122:697–707.

67. Ware JH, Dockney DW, Spiro A, Speizer FE, Ferris BG. Passive smoking, gas cooking, and respiratory health of children living in six cities. Am Rev Respir Dis 1984; 128:366–374.

68. Burchfiel CM, Higgins MW, Keller JB, Howatt WF, Butler WJ, Higgin ITT. Passive smoking in childhood: respiratory conditions and pulmonary function in Tecumseh, Michigan. Am Rev Respir Dis 1986; 133:966–974.

69. Tager IB, Segal MR, Monoz A, Weiss ST, Speizer FE. The effect of maternal cigarette smoking on the pulmonary function of children and adolescents. Am Rev Respir Dis 1987; 136:1366–1370.

70. Hasselblad V, Humble OG, Graham MG, Anderson HS. Indoor environmental determinants of lung function in children. Am Rev Respir Dis 1981; 123: 479–485.

71. Murray AB, Morrison BH. The effect of cigarette smoke from the mother on bronchial responsiveness and severity of symptoms in children with asthma. J Allergy Clin Immunol 1986; 77:575–581.

72. Fergusson DM, Horwood LJ. Parental smoking and respiratory illness during early childhood: a 6 year longitudinal study. Pediatr Plumonol 1985; 1: 99–106.

73. Weitzman M, Gortmaker S, Walker DK, Sobol A. Maternal smoking and childhood asthma. Pediatrics 1990; 85:505–511.

74. Frischer R, Kuehr R, Meinert R, Karmaus W, Barth R, Hermann-Kuna E, Urbanek R. Maternal smoking in early childhood: a risk factor for bronchial responsiveness to exercise in primary-school children. J Pediatr 1992; 121: 17–22.

75. Tashkin DP, Clark VA, Simmons M, Reems C, Coulson AH, Bourque LB, Sayre JW, Detels R, Rokaw S. The UCLA population studies of chronic obstructive respiratory disease: VII. Relationship between parental smoking and children's lung function. Am Rev Respir Dis 1984; 129:891–897.

76. Vedal S, Schenker MB, Samet JM, Speizer FE. Risk factors for childhood respiratory disease: analysis of pulmonary function. Am Rev Respir Dis 1984; 130:187–192.

77. O'Connor GT, Weiss ST, Tager IB, Speizer FE. The effect of passive smoking on pulmonary function and nonspecific bronchial responsiveness in a population based sample of children and young adults. Am Rev Respir Dis 1987; 135:800–804.

78. Colling MH, Moessinger AC, Kleinerman J, Bassi, Rosso P, Colling Am, James LS, Blanc WA. Fetal lung hypoplasia associated with maternal smoking: a morphometric analysis. Pediatr Res 1985; 19:408–412.

79. Magnusson CGM. Maternal smoking influences cord serum IgE and IgD levels and increases the risk for subsequent infant allergy. J Allergy Clin Immunol 1986; 78:898–904.

80. Martinez FD, Antognoni G, Marci F. Parental smoking enhances bronchial responsiveness in nine-year-old children. Am Rev Respir Dis 1988; 138: 518–523.

81. Schwartz J, Gold D, Dockery DW, Weiss ST, Speizer FE. Predictors of asthma and persistent wheeze in a national sample of children in the United States. Am Rev Respir Dis 1990; 142:566–572.

82. Chan KN, Noble-Jamieson CM, Elliman A, Bryan EM, Silverman M. Lung function in children of low birth weight. Arch Dis Child 1989; 64: 1284–1293.

83. Coates Al, Bergsteinsson M, Desmond K, Outbridge FW, Beaudry PH. Long-term pulmonary sequelac of premature birth with and without idiopathic respiratory distress syndrome. J Pediatr 1979; 90:611–616.

84. Holberg CJ, Wright AL, Martinez FD, Morgan WJ, Taussig LM, Group Health Medical Associates. Child day care, smoking by caregivers, and lower respiratory tract illness in the first 3 years of life. Pediatrics 1993; 91: 885–892.

85. Horwood LJ, Fergusson DM, Shannon FT. Social and familial factors in the development of early childhood asthma. Pediatrics 1985; 75:859–868.

86. Murray AB, Morrison BJ. It is children with atopic dermatitis who develop asthma more frequently if the mother smokes. J Allergy Clin Immunol 1990; 86:732–739.

87. Ryssing E, Flensborg EW. Prognosis after puberty for 442 asthmatic children examined and treated on specific allergologic principles. Acta Paediatr 1963; 52:97–105.

88. Buffum WP. The prognosis and asthma in infancy. Pediatrics 1963; 32: 453–455.

89. Barr LW, Logan GB. Prognosis of children having asthma. Pediatrics 1964; 34:856–860.

90. Whatley JW, Guerrant JL. The prognosis of asthma in children. NC Med J 1965; 26:242–243.

91. Buffum WP, Settipane GA. Prognosis of asthma in childhood. Am J Dis Child 1966; 112:214–218.

92. Blair H. Natural history of childhood asthma: 20 year old follow-up. Arch Dis Child 1977; 52:613–619.

93. Jonsson JA, Boe J, Berlin E. The long-term prognosis of childhood asthma in predominantly rural Swedish county. Acta Paediatr Scand 1987; 76: 950–954.

94. Mosfeldt Laursen E, Kaae Hansen K, Backer V, Bach-Mortensen N, Prahl P, Kock C. Pulmonary function in adolescents with childhood asthma. Allergy 1993; 48:267–272.

95. Friberg S, Bevehard S, Graff-Lonnevig V. Asthma from childhood to adult age. Acta Paediatr Scand 1988; 77:424–431.

96. Martin AJ, McLennan LA, Landau LI, Phelan PD. The natural history of childhood asthma to adult life. Br Med J 1980; 280:1897–1400.

97. Kelly WJW, Hudson I, Phelan PD, Pain MCF, Olinsky A. Childhood asthma in adult life: a further study at 28 years of age. Br Med J 1987; 294:1059–1062.

98. Strachan DP, Anderson HR, Bland JM, Peckham C. Asthma as a link between chest illness in childhood and chronic cough and phlegm in young adults. Br Med J 1988; 296:890–893.

99. Giles GG, Lickiss N, Gibson HB, Shaw K. Respiratory symptoms in Tasmanian adolescents: a follow up of the 1961 birth cohort. Austral NZ J Med 1983; 14:631–637.

100. Johnstone DE. A study of the natural histlory of bronchial asthma in children. Am J Dis Child 1968; 115:213–216.

101. Sherrill D, Sears MR, Lebowitz MD, Holdaway MD, Hewitt CJ, Flannery EM, Herbospm GP, Silva PA. The effects of airway hyperresponsiveness, wheezing, and atopy on longitudinal pulmonary function in children: A 6-year follow-up study. Pediatr Pulmonol 1992; 13:78–85.

102. Martin AJ, Landau LI, Phelan PD. Lung function in young adults who had asthma in childhood. Am Rev Respir Dis 1980; 122:609–616.

103. Burrows B, Bloom JW, Traver GA, Cline MG. The course and prognosis of different froms of chronic airways obstruction in a sample from the general population. N Engl J Med 1987; 317:1309–1314.

104. Blackhall M. Ventilating function in subjects with childhood asthma who have become symptom free. Arch Dis Child 1970; 45:363–366.

105. Watanabe H. The effecdt of disodium cromoglycate against bronchial hyperresponsiveness in asthmatic children. J Asthma 1992; 29:117–120.

106. Geller-Bernstein G, Kenett R, Weisglass L, Tsur S, Lahav M, Levin S. Atopic babies with wheezy bronchitis. Allergy 1987; 45:363–366.

107. Kelly WJW, Hudson I, Phelan PD, Pain MCF, Olinsky A. Atopy in subjects with asthma followed to the age 28 years. J Allergy Clin Immunol 1990; 85:548–557.

108. Sims DG, Gardner PS, Weightman D, Turner MW, Soothill JF. Atopy does not predispose to RSV bronchiolitis or postbronchiolitic wheezing. Br Med J 1981; 282:2086–2088.

109. Loren ML, Leung PK, Cooley R, Chai H, Bell RD, Buck VM. Irreversibility of obstructive changes in severe asthma in childhood. Chest 1978; 74:126–129.

110. Kuzemkjo JA. Natural history of childhood asthma. J Pediatr 1980; 97:886–894.

111. Konig P, Shaffer J. Long-term (2–16 yrs) outcome of childhood asthma is influenced by drug therapy: A preview of the international guidelines? (abstr) J Allergy Immunol 1995; 95:223.
112. U.S. Department of Health and Human Services. International Consensus Report on Diagnosis and Treatment of Asthma. Bethesda, MD: National Institutes of Health, 1992.
113. Haahtela T, Jarvinen M, Kava T, Kiviranta K, Koskinen S, Lehtonen D, Nikander K, Persson T, Selroos O, Sovijariv A, Steniu-Aarniala B, Svahn T, Tammivaara R, Laitinen LA. Comparison of B2-agoinst, terbutaline, with an inhaled corticosteroid, budesonide, in newly detected asthma. N Engl J Med 1991; 325:388–392.
114. Haahtela T, Jarvinen M, Kava T, Kiviranta K, Koskinen S, Lehtonen D, Nikander K, Persson T, Selroos O, Sovijariv A, Steniu-Aarniala B, Svahn T, Tammivaara R, Laitinen LA. Effects of reducing or discontinuing inhaled budesonide in patient with mild asthma. N Engl Med 1994; 331:700–705.
115. Johnstone DE, Dutton A. The value of hyposensitization therapy for bronchial asthma in children. A 14 year old study. Pediatrics 1986; 42:793–796.
116. Rackemann FM, Edwards MC. Asthma in children: a follow-up study of 688 patients after an interval of twenty years. N Engl J Med 1952; 246:815–823.
117. Kraepelien S. Prognosis of asthma in childhood with special reference to pulmonary function and the value of specific hyposensitization. Acta Paediatr Scand (suppl) 1963; 140:92–96.
118. Platts-Mills TAE, Tovery ER, Mitchell EB. Reduction of bronchial hyperreactivity during prolonged allergen avoidance. Lancet 1982; 2:675–678.
119. Kaplan BA, Mascie-Taylor CGN. Predicting the duration of childhood asthma. J Asthma 1992; 29:39–48.
120. Stokes GM, Milner AD, Hodges IGC, Groggins, RC. Lung function abnormalities after acute bronchiolitis. J Pediatr 1981; 98:871–874.
121. Welliver RC, Sun M, Rinaldo D, Ogra PL. Predictive value of respiratory syncytial virus-specific IgE responses for recurrent wheezing followiung bronchiolitis. J Pediatr 1986; 109:776–780.
122. Sly PD, Hibbert ME. Childhodd asthma following hospitalization with acute viral bronchiolitis in infancy. Pediatr Pulmonol 1989; 7:153–156.
123. Mok JYO, Simpson H. Symptoms, atopy, and bronchial reactivity after lower respiratory infection in infancy. Arch Dis Child 1984; 59:299–305.
124. NcConnochie KM, Roghmann KL. Bronchiolitis as a possible cause of wheezing in childhood: new evidence. Pediatrics 1984; 74:1–10.
125. Duivermann J, Niejens HF, van Strik R, Affourti MJ, Kerrebijn KF. Lung function and bronchial responsiveness in children who had infantile bronchiolitis. Pediatr Pulmonol 1987; 3:38–44.
126. Pullan CR, Hey EN. Wheezing, asthma, and pulmonary dysfunction 10 years after infection with respiratory syncytial virus in infancy. Br Med J 1982; 284:1065–1069.

127. Kattan M, Keens TG, Lapierre JG, Levison H, Bryan AC. Pulmonary function abnormalities in symptom-free children after bronchiolitis. Pediatrics 1977; 59:683–688.
128. Johnston IDA, Anderson HR, Lambert HP, Patel S. Respiratory morbidity and lung function after whooping-cough. Lancet 1983; 2:1104–1108.
129. Loughlin GM, Taussig LM. Pulmonary function in children with a history of larygotracheobronchitis. J. Pediatr 1979; 59:365–369.
130. Weiss ST, Tager IB, Monoz A, Speizer FE. The relationship of respiratory infections in early childhood to the occurrence of increased levels of bronchial responsiveness and atopy. Am Rev Respir Dis 1985; 131:573–578.
131. Smyth JA, Tabachrick E, Duncan WJ, Reilly BJ, Levison H. Pulmonary function and bronchial hyperreactivity in long-term survivors of bronchopulmonary dysplasia. Pediatrics 1981; 68:333–340.
132. Milligan SWA, Levison H. Lung function in children following repair of tracheo-oesophageal fistula. J Pediatr 1979; 95:24–27.
133. Givan D, Scott P, Jeglum E, Eigen H. Lung function and airway reactivity of children 3 to 10 years after foreign body aspiration. Am Rev Respir Dis 1982; 123 (suppl):158S.
134. Shohat M, Levy G, Levy I, Schonfeld T, Merlob P. Transient tachypnoea of the newborn and asthma. Arch Dis Child 1988; 64:277–279.
135. Rooney JC, Williams HE. The relationship between proved viral bronchiolitis and subsequent wheezing. J Pediatr 1971;78:397–406.
136. Fergusson DM, Horwood LJ, Shannon FT. Parental smoking and respiratory illness in infancy. Arch Dis Child 1980; 55:358–361.
137. Barker DJP, Osmond C. Childhood respiratory infection and adult chronic bronchitis in England and Wales. Br Med J 1986; 293:1271–1275.
138. Rystedt I. Prognostic factors in atopic dermatitis. Acta Derm Venereol 1985; 65:206–213.
139. Roth HL, Kierland RR. The natural history of atopic dermatitis. Arch Dermatol 1964; 89:209–214.
140. Musgrove K, Morgan JK. Infantile eczema: a long term follow-up study. Br J Dermatol 1976; 95:365–372.
141. Quarant JH, Rohr AS, Rachelefsky GS, Siegel SC, Katz RM, Spector SL, Mickey MR. The natural history and response to therapy of chronic urticaria and angioedema. Ann Allergy 1989; 62:421–428.
142. Kauppinen K, Juntunen K, Lanki J. Urticaria in children: retrospective evaluation and follow-up. Allergy 1984; 39:469–472.
143. Smith L, Wray BB, Stafford CT. Outcome of patients with chronic urticaria and angioedema (abstr). J Allergy Clin Immunol 1983; 71(5):159.
144. Pecourd AR, Genton C. Outcome of 83 adults with chronic urticaria and angioedema. J Allergy Clin Immunol 1983; 71:128–133.
145. Harris A, Twarog FJ, Geha RS. Chronic urticaria in children: natural course and etiology. Ann Allergy 1983; 51:161–164.
146. Champion RH, Roberts SOB, Carpenter RG, Roger JH. Urticaria and angioedema: a review of 554 patients. Br J Dermatol 1969; 81:588–593.

147. Dannaeus A, Inganas N. A follow-up study of children with food allergy. Clinical course in relation to serum IgE- and IgG-antibody levels to milk, egg, and fish. Clin Allergy 1981; 11:533–539.

148. Dannaeus A, Johansson SGO. A follow-up study of infants with adverse reaction to cow's milk. Acta Paediatr Scand 1979; 68:377–382.

149. Bock SA, Atkins FM. Patterns of food hypersensitivity during sixteen years of double-bind, placebo-controlled food challenges. J Pediatr 1990; 17: 561–567.

150. Bock SA. Prospective appraisal of complaints of adverse reactions to foods in children during the first 3 years of life. Pediatrics 1987; 79:683–688.

151. Sampson HA. Late-phase response to foods in atopic dermatitis. Hosp Pract 1987; 22:111–128.

152. Bock SA. Natural history of severe reactions to food in young children. J Pediatr 1985; 107:676–680.

153. Ford RPK, Taylor B. Natural history of egg hypersensitivity. Arch Dis Child 1982; 57:649–652.

154. Burrows B, Earle RH. Course and prognosis of chronic obstructive lung disease. N Engl J Med 1969; 280:397–404.

155. Burrows B, Knudson RJ, Camilli AE, Lyle SK, Lebowitz MD. The "horse-racing effect" and predicting decline in forced expiratory volume in one second from screening spirometry. Am Rev Respir Dis 1987; 135:788–793.

156. Van Schayck CP, Dompeling E, Van Herwaarden CLA. Interacting effects of atopy and bronchial hyperresponsiveness on the annual decline in lung function and the exacerbation rate in asthma. Am Rev Respir Dis 1991; 144: 1297–1301.

157. McFadden ER Jr. Pathogenesis of asthma. J Allergy Clin Immunol 1984; 73: 413–424.

158. Lundgren R, Soderberg M, Horstedt P, Stenling R. Morphological studies of bronchial mucosal biopsies from asthmatics before and after ten years of treatment with inhaled steroids. Eur Respir J 1988; 1:883–889.

30

Prevention of Allergic Disease in Infancy

ROBERT S. ZEIGER

Kaiser Permanente Medical Center, San Diego
and University of California, San Diego, School of Medicine
La Jolla, California

I. Overview of Allergy Prevention

An urgency exists to identify and develop effective strategies to prevent allergic disease, owing to the formidable worldwide increase in both the prevalence and morbidity of atopic disorders. Potential approaches in this effort include modulating the primary factors responsible for the atopic state through genetic, immunological, and environmental manipulation. The unraveling of the genetic basis of atopy by identifying candidate genes as detailed in Chapter 27 represents a major scientific effort at the present time and should provide vital knowledge which should aid in allergy prevention in the future. In the very near future, effective immunomodulatory regimens which downregulate, abrogate, or turn off the cellular, cytokine, or humoral (IgE) components of allergy should be available for clinical use. However, the best hope at the present to prevent allergic disease relies on environmental engineering, which refers to active efforts directed at reducing the allergenic and adjuvant load to which an atopic-prone infant may be exposed. Efforts to prevent allergic disease based on IgE-mediated responses can be directed at the three stages of allergic sensitization; primary, secondary, and tertiary (1):

1. Primary prevention: inhibiting IgE sensitization
2. Secondary prevention: blocking disease expression despite prior IgE sensitization
3. Teritiary prevention: suppressing symptoms after disease expression

Strategies to prevent allergic disease have met with considerable difficulty at all of these stages due to limitations in scientific knowledge and societal compliance and resources. Though primary prevention of atopy is optimal, secondary prevention may be required to supplement primary prevention and to serve as a fallback option to families uninterested in allergy prevention until real markers of atopic risk are identified in their offspring. Tertiary prevention, the arena most familiar to practicing allergists, is instituted once manifestations of allergic disease are recognized. For effective allergy prevention, these three stages should be integrated both in the actions of the physician and the minds of the at-risk family. Moreover, the success of prevention programs must be judged by satisfying specific criteria, including the ability to (a) predict those at high risk, (b) demonstrate effectiveness of the intervention strategy, (c) utilize acceptable interventions, (d) minimize adverse effects, and (e) generate cost-effective efforts. Presently, no allergen avoidance intervention study has met all of the above requisites.

Studies suggest that a critical time exists early in infancy in which the genetically programmed atopic-prone infant is at increased risk to become sensitized to allergens when exposed to specific allergens. As such, prompt perinatal identification of such at-risk neonates is important if preventive efforts are to be efficacious, safe, and cost-effective. Research has uncovered several genetic and immunological factors/markers significantly associated with the subsequent development of allergic disease (Table 1); however, at the present time none possesses adequate sensitivity or specificity for practical screening of neonates to reveal those most at risk for atopy (see Chapter 28) (2). Future research efforts may reveal better predictive markers. Such markers could include specific DNA polymorphisms when the genes for atopy are identified (see Chapter 27) (3).

With respect to the institution of antiallergy measures, certain major atopic risk factors, such as atopic heredity, male gender, and nonwhite ethnicity, are completely unmodulatable, while other factors, such as birth month, low socioeconomic status, and urban residence, are relatively unmodulatable. Important atopic risk factors (Chapter 28) which are more modulatable include (a) raising low atopic health consciousness, (b) delaying introduction of allergenic foods during infancy, (c) reducing household dust mite, cockroach, and dander levels, and (d) reducing environmental

Table 1 Risk Factors and Markers for Development of Atopy

Genetic and immunological
  Atopic family history (biparental > uniparental > none, with risk > with
    maternal disease)
  Increased cord blood IgE
  Lambda MS.51 marker on chromosome 11q
  Increased cord IgE-binding factors (soluble FcεRII)
  Increased total serum IgE in infancy and childhood
  Significant specific IgE antibody (skin or serum)
  Decreased T cells (CD8+ subset) in cord blood and in infancy in high-risk
  Decreased cytokine gamma-interferon/IL-4 in high-risk
  Increased blood eosinophilia and nasal basophilia in infancy
  Increased nasal eosinophilia by age 1 year
  Increased monocyte phosphodiesterase activity
  Cord blood thrombocytopenia
  Increased cord blood linoleic acid
  Decreased breast milk long chain polyunsaturated fatty acid levels
  Male gender and low birth weight
Specific environmental stimulation
  Feeding practices
    Brief breast feeding
    Food allergens in breast milk
    Early solid foods
    Time of weaning
  Magnitude of allergen exposure
  Early allergen exposure (foods, mites, pets, month of birth)
Nonspecific environmental stimulation
  Intrauterine exposure to drugs
  Infections (viral and bacterial)
  Passive tobacco smoke pre- and postnatally
  Pollutants
  Tightly ventilated houses
  Household dampness

pollution and environmental tobacco exposure (ETS). A strategy for both
the identification of high-risk infants and the institution of preventive measures directed at all three stages of allergy prevention (4) is presented in
Table 2. This chapter evaluates the successes and failures of investigative
efforts directed at overcoming these atopic risk factors in the context of
the three stages of allergy prevention and offers "practical" guidelines for
the prevention of allergies.

Table 2 Risk Factors Affecting the Development of Atopy from Fetus to Symptomatic Infant and Allergy Prevention Stages to Modulate These Factors

Risk factors	Proband	Prevention stage	Desired outcome
Maternal ETS Low birth weight Male gender Allegens (?) Medications (?)	*High-risk fetus* Atopic parents	*Primary* Encourage ETS cessation Optimize prenatal care Educate on lactation	*Nonsensitized*
Allergens ETS Air pollution Viruses	*High-risk infant* Atopic parents Elevated cord IgE	*Primary* Implement Tables 7 and 9	*Nonsensitized*
Same as above "Atopic march"	*Sensitized infant* Egg (allergen)-IgE Eosinophilia Atopic condition	*Secondary* Active infant screening Impede atopic march Implement Tables 7 and 9 Immunomodulation	*Remission*

Same as above	*Symptomatic infant*
	Atopic disorder
		Tertiary
		Allergen avoidance
		  (Table 9)
		Anti-inflammatory
		  medication
		Immunomodulation
		Virus vaccines
		RSV gamma-globulin
			Asymptomatic

ETS = environmental tobacco smoke.

II. Primary Prevention of Allergy (Table 3)

Grulee and Sanford reported 60 years ago that breast feeding compared to cow's milk feeding reduced the development of eczema sevenfold in a cohort of nearly 20,000 infants (5). Conflicting studies have followed. The failure to appreciate and account for the many routes of food exposure may be responsible for some of these studies' disparate findings. Chicken's egg, cow's milk, and peanut represent those foods in the United States most likely to induce food specific-IgE (sensitization) in infancy. The newborn potentially may become exposed to these and other food allergens through such routes as the placenta, breast milk, formula, solid food, and even inadvertently through airborne droplets or floor dusts. The relative importance of these routes in the development of food allergy and the successes or failures of preventive efforts to interfere with these exposures will be critically evaluated in order to develop useful prevention recommendations.

A. Avoidance of Allergenic Foods During Pregnancy

The fetus has been reported to mount specific IgE responses to foods (6,7) and T-cell responses to milk and egg proteins (8). Specific food IgE responses prenatally probably represent uncommon occurrence or a false positive results, since many studies have detected their presence in less than 0.3% of monitored pregnancies (1). Additional evidence against the existence of clinically meaningful specific-IgE food sensitization in utero emanates from food allergen avoidance studies initiated during pregnancy. These studies showed that food allergen avoidance during pregnancy did not affect the development of atopy in infancy (9–11). Specifically, two randomized studies compared third-trimester-pregnancy maternal diets void of milk, egg, and peanut or with limited ingestion of milk or eggs (12,13) to either normal (9–11) or high (12,13) exposure to these foods. Both food allergen avoidance regimens prenatally failed to reduce the development of atopy in high-risk infants maintained on a hypoallergenic feeding regimen postnatally (breast feeding or casein hydrolysate feeding until 3 months of age, solid foods after 4 months, and cow's milk after 6 months) (Table 3). No differences were found between these infants with respect to (a) cord blood IgE levels, (b) incidence of food sensitization, or (c) development of atopic diseases at 6 to 60 months (9–13). Given the strong experimental evidence that (a) intrauterine food sensitization occurs rarely and (b) restricted third-trimester maternal diets fail to affect atopic disease and IgE sensitization to egg, cow milk, or peanut postnatally, it is inappropriate, contraindicated, and potentially nutritionally harmful to mother and fetus (9–14) to advocate such food avoidance regimens during pregnancy for the purpose of preventing food allergy.

B. Breast Feeding

It should be clearly stated at the onset that breast milk and feeding represents the ideal nutritional, immunological, physiological, and psychological environment for the newborn. As such, breastfeeding should be attempted in all neonates, including those with atopic risk, even though small quantities of food allergens may be present in breast milk.

Table 3 Prospective Randomized Controlled Studies of Food Allergen Avoidance on the

Study (Ref.)	Subjects (*n*)	Mom pregnancy diet	Mom lactation diet	Infant diet
Magnusson et al. (9–11)	197	3rd trimester (No egg, CM) vs. No restriction	None	Breast +/or casein hydrolysate (3 mo); Solids (>4 mo); CM (>6 mo); egg/fish (>9 mo)
Lilja et al. (12,13)	162	3rd trimester (no egg, CM) vs. No restrictions	None	Exclusive breast (5–6 mo) vs. No restrictions
Chandra et al. (79)	71	Entire pregnancy (No egg, CM, fish, peanut, beef) vs. No restrictions	Entire lactation (Same as pregnancy) vs. No restrictions	Exclusive breast (5–6 mo) vs. No restrictions
Zeiger et al. (14,66,80,81)	288	3rd trimester (No egg, CM, peanut) vs. No restrictions	Entire lactation (same as pregnancy) vs. No restrictions	Breast +/or casein hydrolysate (12 mo); Solids (>6 mo); CM, soy, corn (>12 mo); egg, fish, peanut (>24 mo) vs. AAP guidelines
Hattevig et al. (43–45)	115	None	1st 3 Mo of lactation (no egg, CM, fish) vs. No restrictions	Breast +/or casein hydrolysate (6 mo); CM/solids (>6 mo); egg/fish (>9 mo)
Chandra et al. (46)	97	None	Entire lactation (No egg, CM, peanuts, soy, fish) vs. No restrictions	Exclusive breast (~6 mo), Solids (~6 mo)
Chandra et al. (46)	124 (3 groups)	None	None	Exclusive casein hydrolysate vs. CM or soy; No breast feeding
Chandra et al. (54,56)	288 (4 groups)	None	None	Exclusive partial whey hydrolysate (6 mo) vs. CM, soy, or breast-feeding 6 mo
Lucas et al. (18)	75 (preterm)	None	None	Human milk vs. preterm formula 1.5 mo
Vanderplas et al. (70)	67	None	None	Partial whey hydrolysate vs. CM formula 6 mo
Arshad et al. (82,83)	120	None	Entire lactation (No egg, CM, fish, nuts) vs. No restrictions	Breast +/or soy hydrolysate (9 mo); CM/soy (9 mo); egg (11 mo); all others (12 mo) plus mite avoidance (acaracide and encasing) vs. No restriction
Mallet/Henocq (71)	165	None	None	Pregestimil vs. CM formula ± breast milk + no solids 4 mo
Halken et al. (72)	141	None	None	Breast (*n* = 20), Nutramigen (*n* = 59) vs. Profylac (*n* = 62) and delayed solids & CM for 6 mo

Abbreviations: CM (cow's milk), AD (atopic dermatitis), CMA (CM allergy), CMPI (CM protein intol-
yr (year); *p* < .05; **p* < .01.
Source: Ref. 158.

Development of Atopic Disease in Infants of Atopic Parents

Follow-up	SPT/RAST	DBPCFC	Atopic disease	Comments
5 yr.	Not significant	No	Not significant	Pregnancy diet had no effect on infant atopy, SPT, or IgE
1.5 yr	Not significant	No	Not significant	Pregnancy diet had no effect on infant atopy, SPT, or IgE
1 yr	Not determined	No	Reduced AD severity by 1 yr*	No immunological or food challenge confirmation; benefit probably derives from infant diet and/or maternal lactation diet and not pregnancy diet
7 yr	Reduced CM-IgE prevalence at 1* and 2 yr**	Yes; half consented, 80% positive challenges	Reduced current prevalence of AD* & food allergy** at 1 yr; asthma & AR unaffected by 7 yr	Benefits probably derive from infant diet and/or maternal lactation diet and not pregnancy diet (see Magnusson and Lilja above)
4 yr	Reduced # of CM +/or egg-IgE tests at 3 mo**	No	Reduced AD at 3**, 6*, and 48** mo	Groups assigned by hospital rather than by true randomization
1.5 yr	Not determined	No	Reduced AD by 1.5 yr*	No immunological or food challenge confirmation
1.5 yr	Not determined	No	Reduced AD* by 1.5 yr with casein hydrolysate	AD prevalence exceptionally high; no immunological or food challenge confirmation
1.5yr	No difference in CM-IgE at 2 and 6 mo	No	Reduced 6 and 12 mo AD cumulative prevalence*	No immunological or food challenge confirmation; cord blood + CM/Soy-IgE unexplainably high incidence
1.5 yr	Not determined	No	Reduced AD by 1.5 yr*	No immunological or food challenge confirmation; only randomized study of human milk compared to CM feedings
1 yr	No difference in CM-IgE at 2 and 6 mo	Blinded but not DBPCFC	Reduced CMA/CMPI prevalence at 6** and 12* mo	Exceptionally high 6 mo prevalence of AD (77%) and CMA/CMPI (34%) in controls; CMA/CMPI during ($n = 1$) and after ($n = 3$) hydrolsate
2 yr	Not significant at 1 yr, significantly reduced at 2 yr	No	Reduced AD* and asthma* by 1 yr; any atopy at 2 yr	Control group with more smoking mothers ($p = 0.11$), but multivariate analyses confirmed benefit; protective effect seen after exclusion of smokers
4 yr	Not determined	No	Reduced eczema at 4 mo ($p = .07$), 2 & 4 yr ($p < .01$)	Dropout 25% at 1 yr, no specific IgE or accounting for smoking, etc.
1.5 yr	CM-IgE in 4/5 with CMPA/CMPI	Open challenges	CMPA/CMPI = 1/20 vs. 1/59 vs. 3/62, in grps, respectively	Overall CMPA/CMPI = 3.6% vs. 15/75 (20%) in similar 1985 cohort without allergy-preventive efforts

erance), AR (allergic rhinitis), DBPCFC (double-blind, placebo-controlled, food challenge), mo (month),

Protective Effect of Breast Milk on Allergen Exposure and Absorption

By reducing both exposure to and intestinal absorption of food allergens, breast milk may decrease allergic sensitization (2). Specifically, breast milk functions to inhibit the increase in food antigen absorption which occurs early postnatally in newborn animals (15). Similarly, in humans, significantly higher antigen absorption occurs in preterm than in term neonates (16), which may place preterm or low-birth-weight infants at increased risk to develop IgE sensitization to foods, particularly cow's milk formula. In addition, a significant increase in peripheral blood histamine release to cow's milk has been reported in preterm infants fed cow's milk compared to banked breast milk, a response which correlated inversely with birth weight and gestational age (17,18). The specific factor(s) contained in breast milk responsible for these effects remain speculative but include the protective capacity of human breast milk (a) immunoglobulins, especially sIgA, to inhibit intestinal absorption of food antigens (19), although conflicting data exist (20), and (b) mucosal growth factor to facilitate early maturation of the gut (closure) (21).

Regarding the potential protective effect of breast milk sIgA, an uncontrolled study reported that total sIgA and milk-specific IgA antibodies to whole cow's milk and casein were significantly lower in breast milk from mothers of allergic compared to nonallergic infants (22). In contrast to the above study, a prospective controlled study of 123 high-atopic-risk neonates followed from birth and breast fed for at least 4 months noted that maternal breast milk anticow's milk secretory IgA levels were above the median significantly more frequently in those infants developing food allergy by 1 and 2 years (Zeiger and Machtinger, unpublished observations). The discordant findings of these two studies probably cannot arise solely from the study of atopic-prone neonates in the latter and unselected neonates in the former. Studies are needed to resolve these differences.

Effect of Breast Versus Cow's Milk Feeding on Allergic Sensitization and Allergic Disease

Longstanding debate, raised over 60 years ago, exists today regarding whether breast feeding prevents, reduces, delays, or increases the development of allergic disease. Even recent prospective natural history studies note conflicting results (23–29). Such disparate findings may arise from differences in study design, quality, size, and duration. The topic will be discussed only briefly, since several comprehensive reviews of this subject have been published recently (1,2,30). Discussion will concentrate on the prospective studies which compared the effect of breast to cow's milk feeding on the development of atopy. For ease of discussion they have been divided into those studies that reported either that breast feeding was effective (Table 4A) or ineffective (Table 4B) to prevent the development of atopy. Although the quantity of published studies supports the beneficial nature of breast feeding in reducing allergic disease development when compared to cow's milk formula feeding (Table 4A), several recent prolonged exclusive breast-feeding investigations of atopic-prone infants failed to demonstrate any allergy-protective role of breast feeding (Table 4B). The principal design weakness inherent in all but one of these investigations (Tables 4A and Table 4B) was the failure to randomize the study groups, which would tend to bias recruitment and raise several confounding variables. For example, mothers who breast rather formula feed frequently smoke less, attain higher parental educational level, and delay day care, characteristics associated with health consciousness (31). Such behaviors potentially would reduce the risk of developing food and aeroallergent allergies, since they would be expected to delay introduction of solid food, decrease exposure to viruses, and reduce second-hand smoke inhalation (2). In addition to the failure to randomize groups, these breast-versus-cow's milk comparison studies were individually flawed by such shortcomings as (a) nonblinded evaluations, (b) absence of immunological confirmation of diagnoses, (c) failure to document compliance to dietary regimen, (d) inadequate sample size, (e) brief duration of breast feeding, and (f) differences in environmental control measures between groups.

The only prospective randomized study that has compared the effects of human milk versus cow's milk feeding on atopy development studied preterm infants (18), a cohort theoretically at greater risk of allergic sensitization due to enhanced intestinal absorption of dietary antigens (17). Consistent with these findings, a prospective, randomized, and controlled study of 446 preterm neonates demonstrated that early exposure to cow's milk formula compared to banked breast milk increased the risk of developing allergic disease by 18 months (particularly eczema) (odds ratio 3.6 with 95% confidence interval 1.4–9.1) in the subgroup of neonates with an allergic family history (18). Unfortunately, no objective immunological determination of IgE sensitization or food allergy was made.

These limitations of study design preclude reaching definitive conclusions regarding the potential benefits of breast feeding in reducing allergic disease. The detection of dietary allergens in breast milk (1) and the early sensitization of exclusively breast-fed infants to egg and milk (32) add complexity to this situation. These findings indicate that institution of maternal dietary restrictions during exclusive breast feeding might be necessary to prevent food allergy. The design weaknesses of these studies (Tables 4A and 4B) do not permit making definitive conclusions regarding

Table 4 Prospective, Nonrandomized Studies Comparing the Effectiveness of Breast Compared to Cow's Milk Feeding on the Development of Allergic Disease

Study (Ref.)	Year	B(*n*)/CM(*n*)	Interval (yr)	Eczema (E)/ allergy (A)/ asthma (As) outcomes	Design weaknesses[a]
A. Studies supportive of allergy-preventive effect from breast feeding					
Grulee (5)	1936	9749/1707	0.75	E: 0.6% B vs. 4% CM**	2, 3, 4, 5, 6
Matthew (144)	1977	23/19	1	E: 13% B vs. 47% CM*	1, 2, 3, 5, 7, 8, 9
Saarinen (145)	1979	25/19	3	E: 12% B vs. 26% CM*	2, 3, 5, 9
Chandra (146)	1979	37/37	3	E: 11% B vs. 59% CM**	2, 3, 5, 9, 10
Ziering (147)	1979	25/25	2	A: 32% B vs. 65% CM*	2, 3, 5, 9
Gruskay (148)	1982	48/201	15	A: 28% B vs. 53% CM*	2, 3, 5, 6
Businco (7)	1983	34/41	2	A: 18% B vs. 37% CM#	1, 2, 3, 5, 9
Pratt (149)	1984	19/58	5	E: 16% B vs. 38% CM*	2, 5, 6, 9
Chandra (150)	1985	72/48	2	A: 17% B vs. 52% CM**	2, 3, 5, 9
B. Studies nonsupportive of allergy-preventive effect from breast feeding ($p > .1$)					
Kaufman (151)	1972	38/54	2	E: ~50% B and CM	1, 2, 3, 5, 8, 9
Halpern (152)	1973	193/349	0.5–7	A: ~16% B and CM	1, 2, 3, 4, 5, 6
Kaufman (153)	1976	38/56	2	E: 32% B vs. 23% CM	1, 2, 3, 5, 8, 9
Hide (154)	1981	204/62	1	A: 45% B vs. 53% CM	1, 2, 3, 5, 6, 7
Gordon (155)	1982	112/85	2	A: 22% B vs. 13% CM	1, 2, 3, 5
Van Asperen (156)	1984	54/25	1.3	E: 52% B vs. 40% CM	2, 3, 5, 8, 9
Van Asperen (156)	1984	19/60	1.3	E: 58% B vs. 45% CM	2, 3, 5, 8, 9
Hide (157)	1985	35/132	4	E: 17% B vs. 15% CM As: 9% B vs. 11% CM	2, 6, 8

Abbreviations: B = breast feeding; CM = cow's milk feeding.
[a]Design weaknesses: 1 = late solids in B; 2 = not randomized; 3 = unmasked; 4 = unselected sample; 5 = compliance not documented; 6 = no immunological documentation; 7 = differential environmental control in B; 8 = dropout high; 9 = inadequate sample size; 10 = B < 4 months.
#$p = .08$; *$p < .05$; **$p < 0.01$.
Source: Ref. 1.

the relative value of breast feeding in the prevention of food allergy, atopic dermatitis, or asthma. Notwithstanding, the promotion of prolonged breast feeding for all infants must be stressed to provide infants with the ideal source of nutrition, immunological factors, intestinal maturation, and infant–mother bonding. Whether breast feeding prevents food allergy remains to be settled, but the weight of evidence appears to support its protective effect; although, as noted, conflicting data exists. The role of breast feeding in reducing infectious asthma during infancy by transferring neutralizing viral antibodies to the infant has been cited and appears real, particularly those episodes caused by respiratory syncytial virus (RSV) infections (2).

Maternal Avoidance of Allergenic Food During Lactation

Food allergens in human breast milk have been implicated in causing food-specific IgE sensitization and food allergy in about 6% of high-risk infants exclusively breast fed, with initial symptoms occurring at the time of the reported initial direct food exposure (2,33). Moreover, milk-specific IgE has been reported commonly in and even sometimes more often in breast-fed than in formula-fed infants (34). Nanogram concentrations of food allergens in breast milk may be responsible for this phenomenon. Thus far three bovine milk antigens [β-lactoglobulin (BLG), casein, and gamma-globulin] (22,35–38), chicken's egg ovalbumin (OVA) (39), and gliadin (40) have been detected in most samples of breast milk from mothers consuming these foods. These food allergens appear in breast milk within 2 to 6 hr and may persist for days after maternal ingestion of 4 oz of cow's milk, 1 raw egg, or 1 slice of bread. Food antigens were rarely detected in breast milk from mothers avoiding these food substances. Maternal handling of food antigens generally has been found to be similar whether mother or infant are atopic or nonatopic (22,38,40), although other studies report higher breast milk levels of cow's milk protein in infants who develop "atopiclike" symptoms (37) and colic (38). The wide overlap of values suggests that these findings may not be clinically relevant. Molecular sizing of the food antigens in breast milk suggests that these antigens may maintain their potential for infant sensitization (41,42). However, though the levels of food allergens in breast milk exist in sufficient quantities to trigger allergic reactions in sensitized infants, it is unknown whether such quantities can *prime* the infant's immune system to produce food-specific IgE.

Recognition of the existence of potentially allergenic food antigens in breast milk led to attempts to evaluate the effect of maternal diets during lactation on the development of atopy (Table 3) (43–46). Avoidance of egg, cow's milk, and fish was compared to an unrestricted diet during the first 3 months of lactation. Mothers on the lactation diet were at one hospital while mothers on an unrestricted diet were at another hospital providing their health care in Sweden. Infants in both groups were placed on hypoallergenic diets for 6 months. This prospective 48-month study noted a reduction in eczema at 3, 6, and 48 months but not at 18 months in infants in the lactation diet group (43–45). The incidence of IgE antibodies to milk or egg at 3 months was significantly higher in the group with unrestricted lactation. Infants in both the restricted and unrestricted lactation groups developed similar levels of total serum IgE and specific-IgG antibodies to OVA and BLG from birth to 18 months (44). Moreover, restriction of milk and egg during lactation for only 3 months failed to suppress the IgG OVA or BLG responses after these foods were introduced to the infant after 6 months of life. The observation that serum levels of IgG antibodies to OVA increased in infants prior to introduction of eggs into the infants' diet suggests that the ng/mL quantities of egg white antigen in breast milk might be sufficient to induce an IgG antibody response in infants. The association of an augmented IgG OVA response noted concomitant with an increased specific IgE response to egg white suggests that IgG OVA, rather than protecting against the development of an IgE response, merely represents the inherent immunological response of high-responder infants. The failure to randomize the groups weakens the study to some uncertain degree.

Confirmation of the above findings was reported from a prospective, controlled study of 97 infants born to atopic parents (46). Mothers planning to breast feed exclusively for 6 months received random allocation to either a lactation diet avoiding milk products, eggs, fish, peanuts, and soy or a diet with *no* restrictions. The lactation restricted diet appeared to halve the cumulative incidence of eczema by 18 months (Table 3) (46). Since the relationship of the eczema to food sensitization was not investigated immunologically or by food challenge, the results of this study must be considered with reservations.

It is essential to confirm the above findings by more definitive randomized studies that correlate disease occurrence to food sensitization before maternal lactation avoidance diets are universally recommended for the purpose of preventing food allergy and atopic dermatitis in infancy.

C. Effect of Soy Feeding on Development of Atopy (Table 5)

Initial retrospective studies (47–49) extolled the value of soy formula feeding in reducing atopy. A subsequent prospective randomized study by the same group (50) reported that soy feeding reduced asthma and perennial

Table 5 Prospective Randomized Studies of Soy (S) Versus Cow's Milk (CM) Feedings on Development of Allergy in Infancy

Study [yr] (Ref.)	S(n)/CM(n)	Allergy outcome
Johnstone and Dutton [1966] (50)	115/120	Asthma <3 yr ($p < .05$) Chronic rhinitis <6 yr ($p < .01$) No difference in eczema or hay fever by 10 yr
Brown et al. [1969] (51)	85/196	No difference in allergies by 1.5 yr
Kjellman and Johansson [1979] (52)	23/25	No difference in allergies by 3 yr (S = 74%; CM = 60% in infants of biparental atopy)
Miskelly et al. [1988] (53)	228/233	No difference in allergies by 1 yr
Chandra et al. [1989] (46)	40/41	No different in eczema by 1.5 yr

Source: Ref. 1.

rhinitis by 3 years without affecting the development of atopic dermatitis in infancy or hay fever during childhood. Subsequent randomized prospective studies of infants, generally from atopic families, uniformly failed to demonstrate any reduction in the development of atopy in infancy and childhood derived from soy compared to cow's milk feeding (46,51–54). These findings are consistent with studies that verified the immunogenic and allergenic capacity of soybean protein (55). These results suggest that intact soybean protein formulas should not be considered hypoallergenic nor used in attempts to prevent food allergy in infancy.

D. Effect of Hypoallergenic Protein Hydrolysate Formula Feeding on Development of Allergic Disease

Allergenicity / Immunogenicity

Protein hydrolysate (PH) formulas such as Nutramigen and Presgestimil were developed over 50 years ago to treat infants with gastrointestinal food intolerances, food allergies, and malabsorption who were unable to tolerate ingested proteins. The first PH formulas were extensively hydrolyzed to peptides typically below 1500 Da by sequential chemical (mixed pancreatic proteases) hydrolysis of casein protein followed by activated-charcoal absorption. The objective of this process was to obtain low-molecular-weight peptides with from 6 to 9 amino acids, since such peptides behave nonimmunologically upon injection into animals (56). Extensive hydrolysis of proteins for infant formula attempts to reduce/eliminate allergenicity and immunogenicity but retain nutritional adequacy and palatability at reasonable cost. Preclinical screening of these hydrolysates revealed (a) absence of animal anaphylaxis by PCA (suggesting molecular weight <3400 Da), (b) absence of any intact proteins, (c) over 99% of the peptides less than 1500 Da in molecular weight, and (d) less than 1 millionth of the protein determinant equivalence of the original protein (57).

Commercially available protein hydrolysates in the United States reveal different biological and immunological characteristics (Table 6). The two casein hydrolysates, Nutramigen and Alimentum, represent extensively hydrolyzed formulations (58,59). On the other hand, the whey hydrolysate, Good Start, is only partially hydrolyzed, containing large amounts of peptides greater that 4000 Da and more than 2–3 logs higher levels of immunologically identifiable cow's milk proteins than either of the casein hydrolysates (58–60). Recently, the two extensively hydrolyzed casein PH hydrolysates (Nutramigen and Alimentum) were demonstrated to be hypoallergenic as defined by the American Academy of Pediatrics (95% con-

Table 6 Characteristics of Several Commercial Protein Hydrolysate (PH) Formulae

Characteristic	Nutramigen	Alimentum	Good Start
Introduced in United States	1942	1989	1989
Formula	CM casein PH	CM casein PH	CM whey PH
Oil	Corn	Safflower	Coconut/ palm
Carbohydrate	Corn syrup solids	Sucose tapioca	Lactose
Peptides >1500 Da	Rare	Rare	Frequent
CM antigen $<10^{-6}$ of original CM	Yes	Yes	No
+ DBPCFC in IgE-CMA patients	Rare	Rare	Frequent
Hypoallergenic	Yes	Yes	No
Recommended in CMA	Yes	Yes	No
Recommended in allergy prevention	Yes	Yes	?

CM = cow's milk; CMA = cow's milk allergy; DBPCFC = double-blind, placebo-controlled food challenge.
Source: Ref. 1.

fidence that at least 90% of cow's milk-allergic children will tolerate the PH formula) by double-blind, placebo-controlled food challenges (DBPCFC), the gold standard in food testing (58). In contrast, the partially hydrolyzed whey hydrolysate, Good Start, possesses an inadequate immunochemical profile and too frequently induces allergic reactions in quantities from 1 to 15 mL in infants with cow's milk allergy (1,2,61). Although the casein hydrolysates have received hypoallergenic labeling and the safety and hypoallergenicity of Nutramigen has been documented in more than 50 years of safe commercial use in milk-sensitive infants and children (1), they *are not* completely nonallergenic since in rare instances they have been implicated in allergic reactions (62) or intolerances (63) in cow's milk-sensitive subjects. [An extensively hydrolyzed whey PH formula (Profylac), unavailable in the United States, has recently been shown also to be hypoallergenic (64).] It remains prudent, therefore, to introduce these extensively hydrolyzed PH formulas for the first time in cow's milk-allergic patients under the direct supervision of physicians experienced and equipped to treat anaphylaxis (1). These findings should dissuade clinicians from using partially hydrolyzed milk protein formulas in cow's milk-allergic patients (1,59).

Prevention of Atopy

After breast milk, the formula with the least immunogenic and allergenic potential should be fed to high-risk infants in the attempt to prevent food allergy. As noted above, early studies demonstrated in animal sensitizing models that extensive PH evidenced no sensitizing capacity, while formulas such as evaporated milk, purified intact lactose-free casein, chicken, and soy led to sensitization in from all to half of the animals, respectively (65). These data prompted the hypothetical use of protein hydrolysates such as Nutramigen for infant feeding or supplementation in studies evaluating the capacity of various dietary regimens to prevent the development of allergic disease in infants at high risk for atopy (1). Zeiger et al. (14) noted that Nutramigen (as part of a hypoallergenic dietary regimen) compared to cow's milk feeding from birth in non-breast-fed infants or as a supplement to breast feeding was associated with a low prevalence of formula allergy and specific-milk IgE by 1 year in infants at risk for atopy (14). In addition, the hypoimmunogenicity of Nutramigen was documented by its capacity compared to cow's milk formula to inhibit the IgG BLG response prior to and following cow's milk introduction (66). In addition, casein hydrolysate-fed infants demonstrated a decreased BLG IgG response similar to that observed in infants solely breast fed until 1 year, whether or not a maternal lactation diet free of cow's milk was adopted (1). Such findings confirm an earlier preliminary study (67) which reported that infants fed for 3 months casein hydrolysate (Nutramigen) compared to cow's milk formula developed significantly lower whey hemagglutinins prior to and after cow's milk intake. Moreover, the above studies (1,66) extend those which noted that infants solely breast fed for 3 months had reduced cow's milk IgG responses and suppression of the peak response after addition of cow's milk, compared to a group fed cow's milk from birth (68). These findings reveal reduced immunogenicity of casein hydrolysate formula (Nutramigen) and exclusive breast feeding in unselected infants (67,68) and also in high-risk atopic infants (1,66), those most expected to mount strong immunological responses.

Confirming the above beneficial effect of protein hydrolysate formulas, Chandra et al. noted, in two prospective, randomized controlled studies in non-breast-fed atopic-prone infants, that casein (46), or whey (54,69) hydrolysate, compared to cow's milk or soy feeding, was associated with a lower cumulative incidence of eczema in infancy (46,54,69) (Table 3). Unfortunately, immunological and food challenge confirmation was omitted (46) or incomplete (54,69) in these studies. Though several other studies have attempted to determine the effectiveness of protein hydrolysates in allergy prevention (70–72), none has proven definitive (Table 3).

These studies require confirmation with a definitive prospective, randomized, masked, food-challenged study which determines whether protein hydrolysates prevent cow's milk allergy before protein hydrolysate formulas are proclaimed effective and safe for the prevention of atopy in high-atopic-risk infants when breast feeding is not a choice or formula supplementation is desired. Casein hydrolysates are hypoallergenic (58) and hypoimmunogenic (1,66), while the partial whey hydrolysates may induce milk-specific IgE (70) and are more likely to cause anaphylaxis in an infant who has become sensitized to cow's milk from other sources (59,61). The extensively hydrolyzed hypoallergenic protein hydrolysates (Nutramigen and Alimentum in the United States) may be the preferred choice compared to the partial whey hydrolysates for purposes of allergy prevention, as recently recommended by the European Society Pediatric Allergy and Clinical Immunology (59).

E. Delayed Introduction of Solid Foods

The effect of solid food ingestion on the development of eczema by ages 2 and 10 years and asthma by age 4 years was analyzed in an unselected, uncontrolled, prospective birth cohort study of 1265 New Zealand neonates in which 1067 or 84% were evaluated at 10 years (73,74). The prevalence of eczema related significantly to parental atopy and solid feeding patterns.

A 2.5-fold greater incidence of eczema by 2 years occurred in infants of atopic parents. On the other hand, the development of asthma was not related to solid food feeding (75). A statistically significant linear relationship existed between the number of solid foods introduced during the first 4 months of life and the ensuing incidence of 1 episode of eczema by 2 years (73) and recurrent/chronic eczema by 10 years (74). Moreover, there was an almost threefold increase in the risk of recurrent/current eczema by 10 years in infants ingesting 4 or more solid foods compared to infants not receiving solid foods by 4 months (74). Limitations of this series of reports are chart review rather than objective determination of disease etiology either immunologically or by food challenge.

A prospective nonrandomized study of 115 infants from atopic families evaluated the effect of delaying solid food introduction on the development of eczema and food allergy (76,77). Eczema at 1 year (14% versus 35%, $p < .01$) (76) was reduced in infants exclusively breast fed for 6 months compared to a group of breast-fed infants in whom solid foods were introduced at 3 months of age. Atopic disorders and atopic eczema were similar at 5 years in both groups despite the delay in solid food introduction. The failure to randomize groups weakens the impact of the study's findings but suggests that dietary intervention in infancy probably does not provide an avenue to prevent atopy later in childhood when aeroallergens rather than foods represent the major allergens responsible for atopic disease.

Taken together, such findings suggest that early exposure to multiple foodstuffs may predispose infants, particularly those at risk for atopy, to recurrent or chronic eczema. In contrast, it has been reported that the benefit of delaying the introduction of solid foods may merely postpone the development of food allergy (78). Nevertheless, the weight of evidence suggests that the neonate with its immature gastrointestinal system poorly excludes multiple allergens or large quantities of allergens which may prime the IgE sensitizing system in atopic-prone infants. Delaying solid food feeding until after 6 months has many advocates; additional confirmatory studies would solidify such pronouncements.

F. Maternal and Infant Avoidance of Allergenic Foods

The existence of multiple potential sources of food exposure (placenta?, breast, formula, and solid foods) in infants led to two prospective, randomized, controlled studies from Canada (79) and the United States (14,66, 80,81), which attempted to interfere with the ingestion of food allergens by mother and her fetus and infant from these many potential sources in an attempt to reduce the development of atopy—knowing full well the inability to determine which, if any, of the interventions was responsible for any derived benefits. Moreover, these studies were initiated prior to the Swedish prospective studies which failed to demonstrate any allergy-preventive effect from food allergen avoidance during the third trimester of pregnancy (Table 3) (9–13).

Maternal Avoidance Diet Throughout Pregnancy and Lactation, with 6 Months Exclusive Breast Feeding

In a prospective, randomized, controlled study of atopic-prone infants exclusively breast fed for 6 months, Chandra et al. (79) reported a significantly reduced severity and marginally reduced incidence of eczema by 1 year in the group whose mothers excluded milk, egg, peanut, fish, and beef throughout *pregnancy and lactation* compared to a group whose mothers maintained an unrestricted diet (Table 3). BLG, casein, and OVA were rarely detected in the breast milk of mothers practicing dietary restriction compared to control mothers, demonstrating relative compliance in the diet-restricted group. No food challenge or immunological evaluation was done to relate the eczema to atopy.

Effect of Combined Maternal and Infant Food Allergen Avoidance During the Perinatal Period on Atopy from Birth to 7 Years in High-Risk Offspring

We conducted a prenatally randomized, physician-blinded, parallel controlled food allergen avoidance trial on infants born to documented allergic parents. We compared the effect of combined maternal and infant food allergen avoidance (prophylaxis group) to currently recommended maternal and infant feeding practices on the development of allergic disease from birth to 7 years. The diet regimen of the prophylaxis group ($n = 103$) included (a) maternal avoidance of milk, egg, and peanut during both the third trimester of pregnancy and lactation, and (b) infant breast and/or Nutramigen feedings and avoidance of solid foods for 6 months; milk, corn, soy, citrus, and wheat for 1 year; and egg, peanut, and fish for 2 years. The control group ($n = 185$) followed standard pregnancy diets and the American Academy of Pediatrics recommendations for infant feeding. The prevalences of atopic disorders were reduced at 1 year due to lower prevalences of food allergy in the prophylaxis group (Fig. 1). Specific IgE sensitization to foods determined by skin-prick tests was reduced significantly in infants in the prophylaxis group at 1 year due to a lower prevalence of milk-specific IgE ($p = .01$). Serum IgE was marginally lower only at 4 months in the prophylaxis compared to the control group ($p = .07$) (Table 3). The development of food allergy by 4 years was associated with

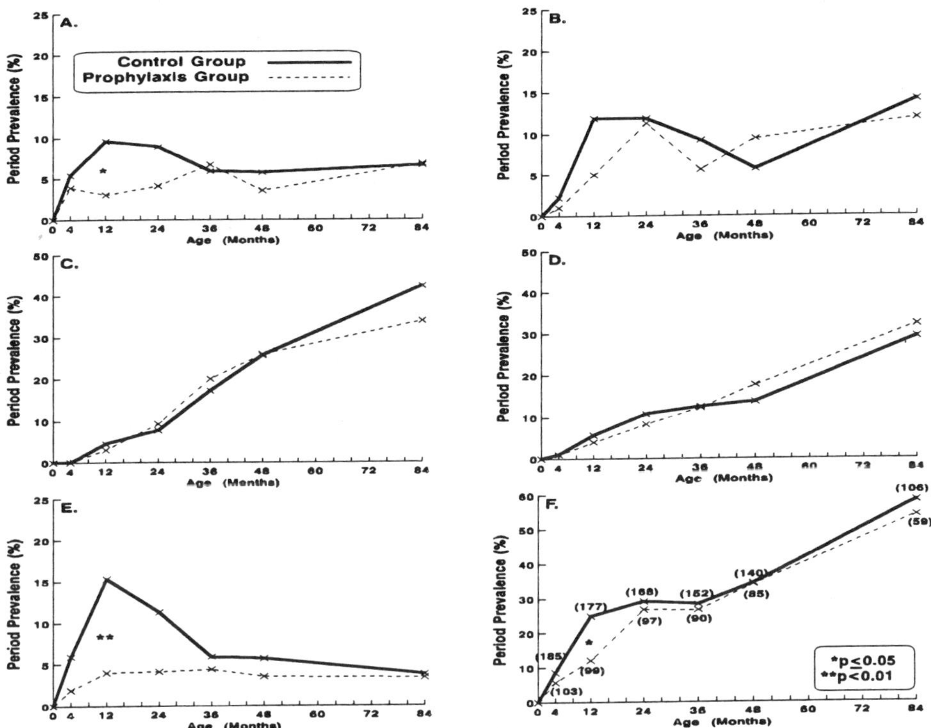

Figure 1 Period (current) prevalences of atopic disorders from birth to 7 years in prophylactic-treated and control groups in combined maternal and infant food allergen avoidance perinatally: (A) atopic dermatitis; (B) urticaria; (C) allergic rhinitis; (D) asthma; (E) food allergy; (F) any allergy.

twofold significant increases in both the prevalences of allergic rhinitis and asthma at 4 and 7 years in analyses combining data from both study groups (66,81). The prevalences of allergic rhinitis, asthma, and aeroallergen sensitization to mite, dander, mold, and pollen were similar in both groups from 4 months to 7 years (Fig. 1 and Table 3) (14,66,81).

During the course of this longitudinal study, atopic diseases (atopic dermatitis, allergic rhinitis, and asthma) and parameters (food and aeroallergen sensitization and nasal eosinophils and basophilic cells) at age 7 years were shown by multivariate analyses to be associated with several genetic and environmental risk factors (male gender, maternal nonwhite ethnicity, maternal asthma, and household smoking), as well as predictive atopic markers during infancy (elevated serum IgE level; egg, cow's milk, and peanut sensitization; and nasal eosinophils and nasal basophilic cells) (81).

In summary, strict prolonged food avoidance perinatally by mother and infant for more than 6 months appears to reduce the development of food allergy during early infancy, but not allergic respiratory disorders from birth to 7 years. The benefit of food allergy prevention may be brief and limited to the first year or two of life, due to the frequent remissions in food allergy by 2 years and the elimination of the responsible foods from the diets of food allergic infants. The benefits attained by the combined maternal and infant avoidance regimens cannot be attributed to the pregnancy diet since, as discussed above, prenatal sensitization to foods is rare (1) and prenatal maternal dietary restrictions, when examined separately in prospective randomized studies, fails to prevent food allergy in infancy (9–13). The relative benefits of maternal lactation diet, use of protein hydrolysate feedings, and/or delay in feeding solid foods on the reduction in food allergy and particularly cow's milk allergy and sensitization can only be unraveled by future studies.

G. Combined Maternal and Infant Food Allergen Avoidance Postnatally and Household Mite Avoidance

Expanding upon the above, Hide and his group on the Isle of Wight added household dust mite avoidance regimen (mite-retardant pillow and mattress zippered encasements and acaricide treatments of household furnishings and carpeting) to the combined postnatal maternal and infant food allergen avoidance protocols in the primary prevention of food and respiratory allergic disease (82,83). This prospective, randomized, controlled study in high-risk infants reported that the combined food allergen and dust mite avoidance regimen in early infancy led to a significant reduction in any atopy, eczema, and asthma at 1 year of age in the prophylaxis group (Table 3) (82). Mite levels as assayed by determining *Der p* I levels were significantly lower in the prophylaxis group only at 9 months (82). [Reduced levels in the prophylaxis group were still at levels greater than the 2 μg/ g of dust level, considered to be the threshold required for mite sensitization (see below).] Unrestricted infancy diet, parental smoking, maternal atopy, and lower socioeconomic status were identified risk factors for the development of atopy. Odds ratios for asthma and eczema were about fourfold lower in the prophylaxis group. By age 2 years, atopy and food and/ or aeroallergen sensitization by skin test were significantly less in the prophylaxis group, but differences in asthma were only marginally lower (83). At the present time this study represents the first approach to the primary prevention of respiratory allergic disease and as such requires confirmation and expansion.

H. Cautions, Implications, and Recommendations for Primary Prevention

Despite the recent flourish of prospective, controlled, and randomized primary allergy-prevention studies, uncertainty still remains with respect to the degree of benefit attainable by such interventions, due to the paucity of definitive studies. What is needed are well-designed, masked, multicenter primary prevention trials with clearly defined singular interventions that determine the development of atopic disorders by precise clinical and immunological criteria. Only provisional recommendations can be offered at this time for the primary prevention of allergic disease, and these should be rapidly updated when new data are reported. These recommendations, which are clearly noted in Table 7, should be directed only at high-risk offspring with highly motivated parents and should not be proselytized universally.

III. Secondary Prevention of Allergy

Secondary prevention of allergic disorders or the blocking of disease expression after the development of specific IgE sensitization to a food or aeorallergen has received only meager attention. Though primary prevention of allergy represents the optimal objective, secondary prevention may be a useful supplementary or alternative for families who need stronger and more immediate evidence of atopic risk before pursuing allergy-prevention measures. Strategies proven effective in primary and tertiary allergy prevention could be adapted for secondary prevention.

A. Prediction of the High-Risk Atopic Postnatally

The scientific basis for secondary allergy prevention derives from knowledge of the natural history of allergy, which conclusively demonstrates the progressive and relentless nature of allergic phenomena or the "atopic march" (see Chapter 29). The "atopic march" predicts that several, sometimes transient, atopic conditions or events often precede the development of other, more permanent atopic situations or disorders, as emphasized by the following situations: (a) food allergy and food and inhalant sensitization precede allergic rhinitis and atopic asthma (84–87); (b) atopic dermatitis precedes atopic asthma (88–90); (c) infectious asthma with concomitant elevated IgE in infancy precedes asthma at age 6 years (91); (d) peripheral

Table 7 Provisional Recommendation for the Primary Prevention of Food
and Aeroallergen-Related Allergic Disorders in Newborns/Infants at
High-Risk for Atopy (159,160)

Strategy	Method or measure
1. Identify high-risk infant prenatlly or early postnatlly	Atopic family (biparental, parent and sibling) or elevated cord blood IgE level
2. Avoid infant exposure to:	
a. Food allergens	
In breast milk	Consider maternal lactation diet with no egg, CM, peanut investigational; supplement maternal diet with 1500 mg calcium daily
In infant diet	Breast feed for at least 4–6 months, preferably the latter
	Supplement or wean with nutritious and hypoallergenic protein hydrolysate formula
	Delay solid foods for 6 months, then add least allergenic first
	After 1 year, add biweekly or monthly, if tolerated: CM, wheat, soy, citrus, egg, peanut, fish; delay egg, peanut, and fish longer in food-atopic infants
b. Aeroallergens	Reduce household dust mite, mold, pet exposure
	Use air conditioners, air purifiers, carpetless floors, petless homes, maintain lowered home humidity
c. Nonspecific environmental adjuvants	No smoking prenatally or postnatally by caretakers/subject
	Reduce air pollution

Source: Ref. 1.

blood eosinophilia at 3 months of age (92) or nasal eosinophils at age 1
year precede allergic rhinitis (81). Based on the above features of the
"atopic march," infants at high risk for the development of atopic disease
could be identified for the purposes of instituting secondary allergy prevention after the onset of one of the following conditions: (a) an indicator
atopic marker [specific food (egg, milk, or peanut)-IgE, aeroallergen-IgE,
elevated asthma IgE, or blood or nasal eosinophilia] and/or (b) an indicator
atopic disorder (food allergy, atopic dermatitis, infectious asthma and elevated serum IgE). A documented or strong parental history of allergies,

particularly on the maternal side (maternal asthma), given its predictive capacity for atopy and asthma, could also supplement the above atopic parameters in identifying high-risk infants postnatally.

For example, a RAST $\geq$ 1+ to egg at 8 months in an unselected cohort indicated 32% and 50% sensitivities and 95% specificities for atopy, respectively, at 1.5 and 7 years. These results were better predictors of atopy than previously determined elevated cord blood IgE levels among the same cohort (85,86). Moreover, a positive OVA-SPT at age 6 months showed a 40% sensitivity and 95% specificity for 18-month atopic disease (93). These studies confirmed earlier findings which demonstrated that a positive egg SPT in infancy predicted more severe atopic diseases and higher prevalences of allergic rhinitis and other food SPTs by 15 years (88). In a 7-year prospective study of the development and prevention of atopy in high-risk infants, we noted that a positive egg SPT at or before age 1 year was significantly predictive for the 7-year current prevalence of atopic dermatitis (sensitivity $-$ 73% and specificity $=$ 89%), allergic rhinitis, and asthma. In this same study, the presence, compared to the absence, of food allergy by age 4 years was associated with significantly higher 7-year current prevalances of allergic rhinitis (odds ratio $=$ 2.8), any atopy (odds ratio $=$ 3.9), and aeroallergen sensitization (odds ratio $=$ 3.1) (66,81). Family history of atopy with its 40% sensitivity and 80% specificity for predicting atopy at ages 7 and 11 years can also be used as an atopic predictor marker for secondary prevention identification (94).

Sensitization to House Dust Mite Allergens

Exposure to elevated levels of *Der p* I in concentrations exceeding 2 μg/ g of dust in carpets and bedding measured during infancy has been related to both an increased prevalence of positive SPT and increased concentrations of *Der p* I specific IgE by age 5 in high-risk infants. Additionally, *Der p* I levels in excess of 10 μg/g of household dust measured during infancy was associated with a fivefold greater risk of developing asthma by age 11 (95). In this study, the age of the initial wheezing episode was inversely related to the level of *Der p* I exposure at age 1 year in all subjects, particularly those found atopic. Moreover, sensitization to mite allergen represents a major risk factor for both early and late-onset asthma and for the persistence of asthmatic signs during childhood, since such sensitization antedates the onset of asthma (87). Other studies appear to support these findings with respect to increased mite sensitization with greater mite exposure (96); however, unexplained is the absence of mite specific IgE in most of these subjects prior to age 2. It is proposed that early exposure primed these infants to develop sensitization later with continued exposure to mite in childhood. These studies demand the medical community to implement mite avoidance measures to prevent sensitization as in primary prevention, or shortly after sensitization as in secondary prevention.

Sensitization to Other Aeroallergens

Cat, dog, and cockroach represent other important indoor allergens whose sensitization appears related to the subsequent development of asthma (97). Cat and dog exposure or cat *Fel d* I in homes during infancy is associated with sensitization to cat by age 1 year (98), dog by 9 years (99), and cat during childhood (100). When cat allergen levels are low (<1 μg *Fel d* I/g dust), as in communities where cats were kept outdoors (San Paulo or inner-city Atlanta), cat sensitization remains low (<10%). In contrast, in localities in which mite exposure and sensitization are low, and in which cats are permitted indoors (Los Alamos, NM), cat concentrations soar (~80 μg *Fel d* I/g dust) and cat sensitization among asthmatics reaches 68% (101). Cat allergen concentrations are still substantial in homes without cats (~3 μg *Fel d* I/g dust), allowing cat sensitization to reach 20% among asthmatics (101). Aside from homes, exposure and potential sensitization to cat allergens may occur through reservoirs on upholstered seats in public buildings and public transport facilities (*Fel d* I > 8 μg/g dust in ~80% of samples) (102). Such reservoirs in public places could thwart allergen control measures instituted only in homes. Cockroach exposure and sensitization are important issues in the development of asthma in communities with high cockroach infestations, such as occurs in the inner city (103). Pollens and molds are also important allergens which both sensitize and are associated with causing and exacerbating asthma in certain communities; however, less definitive studies are available at this time (3). We have recently noted in atopic asthmatics a direct relationship of asthma symptom severity and diminished peak flow rates to aeroallergen concentrations of molds in San Diego (104).

B. An Approach to Secondary Allergy Prevention

One could propose from the above data that an efficient and cost-effective approach to allergy prevention could involve periodic prospective surveillance of infants (young children) for the clinical and immunological expression of atopic sensitization (markers) or disease. The high-risk infant during well-baby visits could be identified by the responsible primary health-care provider by ascertaining (a) atopic sensitization by performing SPT or CAP ELISAs to foods such as egg and milk twice during infancy (4 and 12 months) and yearly to aeroallergens such as dust mite (*Der p*

1/*Der f* I mix), alternaria/cladosporium mix, cat (or dog), and grass mix beginning at age 1 year and (b) atopic disease expression by recognizing recurrent infectious wheezing, eczema, and food allergy. These high-risk infants could then be referred to allergy specialists for allergy-prevention instruction and follow-up. Allergy-preventive regimens that have proven effective for primary and tertiary prevention could be instituted in these high-risk infants. This approach would direct intensive preventive efforts only to those infants who have demonstrated atopic sensitization or atopic disease, in an attempt to prevent the "atopic march." Prospective studies will need to assess the efficacy and cost of instituting such a secondary allergy-prevention program.

C. Preventing the "Atopic March"

Secondary prevention measures could play a modulatory role in the "atopic march," as noted above. Aeroallergens, ETS, and pollution avoidance, as discussed later with tertiary allergy prevention, could be utilized during secondary prevention. Additionally, modulation may be possible pharmacologically. Recently, a report noted that ketotifen administration to infants less than age 3 years with atopic dermatitis appeared to reduce the incidence of asthma over the subsequent 12 months from 42% to 14% in a randomized, double-blind, placebo-controlled study, with an effect seen predominately in those with serum IgE levels >50 IU/mL (105). Current studies in Sweden and England [Early Treatment of the Atopic Child (ETAC)] are attempting to confirm these findings. The use of immunotherapy for allergic rhinitis in children has been recommended (106) but not proven to prevent the progression of allergic rhinitis to allergic asthma. Results from current investigations in Europe on this form of secondary prevention by immunomodulation should be available soon.

D. Advantages and Disadvantages of Primary and Secondary Allergy Prevention

A critical evaluation of both primary and secondary allergy prevention reveals relative advantages and disadvantages of each preventive stage. Each stage complements the other and both should be invoked together to successfully counter the worldwide increase in allergic disease (Table 8).

IV. Tertiary Allergy Prevention

Preventing clinical manifestations of allergic disease is the objective of tertiary allergy prevention, the state in which clinicians are most familiar.

Table 8 Advantages and Disadvantages of Primary and Secondary Prevention of Atopy

Primary prevention	Secondary prevention
Advantages	Advantages
Permits perinatal advice	Better capacity to predict atopic disease
Optimizes early prenatal commitment	More convincing to certain parents
Potential to prevent sensitization or early atopy	Prospective follow-up for atopy encouraged
Bridges atopy's "critical period"	Pediatrician's atopy knowledge improves
Disadvantages	Disadvantages
Predictive markers possess low sensitivity	May miss "critical period" of sensitization
Involves many families not at real risk for atopy	Atopy disease may have developed
Minimal effective preventive efforts unknown	Usual medical care may not allow prospective follow-up
Costs, QOL, aeroallergen effectiveness undetermined	Costs, QOL, effectiveness undetermined

QOL = quality of life.
Source: Ref. 158.

All too often mere lip service rather than detailed advice and support is given to patients, who are too often left on their own to "cope" with the consequences of allergic disease.

A. Role of the Generalist

Generalists, whether pediatricians or primary-care providers, represent the first link in tertiary allergy prevention, in that they potentially are the initial care givers to recognize and diagnose atopic disease. The earlier that diagnosis occurs, the earlier appropriate prevention strategies can be instituted. Next the generalist should seek an expedited referral of newly diagnosed atopic infants and children to allergy specialists skilled in delivering preventive allergy care.

B. Role of the Allergy Specialist

Allergists, specialists in the diagnosis, treatment, and prevention of food allergy, eczema, allergic rhinitis, asthma, venom hypersensitivity, and anaphylaxis, must provide generalists with accurate and timely confirmation or diagnosis of referred atopic children. A major role of the allergist must be to provide comprehensive guidelines on allergen, irritant, and adjuvant avoidance measures to families of the atopic. These guidelines should include measures to (a) reduce mite, dander, and animal emanations in the home; (b) decrease mold and pollen exposure; (c) promote smoking cessation and ETS avoidance; (d) encourage safe occupations and occupation safety; and (e) reduce air pollution contact. The allergist should administer appropriate preventive pharmacological medication (cromolyn, nedocromil, inhaled corticosteroids, and immunotherapy) for asthma and allergic rhinitis according to recent national and international recommendations (107).

C. Modulation of Major Atopic Risk Factors

Modulation of major atopic risk factors includes the reduction/elimination of the following: (a) early food allergen exposure; (b) household dust mite, cockroach, and dander levels; (c) environmental tobacco smoke (ETS) and air pollutants; and (d) RVS infections. As noted earlier, we are approaching an exciting era in allergy prevention in which novel, effective, and safe immunomodulatory therapies will be part of the allergists' arsenal.

Early Food Allergen Exposure

Food ingestion postnatally elicits a brisk humoral immunological response involving specific antibodies of all the immunoglobulin classes, including IgE. Early ingestion of potentially allergenic foods in the high-risk infant triggers a higher and more persistent specific and total IgE response, which often leads to disorders including food allergy, atopic dermatitis, and GI allergy (2). Development of food allergy in infancy should alert the health provider of a high-risk infant in whom it would be indicated to initiate tertiary allergy prevention. Institution of some of the food allergen avoidance measures recommended in primary allergy prevention could be considered, including hypoallergenic protein hydrolysate supplementation and delaying solid food introduction, particularly the more allergenic such as milk, egg, and peanut, until after age 1 year or later (see Appendix).

Early Aeroallergen Exposure

The mechanisms responsible for primary sensitization to inhalant allergens during infancy has been reviewed recently (108). Mite allergen levels are lower at higher altitudes (109) and within day nurseries (110), hospitals (111), and specially designed, mechanically ventilated homes (112). Residence in such environments (109–112), use of allergen-proof encasings for the bedding (113), and application of acaricides in some studies (114) led to improvements in asthma (115) and BHR (116,117), and reduction in inflammatory and immunological atopic markers (Table 9) (118–120). Mite-retardant encasements of pillow and mattress/boxspring may serve as a particularly inexpensive and efficient measure to reduce mite reservoirs within the atopic's bedroom. Washing all bedding and stuffed toys in hot cycle (~130°F) weekly appears to kill and remove mites. Although partially effective for short-term reduction of house dust-mite allergen levels, vacuuming is of only limited value in reducing mite allergen exposure, due to rapid reinfestation (121). Acaricides (mite-cidal chemicals such as benzyl benzoate, pyrethoids, pirimiphos methyl, and liquid nitrogen) and denaturants (3% tannic acid), though effective in vitro against mites, have

Table 9 Effect of Various Environmental Factors on Dust-Mite Levels and Sensitization

Residential factors increasing mite levels (161)
    Use of animal hair blankets
    Use of bed covers, underblankets, or older mattresses
    Dampness and high relative humidity
    Ground floor inhabitance
    Poor ventilation
Effect of altitude (108,116,118,119)
    Mite concentration varies inversely with altitude
    Mite concentration 90% lower at 1 km
    Serum IgE level and mite-IgE 50% lower at 1.4 km residence for 9 months
    Mite specific basophil histamine release reduced
    PD_{20} histamine improves after 1 year residence at Davos
    Serum markers of eosinophil activation decline at 1.8 km
Effect of hospitalization (115)
    Mite antigen levels 98% lower in hospital
    Serum IgE level and mite-IgE decline
    Peak flow rate and symptoms improve
    Asthma medication requirements decline
    PD_{30} histamine improves in majority of mite-allergic asthma patients
Sensitization (95,96)
    Risk level for development of mite-IgE and asthma: 2 µg *Der p* I/g dust
    Risk level for acute asthma: 10 µg *Der p* I/g dust
    Age of first wheezing episode inversely correlated with highest mite antigen exposure in infancy
    Goal: reduce home mite levels below 2 µg *Der p* I (100 mites or 0.6 mg guanine)/g dust

Source: Ref. 158.

shown very mixed success in clinical studies, due in part to difficulty of application, poor carpet penetration, and the necessity for repeat application (122–124). In trials which failed to demonstrate clinical improvement in asthmatic subjects using acaricides or denaturants in their bedrooms, reductions in house dust mite burden were not achieved or were not maintained. Carpet removal appears to be more effective in this regard, leading to long-term reduction in allergen levels and clinical improvement (121). Smooth flooring also appears to reduce levels of other indoor allergens (125).

Control of household dander (particularly cat and dog) and cockroach allergen exposure remains an almost insurmountable task, and few studies are available to help in this area. Vacuuming with central, microfilter, and high-efficiency particulate air (HEPA) filtration systems failed to reduce cat and dog allergens in homes (126). Tannic acid application reduced cat and dog allergens for only 1 week, with levels returning to normal within 2 weeks (124). While initial studies suggested that weekly washing of cats effectively reduced *Fel d* I levels on the cat (127), a recent more comprehensive, blinded, controlled, 2-month investigation of 24 cats failed to demonstrate any benefit from such washings, Allerpet-C spray, or acepromazine (128). Concerted efforts should be made to keep cats and dogs out of the households of high-risk atopics and those with allergic disease. Efforts to eradicate cockroaches have been formidable. Though not specifically studied in atopic households, chemical extermination and "roach motels" may provide some benefit in reducing exposure to cockroach. Practical allergen reduction measures have been successful in reducing mite and dander levels in households during tertiary prevention (Table 10) (129,130).

Environmental Tobacco Smoke Exposure

Environmental tobacco smoke (ETS) exposure prenatally and postnatally causes major adverse atopic consequences which have led to an EPA indictment of its danger (Table 11). Recent disturbing facts concerning ETS have emerged, including (a) adolescent ex-asthmatics harbor strong intentions to smoke (131), (2) 46% of asthmatics versus 28% of nonasthmatics smoke during pregnancy (132), (3) usual advise fails to curtail smoking substantially during pregnancy, and (d) worldwide smoking continues strong despite decreases in some countries (133).

International, national, and community strategies are required to combat ETS. In the United States, aggressive efforts including (a) public educational campaigns on the hazards of ETS, (b) taxation on tobacco, and (c) prohibition of smoking in public and workplaces has led to reductions

Table 10 Practical House Dust Mite and Animal Allergen Reduction Measures

House dust mite avoidance (121,122,124,129)	Animal emanation and danders (126,127,162)
Encase mattress and pillow with impermeable mite-retardant covers	Discourage indoor furry/feathery pets
Wash bedding weekly at 130°F	Wash bedding weekly and use 3% tannic acid sprays for carpet and furniture (controversial)
Remove stuffed toys and clutter from bedroom	Remove carpets
Remove carpets from bedroom and replace with tile, vinyl, or wood	Use vacuum cleaners with HEPA filters or double-thickness bags
Remove upholstered furniture	Exterminate cockroaches (monitor with "roach motels")
Replace nonwashable curtains/drapes with venetian/slat blinds	
Maintain home <68°F and <50% humidity with air conditioning and dehumidifiers	
Expose carpets to intense sunlight	
Improve home exhaust and ventilation	
Avoid basements, upholstered furniture, and lying on carpets	
Consider HEPA filtration cleaining device	

Source: Ref. 158.

in per-capita consumption of cigarette packs per year from 1981 to 1990 in the United States of 23% (from 15.4 to 11.9) and in California of 34% (from 13.1 to 8.6) (134).

Exposure of the high-risk atopic to home ETS can be approached with structured counseling of smoking families. In collaboration with the San Diego State University School of Public Health, we have recently completed a randomized and controlled study which compared behavioral counseling intervention with usual care and measurement control groups in 91 asthmatic children of smoking parents. The study reveals that intensive behavioral modification can successfully reduce the daily exposure of children to their parents' smoke (135). Counseling parents on the hazards of ETS and actions to modulate at home led to reductions in (a) parental smoking rates, (b) children's exposure to ETS, and (c) asthma symptoms at 2 months during the most intensive counseling intervention (135).

Table 11 Adverse Effects of Pre- and Postnatal Passive ETS Exposure on Children

Prenatal passive ETS
Increase in low-birth-weight and small-for-gestational-age newborns
Higher infant mortality
Reduced infant lung function
Higher incidence of infectious wheezing by age 1 year
Postnatal passive ETS
Reduced lung growth and FEV_1
Greater prevalence of bronchial hyperresponsiveness
Higher prevalence of persistent wheeze
More frequent exacerbations of asthma
Higher serum IgE levels
Greater prevalence of aeroallergen specific-IgE
1993 EPA report on passive ETS
Causes annually $1.5-3.0 \times 10^5$ lower respiratory illnesses in infants <18 months
Increases both incidence and severity of asthma
Increases risk of new onset of asthma
Increases risk of serous otitis media

Source: Ref. 158.

Atmospheric Pollution Exposure

Although it is not yet proven, it is quite probable that urbanization, with its associated pollution, holds some degree of responsibility for the increase in the worldwide severity and perhaps even prevalence of atopic disease. Just a short list of associations of pollution to atopy raise the specter of its impact or danger: (a) high concentrations of ozone increases bronchial hyperresponsiveness (BHR) (136), (b) ozone in concentrations of 120 ppb increases BHR to allergen (137); (c) diesel fumes increase cedar pollinosis in Japan (138); (d) polluting paper pulp plants increases BHR and asthma (139); and (e) oxides of ozone increase sensitization to allergen in guinea pigs (140).

Similar to anti-ETS strategies, antipollution measures need to be adopted internationally, nationally, and regionally. Measures in California which have led to reductions in ozone include (a) establishment of air quality control districts and boards, (b) legislation to promote clean air (California and Federal Clean Air Acts of 1988 and 1990), (c) emission controls on automobiles, (d) car pooling, and (e) control or restriction of polluting manufacturing plants. These measures have led to significant re-

                                                              Zeiger

ductions in days of pollution in excess of U.S. and California standards in San Diego from 1980 to 1992 (141). Implementation of antipollution measures reduced both SO_2 levels and cough prevalence in atopic children in whom installation of a polluting power station had aggravated both parameters (142).

Viral Infections

Viral infections may affect atopic disease by (a) acting as polyclonal B-cell activators of IgE antibodies (Epstein-Barr virus), (b) increasing BHR and lower respiratory illnesses in dogs and humans (canine adenovirus and parainfluenza virus), (c) priming for recurrent wheezing in infancy (RSV), and (d) increasing atopic sensitization during infancy (2).

Prevention of RSV infection in high-risk infants would probably reduce the prevalence of viral-induced wheezing in infancy and potentially affect the development of asthma. High-titer RSV immunoglobulin administration preventively in high-risk respiratory and cardiac infants successfully reduced lower respiratory tract infections caused by RSV (143). Several potential measurers to reduce/prevent RSV virus in addition to high-titer RSV-IgG include RSV-Fab infusions and immunization to specific RSV proteins. Until these therapies materialize, high-risk atopies would best benefit from receiving transferred IgA and IgG specific RSV antibodies from breast milk.

V. Future of Allergy Prevention

Future scientific advances which identify the genetic and immunological basis of atopy more precisely will surely lead to monumental new strategies to prevent atopic disease. Some of these strategies are noted in Table 12. For the time being, in addition to the above proposed recommendations for allergy prevention, it would not hurt to have a bit of assistance from the friendly gods. In the interim, families should be provided with an "Allergy prevention bill of rights" to protect them from the ravages of atopic disease. These Rights could include (a) the right to be breast, not formula fed; (c) the right to live in dust-miteless homes; (c) the right to be free from indoor pets, (d) the right to be free from ETS, (e) the right to breathe clean, not polluted air; and (f) the right to be screened for/advised of allergy prevention as part of child care.

Over the past two decades, there appears to have been an alarming increase in the prevalence and morbidity of most, if not all, atopic diseases, particularly asthma. This increase probably reflects (a) increased urbanization (encouraging ornamental pollinating plants/grasses and spewing

Table 12 Lobbying for an International Consciousness for Allergy Awareness
and Prevention

A. Rationale
    Unrelenting increase in atopy and asthma
    Increasing asthma morbidity and mortality despite pharmacologic advances
    Occupational allergy rising
    U.S. cost: $6 billion annually
B. Community factors
    Poor public allergy education and awareness
    Breast feeding not optimized
    ETS and air pollution still high
    High-risk atopic and low SES underserved
C. Identify high-risk atopic
    Future genetic markers
    Atopic parentage and elevated cord blood IgE levels
    Postnatal atopic markers
    Low SES and ethnic clusters
    High-risk occupations
D. Universal prevention strategy
    Promote lengthy breastfeeding
    Discourage early solid foods
    Screen for simple atopic markers during well-baby visits
    Recognize atopy early and advise or refer for prevention guidelines
    Construct mite retardant homes
    Campaign for ETS control/cessation
    Stop pollution and pollutants
    Institute atopic work safeguards
    Screen preemployment for atopy
    Encourage support organizations
E. Individual high-risk prevention strategy
    Supplement/wean with hypoallergenic protein hydrolysate
    Promote mite avoidance (encasings, bare floors)
    Discourage indoor allergenic pets
    Delay daycare
    Avoid atopic high-risk occupations
F. Future strategies
    Prevent RSV infections
    Oral tolerance to aeroallergens
    Recombinant human monoclonal antibody to IgE
    Modulate T cells (peptide antigens)
    Modulate cytokines (monoclonal antibodies, antagonists)
    DNA vaccination with allergen cDNA
    Modulate atopic genes (science fiction?)

Source: Ref. 158.

pollution wantonly), (b) excessive ETS, (c) increased exposure to occupational allergens, (d) poorly ventilated homes with carpeting/wool blankets which encourage warmth/humidity, leading to mite proliferation, and (e) increased survival of critically ill neonates with respiratory disease, as well as other factors not yet identified. To counteract these atopic-promoting factors, a national and international consciousness directed toward allergy prevention must be developed. Otherwise, atopy will become more pervasive, unmanageable, and severe. Measures which could help to stimulate a worldwide allergy consciousness are described in Table 12.

VI. Implications and Recommendations for the Prevention of Atopy

From the above discussion it is clear that more definitive data must be obtained before universal prevention recommendations are pronounced. Randomized, prospective, controlled studies, preferably double-bind, should be directed toward determining the relative efficacy, practicality, and cost of implementing preventive measures such as protein hydrolysate feeding, maternal lactation diet, and delay in introduction of allergenic foods in the attempt to reduce food allergy. In addition, well-designed studies should determine whether elimination of environmental pollutants (parental smoking pre- and postpartum) and aeorallergens such as dust mites and danders (postnatally) will affect such atopic disorders as asthma, allergic rhinitis, and atopic dermatitis. Parental compliance, motivation, and resources will present major obstacles to the success of these preventive efforts. Specifically, the well-controlled studies discussed above emphasized that parental compliance was far from optimal despite apparent motivation and resources provided by the studies. One can anticipate less success when preventive efforts are implemented in uncontrolled, unstructured settings such as are seen in clinical practice. With this in mind, both primary and secondary allergy prevention may generate less success, practicality, and appeal than first envisioned. Given the multiple obstacles encountered during environmental engineering, dietary and inhalant avoidance efforts can only serve, at best, as stopgap measures until more effective and universally acceptable genetic or cellular engineering methods are developed. Future scientific breakthroughs will identify and isolate the essential allergic gene(s), which then could be altered or switched off by directed genetic engineering. In addition, immune/inflammatory cells, cytokines instrumental in IgE synthesis, mediator release, and target organ sensitivity are realistic areas for modulation and preventive efforts within this decade. However, at the present time, clinicians interested in preventing allergic disorders must direct their efforts to manipulating the environmental factors responsible for sensitization and disease expression.

Therefore, only preliminary dietary and environmental recommendations are available for the prevention of allergic disease. These recommendations are based on and modified from the more stringent measures found beneficial in the aforementioned studies. As more compelling evidence emerges, these recommendations will be revised. These recommendations must not be promulgated or proselytized universally but rather, if indicated, given to highly motivated parents of infants at high risk for developing allergic disease (Tables 2, 7, 10, and 12 and Appendix).

Appendix I: Southern California Permanente Medical Group Allergy Department

Introduction of Foods to Infants at High Risk for Food Allergy

Introduction

Allergists have desired to prevent, reduce, or delay the onset of allergic illnesses caused by foods and other allergens for decades. Although no foolproof method exists, recent studies suggest that delaying the introduction of allergenic food to infants at risk for allergies may reduce food allergy within the first year of life. Unfortunately, food avoidance appears to have no effect on the development of asthma or inhalant allergies.

One problem with strict diets is the potential development of nutritional deficiencies if adequate food substitutions are not eaten. Therefore, such diets must be undertaken only with professional supervision. The benefits and risks of such a food avoidance program must be determined for each individual family, depending on specific considerations such as the degree of risk of developing allergies and overall parental compliance.

Description

The diet of infants with a high risk of developing allergy should avoid highly allergenic foods, such as milk, egg, peanut, nuts, soy, corn, and fish, during the first 1–2 years. Breast feeding is encouraged. Nursing mothers may avoid milk, egg, and peanut consumption but this is still investigational. If formula is preferred, hydrolyzed infant formulas such as Nutramigen and Alimentum are recommended; soybean and cow's milk formulas are avoided.

Indication

Studies have shown that this avoidance diet may reduce food allergies in infants of documented allergic parents. This diet does not appear to reduce chronic asthma, chronic rhinitis, or inhalant allergies.

Adequacy

This diet is nutritionally adequate for infants if breast milk or recommended formula and a variety of allowed foods are provided in adequate amounts. Fluoride is suggested after 3 months of age when local water levels of fluoride are low. Nursing women on milk restriction require calcium supplementation of 1500 mg calcium daily.

Nursing Mother

1. Avoid milk, egg, and peanuts during lactation, if physician recommended.
2. 1500 mg supplement calcium daily.

Infant

1. Prolong breastfeeding for at least 4–6 months.
2. Hydrolyzed milk formula is recommended if infant is supplemented or not breast fed.
3. Add solids as follows:
    Birth to 6 months, breast milk or hydrolyzed formula (Nutramigen or Alimentum)
    6–12 months, vegetables, rice, meat, fruit
    12–18 months; add the following food groups if tolerated every 2–4 weeks: milk, wheat, corn, citrus, soy
    After the above foods have been tolerated, and depending on your physician's recommendations, then egg, peanut, and fish may be added.
4. Avoid any foods suspected of causing food allergy. Notify physician of these foods so that he or she may evaluate the situation relative to further consumption.

Food group	Foods allowed	Foods to avoid
6–12 months		
Baked goods	Plain rice cakes	All others
Cereal	Beech-Nut rice cereal	All others
Dessert	None	All
Fats	Safflower oil	Mayonnaise, peanut oil, soy oil, all others
Fruit	Strained, fresh, canned, or frozen without added citrus	All citrus fruits and berries
Fruit juice	Any without added citrus orange juice	Orange or citrus juices

Food group	Foods allowed	Foods to avoid
Meat	Strained, junior or fresh liver, chicken, ham, pork, turkey, veal; fresh-cooked beef, lamb	[a]Strained and junior beef, lamb; any mixed or high meat dinners, breaded meats; chicken or meat sticks; fish; shellfish
Meat substitutes	None	Tomato or tomato products; corn; eggs, peanut butter; tofu; cheese; legumes; soy
Vegetables	[a]Most single-ingredient strained and junior vegetables; fresh vegetables; [a]Most canned or frozen vegetables	Creamed corn, creamed spinach, creamed green beans, creamed peas,[a] some mixed vegetables, legumes, soy, tofu
12–18 months		
Baked goods	Arrowroot cookies, Toddler biscuits, animal cookies, baby pretzels, Zwieback; [a]commercial or home-made baked goods without eggs or peanut products	Any containing egg or peanut products; be aware of type of vegetable oil used
Beverages	Cow's milk or soy-based formulas; whole cow's milk, Gatorade, fruit drinks	[a]Powdered fruit beverages containing egg; Orange Julius
Bread	Homemade or commercial egg-free breads, pita bread, rice cakes	Breads with egg as an ingredient; challah; egg bagels
Cereal and breakfast foods	Dry or jarred cereals, toasted oat rings	Prepared mixes for pancakes, waffles, biscuits, muffins
Dessert	[a]Most strained and junior desserts; popsicles; gelatin; [a]Commercial or home-made desserts without egg or peanut products	Junior puddings; any containing egg or peanut products
Fats	[a]Most margarines, butter, corn or safflower oil, sour cream, cream cheese, non-diary creamer, avocado	Peanut oil; [a]margarine containing peanut oil, mayonnaise
Fruit juice	All	None
Juice	All	None
Meat	Strained, junior, or fresh meat; poultry; high meat dinners	Strained and junior dinners (avoid eggs, egg noodles); fish, shellfish

Food group	Foods allowed	Foods to avoid
Meat substitute	Tofu; cheese	Eggs; peanut butter
Vegetables	Strained, junior, fresh, frozen, canned	Any prepared with an egg batter or cream sauce made with egg; fried in peanut oil

After 18 months

Egg and egg products may be added to the diet if infant does not demonstrate allergies to these products. Fish and peanut products may be added to the diet at your physician's recommendations if infant does not demonstrate allergies to these products. Avoid whole peanuts because of possibility of choking.

[a]These foods may not be allowed on this diet depending on the ingredients. Read the label or contact the manufacturer for product information.

Source: Special thanks given to Barbara Gordon, R.D., Children's Hospital & Medical Center, San Diego, California, from whose diet form the above was modified.

Appendix II: Representative Potentially Allergenic Foods: Identification and Avoidance

Foodstuff	Hidden ingredients listed on label	Foods to avoid	Substitutes
Milk	Casein Caseinate Whey Lactalbumin Sodium caseinate Lactose Nonfat milk solids Cream Calcium caseinate	Cheese Cottage cheese Ice cream, yogurt Creamed soups and sauces Butter and many margarines Baked goods made with milk Some "nondairy" products Candy (creams and milk chocolate) Custards and puddings	Mocha Mix Coffee Rich Nutramigen Soy formulas (Isomil, Prosobes) Tofu Milk-free baked goods (often french bread) Pareve foods Supplement for calcium and vitamin D

Foodstuff	Hidden ingredients listed on label	Foods to avoid	Substitutes
Egg	Albumin Egg whites Egg yolks Eggnog Mayonnaise Ovalbumin Ovumcoid	Many baked goods Egg noodles Custards, pudding Mayonnaise, some salad dressings Hollandaise sauce Meringues Many egg substitutes (Egg-beaters) Some batter-fried foods	Egg-free baked goods[a] Spaghetti Rice Some egg substitutes[a] (read label)
Wheat	(Enriched) flour Wheat germ Wheat bran Wheat starch Gluten Food starch Vegetable starch Vegetable gum Rye Oatmeal Barley Buckwheat	Baked goods made with wheat flour Crackers Macaroni Spaghetti Noodles Gravies, thickened sauces Fried food coating Baking mixes Soy sauce Hot dogs with wheat filler Batter-fried foods Some sausages	Wheat-free breads,[a] crackers (rice cakes, special breads) Certain cold cereals (corn, rice flour, tapioca) Flours: rice, potato

Foodstuff	Hidden ingredients listed on label	Foods to avoid	Substitutes
Soy	Soy flour Soybean oil Vegetable oil Soy protein Soy protein isolate Textured vegetable protein (TVP) Vegetable starch Vegetable gum	Soy sauce Teriyaki sauce Worcestershire sauce Tuna packed in vegetable oil Tofu Baked goods or cereals that include soy	Nutramigen Alimentum
Corn	Cornmeal Corn starch Corn oil Corn syrup (solids) Corn sweetner Corn alcohol Vegetable oil Vegetable starch Vegetable gum Food starch	Some baked goods Corn tortillas (chips, tacos) Popcorn Some cold cereals Corn syrup Pancake syrup Many candies Most baking powders	Wheat flour tortillas Thickeners: wheat, potato or rice flour Beet or cane sugar Maple syrup or honey Baking soda and cream of tartar (for leavening agent)
Chocolate	Cocoa Cocoa butter	Candy Baked goods Colas	Carob products
Beef	Animal shortening Animal lard Animal gelatin	Soups Bouillon Beef gravies and sauces Hot dogs Cold cuts	Pure vegetable shortening
Pork	Animal shortening Animal lard	Bacon Sausage Hot dogs Baked beans and soups with pork	All-beef hot dogs and cold cuts Vegetarian baked beans Pure vegetable shortening

[a]Products available from Ener-G Foods, P.O. Box 84487, Seattle, WA 98124-5787 (1-800-331-5222).

Source: Adapted from Ref. 163.

References

1. Zeiger RS. Prevention of food allergy in infancy. Ann Allergy 1990; 65: 430–441.
2. Zeiger RS. Development and prevention of allergic disease in childhood In: Middleton E Jr, Reed CE, Ellis EE, Adkinson Jr. NF, Yunginger JW, Busse WW, eds. Allergy Principles and Practice, 3d ed. St. Louis: Mosby, 1993; 1137–1171.
3. Cookson WOCM, Faux J, Sharp PA, Hopkin JM. Linkage between immunologlobin E responses underlying asthma and rhinitis and chromosome 11q. Lancet 1989; 1:1292–1294.
4. Clough JB. Pre- and post-natal events leading to allergen sensitization. Clin Exp Allergy 1993; 23:462–465.
5. Grulee CG, Sanford HN. The influence of breast and artificial feeding on infantile eczema. J Pediatr 1930; 9:223–225.
6. Michel FB, Bousquet J, Greillier P, Robinet-Levy M, Coulomb Y. Comparison of cord blood immunoglobulin E and maternal allergy for the prevention of atopic disease infancy. J Allergy Clin Immunol 1980; 65:422–430.
7. Businco L, Marchetti F, Pelligrini G, Berlini R. Predictive value of cord blood IgE levels in "at-risk" newborn babies and influence of type of feeding. Clin Allergy 1983; 13:503–508.
8. Warner JA, Miles EZ, Jones AC, Quint DJ, Colwell BM, Warner JO. Is deficiency of interferon gamma production by allergen triggered cord blood cells a predictor of atopic eczema? Clin Exp Allergy 1994; 24:423–430.
9. Falth-Magnusson K, Kjellman NIM. Development of atopic disease in babies whose mothers were receiving exclusion diet during pregnancy—a randomized study. J Allergy Clin Immunol 1987; 80:868–875.
10. Falth-Magnusson K, Kjellman NIM, Magnusson KE. Antibodies IgG, IgA, and IgM to food antigens during the first 18 months of life in relation to feeding and development of atopic disease. J Allergy Clin Immunol 1988; 81:743–749.
11. Falth-Magnusson K, Kjellman NIM. Allergy prevention by maternal elimination diet during pregnancy—a 5-year follow-up of a randomized study. J Allergy Clin Immunol 1992; 89:709–713.
12. Lilja G, Dannaeus A, Foucard T, Graff-Lonnevig, Johannsson SGO, Oman H. Effects of maternal diet during late pregnancy and lactation on the development of atopic diseases in infants up to 18 months of age—in vivo results. Clin Exp Allergy 1989; 19:473–479.
13. Lilja G, Dannaeus A, Foucard T, Graff-Lonnevig, Johannson SGO, Oman H. Effects of maternal diet during late pregnancy and lactation on the development of IgE and egg- and milk-specific IgE and IgG antibodies in infants. Clin Exp Allergy 1991; 21:196–202.
14. Zeiger RS, Heller S, Mellon MH, Forsythe AB, O'Connor RD, Hamburger RN, Schatz M. Effect of combined maternal and infant food-allergen avoid-

ance on development of atopy in early infancy: A randomized study. J Allergy Clin Immunol 1989; 84:72–89.

15. Udall JN, Colony P, Fritze L, Kleinman R, Walker WA. Development of gastrointestinal mucosal barrier. II. The effect of natural versus artificial feeding on intestinal permeability to macromolecules. Pediatr Res 1981; 15: 245–249.

16. Axelsson I, Jakobsson I, Lindberg T. Macromolecular absorption in preterm and term infants. Acta Paediatr Scand 1989; 78:532–537.

17. Lucas A, McLaughlan P, Coombs RRA. Latent anaphylactic sensitization of infants of low birth weight to cow's milk protein. Br Med J 1984; 289: 1254–1256.

18. Lucas A, Brooke OG, Morley R, Cole TJ, Bamford MF. Early diet of preterm infants and development of allergic or atopic disease: randomized prospective study. Br Med J 1990; 300:837–840.

19. Walker WA, Hanson D. The mechanisms of allergic reactions and local antibody production in infancy. Clin Dis Pediatr Nutr 1985; 4:75–95.

20. Savilahti E, Jarvenpaa AL, Raiha N. Serum immunoglobulin in preterm infants. Comparison of human milk and formula feeding. Pediatrics 1983; 72: 312–316.

21. Kleinman RE, Walker WA. Antigen processing and uptake from the intestinal tract. Clin Rev Allergy 1984; 2:25–37.

22. Machtinger S, Moss R. Cow's milk allergy in breast-fed infants: the role of allergen and maternal secretory IgA antibody. J Allergy Clin Immunol 1986; 77:341–347.

23. Aberg N, Engstrom I, Lindberg U. Allergic diseases in Swedish school children. Acta Paediatr Scand 1989; 78:246–252.

24. Cogswell JJ, Mitchell EB, Alexander J. Parental smoking, breast feeding, and respiratory infection in development of allergic diseases. Arch Dis Child 1987; 62:338–344.

25. Kramer M, Moroz B. Do breast-feeding and delayed introduction of solid foods protect against subsequent atopic eczema? J Pediatr 1981; 98:546–550.

26. Taylor B, Wadsworth J, Golding J, Butler N. Breast feeding, eczema, asthma, and hayfever. J Epidemiol Community Health 1983; 37:95–99.

27. Savilahti E, Tainio VM, Salmenpera L, Siimes MA, Perheentupa J. Prolonged exclusive breast feeding and heredity as determinants in infantile atopy. Arch Dis Child 1987; 62:269–273.

28. Poysa L, Remes K, Korppi M, Juntunen-Backman K. Atopy in children with and without a family history of atopy. 1. Clinical manifestations, with special reference to diet in infancy. Acta Paediatr Scand 1989; 78:896–901.

29. Poysa L, Korppi M, Remes K, Juntunen-Backman K. Atopy in childhood and diet in infancy. A nine-year study. I. Clinical manifestations. Allergy Proc 1991; 12:107–111.

30. Kramer MA. Does breast feeding help protect against atopic disease? Biology, methodology, and a golden jubilee of controversy. J Pediatr 1989; 112: 181–190.

31. Myers MG, Fomon SJ, Koontz FP, McGuinness GA, Lachabruch A, Hollingshead R. Respiratory and gastrointestinal illnesses in breast and formula fed infants. Am J Dis Child 1984; 138:629–632.
32. Zeiger RS, Heller S, Mellon M, O'Connor R, Hamburger RN. Effectiveness of dietary manipulation in the prevention of food allergy in infants. J Allergy Clin Immunol 1986; 78(part 2):224–238.
33. Van Asperen PP, Kemp SS, Mellis CM. Immediate food hypersensitivity reactions on the known exposure to the food. Arch Dis Child 1983; 58:253–256.
34. Hattevig G, Kjellman B, Johansson SGO, Bjorksten B. Clinical symptoms and IgE responses to common food problems in atopic and healthy children. Clin Allergy 1984; 14:551–559.
35. Stuart CA, Twiselton R, Nicholas MF, Hide DW. Passage of cow's milk protein in breast milk. Clin Allergy 1984; 14:533–535.
36. Jakobsson I, Lindberg R, Benediktsson B, Hansson BG. Dietary bovine beta-lactoglobulin is transferred to human milk. Acta Paediatr Scand 1985; 74:342–345.
37. Axelsson I, Jakobsson I, Lindberg T, Benediktsson B. Bovine beta-lactoglobulin in the human milk. A longitudinal study during the whole lactation period. Acta Paediatr Scand 1986; 75:702–707.
38. Clyne PS, Kulczycki A. Human breast milk contains bovine IgG. Relationship to infant colic? Pediatrics 1991; 87:439–444.
39. Cant A, Narsden RA, Kilshaw PJ. Egg and cow's milk hypersensitivity in exclusively breast-fed infants with eczema, and detection of egg protein in breast milk. Br Med J 1985; 291:932–935.
40. Troncone R, Scarcella A, Donatiello A, Cannataro P, Tarabuso A, Auricchio S. Passage of gliadin into human breast milk. Acta Paediatr Scand 1987; 76:453–456.
41. Cavagni G, Paganelli R, Caffarelli C, D'Offizi G, Bertolini P, Aiutia F, Giovannelli G. Passage of food antigens into circulation of breast-fed infants with atopic dermatitis. Ann Allergy 1988; 61:361–365.
42. Kilshaw PJ, Cant J. The passage of maternal dietary proteins in human breast milk. Int Arch Allergy Appl Immunol 1984; 75:8–15.
43. Hattevig G, Kjellman B, Sigurs N, Bjorksten B, Kjellman NIM. Effect of maternal avoidance of eggs, cow's milk and fish during lactation upon allergic manifestations in infants. Clin Exp Allergy 1989; 19:27–32.
44. Hattevig G, Kjellman B, Sigurs N, Grodzinsky E, Hed J, Bjorksten B. The effect of maternal avoidance of eggs, cow's milk, and fish during lactation on the development of IgE, IgG, and IgA antibodies in infants. J Allergy Clin Immunol 1990; 85:108–115.
45. Sigurs N, Hattevig G, Kjellman B. Maternal avoidance of eggs, cow's milk, and fish during lactation: effect on allergic manifestations, skin-prick tests, and specific IgE antibodies in children at age 4 years. Pediatrics 1992; 89:735–739.

46. Chandra RK, Shakuntla P, Hamed A. Influence of maternal diet during lactation and use of formula feeds on development of atopic eczema in high risk infants. Br Med J 1989; 299:228–230.

47. Glaser J, Johnstone DE. Soybean milk as a substitute for mammalian milk in early infancy with special reference to prevention of allergy to cow's milk. Ann Allergy 1952; 10:433–439.

48. Glaser J, Johnstone DE. Prophylaxis of allergic disease in the newborn. JAMA 1953; 153:620–622.

49. Johnstone DE, Glaser J. Use of soybean milk as an aid in prophylaxis of allergic disease in children. J Allergy 1953; 24:434–436.

50. Johnstone DE, Dutton AM. Dietary prophylaxis of allergic disease in children. N Engl J Med 1966; 274:715–719.

51. Brown EB, Josephson BM, Levine HS, Rosen MA. A prospective study of allergy in a pediatric population. Am J Dis Child 1969; 63:388–393.

52. Kjellman NIM, Johansson SGO. Soy versus cow's milk in infants with a biparental history of atopic disease: development of atopic disease and immunoglobulins from birth to 4 years of age. Clin Allergy 1979; 9:347–358.

53. Miskelly FG, Burr ML, Vaughan-Williams E, Fehily AM, Butland BK, Merrett TG. Infant feeding and allergy. Arch Dis Child 1988; 63:388–393.

54. Chandra RK, Singh G, Shridhara B. Effect of feeding whey hydrolysate, soy, and conventional cow milk formulas on incidence of atopic disease in high risk infants. Ann Allergy 1989; 63:102–106.

55. Mortimer ER. Anaphylaxis following ingestion of soybean. J Pediatr 1961; 58:90–92.

56. Singh B, Lee KC, Fraga E, Wilkinson A, Wong M, Barton M. Minimum peptide sequences necessary for priming and triggering of humoral and cell-mediated immune responses in mice: use of synthetic peptide antigens of defined structure. J Immunol 1980; 124:1336–1343.

57. Knights RJ. Processing and evaluation of the antigenicity of protein hydrolystates. Clin Dis Pediatr Nutr 1985; 4:105–115.

58. Sampson HA, Bernhisel-Broadbent J, Yang E, Scanlon SM. Safety of casein hydrolysate formula in children with cow milk allergy. J Pediatr 1991; 118: 520–525.

59. Businco L, Dreborg S, Einarsson R, Giampietro PG, Host A, Keller KM, Strobel S, Wahn U, Bjorksten B, Kjellman NIM, Sampson H, Zeiger R. Hydrolysed cow's milk formulae: Allergenicity and use in treatment and prevention. An ESPACI position paper. Pediatr Allergy Immunol 1993; 4: 101–111.

60. Pahud JJ, Monti JC, Jost R. Allergenicity of whey protein: its modification by tryptic in vitro hydolysis of the protein. J Pediatr Gastroenterol Nutr 1985; 4:408–413.

61. Businco L, Cantani A, Longhi AL, Giampietro PG. Anaphylactic reactions to a cow's milk whey protein hydrolysate (Alfa-Re, Nestle) in infants with cow's milk allergy. Ann Allergy 1989; 62:333–335.

62. Lifschitz CH, Hawkins HK, Guerra C, Byrd N. Anaphylactic shock due to cow's milk protein hypersensitivity in a breast-fed infant. J Pediatr Gastroenterol Nutr 1988; 7:141–144.

63. Rosenthal E, Schlesinger Y, Birnbaum Y, Goldstein R, Benderly A, Freier S. Intolerance to casein hydrolysate formula: clinical aspects. Acta Paediatr Scand 1991; 80:958–960.

64. Halken S, Host A, Hansen LG, Osterballe O. Safety of a new, ultrafiltrated whey hydrolysate formula in children with cow milk allergy: a clinical investigation. Pediatr Allergy Immunol 1993; 4:53–59.

65. McLaughlan P, Anderson KJ, Coombs RRA. An oral screening procedure to determine the sensitizing capacity of infant feeding formulae. Clin Allergy 1981; 11:311–318.

66. Zeiger RS, Heller S, Mellon MH, Halsey JH, Hamburger RN, Sampson HA. Genetic and environmental factors affecting the development of atopy through age 4 in children of atopic parents: a prospective randomized study of food allergen avoidance. Pediatr Allergy Immunol 1992; 3:110–127.

67. Eastham EJ, Lichauco T, Grady MI. Antigenicity of infant formulas: role of immature intestine on protein permeability. J Pediatr 1978; 93:561–564.

68. Kletter B, Gery I, Freier S, Davies AM. Immune response of normal infants to cow milk. II. Decreased immune reactions in initially breast fed infants. Int Arch Allergy 1971; 40:667–671.

69. Chandra RK, Hamed A. Cumulative incidence of atopic disorders in high risk infants fed whey hydrolysate, soy, and conventional cow milk formulas. Ann Allergy 1991; 67:129–132.

70. Vandenplas Y, Hauser B, Van den Borre C, Sacre L, Dab I. Effect of a whey hydrolysate prophylaxis of atopic disease. Ann Allergy 1992; 68:419–424.

71. Mallet E, Henocq A. Long-term prevention of allergic diseases by using protein hydrolysate formula in at-risk infants. J Pediatr 1992; 121:S95–S100.

72. Halken S, Host A, Hansen LG, Osterballe O. Preventive effect of feeding high-risk infants a casein hydrolysate formula or an ultrafiltrated whey hydrolysate formula. A prospective, randomized comparative clinical study. Pediatr Allergy Immunol 1993; 4:173–181.

73. Fergusson DM, Horwood LJ, Beautrais AL, Shannon FT, Taylor B. Eczema and infant diet. Clin Allergy 1981; 11:325–331.

74. Fergusson DM, Horwood LJ, Shannon FT. Early solid feeding and recurrent childhood eczema: a 10-year longitudinal study. Pediatrics 1990; 86:541–546.

75. Fergusson DM, Horwood LJ, Shannon FT. Asthma and infant diet. Arch Dis Child 1983; 58:48–51.

76. Kajosaari M, Saarinen UM. Prophylaxis of atopic disease by six months total solid elimination. Arch Paediatr Scand 1983; 72:411–414.

77. Kajosaari M. Atopy prophylaxis in high-risk infants: prospective 5-year follow-up study of children with six months exclusive breastfeeding and solid food elimination. Adv Exp Med Biol 1991; 310:453–458.

78. Saarinen UM, Kajosaari M. Does dietary elimination in infancy prevent or only postpone a food allergy? A study of fish and citrus allergy in 375 children. Lancet 1980; 1:166–167.

79. Chandra RK, Puri S, Suraiya C, Cheema PS. Influence of maternal food antigen avoidance during pregnancy and lactation on the incidence of atopic eczema in infants. Clin Allergy 1986; 16:563–571.

80. Zeiger RS, Heller S. Development of nasal basophilic cells and nasal eosinophils from age 4 months through 4 years in children of atopic parents. J Allergy Clin Immunol 1993; 91:723–734.

81. Zeiger RS, Heller S. The development and prediction of atopy in high-risk children: follow-up at age 7 years in a prospective randomized study of combined maternal and infant food allergen avoidance. J Allergy Clin Immunol 1995; 95:1179–1190.

82. Arshad SH, Matthews S, Gant C, Hide DW. Effect of allergen avoidance on development of allergic disorders in infancy. Lancet 1992; 339:1493–1497.

83. Hide DW, Matthews S, Matthews L, Stevens M, Ridout S, Twiselton R, Gant C, Arshad SH. Effect of allergen avoidance in infancy on allergic manifestations at age two years. J Allergy Clin Immunol 1994; 93:842–846.

84. Roundtree S, Cogswell JJ, Platts-Mills TAE, Mitchell EB. Development of IgE and IgG antibodies to food and inhalant allergens in children at risk of allergic disease. Arch Dis Child 1985; 60:727–735.

85. Hattevig G, Kjellman B, Bjorksten B. Clinical symptoms and IgE responses to common food proteins and inhalants in the first 7 years of life. Clin Allergy 1987; 17:571–578.

86. Sigurs N, Hattevig G, Kjellman B, Kjellman NIM, Nilsson L, Bjorksten B. Appearance of atopic disease in relation to serum IgE antibodies in children followed up from birth for 4 to 15 years. J Allergy Clin Immunol 1994; 94: 757–763.

87. Kuehr J, Frischer T, Meinert R, Barth R, Schraud S, Urbanek R, Karmaus W, Forster J. Sensitization to mite allergens is a risk factor for early and late onset of asthma and for persistence of asthmatic signs in children. J Allergy Clin Immunol 1995; 95:655–662.

88. Langeland T. A clinical and immunological study of allergy to hen's egg white. I. A clinical study of egg allergy. Clin Allergy 1983; 13:371–382.

89. Aberg N, Engstrom I. Natural history of allergic diseases in children. Acta Paediatr Scand 1990; 79:206–211.

90. Croner S, Kjellman NIM. Natural history of bronchial asthma in childhood. A prospective study from birth up to 12–14 years of age. Allergy 1992; 47: 150–157.

91. Martinez FD, Wright AL, Taussig LM, Holberg CJ, Halonen M, Morgan WJ, and the Group Health Medical Associates. Asthma and wheezing in the first six years of life. N Engl J Med 1995; 332:133–138.

92. Borres MP, Odelram H, Irander K, Kjellman NIM, Bjorksten B. Peripheral blood eosinophilia in infants at 3 months of age is associated with subsequent

development of atopic disease in early childhood. J Allergy Clin Immunol 1995; 95:694–698.

93. Lilja G, Oman H. Prediction of atopic disease in infancy by determination of immunological parameters: IgE, IgE- and IgG-antibodies to food allergens, skin prick tests and T-lymphocyte subsets. Pediatr Allergy Immunol 1991; 2:6–13.

94. Croner S, Kjellman NIH. Development of atopic disease in relation to family history and cord blood IgE levels. Eleven-year follow-up in 1654 children. Pediatr Allergy Immunol 1990; 1:14–20.

95. Sporik R, Holgate ST, Platts-Mills TA, Cogswell JJ. Exposure to house-dust mite allergen (*Der p* I) and the development of asthma in childhood. A prospective study. N Engl J Med 1990; 323:502–507.

96. Lau-Schadendorf S, Wahn U. Exposure to indoor allergens and development of allergy. Pediatr Allergy Immunol 1991; 2:63–69.

97. Platts-Mills TAE, Sporik RB, Ward GW, Heyman PW, Chapman MD. Dose-response relationships between asthma and exposure to indoor allergens. Prog Allergy Clin Immunol 1995; 3:90–96.

98. Arshad SH, Stevens M, Hide DW. The effect of genetic and environmental factors on the prevalence of allergic disorders at the age of two years. Clin Exp Allergy 1993; 23:504–511.

99. Wickman M, Nordvall SL, Pershagan G. Risk factors in early childhood for sensitization to airborne allergens. Pediatr Allergy Immunol 1992; 3:128–133.

100. Warner JA, Little SA, Pollock I, Longbottom JL, Warner JO. The influence of exposure to house dust mite, cat, pollen, and fungal allergens in the home on primary sensitization in asthma. Pediatr Allergy Immunol 1990; 1:79–86.

101. Sporik R, Ingram JM, Price W, Sussman JM, Honsinger RW, Platts-Mills TAE. Association of asthma with serum IgE and skin test reactivity to allergens among children living at high altitude. Tickling the dragon's breath. Am J Respir Crit Care Med 1995; 151:1388–1392.

102. Custovic A, Taggart SCO, Woodcock A. House dust mite and cat allergen in different indoor environments. Clin Exp Allergy 1994; 24:1164–1168.

103. Call RS, Smith TF, Morris E, Chapman MD, Platts-Mills TAE. Risk factors for asthma in inner city children. J Pediatr 1992; 121:862–866.

104. Delfino RJ, Matteucci RM, Anderson R, Zeiger RS, Seltzer JM, Street DH, Koutrakis R. Relationships of symptom severity and peak expiratory flow rates to personal ozone and aeroallergens in a panel of asthmatics. Am J Respir Crit Care Med 1996; 154:633–641.

105. Ikura Y, Naspitz CK, Mikawa H, Talaricoficho S, Baba M, Sole D, Nishima S. Prevention of asthma by ketotifen in infants with atopic dermatitis. Ann Allergy 1992; 68:233–236.

106. Johnstone DE, Dutton A. The value of hyposensitization therapy for bronchial asthma in children. A 14 year old study. Pediatrics 1968; 42:793–802.

107. National Heart, Lung, and Blood Institute: National Asthma Education Program Expert Panel Report: guidelines for the diagnosis and management of asthma. J Allergy Clin Immunol 1991; 88:425–533.

108. Holt PG, McMenamin C, Nelson D. Primary sensitization to inhalant allergens during infancy. Pediatr Allergy Immunol 1990; 1:3–13.

109. Vervloet D, Penaud A, Razzouk H, Senft M, Arnaud A, Boutin C, Charpin D. Altitude and house dust mites. J Allergy Clin Immunol 1982; 69:290–296.

110. Dornelas de Andrade A, Charpin D, Birnbaum J, Lanteaume A, Chapman M, Vervloet D. Indoor allergen levels in day nurseries. J Allergy Clin Immunol 1995; 95:1158–1163.

111. Babe KS, Arlian LG, Confer PD, Kim R. House dust mite (*Dermatophagoides farinae* and *Dermatophagoides pteronyssinus*) prevalence in the homes and hallways of a tertiary care hospital. J Allergy Clin Immunol 1995; 95:801–805.

112. Harving H, Korsgaard J, Dahl R. House-dust mite exposure reduction in specially designed, mechanically ventilated "healthy" homes. Allergy 1994; 49:713–718.

113. Ehnert B, Lau-Schadendorf S, Weber A, Buettner P, Schou C, Wahn U. Reducing domestic exposure to dust mite allergen reduces bronchial hypersensitivity in sensitive children with asthma. J Allergy Clin Immunol 1992; 90:135–138.

114. Kniest FM, Young E, Van Pragg MCG, Vos H, Helianthe S, Kort M, Koers J, De Maat-Bleeker F, Van Bronswijk JEMH. Clinical evaluation of a double-blind dust-mite avoidance trial with mite-allergic rhinitic patients. Clin Exp Allergy 1991; 21:39–47.

115. Platts-Mills TAE, Tovey ER, Mitchell EB, Moszoro H, Nock P, Wilkins SR. Reduction of bronchial hyperreactivity during prolonged allergen avoidance. Lancet 1982; 2:675–678.

116. Peroni DG, Boner Al, Vallone G, Antolini I, Warner JO. Effective allergen avoidance at high altitude reduces allergen-induced bronchial hyperresponsiveness. Am J Resp Crit Care Med 1994; 149:1442–1446.

117. Sette L, Comis A, Marcucci F, Sensi L, Piacentini GL, Boner AL. Benzylbenzoate foam: effects on mite allergens in mattress, serum and nasal secretory IgE to *Dermatophagoides pteronyssinus*, and bronchial hyperreactivity in children with allergic asthma. Pediatr Pulmonol 1994; 18:218–227.

118. Piacentini GL, Martinati L, Fornari A, Comis A, Carcereri L, Boccagni P, Boner AL. Antigen avoidance in a mountain environment: influence on basophil releasibility in children with allergic asthma. J Allergy Clin Immunol 1993; 92:644–650.

119. Boner Al, Peroni DG, Piacentini GL, Venge P. Influence of allergen avoidance at high altitude on serum markers of eosinophil activation in children with allergic asthma. Clin Exp Allergy 1993; 23:1021–1026.

120. Simon HU, Grotzer M, Nikolaizik WH, Ser K, Schoni MH. High altitude climate therapy reduces peripheral blood T lymphocyte activation, eosino-

philia, and bronchial obstruction in children with house dust allergic asthma. Pediatr Pulmonol 1994; 17:304–311.

121. Colloff MJ, Ayres J, Carswell F, Howarth PH, Merrett TG, Mitchell EB, Walsha MJ, Warner JO, Warner JI, Woodcock AA. The control of allergens of dust mites and domestic pets: a position paper. Clin Exp Allergy 1992; 22(suppl 2):1–28.

122. Deitemann A, Bessof JC, Hoyet C, Ott M, Verot A, Pauli G. A double blind, placebo controlled trial of solidified benzyl benzoate applied in dwellings of asthmatic children sensitive to mites: clinical efficacy and effect on mite allergens. J Allergy Clin Immunol 1993; 91:738–746.

123. Marks GB, Tovey ER, Green W, Shearer M, Salome CM, Woolcock AJ. House dust allergen avoidance: a randomized controlled trial of surface chemical treatment and encasement of bedding. Clin Exp Allergy 1994; 24: 1078–1083.

124. Naspitz CK, Rizzo MC, Arruda LK, Fernandez-Caldas E, Sole D, Chapman MD, Platts-Mills TAE. Environmental control of mite allergy. Prog Allergy Clin Immunol 1995; 3:334–339.

125. Dybendal T, Vik H, Elsayed S. Dust from carpeted and smooth floors. II. Antigenic and allergenic content of dust vacuumed from carpeted and smooth floors in schools under routine cleaning schedules. Allergy 1989; 44: 401–411.

126. Munir AKM, Einarsson R, Dreborg SKG. Indirect contact with pets can confound the effect of cleaning procedures for reduction of animal allergen levels in house dust. Pediatr Allergy Immunol 1994; 5:32–39.

127. deBlay R, Chapman MD, Platts-Mills TAE. Airborne cat allergen (*Fel d* I): environmental control with the cat in situ. Am Rev Respir Dis 1991; 143: 1334–1339.

128. Klucks CV, Ownby DR, Green J, Zoratti E. Cat shedding of *Fel d* I is not reduced by washings, Allerpet-C spray, or acepromazine. J Allergy Clin Immunol 1995; 95:1164–1171.

129. Warner JA. Creating optimal home conditions for the house dust mite. Clin Exp Allergy 1994; 24:207–209.

130. Tovey ER, Woolcock AJ. Direct exposure of carpets to sunlight can kill all mites. J Allergy Clin Immunol 1994; 93:1072–1074.

131. Brook U, Shiloh S. Attitudes of asthmatic and nonasthmatic adolescents toward cigarettes and smoking. Clin Pediatr 1993; 32:642–646.

132. Dombrowske MP, Bottoms SF, Bolke GM, Wald J. Incidence of preeclampsia among asthmatic patients lower with theophylline. Am J Obstet Gynecol 1986; 155:265–267.

133. MacKenzie TD, Bartecchi CE, Schrier RW. The human costs of tobacco use (part 2). N Engl J Med 1994; 330:975–980.

134. Burns DM. Positive evidence on effectiveness of selected smoking prevention programs in the United States. J Natl Cancer Inst Monagr 1992; 12: 17–20.

135. Hovell MF, Meltzer SB, Zakarian JM, Wahlgren DR, Leaderer BP, Meltzer EO, Zeiger RS, O'Connor RD, Mulvihill MM, Atkins CJ. Reduction of environmental tobacco smoke exposure among asthmatic children: a controlled trial. Chest 1994; 106:440–446.

136. Zwick J, Popp W, Wagner C, Reiser K, Schmoger J, Bock A, Herkner K, Radunsky K. Effects of ozone on the respiratory health, allergic sensitization, and cellular system in children. Am Rev Respir Dis 1991; 144:1075–1079.

137. Molfino NA, Wright SC, Katz I, Tarlo S, Silverman F, McClean PA, Szalai JP, Raizenne M, Slutsky AS, Zamel N. Effect of low concentration of ozone on inhaled allergen responses in asthmatic subjects. Lancet 1991; 338: 199–203.

138. Ishizaki T, Koisumi K, Ikemore R, Ishiyama Y, Kushibiki E. Studies of prevalence of Japanese cedar pollinosis among residents in a densely cultivated area. Ann Allergy 1987; 58:265–270.

139. Andrae S, Axelsson O, Bjorksten B, Fredricksson M, Kjellman NIM. Symptoms of bronchial hyperreactivity and asthma in relation to environmental factors. Arch Dis Child 1988; 63:473–478.

140. Matsumara Y. The effects of ozone, nitrogen dioxide, and sulfur dioxide on the experimentally induced allergic respiratory disorder in guinea pigs. Am Rev Respir Dis 1978; 102:430–447.

141. Air Pollution Control District County of San Diego Annual Report 1992.

142. Kagamimori S, Katoh T, Naruse Y, Watanabe M, Kasuya M, Shinkai J, Kawano S. The changing prevalence of respiratory symptoms in atopic children in response to air pollution. Ann Allergy 1986; 16:299–308.

143. Groothuis JR, Simoes EAF, Levin MJ, Hall CB, Long CE, Rodriguez WJ, Arrobio J, Meissner HC, Fulton DR, Welliver RC, Tristram DA, Siber GR, Prince GA, Raden MV, Hemming VG, and the Respiratory Syncytial Virus Immune Globulin Study Group. Prophylactic administration of respiratory syncytial virus immune globulin to high-risk infants and young children. N Engl J Med 1993; 329:1524–1530.

144. Matthew DJ, Norman AP, Taylor B, Turner MW. Prevention of eczema. Lancet 1977; 1:321–324.

145. Saarinen UM, Backman A, Kajosaari M, Siimes MA. Prolonged breastfeeding as prophylaxis for atopic disease. Lancet 1979; 1:163–166.

146. Chandra RK. Prospective studies of the effect of breast feeding on incidence of infection and allergy. Acta Paediatr Scand 1979; 68:691–694.

147. Ziering RW, O'Connor R, Mellon, Hamburger R. University of California in San Diego prophylaxis of allergy in infancy study: an interim report. J Allergy Clin Immunol 1979; 63(part 2):199.

148. Gruskay FL. Comparison of breast, cow, and soy feedings in the prevention of onset of allergic disease. Clin Pediatr 1982; 21:486–491.

149. Pratt HF. Breastfeeding and eczema. Early Human Dev 1984; 9:283–290.

150. Chandra RK, Puri S, Cheema PS. Predictive value of cord blood IgE in the development of atopic disease and role of breast feeding in its prevention. Clin Allergy 1985; 15:517–522.

151. Kaufman HS. Diet and heredity in infantile atopic dermatitis. Arch Dermatol 1972; 105:400–404.

152. Halpern SR, Sellers WA, Johnson RB, Anderson DW, Saperstein S, Reisch JS. Development of childhood allergy in infants fed breast, soy, or cow milk. J Allergy Clin Immunol 1973; 51:139–151.

153. Kaufman HS, Frick OL. The development of allergy in infants of allergic parents: a prospective study concerning the role of heredity. Ann Allergy 1976; 37:410–415.

154. Hide DW, Guyer BM. Clinical manifestations of allergy related to breast- and cow's milk-feeding. Arch Dis Child 1981; 56:172–175.

155. Gordon RR, Ward AM, Noble DA, Allen R. Immunoglobulin E and the eczema-asthma syndrome in early childhood. Lancet 1982; 1:72–74.

156. Van Asperen PP, Kemp AS, Mellis CM. Relationship of diet in the development of atopy in infancy. Clin Allergy 1984; 14:525–532.

157. Hide DW, Guyer BM. Clinical manifestations of allergy related to breast- and cow's milk-feeding. Pediatrics 1985; 76:973–975.

158. Zeiger RS. Secondary prevention of allergic disease: an adjunct to primary prevention. Pediatr Allergy Immunol 1995; 6:127–138.

159. Zeiger RS. Breast-feeding and dietary avoidance. In: de Weck AL, Sampson HA, eds. Intestinal Immunology and Food Allergy, Nestle Nutrition Workshop Series. Vol. 34. New York: Raven Press, 1995: 203–222.

160. Zeiger RS. Dietary manipulations in infants and their mothers and the natural course of atopic disease. Pediatr Allergy Immunol 1994; 5(suppl):33–43.

161. Kuehr J, Frischer T, Karmaus W, Meinert R, Barth R, Schraub S, Daschner A, Urbanec R, Forster J. Natural variation in mite antigen density in house dust and relationship to residential factors. Clin Exp Allergy 1994; 24: 229–237.

162. Woodfolk JA, Luczynska CM, de Blay F, Chapman MD, Platts-Mills TAE. The effect of vacuum cleaners on the concentration and particle size distribution of airborne cat allergen. J Allergy Clin Immunol 1993; 91:829–837.

163. Adams EJ, Mahan Lk. Nutritional care in food and allergy intolerance. In: Krause KMV, Mahan, eds. Food, Nutrition, and Diet Therapy. Philadelphia: Saunders, 1984.

Part Seven

ALLERGIC AND IMMUNOLOGICAL DISEASES
DURING INFANCY

31

The Wheezing Infant

**ALAN F. ISLES and
CLAIRE E. WAINWRIGHT**

Royal Children's Hospital
Brisbane, Queensland, Australia

CHRISTOPHER J. L. NEWTH

University of Southern California School of
Medicine, Children's Hospital of Los
Angeles
Los Angeles, California

I. Introduction

Wheezing is one of the most frequently encountered respiratory symptoms of childhood. It causes great concern to parents and frequently causes diagnostic and therapeutic confusion for those treating the infants. Although asthma is the most common cause of wheezing in older children, it is inappropriate to label every wheezy infant as having asthma without considering other possibilities, especially in the very young.

About 30% of infants wheeze with lower respiratory infections during the first 3 years of life and, by age 6 years, almost half of all children have had at least one episode of wheezing (1). In addition, there is mounting evidence that the prevalence of and morbidity from asthma are increasing (2). The reasons for these trends are not immediately obvious and are probably the result of a complex interaction of factors. Hospital admission rates for wheeze in children up to the age of 4 years have increased fourfold in the United Kingdom over the last 2 decades (3). The relationship between wheezy illnesses in infancy and a subsequent risk of asthma has been the subject of much debate over the years. The use, in the past, of diagnostic terms such as "wheezy bronchitis" and "recurrent bronchiolitis" caused much confusion and led to both underrecognition and under-treatment of asthma in the younger age groups (4). The eventual reaction to this was to regard all wheezy children as having asthma. However, several recent birth cohort studies suggest that this approach has been incorrect and those previously "lumped" together as having asthma are again being "split" into different groups (1).

Epidemiological and birth cohort studies have provided an improved understanding of the influence of genes, prenatal events, and early life influences on the causation of asthma. These studies have given some insight into such fundamental issues as whether wheezing illnesses that resolve in early childhood and wheezing which persists into adolescence are the same disease or whether they are manifestations of etiologically distinct disease processes (5–7). Although our understanding of the pathophysiology of asthma has improved, we are still unable to predict why one individual becomes asthmatic and another does not (8).

II. Predisposing Factors

A. Anatomical and Physiological Factors

A variety of anatomic and physiologic factors combine to make the infant uniquely susceptible to respiratory illness (9). Peripheral airway resistance is greater in infants than in adults, as the peripheral airways are disproportionately narrow (10). This explains, in part, why diseases such as bronchiolitis, which predominantly affect the small airways, have such a serious impact on infants. The relative lack of elastic recoil in the infant lung predisposes to early airway closure even during tidal breathing (11). In disease states, this has the effect of predisposing to airway closure at relatively high lung volumes, resulting in ventilation-perfusion mismatching and a more profound disturbance of gas exchange than might be expected in older children. In addition, the pores of Kohn and the bronchoalveolar canals of Lambert (12) are either not present or deficient in both number and size, depriving infants of collateral ventilation and predisposing them to atelectasis during respiratory illness, further aggravating ventilation-perfusion mismatching and hypoxemia.

In infants the angle of the ribs is almost horizontal, in contrast to the more oblique insertion in adults. The horizontal insertion decreases the efficiency of "bucket-handle" outward motion of the thoracic cage during inspiration. Subsequently, there is a greater tendency for the more compliant ribcage of the infant to distort, further decreasing the efficiency of diaphragmatic contraction during inspiration and increasing the work of breathing. In addition, the diaphragm of the infant has fewer type I (fatigue-resistant) muscle fibers than the adult diaphragm, further predisposing the infant to respiratory failure in any condition which increases the respiratory load (13). Gaultier has reviewed respiratory muscle function in infants and discussed in detail the mechanical properties of the chest wall, respiratory muscle function, and thoraco-abdominal coupling, especially in relation to sleep state (14). All of these factors combine to predispose the infant to ventilatory failure.

In normal infants, the number of mucus-secreting cells in the airway epithelium is proportionately greater than in adults (15). Airway inflammation in infants is therefore more likely to result in mucus plugging, atelectasis, and hypoxemia in infants. The latter is also likely to further aggravate the already raised potential for increased pulmonary vascular resistance.

The developmental pharmacology of the respiratory system has been reviewed in detail by Isles and Newth (16). From a practical standpoint, the single most important issue relates to the bronchodilator responsiveness of infants compared to older children (17). It has been said that infants lack bronchial smooth muscle (18) or beta$_2$-adrenergic receptors and are therefore unresponsive to bronchodilators. Studies on children with bronchopulmonary dysplasia have shown an airway response to bronchodilator as early as 25 weeks gestational age (19). Clinical studies of wheezy infants suggest a beneficial response to bronchodilator (20,21). Other studies, using more objective measures of lung function, have produced conflicting results. Hughes et al. found that salbutamol caused no improvement (22), while other studies have shown either deterioration (23) in respiratory mechanics or improvement in spirometry (24) in bronchiolitis. These differences may, in part, be methodological. The clinical studies generally assess response after several or multiple drug treatments, whereas the studies using objective measures of lung function are usually single-dose studies because of the inherent limitations of the measurement technique (16, 25,26). Only one study has been done with objective measures of lung function in the most acute phase of the illness (26). While 50% of the infants improved, the improvement had marginal clinical significance. The age of the infants studied and the cause of their wheezing is also likely to affect their response to medication. Many of the studies of bronchodilator responsiveness in infants have been performed during the recovery phase from acute bronchiolitis, a disease in which the airflow obstruction is due predominantly to edema and airway inflammation and not necessarily reflective of the pathology in infants with recurrent wheeze for other reasons.

O'Callaghan et al. demonstrated that salbutamol (albuterol) protected against bronchoconstriction induced by hypotonic airway challenge in infants less than a year of age with recurrent wheezing (27). The same group had previously published data showing wheezy infants under 18 months of age had no bronchodilator response to the same drug, but did to ipratropium (28).

Recent observations suggest that the airways of wheezy infants differ from those of infants without respiratory symptoms and perhaps give some explanation for the conflicting results from previous studies, these have been the subject of a recent editorial review by Clough (3). Henderson et al. demonstrated that salbutamol produced a significantly faster rate of recovery than saline following histamine-induced bronchoconstriction in infants with no history of airway disease. Clough (3) suggests that this study gives proof for the functional existence of beta$_2$-adrenergic receptors in infants and supports the view that the failure of salbutamol (albuterol) to improve airflow in wheezy illnesses in this age group is due to airflow obstruction caused by airway inflammation and mucus, intrinsic airway narrowing, and increased dynamic compression during forced expiration, rather than bronchospasm alone.

B. Other Predisposing Factors

Although the etiology of childhood wheezing illness is not fully understood, evidence from epidemiological and birth cohort studies suggests that susceptibility to wheezing, and more specifically to asthma, may be determined by events during pregnancy or very early in life. The occurrence of wheeze or documented asthma has been shown to be increased in relation to low birth weight (29,30), preterm birth (31), low maternal age (32,33), and maternal smoking. Feeding practices also influence the risk of subsequent wheeze, as do season of birth (34) and a range of other environmental factors.

Genetic Factors

Population and family studies clearly show that the predisposition to asthma and allergy is inherited. This may involve a single gene, although the mode of inheritance has not yet been clearly defined. However, the relations among the genetics of asthma, atopy, and bronchial responsiveness remain unclear (35). The role of heredity in the development of allergic disease has been reviewed by Zeiger (36). Both retrospective and prospective studies have shown an increased risk of allergic disease when one or both parents have an allergic history. Zeiger reviewed 8 prospective studies. About 50% of the offspring have allergic disorders when one parent has an allergic history, and 70% do when both parents have an allergic history (36). One of these studies also demonstrated that parental atopic disease affects not only the incidence but also the age of onset and type of atopic disease in their offspring. Forty-two percent of children with a double parental history of allergic disease develop atopic disease by 18 months of age. Moreover, in families in whom both parents have an identical type of allergy (respiratory or cutaneous), the total incidence of atopic disease in their children was as high as 72% and the offspring manifested the same disease (37).

There is, however, a complex interaction between genetic predisposition and environmental factors, as children usually inherit more than their genes from their parents; they also share the same environment. Environmental factors may be important in inducing or "switching on" asthma in genetically predisposed individuals (35).

Gender and Reduced Lung Function

Gender and reduced lung function are interrelated risk factors for wheezing. A number of studies have reported gender differences in both the prevalence of atopy and of asthma, with more males than females being affected. Sears et al. (38) reported data from a birth cohort study at age 13 years. A history of current asthma was 1.6 times more common in boys than girls. The authors attributed the increased prevalence of asthma in boys to their higher incidence of atopy. These findings are similar to the original study from Melbourne (39), where wheeze of all but the mildest grade was more common in males. In the most severely affected group, boys outnumbered girls by almost fourfold. With age, however, more males improved than females, and by age 21 the ratio of males to females had decreased to 1.5:1.

Several studies suggest that male children suffer more respiratory illness of all kinds than females do (8). Hospital admission for asthma in children less than 10 years of age is more common in males than in females (40,41). The increased respiratory morbidity in males in early life is associated with and, perhaps caused by, differences in spirometric indices (8).

Several retrospective studies of children hospitalized with bronchiolitis showed significantly lower mean values for several indices of lung function when the children were assessed years later (42–44). Strope (45) reported similar findings for children who had had wheezy episodes but not required hospitalization. In that study, boys who had experienced two or more wheezy episodes during the preschool years had lower FEV_1 and FEF_{25-75} than boys with one or no wheezy episodes. The development of techniques to measure lung function in infants has facilitated further investigation in this field. Three prospective studies of infants (46–48) have shown that maximal expiratory flow at end tidal expiration ($\dot{V}max_{FRC}$) is significantly reduced in infants who subsequently develop wheezy illnesses and that these changes antedate the development of such illnesses, suggesting that they are the cause of, rather than the result of, the wheezy illness.

Environmental Factors

Exposure to allergens in early life may be important in the development of subsequent asthma and atopic disease. A high incidence of asthma has been found in children born in certain months of the year, although the pattern is variable (34). Aeroallergens appear to be the most important environmental triggers (49). Sporik et al. reported higher levels of house dust mite allergen in the homes of those who subsequently develop asthma (50).

The role of both external and indoor environmental pollution is the subject of ongoing investigation. Several studies have compared the prevalence of asthma and other respiratory symptoms in matched populations from regions of high and low air pollution and found no evidence to support the usually held view that air pollution and asthma are linked (51,52).

Asthma prevalence is greater in more affluent countries (53), and a link to indoor environmental or dietary factors has been suggested. It is currently unclear whether the increased prevalence of asthma and allergic symptoms in the past decade is a function of increased exposure to potent allergens or of increased susceptibility to allergens already present (53). There is speculation about the rule of various dietary factors, including a high dietary sodium intake, chemical additives, and preservatives, but firm conclusions as to their role cannot yet be drawn (53).

Smoking

A wide range of respiratory tract morbidity has been attributed to the exposure of infants and children to parental (especially maternal) smoking (54). Martinez et al. (55) demonstrated a conclusive link between parental smoking and childhood asthma. Asthmatic children with smoking parents had increased airway responsiveness when compared to asthmatic children with nonsmoking parents. Other studies, which have not been confirmed, have shown cord blood IgE concentrations to be increased in infants born to mothers who smoked during pregnancy, and infants born to mothers who smoked in pregnancy had a fourfold increased risk of developing a clinically manifest allergic state (56). In addition, Young et al. have shown that elevated levels of airway responsiveness are related to parental smoking and a family history of asthma (57). Male children from smoking parents were found to have increased skin-test reactivity when compared to children from nonsmoking parents (58). Maternal smoking has also been shown to be associated with reduced lung function during childhood (591–61). Lewis et al. have recently demonstrated smoking to be an independent risk factor for a subsequent risk of wheezing in childhood (62). On the basis of the above data, it seems reasonable to postulate that early (even intrauterine) passive exposure to products of tobacco combustion may make an important contribution to the occurrence of bronchial hyperreactivity, atopy, and asthma (63). Passive smoking has documented effects on IgE-mediated immune responses and may represent a pathway by which an environmental trigger could contribute to the pathogenesis of asthma and other respiratory disorders (64).

The evidence from these studies suggests that passive exposure to cigarette smoke in utero results in small airways at birth. In addition, exposure to maternal cigarette smoke after birth might increase the risk of childhood wheezing by increased sensitization to environmental allergens, perhaps through increased mucosal permeability or impaired lung development.

Low Birth Weight

Lewis et al. (62), in a recent birth cohort study, identified low birth weight (<2.5 kg) as being associated with a 1.26-fold increased risk of wheezing.

Viral Respiratory Infection

Viral respiratory infections have long been recognized as a common trigger of wheezy episodes in children. The epidemiological evidence for virus-induced airway obstruction and airway hyperresponsiveness has been reviewed in detail by Busse (65) and by Stark and Graziano (66). The latter report also reviews the evidence that viral infections can alter beta-adrenergic function and neural control of airways through alterations in both cholinergic and nonadrenergic, noncholinergic pathways as well as damaging the airway epithelium. The airway epithelium plays a central role in regulating airway tone by metabolism of tachykinins, production of an endogenous bronchodilator substance, and production of adhesion molecules for airway inflammatory cells. Damage to the respiratory epithelium by respiratory viruses can alter these functions and lead to subsequent airway obstruction and hyperresponsiveness (66).

Martinez has also raised the possibility that early exposure to viral respiratory infections might be protective against asthma by promoting immunological changes which reduce the risk of allergy (67). Viral infections activate TH-1 lymphocytes, thus preventing the proliferation of TH-2 lymphocytes which are associated with allergic sensitization (68). There are data from population studies which support this hypothesis. Family size has been shown to alter the risk of allergy during childhood. In large families the younger children have a lower risk of hayfever and atopy than the older children (53,69,70).

The relationship between bronchiolitis and the subsequent risk of asthma remains a controversial area. The relevant studies have been reviewed by Landau (35). It is unclear whether those who develop the clinical syndrome of bronchiolitis followed by subsequent wheezing are in some way different from those who do not have recurrent wheeze.

Viral respiratory infection accounts for 26–49% of asthma attacks in children, compared to 10% in adults (71). Atopy is apparently not an independent risk factor for the development of wheezing during a respiratory tract infection (71). Approximately 55–75% of symptomatic respiratory infections in asthmatic children result in exacerbation of asthma (72). Rhinovirus is an important precipitant of asthma in asthmatic individuals of all ages. In childhood, approximately 85% of rhinovirus infections trigger an episode of asthma (73). The importance of RSV as a cause for acute bronchiolitis and subsequent episodes of wheezing has already been discussed. Between 6 and 11 cases of virus-induced wheezing will be observed annually for each 100 children followed during the first 24 months of life (74). Other host factors, such as the number of siblings, socioeconomic status, and day-care attendance, alter the prevalence of viral infection in this age group (75). A longitudinal study has demonstrated an increased frequency of viral respiratory infection in asthmatic children when compared to their nonasthmatic control siblings. Infection rates were 85.7% in the asthmatics compared to 56.3% in the controls (76,77). This increased susceptibility to infection was not found in nonasthmatic atopic individuals.

Breast or Artificial Feeding

Breast feeding has been shown to be protective against wheezy lower respiratory tract illness early in life, particularly in those at higher risk because of poor socioeconomic status (78). Similarly, Lewis et al. (62) identified early artificial feeding as a risk factor for subsequent wheezing. Studies evaluating the role of artificial feeding and early use of solids have provided conflicting conclusions, and there is no clear consensus as to whether they are harmful. Zeiger has recently provided a comprehensive review of this literature (79) and provided some dietary guidelines for infants identified as "at risk" on the basis of family history.

III. An Approach to the Differential Diagnosis of Wheeze in Infancy

Asthma is by far the most common cause of wheezing in older children and adults. In infants, however, the differential diagnosis is much broader and includes a wide range of congenital and acquired disorders (Table 1).

A. Age of Onset

Symptoms that begin in the first few weeks or months of life should arouse suspicion of an underlying congenital abnormality. A chest radiograph should always be obtained.

Table 1 Causes of Wheezing in Infants

1.	Congenital		
	A. Extramural	(a)	Lobar emphysema
		(b)	Bronchogenic cyst
		(c)	Vascular ring
	B. Intramural	(a)	Primary tracheomalacia
		(b)	Tracheomalacia associated with tracheo-esophageal fistula and vascular ring
		(c)	Tracheal stenosis
		(d)	Bronchial stenosis
	C. Intraluminal	(a)	Tracheal web
		(b)	Cystic fibrosis
2.	Acquired causes		
	A. Extramural	(a)	Cystic or mass lesions compressing trachea or bronchi
		(b)	Enlarged lymph nodes (e.g., tuberculosis)
	B. Intramural	(a)	Infections, e.g., bronchiolitis
		(b)	Acquired tracheo-bronchial stenosis
		(c)	Tumors, e.g., hemangioma
		(d)	Asthma
		(e)	Bronchopulmonary dysplasia
	C. Intraluminal	(a)	Foreign body
		(b)	Mucus plugging secondary to infection or asthma
		(c)	Aspiration (gastro-esophageal reflux)
		(d)	Parental smoking

B. Nature of Symptoms

The nature of the symptoms often provides important clues as to the likely underlying problem. A harsh, brassy-sounding cough, if present, is suggestive of tracheal pathology such as tracheomalacia. Wheezing which is both inspiratory and expiratory suggests fixed airway obstruction. Stridor in association with wheezing should always suggest an underlying congenital abnormality. Cyanotic spells can be due to recurrent aspiration or severe tracheomalacia.

C. Preceding History

Prematurity, especially if associated with intubation, mechanical ventilation, and repeated suctioning, may indicate an underlying airway problem such as tracheal or bronchial stenosis secondary to granulation tissue or scarring. Airway obstruction and recurrent or persistent wheeze are typical features of bronchopulmonary dysplasia. A history of gastro-esophageal reflux should also be sought. Previous repair of a tracheo-esophageal fistula introduces tracheomalacia, gastro-esophageal reflux, and recurrent fistula into the differential diagnosis.

D. Chest Radiograph

Careful inspection of the chest radiograph can provide important clues as to the underlying diagnosis. The lung fields should be inspected carefully for evidence of generalized or lobar hyperinflation. The vascularity of the lungs and the individual lobes within should be examined carefully. The descending aorta should be identified, as a right-sided aortic arch may indicate a vascular ring. Both the antero-posterior and lateral chest radiographs should be examined for evidence of tracheal displacement. The hilar region should be examined carefully in the lateral view, as this is the typical site for bronchogenic cysts and enlarged hilar lymph nodes. The tracheal outline should be inspected, especially in the lateral view, for evidence of narrowing that might suggest tracheomalacia or tracheal stenosis.

E. Investigation

The plain chest radiograph is the most useful initial investigation. Depending on the history and other suggestive features outlined above, a barium swallow and cine-screening of the airway may be indicated. Where intrinsic airway pathology is suspected, more invasive investigation such as bronchoscopy and conventional or ultrafast CT examination may be indicated (80).

IV. Specific Conditions

A. Lobar Emphysema

Lobar emphysema is an important cause of respiratory distress in the first few months of life (81). Infants are usually symptomatic within the first few weeks of life, and almost all present within the first three months. Symptoms include tachypnea, lower rib cage retraction, and expiratory wheeze. Breath sounds may be diminished over the affected lobe, and the chest may be asymmetric in shape. There may also be evidence of mediastinal displacement.

Typically the left upper lobe is most often affected, but any lobe can be involved. The chest radiograph typically shows marked hyperinflation and lucency of the affected lobe, with herniation across the anterior mediastinum. Radiographs in the newborn period may be confusing, as the affected lobe may be fluid-filled and therefore radioopaque. With those that present early, progressive respiratory compromise usually occurs. Treatment of congenital lobar emphysema is surgical excision of the affected lobe for those with significant respiratory compromise, or for repeated pulmonary infections for those who present later with little or no respiratory difficulty.

Bronchogenic Cysts

Bronchogenic cysts are usually found in close association with the trachea and major bronchi, the most common site being the region of the carina. Cough and wheeze are the usual symptoms. If tracheal or bronchial compression is severe, the infant may present with respiratory distress or failure. Typical radiographic findings are hyperinflation of one lung. The cyst itself is usually not visible. Compression or displacement of the esophagus is commonly evident on a barium swallow. The diagnosis is usually obvious on CT scan. Treatment is surgical removal of the cyst.

Vascular Ring

Tracheal compression from vascular anomalies can be divided into three main types:

1. Double aortic arch
2. Rings in which the aorta and a combination of other vessels and rudimentary structures such as the ligamentum arteriosum cause the obstruction
3. A major artery of anomalous origin

The symptoms which result depend on the degree of tracheal narrowing and compression. There is usually an inspiratory stridor or wheeze with associated expiratory wheezing. The cough is usually abnormal, being harsh or brassy sounding, and swallowing (feeding) difficulties may also be a feature.

The diagnosis is usually be made by barium swallow. Angiography may be necessary to define the vascular anatomy accurately prior to surgery, although this can often be done by echocardiography. If an aberrant left pulmonary artery is present, bronchoscopy is indicated to exclude associated tracheal stenosis.

B. Intramural Conditions

Tracheomalacia

Tracheomalacia may occur as a primary disorder or secondary to other conditions such as tracheo-esophageal fistula or vascular ring. The tracheomalacia may be localized to one segment of the trachea or may be more generalized and may, on occasion, extend into the major bronchi as well. The symptoms which result obviously depend on the extent and severity of the tracheomalacia. Infants with localized tracheomalacia will usually have a harsh, brassy-sounding cough, a mucousy or rattly chest with retained secretions, and a degree of expiratory wheeze. Wheezing may be minimal with quiet breathing but usually increases with activity or during intercurrent infection. When generalized tracheomalacia is present, the wheezing is usually more prominent and may, on occasion, be associated with cyanotic spells. The tracheomalacia can be confirmed by cineradiography. Interpretation may not be easy, as a degree of dynamic collapse of the trachea during crying is normal. Bronchoscopy may be required to fully assess the extent of the tracheomalacia. Again, considerable experience is required, as anesthesia may obscure the diagnosis, particularly if a rigid ventilating bronchoscope is used. Anesthesia with neuromuscular blockade causing paralysis makes the diagnosis almost impossible. Flexible fiber-optic bronchoscopy in the spontaneously breathing, sedated infant is generally preferred in this situation, if available. In the majority of cases, no specific treatment is required and improvement can be expected during the first 12–18 months of life. Children with repaired tracheo-esophageal fistula retain an abnormal cough and impaired mucociliary clearance and frequently have detectable abnormalities on pulmonary function testing (82). On occasions, life-threatening cyanotic spells can require surgical intervention such as aortopexy or external splinting of the trachea in the region of the tracheomalacia (83,84).

C. Intraluminal Conditions

Tracheal Web, Tracheal Stenosis, and Bronchial Stenosis

Tracheal web and strictures are uncommon anomalies and usually present with both inspiratory and expiratory wheeze. As with tracheomalacia, symptoms are increased by activity and intercurrent infection. Tracheal stenosis is often associated with other abnormalities such as pulmonary agenesis or aberrant left pulmonary artery or pulmonary sling. Tracheal stenosis may be a localized disorder or, more frequently, it is associated with complete or circumferential tracheal rings which narrow distally (the so-called "rat-tailed" trachea). Esophagograms and/or bronchoscopy are required to define the nature and extent of the stenosis. Separate cardiac investigations, including angiography, may also be required. Bronchoscopy is usually indicated when the wheeze is both inspiratory and expiratory. Bronchial stenosis will cause inspiratory and expiratory wheeze and may be associated with focal hyperinflation or collapse on the chest radiograph.

Cystic Fibrosis

Cystic fibrosis is a common inherited condition affecting approximately 1:2000 Caucasian children, with a lesser incidence in other population groups. In many areas, infants with cystic fibrosis are diagnosed shortly after birth in newborn screening programs. If not diagnosed at birth, most will present in the first year of life with recurrent respiratory symptoms and failure to thrive. A small percentage of these children have recurrent or persistent wheezing due to diffuse small airway disease. Sometimes the wheezing may be a major management problem and infrequently even leads to respiratory failure. Mechanical ventilation in this situation is usually justified, as most infants can be subsequently weaned from the ventilator after clearance of thick secretions. The wheezing often resolves in the first 1–2 years of life.

D. Acquired Lesions

Intramural Lesions

Bronchiolitis

Bronchiolitis is a disease of infants during the first year of life, being most common in those aged 6–12 months. It is characterized by inflammation and edema in bronchioles. Airflow obstruction results from accumulation of inflammatory mucus and cellular debris within the lumen of bronchioles, edema of the bronchiolar wall, and, at least in some cases, a degree of bronchiolar spasm (26,85). Partial airway obstruction causes gas trapping and hyperinflation, resulting in an increased work of breathing. Ventilation-perfusion mismatching causes hypoxia, the extent of which is dependent on the severity of the illness. Respiratory syncytial virus (RSV) and para-influenza virus are the most common etiological agents, with RSV causing more than 90% of infections. Rarely, infection with adenovirus results in a more severe illness characterized by obliterative bronchiolitis (81). Infection with RSV can occur at any time, but is most prevalent during the winter months, often occurring in epidemics. Parental smoking is a recognized risk factor for bronchiolitis (86).

Patients usually present with a history of an antecedent coryzal illness with a mild fever. This is followed by the onset of a harsh cough, tachypnea, chest retraction, and hyperinflation. Auscultatory findings include an expiratory wheeze and inspiratory crackles. The radiographic changes include hyperinflation, patchy consolidation, and atelectasis. Hypoxia is usually present, with the severity of the hypoxia being dependent on the severity of the illness. Apnea is a recognized complication during the initial phase of the illness (81).

The acute phase of bronchiolitis typically lasts 5–10, days but it may be some weeks before symptoms fully resolve. On occasion, a more severe and protracted course is encountered (87). Mortality is rare in previously healthy children if appropriate intensive-care facilities are readily available, but is a major risk in those with preexistent respiratory problems such as bronchopulmonary dysplasia or congenital heart disease (88). The diagnosis of bronchiolitis is a clinical one and dependent on a history of a prodromal illness followed by an illness with typical clinical and radiographic findings. Identification of a viral pathogen in respiratory secretions by immunofluorescence provides additional confirmatory evidence.

Treatment of the hospitalized infant includes monitoring of oxygenation and use of humidified oxygen to maintain an oxygen saturation in excess of 92–94%. Feeding problems are common and will often necessitate the use of intravenous fluids, as nasogastric feeding tubes increase respiratory resistance and may aggravate incipient respiratory failure. Antibiotics are rarely necessary. The role of bronchodilator drugs in the treatment of bronchiolitis remains controversial. Most reports discourage their use because of a lack of proven efficacy. Sly et al., in a study of infants recovering from bronchiolitis, showed no improvement in lung mechanics from a single dose of salbutamol (89). In contrast, Schuh et al. (21), in a placebo-controlled study of infants aged 6 weeks to 24 months with bronchiolitis, demonstrated an improvement in clinical score, oxygen saturation, and respiratory rate after two doses of nebulized salbutamol. Corticosteroids are not beneficial. The role of ribavirin in the treatment of bronchiolitis remains controversial and was the subject of a symposium in which the safety and efficacy were extensively reviewed (90). The American Academy of Pediatrics has published recommendations for the use of ribavirin in patients with RSV infection. These include patients with congenital heart disease, bronchopulmonary dysplasia and other forms of chronic neonatal lung disease, prematurity, immunodeficiency, multiple congenital anomalies, and progressive respiratory failure (91). Groothius et al. showed that ribavirin administered early in the course of infection in high-risk patients significantly reduced the morbidity from RSV infection (92), but Meert et al. were unable to confirm this advantage in critically ill, mechanically ventilated infants. Ribavirin is potentially teratogenic, so special care must be taken when using it to ensure the safety of care givers.

A high percentage (50–90%) of infants who have an episode of bronchiolitis have recurrent episodes of wheezing (93). There are a number of possible explanations. First, the initial viral infection may trigger bronchial hyperreactivity. Second, there may be an inherited predisposition to bronchiolitis through inherited bronchial reactivity. Some studies have shown a higher incidence of atopy in first-degree relatives of infants with bronchiolitis, compared to controls (35). There is additional evidence that those who develop wheezing subsequent to bronchiolitis may have an immunological response different to other children. Welliver found RSV-specific IgE antibodies in nasopharyngeal secretions at the time of the initial episode (94). Importantly, those with smaller airways at birth may be predisposed to wheeze with viral infections (35).

Bronchiolitis may be associated with long-term sequelae other than asthma. Abnormalities in various measures of lung function have been described 8–10 years after bronchiolitis (87).

In general, the first episode of wheezing in an infant is called bronchiolitis, the second should be viewed suspiciously, and the third labeled as asthma, particularly when there is a supporting family history (95).

Gastro-Esophageal Reflux

Gastro-esophageal reflux must always be considered in the differential diagnosis of wheezing and other respiratory symptoms in infants. Significant reflux can be present with little in the way of typical symptoms such as vomiting. Gastro-esophageal reflux should be considered where there are prominent nocturnal respiratory symptoms. The relationship between reflux and respiratory symptoms has recently been reviewed by Orenstein and Orenstein (96). Reflux may be the primary cause of respiratory symptoms (97). Possible mechanisms include gross or micro-aspiration, reflex bronchoconstriction and increased bronchial reactivity, reflex bronchospasm, reflex central apnea, and reflex bradycardia (96). Reflex bronchoconstriction secondary to reflux is likely to occur only in the presence of esophagitis (98). In other circumstances, a primary respiratory condition (e.g., bronchopulmonary dysplasia) may be complicated by reflux. Coughing, increased negative intrathoracic and positive intraabdominal pressures with increased respiratory effort, and hyperinflation with diaphragm flattening from the primary respiratory disease, will all predispose the affected infant to reflux. Medications such as theophylline and, to a lesser extent, beta-agonists when used in the treatment of the primary disorder, may precipitate or aggravate gastric reflux by causing relaxation of the lower esophageal sphincter and increased gastric acid secretion.

Because reflux is a common condition, affecting about 20% of all infants, it can be difficult to establish an exact causal relationship between reflux and respiratory symptoms in an individual patient (96). The presence of reflux can be defined by radiography, endoscopy, pH probe, or scintigraphy. No method is without its deficiencies, and the diagnosis of pathologic gastro-esophageal reflux is often a clinical decision weighing the clinical features with the other supporting evidence. The presence of fat-laden alveolar macrophages in tracheo-bronchial secretions may be helpful, but there is a high false positive rate (98).

Treatment of gastro-esophageal reflux includes conservative measures such as posturing, and thickening of feeds. The seated posture increases reflux and should be avoided (96). Pharmacological treatment includes prokinetic agents such as domperidone and cisapride and gastric acid suppressant therapy. Fundoplication must be considered in children with complex respiratory problems such as bronchopulmonary dysplasia complicated by reflux which does not respond to medical management.

E. Asthma

Asthma affects 10% or more of all young children. About 30% have the onset of their symptoms in the first year of life and 50% by 2 years of age (99). There is also significant evidence that the frequency of asthma is increasing. Burr et al., in two identical surveys 15 years apart, showed that a history of current asthma symptoms increased from 5.2% to 12% over the time and a history of wheeze at any time increased from 17% to 22% (100). Hospital admission rates, especially for males, have also increased during recent years (101).

In infancy, asthma is twice as common in males as in females (41). Schwartz et al. showed that for children 6 months to 11 years of age, the prevalence of asthma was 3% among white children and 7.2% among blacks. The prevalence of frequent wheeze was 6.2% among whites and 9.3% among blacks. They also identified other factors such as young maternal age and central-city birthplace as being independent risk factors, suggesting that the intrauterine environment may play a priming role in the development of asthma (102).

Atopy or the genetic predisposition to asthma remains a major causative factor. Progress is being made in unraveling the underlying genetic defect, but this work is not yet complete (103). The relationship between genetic predisposition and environmental factors remains poorly understood. In a 1985 study, Bertrand et al. showed that prematurely born children in whom respiratory disease did not develop during the neonatal period have evidence in later childhood of airflow limitation that is related to maternal airway hyperreactivity and not to their prematurity (104). A retrospective study in Israel demonstrated that infants with transient tachypnea of the newborn had a much higher incidence of symptoms consistent with asthma and signs consistent with atopy (105).

Food allergies are common in infants. However, respiratory symptoms are the least common manifestation of allergic problems in this age group and are rarely the sole symptom of a positive food challenge (106). The widely held view that milk causes mucus secretion has no scientific basis. Milk is the major source of calories, calcium, and the other essential nutrients in infants, and dairy products should not be withdrawn from the diet without nutritional advice from a pediatric dietitian. In short, for the vast majority of infants with respiratory symptoms, dietary manipulation is totally unwarranted (106).

Viral respiratory infection is perhaps the single greatest risk factor for the development of asthma in infancy. Both clinical and epidemiological observations support the hypothesis that viral respiratory tract infection has a definite causal relationship in the development of airway reactivity and particularly in the causation of wheeze with subsequent viral infection. Microbiological studies of patients with acute asthma have shown no association between asthma and bacterial infection in childhood (107). Therefore, although antibiotics are frequently prescribed to wheezy infants, they are of no value unless there is an associated bacterial infection such as otitis media.

Pathology and Pathophysiology

Current concepts of the pathogenesis of bronchial hyperresponsiveness and asthma have been reviewed recently by Barnes (108) and by de Jongste et al. (109). The pathology and pathophysiology of asthma in infancy have been reviewed by Tabachnik and Levison (95). Airway inflammation, epithelial damage, mucosal edema, mucus secretion, and bronchial smooth muscle spasm contribute to the causation of airflow obstruction. The relative contribution of each of these factors may vary from time to time within individual patients. The role of smooth muscle spasm in infants remains a controversial area. There is also a very strong association between asthma in infants and recurrent or persistent otitis media (110).

Clinical Presentation

In infancy, the majority of episodes of wheezing are preceded by an upper respiratory infection which is then followed by wheeze or cough or both. Depending on the severity of the airflow obstruction, there may be hyperinflation, tachypnea, subcostal, intercostal, and suprasternal retraction. Occasionally, coughing, especially at night, may be the only asthmatic symptom. A small percentage of infants have rapidly progressive episodes which lead to respiratory failure. This group of asthmatic infants can be among the most difficult of all asthmatics to treat (Table 2).

Investigation

Investigations should be kept to an absolute minimum. An initial chest radiograph should be obtained. Further radiographs are not usually required unless there is some specific indication. If the child has atypical or recurrent symptoms, a sweat test may be indicated. Skin tests, IgE levels, and so on, are rarely helpful and should never be ordered routinely. Alpha-1 antitrypsin disease rarely causes symptoms in childhood, and measurement of serum levels should not be requested routinely. Some measures of pulmonary function can now be made routinely (111).

Numa and Newth (112) recently provided an approach to the assessment of respiratory function in the intensive-care unit. Their extensive review examines the value and problems associated with the various physiological measurements and monitoring techniques.

Measurement of Lung Function

Measuring lung function in wheezy infants is done to answer both research and clinical questions. These are many different ways of measuring lung function in infants, most of which require specialized equipment and may require sedation, so it is not surprising that the literature reflects a great diversity of approaches.

Pulmonary function testing may be helpful in diagnosis, in predicting outcome, in assessing response to treatment, and in monitoring wheezy infants over time.

Table 2 Estimation of Severity of Exacerbations of Asthma in Infants

Sign/symptom	Mild	Moderate	Severe
Respiratory rate, resting or sleeping	Normal to 30% increase above the mean	30–50% increase above the mean	Increase over 50% above the mean
Alertness	Normal	Normal	May be decreased
Dyspnea[a]	Absent or mild; normal suckling and feeding	Moderate; speaks in phrases or partial sentences; infant's cry softer and shorter, infant has difficulty suckling and feeding	Severe; speaks only in single words or short phrases; infant's cry softer and shorter, infant stops suckling and feeding
Accessory muscle use	No intercostal to mild retractions	Moderate intercostal retractions with tracheosternal retractions; use of sternocleidomastoid muscles; chest hyperinflation	Severe intercostal retractions, tracheosternal retractions with nasal flaring during inspiration; chest hyperinflation
Color	Good	Pale	Possibly cyanotic
Auscultation	End expiratory wheeze only	Wheezing during entire expiration and inspiration	Breath sounds becoming inaudible
Oxygen saturation	>95%	90–95%	<90%
P_{CO_2}	<35	<40	>40

Note: Within each category, the presence of several parameters, but not necessarily all, indicate the general classification of the exacerbation

[a]Parent's or physician's impression of degree of child's breathlessness.

It is helpful to separate infant lung function assessment into three broad though related groups. Lung function is often measured using a range of techniques from each group to maximize the information obtained.

Flow Measurements

In older children and adults, airways obstruction is often diagnosed and monitored using standard maximal expiratory flow parameters. Three methods have evolved which allow examination of forced expiratory flow volume characteristics in infants.

1. The rapid thoraco-abdominal compression (RTC) method was described in 1978 (113) and later modified (114). This technique involves applying compressive pressure to the thorax and abdomen at the end of tidal inspiration. The compressive pressure is increased until flow limitation is achieved. The maximum flow at functional residual capacity ($Vmax_{FRC}$) is measured. This technique has been widely used in many studies but has the disadvantage of producing only a partial expiratory flow volume curve (PEFV) and in practice there is some doubt about whether flow limitation is achieved.

Bronchial responsiveness has been measured in infants by finding the provocative concentration of inhaled histamine or methacholine that induces a 30% fall in $Vmax_{FRC}$.

2. A new technique recently described (115) allows forced expiratory flow-volume curves to be produced by RTC after infant lung volumes have been raised by a pump. Forced expiratory volume-time (FEVt) parameters are used and have been found to be reproducible, adequately detect reduced lung function during histamine challenge testing in infants, and detect differences between wheezy and normal infants. This techniques appears very promising but still requires sedation.

3. The forced deflation technique (116) requires endotracheal intubation, deep sedation, and muscle relaxation, and so is possible only in an intensive-care situation. The lungs are inflated to a standard pressure (+40 cm H_2O) and then rapidly deflated to residual volume by sudden exposure to a negative pressure (−40 cm H_2O). This method does allow increased flows over the entire vital capacity, and flow limitation is always achieved.

There has been much interest in the examination of tidal breathing flow-volume curves (TBFV), and parameters from these curves have been shown to predict wheezing in infancy (46) and correlate with clinical findings in wheezing infants treated aggressively for severe gastro-esophageal reflux (97). These curves may be obtained without resort to sedation, which makes them an attractive alternative if frequent assessments are needed. However, Silverman's group have shown tidal indices to be an insensitive measure of airway function in infants compared with $Vmax_{FRC}$ (117), and there is also a question as to how the indices vary with respiratory rate.

Lung Volumes

The only lung volume which can be measured reliably and reproducibly in infants is functional residual capacity (FRC), which is defined as the volume of air contained in the lungs at end-tidal expiration. As lung mechanics can vary depending on the lung volume at which they are measured, it is important to measure the FRC so that mechanics measurements can be reliably interpreted. In wheezy infants the degree of gas trapping associated with airways obstruction is important, as are changes in lung mechanics due to therapy. There are two widely used techniques for measuring FRC in infants.

> *Whole-body plethysmography*, as adapted for infants (118), measures thoracic gas volume (Vtg), which is all the gas in the thorax including gas which is trapped in obstructive airways disease. In infants this method usually requires sedation. Boyle's law governs the change in volume of a gas which undergoes isothermal compression. The subject is placed in a rigid, sealed plethysmograph, and respiratory efforts are made against an occlusion at the airway opening which will rarefy and compress thoracic gas. The change in the body volume and opening airway pressure during the occlusion can be measured, and V_{tg} can be calculated by substituting in the Boyle's law equation, $P_1V_1 = P_2V_2$. This technique has been more applicable to research laboratories, as the equipment is cumbersome and expensive and requires considerable training to use, but there are now some commercially available infant whole-body plethysmographs.
>
> *Gas dilution* methods are widely used, as they are relatively simple to do. There are commercially available, mobile systems which give reproducible results and do not necessarily require sedation. Gas dilution methods measure gas volume in direct communication with the central airways during tidal breathing and so will not measure trapped gas. The measurement of FRC is based on mass balance. The initial and final concentrations of the dilutional gas are measured and the amount of the dilutional gas is either initially known (closed-circuit helium dilution) or measured (open-circuit nitrogen washout). Both helium dilution and nitrogen washout techniques give similar values for FRC (119), but the volume measured is less than that from the infant body plethysmograph.

There has been recent research interest in the analysis of nitrogen washout curves. Analysis of the shape of the washout curve appears to differentiate healthy infants and infants with obstructive airways disease (120). However, there is some controversy over the best index to use, and work needs to be done to derive useful standards for this type of measure of lung ventilation.

Lung Mechanics

Many different techniques, both passive and dynamic, have been used to assess compliance and resistance in infants. Some commercially available systems have made some of these measurements easier to perform in the clinical setting. Some of the methods commonly used to assess wheezy infants are described below. The reciprocal of the resistance, conductance, is often given and divided by the FRC value to give specific conductance. Conductance is related to the fourth power of the airway radius and so gives an index of airway calibre.

Plethysmographic Measurement of Airways Resistance

Plethysmographic measurement of airways resistance involves the infant being placed in a rigid sealed plethysmograph and a satisfactory pressure–flow loop obtained. To avoid potential confounding variables such as temperature differences between inspiration and expiration and changes in lung volume, a warmed, humidified, oxygen-enriched gas at BTPS in a rebreathing bag is used. This method offers the advantages of measuring changes in airways resistance at different parts of the respiratory cycle. However, it is only really applicable to the research laboratory at this time, as it requires highly specialized equipment and considerable training. It is also not a method which can be applied to critically sick infants, and so its clinical usefulness is somewhat limited. There are also some concerns that CO_2 levels inevitably will rise using a rebreathing bag, and this will lead to changes in ventilatory drive and lung mechanics.

The Single-Breath Technique

The single-breath technique (SBT) measures the resistance, compliance, and time constant of the respiratory system, including components due to chest wall, lung, and airways, during a passive expiration following a brief airway occlusion at end-inspiration. When the airway is occluded there is a rise in the pressure trace to a plateau which represents equilibration of pressure at the mouth with airway pressure. The expiratory flow–volume curve following the occlusion is analyzed. A linear portion of the expiratory flow–volume curve over approximately 40% of the tidal volume is used, and the compliance, resistance, and time constant of the respiratory system can be calculated from the plateau pressure and the intercepts and slope of the linear portion of the curve. The validity of the SBT is dependent on there being a passive expiration and an adequate and truly linear portion of the expiratory flow–volume trace. There are some criticisms of this technique, including its failure to detect the important dynamic changes in resistance throughout a breath. However, it is easy, quick, and noninvasive to perform, does not necessarily require sedation, and can safely be used in intubated infants, which makes it an attractive, clinically applicable technique. A recent comparison of SBT and plethysmographic measurements of resistance in infancy showed statistically significant differences between the two techniques, but the differences were too small to be of any probable physiological significance (121).

Forced Oscillation

Forced oscillation is a method which also measures total respiratory resistance from the oscillatory relationship of flow and pressure when flow oscillations generated by a loudspeaker are delivered through a face mask and pneumotachograph. Upper airway contribution to the results may be high using this technique unless great care is taken to support the cheeks.

Many other methods of measuring lung mechanics have been developed, and there are valid criticisms and advantages to all these different techniques. Unlike methods for assessing obstructive airways disease in older children, there is as yet no accepted, standard method for assessment in infants and young children.

Treatment

Treatment must encompass both preventive measures and pharmacological treatment.

Environmental control: Every effort must be made to control the environment of the susceptible infant. Parents should cease smoking, and dust and other inhaled irritants should be kept to a minimum.

Diet: Controversy exists as to whether breast feeding has a protective effect or not in the potentially atopic child (see earlier discussion). Until a more definitive answer is available, it seems reasonable to recommend breast feeding until 6 months of age, at least in infants thought by way of family history to be at risk of asthma.

Antibiotics: Although antibiotics are widely prescribed for intercurrent respiratory symptoms, there are no grounds at all for their routine use in asthma, even in infants. An associated otitis media or persisting muco-purulent nasal discharge for more than 4–5 days may be reasonable grounds for the introduction of antibiotics.

Immunotherapy: Immunotherapy has no role at all in the management of allergy and respiratory symptoms in infants (122). Acute insect allergy might be the only exception, and then only after specialist opinion from a pediatric allergist.

Pharmacological treatment: Pharmacological treatment remains the mainstay of treatment and should be individualized according to the frequency and severity of the patient's symptoms. Isles and Newth have recently reviewed the cellular mechanism of action of antiasthmatic medications (123) and reviewed the treatment of acute asthma in children (Table 3).

Specific Pharmacological Agents

Beta-Adrenergic Agonists. The selective beta-adrenergic agonists salbutamol (albuterol) and terbutaline remain the agents of choice for the treatment of asthma in children. Their pharmacology has been reviewed by Isles and Newth (123). The various immediate-acting $beta_2$-adrenergic agonists should be regarded as effectively equipotent. Nonselective adrenergic agents such as adrenaline have a role in the management of acute anaphylaxis and acute severe status asthmaticus not responsive to $beta_2$-adrenergic agonists, and croup. $Beta_2$-adrenergic agonists may be administered orally, by wet nebulization, or by metered-dose aerosol with face mask. Wet nebulization and metered-dose aerosol deliver the drug direct to the lung, providing rapid relief of symptoms with few side effects. Oral administration, although often easier in the infant, takes longer to attain its maximal effect (typically 30–60 min) and is associated with a much higher incidence of side effects such as hyperactivity and sleep disturbance. The choice for the route of administration depends on the frequency and severity of the child's symptoms. The clinical use of $beta_2$-adrenergic agonists in the treatment of acute asthma has been reviewed by Isles and Newth (123).

Theophylline. Despite its continued widespread use in the United States, theophylline is receding in importance in other countries. Side effects such as mood and behavior disturbance and sleep disturbance are so common as to be a major limiting factor in using the drug. However, sustained-release formulations are useful for treatment of nocturnal asthma. Theophylline also has major practical benefits when a child has difficulty taking drugs in other forms, or when compliance needs to be monitored (serum drug concentrations). In the United States, theophylline is often used as a prophylactic or preventive drug. Recent progress in understanding the anti-inflammatory effects of theophylline provide some basis for this treatment and have provoked a reexamination of the role of theophylline in asthma therapy (124). Weinberger has provided many extensive reviews of theophylline pharmacology, dosing guidelines, and interpretation of serum levels (63). Hendeles et al. have reviewed the safety and efficacy of theophylline in children with asthma (125). Isles and Newth (123) have recently reviewed the role of aminophylline in acute asthma and recommended restricting its use to the subset of patients with severe acute asthma unresponsive to maximal doses of inhaled $beta_2$-adrenergic agonist.

Table 3 Dosages of Drugs in Acute Exacerbations of Asthma in Infants

Drug	Available form	Dosage	Comment
Inhaled beta-agonist Albuterol Nebulizer solution	0.5% (5 mg/mL)	0.1–0.15 mg/kg/dose up to 5 mg every 20 min for 1–2 hr (minimum dose 1.25 mg/dose)[a] 0.5 mg/kg/hr by continuous nebulization (maximum 15 mg/hr)	If improved, decrease to 1–2 hr; if not improved, use by continuous inhalation
Metraproterenol Nebulizer solution	5% (50 mg/mL)	0.1–0.3 mL (5–15 mg); do not exceed 15 mg	
	0.6% unit-dose vial of 2.5 mL (15 mg)	As above 5–15 mg; do not exceed 15 mg	
Corticosteroids Outpatients	Oral prednisone, prednisolone, or methylprednisolone	1–2 mg/kg/day in single or divided doses	Reassess at 3 days as only a short burst may be needed; no need to taper dose
Hospitalized patients	Methylprednisolone IV or PO	1–2 mg/kg/dose q6 hr for 24 hr, then 1–2 mg/kg/day in divided doses q 8–12 hr	Length depends on response; may only need a few days
Systemic beta-agonist Epinephrine HCl	1:1000 (1 mg/mL)	0.01 mg/kg up to 0.3 mg subcutaneously every 20 min for 3 doses	Inhaled beta$_2$-agonist preferred

Table 3 Continued

Drug	Available form	Dosage	Comment
Terbutaline	(0.1%) 1 mg/mL in solution for injection in 0.9% NaCl	Subcutaneous: 0.01 mg/kg up to 0.3 mg every 2–6 hr as needed; intravenous: 10 μg/kg over 10 min loading dose; maintenance: 0.4 μg/kg/min: increase as necessary by 0.2 μg/kg/min and expect to use 3–6 μg/kg/min (74).	Inhaled beta$_2$-agonist preferred
Methylxanthines Theophylline	Aminophylline (80% anhydrous theophylline)	Loading dose:[a] If theophylline concentration known: every 1 mg/kg theophylline will give 2 μg/mL increase in concentration. Loading dose:[a] If theophylline concentration is unknown:	

No previous theophylline:
  6 mg/kg/aminophylline
Previous theophylline:
3 mg/kg aminophylline
Constant infusion rates:[a]
  Infusion rates to obtain a
  mean steady-state
  concentration of
15 μg/mL:
  Age

Age	
1–6 mo	0.5 mg/kg/hr aminophylline
6 mo–1 yr	1.0 mg/kg/hr aminophylline
1–9 yr	1.5 mg/kg/hr aminophylline
10–16 yr	1.2 mg/kg/hr aminophylline

[a]Check serum concentration at approximately 1, 12, and 24 hr after the infusion.

Ipratropium Bromide.   The combination of albuterol and ipratropium is more effective than albuterol alone in the management of acute wheezing (126,127). It has few side effects and is also helpful in providing symptomatic relief for the coughing which can be so troublesome in asthma. Its peak effect is 30–60 min after administration, so it should always be administered in combination with a beta-adrenergic agonist.

Cromolyn.   For children who require regular preventive treatment, cromolyn remains the drug of first choice (122). It has the major advantage of being free of significant side effects, is anti-inflammatory, and it also reduces airway reactivity with long-term use. Newth et al. demonstrated its effectiveness in reducing asthma symptoms in a cohort of preschool children (128).

Inhaled Steroids.   The introduction of nebulized budesonide has been a major advance in this age group, as has been the use of valved spacers with attached face masks for aerosol administration. The current indication for long-term inhaled steroid use is persistent asthma not adequately controlled with nonsteroid agents. Budesonide and beclomethasone are effectively equipotent, but budesonide has the advantage of rapid clearance and a shorter half-life with fewer systemic side effects. Its topical-to-systemic ratio of activity is therefore superior to that of beclomethasone. Russell has recently reviewed the use of topical corticosteroids in the treatment of childhood asthma with particular emphasis on the potential for side effects (129) and concluded that, within the recommended range, inhaled corticosteroid therapy has an excellent record in children. However, on a cautionary note, he also noted increasing evidence of dose-related side effects. The potential effect of inhaled steroids on growth is a cause for concern but must be viewed in the context of the effects of asthma itself on growth (130).

Bisgaard et al. reported a study of 77 children aged 11–36 months in which budesonide by aerosol and mask resulted in significant clinical improvement, less oral steroid use, and fewer admissions to hospital (131). Freigang and Ashford assessed the effect of inhaled steroid (400 μg/day) administered by face mask to 17 children 12–26 months of age. All infants showed improvement in symptoms after 1 year, and all showed a decrease in the use of concomitant medication. Measures of adrenal function after 1 year showed no change (132). There remain concerns about the effect of inhaled steroids on growth, but the dysphonia and oral thrush reported frequently in adults seem not to be problems in infants and young children.

Oral Steroids.   Oral steroids are now used earlier and more aggressively in the treatment of acute exacerbations of asthma. The mechanism of action at a cellular level has been reviewed by Isles and Newth (123). Weinberger has provided an extensive literature review focusing especially on safety aspects (133). Storr et al. (134) demonstrated that a large dose of prednisone administered early in an acute attack was effective at aborting many episodes and preventing admission to hospital. Extended tapering courses are generally not necessary. A short (3–5 day) course of high-dose (1–2 mg/kg) is effective for most acute episodes (123). Longer courses may be necessary when the acute attack occurs on a background of pre-existing subacute asthma. Fewer than 5% of patients require continuing long-term treatment with oral corticosteroids. The dose should be titrated to provide optimal symptom control with the fewest possible side effects. The dose should fluctuate according to the patient's symptoms and, where possible, alternate-day steroid therapy should be the goal.

Administration of Treatment. The age of the child, the severity of symptoms, and the child's level of cooperation all influence decisions about the route of drug administration. The relative merits and disadvantages of the various routes for drug delivery in children have recently been reviewed by Isles and Newth (123). Although the oral route is easiest, it has the most side effects and is the least effective way of giving medication, particularly if symptoms are severe. The nebulizer has traditionally been seen as the most effective way of giving medication to children and, during an acute symptomatic phase this view is probably correct, at least for beta-adrenergic agonists. The amount of medication delivered depends on the efficiency of the nebulizer system and can vary enormously (135). There are now a number of reports of administering aerosols by spacer and face mask to young children (136,137). These devices are an alternative for the uncooperative child who refuses nebulizer therapy and, even for the co-operative patient, they can often replace the nebulizer for much of the daily medication during asymptomatic phases, increasing parental freedom and mobility. Compliance with therapy is thus encouraged. Administration of an inhaled steroid by aerosol and mask rather than nebulizer also avoids the potential risks of deposition of the steroid in the eyes and on the skin. Parents are no longer dependent on the nebulizer for drug administration and have an effective way of giving beta-adrenergic agonists as well if they are away from home and the child becomes symptomatic.

V. An Approach to Treatment of the Individual Patient

As previously stated, treatment must be individualized according to the frequency and severity of the patient's symptoms. A systematic approach and specific guidelines can be found in the International Consensus statement (122) and in the review of Isles and Newth (123,138). A suggested approach to the management of infants with either episodic asthma (episodes of acute symptoms with no interval symptoms) and those with persistent asthma (intermittent acute exacerbations with frequent symptoms between) is given in Table 4 and Figs. 1–3 (modifications of the National Asthma Education Program).

The studies of Martinez and others (reviewed earlier) show that many infants, especially males, wheeze because of smaller airways, with dynamic airway narrowing during expiration. Not all such infants require treatment, and the response to treatment is often disappointing. Long-term use of inhaled corticosteroids should be avoided unless there is an obvious beneficial response.

A. Acute Episodes

The management of acute asthma in children has been reviewed by Isles and Newth (123). The treatment of acute asthma in infants is little different

Table 4 Classification of Asthma Severity in Infants

Classification of severity	Common features	Maintenance therapy
Infrequent episodic	Episodes >6–8 wks apart Exacerbations generally not severe Symptoms rare between exacerbations Physical exam. normal between episodes	Preventive treatment generally not required Parenteral use of beta-agonist when symptomatic
Frequent episodic	Attacks <4–6 wks apart Attacks more troublesome Increasing frequent symptoms between attacks	Begin with sodium cromoglycate, either nebulized or pMDI with spacer and face mask If not effective use low-dose inhaled steroid
Persistent asthma	Symptoms most days Nocturnal symptoms >2/wk Exacerbations <4–6 wks apart Beta-agonist needed daily Abnormal lung function (if measured) History of hospital admissions	Inhaled steroids usually required If continuing treatment with inhaled steroids is required, specialist supervision is strongly recommended

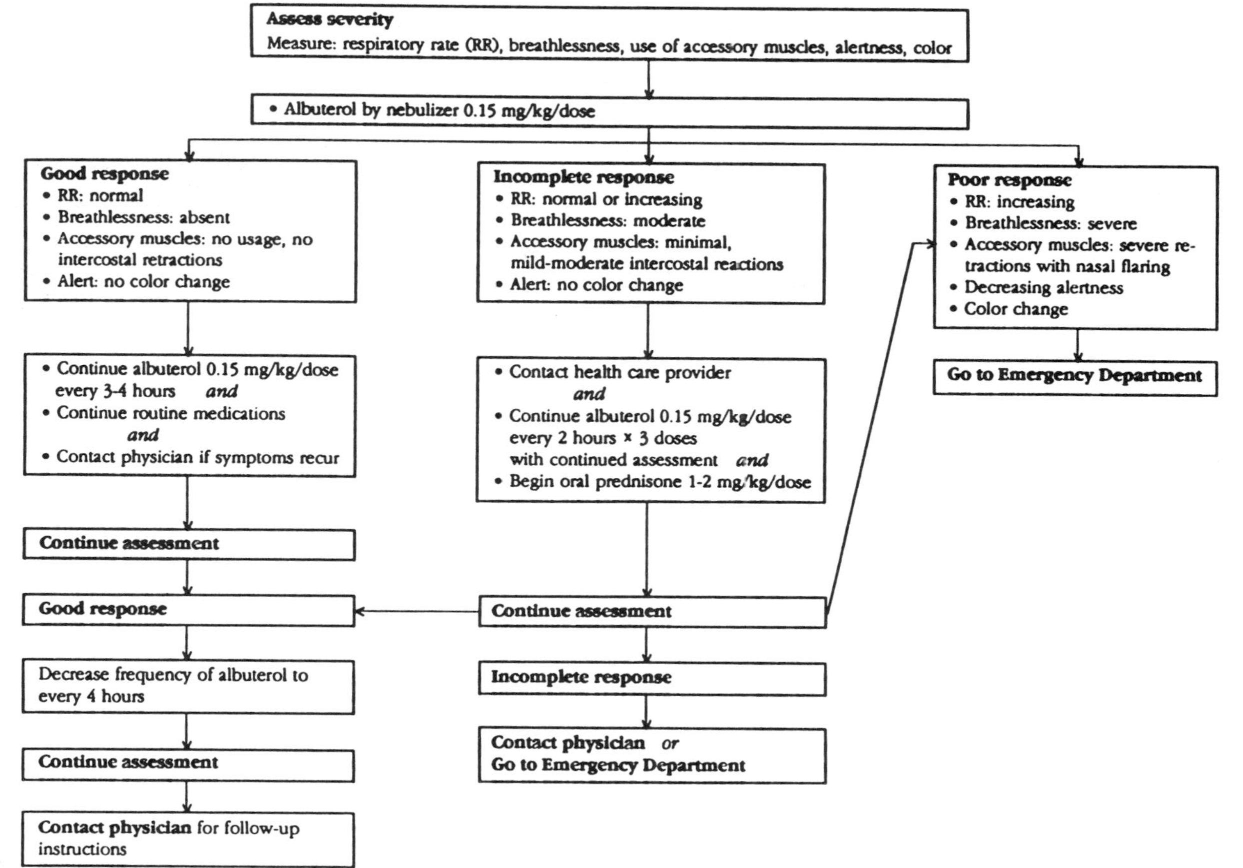

Figure 1 Acute exacerbations of asthma in infants: home management.

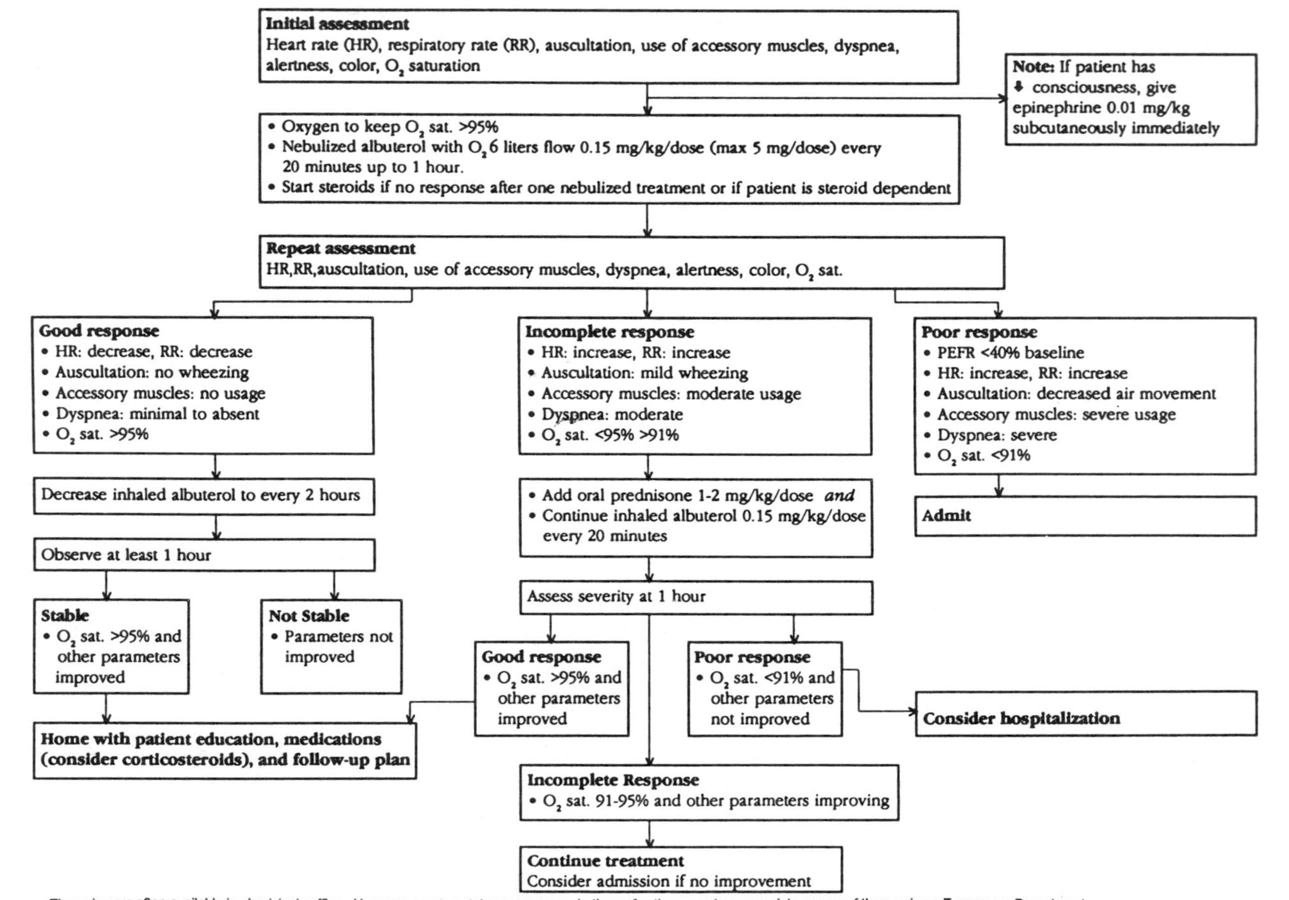

Figure 2 Acute exacerbations of asthma in infants: emergency department management.

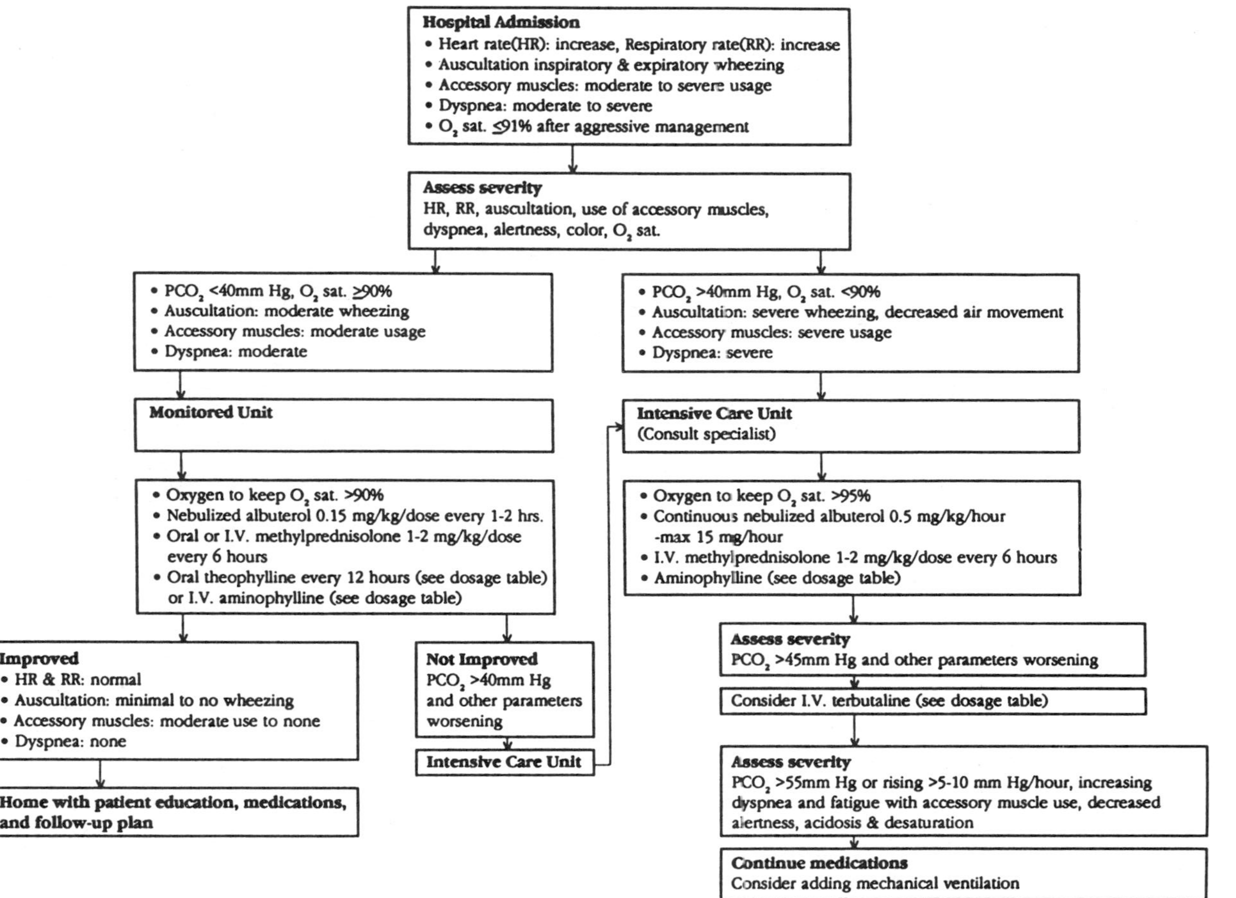

Figure 3 Acute exacerbations of asthma in infants: hospital management.

from that in older children, except that medication doses are different and their overall response is often dramatic. Oxygenation should be carefully monitored and supplemental oxygen given to maintain the oxygen saturation at greater than 94%. Inhaled beta-adrenergic agonists remain the mainstay of treatment. There has been a trend in recent years to use these agents more and more aggressively as their safety has been better understood. With appropriate monitoring, nebulizer therapy every 30–60 min is now commonplace, and in the critically ill infant, continuous nebulized beta-adrenergic agonist may be given safely (139). Intravenous beta-adrenergic agonists may be administered if the infant is unresponsive to inhaled agents. Hypokalemia is a common side effect, and potassium supplementation and monitoring are essential (123). The addition of ipratropium may be useful (64) but, if used often, signs of atropinism may develop. Corticosteroids should be administered, either orally or parenterally, with the expected time course of action being about 3–12 hr. There is a limited role for the use of intravenous aminophylline in incipient respiratory failure, as it has a stimulation effect on the diaphragm (140) as well as the respiratory center. For the critically ill infant there can be no substitute for care in an appropriate pediatric intensive-care facility with the capacity for routine respiratory monitoring and assisted ventilation when necessary. A full review of the intensive-care management of acute asthma in children is beyond the scope of this discussion but can be found in the review by Isles and Newth (123).

Overall Prognosis

The best data on long-term prognosis come from the longitudinal study of asthma morbidity initiated by Williams et al. in the 1960s (141). A cohort of children have now been followed for close to 30 years. Briefly, the important observations are that there is a general trend for asthma to improve with age. For those with mild symptoms in childhood, there is about a 75% chance that they will "grow out" of their asthma as they grow older. For those with more severe childhood asthma, the prospect of growing out of their asthma is reduced to about 50%. Those with multiple admissions to hospital in the first 1–2 years, chest deformity, and severe eczema are more likely to carry their disease through to adult life.

Although Williams and McNicoll in their prospective study were unable to show that infants who wheezed only with infection had a different prognosis, other studies have suggested that there may be two distinct groups. Parkes et al., in a long-term follow-up study over 10 years, identified two groups (142). The first is a large favorable-prognosis group who have recurrent episodes of cough and wheeze with viral infection, who come from a nonatopic family and have no other clinical or laboratory evidence of atopy. Such children can be expected to outgrow their asthma by school age or shortly after. The second group is smaller, and the children in this group have features considered unfavorable. These include coexistent eczema, allergic rhinitis and positive skin tests, asthma in one or both parents, and frequent severe wheeze in the first 2 years of life. It is possible that the two groups are not distinct but are part of the same continuum.

Data from several prospective birth cohort studies has led to a revision of thinking about wheezy episodes in infants and the subsequent risk of asthma. The study of Martinez et al. suggests that within the population of wheezy babies there are almost certainly at least two groups, those with a transient predisposition to wheezing, probably due to small airways, and a second group who have continuing asthma (1). Of those with early-onset wheezing, only a third continue to have asthma at age 6 years. While symptomatic use of asthma medications may well be appropriate in infants, the prospective studies suggest that we should be cautious about extending this to mean that the infants have an established diagnosis of asthma. The data of Martinez et al. (1) suggest that the group of infants with early-onset wheezing comprises two subpopulations; those with transient early-onset wheezing and those with early-onset asthma. Wilson (6) has reversed the entire cycle of thinking in this area by suggesting that the term "wheezy bronchitis" might again be a suitable diagnostic term.

B. Bronchopulmonary Dysplasia

With the increasing availability of neonatal intensive care and the aggressive treatment offered to very small premature infants, bronchopulmonary dysplasia (BPD) and other forms of chronic neonatal lung disease are an increasing part of pediatric pulmonary practice. A full review of BPD is beyond the scope of this review (143,144). In survivors of the acute phase of BPD, airway reactivity is very common (145), and wheezing may be a major management problem in these infants. Airway reactivity appears to be a common component of the resolving airway injury in these infants. Gastro-esophageal reflux is so common in infants with BPD that it must always enter into the differential diagnosis of continuing respiratory symptoms in this age group.

Infants with severe BPD who are chronically oxygen-dependent and hospitalized are at special risk because of the high incidence of nosocomial viral infection in this situation. Many of these infants are so precariously poised physiologically that it takes little additional stress to precipitate acute respiratory failure. In this situation, respiratory failure is often a complex interaction between cardiac and respiratory factors. Treatment of these exacerbations should ideally be carried out in a pediatric intensive-care facility. Treatment involves adequate oxygenation, a trial of nebulized or intravenous beta-adrenergic agonist, and steroids.

In children with BPD who have a continuing "asthma" syndrome, a trial of nebulized cromolyn or budesonide is certainly warranted. Some may require intermittent or continuous oral steroids. Treatment of other potential aggravating factors such as gastro-esophageal reflux may also need to be vigorous.

C. Foreign Body

In young children, an inhaled foreign body (either tracheal or esophageal) must always enter into the differential diagnosis of acute or persistent wheezing. In the very young infant, an esophageal foreign body may present with respiratory symptoms from tracheal pressure. Questioning about the possibility of an inhaled foreign body should be a routine part of the initial evaluation of a wheezy infant. Regional differences in breath sounds or evidence of collapse or ball-valve obstruction on the chest radiograph are suggestive features. When a foreign body is seriously suspected, bronchoscopy (and often esophagoscopy) are indicated.

References

1. Martinez FD, Wright AL, Taussig LM, et al. Asthma and wheezing in the first six years of life. N Engl J Med 1995; 332:133–138.
2. Peat JK, Toelle BG, Gray E, et al. Prevalence and severity of childhood asthma and allergic sensitisation in seven climatic regions of New South Wales. Med J Austral 1995; 163:22–26.
3. Clough JB. Bronchodilators in infancy (editorial). Thorax 1993; 48:308.
4. Helms PJ. Wheezing infants (editorial). Clin Exp Allergy 1994; 24:97–99.
5. Williams H, McNichol KN. Prevalence, natural history, and relationship of wheezy bronchitis and asthma in childhood. Br Med J 1969; 4:321–325.
6. Wilson NM. Wheezy bronchitis revisited. Arch Dis Child 1989; 64:1194–1199.
7. Silverman M. Out of the mouths of babes and sucklings: lessons from early childhood asthma. Thorax 1993; 48:1200–1204.
8. Clough JB. The effect of gender on the prevalence of atopy and asthma. Clin Exp Allergy 1993; 23:883–885.
9. Newth CJL. Recognition and management of respiratory failure. Pediatr Clin N Am 1979; 26:617–644.
10. Hogg JC, Williams J, Richardson JB, et al. Age as a factor in the distribution of lower airway conductance and in the pathologic anatomy of obstructive lung disease. N Engl J Med 1970; 282:1283–1287.

11. Bryan AC, Mansell AL, Levison H. Development of the mechanical properties of the respiratory system. In: Hodson W, ed. Development of the Lung. New York: Marcel Dekker, 1977.

12. Boyden EA. Notes on the development of the lung in infancy and early childhood. Am J Anat 1967; 121:749–762.

13. Keens T, Bryan AC, Levison H, et al. Development of fatigue resistant muscle fibers in the human diaphragm and intercostal muscles. Physiologist 1977; 20:50–54.

14. Gaultier C. Respiratory muscle function in infants. Eur Respir J 1995; 8: 150–153.

15. Matsuba K, Thurlbeck WM. Increased mucus glands in normal children compared to adults. Am Rev Respir Dis 1972; 105:708–710.

16. Isles AF, Newth CJL. Respiratory pharmacology. In: MacLeod S, Radde IC, eds. Textbook of Pediatric Clinical Pharmacology. Massachusetts: PSG Publishing Company, 1985: 188–208.

17. Lenny W, Milner AD. At what age do bronchodilators work? Arch Dis Child 1980; 58:279–283.

18. Polgar G, Weng TR. Functional development of the respiratory system. Am Rev Respir Dis 1979; 1120:625–695.

19. Rotschild A, Solimano A, Puterman M, Smyth J, Sharma A, Albersheim S. Increased compliance in response to salbutamol in premature infants with developing bronchopulmonary dysplasia. J Pediatr 1989; 115:984–991.

20. Mallol J, Barrueto L, Girardi G, et al. Use of nebulized bronchodilator in infants under 1 year of age: analysis of four forms of therapy. Pediatr Pulmonol 1987; 3:298–303.

21. Schuh S, Canny G, Reisman J, et al. Nebulized albuterol in acute bronchiolitis. J Pediatr 1990; 117:633–637.

22. Hughes DM, LeSouëf PN, Landau LI. Effect of salbutamol on respiratory mechanics in bronchiolitis. Pediatr Res 1987; 22:83–86.

23. Prendiville A, Green S, Silverman M. Paradoxical response to nebulised salbutamol in wheezy infants assessed by partial expiratory flow volume curves. Thorax 1987; 42:86–91.

24. Mallory GB Jr, Motoyama EK, Koumbourlis AC, Mutich RL, Nakayama D. Bronchial reactivity in infants with respiratory failure with viral bronchiolitis. Pediatr Pulmonol 1989; 6:253–259.

25. Gupta SK, Wagener JS, Erenberg A. Pulmonary mechanics in healthy term neonates; variability in measurements obtained with a computerized system. J Pediatr 1990; 117:603–606.

26. Hammer J, Numa A, Newth C. Albuterol responsiveness in infants with respiratory failure caused by respiratory syncytial virus infection. J Pediatr 1995; 127:485–490.

27. O'Callaghan C, Milner AD, Swarbrick A. Nebulised salbutamol does have a protective effect on airways in children under 1 year of age. Arch Dis Child 1988; 63:479–483.

28. Lenny W, Milner AD. Alpha and beta adrenergic stimulants in bronchiolitis and wheezy bronchitis in children under 18 months of age. Arch Dis Child 1978; 53:707–709.

29. Seidman DS, Laor A, Gale R, Stevenson DK, Danon YL. Is low birth weight a risk factor for asthma during adolescence? Arch Dis Child 1991; 66: 584–587.

30. Schwartz J, Gold D, Dockery DW, Weiss ST, Speizer FE. Predictors of asthma and persistent wheeze in a national sample of children in the United States. Am Rev Respir Dis 1990; 142:555–562.

31. Rona RJ, Guiliford MC, Chinn S. Effects of prematurity and premature growth on respiratory health and lung function in childhood. Br Med J 1993; 306:817–820.

32. Anderson HR, Bland JM, Peckham CS. Risk factors for asthma up to 16 years of age. Chest 1987; 91:127s–130s.

33. Anderson HR, Bland JM, Patel S, Peckham C. The natural history of asthma in childhood. J Epidemiol Community Health 1986; 40:121–129.

34. Haberg N. Birth season variation in asthma and allergic rhinitis. Clin Exp Allergy 1989; 19:643–648.

35. Landau LI. Bronchiolitis and asthma: are they related? Thorax 1994; 49: 293–296.

36. Zeiger RS. Development and prevention of allergic disease in childhood. In: Middleton E Jr, Reed CE, Ellis EF, et al., eds. Allergy: Principles and Practice. 4th ed. St. Louis: Mosby, 1137–1171.

37. Kjellman NM, Johansson SGO. Soy versus cow's milk in infants with a biparental history of atopic disease: development of atopic disease and immunoglobulins from birth to 4 years of age. Clin Allergy 1979; 9:347.

38. Sears MR, Burrows B, Herbison GP, Flannery EM, Holdway MD. Atopy in childhood I: gender and allergen related risks for development of hayfever and asthma. Clin Exp Allergy 1993; 23:957–963.

39. Martin AJ, McLennan LA, Landau LI, Phelan PD. The natural history of childhood asthma to adult life. Br Med J 1980; 280:1397–1400.

40. Eliasson O. The male–female ratio of hospital admissions for asthma. Am Rev Respir Dis 1985; 131(Part 2):A110.

41. Skobeloff EM, Spivey WH, St Clair SS, Schoffstall JM. The influence of age and sex of asthma admissions. JAMA 1992; 268:3437–3440.

42. Sims DG, Downham MAPS, Gardner PS, et al. Study of 8 year old children with a history of respiratory syncytial virus bronchiolitis in infancy. Br Med J 1978; 1:11–14.

43. Pullen CR, Hey EN. Wheezing, asthma and pulmonary dysfunction 10 years after infection with respiratory syncytial virus in infancy. Br Med J 1982; 84:1165–1169.

44. Mok JYO, Simpson H. Outcome of acute lower respiratory tract infections in infants: preliminary report of seven year follow-up study. Br Med J 1982; 285:333–337.

45. Strope GL, Stewart PW, Henderson FW, et al. Lung function in school age children who had mild lower respiratory illnesses in early childhood. Am Rev Respir Dis 1991; 147:811–817.

46. Martinez FD, Morgan WJ, Wright AL, et al. Initial airway function is a risk factor for recurrent wheezing respiratory illnesses during the first 3 years of life. Am Rev Respir Dis 1991; 143:312–316.

47. Tager IB, Hanrahan JP, Toseson TD, et al. Lung function, pre-natal smoke exposure and wheezing in the first year of life. Am Rev Respir Dis 1993; 147:811–817.

48. Young S, Arnott J, LeSouëf PN, et al. Flow limitation during tidal expiration in symptom-free infants and the subsequent development of asthma. J Pediatr 1994; 124:811–817.

49. Sears M, Herbson G, Holdway M, et al. The relative risk of sensitivity to grass pollen, house dust mite and cat dander in the development of childhood asthma. Clin Exp Allergy 1989; 19:419–424.

50. Sporik R, Holgate ST, Platts-Mills TAE, Cogswell JJ. Exposure to house-dust mite allergen (*Der p*) and the development of asthma in childhood. N Engl J Med 1990; 323:502–507.

51. Braback L, Breborowicz A, Dreborg S, et al. Atopic sensitisation and respiratory symptoms among Polish and Swedish school children. Clin Exp Allergy 1994; 129:366–374.

52. von Mutius E, Fritzsch C, Weland SK, Roll G, Magnussen H. Prevalence of asthma and allergic disorders among children in United Germany: a descriptive comparison. Br Med J 1992; 305:1395–1399.

53. Peat J. The rising trend in allergic illness: which environmental factors are important? Clin Exp Allergy 1994; 24:797–800.

54. Passive smoking—bronchial responsiveness and atopy (editorial). Am Rev Respir Dis 1988; 138:507–509.

55. Martinez FD, Antognoni G, Macri F, Bonci E, Midulla F, DeCastro G, Ronchetti R. Parental smoking enhances bronchial responsiveness in 9 year old children. Am Rev Respir Dis 1988; 138:518–523.

56. Magnussen CG. Maternal smoking influences cord serum IgE and IgD levels and increases the subsequent risk for allergy. J Allergy Clin Immunol 1986; 78:898–904.

57. Young S, LeSouëf PN. Geelhoed GC, et al. The influence of a family history of asthma and parental smoking on airway hyperresponsiveness in early infancy. N Engl J Med 1991; 324:1168–1178.

58. Martinez FD, Antigoni G, Macri F, et al. Parental smoking enhances bronchial responsiveness in 9 year old children. Am Rev Respir Dis 1988; 138: 518–523.

59. Rona RJ, Guillford MC, Chinn S. Effects of prematurity and intrauterine growth on respiratory health and lung function in childhood. Br Med J 1993; 306:817–820.

60. Hanrahan JP, Tager IB, Segal MR, Tosteson TD, Castile RG. The effect of maternal smoking during pregnancy on early lung function. Am Rev Respir Dis 1992; 145:1129–1135.

61. Tager IB, Weiss ST, Muñoz A, Roser B, Speizer FE. Longitudinal study of the effects of maternal smoking on pulmonary function in children. N Engl J Med 1983; 309:699–703.

62. Lewis S, Richards D, Bynner J, Butler N, Britton J. Prospective study of risk factors for early and persistent wheezing in childhood. Eur Respir J 1995; 8:349–356.

63. Passive smoking—bronchial responsiveness and atopy (editorial). Am Rev Respir Dis 1988; 138:507–509.

64. Magnussen CG. Maternal smoking influences cord serum IgE and IgD levels and increases the subsequent risk for allergy. J Allergy Clin Immunol 1988; 78:898–904.

65. Busse WW. The role of respiratory infections in airway hyperresponsiveness and asthma. Am J Crit Care Med 1994; 150:S77–S79.

66. Stark JM, Graziano FM. Lower airway response to viruses. In: Busse W, Holgate ST, eds. Asthma and Rhinitis 1995. Boston: Blackwell. 1229–1247.

67. Martinez F. Role of viral infections in the inception of asthma and allergies during childhood: could they be protective? Thorax 1994; 49:1189–1191.

68. Romagnani S. Human TH1 and TH2 sub-sets: regulation of differentiation and the role in protection and immunopathology. Int Arch Allergy Immunol 1992; 98:279–285.

69. von Mutius E, Martinez FD, Fritzsch C, et al. Skin test reactivity and number of siblings. Br Med J 1994; 308:692–695.

70. Strachan DP. Hay fever, hygiene and household size. Br Med J 1989; 299: 1259–1260.

71. Li TC, O'Connell E. Viral infection and asthma. Ann Allergy 1987; 59: 321–331.

72. Minor TE, Dick EC, deMeo AN, et al. Viruses as precipitants of asthmatic attacks in children. JAMA 1974; 227:292–298.

73. Minor TE, Dick EC, Baker JW, et al. Rhinovirus and influenza type A infection as precipitants of asthma. Am Rev Respir Dis 1976; 113:149–153.

74. Henderson AT, Clyde WA. The etiologic and epidemiologic spectrum of bronchiolitis in pediatric practice. J Pediatr 1978; 95:183–190.

75. Skoner D, Calliguri L. The wheezy infant. Pediatr Clin N Am 1988; 35: 1011–1030.

76. Minor TE, Baker JW, Dick EC, et al. Greater frequency of viral respiratory infection in asthmatic children compared to non-asthmatic siblings. J Pediatr 1974; 85:472–477.

77. Cogswell JJ, Halliday DF, Alexander JR. Respiratory infections in the first year of life in children at risk of developing atopy. Br Med J 1982; 284: 1011–1013.

114. Taussig L, Landau LI, Godfrey S, Arad I. Determinants of forced expiratory flows in newborn infants. J Appl Physiol 1982; 53:1220–1227.

115. Turner DJ, Stick SM, LeSouef PN, Sly PD. A new technique to generate and assess forced expiration from raised lung volume in infants. Am J Respir Crit Care Med 1995; 151:1441–1450.

116. Motoyama EK. Pulmonary mechanics during early post-natal years. Pediatr Res 1977; 11:220–223.

117. Clark JR, Aston H, Silverman M. Evaluation of a tidal expiratory flow index in healthy and diseased infants. Pediatr Pulmonol 1994; 17:285–290.

118. Auld PAM, Nelson NM, Cherry RB, Rudolph AJ, Smith CA. Measurement of thoracic gas volume in the newborn infant. J Clin Invest 1963; 42: 476–482.

119. Tepper RS, Asdell S. Comparison of helium dilution and nitrogen washout measurements of functional residual capacity in infants and very young children. Pediatr Pulmonol 1992; 13:250–254.

120. Watts JL, Ariagno RL, Brady JP. Chronic pulmonary disease in neonates after ventilation: distribution of ventilation and pulmonary interstitial emphysema. Pediatrics 1977; 60:273–281.

121. Dundas I, Dezateux CA, Fletcher ME, Jackson EA, Stocks J. Comparison of single-breath and plethysmographic measurements of resistance in infancy. Am J Respir Crit Care Med 1995; 151:1451–1458.

122. Warner JO, Götz M, Landau LI, et al. Asthma: a follow-up statement from an international paediatric asthma consensus group. Arch Dis Child 1992; 67:240–248.

123. Isles A, Newth CJL. Acute asthma in children. In: Phelan PD, ed. Asthma, Baillière's Clinical Paediatrics. Vol. 3. London: Baillière Tindall, 1995: 341–378.

124. Barnes PJ, Pauwels RA. Theophylline in the treatment of asthma: time for reappraisal? Eur Respir J 1994; 7:579–591.

125. Hendeles L, Weinberger M, Szefler S, Ellis E. Safety and efficacy of theophylline in children with asthma. J Pediatr 1992; 120:177–183.

126. Reismann J, Galdes-Sebalt M, Kazim F, Canny G, Levison H. Frequent administration by inhalation of salbutamol and ipratropium bromide in the management of acute severe asthma in children. J Allergy Clin Immunol 1988; 81:16–20.

127. Schuh S, Johnson DW, Callahan S, Canny G, Levison H. Efficacy of frequent nebulized ipratropium bromide added to frequent high-dose albuterol therapy in acute severe childhood asthma. J Pediatr 1995; 126:639–645.

128. Newth CJL, Newth CV, Turner JAP. Comparison of nebulised sodium cromoglycate and oral theophylline in controlling symptoms of chronic asthma in preschool children. Austral NZ J Med 1982; 12:232–238.

129. Russell G. Inhaled corticosteroid therapy in children: an assessment of the potential for side-effects. Thorax 1994; 49:1185–1188.

130. Russell G. Childhood asthma and growth—a review of the literature. Respir Med 1994; 88(Suppl A):31–37.

131. Bisgaard G, Munch SL, Nielson JP, et al. Inhaled budesonide for the treatment recurrent wheezing in early childhood. Lancet 1990; 336(8716): 649–651.

132. Freigang B, Ashford DR. Adrenal cortical function after long term aerosol ste therapy in early childhood. Ann Allergy 1990; 64:342–344.

133. Weinberger M. Anti-asthmatic therapy in children. Pediatr Clin N Am 1989; 36:1251–1284.

134. Storr J, Barry W, Barrell E, Lenney W. Effect of a single oral dose of prednisolone acute childhood asthma. Lancet 1987; 8538:879–881.

135. Bisgaard H. Aerosol treatment of young children. Eur Respir Rev 1994; 4: 15–20.

136. Connor WT, Dolovich MB, Frame RA, Newhouse MT. Reliable salbutamol administration in 6–36 month old children by means of a metered dose inhaler and aerochamber with mask. Pediatr Pulmonol 1989; 6:263–267.

137. O'Callaghan C, Milner A, Swarbrick A. Spacer device with face mask attachment for giving bronchodilator to infants with asthma. Br Med J 1989; 289:160–161.

138. Canny G, Levison H. Childhood asthma: a rational approach to treatment. Ann Allergy 1990; 64:406–416.

139. Portnoy L, Aggarwal J. Continuous terbutaline nebulization for the treatment of severe exacerbations of asthma in children. Ann Allergy 1988; 60: 368–371.

140. Aubier M, DeTroyer A, Sampson M. Aminophylline improves diaphragmatic contractility. N Engl J Med 1981; 305:249–252.

141. Williams H, McNicoll KN. Prevalence, natural history, and relationship of wheezy bronchitis and asthma in children: an epidemiological study. Br Med J 1969; 4:321–333.

142. Parkes ES, Golding J, Carswell F, et al. Pre-school wheezing and prognosis at 10 years of age. Arch Dis Child 1986; 61:642–646.

143. O'Brodovich H, Mellins RB. Bronchopulmonary dysplasia: unresolved neonatal acute lung injury. Am Rev Respir Dis 1985; 132:694–709.

144. Blanchard PW, Brown TM, Coates AL. Pharmacotherapy in bronchopulmonary dysplasia. Clin Perinatol 1987; 14:881–909.

145. Northway WH, Moss RB, Carlisle KB, et al. Late sequelae of bronchopulmonary dysplasia. N Engl J Med 1990; 323:1793–1799.

32

Food Hypersensitivity in Infancy

S. ALLAN BOCK

National Jewish Medical and Research
  Center
Denver, Colorado

HUGH A. SAMPSON

Johns Hopkins University School of
  Medicine
Baltimore, Maryland

I. Introduction and Definition of Terms

For eons the topic of food allergy has been the subject of mythology and misunderstanding. Practitioners, both medical and nonmedical, have had strongly held opinions about the effect of foods on people. The first adverse interaction between food and man is described in *Genesis* (1). Throughout the centuries, where records remain, adverse reactions to foods have been offered as an explanation for many of man's ills (2). This chapter is devoted to examining the scientific basis of food hypersensitivity (allergy) and endeavors to separate the information that is currently extant based on properly controlled research from the opinions and impressions of practitioners whose claims often have an unhappy effect on the laity.

The first problem encountered in discussions of food hypersensitivity is the definition of the word *allergy*. The term has been abused for so long that many authors in the field have chosen to substitute the term *hypersensitivity* when discussing adverse reactions to foods that can be proved to involve the immune system. When patients initially complain of symptoms associated with food ingestion, it seems wise to counsel them to describe their symptoms as adverse reactions to the suspected food. Then one may attempt to prove unequivocally that food is responsible for the reaction and attempt to find the mechanism involved. A number of mechanisms are clearly associated with adverse symptoms following food ingestion, and greater precision of terminology must be established when trying to understand those reactions. This chapter examines those symptoms that have been proved to involve or are highly likely to involve immunological events precipitated by food ingestion, and this may properly be termed *food hypersensitivity* or *food allergy* (3,4).

Several additional terms have been applied to adverse reactions to foods. *Food intolerance* is often used as a generic synonym for adverse reactions to food. However, the carbohydrate intolerances (e.g., lactose, sucrose, isomaltose intolerance) are illnesses for which the specific biochemical but nonimmunological mechanism, dissacharidase enzyme deficiencies, have been identified. Therefore, it seems most appropriate to reserve the term *intolerance* for the disaccharidase deficiencies.

Toxic reactions may have two sources (5–7). There are natural toxins in our diet, including many natural carcinogens. There are endless examples, including toxins in "organically" grown food, such as the oxalates in rhubarb or the cyanides in the stones of apricots. Other intoxicants include contaminants such as aflatoxin, which is present only in low levels unless foods have been inappropriately stored and the mold that produces aflotoxin has been allowed to produce copious amounts of the intoxicating substance. Accidental intoxication may occur when foods are contaminated during the processing. Attention has been given to the possible effect of pesticides, especially on young children. Some of these compounds may be passed to infants through breast milk (8–10).

The term *idiosyncratic* has been applied to many food reactions, but it does not have a clearly associated biochemical mechanism and therefore will not be used in this discussion. Strongly held beliefs about symptoms produced by certain foods under diverse circumstances may be classified as psychological reactions. Unfortunately, at this time, in our culture, this may be the largest group of "adverse reactions to foods." Notions such as the production of behavioral aberrations by sugar ingestion are so rampant among the population that even the medical profession has succumbed to perpetuation of these beliefs.

II. Prevalence

The exact frequency of occurrence of adverse reactions to foods, let alone determination of the frequency of true food hypersensitivity, has been an elusive figure. Methodological problems have complicated the acquisition of a definitive value for the incidence or prevalence of food hypersensitivity. A number of studies throughout the world have attempted, in various ways, to approach the determination of these figures, and the results of these studies have led to estimates from less than 1% up to 30% (11–20). (Of course, there is a group of enthusiasts who feel that food hypersensitivity affects 100% of children).

Most of these studies suffer from one or more methodological deficiencies. Many of them investigate only one aspect of the problem, e.g., development of "allergy" to one or two foods. Although few foods cause adverse reactions during the first 2 years of life (primarily milk and soy), examination of all foods is needed to gain a true picture of the problem. A second major flaw in the cited studies (and others not listed) is definitions of symptoms. Persistent rhinitis in young children is often termed allergic without any proof that the immune system is involved. Wheezing in infants has been attributed to foods by association rather than by objective food challenge. Atopic dermatitis, an illness notorious for symptomatic fluctuation, has been blamed on foods because of improvement when the diet has been altered. This imprecision points to a major problem in most prevalence studies: lack of confirmation of the link between food and symptoms by properly controlled, double-blind, placebo-controlled food challenge. Without this rigorous proof it is hard to know if the true prevalence is closer to 1% or 30%. Certainly it is unacceptable to use such widely disparate figures to counsel families. One of the most useful pieces of numerical data concerning prevalence has been the finding by Burks that one-third children presenting to university dermatology and allergy clinics with atopic dermatitis have food hypersensitivity (21).

Perhaps of assistance to physicians caring for infants is Bock's observation that 208 of 480 children had some symptom attributed to food during the first 3 years of life (19). Eighty percent of the initial complaints occurred during the first year of life. A second observation from the same study was the brief period of time during which the reactions persisted. For the majority of children with previously confirmed reactions due to food, the culprit was reintroduced into the diet within a mean of 6 months. Few of these reactions could be shown to be "allergic," that is, could be shown to be associated with immune mechanisms. Thus, primary-care practitioners caring for infants were frequently told about foods "causing symptoms" by the parents of their patients. These parents may be reassured that if the problem is real, it should not persist for more than a few months and careful systematic reintroduction of the food into the diet may promptly demonstrate the resolution of the problem. Symptoms caused by

Table 1 Estimated Prevalence of Cow Milk Allergy (CMA) in the First 3 Years of Life

Author	No. subjects	% CMA
Hide 1983 (22)	609	2.5
Bock 1987 (19)	480	2.3
Host 1990 (23)	1749	2.3
Schrander 1993 (24)	1386	2.8

foods that appear to persist may require further evaluation either by the primary-care practitioner or by referral to an allergist familiar with food hypersensitivity in infants.

Bock's study and three others (22–24), Table 1, allow an estimate of the prevalence of cow milk allergy in the first 3 years of life. The estimated prevalences are remarkably similar, ranging from 2.3% to 2.8%. Based on all the studies in the literature, we estimate that the incidence of true food allergy in children does not exceed 1–2% of children. This prevalence decreases as the children mature.

III. Clinical Presentation of Food Hypersensitivity

A. Symptoms and Signs

Gastrointestinal

Gastrointestinal symptoms (Table 2) are the first or second most common symptoms of an adverse reaction to food in children during the first 2 years of life (4,13,20). Gastrointestinal symptoms include acute vomiting and diarrhea as well as chronic prolonged diarrhea. Abdominal pain and nau-

Table 2 Symptoms Confirmed During DBPCFC[a]

Gastrointestinal: nausea, vomiting, abdominal pain (colic?), diarrhea, colitis
Cutaneous: urticaria, angioedema atopic dermatitis, erythema
Respiratory: rhinorrhea, sneezing, tearing, conjunctival swelling, laryngospasm, wheezing
Cardiovascular: hypotension, collapse, shock
CNS: migraine (unproven in children), "hyperactivity/irritability" (rarely only symptom)

[a]DBPCFC = double-blind, placebo-controlled food challenge.

sea, about which young children cannot complain, are often suspected by observation of their behavior, which often mimics the behavior of older children in whom these complaints can be verbalized. Acute vomiting and diarrhea are often easy to observe in relation to food ingestion, because there is a prompt onset of a rather impressive symptom and then often very prompt resolution. Vomiting and diarrhea due to food hypersensitivity may be distinguished from intoxications and gastrointestinal infections by the prompt resolution of symptoms and prompt return of the young child's appetite. Some children with food allergy may often appear quite ill, with pallor and some lethargy developing; however, these symptoms usually resolve within minutes. When pallor persists, shock should be suspected, blood pressure measured, and epinephrine (adrenalin) administered.

Children with chronic diarrhea are more troublesome to evaluate because of the multiple pathogenic causes of chronic diarrhea. The differential diagnosis of chronic diarrhea in infancy comprises numerous conditions, especially infectious etiologies, which are beyond the scope of this review. However, food-associated chronic diarrheas are important considerations once some of the more common etiologies have been eliminated by the initial evaluation. A variety of syndromes have been characterized in which diarrhea is often a major component.

Food Protein-Induced Enterocolitis

Food protein-induced enterocolitis is most frequently seen as adverse reaction to cow's milk or soy protein formulas in young infants (25–36). Symptoms consist primarily of vomiting and/or diarrhea and generally develop within the first 3 months of life. Not uncommonly, the infant will present dehydrated and quite ill. Diarrheal stools usually contain blood and increased numbers of eosinophils and polymorphonuclear neutrophils (PMNs). A jejunal biopsy characteristically reveals flattened villi, edema, and increased number of lymphyocytes, eosinophils, and mast cells. Elimination of cow's milk or soy from the diet frequently results in resolution of symptoms within 72 hr. Vomiting and/or diarrhea generally occur within one to several hours after ingesting the offending food, but rarely may be delayed for as long as 20 hr (37). If peripheral blood white blood cell counts are monitored, they may rise 3500 cells/mm^3 by 4–6 hr. Polymorphonuclear leukocytes and eosinophils may be found in stools. Serum antibody titers to the offending antigen may increase in response to the milk challenge (38), and there is an increase in the number of IgA- and IgM-containing cells in the jejunal mucosa (28,30,32,39). Secondary disaccharidase deficiency is not uncommon, presumably because of damage to the intestinal mucosa (36,40).

Food-Induced Colitis Syndrome

Food-induced colitis syndrome is also most commonly due to adverse reactions to cow's milk or soy protein formulas or to food antigens passed in maternal breast milk (e.g., cow's milk, egg, peanut), but involves primarily the colon rather than upper small bowel (35,41–43). Similar to infants with the enterocolitis syndrome, these infants present in the first 3 months of life with diarrhea, but generally do not appear ill. They are frequently detected because of the presence of gross or occult blood in the stool, and in many cases these infants have no other evidence of bowel disease. Hematochezia usually clears within 72 hr of eliminating the offending food, but the length of time required for resolution of mucosal findings is highly variable and may take up to 1 month (35). Sigmoidoscopy will reveal mild patchy injection of the mucosa to severe friability with small aphthoid ulcerations. Colonic biopsy reveals infiltration of eosinophils within the lamina propria and into the surface and crypt epithelia (44). In severe cases with crypt destruction, PMNs are also prominent.

Food-Induced Malabsorption Syndrome

Food-induced malabsorption syndrome (excluding celiac disease) may present in the first several months of life with poor weight gain and diarrhea and, not infrequently, steatorrhea (27). Most infants will have some vomiting, and about 20% are reported t have atopic dermatitis and recurrent respiratory infections. Laboratory studies frequently reveal elevated serum IgA concentrations and elevated levels of IgG antibodies to cow's milk, proteins. Endoscopy and intestinal biopsy reveal patchy villous atrophy with a prominent mononuclear round cell infiltrate of the epithelium and lamina propria and some eosinophils, not unlike celiac disease but generally less severe (45). Elimination of cow's milk (soy, egg, and wheat also implicated) leads to resolution of clinical symptoms within days to several weeks and complete normalization of intestinal mucosa in 0.5 to 1.5 years.

Gluten-Sensitive Enteropathy (Celiac Disease)

Celiac disease is the best-studied form of malabsorption syndrome. It is a mucosal disease of the small intestine precipitated in susceptible individuals by gliadin, the alcohol-soluble portion of gluten found in wheat, oats, rye, and barley. Diarrhea, or frank steatorrhea, growth failure in children, abdominal distention or flatulence, malaise, and irritability are the most common forms of presentation. Mouth ulcers and a variety of extraintestinal manifestations primarily secondary to malabsorption are not infrequent. In some children the diarrhea is not impressive, but they fail to thrive. Occasionally the weakness and poor growth is reminiscent of neuromuscular disease. In patients with untreated celiac disease, intestinal biopsy reveals subtotal or total villous atrophy with marked increase in intraepithelial lymphocytes. This disease itself has occupied volumes, and a complete review here is not possible, but the interested physician may profitably review several of the cited references on this subject (46–50).

Allergic Eosinophilic Gastroenteritis

Allergic eosinophilic gastroenteritis is a rare form of enteropathy which may present in the infant as abdominal pain, vomiting, diarrhea, and failure to thrive (51–55). In the mucosal form, patients often have atopic disease elevated serum IgE, positive prick skin tests to a variety of foods, and peripheral blood eosinophilia in about 50% of patients. Clinical symptoms correlate with the extent of eosinophil infiltration of the bowel wall. Infiltration of the mucosal layer corresponds to a syndrome of malabsorption, while infiltration of the muscular layer presents a clinical picture of obstruction. Rarely, infants with this syndrome may present with pyloric stenosis and outlet obstruction (56) or severe protein-losing enteropathy with anasarca (57).

Recently, a group of 10 children were described with postprandial abdominal pain (colic), early satiety (or food refusal), vomiting (frequently with thick, stringy mucus), occasionally diarrhea, and failure to thrive (58). All these children had been diagnosed with gastroesophogeal reflux and had failed standard medical therapy, and 6 of 10 had continued symptoms and failure to thrive despite Nissen fundoplication. Endoscopy and biopsies of the esophagus, stomach, and proximal intestine are consistent with a diagnosis of allergic eosinophilic gastroenteritis. Symptoms completely resolved in 8 or 10 children and substantially improved in the remaining 2 following 6–8 weeks of an amino acid-based elemental diet (Neocate). Postdiet biopsies of the esophagus showed marked reduction or clearing of infiltrating eosinophils. Utilizing elemental diets and blinded food challenges, both IgE-mediated and non-IgE-mediated mechanisms were implicated in the pathogenesis of the food-induced symptoms. Unfortunately, the predictive accuracies (both positive and negative) of skin tests in these children was poor.

Food-Induced Pulmonary Hemosiderosis (Heiner's Syndrome)

Heiner's syndrome is a rare disorder characterized by recurrent episodes of pneumonia associated with pulmonary infiltrates, hemosiderosis, anemia, and failure to thrive (59–61). These infants tend to have high precipitin titers to several cow's milk proteins. In other studies of patients with this syndrome, deposits of IgG, IgA, and C3 have been identified in lung biopsy material (62). Both antigen-antibody complexes and lymphocytes-mediated hypersensitivity responses to milk are postulated in the immunopathogenesis of this disorder. However, this is based primarily on the presence of elevated serum levels of milk-specific IgG antibodies and the in-vitro proliferative response of patient lymphocytes to milk antigen. Much more information is needed concerning the true incidence of this syndrome and particularly the natural history of disease in these children.

Other Syndromes

Another, more subtle condition appears in children with large volumes of milk intake, protein loss in the stool, blood loss in the stool, anemia, and sometimes failure to thrive (63–65). The studies cited concerning this condition suffer from a lack of immunological data, and they do not explore the mechanism whereby the food produces the symptoms; thus there is substantial data missing, the presence of which might enable more specific classifications of these "syndromes." One study examined biopsy specimens in children with the iron deficiency and problem loss syndromes but did not find immunological changes similar to those found in protein enteropathy, suggesting that hypersensitivity is not involved in this syndrome (66).

A final and common, albeit unexplained, cause of chronic diarrhea, especially in the second year of life, is diarrhea associated with fruit juice ingestion. Along with the infectious diarrheas, this seems to be one of the most common causes of diarrhea in young children (19). Removal of fruit from the diet results in complete resolution of the symptoms. The adverse reaction usually does not persist, and small amounts of juice and fruit may often be immediately reintroduced into the diet. In the 1950s, oil in the peel of orange was felt to be toxic to the intestines of young children (67). More recently, Hyams has proposed and demonstrated that malabsorption of natural carbohydrates may be the mechanism responsible (68–70).

Cutaneous

Cutaneous signs and symptoms are the other most common presentations of food hypersensitivity (see Table 2).

Urticaria/Angioedema

Urticaria of abrupt onset and usually lasting only hours is common in young children with food hypersensitivity and may be rather dramatic. The urticaria may be accompanied by angioedema. Recurring outbreaks of urticaria are uncommon unless the offending food is eaten frequently. Urticaria may be triggered by ingestion or contact or by both. Chronic urticaria, rarely seen in children less than 2 years of age, is rarely due to food hypersensitivity.

Atopic Dermatitis

By contrast, atomic dermatitis is very common in children less than 2 years of age, and 60% of individuals developing atopic dermatitis will do so in the first year of life. At times it presents a severe management problem. Atopic dermatitis is usually characterized by extreme pruritus but occasionally in very young children it seems not to itch or otherwise disrupt their apparent well-being. The rash is usually an erythematous, papulovesicular eruption, often with crusting. It may progress to scaling and lichenification, but it is not unusual for infants even with severe involvement to experience complete resolution without detectable stigmata of the skin disease. In infancy the rash is often distributed initially over the cheeks, neck, and extensor surfaces. With age the flexor surfaces become more involved, with less eruption on the face. Much of the skin alteration seen by the physician is due to excoriation; in fact, atomic dermatitis has no primary skin lesion but is identified by a constellation of symptoms (71,72). The incidence of atopic dermatitis (with or without) food hypersensitivity has apparently been worsening over the past 40 years and is now estimated to affect 10–12% of children (73).

The intensity of the evaluation of the young child with atopic dermatitis depends on the severity and extent of involvement of the skin. In the mild situation in which few areas of the body are slightly involved, the history may be used as a guide to the initial plan recommended by the physician. If the mother or caretaker does not suspect any food to be causing an exacerbation of symptoms, then the youngster may be treated with topical medication; if the skin responds promptly to minimal medication, further evaluation may be unnecessary and not cost-effective.

At the opposite end of the spectrum is the youngster with severe and generalized skin involvement. A food hypersensitivity evaluation may be helpful, even in the absence of any history of foods suspected of causing a reaction. At least 30–50% of these severely affected children may be expected to have food hypersensitivity (21). Conversely, a significant number will not have detectable food hypersensitivity; hence, the evaluation must be cost-effective in terms of expense and also the degree of dietary manipulation required of the family. Although firm rules cannot be proposed from the existing data, some suggestions may be helpful. When specific foods are suspected, skin testing for those foods may be undertaken. Given the results, the physician may suggest pursuit of an elimination diet or elect to postpone dietary manipulation and attempt topical measures to determine the response. In circumstances in which no foods are suspected, skin tests can be undertaken for the food allergens known to be most likely to exacerbate atopic dermatitis (egg, milk, peanut, wheat, soy). Alternatively, the child may be placed on a strict elimination diet or an elemental diet for a few days. In our experience, when food hypersensitivity is a part of the problem, a very limited diet often makes the skin much easier to manage, and less medication is required. When a child presents with very severe atopic dermatitis that may include infected skin, it is often necessary to make multiple changes concurrently and determine the effective ones as the evaluation proceeds. For example, to control severely involved skin it may be necessary to apply aggressive topical skin treatment (wet wraps over steroid cream), oral antibiotics, and an elimination diet. Then, as the skin improves, the important components of the management may be identified. As discussed elsewhere in this chapter, we have found the elemental formulas to be very helpful in managing these youngsters.

The breast-feeding mother presents a particular challenge because it is often difficult to provide a nutritionally adequate diet to both mother and baby if many food groups are eliminated from the mother's diet. Occasionally, we have had to ask the mother to discontinue breast feeding for a few days while the elemental formula is used. During this time the mother will need to use a breast pump to maintain her comfort and assure her milk supply so that breast feeding can be resumed when appropriate. Rarely, the nursing mother may be placed on the elemental formula. If the baby shows substantial skin improvement while on the elemental diet, then foods in the mother's diet may be suspected and eliminated if documented to cause repeat exacerbations; if not, then breast feeding may be reintroduced and the mother does not have to be concerned about limiting her own diet.

Other Dermatoses

Less specific dermatoses have been noted in youngsters with food hypersensitivity, including erythema which does not have a pattern typical of either urticaria or atopic dermatitis and is not accompanied by a discreet eruption. The mechanism of these reactions is unclear, however, they are often closely associated with the presence of IgE as detected by skin testing or RAFT (3). Finally, it is extremely common for cutaneous and gastrointestinal manifestations to occur simultaneously, especially in infancy (19).

Respiratory

In infancy, respiratory symptoms, either as the sole manifestation of an adverse reaction to food, or in concert with other manifestations, are much less common than cutaneous and gastrointestinal symptoms, yet respiratory symptoms are frequently attributed to foods (19). In the first 2 years of life, upper respiratory symptoms, particularly continuous rhinorrhea, or nasal airway congestion, are common childhood problems. However, the frequency with which these symptoms have been proven to be caused by foods is quite low. Several different studies have sought to attribute upper respiratory manifestations, including chronic rhinitis, rhinorrhea, and otitis media, to food hypersensitivity. Even in situations in which youngsters with these conditions are sensitized to foods identified by skin testing, elimination of food from the diet and challenge to the foods have not regularly reproduced the incriminated symptoms (4,19). Examination of the data from the major centers studying food hypersensitivity in large numbers of children shows that the occurrence of upper respiratory symptoms due to foods is much less common than either cutaneous or gastrointestinal symptoms (3,4,19–21,74–78). Moreover, respiratory tract symptoms typically are acute, rather than chronic, when triggered by foods (19–21,74–78).

Occasionally, when children have significant cutaneous and gastrointestinal manifestations due to food hypersensitivity, they will also exhibit ocular signs and symptoms including tearing and swelling of both the conjunctiva and the upper and lower eyelids. At times these symptoms are accompanied by profuse rhinorrhea and sneezing. Contact reactions may produce ocular symptoms. For example, youngsters who have milk hypersensitivity and in whom milk comes in contact with the eye exhibit very impressive ocular swelling, chemosis, and eyelid edema. This has also been noted with contact from eggs, various nuts, and peanuts.

As with upper respiratory symptoms, lower respiratory symptoms including cough, wheezing, breathlessness, "bronchitis," and bronchospasm have been reported as manifestations of adverse food reactions. Perusal of the studies of several authors who have sought wheezing and asthma as manifestations of food hypersensitivity in young children have shown this to be an uncommon event (3,4,19,20,74–80). However, although wheezing in a child younger than 2 years of age usually occurs secondary to viral infections, acute wheezing may occasionally be due to food hypersensitivity. As a result, food hypersensitivity should be considered as a possible cause of intermittent acute and brief wheezing in infancy. Nevertheless, it is highly unlikely that wheezing will be the sole manifestation of food hypersensitivity. Furthermore, the connection between the food ingestion and the onset of wheezing is likely to be obvious, and the duration between ingestion and onset of wheezing will almost always be brief.

Behavioral

In children under 2 years of age, who are unable to communicate their discomfort, it is often frustrating for parents and primary-care practitioners to help the fussy, unhappy, sleepless, "colicky" infant. It would certainly be attractive to find that the majority of these youngsters do have food hypersensitivity. Studies examining colic in young children have shown promising responses to food elimination in a small number of subjects (81–84). These studies have been faulted for methodological errors, but the weight of the evidence supports improvement in some children. One study of sleep disturbance in children, using double-blind, placebo-controlled food challenge, supports the contention that a few sleepless infants will experience improvement of their sleep disturbance if milk is removed from the diet (85). This study needs to be confirmed by other investigators. Removal of foods from the diet or feeding the infant an elimination diet for a few days should identify those youngsters in whom food is affecting sleep; if successful, it will be helpful to those families. It is not recommended that youngsters with these symptoms be placed on prolonged elimination or elemental diets. When more is learned about the biochemical mechanisms of food hypersensitivity, it may be possible to be more precise about which of these infants would benefit from a food elimination diet.

Anaphylaxis

Fortunately, anaphylaxis in infancy due to foods or any other cause is extremely rare; however, when it occurs, it is potentially catastrophic. When an infant presents with cardiovascular collapse it is often difficult to immediately identify food as a possible inciting factor. Most of these children exhibit pallor and lethargy. Epinephrine administration under these circumstance is crucial and should be done immediately. Moreover, it is mandatory that the physician attempt to measure a blood pressure; emergency rooms where infants are seen should have infant blood pressure monitoring devices. If the youngster's blood pressure is below normal, then prompt administration of intravenous fluids may be crucial and life-saving. Laryngospasm does occur in these youngsters, but the cardiovascular alterations produce the more prominent and probably more difficult to treat problem. Fatalities in this age group, even in situations where anaphylaxis has been precipitated, are exceedingly rare (86). Recently, Platt et al. (87) reported elevated serum tryptase in 40% of infants dying of sudden infant death syndrome (SIDS). Tryptase is released from mast cells during an anaphylactic reaction. Interestingly, 40% of infants with SIDS had IgE antibodies to B-lactoglobulin, whereas only 10% of control subjects were found to have such antibodies, leading the authors to speculate that food-induced anaphylaxis might be a cause of SIDS in some infants.

B. Timing

Prompt Onset

Currently, most research on food hypersensitivity in infancy suggests that the majority of symptoms occur promptly after the ingestion of the food (Table 3). In fact, the majority of youngsters will react within 2 hr and often within a few minutes of ingestion of the food. All the aforementioned symptoms will usually be characterized by their prompt onset and fairly rapid disappearance.

Delayed Onset

Children younger than 2 years are also the group in whom delayed-onset or late-onset symptoms have been demonstrated by controlled challenge. In some of these infants, particularly those with atopic dermatitis, there is an immediate onset of symptoms, with prolongation of the eruption. Research in progress is demonstrating that this eruption has the characteristics of the late-phase reaction which has been well demonstrated in older patients with allergic rhinitis and asthma after challenges with inhalant allergens and occupational exposures. Young children exhibit the delayed-onset chronic diarrhea patterns which have been well documented to be initiated by the gliadin fraction of wheat gluten, cow milk protein, and soy protein. It is characteristic of the protein enteropathies that it may take a number of days for the symptoms to begin and also a number of days for the diarrhea to resolve once the food is removed from the diet. It is also important to know that soy protein and cow milk protein enteropathies are self-limited illnesses of young children; rarely does one find these conditions in older children. In contrast, gluten-sensitive enteropathy is a life-long disease, and there are data which suggest that the failure of patients to adhere to their gluten-free diet could result in chronic bowel problems and malignancy later in life.

C. Specific Foods

During the early years of life the list of foods demonstrated to elicit symptoms (Table 4) expands as the diversity of the diet widens. Initially, the incriminated foods are usually formulas composed of cow's milk and soy. Foods tend to be added to the diet of American children in a fairly predictable fashion, with grains and fruits added to the diet in the latter part of the first year. By the second birthday, most American children have a fairly diverse diet and, therefore, almost any food that might be ingested may be a putative culprit. In one study for which the foods were tabulated,

Table 3 Onset of Reactions Observed During DBPCFC

Many reactions within minutes
Most reactions within 2 hr
Rare IgE-mediated reactions over 2 hr
Non-IgE-mediated reactions (gastroenteropathy) hours to days

the list of incriminated foods included milk, egg, soy, peanut, chocolate, corn, rice, wheat, and a multitude of fruit and fruit juices, with orange, tomato, and apple being the most frequently suspected (19).

In contrast to the list of incriminated foods, the list of foods shown by double-blind, placebo-controlled food challenge to be responsible for the production of any of the symptoms discussed above is much shorter. Examination of several studies using double-blind, placebo-controlled food challenges to confirm histories in children under the age of 2 has shown that in over 80% of children, the offenders are milk, egg, peanut, soy, and wheat. Although other foods have been shown to produce reactions in this age group, they are much less common, and two popular culprits, chocolate and corn, are rarely proven to cause food reactions (3,4,17, 19–21,76–79,86).

Foods that pass through breast milk may assume importance in this age group. There is as yet no evidence that infants have ever reacted to proteins produced by the mother. By contrast, there are numerous reports of youngsters reacting to proteins ingested by their mothers (88–90). With the results of well-controlled studies as a basis for examination of this question, the major foods responsible for producing symptoms when passed through the breast milk are egg, milk, peanut, and soy. It has been most interesting to find that symptoms may be produced rapidly in the infant following ingestion of the protein by the mother and then breast feeding the infant. It would appear that as little as 15 min is sufficient to allow maternal absorption of peanut protein and passage into the breast

Table 4 Foods Proved to Cause Food Hypersensitivity

Egg, peanut, milk, soy, wheat (80–85%)
Tree nuts, fish, shellfish (10%)
Pea, chicken, turkey, banana, other grains, other vegetables
Fruits and juice (especially in small children, non-IgE)
(Corn and chocolate rarely confirmed food villains)

milk; then, when the infant is breast fed, the prompt onset of symptoms is noted (S.A. Bock, unpublished observation).

IV. Pathogenesis and Immunology

A. Differential Diagnosis

The differential diagnosis of food hypersensitivity includes a number of categories (Table 5). Probably the most common cause of adverse reactions to foods in North America, and a very common cause of adverse food reactions in young children, is carbohydrate intolerance. For most children under the age of 2, the most important carbohydrate intolerance is lactase deficiency, leading to lactose intolerance. This usually occurs following a gastroenteritis when there is damage to the brush border enzyme-producing apparatus, leading to a secondary deficiency of lactase. The problem is transient but in some youngsters does require the administration of a di-saccharide-free formula for a period of time. Sucrase-isomaltose deficiency, which is much less common, also occurs in this age group. In youngsters with chronic diarrhea, especially following gastroenteritis, the possibility of carbohydrate intolerance should be considered.

Toxic reactions due to materials in infant foods have been reported. In the early 1990s there was substantial public concern about the pesticide Alar contaminating children's apple juice. (This proved to be of little consequence.) Some of these intoxications are natural and others are due to contamination of food as mentioned earlier in this chapter.

One of the most common causes of putative adverse food reactions are strongly held beliefs influencing feeding patterns. Coincidental observation associating the onset of symptoms and the administration of new foods is all too common in North America. Fads in feeding habits and the influence of "alternative practitioners" also have a significant impact in this area. Suffice to say that many primary-care physicians will be confronted with dietary alterations which have been made because symptoms

Table 5 Differential Diagnosis of Adverse Reactions to Foods

Deficiencies of intestinal enzymes (disaccharides)
Hypersensitivity/allergy (immunological)
Psychological (strongly held beliefs)
Noxious natural constituents (poisons)
Contaminants (microorganisms, parasites, toxins, and chemicals)

have been attributed to observations which have not been confirmed through objective challenge.

Hypersensitivity or allergic mechanisms constitute the major mechanism and differential diagnostic category to which this chapter is devoted. In immunology over the past couple of decades it has been common to consider hypersensitivity disorders in terms of the Gell and Coombs classification (types I, II, III, IV) (91). While this classification system has been extremely useful for categorizing and investigating hypersensitivity reactions, it now seems likely that most hypersensitivity reactions involve combinations of more than one type of Gell and Coombs interaction, based on present knowledge that most hypersensitivity reactions involve humoral and cellular components of the immune/inflammatory system.

B. Immunological Mechanisms

Immunoglobulin E (IgE)-Mediated Reactions

IgE-mediated hypersensitivity is the immune mechanism (Table 6) most strongly associated with adverse reactions to foods in young children. A reasonably pure example of an IgE-mediated reaction with mediators being

Table 6 Proposed Immune-Mediated Adverse Food Reactions in Infants

Type I, IgE-mediated	
Cutaneous	Urticaria/angioedema, atopic dermatitis
Respiratory	Rhinoconjunctivitis, asthma
Gastrointestinal	GI anaphylaxis (nausea, colic, vomiting, diarrhea), infantile colic, allergic eosinophilic gastroenteritis, ? food-induced enterocolitis syndrome
Type III, antigen–antibody complexes	
? Food-induced enterocolitis syndrome	
? Food-induced colitis syndrome	
? Food-induced malabsorption syndrome	
? Celiac disease	
? Food-induced pulmonary hemosiderosis	
Type IV, cell-mediated hypersensitivity	
Celiac disease	
? Food-induced enterocolitis syndrome	
? Food-induced colitis syndrome	
? Food-induced malabsorption syndrome	
? Food-induced pulmonary hemosiderosis	

released from tissue mast cells is the immediate-hypersensitivity skin test. When a food allergen is placed into the skin, there is cross-linking between IgE molecules which are bound to cell membranes by high-affinity receptors for IgE. Ensuring membrane and cellular interactions result in immediate release of histamine as well as other preformed mediators. The histamine is responsible for the wheal-and-flare reaction via vasodilatation and fluid leakage from blood vessels. The importance of other mediators, both preformed and those produced after cellular activation, are under intense investigation to determine their role in both the immediate and late-phase reaction. We should probably adopt the notion that IgE is necessary but not sufficient to produce these responses.

Immunoglobulin E (IgE)-Mediated Cutaneous Late-Phase Reactions

It has now been shown repeatedly that the reaction described above is only the first part in the role IgE plays in a sequence of events which are termed the late-phase reaction. Within 2–4 hr after the immediate reaction, the late-phase changes begin with an influx of neutrophils and eosinophils. The cellular influx is promoted by neutrophil and eosinophil chemotactic factors released from mast cells, endothelial cells, and probably other sources. The response is then protracted due to the presence and ongoing production of all the recently described mediators of inflammation, viz., adhesion molecules, cytokines, platelet-activating factor (PAF), prostaglandins, leukotrines, major basic protein and eosinophilic cationic protein (both from eosinophils), oxygen free-radical metabolites, and others. After 6–8 hr the cellular infiltrate contains predominantly mononuclear cells and eosinophils, with smaller numbers of neutrophils, basophils, and mast cells. Later biopsies, between 24 and 48 hr, detect a mononuclear cell infiltrate which appears identical to the classic type IV cell-mediated response (92–95). Recently it has been shown that food-antigen specific lymphocytes with "homing receptors" to specific target organs are selectively activated in vitro in the presence of the food allergen (96).

The eosinophil has now been incriminated in the pathophysiology of atopic dermatitis, due to the detection of major basic protein, the major protein of eosinophilic granules, in active eczematous lesions. The major basic protein is able to damage skin epithelial cells and promote further mast cell degranulation (97).

Non-Immunoglobulin E (IgE)-Mediated Reactions

There are some well-documented adverse reactions to foods which appear to involve the immune system and are either not IgE-mediated or IgE is only a limited component in the production of the symptoms. The protein enteropathies were mentioned earlier and include milk, soy, and gluten-sensitive enteropathies (celiac disease).

The histological characteristic of the protein enteropathies is a flattening of the intestinal mucosa. This appears to occur because of the rapid turnover of the upper layers of epithelial cells. The reproducing crypt cells are unable to replace the lost villous mucosal epithelial cells rapidly enough. At this time there is still debate concerning the exact manner in which the immune system participates in the production of this lesion. The reason that this lesion is transient for milk and soy proteins but is life-long for gluten protein is unknown (46–50).

The presence of increased IgG antibodies to cow's milk (or soy) compared to normal controls has led some to speculate that a type III hypersensitivity mechanism is responsible for this disorder. Others have suggested a type IV mechanism based on the presence of increased lymphocyte proliferation in vitro in most patients with this disorder (29). Skin-prick tests and RAST are generally negative in affected infants. However, in investigating two infants with this syndrome, Shiner et al. found increased mucosal IgE-containing plasma cells, degranulation of mast cells in response to milk challenge, and deposition of IgG and C3 in intestinal connective tissue and basement membrane (98). More recently, Nolte demonstrated histamine release in response to milk antigen from dispersed intestinal mast cells of infants with this disorder (99). Taken together, these studies suggest a localized IgE-mediated mechanism is at least partly responsible for this disorder.

In infants with the food-induced colitis syndrome, an oral challenge with the offending antigen will induce symptoms within hours to a few days. Sigmoidoscopy reveals an acute colitis. Histopathologically, glandular and epithelial architecture appear intact, with PMNs and eosinophils infiltrating the lamina propria. Both type III and type IV hypersensitivities are suggested as pathological mechanisms because of increased serum antibodies and lymphocyte proliferative responses to food antigens (100).

Both type III and type IV hypersensitivity mechanisms are suggested in the etiology of the food-induced malabsorption syndrome, but no clear immunological mechanisms have been demonstrated. Morphological evidence and information generated in experimental animal models strongly implicates a type IV, cell-mediated mechanism in the pathogenesis of the intestinal lesion in celiac disease (100,101). However, experimental evidence in some patients and rodent models suggests that a cell-mediated response to gliadin alone is not sufficient for full expression of the enteropathy (102). Evidence suggests that a defect in mucosal digestion of gliadin in celiac patients may be responsible for the production of toxic peptides which contribute to the development of the intestinal lesion (103). Whether the elevated IgE and IgA antibodies to gliadin contribute to the pathogenesis of celiac disease is unclear. The increased levels of IgG-, IgA-, and IgM-containing immune complexes do not appear to correlate with disease activity in patients (104).

Studies of gluten-sensitive enteropathy have provided most of the available information about protein-induced malabsorption. The recommended procedure has involved placing the patient on a gluten-free diet, observing resolution of symptoms, performing a biopsy which is found to be normal, and performing a biopsy following a gluten challenge when the chronic diarrhea has returned. The a-gliaden fraction of gluten is clearly able to stimulate the immune system, as shown by the detection of antigliadin (or antireticulin) antibodies in patients who have the disease (105). It is hypothesized that the antibodies, through interaction with the antigen, can then produce a cellular immune reaction which is responsible for inflammation and for the pathological lesion. Elegant organ culture studies were undertaken by several investigators and at that time it was shown that immunological interactions were detectable at the time the abnormal histology was noted (46–48,106,107).

The role of IgE and atopy in general in the production of gluten-sensitive enteropathy has long been debated. A recent case controlled study strongly suggests that there is not an increased prevalence of atopy in subjects with gluten-sensitive enteropathy and their relatives, compared to controls and their relatives. Despite some problems with precision in definition of terms, this is one of the best-controlled studies on this subject (108).

The immunopathogenetic mechanism(s) responsible for allergic eosinophilic gastroenteritis are not known. A subset of patients have exacerbation of symptoms following the ingestion of food to which they have specific IgE antibodies, thus implicating a role for an IgE-mediated mechanism in some patients. Other evidence supporting this mechanism includes the presence of IgE-staining cells in jejunal tissue, elevated IgE in duodenal fluids, and the resolution of symptoms with removal of the implicated food from the diet (104). However, immune complex-mediated complement activation or lymphokine release from activated lymphocytes could also account for the massive influx of eosinophils into the bowel wall.

A rare and somewhat controversial syndrome is that of chronic lower respiratory disease associated with antibodies to cow's milk in the serum. This syndrome is known as Heiner's syndrome and has been reported with variable consistency. These infants exhibit pulmonary infiltrates and pulmonary hemosiderosis. They have been reported to present with anemia, failure to thrive, and chronic lung disease. Hemosiderin-laden macrophages have been found in gastric material aspirated from the stomach in the early morning, and they have been found in lung biopsy specimens. The detection of precipitating antibodies to cow's milk led the original observers to remove cow's milk from the diet and notice a prompt improvement. IgE has not been shown to have any role in this condition. This illness would be better understood if a group of these youngsters were subjected to systematic and prolonged observation and study to determine the true role of the milk proteins. Case reports of this problem are so sporadic that it has been difficult to draw firm conclusions about the youngsters reported. Also, the question arises concerning the possibility that other food proteins might produce chronic pulmonary changes in youngsters with "idiopathic" lung diseases (59–62).

V. Laboratory Diagnosis

A. Skin Testing

Currently, the most useful laboratory test for identifying IgE-mediated food hypersensitivity in children of any age, including young children, is the prick/puncture skin test. Skin tests for foods have always had a bad reputation. This is primarily because of misinterpretation of skin testing and, therefore, a lack of understanding of the usefulness of the results. Skin tests merely detect antibody. This is true at any age and it is true for any allergen. Skin-test extracts must be verified; that is, they must be shown to detect antibody in those persons who have it, and they must be shown not to be nonspecifically irritating. This has been demonstrated to be true for foods often proved to cause symptoms. It has also frequently been said that skin testing in young children does not give useful information. On the contrary, a number of studies have shown that beyond several months of age, skin tests have a high negative predictive accuracy. Skin testing for any food at any age has a lower positive predictive accuracy because of the ability of the skin test to detect the presence of antibody in patients in whom no symptoms occur when the food is ingested. This set of conditions, that is, the presence of IgE antibodies as detected by skin testing without concomitant symptoms during food ingestion, is properly termed *asymptomatic hypersensitivity.* These positive tests are not incorrect, nor are they "false positive." If persons with IgE antibodies detected by skin testing, who have no symptoms upon ingestion of food, were given the allergen intravenously, marked symptoms would rapidly appear. At present the search continues for a test for food hypersensitivity with a higher positive predictive accuracy. Nevertheless, since there is such vast overdiagnosis of food "allergy" in our society, and since the negative skin test has a high negative predictive accuracy, it is a useful test for determining which patients are highly unlikely to have an adverse reaction to food upon ingestion and, therefore, are unlikely to have food hypersensitivity (3,4,20,21,74–78,109–111).

In children younger than 1 year of age, an additional point should be considered. In this age group the detection of IgE is unusual. Therefore, when a properly performed skin test is positive for a food under suspicion based on the history, strong consideration should be given to the possibility that the food is truly causing symptoms and a challenge should be arranged. In young children, we recommend the judicious use of a few well-characterized skin tests on a history of specific association between the ingestion of that food and the prompt onset of symptoms.

B. Radioallergosorbent Testing (RAST)

The radioallergosorbent test is a very useful in-vitro method for detection of IgE antibodies in the circulation. The major limitation of the RAST concerns its expense and the requirement for radioisotopes in the use of the original test. A newer version of the RAST, the CAP-RAST, is slightly more sensitive and possibly more predictive, and another version uses enzyme-linked immunosorbent (ELISA) technology for detection of the antibody. It is also important to note that quality control of the RAST is sometimes not optimal. The RAST remains an excellent tool for research, but at the present time it cannot be recommended for regular clinical use.

C. Mediator Levels

Measurement of circulating histamine levels has been undertaken following blinded food challenges. Elevated levels are demonstrable. As yet this and the measurement of other mediators released during food challenge cannot be recommended for routine clinical use (112).

D. Total Serum Immunoglobulin E

Measurement of serum immunoglobulins, particularly total IgE, has limited usefulness in this aged group. Unfortunately, total IgE measurements in any single individual are not optimally predictive of the presence of symptomatic food or inhalant hypersensitivity. Because total IgE production is under strong genetic influence, it is quite common to find youngsters who have a high total IgE with no detectable hypersensitivity. By the same token, it is not unusual to find youngsters with food or inhalant hypersensitivity who also have normal IgE measurements.

E. Intestinal Biopsy

Biopsy of the small bowel or colon for diagnosis of food protein-induced enteropathy or food protein-induced colitis is a test which should receive more attention. The true frequency of these illnesses is unknown but is probably under diagnosed because of our reticence to undertake these biopsies in very young patients with chronic bowel symptoms. The chronic diarrheal syndromes, while transient, probably constitute the major source of non-IgE-mediated adverse reactions to foods that are likely to involve the immune system. Further study might illustrate the presence of IgE-mediated late-phase reactions in the intestines.

F. Food Challenge

The gold standard for identifying an adverse reaction to a food is the *double-blind, placebo-controlled food challenge* (DBPCFC). This procedure consists of administering the food to the child in a blinded fashion so that all observers as well as the patient are unaware of the contents of the challenge. Although this would seem an unnecessary step in children under 2 years of age, it must be remembered that parental observations in this age group often lead to foods being eliminated from the diet because of a coincidental association between the ingestion of a food and the appearance of symptoms. For certain objective symptoms such as vomiting, abrupt-onset skin rashes, and some cases of diarrhea, the open administration of foods can be helpful in demonstrating the presence of absence of the adverse reaction. In particular, open challenges are useful for refuting histories of adverse reactions to foods. This is a particularly common finding in children under 2 years of age (19,113). The reason that blinded challenges are so important is that all of the studies cited which have used DBPCFC have found that 40–60% of the histories of adverse reaction cannot be confirmed. This makes history of adverse food reaction unacceptable as a tool for making an adequate diagnosis, so an unbiased test (DBPCFC) must be employed.

The DBPCFC is particularly easy to accomplish in youngsters less than 2 years of age. Often the foods under suspicion are liquids (soy formula, cow's milk) which may easily be hidden in one of the available elemental formulas. The suspect food is given in incrementally increasing amounts until a reaction occurs, or if no symptoms are elicited the food is returned to the diet in usual and customary portions. One should refer to a practical manual devised for the use of DBPCFC as an office procedure (113).

Food challenges utilized in non-IgE-mediated gastrointestinal food hypersensitivity are frequently modified, often eliminating the blinding and including a postchallenge bowel biopsy. In the cow's milk-induced enterocolitis syndrome, a challenge with milk (up to 0.6 g protein/kg body weight) provokes adverse clinical manifestations, increased PMNs and eosinophils in the stool, peripheral leukocytosis 6–8 hr after milk ingestion (increase of >3500 cells/min^3), and villus atrophy of the duodenum and jejunum (22,36,114). Protracted vomiting and hypotension may occur in about 15% of infants, so care must be excerised in performing these challenges. Similar reactions may occur to soy protein (31,32,36,115,116), and up to 50% of patients sensitive to cow's milk will also react to soy protein depending on the population under study (4,117).

Diagnosis of food-induced colitis similarly is dependent on an oral food challenge and postchallenge colonic biopsy to demonstrate the characteristic intestinal lesions, which may require 3–4 weeks to develop.

The diagnosis of the malabsorption syndrome is made by demonstrating biopsy evidence of small intestinal mucosal injury, resolution with elimination of the responsible antigen from the diet, and recurrence of intestinal injury after challenge with the implicated antigen. Immunoglobulin A antibodies to gluten are present in over 80% of children with untreated celiac disease (118). In addition, patients with celiac disease frequently have high levels of IgG antibodies to a variety of foods, presumably reflecting their response to increased antigen absorption. Recently, measurement of intraepithelial lymphocytes within the rectal mucosa 6 hr after rectal challenge with 2 g of a peptic-tryptic digest of gluten served as a simple, safe, and reliable test of gluten sensitivity. This test may obviate the need for oral gluten challenge if confirmed by further studies (119).

VI. Treatment

A. Avoidance

With young children in whom a definite diagnosis of food hypersensitivity has been made, two questions concerning treatment arise. First, is any treatment needed? Second, if treatment is needed, what treatment should be applied? For some young children, the only adverse symptom they have to food is the repeated development of erythema or urticaria upon contact with that food. In these youngsters, no treatment need necessarily be prescribed as long as the rash that develops is merely an aesthetic problem.

The major treatment for confirmed food hypersensitivity is manipulation of the diet so that the food culprit can be avoided while providing a nutritionally adequate diet. In infancy, food avoidance often means removal of one or more major foods, such as cow's milk and/or soy from the child's diet. In this situation, alternatives must be provided. When the youngster exhibits milk hypersensitivity but can tolerate soy, then soy formula can be provided. On the other hand, when both foods have been incriminated, the child must be fed a "hypoallergenic" formula (extensively hydrolyzed milk protein-based formula or an elemental formula). In the situation where an elemental formula is employed, these formulas are nutritionally complete and therefore do not require additional dietary supplementation. Youngsters on a dairy product-free diet who are not receiving an alternative formula do need to have supplemental calcium in accordance with current dietary recommendations of elemental calcium (birth to 6 months, 360 mg; 6–12 months, 540 mg; 1–10 years, 800 mg. It is important to note that reactions to hypoallergenic diets are extremely rare but have been reported and should be suspected if the child appears not to tolerate the hypoallergenic diet (120–122).

In infants who are nursing, particularly during the first few months of life, maternal dietary manipulation may be required and must be done with care. Several dietary proteins rapidly cross into breast milk. If dairy products are removed from the mother's diet, it is crucial that her calcium intake be monitored; if it is insufficient then supplementation must be provided to a maximum of 1500 mg daily. Rarely, we have been confronted with a situation in which the maternal diet has been so limited that both the child and the mother are receiving inadequate nutrition. This is a circumstance that certainly must be avoided.

B. Medication

A number of medications have been used to treat youngsters with adverse food reactions caused by food hypersensitivity. Studies of their efficacy have been either inadequately controlled or have shown the medications to be ineffective. Particularly in the infant age group, medication treatment is rarely required. Specifically, cromolyn sodium has not yet been shown to be effective in properly controlled studies for treatment of food hypersensitivity (123). Since an oral form of cromolyn is now available in the United States for treating mastocytosis, it may be tempting to try applying this treatment to youngsters who seem to have food hypersensitivity, especially if they seem to react to multiple foods. This temptation should be resisted unless it can be shown that the drug is effective. In all cases, it must first be proved that the child has food hypersensitivity. The same comments and criticisms apply to the use of antihistamines in children with food hypersensitivity.

The immediate treatment of a patient experiencing an allergic reaction to a food is the same as the treatment for any other allergic reaction. During an acute allergic or anaphylactic reaction, the usual medical assessment measures include examination of airway patency, breathing effort, and circulatory status. The most immediate and important medication is epinephrine. In children younger than 2 years of age, a dose of 0.1–0.2 mL is appropriate. Some authors have recommended a per-kilogram dose, but the dose suggested is not really based on controlled studies and it is more important to administer quickly the medication and to constantly monitor the child. Diphendydramine given orally or intramuscularly may be given in addition to the epinephrine during the immediate reaction. Most often, oral antihistamine is all that is required because the reaction is not life-threatening. For young children, a dosage of diphenhydramine of 5 mg/ kg per day is recommended. This may be divided into four doses and continued until the reaction subsides. For the rare severe and prolonged reaction, the usual resuscitative measures should be employed, including intravenous support and ventilatory management if needed. In the rare patient with a reaction severe enough to require these tools, intravenous corticosteroids should be added to the program, realizing that they will require hours before they are of assistance.

There are rare diagnoses such as secretory diarrheas and eosinophilic gastroenteritis which may occur in infants and do require treatment with corticosteroids. In particular, severe eosinophilic gastroenteritis, which can be quite threatening to a youngster's health and nutrition, will respond dramatically to treatment with corticosteroids. The recommended starting dose is 2 mg/kg per day and then, when the symptoms subside and eosinophilia has disappeared, the dose can be slowly tapered and discontinued. Usually the youngster's course can be monitored by following the peripheral eosinophil count.

Injection therapy for food hypersensitivity has never been shown to be effective in any age patient in properly controlled trials. Injections have been inflicted by a number of different techniques, but none has been shown to be efficacious. There is no justification whatever for giving allergy injections for foods to infants. Any use of allergy injection treatment should be viewed as experimental and should be administered only under properly supervised protocols. (124).

VII. Natural History and Prognosis

The natural history of food hypersensitivity (Tables 7–9) has two components, the development of the symptoms due to food and the loss of the reactivity. The former subject is covered in Chapter 27 and the latter in Chapter 29. A number of studies over the years have demonstrated that

Table 7 Managing the Child Presenting with Adverse Food Reaction[a]

Eliminate food(s), use elimination diet to see if symptoms resolve.
Reintroduce food in small amount to see if tolerated or if reaction.
Rechallenge suspected foods at regular intervals.
Arrange for blinded flood challenge if problem persists.

[a]This approach is not for anaphylaxis or severe reactions.

children with DBPCFC-proven food hypersensitivity do lose their reactivity with time (125–128). Particular patterns of predictable loss of symptoms are becoming clear from the studies. It is important to begin with children in whom DBPCFC have been used to prove that the problem exists so that the data on which conclusions are drawn have validity. In studies where this precaution is not followed, the results are often similar but more difficult to interpret, because the initial status of the subjects is not known with certainty (129,130).

Loss of clinical reactivity appears to be more rapid in proximity to the initial diagnosis. Up to one-third of children will "lose" their clinical sensitivity over the first 1–3 years, and then at a slower rate of resolution thereafter. Hypersensitivity to milk, egg, soy, and wheat are more likely to disappear, while reactivity to peanut seems to persist indefinitely in many children. Problems with fish and other nuts are less troublesome in infants, from whom these foods are usually withheld. Even in children in whom reactions are severe, it has been shown that loss of anaphylactic reactivity may disappear over time (86). These comments apply to children in whom DBPCFC has been found to be positive and in whom IgE has been implicated in the pathogenesis. In infants in whom adverse reactions can be

Table 8 Some Conclusions Based on Natural History Studies

Prolonged elimination of most foods is unnecessary, regular confirmation is important.
Cross-reactions between food families are rare—each food stands alone.
Food reactions may be lost at the rate of about 25% per year for foods listed.
Positive skin tests may persist for years, despite lack of symptoms during ingestion.
Life-threatening (anaphylactic) reactions in young children may be outgrown (egg, milk, soy); less likely in older children.

Table 9 Natural History of Food Allergy

Egg, milk, soy, and wheat likely to stop producing symptoms.
Peanut and tree nuts unlikely to stop producing symptoms.
Fish and shellfish probably unlikely to stop (little data in children).
Fruit and fruit juice: non-IgE-mediated reactions very likely to
  remit.
Other grains and less common foods: little data available.

documented but in whom no mechanism has been found, the loss of clinical reactivity may occur even more quickly (19). However, all the studies in which IgE is detected demonstrate that its presence remains detectable long after clinical reactivity may have disappeared. Thus, skin testing may not be used to determine whether or not clinical symptoms persist over time.

These observations have led to the development of recommendations for regular reintroduction of foods which produce reactions into the diet of food-allergic children (see Table 6). While there is not universal agreement among investigators, the following guidelines may be found to be helpful for the management of children who *do not* exhibit life-threatening food allergic symptoms. In children between the age of 1 and 2 years in whom reactions to milk have occurred, reintroduction could be undertaken every 6–12 months. For soy and wheat the interval could be every 3–6 months depending on the character and severity of the preceding reaction. If a reaction to peanut occurs during the first 2 years and the association between peanut and the symptoms makes peanut the likely culprit, then peanut should be avoided until after the third birthday. (*We strongly recommend that no children, especially in atopic families, be fed peanut or peanut butter during the first 3 years of life.*) The same recommendation should be followed for egg, tree nuts (almonds, pecans, walnuts, etc.), shellfish, and fish. For other foods little or no data exist and thus useful recommendations are harder to evaluate. The recommended intervals may be altered by observations during accidental ingestion. Particular concerns of parents, such as likely exposure to incriminated food in day-care settings, may result in challenges under observation earlier than the recommended intervals (19,125–128).

VIII. Vaccine Administration in Egg-Hypersensitive Children

A significant problem for primary-care practitioners caring for infants is the administration of measles, mumps, and rubella vaccine (MMR), and influenza vaccine in egg-allergic children. Both of these vaccines used to be grown in avian embryos and contained measurable amounts of egg protein (131), but MMR constituents are now grown on chicken embryo fibroblasts and contain virtually no egg protein. Nevertheless, controversy remains about the safest manner in which to screen egg-allergic patients and how best to administer the vaccine. The American Academy of Pediatrics makes specific recommendations for skin testing in a rather cumbersome three-step procedure and then for administration of the vaccine if the skin test is positive (132). This will reportedly be changed in the next edition. Several recent studies using MMR vaccine (133–136) and influenza vaccine (137) have tested variations of the "official" recommendations. Each of these studies has suffered from one main fault and a few minor ones. The major fault has been the absence of DBPCFC-proven egg hypersensitivity at the time of evaluation, with reliance instead on history of egg-induced symptoms and egg skin tests. The reader of this chapter will by now realize the potential pitfalls of basing conclusions on history and skin tests in the absence of DBPCFC. Since severe reactions to the small amount of egg in these vaccines is rare even in egg-allergic children, studies of this nature require large numbers of patients in order to provide accurate conclusions. The study of Lavi (136) best supports the recommendations of the American Academy of Pediatrics.

There is growing evidence that this cumbersome and uncomfortable procedure is unnecessary. Three lines of evidence suggest that the MMR currently available is safe for use in children allergic to eggs. One hundred twenty children with egg allergy documented by DBPCFC have been immunized with vaccine without difficulty (138). Of this group, 60 were prick skin tested with full-strength MMR and only 2 were considered positive (mean wheal diameter >3 mm) while 5 demonstrated erythema only. Initially, intradermal skin testing was performed with 0.02–0.03 mL of MMR vaccine (1:100 dilution) prior to immunization. However, this practice was discontinued because it provoked sharp burning pain in most patients and controls and was found to yield many false positive responses. Second, 2 patients were identified who had anaphylactic reactions to MMR. Neither patient had a history of egg hypersensitivity, prick skin test positivity to egg, nor evidence of egg-specific IgE antibodies. Finally, the MMR vaccine was analyzed with sensitive ELISAs capable of detecting picogram quantities of ovalbumin. This analysis indicated that <50 pg/dose of immunologically recognizable ovalbumin was present, a quantity unlikely to provoke any response. Similar data has been collected by Beck et al. (139). Most recently, James et al. (140) reported that over 1200 egg-allergic children have been immunized in the routine fashion, regardless of MMR vaccine skin test results or the severity of their previous egg allergic reactions. Combining these observations, it seems unlikely that egg-allergic children are at any greater risk of anaphylaxis from MMR than the general population.

One must conclude that precautions must be taken when administering egg-containing vaccines to egg-allergic youngsters because there are rare children who may have systemic reactions to the vaccine. However, it is also important to know that there have been rare but serious reactions to some component of the vaccine in non-egg-allergic children (141). Therefore administration of these vaccines should only be undertaken by persons familiar with treatment of acute allergic reactions. However, the current recommendations are cumbersome and, if followed exactly, produce a great deal of discomfort in the child being inoculated. Thus, further research in this area is needed to derive a more efficient and less painful procedure.

IX. Unproved Diagnostic and Therapeutic Practices

A. Tests

Over the last several decades there has been an evolution of testing methods which have no proven efficacy. These procedures have involved methods such as the cytotoxic food test, including the automated ALCAT, dilution neutralization skin testing, and sublingual testing. For the most part these methods have not been applied to infants; however, the cytotoxic food test has been used in children of all ages. Since this test has generally become debunked it has been replaced by ever more sophisticated but equally unsubstantiated methods. The latest testing methods involve measurements of circulating antibodies of IgG, the IgG4 subclass, and of "food immune complexes." Although these tests do measure the presence of antibody, and of immune complexes, they suffer from having never been correlated with double-blind, placebo-controlled food challenges. Therefore, almost all the claims made for the tests are based merely on the detection of circulating antibodies and cannot be relied upon to diagnose food hypersensitivity (142). These tests should be used only in experimental situations until their efficacy (or lack thereof) can be demonstrated. In the meantime, extravagant claims based on their use should be countered by reference to the absence of application of the scientific method in their evaluation and application. Even in infants, observations may be subject to the placebo effect.

B. Diets

Over the years a number of diets have been popularized for use in children with food hypersensitivity. Rarely are these diets applied to children under 2 years of age. However, readers should be aware of their availability, and that in certain areas of the country, enthusiasm for these diets does extend to young children. The most well known of these is the so-called "rotation" or "rotary-diversified diet." Since most young children with food hypersensitivity have a self-limited course, as pointed out in an earlier section, the application of any diet which tends to keep foods out of the diet, or maintains quantities at a minimum, is likely to appear efficacious. At this time these diets should be considered experimental and should not be used for the treatment of true food hypersensitivity.

As discussed in Chapter 30, hypoallergenic formulas may be used in an attempt to prevent milk allergy and some atopic symptoms. In addition, formulas meeting the FDA-recommended definition of "hypoallergenic" may be used to treat almost all milk-allergic patients. In order to be approved as hypoallergenic, a manufacturer needs to demonstrate with 95% confidence that 90% of subjects with milk allergy documented by DBPCFC will not react to a given formula (122). From this definition it is clear that some caution must be exercised when giving a highly sensitive infant a hypoallergenic formula. *Hypoallergenic* does not mean *nonallergenic*, and there may be rare infants who react to a hypoallergenic formula (122). There are now four formulas available in the United States that appear to meet the definition of hypoallergenicity (although none has received that FDA designation at this time): Alimentum (Ross Laboratories); Nutramigen and Pregestemil (Mead Johnson), which are casein hydrolysates; and Neocate (Scientific Hospital Supplies), an elemental formula. Theoretically, Neocate should be the least allergenic, since it is formulated from amino acids, vitamins, and minerals to mimic the composition of human breast milk, whereas the hydrolysate formulas are generated from enzymatically degraded cow's milk casein. Tolerex (Vivonex) is a completely elemental formula which has been used as the sole source of nutrition in persons of all ages.

X. Future Considerations

The critical reader of this chapter will be able to see a number of lacunae in our current knowledge. The real prevalence of food-induced disease requires objective determination. The recent observation that cow's milk protein intolerance appears on the wane in Spain (possibly from the use of adapted formulas) is encouraging, but requires confirmation (143). More information about the pathogenesis of food hypersensitivity is certainly needed. There are several areas in which some preliminary data have been gathered, but further elucidation is needed of observations such as the importance of high spontaneous release of histamine and the role of histamine-releasing factors in food hypersensitivity (144,145). It is of great interest to investigators in this field to try to determine which biochemical mediators of inflammation are involved in food hypersensitivity, especially when compared to the biochemistry now unfolding from studies of allergic rhinitis and asthma. In particular, it would be most helpful if we could demonstrate the presence or absence of late-phase reactions in the pathogenesis of food hypersensitivity. Do protein enteropathies involve IgE, and do they have a late-phase component? Does inflammation of the upper respiratory tract occur from food hypersensitivity with a greater frequency than has been identified?

Another area where we need further understanding is in the area of non-IgE-mediated food hypersensitivity. Despite the great claims made about late and delayed food reactions, and the involvement of foods in the production of arthritis, kidney disease, epilepsy, and migraine headache, there remains a great deal of anecdotal and testimonial information with precious little confirmable science in this area. Understanding of the pathogenesis of "delayed" food reactions, if they exist, might improve our ability to diagnose and treat the condition and to bring an end to some of the speculative diagnostic procedures and questionable treatments that are currently being prescribed, especially by "alternative practitioners."

A major area where important advances would be helpful is in the diagnosis of food hypersensitivity. The skin test is certainly a useful test, particularly for eliminating the probability of IgE-mediated food hypersensitivity. This is true in older children, and equally true in many infants. The RAST and ELISA remain useful as adjuncts in clinical diagnosis and as research procedures. The small-bowel biopsy, which has been mentioned in previous sections, can be extremely helpful, but in many centers there is resistance to undertaking small-bowel biopsies in young children for conditions that may be self-limited. Newer, noninvasive techniques and biochemical measurements which can be developed and obviate the use of the double-blind, placebo-controlled food challenge would certainly be welcome. In the meantime, more practitioners need to become skilled in the use of the double-find food challenge, which is a technique that, after limited practice, becomes as routine as any other general office procedure. Certainly we do not find this a cumbersome technique to apply for either routine clinical purposes or for research purposes.

The area for which there is the least information is the relative merit of active pharmacological prevention as opposed to avoidance and reintroduction of foods into the diet. Certainly for most children younger than 2 years of age, this is all that is needed because of the self-limited nature of this problem. However, there are youngsters in this age group who do have true multiple food hypersensitivity and for whom some kind of treatment that would either hasten the natural history or block the biochemical reaction would be most helpful.

In conclusion, we hope that the reader of this chapter will have found that a useful approach can be developed to handle in an efficient and timely manner those children who present with a history of adverse reactions to foods. In the last two decades a great deal of information has been learned in this field and has allowed a systematic approach to be developed which aids the practitioner in coping with this frequent complaint.

References

1. *Genesis* 3.
2. Cohen SG, Saaredra-Delgado AM. Through the centuries with food and drink, for better or worse. Allergy Proc 1989; 10:281–290.
3. Sampson HA. Role of immediate food hypersensitivity in the pathogenesis of atopic dermatitis. J Allergy Clin Immunol 1983; 71:473–480.
4. Bock SA, Atkins FM. Patterns of food hypersensitivity during sixteen years of double blind placebo controlled food challenges. J Pediatrics 1990; 86: 387–392.
5. Bryan F. Diseases transmitted by foods: a classification and summary. US Dept HHS, Public Health Service, Center for Disease Control, HAS publication no. (CDC) 81-8237, 1981.
6. National Research Council, Committee on Food Protection. Toxicants Naturally Occurring in Foods. Washington, DC: National Academy of Sciences, 1973.
7. Anderson JA, Sogn DD. Adverse reactions to foods. US Dept HHS, Public Health Service, NIH, NIH pub no. 84-2442, 1984.
8. Committee on Drugs, American Academy of Pediatrics. Transfer of drugs and other chemicals into human milk. Pediatrics 1989; 84:924–936.
9. Rogon WJ, Bagniewski W, Damstra T. Pollutants in human milk. N Engl J Med 1980; 302:1450–1453.
10. Bakken AF, Seip M. Insecticides in human milk. Acta Paediatr Scand 1976; 65:535–539.
11. Halpern SR, Sellers WA, Johnson RB. Development of childhood allergy in infants fed breast, soy or cow milk. J Allergy Clin Immunol 1973; 51: 139–151.
12. Gerrard JW, MacKenzie JWA, Goluboff N. Cow's milk allergy: prevalence and noninfestations in an unselected series of newborns. Acta Paediatr Scand 1973; 234(suppl 27):3–21.

13. Jakobsson I, Lindberg T. A prospective study of cow's milk protein intolerance in swedish infants. Acta Pediatr Scand 1979; 68:853–859.

14. Stintzing G, Zetterstrom R. Cow's milk allergy, incidence and pathogenetic role of early exposure to cow's milk formula. Acta Pediatr Scand 1979; 68: 383–387.

15. Heiner DC. Allergy to cow's milk. N Engl Soc Allergy Proc 1981; 2: 198–203.

16. Kajosaari M. Food allergy in Finnish children aged 1 to 6 years. Acta Pediatr Scand 1982; 71:815–819.

17. Hattevig G, Kjellman B, Johansson SGO, Björkstén B. Clinical symptoms and IgE responses to common food proteins in atopic and healthy children. Clin Allergy, 1984; 14:551–559.

18. Hattevig G, Kjellman B, Björkstén B. Clinical symptoms and IgE responses to common food proteins and inhalants in the first 7 years of life. Clin Allergy, 1987; 17:571–578.

19. Bock SA. Prospective appraisal of complaints of adverse reactions to foods in children during the first 3 years of life. Pediatrics 1987; 79.683–688.

20. Zeiger RS, Heller S, Mellon MH, Forsythe AB, O'Connor RD, Hamburger RN, Schatz M. Effect of combined maternal and infant food-allergen avoidance on development of atopy in early infancy: a randomized study. J Allergy Clin Immunol 1989; 84:72–89.

21. Burks AW, Mallory SB, Williams LW, Shirrell MA. Allergic dermatitis: clinical relevance of food hypersensitivity reactions. J Pediatrics 1988; 113: 447–451.

22. Hide DW, Guyer BM. Cow's milk intolerance in Isle of Wight infants. Br J Clin Prac 1983; 37:285–287.

23. Host A, Halken S. A prospective study of cow milk allergy in Danish infants during the first three years of life. Allergy 1990; 455:587–596.

24. Schrander JJP, van den Bogart JPH, Forget PP, Schrander-Stumple CT, Juijten RH, Kester AD. Cow's milk protein intolerance in infants under 1 year of age: a prospective epidemiological study. Eur J Pediatr 1993; 152: 640–644.

25. Iyngkaran N, Robinson MJ, Prathap K, Sumithran E, Yadav M. Cow's milk protein-sensitive enteropathy. Combined clinical and histological approach to diagnosis. Arch Dis Child 1978; 53:20–26.

26. Iyngkaran N, Robinson MJ, Sumithran E, Lam SK, Puthucheary SD, Yadav M. Cow's milk protein-sensitive enteropathy. Arch Dis Child 1978; 53: 150–153.

27. Kuitunen P, Visakorpi JK, Savilahti E, Pelkonen P. Malabsorption syndrome with cow's milk intolerance: clinical findings and course in fifty-four cases. Arch Dis Child 1975; 50:351–356.

28. Savilahti E. Immunochemical study of the malabsorption syndrome with cow's milk intolerance. Gut 1973; 14:491–501.

29. Fontaine JL, Navarro J. Small intestinal biopsy in cow's milk protein allergy in infancy. Arch Dis Child 1975; 50:357–363.

30. Bock SA, Remigio LK, Gordon B. Immunochemical localization of proteins in the intestinal mucosa of children with diarrhea. J Allergy Clin Immunol 1983; 72:262–268.

31. Ament ME, Rubin C-E. Soy protein–another cause of the flat intestinal lesion. Gastroenterology 1972; 62:227–234.

32. Perkkiö M, Savilahti E, Kuitunen P. Morphometric and immunohistochemical study of jejunal biopsies from children with intestinal soy allergy. Eur J Pediatr 1981; 137:63–69.

33. Halpin TC, Byrne WJ, Ament ME. Colitis, persistent diarrhea and soy protein intolerance. J Pediatr 1977; 91:404–407.

34. Vitoria JC, Camareno C, Sojo A, Ruiz A, Rodriguez-Soriano J. Enteropathy related to fish, rice, and chicken. Arch Dis Child 1982; 57:44–48.

35. Gryboski JD. Gastrointestinal milk allergy in infants. Pediatrics 1967; 40:354–362.

36. Powell GK. Milk and soy induced enterocolitis of infancy. J Pediatr 1978; 93:553–560.

37. Hill DJ, Shelton MJ, Hosking CS. Manifestations of milk allergy in infancy: clinical and immunologic findings. J Pediatr 1986; 109:270–276.

38. McDonald PJ, Goldblum RM, Van Sickle GJ, Powell GK. Food protein-induced enterocolitis: altered antibody response to ingested antigen. Pediatr Res 1984; 18:751–755.

39. Pearson JR, Kingston D, Shiner M. Antibody production to milk proteins in the jejunal mucosa of children with cow's milk protein intolerance. Pediatr Res 1983; 17:406–412.

40. Iyngkaren N, Abdin Z, Davis K, Boey CG, Prathap I, Yadav M, Lam SK, Puthucheary SD. Acquired carbohydrate intolerance and cow milk protein-sensitive enteropathy in young infants. J Pediatr 1979; 95:373–378.

41. Lake AM, Whittington F, Hamilton SR. Dietary protein-induced colitis in breast fed infants. J Pediatr 1982; 101:906–910.

42. Berezin S, Schwarz SM, Glassman M, Davidian M, Newman LJ. Gastrointestinal milk intolerance of infancy. Am J Dis Child 1989; 143:361–362.

43. Jenkins HR, Pincott JR, Soothill JF, Milla PJ, Harries JT. Food allergy: the major cause of infantile colitis. Arch Dis Child 1984; 59:326–329.

44. Goldman H, Proujansky R. Allergic proctitis and gastroenteritis in children. Am J Surg Pathol 1986; 10:75–86.

45. Kosnai I, Kuitunen P, Savilahti E, Sipponen P. Mast cells and eosinophils in the jejunal mucosa of patients with intestinal cow's milk allergy and celiac disease of childhood. J Pediatr Gastroenterol Nutr 1984; 3:368–372.

46. Strober W, Falchuk ZM, Rogentine GN, Nelson DL, Klaeveman HL. The pathogensis of gluten-sensitive enteropathy. Ann Intern Med 1975; 83:242.

47. Falchuck ZM, Katz AJ, Shwachman H. Gluten-sensitive enteropathy: genetic analysis and organ culture study in 35 families. Scand J Gastroenterol 1978; 13:839–843.

48. Jos J, Labbe F, Geny B, Griscelli C. Immunoelectron microscopic localization of immunoglobulin A and secretory component in jejunal mucosa from children with coeliac disease. Scand J Immunol 1979; 9:441–450.

49. Aurricchio S, Greco L, Tronccone R. Gluten-sensitive enteropathy in childhood. Ped Clin N Am 1988; 35:157–187.

50. Kagnoff M. Immunopathogenesis of celiac disease. Immunol Invest 1989; 18:499–507.

51. Kettlehut BV, Metcalfe DD. Adverse reactions to foods. In: Middleton E Jr, Reed CE, Ellis EF, Adkinson NF Jr, Yunginger JW, eds. Allergy. Principles and Practice. Vol. II. 3d ed. St. Louis: Mosby, 1988:1481–1502.

52. Katz AJ, Goldman H, Grand R. Gastric mucosal biopsy in eosinophilic (allergic) gastroenteritis. Gastroenterology 1977; 73:705–709.

53. Katz AJ, Twarog FJ, Zeiger RS, Falchuk M. Milk-sensitive and eosinophilic gastroenteropathy; similar clinical features with contrasting mechanisms and clinical course. J Allergy Clin Immunol 1984; 74:72–78.

54. Vandenplas Y. Milk-sensitive eosinophilic gastroenteritis in a 10 day old boy. Eur J Pediatr 1990; 149:244–245.

55. IIill SM, Miller PJ. Colitis caused by food allergy in infants. Arch Dis Child 1990; 65:132–133.

56. Snyder JD, Rosenblum N, Wershil B, Goldman H, Winter HS. Pyloric stenosis and eosinophiic gastroenteritis in infants. J Pediatr Gastroenterol Nutr 1987; 6:543–547.

57. Waldman TA, Wochner RD, Laster L, Gordon RS. Allergic gastroenteropathy. N Engl J Med 1967; 276:761–769.

58. Kelly KJ, Lazenby AJ, Rowe PC, Yardley JH, Perman JA, Sampson HA. Eosinophilic esophagitis attributed to gastroesophageal reflux: improvement with an amino acid-based formula. Gastroenterol 1995; 109:1503–1512.

59. Heiner DC, Sears JW, Kniker WT. Multiple precipitins to cow's milk in chronic respiratory disease. Am J Dis Child 1962; 103:634–654.

60. Holland NH, Hong R, Davis NC, West CD. Significance of precipitating antibodies to milk proteins in the serum of infants and children. J Pediatr 1962; 61:181–195.

61. Boat TF, Polmar SH, Whitman V, Kleinerman JI, Stern RC, Doershuk CF. Hyperreactivity to cow milk in young children with pulmonary hemosiderosis and cor pulmonale secondary to nasopharyngeal obstruction. J Pediatr 1975; 87:23–29.

62. Lee SK, Kniker WT, Cook CD, Heiner DC. Cow's milk-induced pulmonary disease in children. Adv Pediatr 1978; 25:39–57.

63. Wilson JF, Lahey NE, Heiner DC. Studies on iron metabolism V. Further observations on cow's milk induced gastrointestinal bleeding in infants with iron deficiency anemia. J Pediatr 1974; 84:335–343.

64. Woodruff CW, Clark JL. The role of fresh cow's milk in iron deficiency. I. Albumin turnover in infants with iron deficiency anemia. Am J Dis Child 1972; 124:18–23.

65. Ziegler RE, Fomon SJ, Nelson SE, Rebouche CJ, Edwards BB, Rogers RR, Lehman LJ. Cow milk feeding in infancy: further observations on blood loss from the gastrointestinal tract. J Pediatr 1990; 116:11–18.
66. Lundstrom U., Perkkio M., Savilahti E., Siimes M. Iron deficiency anemia with hyproteinemia. Arch Dis Child 1983; 58:438–441.
67. Ratner B., Untracht S, Malone J. Allergenicity of modified and processed food stuffs in oranges. Allergenicity of orange studied in man. J Pediatr 1953; 43:421–428.
68. Hyams JS, Leichter AM. Apple juice: an unappreciated cause of chronic diarrhea. Am J Dis Child 1985; 139:503–505.
69. Hyams JS, Etienne NL, Leichter AM, Thever TC. Carbohydrate malabsorption following fruit juice ingestion in young children. Pediatrics 1988; 88: 64–68.
70. Lifshitz F, Ament ME, Kleinman RE, Klish W, Lebenthal E, Perman J, Udall JN. Role of juice carbohydrate malabsorption in chronic nonspecific diarrhea in children. J Pediatr 1992; 120:825–829.
71. Blaylock WK. Atopic dermatitis: diagnosis and pathobiology. J Allergy Clin Immunol 1976; 57:62–79.
72. Hanifin JM, Rajka G. Diagnostic features of atopic dermatitis. Acta Dermatol Venerol 92(suppl) 1980:44–47.
73. Hanifin JM. Epidemiology of atopic dermatitis. Monogr Allergy 1987; 21: 116–131.
74. May CD. Objective clinical and laboratory studies of immediate hypersensitivity reactions to foods in children. J Allergy Clin Immunol 1976; 58: 500–515.
75. Bock SA, Lee WY, Remigio LK, May CD. Studies of hypersensitivity reactions to foods in infants and children. J Allergy Clin Immunol 1978; 62: 327–334.
76. Sampson HA, McCaskill CM. Food hypersensitivity and atopic dermatitis: evaluation of 113 patients. J Pediatr 1985; 107:669–675.
77. Sampson HA. The role of food allergy and mediator release in atopic dermatitis. J Allergy Clin Immunol 1988; 81:635–645.
78. Burks AW. Antibody response to milk proteins in patents with milk protein intolerance documented by challenge. J Allergy Clin Immunol 1990; 85: 921–927.
79. Onorato J, Merland N, Terral C, Michel FB. Placebo-controlled double-blind food challenge in asthma. J Allergy Clin Immunol 1986; 78:1139–1146.
80. Novembre E, de Martino M, Vierucci A. Food and respiratory allergy. J Allergg Clin Immunol 1988; 81:1059–1065.
81. Jakobsson I, Lindberg T. Cow's milk proteins cause infantile colic in breast-fed infants: a double-blind crossover study. Pediatrics 1983; 71:268–271.
82. Lothe L, Lindberg T. Cow's milk whey protein elicits symptoms of intractable colic in colicky formula-fed infants: a double-blind crossover study. Pediatrics 1989; 83:262–266.

83. Forsythe BWC. Colic and the effect of changing formulas: a double-blind multiple crossover study. J Pediatr 1989; 115:521–526.
84. Sampson HA. Infantile colic and food allergy: fact or fiction. J Pediatr 1989; 115:583–584.
85. Kuhn A, Mozin MJ, Rebuffat E, Sottiaux M, Muller MF. Milk intolerance in children with persistent sleeplessness: a double-blind crossover evaluation. Pediatrics 1989; 84:595–603.
86. Bock SA. Natural history of severe reactions to foods in young children. J Pediatr 1985; 107:676–680.
87. Platt MS, Yunginger JW, Sekula-Perlman A, Irani AA, Smialek J, Mirchandani HG, Schwartz LB. Involvement of mast cells in sudden infant death syndrome. J Allergy clin Immunol 1994; 94:250–256.
88. Jakobsson I, Lindberg T, Benediktsson B, Hansson B-G. Dietary bovine B-lactoglobulin is transferred to human milk. Acta Pediatr Scand 1985; 74:342–345.
89. Machtinger S, Moss R. Cow's milk allergy in breast fed infants; the role of allergen and maternal secretory antibody. J Allergy Clin Immunol 1986; 77:541–547.
90. Host A, Husby S, Osterballe O. Prospective study of cow's milk allergy in exclusively breastfed infants. Acta Paediatr Scand 1988; 77:663–670.
91. Strobel S. Immunologically-mediated damage to the intestinal mucosa. Acta Paediatr Scand 1990; 365(suppl):46–57.
92. Dolovich J, Hargreave FE, Chalmers R, Shier KJ, Gauldie J, Bienenstock J. Late cutaneous allergic responses in isolated IgE-dependent reactions. J Allergy Clin Immunol 1973; 52:38–46.
93. Solley GO, Gleich GJ, Jordan RE, Schroeter AL. Late phase of the immediate wheal and flare skin reaction: its dependence on IgE antobodies. J Clin Invest 1976; 58:408–420.
94. Sampson HA. Late phase response to food in atopic dermatitis. Hospital Practice 1987; 22:91–106.
95. Sampson HA. Pathogenesis of eczema. Clin Exp Allergy 1990; 20:459–467.
96. Abernathy-Carver KJ, Sampson HA, Picker LJ, Leung DYM. Milk-induced eczema is associated with the expansion of T cells expressing cutaneous lymphocyte antigen. J Clin Invest 1995; 95:913–918.
97. Leiferman KM, Ackerman SJ, Sampson HA, Haugen HS, Venenice PY, Gleich GJ. Dermal deposition of eosinophil granule major basic protein in atopic dermatitis. Comparison with onchocerciasis. N Engl J Med 1985; 313:282–285.
98. Shiner M., Ballard J., Smith ME. The small intestinal mucosa in cow's milk allergy. Lancet 1975; 1:136–140.
99. Nolte H, Skov PS, Kruise A, Schiotz PO. Histamine release from dispersed human intestinal mast cells. Allergy 1989; 44:543–553.
100. McDonald TT. The role of activated T-lymphocytes in gastrointestinal disease. Clin Exp Allergy 100; 20:247–252.

101. Ferguson A. Models of immunologically driven small intestinal damage. In: Marsh MN, ed. Immunopathology of the small intestine. Chichester: Wiley, 1987:225–252.

102. Troncone R, Ferguson A. Induction of intestinal cell-mediated immunity to gliadin in mice. In: Kumar P, Walker-Smith J, eds. Proceedings of the International Symposium of Coeliac Disease. Leeds: University Printing Service, 1990.

103. Cornell HJ. Amino acid composition of peptides remaining after in vitro digestion of a gliadin sub-fraction with coeliac disease. Clin Chim Acta 1988; 176:279–290.

104. Saavedra-Delgado AM, Metcalfe DD. Interactions betweens food antigens and the immune system in the pathogenesis of gastrointestinal diseases. Ann Allergy 1985; 55:694–702.

105. Lycke N, Kilander A, Milsson LA, Torkowksi A, Werner N. Production of antibodies to gliadin in intestinal mucosa of patients with celiac disease: a study at the single cell level. Gut 1989; 30:72–77.

106. Falchuk ZM, Gebhard RL, Sessams C, Strober WL. An in vitro model of gluten sensitivity enteropathy: effect of gliaden on intestinal epithelial cells of patients with gluten sensitive enteropathy in organ culture. J Clin Invest 1974; 53:487–500.

107. Fluge G, Andersen KJ, Aksnes L, Thunold K. Brush border and lysomal marker enzyme profiles in duodenal mucosa of coeliac patients before and after organ culture. Scand J Gastroenterol 1982; 17:465–472.

108. Greco L, DeSeta L, D'Adamo G, Baldassarne C, Mayer M, Siani P, Lojodice D. Atopy and celiac disease: bias or true relation? Acta Pediatr Scand 1990; 79:670–674.

109. Bock SA, Buckley J, Holst A, May CD. Proper use of skin tests with food extracts in diagnosis of hypersensitivity to food in children. Clin Allergy 1977; 7:375–383.

110. Bock SA, Lee WY, Remigio LK, Holst A, May CD. Appraisal of skin tests with food extracts for diagnosis of food hypersensitivity. Clin Allergy 1978; 8:559–564.

111. Sampson HA, Albergo R. Comparison of results of skin tests, RAST and double-blind, placebo-controlled food challenges in children with atopic dermatitis. J Allergy Clin Immunol 1984; 74:26–33.

112. Sampson HA, Jolie PL. Increased plasma histamine concentrations after food challenges in children with atopic dermatitis. N Engl J Med 1984; 31:372–376.

113. Bock SA, Sampson HA, Atkins FM, Zeiger RS, Lehrer S, Sachs M, Bush RK, and Metcalfe DD. Double blind placebo controlled food challenge (DBPCFC) as an office procedure: a manual. J Allergy Clin Immunol 1988; 82:986–997.

114. Wilson SJ, Walzer M. Absorption of undigested proteins in human beings. IV. Absorption of unaltered egg protein in infants. Am J Dis Child 1935; 50:49–54.

115. Butler HL, Byrne WJ, Marmer DJ, Eulaer AR, Steele RW. Depressed neutrophil chemotaxis in infants with cow's milk and/or soy protein intolerance. Pediatrics 1981; 67:264–268.

116. Van Sickle GJ, Powel GK, McDonald PJ, Goldblum RM. Milk- and soy protein-induced enterocolitis: evidence for lymphocyte sensitization to specific food proteins. Gastroenterology 1985; 88:1915–1921.

117. Burks AW, Casteel HB, Fiedorek SC, Williams LW, Pumphrey CL. Prospective oral food challenge study of two soybean protein isolates in patients with possible milk or soy protein enterocolitis. Pediatr Allergy Immunol 1994; 5:40–45.

118. Scott H, Fausa V, Ek J, Brandtzaeg P. Immune response patterns in coeliac disease: serum antibodies to dietary antigens measured by an enzyme linked immunosorbent assay. Clin Exp Immunol 1984; 57:25–32.

119. Loft DE, Marsh MH, Crowe PT. Rectal gluten challenge and diagnosis of celiac disease. Lancet 1990; 335:1293–1295.

120. Bock SA. Probable allergic reaction to casein hydrolsate formula. J Allergy Clin Immunol 1989; 84:272.

121. Lipshitz CH, Hawkins HK, Guera C, Byrd N. Anaphylactic shock due to cow's milk protein hypersensitivity in a breast fed infant. J Pediatr Gastroenterol Nutr 1988; 7:141–144.

122. Sampson HA, Bernhisel-Broadbent J, Yang E, Scanlon S. Safety of casein hydeolysate formula in children with cow milk allergy. J Pediatr 1991; 118:520–525.

123. Burks AW, Sampson HA. Double blind placebo controlled trial of oral cromolyn sodium in children with documented food hypersensitivity. J Allergy Clin Immunol 1988; 77:417–423.

124. Oppenheimer JJ, Nelson HS, Bock SA, Christensen F, Leung DYM. Treatment of peanut allergy with rush immunotherapy. J Allergy Clin Immunol 1992; 90:256–262.

125. Sampson HA, Scanlon S. Natural history of food hypersensitivity in children with atopic dermatitis. J Pediatr 1989; 115:23–27.

126. Bock SA, Atkins FM. The natural history of peanut allergy. J Allergy Clin Immunol 1989; 83:900–904.

127. Bock SA. The natural history of food hypersensitivity. J Allergy Clin Immunol 1982; 69:173–177.

128. Ford RPK, Taylor B. The natural history of egg hypersensitivity. Arch Dis Child 1982; 57:649–652.

129. Danaeus A, Inganäs M. A follow up study of children with food allergy, clinical course in relation to serum IgE and IgG antibody levels to milk, egg, and fish. Clin Allergy 1981; 11:537–539.

130. Bishop JM, Hill DJ, Hosking CS. Natural history of cow milk allergy: clinical outcome. J Pediatr 1990; 116:862–867.

131. O'Brien TC, Maloney CJ, Tauraso NM. Quantitation of residual host protein in chicken embryo derived vaccines by radial immunodiffusion. Appl Microbiol 1971; 21:780–782.

132. American Academy of Pediatrics. Report of the Committee of Infectious Disease (red book). Elk Grove Village, IL: American Academy of Pediatrics, 1988.

133. Herman JJ, Radin R, Schneiderman BS. Allergic reactions to measles (rubeola) vaccine in patients hypersensitive to egg protein. J Pediatr 1983; 102: 196–199.

134. Greenberg MA, Birx DL. Safe administration of mumps-rubella vaccine in egg-allergic children. J Pediatrics 1988; 113:504–506.

135. Kemp A, VanAsperen P, Mukhi A. Measles immunization in children with clinical reactions to egg protein Am J Dis Child 1990; 144:33–35.

136. Lavi S, Zimmerman B, Koren G, Gold R. Administration of measles, mumps, and rubella virus vaccine (live) to egg-allergic children. JAMA 1990; 263: 269–271.

137. Murphy KR, Strunk RC. Safe administration of influenza vaccine in asthmatic children hypersensitive to egg proteins. J Pediatrics 1985; 106: 931–933.

138. Fasano MB, Wood RA, Cooke SK, Sampson HA. Egg hypersensitivity and adverse reactions to measles, mumps, and rubella vaccine. J Pediatr 1992; 120:878–881.

139. Beck SA, Williams LW, Shirrell MA, Burks AW. Egg hypersensitivity and measles-mumps-rubella vaccine administration. Pediatrics 1991; 88: 913–917.

140. James JM, Burks AW, Roberson PK, Sampson HA. Safe administration of measles vaccines to egg-allergic patients. N Engl J Med 1995; 332: 1262–1266.

141. Kelso JM, Jones RT, Yunginger JW. Anaphylaxis to measles, mumps, and rubella vaccine mediated by IgE to gelatin. J Allergy Clin Immunol 1993; 91:867–872.

142. Sheffer AL, Lieberman PL, Aaronson DW, Anderson JA, Kaplan AP, Pierson WE, Ellis EF, Lichtenstein LM, Lockey RF, Salvaggio JC, Zweiman B, Zimmerman B. Measurement of circulating IgG and IgE food immune complexes. J Allergy Clin Immunol 1988; 81:758–759.

143. Victoria JC, Sojo A, Rodriquez-Soriano J. Changing pattern of cow's milk protein intolerance. Acta Pediatr Scand 1990; 79:566–567.

144. May CD, Remigio L. Observation on high spontaneous release of histamine from leukocytes in vitro. Clin Allergy 1982; 12:229–241.

145. Sampson HA, Broadbent KR, Bernhisel-Braodbent, J. Spontaneous release of histamine from basophils and histamine-releasing factor in patients with atopic dermatitis and food hypersensitivity. N Engl J Med 1989; 321: 228–257.

33

Atopic Dermatitis and Other Immunological Dermatoses of Infancy

MICHAEL H. MELLON

Kaiser Permanente Medical Center, San Diego
and University of California, San Diego,
   School of Medicine
La Jolla, California

I. Atopic Dermatitis

A. Background

The condition of infantile atopic dermatitis (AD) is often a source of confusion and frustration for physicians and parents. Confusion arises from the term itself since, while many patients have a personal or family history of atopy, a type I, or IgE-mediated, immunological reaction does not explain all the observations seen in this disorder. Furthermore, the term AD is often used interchangeably with eczema, which is actually a symptom complex of papules, erythema, vesicles, serous discharge, and pruritus, of which atopic dermatitis is but one type (as are contact dermatitis, seborrheic dermatitis, and nummular dermatitis). Finally, because this condition is variable but can be associated with immunodeficiencies, food sensitivities, and, subsequently, other atopic conditions, the need for extensive diagnostic evaluation and therapeutic trials for an infant may be unclear.

AD is primarily a disease of infancy but rarely presents before age 2 months. Most affected individuals have onset within the first year and 85% within the first 5 years (1). The incidence is thought to be increasing to 10% of the population, with much less frequency in adults. All races are affected, with Asians having an increased susceptibility; males experience it more commonly, at a ratio of 3:2 (2). This disorder appears to have a strong genetic basis, as evidenced by high concordance in monozygotic twins and a family history of allergy in over two-thirds of patients with AD (3). While both autosomal dominant and recessive modes of inheritance have been proposed, other studies have suggested a multifactorial pattern. Because over 80% of AD patients have elevated IgE levels and positive skin tests, work showing an association between IgE production and genetic polymorphisms may provide a new approach to this disease (4).

The natural course of AD is variable but tends toward improvement. Initially presenting as an erythematous, pruritic eruption of the cheeks, it may progress to a brawny, fissured appearance of the extensor surfaces of the arms, legs, and wrists and, as the child matures, it may spread to flexural and collar regions and spare the face. Spontaneous resolution may occur by age 2–3 years, but unexplained remissions and exacerbations are a hallmark of AD. Severe disease in infancy and positive skin tests to foods are prognostic for persistence of skin involvement through age 5 and for development of other atopic symptoms. It is estimated that 30–50% of infants with significant AD will eventually develop symptoms of allergic rhinitis or asthma (5).

Epidemiological considerations of atopic dermatitis will become more accurate as the diagnostic criteria become more uniform. To this end, an international group in 1979 proposed characteristics for diagnosis of AD in children (Table 1) stressing the morphology and distribution of the lesions, the chronicity of the condition, and the atopic nature of the patients and their families.

B. Pathogenesis

Despite the fact that no unifying coherent theory completely explains the vast spectrum of AD, many physiological abnormalities have been identified and often guide therapeutic as well as etiological inquiries. The areas of most interest have been immunology and dermatophysiology.

The immunological basis of AD has been suggested by observations that patients with primary T-cell abnormalities, such as Wiskott Aldrich syndrome, often have elevated serum IgE levels and the skin rash of AD. When the immunological abnormalities are corrected in these patients by bone marrow transplantation, the eczematoid rash clears. This observation implicates a bone marrow-derived cellular dysfunction as the cause of AD and relegates a lesser role to an innate skin defect. More likely is an interrelated defect or an underlying immunoregulatory abnormality, sug-

Table 1 Characteristics for Diagnosis of Atopic Dermatitis in Infants

Major features (must have three)
  Pruritus
  Typical morphology and distribution
    Facial and extensor involvement during infancy and early childhood
  Chronic or chronically relapsing dermatitis
  Personal or family history of atopy (asthma, allergic rhinoconjunctivitis, atopic
    dermatitis)
Minor or less specific features
  Xerosis
  Periauricular fissures
  Ichthyosis/palmar hyperlinearity/keratosis pilaris
  IgE reactivity (increased serum IgE, RAST, or prick test positivity)
  Hand/foot dermatitis
  Cheilitis
  Scalp dermatitis (e.g., cradle cap)
  Susceptibility to cutaneous infections (especially *S. aureus* and herpes simplex)
  Perifollicular accentuation (especially in pigmented races)

Source: Modified from Hanifin JM. Atopic dermatitis in infants and children. Pediatr Clin N Am 1991; 38:763–789.

gested by the following immunological observations in AD patients (6): (a) increased IgE production, (b) positive immediate skin tests to allergens, (c) increased basophil histamine release, (d) frequent skin infections, (e) decreased numbers of CD8 suppressor/cytotoxic cells, (f) increased production of IL-4, decreased production of interferon gamma, and (g) decreased sensitivity to rhus dermatitis. These aberrations in the T-cell-directed areas of IgE production and cell-mediated immunity with accompanying IL-4 overproduction and recently described eosinophil granule proteins in skin lesions add to our understanding of AD.

The skin of the AD infant is characterized by excessive dryness, lowered threshold to pruritic stimuli, and easy damagibility to physical stimuli such as itching. This sequence appears to be a key to the development of the typical eczematoid lesions of AD, as the sites of predilection for this rash are those areas most easily reached by the infant to scratch or rub and inaccessible areas such as the back or diaper area are spared. Development of added palmar creases and atopic pleats of the lower eyelid may be related to xerosis and thickening of localized skin and indicate poor prognosis. Keratosis pilaris, a cornification of the hair follicles, gives the skin a gooseflesh appearance, especially on the outer arms and legs. This continual piloerectile state has been explained by a possible high level of alpha-adrenergic activity due to beta-adrenergic blockade as postulated to be an underlying cause of atopy. Abnormal vascular responses are also seen in AD skin, as manifested by generalized pallor, abnormal white blanching in response to acetylcholine injection, and white dermographism. The normal dermographic response is a red line at the site of stroking, followed by an erythematous flare which becomes a wheal 1–3 min later. In white dermographism the red line is replaced quickly by a white line with no wheal formation. This phenomenon is not pathognomonic of AD alone, but may aid in its diagnosis. Patients with atopic dermatitis also secrete more sweat in response to acetylcholine injection than control patients, and their skin contains less total lipid than does normal skin, partial explanations for the excessive dryness associated with this disorder.

C. Triggering Factors

Identification and reduction of known exacerbating factors of AD are essential to the management of these patients. The generally accepted group of triggers includes irritants, xerosis, heat and sweating, emotional upset, infection, and allergens (2). Members of this group are linked by their ability to cause itching in susceptible skin and thus initiate the spreading itch of AD which leads to eventual skin damage.

Irritants may take the form of prickly wool clothing or overwashing or bathing with drying soaps. The paradox of bathing can be resolved if parents are taught to apply moisturizer within 3 min of bathing to maintain the hydration of the bath and prevent the evaporation which leads to the contraction and cracking of the stratum corneum. Cleaning with nonlipid lotions such as Cetaphil is an alternative. Conditions that increase sweating may be thermal or emotional in nature, but both may cause increased itching in children and need to be recognized. The condition of cholinergic urticaria often accompanies or precedes a flare of AD in these children.

The skin of AD infants is particularly prone to develop *infection* because of immune dysfunction and partly because of excoriated areas. While infections can be considered a sequelae or complication of AD, certain infectious agents can act as allergens themselves (7). The most common infections are with *Staphylococcus aureus* (*S. aureus*), wart viruses, herpes simplex, molluscum contagiosum, and *Pityrosporium ovale.* The latter is a common yeast that inhabits the skin of all individuals but, compared to normals, some AD children have high levels of IgE specific for this organism and experience clinical improvement of skin lesions when treated with ketoconazole. Likewise, *S. aureus* is also found in high concentrations on eczematoid skin lesions, and several studies have shown the existence of *S. aureus*-specific IgE antibody in the serum and the skin lesions of AD patients (8). Furthermore, histamine release occurs from basophils from these patients when exposed to specific exotoxins and not from control patients or AD patients without *S. aureus* IgE. These observations may help to explain the marked improvement some AD patients experience with antistaphylococcal antibiotics.

The role of *allergens* in infantile AD may have been unsubstantiated in the past, but elevated IgE levels and increased immediate skin-test reactivity observed in infants have fueled the search for relevant allergens in AD and has proven a role for allergy, especially to foods, in up to 35% of severely affected infants (9). The importance of *food allergy* in AD has been hotly debated among the different specialists who treat this disease, and estimates of incidence vary from 10% to 50% (5,10), depending on the severity of the patients and the type of referral clinic involved. Burks and Mallory (11) used double-blind, placebo-controlled food challenges (DBPCFC) to demonstrate food allergy in approximately one-third of AD children seen in an allergy clinic. Other investigators, including dermatologists, estimate the incidence at closer to 10%, and this may reflect a population referred by virtue of its poor response to elimination-diet therapy. The importance of IgE-mediated food reactions to the pathogenesis of AD lesions has been shown by increases in serum histamine following oral food challenges in food-sensitive AD patients compared to nonsensitive patients and controls. Sampson (12) showed increased spontaneous histamine release from the basophils of these patients, an abnormality that improves after strict adherence to an avoidance diet for an extended period of time. In addition, a histamine-releasing factor (HRF) (13) is produced by the mononuclear cells of these sensitive patients which is capable of provoking mediator release from basophils of other food-sensitive patients by an IgE mechanism. This reaction may involve IgE-bearing Langerhans cells which present antigen to TH$_2$ lymphocytes, CD4$^+$ T cells capable of secreting potent cytokines which upregulate IgE production and receptor activity leading to the cellular infiltration of lymphocytes and mast cells (14). Beside this "immediate" reaction, a late IgE-mediated sequence is often observed 6–8 hr after positive DBPCFCs. This cascade produces an increase in circulating polymorphonuclear cells and a drop in circulating eosinophils which are replaced by hypodense eosinophils (15). The skin lesion induced by the challenge can be shown to contain these activated eosinophils and their major basic protein deposits by 8–14 hr after the DBPCFC (16). The complex interrelationships of these immune pathways and their contribution to the immunopathology of AD continues to be investigated.

The significance of pollen and mold allergy, which has been shown in older patients with AD to vary with seasonal change and improve with environmental modification, has yet to be documented in infants. However, in the case of the dust mite *Dermatophagoides*, which is often the first aeroallergen to sensitize infants, strong proof has emerged of its ability to induce eczematoid lesions on the abraded skin of AD patients. These lesions have the typical cellular infiltrates of AD, and 90% of the patients involved show basophil histamine release following incubation with the dust-mite allergen Der P1. Other studies have shown the presence of T cells sensitized to antigen Der P1 in AD patients with positive skin tests to dust mite. These cells have been shown to accumulate in the skin lesions of AD and may direct production of large amounts of IL-4 and other cytokines capable of inducing IgE production and causing cellular infiltration, leading to disruption of normal skin (17,18). Finally, Beck and Korsgaard (19) conducted an epidemiological study showing a clear relationship between AD severity and dust mite exposure and clinical improvement after environmental control in 26 patients with the disease.

D. Clinical Considerations

AD may be divided into infantile, childhood, and adult stages. The infantile stage presents between 2 and 6 months of age and usually clears by age 3. Intensely pruritic and consisting of erythema and papules with vesicular and crusting stages, the rash in infants usually begins on the face and scalp and spreads to the trunk and extremities, often sparing the diaper area (Figs. 1–4). Older infants may develop the sharply demarcated, oval lesions

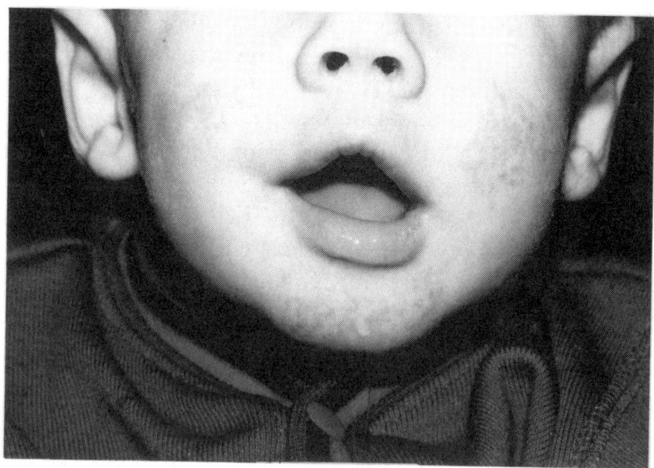

Figure 1 Facial rash of infantile atopic dermatitis.

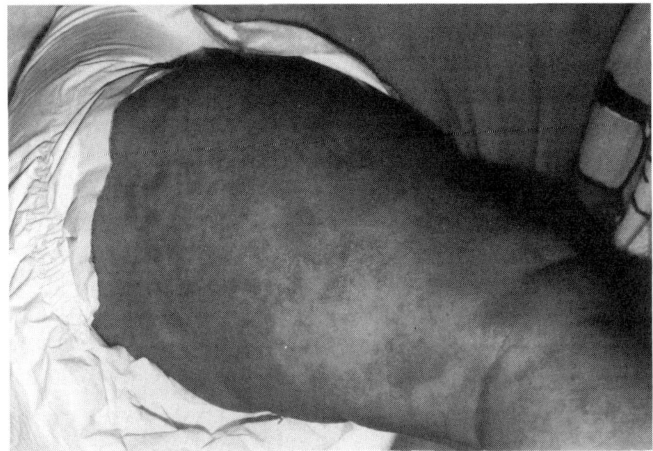

Figure 2 Eczema involving the trunk and extensor surfaces of the extremities.

on the face and trunk consistent with nummular eczema. A particularly virulent form of infantile AD is erythroderma characterized by a generalized, diffuse, extremely pruritic and erythematous rash without much vesiculation. The skin is smooth and lymph nodes are prominent. These infants are more susceptible to infection, and some with increased eosin-

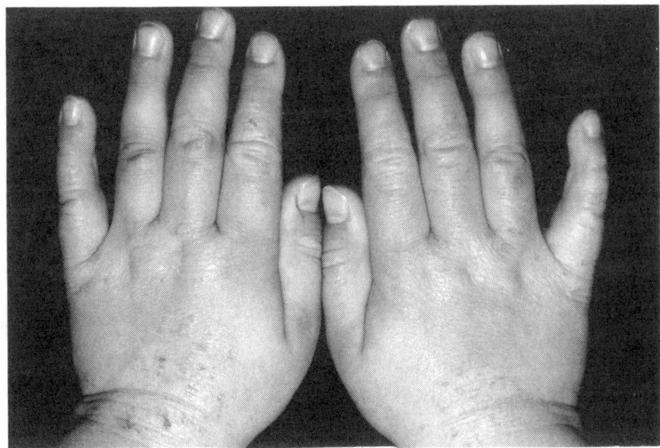

Figure 3 Lichenified eczema of the extensor areas of the wrist and hands.

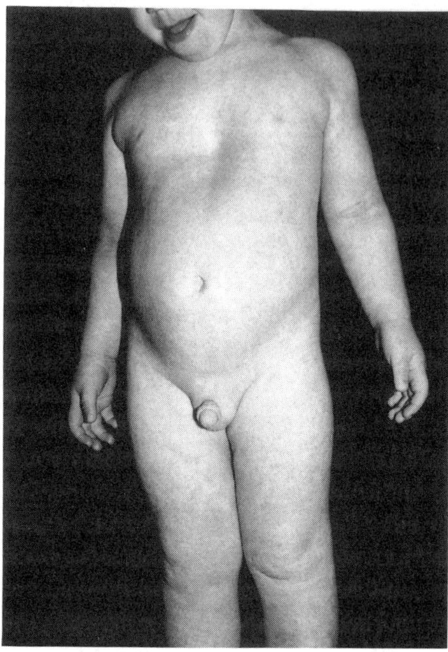

Figure 4 Acute atopic dermatitis with erythrodermatous changes.

ophilia and serum IgE levels may exhibit degrees of immuno-deficiency.

The typical infant with AD is easily diagnosed because of the chronicity, pruritus, and appearance and location of the lesions. The major and minor criteria for diagnosis are outlined in Table 1. The need for further evaluation is determined by the severity and responsiveness of the skin rash. Mild cases with localized involvement are easily controlled with topical medications, and further investigation is unnecessary and not cost-effective. The infant with generalized and refractory disease needs evaluation for food hypersensitivity, guided by historical clues and aimed at egg, milk, peanut, wheat, soy, and fish, which are responsible for 95% of the positive DBPCFCs in these infants (20). Immediate allergy skin testing and RAST testing appear to be comparable in their accuracy to diagnose food allergy. Negative tests virtually exclude the food tested as a trigger. On the other hand, a positive test indicates the need for the more definitive, physician-monitored food challenge, as described in Chapter 32. This objective diagnostic tool is essential at this stage because only strict avoidance of the offending food is acceptable therapy at this time. Up to 50% of severe AD infants may be expected to be food allergic. Positive food challenges result in cutaneous symptoms, especially morbilliform rash at the predilection sites, about 75% of the time, and gastrointestinal and respiratory symptoms 51% and 45% of the time, respectively. While many infants demonstrate cross-sensitivity within food families by skin or in-vitro testing, they often react clinically to single members of these groups, stressing the need for food challenges or controlled elimination diets to structure nutritionally sound but allergen-free diets. About 33% of these food-allergic infants with AD will lose this sensitivity, as shown by a negative food challenge by the second year of a restrictive or elemental diet treatment. Children sensitive to egg, milk, soy, and wheat are more likely than those allergic to nuts, peanuts, and seafoods to "outgrow" these allergies.

The nccd for inhalant allergen hypersensitivity testing is indicated by the presence of concomitant allergic rhinitis symptoms and nasal eosinophilia (21). Markedly elevated serum IgE levels are seen in infants with severe AD or accompanying immunodeficiency. Other quantitative immunoglobulins may be measured, but one should remember that the lesions of atopic dermatitis rarely accompany antibody deficiency syndromes when T-cell function is intact. Therefore, in the absence of systemic infections, costly immune workups are usually unnecessary.

Infants with phenylketonuria, ahistidinemia, gluten-sensitive enteropathy, and ectodermal dysplasia may exhibit an atopiclike dermatitis, and specific tests for these disorders should be considered when symptoms are suggested in infants. Finally, skin biopsy can ascertain the true nature of the eruption in doubtful cases. The acute lesion of infantile AD consists of hyperkeratosis and hyperplasia of the epidermis with a diminution of the granular cell layer, but increased fluid accumulation (spongiosis) and migration of leukocytes.

The complications most often affecting infants with AD are dermal infections due to bacteria, fungi, and viruses, with the latter being potentially the most lethal. Pyoderma due to *S. aureus* and less often to beta-hemolytic streptococci is difficult to distinguish from primary impetigo.

Abscess formation is rare in AD and occurs more often in erythroderma or hyper-IgE syndrome. AD patients are highly susceptible to vaccinia, herpes simplex, and molluscum contagiosum infections. Vaccinia causes eczema vaccinatum, herpes simplex causes eczema herpeticum (Fig. 5), and the two conditions are referred to collectively as Kaposi's varicelliform eruption. The lesions are vesicular and pustular; the patients are

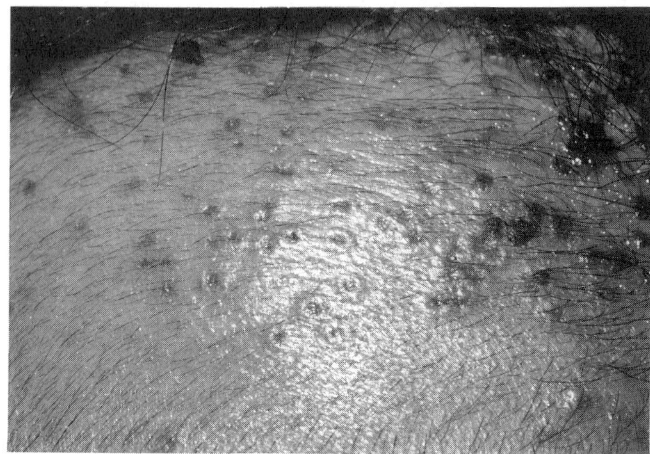

Figure 5 Eczema herpeticum.

febrile and usually quite ill and require treatment with intravenously administered antiviral agents. These infections may occur even when the AD is in a mild stage.

Ocular abnormalities, seen in about 5% of AD patients, are cataracts, keratitis, and kerataconus. These complications are rarely seen in infantile AD (22).

E. Differential Diagnosis

The typical infant with AD will present with a chronic or recurrent rash, intense pruritus, and a personal or family history of atopy, and will rarely be a diagnostic dilemma. There are, however, other skin conditions which may resemble AD. *Seborrheic dermatitis* is the rash most often confused with AD. The salient differentiating features are found in Table 2 and include earlier onset, characteristic greasy lesions, and predilection for intertriginous areas, sparing the hands and feet. Pruritus is usually absent, and the course of seborrheic dermatitis is often truncated. Atopy in the infant and his family is variable. The conditions may coexist in the same infant, but time will reveal the chronic nature of AD.

The infestation of *scabies* may resemble AD because of eczematoid skin changes caused by excessive rubbing and harsh topical agents. The axillary and genital distribution, as well as involvement of the hands and feet, typify this condition. In the absence of the pathognomonic linear burrowing lesions or family members with similar rashes, microscopic ex-

Table 2 Features Distinguishing Seborrheic and Atopic Dermatitis in Infancy

	Seborrheic dermatitis	Atopic dermatitis
Family history for atopy	Variable	Usually positive
Age of onset	Usually under 2 months	Usually over 2 months
Distribution	Scalp; any flexures, especially genitoanal; in older child eyebrows, eyelids	Cheeks, forehead, extensor surfaces of limbs (flexural involvement in older patients)
Lesions	Erythema with greasy, yellowish scales. Sharply demarcated flexural lesions	Erythema, papules, vesicles No scales (may be *crusted*) Tapering
Pruritus	Minimal	Severe (a hallmark of the disease)
Laboratory findings	Eosinophilia absent; negative skin test reactions	Eosinophilia; positive skin test reactions frequent
Prognosis	Usually clears in 3 to 4 weeks, up to 2 months. No associated allergy	Prolonged course. High incidence of associated allergic rhinitis and asthma development

Source: Modified from Jacobs AH, Goldsobel AB. Atopic dermatitis. In: Bierman CW, Pearlman DS, eds. Allergic Diseases from Infancy to Adulthood. Philadelphia: Saunders, 1988:385–404.

amination for positive identification of the scabies mite might be necessary for proper diagnosis, especially in situations where topical corticosteroid therapy does not improve the rash.

Contact dermatitis in infants is usually of the primary irritant type and is caused by saliva, harsh soaps, urine, or talcum powders, with the site of the eczema varying with the etiological agent involved. This rash tends to be less pruritic and milder in terms of skin disruption than infantile AD.

Although *nummular dermatitis* is sometimes considered a variant of AD, its existence without elevated IgE levels and accompanying atopy suggest that it may be a separate entity, especially in older children and adults. The lesions of nummular eczema are coin-shaped, vesiculo-papular eruptions found usually on dry skin areas of the extensor surfaces of the arms and legs. Itching is less intense than that seen in AD, and allergic management is ineffective for this disorder.

Some inherited diseases of immunodeficiency or metabolism may present in part with eczematoid rashes indistinguishable from AD. *Letterer-Siwe disease* (histiocytosis X) is a lethal condition of the reticulo-endothelial system with a rash that contains elements of both AD and seborrheic dermatitis but is distinguished by purpuric papules which may be vesicular and crusted and appear on the scalp in infants. Petechiae, failure to thrive, hepatosplenomegaly, and lymphadenopathy are common findings, and the skin biopsy showing abnormal reticulum is diagnostic. The X-linked recessive disorder *Wiskott-Aldrich syndrome* is characterized by severe eczema, thrombocytopenia, impaired antibody formation to polysaccharide antigens, and increased susceptibility to infections. The marked IgE elevations and T-cell dysfunction seen in these patients are also common to other immunodeficiency diseases which may produce eczematous dermatitis (e.g., *Nezelof* and *Di George syndromes*). The lichenified skin lesions, together with pneumonias and multiple abscesses of the skin and other organs, serve to readily differentiate AD from the *hyper-IgE syndrome*; in the former, infections are superficial and impetiginous only, while the latter spares flexural areas and is papular and erythematous on the scalp and face and may progress to furuncle formation of the skin as well as produce pneumatoceles in the lung. A hereditary disorder, *acrodermatitis enteropathica*, is characterized by vesiculobullous eczematoid lesions in the acral and perioral areas. These infants have chronic diarrhea, failure to thrive, low serum zinc levels, alopecia, and nail dystrophy, and, in the full-blown clinical picture, are easily distinguished from AD. In *phenylketonuria*, the extreme devastation of mental retardation and seizures sets apart these blond, photo-sensitive infants who may also have eczema similar to that seen in AD. Serum phenylalanine concentrations of greater than 15 mg/dL confirm the diagnosis of this disease.

F. Treatment

Although there is no cure for AD, commonly employed treatment regimens so often result in improvement that in infants where treatment fails, the diagnosis needs to be reexamined or chronic allergen exposure, such as food allergy, needs to be explored. Therapy is directed at avoiding triggers, reducing pruritus and dryness, providing anti-inflammatory treatment, and preventing the complications of AD. The physician should stress the overall favorable prognosis of AD and help to keep mild cases with local involvement in proper perspective for parents. Feelings of frustration that result in seeking costly alternative therapies need to be discussed and avoided.

Control Pruritus

The most important goal of treatment is *reduction of skin dryness and pruritus and the elimination of scratching* (23). Antihistamines, such as hydroxyzine hydrochloride (2 mg/kg/day), may be used in divided doses or primarily at night to break the itch, scratch, rash cycle. Extremes of temperatures, especially those which promote sweating, should be avoided. Infants should not be exposed to rough bedding or clothing, and their fingernails should be cut short. Contrary to common belief, bathing should not be avoided because it aids in control of infections, removal of crusts, and softening of the skin. It is essential, however, to follow bathing and swimming immediately with generous applications of emollients such as Vaseline or Aquaphor while the skin is still wet. Lubricants should be applied routinely during the day; lanolin-based creams such as Unibase or water-in-oil-based creams such as Eucerin are especially well tolerated. Some dermatologists advise adding Clorox bleach (2 teaspoons per gallon) to baths to prevent infections, and table salt (1 cup) to reduce stinging. Wet compresses with germicidal Burows solution suppress the weeping and oozing of acute AD lesions.

Control Allergens

Allergen control can further reduce pruritus. Avoidance of dust mite, animal dander, and other inhalant allergens becomes more important as the infant grows older and skin test positivity and concomitant allergic rhinitis develop. Injection immunotherapy is generally considered to be of little value in treating AD and is, in fact, often poorly tolerated when given to these patients for respiratory allergies (24). In the infant whose AD is poorly controlled or in whom an inordinate amount of treatment is required, *food allergy* needs to be investigated. The relevance of suspected foods, as suggested by history or positive IgE testing, needs to be documented by food challenge, in the absence of an anaphylactic history (25). Foods giving a positive challenge are strictly eliminated. In lieu of this approach, an infant might be placed on an elemental diet consisting of breast milk alone (with maternal diet surveillance) or an extensively hydrolyzed protein hydrolysate formula (Alimentum or Nutramigen) and, possibly, foods such as carrots, squash, rice cereal, and banana. If clinical improvement occurs, foods which are difficult to avoid may be added one at a time after a 1- to 2-week period. This approach is less definitive than food challenges.

Control Infection

Patients with AD have a poorly understood susceptibility to cutaneous infections by bacteria, viruses, or fungi. The most common are bacterial infections caused by *S. aureus*, which heavily colonizes the skin lesions of most infants with AD. The areas involved become follicular and pustular and often progress to impetiginized crusts. Antibiotics are used to treat the acute infectious episodes of AD and also to reduce the allergenic load of *S. aureus*, which appears to be an important trigger for many infants. Courses of antibiotics or long-term suppressive regimens may be appropriate depending on the clinical response. Erythromycin is a good initial treatment, but dicloxacillin or cephalosporin should be used if resistant organisms are suspected. Topical antibiotics have limited usefulness in AD.

Viral infections such as herpes simplex, vaccinia, molluscum contagiosum, and warts often invade the skin of AD patients, who may experience more spreading and refractoriness with these agents than do normal patients. Fortunately, these infections are usually limited to the skin, but infants with disseminated herpes simplex infection, eczema herpeticum, may have mucous membrane or systemic involvement and require treatment with acyclovir.

Topical dermatophyte infections may appear with generalized flares of AD away from the site of the infection (5). These infections usually respond to topical imidazole creams or oral griseofulvin therapy.

Control Inflammation

The medicinal agents most effective in the *control of inflammation* are the corticosteroids (26). Rarely needed in the systemic form, the topical application of these agents requires attention to potency and vehicle considerations. Potent gels and milder lotions share the disadvantage of increasing dryness and should be avoided. Ointments penetrate effectively and are more potent than equivalent cream formulations. They are occlusive and useful in the management of lichenified areas but are not as well accepted as creams, especially in hot, dry climates and when applied to intertriginous areas. Some urea-steroid combination preparations such as Lacticare help avoid these drying effects. Because striae, telangiectasias, and cutaneous atrophy may occur with long-term use of topical steroids, care must be taken to use the least potent agent needed. Halogenated steroids and other potent steroids should never be applied to the face, and their use should be curtailed when clinical improvement begins. Occlusive steroid dressings can increase steroid penetration in lichenified areas but should be limited to 8- to 12-hr periods to avoid local atrophy. Reports of systemic side effects of topical steroids are extremely rare and should not deter their use for proper control of AD and its complications. Oral steroids, often in combination with antibiotics, arc sometimes needed to control erythroderma or other forms of severe eczema in AD. Tar preparations are a nonsteroidal adjunct to anti-inflammatory therapy. Their mechanism of action is poorly understood and they are often cosmetically unacceptable.

In refractory cases of AD treatment or instances of noncompliance, hospitalization of the infant may be necessary to bring the skin back to normal, investigate the role of diet, and teach parents proper skin care.

When routine care fails, less well established therapies may be tried. The use of ultraviolet light may inhibit antigen processing by Langerhans cells and T-cell response to mitogens (27). In particular, long-wave UVA (340–400 nm) and PUVA (orally ingested psoralen plus UVA radiation) appears to be effective in severely affected children with AD.

The use of *immunomodulators* is gaining interest in AD therapy (28). Cyclosporin A, in a dose of 5 mg/kg/day, reduces severity scores and extent of AD lesions with reduction of pruritus, but causes nausea, paresthesias, hyperbilirubinemia, and renal impairment and should probably be avoided in AD children (29). Thymopentin, the active pentapeptide of thymic hormone, which promotes the differentiation of preferentially the T_{H1} subset, improved the overall severity and specifically the erythema of adults with AD (30).

The agent holding out the most hope for infants and children is interferon-γ. This is a potent lymphokine produced by T-helper cells designated T_{H1}. In AD, the T_{H1} subset is thought to be dominated by the subclass T_{H2}, which directs IL-4 (IgE production) and IL-5 (eosinophilia) formation important in the pathogenesis of AD. Thus, it is postulated that interferon-γ administration might correct the effects of this imbalance. A clinical trial of this agent, delivered by subcutaneous injection, showed improvement in global response scores and specific inflammatory change of AD. The treated group had a reduction of eosinophilia, but no change in IgE production, compared to placebo-treated patients (31). The drug appears to be better tolerated in younger patients. Unfortunately, the effects of interferon-γ are not lasting, and long-term administration would be necessary.

G. Prevention

Allergy prophylaxis by means of hypoallergenic dietary approach during infancy has been studied by Zeiger and colleagues, who followed 288 high-risk-for-atopy children from birth through age 2 and then 165 of these children until age 7 (32,33), as discussed in detail in Chapter 30. The results showed an overall decrease in atopy at age 12 months in the prophylactic group, reflected in a lower incidence of AD and food allergy. This preventive effect on the development of AD in infancy was not apparent as follow-up after age 2. Recommendations for the prevention of allergic disease including AD based on this and other studies (34,35) are detailed in Chapter 30.

II. Urticaria

Unlike AD, the condition of urticaria does not have a special predilection for infants. Urticaria can be classified into three main types, acute, chronic, and physical, with the latter being extremely rare in infants.

A. Acute Urticaria

While the impression is that acute urticaria is common in children, the exact incidence is unknown because it so often goes unreported. Acute urticaria is self-limiting and a cause is usually evident. Often following closely ingestion or contact of an offending food or drug by the sensitive infant, the urticaria may be accompanied by angioedema and the relationship to the agent in question is obvious, precluding the need for further workup. Demonstrating specific IgE antibody to the food or drug (i.e., penicillin) in question is valuable only if the history confirms the etiology. Viral (e.g., herpes simplex) and bacterial (e.g., beta-hemolytic strep A) infections are a leading cause of acute urticaria in infants and children. Finally, urticaria often accompanies other atopic conditions such as AD and allergic rhinitis and may be a manifestation of these processes.

B. Chronic Urticaria

Urticaria lasting longer than 6 weeks is classified as chronic urticaria and rarely occurs in infants. Chronic urticaria is almost never due to an allergy and so if the condition is established, an accompanying systemic illness may be considered (e.g., juvenile rheumatoid arthritis, hepatitis, or rarely, malignancy).

The diagnosis of urticaria with or without visible rash at the time of the examination is usually uncomplicated owing to the abrupt onset and transient nature of the eruption. Urticarial lesions have a clear center of edema with a halo of erythema. They may be localized or coalesce to cover large skin areas. Infants with urticaria may develop swelling of the extremities and acrocyanosis as well as form bullae in the center of the urticarial wheal. The urticarial lesions are transient and rarely persist for more than 24 hr. The differential diagnosis may include dermographism, insect bites, contact dermatitis, erythema multiforme (EM), mastocytosis, and vasculitis (36). Lesions of EM and vasculitis are fixed for several days, with the former distinguished from urticaria by its dark center with surrounding erythema. Urticarial vasculitis may be accompanied by fever, arthralgias, arthritis, and an elevated sedimentation rate. Epinephrine suppresses urticaria but has no effect on the eruption of EM. The more severe nature of EM and its association with Stevens Johnson syndrome make it important not to confuse urticaria with this condition.

Identifying the etiological agent to ensure its avoidance may be frequent in acute and uncommon in chronic urticaria (37). Symptomatic relief is provided with antihistamines, especially hydroxyzine by virtue of its strong suppression of histamine activity in the skin and its tolerance by infants. Subcutaneous epinephrine is useful as a therapeutic trial or in cases of urticaria complicated by acute angioedema or anaphylaxis. Oral steroids are effective but rarely necessary in uncomplicated urticaria.

Studies of the prognosis of urticaria in children are often limited by their short duration but suggest that 30% of infants with acute urticaria will develop chronic urticaria and that chronic urticaria in children under the age of 16 years has an average duration of 16 months (38).

III. Hereditary Angioedema

Hereditary angioedema (HANE), a serious but rare autosomal dominant disorder, occurs in 1 in 150,000 persons and is caused by a deficiency (85% of patients) or a dysfunction (15%) of the enzyme C_1-esterase inhibitor (C1-INH). The immunological consequences and typical clinical presentations of HANE are discussed in Chapter 16. The diagnosis of HANE is made by complement screening finding decreased levels of C4 and C2 and confirmed by demonstrating low levels of C1-INH antigen or, in the presence of normal levels, an absence of C1-INH enzyme activity. A method to perform these tests on umbilical cord blood has recently been described and will allow early diagnosis of HANE in high-risk infants born to affected families (39). This is important because HANE often presents in infants and young children, exacerbates in adolescence, and subsides in the fifth decade. In infants, skin mottling may be the first evidence of the disorder, progressing to a circumscribed erythema marginatum which is nonurticarial and nonpruritic. Recurrent bouts of submucous or subcutaneous edema follow and last for 2 to 5 days, often occurring after episodes of emotional upset, infections, trauma, or dental work, all commonly encountered during childhood. Gastrointestinal involvement in HANE occurs less frequently but is particularly worrisome in infants because it is marked by vomiting, diarrhea, and colic and often mimics a surgical abdomen. The absence of fever and leukocytosis in HANE episodes may help to differentiate the two. Contrast x-rays taken during these acute episodes reveal mucosal edema of the intestine causing separation of loops of bowel and narrowing or obstruction of the lumen. The most serious manifestation of HANE is swelling of the oropharynx and upper airway, which may lead to obstruction and death. This complication is most often seen in the third decade of life.

Treatment of acute episodes of HANE is usually supportive. Antihistamines, epinephrine, and corticosteroids are not generally effective in the management of these patients. Intravenous C1-INH concentrates have terminated HANE attacks and are currently available in the United States under compassionate-use protocols. Whole plasma infusions have been proposed but are currently not recommended. The major concern in acute attacks of angioedema is airway obstruction, and avoiding mortality from this complication sometimes necessitates tracheostomy.

Chronic maintenance therapy is usually unnecessary in infants with HANE. Patients with infrequent or mild attacks may be followed without chronic use of the agents used to prevent attacks, which are particularly toxic for young children. Androgenic agents such as danazol and stanozolol stimulate synthesis of C1-INH, but their masculinizing side effects, while attenuated compared to testosterone, are unacceptable for children over extended periods of time. Alternatively, these patients may receive short-term prophylaxis with attenuated androgens prior to provocations such as surgery or dental work.

IV. Mastocytosis

The group of disorders referred to collectively as mastocytosis is characterized by mast cell hyperplasia in the skin and other organs. In children, the disease usually takes one of three forms: (a) individual lesions termed solitary mastocytosis; (b) the generalized form called urticaria pigmentosa; and, more rarely, (c) diffuse cutaneous mastocytosis (40). Urticaria pigmentosa is the most common form of mastocytosis, often present at birth, but usually presenting between 3 and 9 months of age. Infants have a better prognosis than adults, as the disease is almost always exclusively cutaneous and resolves spontaneously when the onset occurs before age 10 years.

The skin lesions in urticaria pigmentosa are small yellow to red-brown macules, usually involving the trunk and extremities. Physical disruption of these lesions by scratching or rubbing results in erythema and urtication around the macules, a phenomenon known as Darier's sign. Infants have a strong tendency to form bullous or vesicular variants of these lesions, either present at birth or in response to infection or immunization in a condition called bullous urticaria pigmentosa. These blisterlike lesions contain histamine, prostaglandin D_2, and platelet-activating factor. Dermographism is found in up to 50% of patients with urticaria pigmentosa. The skin biopsy of affected areas confirms the diagnosis and shows markedly increased numbers of mast cells in the subpapillary layers and midcutis.

The course of urticaria pigmentosa of infancy is often benign, with less than 5% of patients developing systemic mastocytosis (41). About 50% will resolve their skin lesions by adolescence and another 25% will do so during adulthood. Infants with the rare diffuse cutaneous or erythrodermic forms of mastocytosis are more likely to have persistent or systemic disease. The rare association of leukemias in children with mastocytosis have been associated with these variants which differ from urticaria pigmentosa by the large areas of thickened, doughy skin involved and the tendency to progress to severe bullous lesions and systemic disease. The course of urticaria pigmentosa in infants is normally one of relapsing skin rash unresponsive to treatment but usually resolving with time. Generalized flushing and pruritus occur intermittently. Systemic mastocytosis is characterized by tachycardia, gastrointestinal symptoms, hypotension, syncope, and bone pain determined by the organs involved. In general, only children with diffuse cutaneous mastocytosis or relatively late onset of urticaria pigmentosa (after age 10 years) need be screened for systemic disease by blood counts, clotting studies, bone marrow examination, gastrointestinal studies, or bone scans unless suggested by specific symptoms (42).

There is no specific treatment for mastocytosis in children. Avoidance of mast cell degranulators such as aspirin, codeine, opiates, and radiographic dyes as well as hot baths and vigorous rubbing is important. The use of H1 antihistamines, especially hydroxyzine in infants, is indicated to reduce pruritus, tachycardia, and flushing. H2 receptor antagonists should be added if better control is needed. Topical steroids applied to the lesions of urticaria pigmentosa are variably successful. Oral cromolyn sodium (Gastrocrom) in doses of 20 mg/kg/day for infants has been used to relieve symptoms of gastrointestinal disease and in instances of diffuse cutaneous mastocytosis and urticaria pigmentosa complicated by blistering and bullae (43).

The physician caring for an infant with a dermatosis reflecting an aberration of the immune system is particularly challenged because these rashes may improve with as little influence as the passage of time or may represent serious underlying disorders. Diagnostic acumen and a commitment to chronic care are needed for success with these disorders. An ever-increasing knowledge of immune modulation and genetic control of the immune response hold promise for breakthroughs in these areas.

Acknowledgments

The author would like to thank Ms. Pat Stanwood for secretarial assistance. Dr. Gary White, MD, of San Diego Kaiser Department of Dermatology, provided the photographs used in this chapter.

References

1. Buckley RH. Atopic dermatitis. In: Kaplan AP, ed. Allergy. New York: Churchill Livingstone, 1985:417–438.
2. Hurwitz S. Eczematous eruption in childhood. In: Hurwitz S, ed. Clinical Pediatric Dermatology. Philadelphia: Saunders, 1993:45–59.
3. Schultz-Larsen F, Holm K, Henningsen K. Atopic dermatitis: a genetic-epidemiologic study in a population-based twin sample. J Am Acad Dermatol 1986; 15:487–494.
4. Hamid Q, Boguniewicz M, Leung DYM. Differential in situ cytokine gene expression in acute versus chronic atopic dermatitis. J Clin Invest 1994; 94: 870–876.
5. Hanifin JM. Atopic dermatitis in infants and children. In: Hurwitz S, ed. Pediatric Clinics of North America. Philadelphia: Saunders, 1991:763–790.
6. Leung DYM, Rhodes AR, Geha RS, Schneider L, Ring J. Atopic dermatitis. In: Fitzpatrick TB, Eisen AZ, Wolff K, Freeberg IM, Austen KF, eds. Dermatology in General Medicine. New York: McGraw-Hill, 1993:1543–1564.

7. Lacour M, Hauser C. The role of microorganisms in atopic dermatitis. Clin Rev Allergy 1993; 11:491–522.

8. Leung DYM, Harbeck R, Bina P, Hanifin JM, Reiser RF, Sampson HA. Presence of IgE antibodies to staphylococcal exotoxins on the skin of patients with atopic dermatitis: evidence for a new group of allergens. J Clin Invest 1993; 92:1374–1380.

9. Jones SM, Sampson HA. The role of allergens in atopic dermatitis. Clin Rev Allergy 1993; 11:471–490.

10. Sampson HA. The role of food allergy and mediator release in atopic dermatitis. J Allergy Clin Immunol 1988; 81:635–645.

11. Burks AW, Mallory SB, Williams LW, Shirrell MA. Atopic dermatitis: clinical relevance of food hypersensitivity reactions. J Pediatr 1988; 113:447–451.

12. Sampson HA, Jolie PL. Increased plasma histamine concentrations after food challenges in children with atopic dermatitis. N Engl J Med 1984; 311:372–376.

13. Sampson HA, Broadbent KR, Bernhisel-Broadbent J. Spontaneous release of histamine from basophils and histamine-releasing factor in patients with atopic dermatitis and food hypersensitivity. N Engl J Med 1989; 321:228–232.

14. Van Reijsen FC, Bruijnzeel-Koomen CA, Kalthoff FS, Maggi E, Sromagnani S, Westland JKT, Mudde GC. Skin-derived aeroallergen-specific T-cell clones of the T_{H2} phenotype in patients with atopic dermatitis. J Allergy Clin Immunol 1992; 90:184–193.

15. Leiferman KM. Eosinophils in atopic dermatitis. J Allergy Clin Immunol 1994; 94:1310–1317.

16. Sampson HA. Pathogenesis of eczema. Clin Exp Allergy 1990; 20:459–467.

17. van der Heijden FL, Wierenga EA, Bos JD, Kapfenberg MK. High frequency of IL-4 producing CD4+ allergen-specific T lymphocytes in atopic dermatitis lesional skin. J Invest Dermatol 1991; 97:389–394.

18. Vollenweider S, Saurat J-H, Röcken M, Hauser C. Evidence suggesting involvement of interleuken-4 (IL-4) production in spontaneous in vitro IgE synthesis in patients with atopic dermatitis. J Allergy Clin Immunol 1991; 87:1088–1095.

19. Beck HI, Korsgaard J. Atopic dermatitis and house dust mites. Br J Dermatology 1989; 120:245–251.

20. Sampson HA. Food hypersensitivity and dietary management in atopic dermatitis. Pediatr Dermatol 1992; 9:376–379.

21. Platts-Mills TAE, Chapman MD, Mitchell B, Heymann PW, Deuell B. Role of inhalant allergens in atopic eczema. In: Ruzicka T, Ring J, Przybilla B, eds. Handbook of Allergens in Atopic Eczema. Heidelberg: Springer-Verlag, 1991:192–203.

22. Hanifin JM. Recognizing and managing clinical problems in atopic dermatitis. Allergy Proc 1989; 10:387–402.

23. Leung, DYM. Atopic dermatitis: the skin as a window into the pathogenesis of chronic allergic diseases. J Allergy Clin Immunol 1995; 96:302–318.

24. Glover MT, Atherton DJ. A double-blind controlled trial of hypersensitization to dermatophagoides pteronyssinus in children with atopic eczema. Clin Exp Allergy 1992; 22:440–446.

25. Niggemann B, Beyer K, Wahn U. The role of eosinophils and eosinophilic cationic protein in monitoring oral challenge tests in children with food-sensitive atopic dermatitis. J Allergy Clin Immunol 1994; 94:963–971.

26. Clayton MH, Leung DYM, Surs W, Szefler SJ. Altered glucocorticoid receptor binding in atopic dermatitis. J Allergy Clin Immunol 1995; 96:421–423.

27. Cooper KD. New therapeutic approaches in atopic dermatitis. Clin Rev Allergy 1993; 11:543–560.

28. Chan SC, Hanifin JM. Immunopharmacologic aspects of atopic dermatitis. Clin Rev Allergy 1993; 11:523–542.

29. Sowden JM, Berth-Jones J, Ross JS, Motler RJ, Marks R, Finlay AY, Salek MS, Graham-Brown RAC, Allen BR, Camp RDR. Double-blind, controlled, crossover study of cyclosporin in adults with severe refractory atopic dermatitis. Lancet 1991; 338:137–140.

30. Leung DYM, Hirsch RL, Schneider L, Moody C, Takaoka R, Li SH, Meyerson LA, Mariam SG, Goldstein G, Hanifin JM. Thymopentin therapy reduces the clinical severity of atopic dermatitis. J Allergy Clin Immunol 1990; 85:927–934.

31. Hanifin J, Schneider L, Leung D, Ellis CN, Jaffe HS, Allen EL, Bucalo LR, Hirabayashi SE, Tofte SJ, Cantu-Gonzales G, Milgrom H, Boguniewicz M, Cooper KD. Recombinant interferon gamma therapy for atopic dermatitis. J Am Acad Dermatol 1993; 28:189–197.

32. Zeiger RS, Heller S, Mellon MH, Halsey JF, Hamburger RN, Sampson HA. Genetic and environmental factors affecting the development of atopy through age 4 in children of atopic parents: a prospective randomized study of food allergen avoidance. Pediatr Allergy Immunol 1991; 3:110–127.

33. Zeiger RS, Heller S. The development and prediction of atopy in high risk children: followup at age seven years in a prospective randomized study of combined maternal and infant food allergen avoidance. J Allergy Clin Immunol 1995; 95:1179–1190.

34. Kajosaari M, Saarinen UM. Prophylaxis of atopic disease by six months' total food elimination. Acta Paediatr Scand 1983; 72:411–414.

35. Chandra R, Shakuntla P, Hamed A. Influence of maternal diet during lactation and use of formula feeds on development of atopic eczema in high risk infants. Br J Med 1989; 299:228–230.

36. Hurwitz S. The hypersensitivity syndromes. In: Hurwitz S, ed. Clinical Pediatric Dermatology. Philadelphia: Saunders, 1993:515–538.

37. Bonifazi E, Meneghini CL, Ceci A. Pathogenic factors in urticaria in children. Dermatologica 1977; 154:65–72.

38. Harris A, Twarog FJ, Geha RS. Chronic urticaria in children: course and etiology. Ann Allergy 1983; 51:61–70.

39. Nielsen EW, Johansen HT, Holt J, Mollnes TE. C1 inhibitor and diagnoses of hereditary angioedema in newborns. Ped Res 1994; 35:184–187.

40. Hurwitz S, Mastocytosis. In: Hurwitz S, ed. Clinical Pediatric Dermatology. Philadelphia: Saunders, 1993:663–668.
41. Klaus SN, Winkleman RK. Course of urticaria pigmentosa in children. Arch Dermatol 1962; 86:116–119.
42. Kettelhut BV, Metcalfe DD. Pediatric mastocytosis. J Invest Dermatol 1991; 96:155–156.
43. Frieri M, Alling DW, Metcalfe DD. Comparison of the therapeutic efficacy of cromolyn sodium with that of combined chlorpheniramine and cimetidine in systemic mastocytosis: results of a double-blind clinical trial. Am J Med 1985; 78:9–14.

34

Immunobiology of the Neonate and an Overview of Immune Deficiencies in the Neonatal Period

RICHARD I. SCHIFF

Miami Children's Hospital
Miami, Florida

NOAH J. FRIEDMAN

University of California, San Diego, School
of Medicine, La Jolla
and Kaiser Permanente Medical Center
San Diego, California

I. Immunobiology of the Neonate

A. Introduction

Despite a rapid growth in the number of studies evaluating the host defenses of infants, the explanation for the high incidence of infection and malignancy in the very young has been elusive. The infant is both immunologically immature, that is, the immune system has not fully developed, and immunologically naïve because the child has not been exposed to a wide variety of antigens. Nonspecific host defense mechanisms, such as mucosal barriers and skin integrity, are less well developed compared to older children and adults. Despite the tacit acceptance of these differences, however, our understanding of the specific mechanisms for the poorer response is still incomplete.

On initial evaluation the immune system of the neonate appears to be relatively intact. Absolute numbers of neutrophils, monocytes, and lymphocytes are higher in neonates than in children and adults. Many studies of neutrophil function, such as phagocytosis, killing, and oxidative burst, are functionally equivalent to that of adults. Neonates possess normal numbers of B lymphocytes, but other than IgG that is transplacentally acquired from the mother, the levels of immunoglobulins are extremely low at birth. However, if the fetus is infected in utero, it can respond and make IgM antibodies, and normal infants can respond to a wide variety of antigens in vaccines beginning in the immediate postpartum period. Cellular immunity also appears relatively intact at birth, with normal or elevated numbers of T cells and normal responses to mitogens such as phytohemagglutinin and to allogeneic cells in the mixed leukocyte reaction. Thus, although it appears that most aspects of the neonatal immune system are intact, other studies indicate that neonatal cells are slower, more easily depleted, or less sophisticated compared to adult's cells (Table 1). Not all of these differences are a disadvantage. For example, neonates are more easily made

Table 1 Defects in Neonatal Host Defense

Nonspecific immunity		
Anatomic barriers	Phagocytic system	Complement
Decreased skin thickness	Decreased neutrophil storage pool	Decreased levels, esp. C5–C9
Decreased intracellular adhesion	Decreased adhesion molecules	Decreased factor B
Decreased sebaceous secretions	Decreased deformability	Decreased properdin
Decreased gastric acidity	Decreased complement receptors	Decreased complement receptors
Decreased lactoferrin, lysozyme	Impaired chemotaxis	
Permeable microvillus membrane	Decreased intracellular killing	
	Decreased monokine production	

Specific immunity	
Humoral immunity	Cellular immunity
Decreased IgA and IgM	Decreased helper activity for B cells
Decreased IgG in premature infants	Impaired cytokine production—IL-4, IF-γ, IL-2
Poor response to polysaccharide antigens	Excessive suppressor activity
Lack of memory B cells (naiveté)	Limited T-cell receptor repertoire
Decreased mucosal immunity	
Decreased cytokine production	

tolerant to foreign cells, which leads to a much higher success rate in neonatal recipients of organ and bone marrow transplants. In the past few years a much greater understanding has been gained of the cellular and molecular mechanisms for these differences. This knowledge not only can help explain why infants are more susceptible to infections, but also can help guide development of vaccines and other strategies to enhance the neonate's response and may lead to improvements in transplantation.

B. Fetal Development

Development of the immune system begins early in fetal life (Table 2), suggesting that at least some aspects of immunity are important even to the fetus. Maturation of the specific, or lymphocyte-mediated, immune sys-

Table 2 Development of the Immune System in the Fetus

Fetal age (wk)	Immunological change
4	Hematopoietic progenitors in yolk sac
7	Thymus precursor cells (CD7+) arrive in thymus
8	C4, C2, and C3 in liver; C5 in liver and lung
	B-cell precursors present in liver
8.5	CD3+ cells in thymus, IL-2R+
9–12	Immature B cells (sIgM+) in liver
9.5	Thymic receptor rearrangement
10	Thymic lobulation begins
	CD1+, CD4+, CD8+ T cells in thymus
11	CD2+ T cells in thymus
	B-cell development in liver and spleen
12	Neutrophils present in blood
	Pre-B cells in bone marrow
	T cells begin to appear in blood; express either CD4 or CD8
	Mitogen-responsive T cells in thymus
13	B cells of all isotypes in marrow
14	c1q in spleen
	Thymic corticomedullary distinction
	T cells in blood capable of proliferating to mitogens
16	IgM plasma cells
	Hassal's bodies develop in the thymic medulla
17	Serum IgM plasma cells
20	Lymphoid follicles in spleen and nodes
22	Complement detected in serum
30	Serum IgA detectable

tem is very complex. Not only must the lymphocytes learn to recognize and respond to foreign or non-self antigens, they must recognize self and become tolerant. The fetus also must coexist with the maternal immune system, minimizing sensitization and preventing rejection by the maternal cells. Exposure to an antigen during fetal life is more likely to induce tolerance than an immune response; this tendency does not disappear immediately after birth, which may help explain why it is easier to transplant young children. Fetal T cells and monocytes also are more likely to be suppressive to adult cells, which may be important in preventing rejection by the maternal cells. This may be of benefit before birth, but can be a disadvantage after the baby is born and must be able to respond to assault by a wide variety of microorganisms.

Blood cells are initially produced in the yolk sac, later in the liver, and only around mid-gestation are the majority of hematopoietic cells derived from the bone marrow. Leukocytes are produced in the liver beginning at about 8 weeks gestation, and by 20 weeks significant granulopoiesis is present in the marrow. Lymphocytes are detectable in the fetal blood in significant numbers by 7 weeks gestation. B-cell development begins in the fetal liver between 8 and 9 weeks gestation, with differentiation of progenitor cells to pre-B cells characterized by the presence of CD19, MHC class II antigens, and cytoplasmic μ chains. Between 8 and 13 weeks pre-B cells progress to immature B cells with surface IgM and IgD, and the receptor for C3d or CD21. During this period clonal expansion progresses rapidly to provide the fetus with a diverse antibody repertoire. Under the influence of monokines and T-cell cytokines, these immature cells further develop to B cells expressing only one immunoglobulin class, IgM, IgG, IgA, or IgE. However, despite the apparent development of these cells, immunoglobulin production and the formation of specific antibodies appears much later in gestation. T-cell development parallels that of the B cell. The thymic anlage develops from the third and fourth brachial pouches at about the sixth week of gestation and is populated by blood-borne stem cells beginning in the eighth week. Differentiation of the thymus into cortex and medulla progresses rapidly, so that CD2+ T cells are detectable in the thymus by 11 weeks and in fetal blood by 14 weeks. The T cells are capable of graft-versus-host response by 13 weeks and of responding to phytohemagglutinin by 14 weeks. More specific responses, such as specific cytotoxicity, do not develop until late in the second trimester. Thus, by the beginning of the third trimester, all of the essential elements of the immune system have formed, though further maturation may require weeks, months, or even years.

C. Nonspecific Host Defenses

Physical and Chemical Barriers

Host defenses begin at the interface that separates the individual from the environment (Table 1). The skin and mucosal surfaces provide protection against physical trauma and microbial invasion. The skin of the neonate, and especially that of a premature neonate, is thinner, has fewer intracellular attachments, and produces less sweat and sebaceous secretions (1,2). The skin of the term neonate has a stratum corneum that is similar to that of an adult, with 15 cells or 9.3 μm in thickness, whereas that of a 30-week premature has only a few cells providing a layer of 4.1 μm (2). Similarly, the density of keratin filaments, frequency of desmosomes, number and size of anchoring fibrils and filaments, and papillary dermal collagen are normal in the term infant but significantly reduced in the premature. The term infant has smaller reticular dermal collagen bundles and finer, less mature reticular dermal elastic fibers compared to the adult, but the premature is even more severely affected. Lipid production is minimal in the premature infant's skin, leading to impaired barrier function and xerosis. The neonate's skin also has less enzyme activity that functions to detoxify, deactivate, or modify chemicals, which can lead to greater toxicity and absorption. As a result of these differences, the skin of the neonate, and especially the premature neonate, is more permeable (3), though some contend that the greater absorption of chemicals by term infants is due primarily to the greater surface area-to-body volume ratio (2).

The mucosal surface consists of the microvillus membrane and the mucus layer as well as intraluminal fluids such as saliva, gastric acid, and digestive enzymes (4). The composition of the mucus and intraluminal fluids can affect binding of microorganisms and passage of macromolecules (5). The pH of the secretions markedly affects the ability of microorganisms to grow (6). In addition, proteins such as lactoferrin (7), which is bacteriostatic, lysozyme (8) which is active against the cell wall of gram positive bacteria, and lactoperoxidase (9,10) may serve to limit infection. Interferon appears in secretions within hours of infection and can stimulate the immune response. Carbohydrate moieties of the glycoproteins in mucus can act as binding sites or inhibitors of receptors for ingested antigens, microorganisms, and toxins (11,12).

The influence of these factors in the neonate is incompletely understood, but studies, primarily in experimental animals such as the rat, suggest that these factors are less effective in the neonate (4). Decreased gastric acidity allows bacteria to traverse the stomach into the intestine, thus increasing the risk of infection (13). In the neonatal rat, the glycoproteins in mucus have a lower carbohydrate-to-protein ratio and decreased content of fucose and N-acetylgalactosamine than the adult (5), perhaps indicating a decreased ability to restrict passage of organisms and antigens. The microvillus membrane of neonatal animals is less organized and more permeable than that of adults (5); it has a higher cholesterol and phospholipid content compared to that of the adult, and the sialic acid content is higher and the fucose content lower. As a result, the accessibility of certain carbohydrate side chains and glycolipids within the microvillus membrane differs in neonatal and adult animals and may influence the attachment of antigens and microorganisms (5).

Nonspecific Opsonins

Fibronectin

Fibronectin is a large-molecular-weight glycoprotein that is important in inflammatory responses, cellular activation and adhesion, and vascular integrity (14). It exists in both a soluble form in plasma and extravascular fluids and an insoluble form in many connective tissues and extracellular matrices. Isomeric forms of fibronectins exist and are both cell-specific and tissue-specific. The fibronectins are capable of binding multiple ligands, including some bacteria such as *Staphylococcus aureus*, DNA, heparin, fibrin, IgG, C1q, actin, matrix molecules, and gangliosides. Thus, these dimeric molecules facilitate opsonization and interactions among cells and between cells and the extracellular matrix (15). Binding of fibronectin to neutrophils enhances adhesion, chemotaxis, phagocytosis, and intracellular killing. Fibronectin is not a direct opsonin, but enhances the binding through C3 and Fc receptors. It has affinity for extracellular matrix and is thought to promote vascular integrity at least in part by its regulatory effect on neutrophil adherence to the vascular endothelium.

The serum concentrations of fibronectin in the plasma of term infants is approximately half that of term adults, 220 mg/mL in infants compared to 350 mg/mL in adults (14,16–18). Premature infants have substantially lower plasma levels, with a direct correlation with gestational age (18). Levels fall even further in infants with sepsis or respiratory distress syndrome (14). Although the effects of fibronectin deficiency are clear in in vitro studies, the physiological effects of the decreased levels have not been proven in neonates. If the deficiency is proven to be of clinical importance, then infusions of fibronectin may be of benefit in septic infants.

C-Reactive Protein

C-reactive protein (CRP) is an acute-phase reactant that has structural similarity to the C1q-binding domain of IgG. CRP binds to polysaccharide antigens such as that present in the capsules of pneumococci and other bacteria; it binds to the polysaccharide capsule and activates complement so that the organism is coated with C3 and is opsonized just as though the complement had been activated by IgG binding to the organism. The levels of CRP are similar in neonates and adults (15) and increase appropriately with infection, and thus may serve an especially important role before the infant can generate specific antibodies.

Lactoferrin

Lactoferrin enhances neutrophil-endothelial cell interactions and production of reactive oxygen intermediates and thereby promotes chemotaxis and killing (15). It is a cationic iron-binding protein present in the specific granules of neutrophils. Levels of lactoferrin are profoundly deficient in the granules of resting neutrophils from neonates, but can be raised to near adult levels by stimulation with the synthetic chemoattractant f-MLP. However, release of lactoferrin is impaired when neonatal neutrophils are stimulated to spread on artificial surfaces. Though impaired adherence and directed migration have been reported in patients with inherited deficiency of lactoferrin, the clinical significance of the deficiency in neonates is unclear.

D. Development of the Neutrophil and Macrophage System

Phagocytosis is the most primitive host defense mechanism, but mammalian neutrophils and monocytes have evolved complex functions that go far beyond phagocytosis. In addition to producing an array of enzymes that are capable of killing bacteria and viruses, these cells generate oxygen free radicals that are capable of killing even highly resistant bacteria, produce cytokines that activate lymphocytes, endothelial cells and stromal cells such as fibroblasts, and process and present antigen to B and T lymphocytes. In order to function appropriately, the neutrophils and macrophages must be able to respond to a chemotactic stimulus, adhere to endothelial cells or intracellular matrix, deform to fit between the endothelial cells, bind to the target, and ingest and kill the organism. The phagocytic cells of the neonate are defective to some degree in all of these functions (19).

The first step in the inflammatory response is adhesion of neutrophils to endothelium at the site of inflammation. Adhesion is mediated largely by a family of cell surface glycoproteins, the integrins, that include the iC3b receptor (Mac-1, CR3 or CD11b/CD18), LFA-1 (CD11a/CD18), and p150,95. These receptors interact with ICAM on the endothelial cells that has been upregulated by IL-1 and TNF-α. After adhering to a substrate the phagocyte must be able to recognize and migrate along a concentration gradient of an attractant substance. Stimulation of the cell upregulates receptors and causes ruffling of the membrane and increase in random movement. Receptors for the chemoattractant are concentrated along the leading edge of the cell; after interaction with the ligand, the receptor–ligand complex is moved to the uropod or trailing foot of the cell. There it is ingested and broken down. New receptor is synthesized and fused with the cell membrane to allow further recognition of the gradient. The cell moves by attaching the leading edge using adhesion molecules and then contracting the cytoskeleton, which consists of microfilaments of actin and myosin. The cells must be deformable to fit between endothelial cells and through the extracellular matrix. Once the cell reaches the site of infection, it must attach to the organism or infected cell. Attachment requires that the organism be opsonized with substances such as IgG, complement, or fibronectin; thus, the cell must express specific receptors such as Fcγ III, CR3, CR4, or the fibronectin receptor. The cell engulfs the attached organism by extending pseudopods to surround the particle and forms a phagocytic vesicle that subsequently fuses with the primary granules to form phagolysosomes. Organisms are killed using a variety of methods involving both oxidative and nonoxidative mechanisms. The former require generation of free oxygen radicals through the hexose monophosphate shunt and NADPH oxidase. These are converted to hydrogen peroxide, then ˙OH, and subsequently to hypochlorous acid (OCl$^-$) by myeloperoxidase. Organisms also are killed by numerous enzymes contained within the granules such as lysozyme, cathepsin, defensins, and bactericidal/permeability-inducing protein. Neutrophils and mononuclear phagocytes share most of these functions; in addition, mononuclear phagocytic cells process and present antigen to T lymphocytes. There is evidence that neutrophils and monocytes from preterm neonates, and to a lesser extent term infants, are defective in most of these functions.

Ontogeny of Neutrophils and Monocytes

Precursors of neutrophils can first be detected in the yolk sac and mature neutrophils are detected in the peripheral blood by 12–14 weeks gestation (20). The number of cells rises rapidly during the ensuing 12 weeks (21). Premature infants of birth weight <1000 g have neutrophil counts of approximately 8×10^9/L at birth, whereas small-for-gestational-age infants have neutrophil counts of only 2×10^9/L, which may fall even further during the first few days of life (22). Term infants have much higher counts, averaging 24×10^9/L at 4 hr after birth in one study (23), though others (24,25) found absolute neutrophil counts to be closer to 8×10^9/L at birth, rising over the first 3 days and then declining to approximately 4×10^9/L. Despite these values, which are greater than those for adults, neonates are prone to develop neutropenia when septic (20,26). Neonates have very small storage pools of immature neutrophils in the marrow, only approximately twice the number in the peripheral circulation, compared to 14 times in the adult (27). Once the storage pool is depleted, the infants are at risk for developing overwhelming sepsis that often is fatal.

The development of monocytes and tissue macrophages has not been studied as extensively as that of the neutrophil. Mean monocyte counts ranged from 6 to 9 $\times$ 10^9/L, with a range of 0 to 19.12 $\times$ 10^9/L (24,28).

Neutrophil Function

Adhesion

Early studies indicated that adherence by neonatal neutrophils was significantly diminished compared to those from children and adults (29,30), but these measured adherence to glass beads or nylon wool, which do not require specific receptor interactions. Studies using human umbilical vein endothelial cells (HUVEC) indicated that baseline adherence by neonatal cells, which is dependent on LFA-1, is normal, but adherence through CD11b/CD18 is impaired (31). Chemotactic stimulation greatly increased adhesion of adult but not neonatal neutrophils, perhaps due to both a deficiency in the expression of CR3 (32) and the lack of upregulation when the cells are stimulated (33). On the other hand, CM-CSF primes the neonatal neutrophils so that stimulation with the peptide formyl-methionyl-leucyl-phenylalanine (f-MLP) upregulates CR3 expression and improves adhesion (34). Hence, although the neonatal cells are deficient compared to those from adults, under some circumstances they can be induced to normal activity.

Locomotion and Chemotaxis

As discussed in the previous section, migration across the endothelial membrane is abnormal, at least in part, because of defective expression of adhesion molecules (31). However, the cells are defective in several other ways. Diapedesis requires energy utilization, a contractile system that involves actin and myosin, and regulation of membrane fluidity (35) by proteins such as gelsolin (36). Neutrophils from neonates show abnormal actin polymerization (37) and decreased deformability when measured by elastometry (38). These abnormalities undoubtedly contribute to the impaired random migration (39) as well as response to a chemotactic stimulus which may persist until the child is 6 years old (40–42).

The degree to which the response of neonatal cells to a chemotactic stimulus is abnormal may depend on the assay used (39–43). Using a Boyden chamber, migration of neutrophils from preterm infants was equivalent to that of term infants, about 20% of adult values (44); chemotaxis improved when the infants developed superficial bacterial infections, but was absent when they were septic. Migration through a 3-μm pore filter indicated a greater degree of abnormality than when 8-μm pores were used (43), suggesting that the cells recognized the chemoattractant and began movement but that fluidity of the cell was abnormal. The degree of abnormality was greater if zymosan was used as the stimulant rather than *Escherichia coli* chemotactic factor (40). Binding of the chemotactic stimulant f-MLP was the same in adult and neonatal cells, suggesting that the cells are capable of recognizing the chemoattractant (45); however, fewer receptors are placed on the membrane from the intracellular granules, and signal transduction through the f-MLP receptor is reduced compared to cells from adults (15). In addition, cells from neonates do not upregulate CR3 receptors normally (46) and fail to generate additional levels of actin upon stimulation (47). In summary, the abnormalities in diapedesis, random migration, and directed migration are due to defective upregulation of adhesion and chemoattractant molecules, impaired membrane fluidity, and decreased actin polymerization.

Phagocytosis

Attachment to particulate antigens utilizes receptors for complement C3b and iC3b and the Fc portion of the IgG molecule. Neonatal neutrophils express significantly lower levels of the IgG receptor FcγRIII, though the levels of FcγR1 and FcγRII are normal or elevated (48). However, there may not be a close correlation between the levels of these receptors and phagocytosis. In one study, phagocytic rates and number of *E. coli* ingested was slightly lower in neonates compared to adult neutrophils, but premature infants were significantly impaired (49). Although they confirmed the decreased receptor numbers, they could not find a correlation between the number of receptors and the degree of impairment. Most studies have shown that phagocytosis by neutrophils from term infants of a variety of organisms is equivalent to that of older children and adults (50–53). When neonatal cells are stimulated by infection or artificial stimulants such as f-MLP, phagocytosis is stimulated (52,54). Most studies have demonstrated that even preterm infants' neutrophils have normal phagocytic activity (50,55), though they may be more easily overcome when the number of infectious organisms is high (55).

Killing

The ability of neutrophils to kill microorganisms can be determined directly in bactericidal or fungicidal assays, or indirectly by measuring the ability to generate an oxidative burst using NBT dye reduction, chemiluminescence, or measurement of free radicals. Studies measuring NBT dye reduction in resting leukocytes indicated that term and premature infants were normal, though the percentage of positive cells decreased significantly in septic infants (56). All of the cells increased appropriately when they were stimulated. Chemiluminescence of zymosan-stimulated neutrophils from term infants was significantly reduced compared to that of their mothers' or normal controls (57). Neutrophils from premature infants were abnormal for up to 2 months after birth, and the degree of abnormality correlated with a higher frequency of serious infections (58). Neutrophils from neonates generated higher-than-normal $\cdot O_2^-$ radicals but much less $\cdot OH$ than adults (59). The cause of the defective conversion is unknown but would result in poor production of OCl^-. Generation of superoxide anion was greatly enhanced in neonatal neutrophils after preincubation in recombinant human G-CSF (60), though bactericidal activity was not increased. Others have found that chemiluminesce by neonatal neutrophils was equivalent to that of adults when they were stimulated with f-MLP, but that they did not increase appropriately when primed with lipopolysaccharide (LPS) or TNF-α (61). Binding affinity for LPS and TNF-α was the same for adult and neonatal cells, but the number of binding sites for f-MLP was decreased in neonatal neutrophils. However, although the number of binding sites for LPS, designated CD14, was similar between the adult and neonatal cells, the neonatal cells did not upregulate the number of CD14 receptors on the surface after stimulation with LPS (62).

Intracellular killing of microorganisms by healthy term neonates is considered to be normal (63). Even premature infants showed normal killing if they were healthy (64). However, stressed infants showed a marked impairment of killing of *E. coli* and *Staphylococcus* (29). When high bacteria-to-neutrophil ratios were used, the ability to kill *E. coli* was significantly impaired (57), indicating that the neonatal cells have little reserve. The ability of neutrophils from neonates to kill microorganisms such as group B streptococci also was reduced compared to adults (65). On the other hand, killing of *Candida albicans* was normal in term, healthy infants (66). Thus, killing by infants is equivalent to that of adults as long as the neonates are healthy and the assay system is not stressed by adding a high multiplicity of organisms. The significance of these in vitro findings is not entirely known, but it does suggest that neonates can be more easily overwhelmed by bacterial infection, and once sick they become even more deficient in their ability to resist the infection.

Macrophage Function

The mononuclear phagocytes have similar functions to the polymorphonuclear leukocytes. In addition, they are important sources of cytokines and are crucial as antigen-presenting cells. The function of the mononuclear phagocyte system has been reviewed in detail by Yoder and his colleagues (67).

Chemotaxis, Phagocytosis, and Killing

Studies of monocytes from both preterm and term neonates demonstrate both normal and impaired chemotaxis, phagocytosis, and killing, similar to that of the neutrophil. In one study all of these functions were entirely normal (68). Random movement was normal (41) but chemotaxis in a gradient was significantly decreased and did not achieve adult levels for up to 6 years (42,69). The expression of CD14, the receptor for LPS, was normal in monocytes from term neonates, but the density of the adhesion molecules CD11a, CD11b, and CD11c was less than that of adult monocytes (70). Since the adhesion molecules are important to phagocytosis, the lower density could contribute to impaired ability to ingest particles. Phagocytosis by term neonates has been reported to be both normal (71) and impaired (72,73). Ingestion of polystyrene particles was delayed in neonatal monocytes, though eventually it was equivalent to those from adults (72). Phagocytosis of *Streptococcus agalactiae* was significantly lower in cord blood monocytes (73), but ingestion of a wide variety of particles and microorganisms, including latex particles, opsonized sheep erythrocytes, *Staphylococcus aureus*, *Toxoplasma gondii*, and type II herpes simplex virus was equivalent in cord blood and adult monocytes (71). Cord blood monocytes were capable of killing *Candida albicans* to an equivalent degree as adult monocytes, but did not demonstrate augmentation when stimulated with IFN-γ (74). Similarly, cord blood monocytes can kill a variety of bacteria (71). Others found less efficient killing of *Staphylococcus aureus* and type III group B streptococci by cord blood monocytes (73); the lack of correlation between these finding may be due to differences in assay conditions.

Antigen Presentation

Mononuclear macrophages play a critical role in presenting antigen to T cells. Antigen is processed within the macrophage and presented to CD4 cells in the context of class II (HLA-DR) antigens or to CD8 cells in the context of HLA class I (HLA-A and HLA-B) antigens. Interaction of the T cell and the macrophage induces the macrophage to elaborate IL-1, which subsequently stimulates the T cell to proliferate and produce IL-2. HLA-DR expression is deficient in cord blood monocytes, but is increased to normal levels when the cells are stimulated with lymphokines such as IFN-α (75). Cord blood monocytes co-cultured with maternal or paternal T cells were fully capable of presenting tetanus toxoid (76,77) or *E. coli*

(78) to induce the T cells to proliferate. However, when the monocytes were "pulsed" with antigen, the response was significantly decreased when cord blood monocytes were used compared to those from adults. The significance of this difference in technique is not clear, but it may suggest a difference in the kinetics of antigen presentation by cord blood monocytes.

Monokine Production

Monocytes are important sources of inflammatory cytokines, including IL-1-β, TNF-α, IL-6, and IL-8, as well as leukotrienes. IL-1 activity has been reported to be normal (79) and diminished (80). In the first study, monocytes from 27 infants of gestational age 31–41 weeks produced normal amounts of IL-1 when stimulated with LPS; unstimulated levels were elevated in infants with perinatal stress or infections (79). In the second study, both IL-1 and TNF-α were significantly reduced in term and preterm infants compared to adult controls (80). Both measured IL-1 using an IL-1-dependent mouse T cell line; TNF-α was measured by ELISA. There is no ready explanation for the discrepancy, but several other studies showed similar dichotomy (80), which may be due to selection of the infant populations to be studied. IL-6 is a monocyte-derived cytokine that is produced in response to IL-1 stimulation and is involved in B- and T-cell maturation and cycling of hematopoietic progenitor cells. In one study purified monocytes from term neonates produced only 50% and premature infants only 25% as much IL-6 as adult controls (81). Others did not find a significant difference when using whole blood rather than purified monocytes (82). It is possible that other cells in the mixture bound or degraded the IL-6 in the adult cell suspensions. Both levels of IL-8 and messenger RNA were decreased in purified monocytes from preterm and term infants (83,84). In one study the cells were stimulated with IL-1α, TNF-α, and LPS with similar results (83). In the other study the cells were stimulated with group B streptococci (84). The monocytes also produced less leukotriene-B_4 in response to stimulation with streptococci (84). Both IL-8 and LT-B4 are potent chemoattractants, and the decreased levels may contribute to the poor response of neonates to infection.

Development of the Complement System

The complement system consists of a complex series of proteins that serve two major functions, to lyse cells and microorganisms directly, and to act as potent opsonins (85). C3 is crucial to the complement cascade. Fragments of C3, C3b, iC3b, and C3d attach to target cells and bind to specific receptors on phagocytic cells, thereby greatly enhancing phagocytosis. Another C3 fragment, C3a, serves as a mediator of inflammation, stimulating chemotaxis and increasing vascular permeability. After C3 is activated, it can initiate the rest of the cascade, C5 to C9, which ultimately leads to lysis of red cells and some microorganisms. C3 can be activated through one of two pathways. The so-called classical pathway is initiated by antibody–antigen complexes that fix the complement components C1, C4, and C2, which form an enzyme that cleaves a thioester on the inactive C3 molecule to form the active C3. This pathway is dependent on the presence of specific antibody, especially IgM, so it is less active in the neonate that lacks IgM and has limited amounts of specific IgG. However, some gram-positive and gram-negative bacteria, mycoplasma, and RNA viruses are capable of directly activating C1q and bypassing the need for antibody in the classical pathway. The other pathway to activate C3 is known as the alternative pathway and is independent of antibody. Factor B binds to small amounts of cleaved C3 that are spontaneously generated in the plasma. Normally this C3–factor B complex is degraded, but if the interaction takes place on an appropriate cell surface, the complex is protected, and, in concert with other proteins such as factor D and properdin, acts as a potent enzyme to cleave additional C3 and initiate the remainder of the complement cascade. Most mammalian cells have complement-regulatory proteins on their surface to prevent activation of the alternative pathway. However, if the interaction takes place on a bacterial or fungal cell surface, C3 is activated and the remainder of the complement system is directed against the organism.

Because the complement system is a cascade involving many different proteins, a severe deficiency of one protein or a relative deficiency of many proteins can result in decreased function of the entire system. Complement is present early in fetal development. Most of the complement components have been detected in cultures of fetal tissues: C5 from lung and liver at 8–9 weeks gestation, C4, C2, and C3 in cultures of fetal liver at 8–14 weeks, C1q from spleen at 14 weeks, and C1 from small intestine and colon at 19 weeks (85). None of the complement components crosses the placenta, as shown by studies of allotypic markers on the proteins, so the levels in the infant reflect synthesis (85,86). The concentrations of the various components increase throughout gestation and are approximately 50–90% of adult values by term, though preterm infants have significantly lower levels of all components, especially those of the alternative pathway (15,85). Concentrations of the later components, especially C6, C8, and C9, were more affected, ranging from 10% to 47% of adult values (85). The functional assay, CH50, ranged from 50% to 81% of adult values, depending on whether the infants were compared to normal adults or the higher values found in their postpartum mothers (85). Levels of activation products, C3a-desArg from the classical pathway, and C3bBbP from the alternative, were similar in term infants and adults and increased transiently in infected newborns (87), suggesting that the lower levels were due to low synthesis rather than consumption. This study also showed that the infants were capable of activating complement in response to infection, but only the early steps in the cascade were evaluated. The serum of newborns had decreased opsonic activity (88) and production of chemotactic factors (10). The decreased generation of chemoattractant was not due to lack of specific antibody, since addition of antigen–antibody complexes did not overcome the defect (10). Adding specific antibody did not normalize generation of C5a, but normal levels of the chemoattractant could be achieved by adding C3 (89). Thus, the levels of the complement components are sufficiently low to impair function, especially in premature infants, and together with decreased levels of specific antibodies and impaired levels of other opsonins, are a significant cause for increased infection in young children.

Development of Humoral Immunity

The humoral immune system consists of the B lymphocytes and their secreted products, the immunoglobulins. B cells begin development very early in fetal development, but in humans the humoral system is very immature at birth, and full maturation does not occur until around the time of puberty. Our understanding of B-cell development has been greatly enhanced by molecular biology techniques that have elucidated the complex gene rearrangements that are unique among the genes of the immunoglobulin supergene family. The primary purpose of B cells is to produce immunoglobulins which are specific antibodies. B cells also present antigen to T cells and produce a joining or J chain that helps hold the dimeric IgA and pentameric IgM together.

B-cell development occurs in two stages (15). In the initial stages precursor cells rearrange the heavy-chain μ genes and express cytoplasmic μ chains; these are termed pre-B cells. Next, the light chain rearranges and the cell can express IgM on the surface. At this point the cell is an immature B cell. Up to this point the maturation process is antigen independent and can occur in the total absence of T cells. Indeed, exposure of these immature B cells to antigen, in the absence of T-cell help, leads to clonal deletion. This is a mechanism for eliminating cells that are capable of reacting to self-antigens. Isotype switching occurs and the immature B cell can express IgA and IgG on the surface, though the number of cells is low and these immunoglobulins are co-expressed with IgM and often IgD. This isotype switching is also T-independent, though later T-cell help is required for isotype switching of mature B cells to IgG- or IgA-producing plasma cells. After the mature B cell has formed, further exposure to antigen results in clonal expansion of cells whose surface immunoglobulin binds to that antigen and development of plasma cells producing specific antibody.

Ontogeny of B Cells

B-cell precursors originate in yolk sac and initially develop in the fetal liver (90–95). The first recognizable cell is a large cycling lymphoid cell with cytoplasmic μ heavy chains but no light chains. These cells appear in the human fetal liver at about 8 weeks gestation. By 12 weeks gestation these cells can be identified in fetal bone marrow. The large pre-B cells give rise to small, resting pre-B cells that express HLA-DR and about this time begin to express the receptor for EBV, CD21 (90). The pre-B cell rearranges either a κ or λ light chain, is able to express IgM on the cell surface (91,92), and is an immature B cell. A small proportion of sIgM$^-$ cells have cytoplasmic light chains; these cells represent an intermediate stage in transition between a pre-B and a B lymphocyte. Immature sIgM$^+$ B cells are the predominant type from the 9th to the 12th week of gestation. Pre-B cells are numerous in fetal liver but are far outnumbered by B cells in spleen, blood, and lymph nodes. By the second half of gestation the major site of pre-B cell production shifts from the liver to the bone marrow (93). By the 13th week the majority of cells express both IgM and IgD, and a few sIgA and sIgG cells begin to appear at about this time (90). The frequency of B cells expressing the various isotypes achieves adult proportions by the 15th week, but nearly all coexpress sIgM which is an immature phenotype. The shift toward cells expressing a single isotype does not occur until after birth. For example, IgA-bearing cells that do not co-express sIgM appear at 3–5 months of age (90). The number of IgA-secreting cells is reduced at birth, especially in premature infants, though the number is significantly increased if the neonate is infected (96).

B-cell development can be further characterized using monoclonal antibodies. The pre-B cells and immature B cells in fetal liver express IgM, CD19, CD20, and CD24, but are negative for CD21 and CD22 (94,95). However, CD21, which is the receptor for C3b and Epstein-Barr virus (EBV), develops at about this time since EBV infection of these cells leads to proliferation (90). These early pre-B and some immature B cells are positive for the surface enzyme TdT (terminal deoxynucleotidyl transferase) and CD10 or cALLA (common acute lymphoblastic leukemia antigen) (95). These surface antigens largely disappear early in B cell development, though some CD10$^+$ cells can be found in peripheral blood B lymphocytes. HLA-DR also is present at the pre-B cell stage (97). Greater numbers of HLA-DR cells than HLA-DP or HLA-DQ cells are present at 12 weeks gestation. Expression of HLA-DQ occurs about the same time as expression of sIgD and is coincident with the development of follicles (97). Both lymph node cells at 17 weeks and spleen at 16–21 weeks gestation are positive for all of these antigens but are negative for CD5, an antigen that is shared by T cells. After 17 weeks the B cells in lymph node are positive for CD5 (94). In the fetal spleen, up to 40–60% of the B cells are CD5 positive. CD5$^+$ B cells are increased following bone marrow transplantation, HIV infection, and some autoimmune diseases (98). The percentage and absolute number of CD5$^+$ B cells is markedly elevated in the blood of term or premature infants (96). A late marker of B-cell maturation is the enzyme ecto-5′-nucleotidase (ecto-5′-NT) (99). Activity of ecto-5′-NT is decreased in a variety of B-cell disorders, such as X-linked agammaglobulinemia and common variable immunodeficiency, and is low on neonatal B cells but reaches normal adult levels by 6 months of age (99). Isotype switching is dependent on CD40 ligand (CD40-L) on the T cell interacting with CD40 on B cells. Although CD40 is present on the surface of neonatal B cells, they are unable to switch to IgG or IgA by stimulation with CD40 agonists such as anti-CD40 or soluble CD40-L in the presence of IL-4 or IL-10 (100).

The development of B cells can be evaluated by the ability to synthesize immunoglobulin in response to a variety of stimuli. Some, such as pokeweed mitogen (PWM), require T-cell help and thus are difficult to use in neonates, whose T cells are also immature. Others, such as Nocardia water-soluble mitogen (NWSM) and *Staphylococcus aureus* Cowan I are relatively independent of T cells, and infection with EBV is completely T-independent. Transformation of both sIgM$^+$ and sIgM$^-$ cells from neonatal blood resulted in secretion of IgM, whereas stimulation only of sIgM$^+$ adult cells resulted in IgM production (101). B cells from the peripheral blood of adults produced predominantly IgM, whereas production of other isotypes depended on the tissue source of the B cells; splenocytes produced IgG but B cells from the appendix produced IgA. Cord blood B lymphocytes developed into cells with cytoplasmic IgM but not IgA or IgG, though IgG-secreting cells were detected in the cultures, as shown by a reverse hemolytic plaque assay (102). Nocardia water-soluble mitogen (NWSM) stimulated cord and newborn peripheral blood to produce small numbers of IgM-producing B cells but only rare IgA- or IgG-producing cells (103). The number of IgM-producing cells reached adult levels by 1 month of age, whereas the number of IgG-producing cells was not normal until 5–8 years of age and IgA by 9–12 years. Purified B cells from adults produced immunoglobulins poorly, but were significantly augmented when either adult or neonatal T cells were added. Similar results were obtained using cord blood B cells, though only IgM-secreting cells were produced and the magnitude was much lower than when using adult B cells. The addition of T cells from adults did not increase the number of cells synthesizing IgG or IgA (103). Stimulation of unfractionated cord cells with PWM yielded similar results, though none of the isotypes was normal by 3 years of age (103). The total number of immunoglobulin-producing cells was about 50% of adult values at 3 years of age and was equivalent to that of adults by 5 years. It was found that cord blood T lymphocytes were suppressive and that their removal resulted in greater number of IgM-producing B cells (103). The suppressive effect was absent when infants were tested between 1 and 2 years of age. The addition of hydrocortisone decreased the suppressive activity and enhanced immunoglobulin in a majority of neonates tested (104,105). Depletion of monocytes did not have an effect (105). Substituting adult T cells for cord blood T cells increased the production of Ig plaque-forming cells, particularly of the IgG and IgA classes (106,107).

Staphylococcus aureus Cowan I (SAC) stimulated a subset of B cells that rosette with mouse erythrocytes to proliferate, but these cells did not proceed to immunoglobulin production (108). SAC does not stimulate the nonrosetting B cells in the presence or absence of T cells. The addition of PWM in the presence of T cells resulted in immunoglobulin synthesis by the rosette-negative B cells only (108). The combination of PWM and SAC enhanced the production of immunoglobulin by unfractionated cord cells compared to PWM alone (109). Addition of IL-1 could substitute for the SAC, and various elements of T-cell-conditioned medium, now known to be IL-2, IL-4, and IL-6, could replace the PWM. In a more recent study, B cells form fetal liver, spleen, and bone marrow could be induced to produce IgM, IgG, and IgE, but not IgA, in response to IL-4 and either anti-CD40 or cloned CD4$^+$ T cells (110). The majority of the responding cells had the phenotype CD19$^+$, CD10$^+$, CD5$^+$. Addition of IL-6 did not have an effect. Pre-B cells that were sIgM$^-$ could not be induced to produce immunoglobulin. Thus, poor immunoglobulin production in the neonate is due in part to immaturity of the B cells which produce mainly IgM, but suppressor activity by neonatal T cells and T-cell immaturity also are significant factors.

Immunoglobulin Production

Normally the fetus produces very little immunoglobulin prior to birth. The fetus is capable of producing antibody in response to infection, but nearly all is of the IgM isotype. Maternal antibody is specifically transferred across the placenta beginning at the end of the first trimester, though the majority of IgG enters the fetus in the last 12 weeks, Immunoglobulin production begins at the time of birth, probably as a result of antigen stimulation regardless of whether the child is term or premature (111). However, premature infants do not receive as much IgG from the mother. Thus, premature infants begin life with low IgG levels and remain hypogammaglobulinemic for more than 6 months (112). IgM production is only slightly delayed compared to that of normal full-term children, whereas IgA production is severely impaired (112). In the term infant the levels of IgG approach that of adults by 5 or 6 years of age, IgM by 2 or 3 years, and IgA by 10 to 12 years (113). The secretory IgA system develops slowly after birth (114). There are no IgA plasma cells in the lamina propria at birth, but within a short time IgA^+ cells appear and IgA can be detected by immunofluorescence (115). There was more IgM than IgA antibody in intestinal secretions after peroral immunization with *Escherichia coli* (116). IgA was detectable in the tears of infants as young as 10–20 days of age (117) and in saliva by the second week (118). The concentration of sIgA increased slowly, reaching adult levels by 6–8 years of age (119).

Specific Antibody Formation

The fetus is able to synthesize IgM antibodies in response to infection by the 20th week of gestation (120,121). Immunization of the mother with tetanus toxoid has induced IgM antitetanus antibody in the fetus (122), presumably on the basis of antigen that has crossed the placenta. However, the presence of secretory IgA and IgM antibodies to *E. coli* and poliovirus in neonates suggests that the infant was responding to anti-idiotype antibodies from the mother, since it was unlikely that the mother was exposed to polio antigen and therefore could not have transmitted it to the fetus (123). This interesting observation has not been confirmed in other systems, but it does raise questions about interpretation of antibody responses in neonates.

Neonates are capable of responding to protein antigens such as tetanus toxoid or conjugated *Hemophilus influenzae* vaccine within a few weeks of birth (124–126). However, there is little response to the T-independent polysaccharide antigens until the child is at least 24 months of age (127–129); younger children are capable of producing transient IgG1 antibodies but are unable to develop immunological memory. Premature infants produced antibodies to ingested protein antigens, such as bovine serum albumin (111), and premature infants also produced antibodies to routine immunizations, though the levels were lower than in term infants (130). In the premature infants, IgG antibody to tetanus and diphtheria fell from birth to 4 months of age and then rose significantly by 9 months, 2 months after the third DPT immunization. However, the levels were lower than in term infants. IgG antibody levels to *Staphylococci* were comparable to those of term babies. IgM opsonic activity to *E. coli* was low in both term and preterm infants at birth and rose comparably by 9 months of chronological age. Thus, the preterm infants matured in relation to postnatal chronological age rather than gestational age (130).

E. Development of the Cellular Immune System

The cellular immune system is comprised of the thymus-derived or T lymphocytes. T cells are responsible for protection against viral, fungal, parasitic organisms, and neoplastic cells, and in addition play a crucial role in the regulation of B cells. Development of the thymus and T cells begins early in fetal life, and the early T cells have many of the functions of mature cells; however, at the time of birth the human T cells are functionally immature, with impaired capacity to produce cytokines, poor ability to provide help for B cells, and excessive suppressor activity (131–133).

Ontogeny of T Cells

T cells arise from lymphoid precursors that develop within the thymus. The primitive thymic rudiment forms at about 4 weeks gestation from the ectoderm of the third branchial cleft and the endoderm from the third brachial pouch (134). The right and left rudiments enlarge and fuse by the 8th week, and about that time the first precursors from the fetal liver and bone marrow begin to colonize the epithelial rudiment. Mesodermal cells invade the rudimentary thymus in the 10th week, effecting lobulation and inducing proliferation of the epithelial cells. Corticomedullary distinction is present by 14 weeks and the first Hassal's bodies by 16 weeks. The epithelial cells in the 7-week thymic rudiment express class II determinants and by 8.5 weeks both class I and class II. If the hematopoietic precursors are not normal and cannot interact with the other thymic elements, as occurs in babies with severe combined immunodeficiency disease, development is arrested and the thymus remains epithelial and primitive. Thus, mutual interaction among all of the elements, epithelial, mesenchymal, and hematopoietic, are required for normal thymic development.

The first cells that can be considered pre-T cells are present in the 7-week thymus and are $CD7^+$ but negative for the classical T cell antigens CD3, CD4, or CD8. By 8.5 weeks a subset is positive for the sheep red blood cell receptor CD2; these are at the thymocyte stage I (134). Development proceeds rapidly, and by 10 weeks thymocytes are positive for CD5, CD3, CD25, both CD4 and CD8, and a subset are positive for the transferrin receptor CD71. The IL-2 receptor, CD25 or Tac, is present on both B and T cells, though in higher density on the T cell. The majority of Tac^+ cells in the thymus are present in the medulla (135). Few cells are positive in the fetal liver or spleen at 18–20 weeks gestation. Rearrangements of the T-cell $\alpha\beta$ receptor occurs at about the same time as expression of the CD3 molecule, but some of the CD3$^+$ cells express the $\gamma\delta$ T cell receptor; the percentage of $\gamma\delta^+$ cells peaks at about 15 weeks gestation and then decreases toward adult levels by birth. However, these cells are found in higher proportion in the mucosal lymphoid areas. At 10 weeks, 47% of the CD3$^+$ cells express the β chain of the T-cell receptor and 25% are positive for both α and β (133). CD1, another marker of T cells, also appears shortly after CD3, at about 12 weeks gestation. As the thymocytes mature, the density of CD3 on the surface increases to that seen in peripheral blood T cells (133).

Occasional CD3+ cells are present in the blood from the end of the 12th week, their proportion rising from 20–30% at 14 weeks to 50% by 22 weeks. These cells are positive for either CD4 or CD8, but not both. Nearly all of the T cells are positive for the CD45RA phenotype characteristic of naïve T cells. The appearance of T cells in the blood is paralleled by the presence of T cells in the spleen and liver.

Lymphoid cells obtained from fetal thymus as early as 10–12 weeks or peripheral blood at 14 weeks gestation are capable of responding to mitogens such as PHA or Con A, or to allogeneic cells (136–138). Responses to Con A develop more slowly, as is seen in some animal models (139). Since proliferation of T cells is dependent on production of IL-2, it is clear that fetal cells are capable of synthesizing that cytokine. By the time of birth the cord blood T cells respond to mitogen stimulation as well as those of adults, though some investigators have reported reduced responses in premature infants, perhaps due to excessive suppressor activity (139). The T cells from 15 to 22 weeks are capable of developing specific cell-mediated cytotoxicity following stimulation with alloantigens, though much more poorly than those from term infants or adults (140). Despite the ability of these cells to proliferate, as is discussed in the following sections, these T cells are both naïve and immature.

Post-Natal Development of T-Cell Function

Maturation of the T-Cell Repertoire

Maturation of the T cells. Neonatal T cells express CD3, CD4, and CD8 in proportions that approximate that of the adult, yet the cells are phenotypically and functionally immature. In early studies it was shown that cord-blood T cells had a lower percentage of the helper-inducer phenotype, 2H4$^-$4B4$^+$, whereas the percentage of suppressor-inducer phenotype, 2H4$^+$4B4$^-$, was slightly higher than in the adult (141). More recently it has been shown that the majority of the cord-blood T cells are CD45RA$^+$,

CD45RO⁻, which is characteristic of virgin or naïve T cells (142). Many of these cells displayed a low level of fluorescence when stained with an anti-CD45 antibody; this CD45RO^{dim} population is not seen in older children or adults. The amount of CD45RO could be upregulated by stimulation with PHA or allogeneic cells. The percentage of CD3$^+$ cells with CD45RO increases logarithmically during the first several years of life, from <10% at birth to 40% at 10 years of age and >60% in adulthood. Infants who became atopic in the first years of life tended to have lower levels of the mature CD45RO$^+$ T cells (143), perhaps leading to poorer T-cell regulation.

There is a higher proportion of γδ T cells in the neonate (131,144). The neonatal Tγδ cells are phenotypically and functionally different than γδ T cells in the adult (144). They are weakly cytotoxic for K562, an NK-sensitive line, lectin-mediated cytolysis, and redirected cytolysis. They express lower levels of CD2, LFA-1, and CD45RO than adult cells and are therefore more similar to the small population of CD4$^+$ γδ T cells in the adult. The neonatal T cells express a diverse Vγ and Vδ gene segments rather than the predominant Vγ2Vδ2 commonly seen in adult Tγδ cells. A large proportion of these neonatal cells respond to mycobacterial heat shock proteins, and their numbers can be increased by immunization, especially with pertussis (131).

The T cells from newborns are deficient in their ability to provide B-cell help. It is now known that interaction of CD40 ligand (CD40-L) on T cells with CD40 on B cells is critical for immunoglobulin isotype switch and normal production of antibody. Expression of the CD40 ligand is lower in newborn lymphocytes compared to adult cells after stimulation with phorbol ester and Ionomycin (145,146). The activated cord T cells also had lower amounts of mRNA for CD40-L. Neonatal B cells were able to synthesize IgE when provided with IL-4, and their CD40 receptor was engaged by anti-CD40, indicating that the defect is primarily in the T cell (145). Neonatal cells could not express CD40-L even though they expressed other activation markers such as CD69 (100). CD40-L was expressed on 19- to 28-week fetuses and could be expressed on newborn T-lymphocyte cell lines generated with PHA and IL-2. CD40-L mRNA transcripts and intracytoplasmic protein expression were reduced, indicating a possible transcriptional downregulation of CD40-L expression (100).

Neonatal T cells have reduced expression of the IL-2 gamma chain, which is correlated with decreased IL-2-dependent T-cell activation (147,148). This is in contrast to fetal cells and those from preterm infants, who had high expression of CD25 along with an immature phenotype, CD1$^+$,CD38$^+$CD71$^+$, which is more characteristic of mature thymic cells (149). The immaturity of the cord-blood T cells is further shown by the upregulation of CD38 on neonatal but not adult T cells (150), a higher proportion of double $CD4^+CD8^+$ $CD3^+$ cells (151), and binding to peanut agglutinin characteristic of mature thymocytes (152). Cord-blood lymphocytes also have reduced expression of receptors for IL-2, IL-4, IL-6, IL-7, TNF-α, and IF-γ (153). None of the receptors was absent, but the reduced expression might be responsible for the decreased responsiveness to those cytokines.

Normal Values for T Lymphocytes in Infancy and Childhood. Infants have a marked lymphocytosis at birth. Mean lymphocyte counts for healthy newborn infants was $4185/mm^3$, with a 2 SD range of 2017–7261 (28). By 5 days the number had increased to 5616 with a range of 2856–9125. The normal numbers of lymphocytes, T cells, B cells, and NK cells are summarized in Table 3 (154). The relative percentage of T cells is decreased in neonates, but the absolute number is increased due to the lymphocytosis, and the number remains higher than adult values until nearly 7 years of age. The same is true of B cells and NK cells, although the latter fall within the adult range by 1 year of life (155). CD4 and CD8 counts were determined from a large group of infants from 0 to 4 years of age by the European Collaborative Study (156). Though focused on providing normal values for evaluating children for HIV infection, the resulting graphs are nonetheless useful in evaluating children with suspected primary immunodeficiency diseases. In this study CD4 counts peaked at around 6 months of age, with a 50th percentile of $2000/mm^3$. CD8 counts peaked much later, at around 1 year of age. More extensive evaluation of lymphocyte subsets was done, comparing cord blood values to those obtained from infants at 5 days of age (157). For the majority of children the

Table 3 Absolute Numbers of Lymphocyte Subsets from Birth to Adulthood

Lymphocyte subset	<1 year	1–3 years	3–5 years	5–13 years
CD3	5026 ± 2996	2971 ± 2188	2641 ± 1739	1890 ± 872
CD4	3817 ± 2570	2094 ± 1527	1798 ± 1372	1104 ± 616
CD8	1614 ± 1131	1019 ± 990	1003 ± 779	865 ± 530
CD20	1149 ± 1278	591 ± 811	362 ± 476	233 ± 242
CD57	852 ± 1517	531 ± 704	717 ± 408	599 ± 649
HLA-DR	2337 ± 2266	1625 ± 1363	1189 ± 784	910 ± 556

Mean ± 2 SD. CD 3 = pan T cells; CD4 = helper/inducer T cells; CD8 = suppressor/cytotoxic T cells, subset of NK cells; CD21 = B cells; CD57 = subset of NK cells and subset of activated T cytotoxic cells.
Source: Adapted from Ref. 154.

CD3[+], CD4[+], and CD5[+] counts and percentages were higher in the sample obtained at 5 days compared to their cord blood. B-cell numbers and percentages decreased, as did the number and percentage of NK cells determined by antiCD16[+]/CD56[+]. Another study of 53 newborns reported the normal values of T-cell, B-cell, and NK-cell percentages and absolute numbers, as well as the values for CD71, CD25, TcR$\alpha\beta$, and CD11a (158). The values in this study were comparable to the previous studies. Cytotoxic T cells and NK cells were studied in 12 neonates using two-color flow cytometric analysis (159). Both the percentage and absolute numbers of CD57[+] lymphocytes and non-MHC-restricted cytotoxic T cells (CD3[+]CD56[+]) were reduced. The phenotype of the NK cells was different from that of adults, with higher levels of CD11b[+] and lower levels of CD57[+] among the CD16[+] lymphocytes. The percentages and absolute numbers of CD4+, CD8+, CD3[+], CD16[+], CD19[+], CD20[+], and HLA-DR[+] cells were reported in 72 Japanese infants and children from 2 months to 13 years of age (154). Recently, an extensive study of 429 children from birth to 16 years of age was reported from the Netherlands (160). The large number of individuals studied allowed them to divide the group into much narrower ranges than in previous studies, and improvements in flow cytometry enabled them to evaluate the cells using two-color analysis to identify subsets with greater precision.

Proliferation

Cord-blood T cells from term infants proliferate in response to mitogens such as PHA or allogeneic cells as well as, or even better than, adult T cells (161–164). The responses decrease into the normal adult range late in infancy (163,164). A subpopulation of activated T cells in cord blood that are HLA-DR[+], CD25[+], and co-express both CD4 and CD8 undergo strong IL-2-induced proliferation and may be a mechanism to provide strong responses to an otherwise compromized immune system (165). Although the responses to classical mitogens are normal, the responses to other stimuli, such as anti-CD2 (166) or anti-CD3 (163,167,168) are markedly reduced. The response to anti-CD2 can be augmented by addition of calcium ionophore (166) or IL-1 (169) into the culture, indicating that the poor response is due to defective upregulation of IL-2 production. In contrast to the response to mitogens by T cells from term infants, in most studies T cells from premature neonates have reduced responses (170,171). Half of the infants <1000 g had impaired responses to PHA and Con A, whereas infants from 1251 to 1500 g had normal responses (172). In another study of very-low-birth-weight infants, 700–1300 g, nearly all had significantly reduced responses to PHA which did not rise into the normal range until 8 weeks after birth (170). However, in another study by Herrod and co-workers of 16 healthy premature infants <1350 g, nearly all had responses equivalent to those of healthy term infants (173). The difference between this study and the others may be the health of the infants and that they all received enteral nutritional support. Neonatal cells are much more sensitive to the effects of dexamethasone than are adult cells, but the inhibition can be reversed by adding IL-2 (174). Thus, although responses to routine mitogens or allogeneic cells suggests that neonates are normal, there are several lines of evidence, such as the poor response to anti-CD3 or anti-CD2 and the sensitivity to corticosteroids, that indicate that the cells are functionally immature.

Helper and Suppressor Activity

One of the more interesting aspects of the neonatal immune response is the strong suppressor activity, even within the so-called helper or CD4$^+$ subset of T cells. The first indication of the suppressor function of neonatal cells was the observation by Olding and Oldstone that lymphocytes from neonates strongly decreased proliferation of their mother's cells (175). Suppressor activity was present in fetal liver as early as the 8th week of gestation and in fetal blood by the 14th week, and persisted until the infant was about 1 year of age (176). Supernatants of cord blood T cells were capable of suppressing immunoglobulin production by adult B cells in a PWM-driven system (177). Initially the primary suppressor activity was identified to be within the CD8$^+$ population (178); resting T cells were not suppressive and had to be activated by PWM or allogeneic cells before they could exert their activity (179). These observations are in contrast to a large number of studies that conclusively demonstrated that nearly all of the suppressor activity resided in the CD4$^+$CD8$^-$ population of T cells (180–184). Cord-blood mononuclear cells depleted of CD8$^+$ cells still showed strong suppression of immunoglobulin production by adult B cells, whereas depletion of CD4$^+$ T cells abrogated suppression in a PWM-driven system (180,182). Cord mononuclear cells activated with PWM or allogeneic cells were also capable of suppressing mitogen-induced proliferation of adult cells (181), but Con A, which stimulates predominantly CD8$^+$ cells, did not induce suppressor activity in cord blood (183). The suppressor activity was eliminated by irradiation or hydrocortisone (182,185).

The neonatal cells are relatively resistant to their own suppressive activity (186). Cord-blood CD4$^+$ cells exert their suppressive activity directly, not by inducing adult CD8$^+$ suppressor cells (181). Maternal mononuclear cells depleted of CD4 or CD8 were highly sensitive to suppression by prostaglandin E$_2$ (PGE$_2$), whereas similar cord blood populations were resistant (181,187,188). The mechanism of the PGE$_2$-induced suppression is not known, but it was shown that PGE$_2$ could suppress proliferation by calcium ionophore or various mitogens, but not phorbol ester (189). This differential sensitivity to PGE_2 could provide a mechanism for fetal and neonatal cells to suppress graft-versus-host activity of maternal lymphocytes without inhibiting their own T-cell-mediated functions.

In contrast to the strong suppressor activity exerted by cord blood CD4$^+$ cells, they have poor ability to provide help for either neonatal or adult B cells (180,185,190). This inability to provide help is independent of the suppressor activity and may be due, at least in part, to deficiencies in cytokine production (190), as is discussed in the next section.

Cytokine Production

The majority of studies of cord blood and young infants indicate that production of the cytokines is defective, both TH1 cytokines such as IF-γ and IL-2, and the TH2 cytokines involved in helper activity for B cells. Early studies indicated that the production of immune or gamma-interferon was defective (132,191–194), whereas production of classical or alpha-interferon was normal (191). The defect in IF-γ production may be due to immaturity of the macrophages rather than an intrinsic T-cell defect (195). Production of IF-γ remains abnormal for several months (193), and perhaps years (194) after birth. Production of IF-γ in response to natural infection with herpes simplex virus was significantly impaired in neonates and post-partum women for up to 6 weeks (196). In contrast to these studies, Stephens and co-workers found IF-γ production to be normal in 30 term infants from birth to 9 months of age (197). Wu and colleagues found that the CD45RA or naïve T cells in cord blood could be induced to produce IF-γ when cultured in the presence of IL-12 (198). Production was enhanced in the presence of IL-1 or macrophages, IL-2, and TNF-α. In the presence of IL-12 the T cells become activated and express CD25, CD71, and HLA-DR. The IL-12 enhances the production of IL-2 and IF-γ, but not IL-4, and thus favors maturation into the TH1 phenotype (198).

Cord blood cells stimulated with PHA or phorbol myristate acetate produced less IL-2 and IL-6, and provided less growth and differentiating activity for B cells than T cells from adults (199). Decreased IL-2 production can lead to failure to expand antigen-specific precursor cell populations and hence poor responses to antigens (200). Augmentation of IL-2 production by addition of IL-1 markedly improved the otherwise poor response of neonatal cells to anti-CD2 (169), again indicating that diminished IL-2 production is central to the hyporesponsiveness of neonatal cells. IL-4 production also is reduced, which may, at least in part, be responsible for the poor ability to provide help for B cells (132,194). Other cytokines, such as macrophage inhibiting factor (MIF) and lymphocyte inhibiting factor (LIF), also were decreased, though these factors remain poorly characterized and the early studies have not been confirmed (201).

Natural Killer Cells and Cytotoxicity

Natural killer cells are defined as a population of cells that are capable of spontaneous cytotoxicity against a wide variety of target cells. NK cells resemble large granular lymphocytes, but the exact origin of these cells is unknown. They express the CD2 antigen which is present on the majority of T lymphocytes, but they also express CD16, the Fcγ receptor on granulocytes. Currently they are defined as $CD3\epsilon^-$, $CD16^+$, and/or $CD56^+$ lymphocytes that mediate MHC-unrestricted cytotoxicity. NK cells do not rearrange the T-cell antigen receptor genes and thus differ from T cytotoxic cells. NK cells are active against tumor cells and virally infected cells, regardless of whether they express HLA antigens, and thus may play an important role in immune surveillance. NK activity develops early in fetal life. Activity was detected in the liver as early as 9 weeks gestation (202), though functional NK cells could not be detected in the fetal blood until approximately 27 weeks gestation (203). Cord blood from 3 of 4 premature infants of gestational age 28 to 33 weeks demonstrated activity comparable to that of term infants (202). The fetal NK cells and a subset of cord NK cells differed from adult NK cells in that they expressed substantial amounts of $CD3\delta$ and $CD3\epsilon$ proteins in the cytoplasm (204). The fetal cells also differed from the adult in their response to IL-2 and IFN-γ (203); the activity of adult cells is boosted by both cytokines, whereas the NK cells obtained from early fetuses responded to IL-2 but not the interferon.

The proportion of $CD16^+$ cells in cord blood or the blood of infants is diminished compared to adult values, but the absolute numbers are not significantly different (159). The NK cells from the newborn are phenotypically different, with much higher levels of CD11b and lower levels of CD57. The NK activity of normal term infants has been shown to be diminished in several studies (205–208). Some studies have demonstrated a bimodal distribution, with 12 of 20 cord bloods exhibiting normal activity and the remaining 8 virtually no NK function (205), and a similar proportion in a more recent study (209). Other studies have shown that the overall NK activity of the neonate is significantly reduced, for example, 16% specific activity compared to 36% (206) or 27% compared to 39% in adults (207). NK activity remains lower than adult levels for at least 4 years (210). If the cord blood cells are incubated overnight in interferon-alpha (IF-α), NK activity increases significantly and approximates that of the adult (206,207). Similarly, incubation in IL-2 increases killing by cord blood NK cells to the normal range (211). These observations suggest that the NK cells are present but fail to mature because of lack of T-cell-derived cytokines. It is likely that in premature and even in term infants two populations of NK cells exist (209). Normal activity was associated with cells that were CD16$^+$CD56$^+$. The cord cells were responsive to IL-2, but not to IFN-γ, unlike adult cells which respond to both. Although no study has shown a direct correlation between the reduced NK activity and clinical disease, it may be responsible for the increased incidence of malignancy and overwhelming viral infections in the neonatal period.

The other cytotoxic mechanisms have been less well studied in the neonate. Lectin-dependent T-lymphocyte cytotoxicity was significantly reduced in cord and neonatal blood, whereas lectin-dependent cytotoxicity by non-T cells was normal or even enhanced (208). Similarly, antibody-dependent cellular cytotoxicity was markedly reduced in infants (212,213), improving over the first weeks of life. Others found that NK activity was low in neonates but that antibody-mediated cytotoxicity and NK-like activity generated in mixed lymphocyte cultures were equivalent to that of adults, and lymphokine-activated killer cells (LAK cells) was high in the neonate (214). While these defects may explain the increased susceptibility to viral infections that is observed in neonates, the biological relevance of these assays is far from clear.

II. Immunodeficiency Diseases Presenting in Infancy

A. Approach to the Child with Suspected Immunodeficiency Disease

While it is true that all neonates are immunodeficient to some degree, children with primary immunodeficiency diseases are more severely affected and therefore at risk of developing infections and autoimmune diseases early in life. In general, primary humoral immunodeficiencies do not present in the perinatal period, since the maternal antibodies transferred across the placenta help to protect the newborn infant from infection for the first 3–6 months of life. However, defects in cellular immunity or neutrophils can present within hours to days of birth.

Specific points in the history, physical examination, and laboratory evaluation can be helpful in determining whether a child has an immune defect (Table 4). All children are at risk of developing infections, but the frequency, severity, and infectious agent can give important clues when deciding who should undergo an immunological evaluation. Infections with opportunistic agents such as *Pneumocystis carinii* or *Candida albicans* should always lead to a high index of suspicion. Recurrent or persistent

Table 4 Evaluation of Host Defense in Infants with Suspected Immune Deficiency

General	
Detailed history	Chest x-ray
Physical examination	Sinus x-ray or CT scan
Family history	Tests for allergy

Humoral immunity	
Screening tests	Advanced tests
White blood count and differential	B-cell phenotyping
Quantitative immunoglobulins	Antibodies to vaccine antigens, e.g., tetanus,
Isoagglutinins (anti-A and anti-B)	diphtheria, *H. influenzae*
CH50 or CH100	Specific complement components

Cellular immunity	
Screening tests	Advanced tests
White blood count and differential	Lymphocyte phenotyping
Delayed-hypersensitivity skin tests	Proliferation to mitogens, antigens, allogeneic cells
	In-vitro immunoglobulin synthesis
	Cytokine production
	Cellular cytotoxicity (e.g., NK assay)

Phagocytic system	
Screening tests	Advanced tests
White blood count and differential	Oxidative burst assay
NBT	Quantitative NBT
	Cell surface receptors by flow cytometry
	Chemotaxis
	Phagocytosis
	Bactericidal assay
	Cellular adhesion

infections or infections that are unusually severe also should be an indication for undertaking an evaluation of the immune system. A history of chronic diarrhea, rash, or failure to thrive are all of special concern. As will be discussed in the following sections, many of the immune deficiency diseases are associated with specific abnormalities. Thus, hypocalcemia, congenital heart disease, and abnormal facial features suggest DiGeorge syndrome. Similarly, an eczematous rash, petechiae or bleeding, and sinopulmonary infections in a boy is consistent with the Wiskott-Aldrich syndrome. Babies with severe combined immune deficiency (SCID) can present with thrush, diarrhea, and failure to thrive, but may also have an erythematous morbilliform rash due to graft-versus-host disease from transplacentally acquired maternal T lymphocytes. The constellation of omphalitis, or delayed separation of the umbilical cord, and a marked leukocytosis is very suggestive of LAD or leukocyte adhesion defect. It is important to realize that children can initially present with a very benign history, and thus a very high index of suspicion and a willingness to evaluate children with unusual features is critical if the diagnosis is to be made early, before serious complications can develop. The genetic basis for many of these immunodeficiency diseases has been identified (Table 5) (215,216), making diagnosis possible in utero or at the time of birth.

A careful *family history* for immunodeficiency should be obtained, with special emphasis on a history of recurrent infections or early childhood deaths, especially among male members of the family since many of the primary immunodeficiency diseases are inherited in an X-linked fashion. Risk factors for *AIDS* also need to be explored and in most cases followed by specific testing of the infant and the mother. The *physical exam* should focus on the general health and nutrition of the infant, and include an evaluation of lymphoid tissue, as either absence or hypertrophy of these tissues indicate an immune defect. Properly conducted and interpreted laboratory studies are an important part of the immunological evaluation. The presence of a thymic shadow can be evaluated by a chest roentgenogram. A complete blood count with differential is a crucial and cost-effective screening test. Absolute lymphocyte count can be an important clue as to the presence of SCID, DiGeorge, or other T-cell disorders. A leukocytosis might suggest either a severe infection or LAD. Similarly quantitative immunoglobulins is an inexpensive screening test for B cell and combined immune disorders. It is important to remember that in the first few months of life the IgG is likely maternal in origin. However, a low IgA or IgM can be suggestive. The values must be compared to the age-adjusted normal reference ranges (Table 6). IgG subclasses offer little, especially if the total IgG is low, and have no place as a screening test. Most children can be evaluated for their ability to make specific antibody to vaccine antigens. The tests are readily available through commercial laboratories, but it is necessary to be sure that the same laboratory is used consistently and that it is understood that the "normal" values that are listed in the reports are those considered to be "protective," not necessarily the level achieved by the normal child. Thus, a level that is barely protec-

Table 5 Prenatal Diagnosis and Carrier Detection of Immunodeficiency Diseases

Syndrome	Protein defect	Genetic origin	Prenatal diagnosis
SCID	γ chain	γ chain	(a) Lymphocyte function studies of fetal blood
		X-chromosome	(b) Genetic studies of CVS[a]
			(c) Carrier detection by nonrandom X-chromosome inactivation
XLA	btk	Xq22	(a) Genetic studies of CVS[a]
			(b) Carrier detection by nonrandom X-chromosome inactivation
Hyper-IgM	CD40 ligand	Xq24-27	(a) Genetic studies of CVS[a]
			(b) Carrier detection by nonrandom X-chromosome inactivation
DiGeorge syndrome	? mitochondrial citrate transporter	22q18	(a) Chromosomal analysis by FISH
Wiskott-Aldrich syndrome	WASP	Xp11	(a) Genetic studies of CVS[a]
			(b) Carrier detection by nonrandom X-chromosome activation
Ataxia telangiectasia	ATM	11q23.1	(a) Genetic studies of CVS[a]
Chronic granulomatous disease	(a) gp91-phox	(a) Xp21.1	(a) Genetic studies of CVS[a]
	(b) p47-phox	(b) 7q11.23	(b) Carrier detection by nonrandom X-chromosome inactivation
	(c) p67-phox	(c) 1q25	
	(d) p22-phox	(d) 16q24	
Leucocyte adhesion defect	(a) LFA-1	CD18 gene	(a) Flow cytometry using fetal blood
	(b) Mac-1		
	(c) p150,95		

[a]CVS, chorionic villous sampling.
Source: Adapted from Refs. 215 and 216.

Table 6 Serum Immunoglobulin Concentrations Throughout Childhood

Age	IgG		IgA		IgM	
	Mean	Range	Mean	Range	Mean	Range
Newborn	967	591–1583	0		9	4–20
1–3 mo	297	181–495	14	9–23	37	17–79
4–6 mo	315	192–515	19	12–31	59	39–92
7–9 mo	429	263–703	19	12–31	72	18–191
10–18 mo	582	356–952	29	12–73	86	43–174
2 yr	640	391–1047	38	15–95	131	49–202
3 yr	640	391–1047	43	17–108	88	43–179
4 yr	814	498–1332	52	21–129	63	31–126
5 yr	814	498–1332	61	23–144	80	40–163
6 yr	938	573–1534	56	22–141	88	43–177
7 yr	1051	643–1720	96	38–240	74	37–151
8 yr	850	520–1098	92	36–230	85	42–172
9 yr	806	492–1319	99	40–248	86	43–174
10 yr	895	547–1465	81	32–203	92	45–185
11 yr	857	524–1403	110	44–277	86	43–174
12 yr	857	524–1403	100	40–228	85	42–171
13 yr	902	551–1476	101	40–253	80	40–162
14 yr	831	507–1355	93	37–234	103	103–208
Adult	962	588–1573	114	46–287	117	117–237

Source: Adapted from Ref. 113.

tive might be very abnormal. The CH50 is an adequate screen for congenital defects in the complement system, as all children with a complete absence of one component will have an abnormal CH50 or CH100. Delayed-hypersensitivity skin testing, using recall antigens such as tetanus, diphtheria, or measles, or common antigens such as *Candida*, are a useful screen in infants over a year of age. Even then as much as 20% will respond poorly, especially if only one or two antigens are used. A positive test is reassuring, however. Children under a year of age cannot be tested reliably by intradermal skin tests.

More specific diagnoses can be made through functional studies of the immune system, including lymphocyte subset enumeration by flow cytometry, T-cell proliferative responses to mitogens such as phytohemagglutinin, concanavalin A, and pokeweed, and more exotic tests such as in-vitro immunoglobulin synthesis or cytokine production. However, although many of these assays are available through commercial laboratories, not all are reliable and interpretation requires considerable expertise. Thus, consultation with an immunologist should be undertaken before ordering such tests. Neoantigens such as the bacteriophage ØX174 are very helpful in evaluating the ability to generate a primary immune response, but most are available only in a research setting.

If a primary immunodeficiency disease is suspected in an infant, several precautions should be taken until the diagnosis is clarified. These include the avoidance of live-virus vaccines to minimize the risk of infection and the exclusive use of irradiated blood products in order to preclude transfusion-acquired graft-versus-host disease. Strict isolation is seldom indicated unless SCID is suspected, but removal from day care might be wise. Common respiratory viruses such as RSV, parainfluenza, and adenovirus can be deadly in children with T-cell disorders. Thus, relative isolation until a specific diagnosis can be made is warranted.

Classically, immunodeficiency disorders involving lymphocytes can be thought of as primary B-cell disorders or primary T-cell disorders. It is becoming increasingly clear, however, that most immunological diseases involving lymphocytes probably have their basis, at least in part, at the T-cell level (with the exception of X-linked agammaglobulinemia). For the purposes of this discussion, these disorders will be categorized as disorders primarily affecting either humoral immunity or cellular immunity. In addition, disorders of the immune system can affect primarily granulocyte lines or the complement system. AIDS has already been discussed in Chapter 24 and will not be discussed in depth in this chapter. Disorders of the complement system will also not be considered. In addition, common variable immune deficiency will not be discussed in this chapter, as presentation in infancy is rare. An overview of immunodeficiencies, including AIDS, is presented in Table 7, with emphasis on distinguishing clinical characteristics and laboratory findings.

B. Immunodeficiencies Involving Primarily Humoral Immunity

X-Linked Agammaglobulinemia

First described by Bruton in 1952 (217), X-linked agammaglobulinemia (XLA) is the only clearly defined immunodeficiency to affect B-cell morphogenesis directly. Two and a half decades later, the criteria for diagnosis were codified and are currently defined by the WHO (218): a) male sex, b) onset in early infancy or childhood, c) low IgG, IgA, and IgM, and d) normal cell-mediated immunity. The defect appears to be an inability of B-cell precursors to switch from pre-B cells to B cells. While there are no B cells in the circulation and patients cannot make antibody or clear antigens, pre-B cells can be found in the bone marrow (219).

Table 7 Characteristics of Immunodeficiency Diseases Presenting During the First Year of Life

Disease	Types of infection	WBC #s	T-cell #'s	B-cell #'s
X-linked agamma-globulinemia	High-grade bacterial	Normal	Normal	Absent
Severe combined immunodeficiency	Opportunistic high-grade bacterial, fungal, viral, parasitic	↓ ALC	↓ or absent	↓ absent or normal
HIV disease	Opportunistic high-grade bacterial, fungal, viral, parasitic	Normal or ↓ ALC	Normal or ↓	Normal
Immunodeficiency assoc. with DiGeorge syndrome	Opportunistic, high-grade bacterial fungal, viral	Normal or ↓ ALC	↓ or absent	Normal or ↑
Wiskott-Aldrich syndrome	Opportunistic, high-grade bacterial, fungal, viral	ALC ↓ or normal. AEC ↑ or normal	↓ or normal	Normal
Ataxia telangiectasia	Bacterial and viral	↓ ALC	↓ or normal	No data
Chronic granulomatous disease	Catalase-positive organisms, esp. *Staphylococcus* and *Aspergillus*	Normal	Normal	Normal
Leukocyte adhesion deficiency	High-grade bacteria	Granulocytes increased	Normal	Normal
Hyper-IgM syndrome	High-grade bacteria opportunistic infections	Cyclic neutropenia	Normal or ↓	Normal
Transient hypoagamma-globulinemia of infancy	bacterial	Normal	Normal	Normal
Hyper-IgE syndrome	*Staphylococci* *Candida* *Streptococci*	Total WBC normal or ↑ AEC ↑	Normal	Normal

Serum immunoglobulin	Ig function	T-cell function	Lymph tissue	Other
↓ or absent	Absent	Normal	Absent	Male sex
↓ or absent	Absent	Absent	Absent	Many types; ADA def. X-linked Omenn's
Normal or ↑	↓ or absent	↓ or absent	Present or ↑	HIV titer or culture positive
Normal or ↓	Absent	Absent	Thymic hypoplasia	Hypoparathyroid, cardiac defects
↑, ↓ or normal	Normal or ↓	Normal or ↓	Splenomegaly	Platelets decreased, atopic dermatitis
IgA ↓ in 70%. IgG, IgM, IgG subclasses ↓ IgM ↑	↓ or normal	↓ or normal	Thymic tissue ↓ or absent	Oculocutaneous telangiectasias, ataxia, sensitive to radiation
Normal or ↑	Normal	Normal	Mild lymphadenopathy, splenomegaly	NBT+, elevated ESR
Normal or ↑	Normal	Normal	Normal	CD11/CD18 decreased or absent
IgM ↑ and IgG, IgA, and IgM ↓ or absent	↓	Normal	Lymphoid hyperplasia	Defective isotype switching
↓	↓	Normal	Normal	Infections resolve after 6 mos., immunoglobulins resolve after 2 years.
IgE ↑ IgD ↑ IgG, A, M Normal or ↑	↓ or normal	Normal to mitogens ↓ or normal to antigens	Lymphadenopathy common	Pneumatocoeles, abscess

Abbreviations: ALC = absolute lymphocyte count; AEC = absolute eosinophil count; Ig = immunoglobulin; ADA = adenosine deaminase.

Initially patients were treated with aggressive use of antibiotics and intramuscular immunoglobulin. However, in the early 1980s, the treatment of patients with XLA was revolutionized with the institution of intravenous immunoglobulin (IVIG), which allows much higher doses to be given. In the past few years the gene responsible for XLA, the Bruton tyrosine kinase (BTK), was identified (220,221), and the hope of gene therapy for the treatment of this classical immunodeficiency was raised.

Clinical Features

The clinical hallmark of X-linked agammaglobulinemia is recurrent, severe pyogenic infections. Because of maternal antibodies, clinical symptoms generally do not begin in the first 4–6 months of life. However, 50% of cases present within the first 8 months and 90% within the first 18 months of life (222).

In 1985, Lederman and Winkelstein (222) presented a review of 96 patients with XLA. According to their data, the most frequent infections in XLA involve the sinopulmonary and gastrointestinal tracts, but septicemia, arthritis, and CNS infections are also seen. The sinopulmonary infections presenting in infancy are most often otitis media or pneumonia, with high-grade pathogens such as *S. pneumoniae, H. influenza,* or *S. aureus.* As patients get older, sinusitis remains a persistent problem. Diarrhea can be a presenting feature of XLA in infancy; gastroenteritis can be either bacterial, viral, or parasitic (especially *Giardia*) in origin. Arthritis, either mono- or polyarticular, can also be a feature of XLA on presentation, generally caused by *S. pneumoniae, H. influenza,* or *S. aureus,* though viral pathogens have also been identified. About 15% of patients may have CNS infections at the time of presentation, generally with bacterial organisms, though the danger of live vaccines in these patients is illustrated by numerous cases of acute polio virus encephalitis seen in infants. Older patients are at risk of developing chronic enteroviral meningoencephalitis (CEME), usually with one of the ECHO viruses (223). In a related manner, paralytic polio (224) and vaccinia gangrenosum have also been reported after polio and smallpox vaccines, respectively.

Excluding patients with meningitis, Lederman and Winkelstein reported septicemia at presentation in 10% of patients, associated with pneumonia otitis and cellulitis. They also reported 4 cases of sepsis with *Pseudomonas* species without a focus of infection.

Later, noninfectious complications of XLA include a dermatomyositis like syndrome, secondary to enteroviral infections, and malignancies (222,225,226), particularly those involving the lymphoreticular system or the gastrointestinal tract.

Laboratory Findings

The hallmark of diagnosis of XLA remains the absence of circulating B cells (CD19$^+$ and CD20$^+$ cells) (227–229); T-cell responses to mitogens and antigens are generally normal. Serum IgG is <200 ng/dL and IgA and IgM markedly decreased for age (222). There have been reports of increased T-suppresser activity as well as a deficiency in the numbers of circulating memory T cells (CD4$^+$ CD45RO$^+$ cells) (230). The clinical or etiological significance of these T-cell abnormalities is not known; lymphopenia is not generally present.

Treatment

The mainstay of treatment for XLA remains replacement therapy with IVIG, generally begun at a dose of 400 mg/kg every 3–4 weeks. When this therapy is begun early, the devastating infectious complications of XLA such as CEME and chronic pulmonary disease can be nearly completely ameliorated, though sinusitis and diarrhea can remain particularly vexing problems. Infections require prompt treatment with appropriate antibiotics; prophylactic antibiotics are often required, particularly in patients with chronic sinusitis. Surveillance for malignancy needs to be carried out on a regular basis.

The prognosis of untreated XLA is almost invariably fatal. The success of current treatment of XLA and the hope of gene therapy in the near future demands a prompt diagnosis. Therefore, infants with frequent bacterial infections in the first year of life should be screened, particularly if several organ systems are involved and infections remain refractory to standard treatment.

Hyper-IgM Syndrome

A condition related to XLA is the hyper-IgM syndrome, which can be inherited in either an X-linked or occasionally in an autosomal recessive manner. Patients present clinically in much the same manner as patients with XLA, but the basic molecular defect in the X-linked form of the disease is thought to involve the CD40 ligand on T cells which can effect isotype switching in B cells; without activation of CD40, large amounts of IgM can be produced but not other isotypes (231–233). These patients have normal numbers of B cells, and have low serum levels of IgG, IgA, and IgE but elevated IgM. Also, in contrast to patients with XLA, patients with the hyper-IgM syndrome are prone to opportunistic infections, have marked lymphoid hyperplasia, can develop autoimmune manifestations including neutropenia (234), and are at a high risk of developing lymphoreticular malignancies.

Transient Hypogammaglobulinemia of Infancy

Transient hypogammaglobulinemia of Infancy (THI) is a poorly defined syndrome in which infants less than 2 years of age have one or more major immunoglobulin class below normal for age (235). Usually the ability to form specific antibodies is normal. The incidence of this condition has recently been estimated at 6.1/100,000 population in an Australian study (236). The syndrome is distinguished from other, more serious forms of immunodeficiency by the lack of severe infections after 6 months and a resolution of significant abnormal immunoglobulin levels and function by 2–4 years of age. IgA levels have been noted to remain abnormal in some patients, however, even after resolution of stigmata of immunodeficiency (237).

Clinical findings range from asymptomatic infants to patients with severe recurrent bacterial infections before 6 months of age. While most studies report no increased incidence of allergy in these patients, Walker et al., did report an incidence of either atopic disease, food allergy, or food intolerance in over 50% of infants with either proven or probable THI (236).

Treatment of these patients should be expectant; IVIG should generally not be administered because of theoretical concerns regarding potential delay of natural synthesis of immunoglobulin if passive antibody is infused. Obviously, the diagnosis can only be made over time, after the child has recovered. Immunoglobulin levels and titers of specific antibody should be monitored every 4–6 months and prophylactic antibiotics used for those with a high incidence of infection.

Hyper-IgE Syndrome

In 1972, Buckley et al. described a syndrome of recurrent severe staphylococcal abscesses of the skin and other deep seated sites such as the lungs and joints, associated with very high serum IgE concentration (238). Infections are most frequently caused by *Staphylococcus aureus*, but other frequently implicated bacterial pathogens are *Pneumococcus*, group A strep and gram negative species. Fungal infections are common, generally caused by *Candida* and *Aspergillus*, though disseminated cryptococcal infection (239) has been described. Recurrent pneumonias are the rule in patients with the hyper-IgE syndrome, and pneumatoceles occur in virtually all patients with the disease. The vast majority of patients will develop their first related infection in the first year of life. Prophylactic antibiotics remain the mainstay of treatment in these patients, and while interferonγ has been shown to decrease IgE synthesis in these and other patients, consistent clinical benefit has not yet been shown (240,241).

The typical laboratory findings are summarized in Table 7; it must be emphasized that this syndrome is rare and its diagnosis is based primarily on clinical findings. It needs to be distinguished from much more common conditions such as atopic dermatitis and asthma, which can also lead to recurrent staph infections of the skin and recurrent pneumonias, respectively; these conditions are also frequently associated with a high serum IgE. These allergic conditions can be distinguished from the hyper-IgE syndrome by the severity and deep-seated nature of the infections and particularly by the development of pneumatoceles, seen only in the hyper-IgE syndrome.

C. Immunodeficiencies Involving Primarily Cellular Immunity

Severe Combined Immunodeficiency

Severe combined immunodeficiency (SCID) is a syndrome involving a severe T-cell dysfunction in which both T- and B-cell activity is absent. Both autosomal recessive and X-linked forms exist. Unless diagnosed and treated early, the syndrome leads almost invariably to death within the first year of life. As it is a syndrome rather than a well-defined disease, no single pathophysiological mechanism exists. Initially the various forms of SCID were described by the mode of inheritance and the pattern of B- and T-cell defects. However, in the past 10 years a wide variety of genetic abnormalities have been described; an abbreviated list is shown in Table 8. Two of the molecular defects that have been identified are the autosomal

Table 8 Genetic Forms of Severe Combined Immune Deficiency (SCID)

Inheritance	SCID type
X-linked recessive	IL-2 receptor deficiency (common γ chain)
	SCID with presence of B cells (most cases)
Autosomal recessive	Absence of T and B lymphocytes
	ZAP-70
	JAK-3
	ADA deficiency
	PNP deficiency
	Omenn's syndrome
	Cartilage hair hypoplasia
	Bare lymphocyte syndrome (class I or class II)
Either	SCID with maternal engraftment of T cells
Unknown	Low expression of T-cell receptor complex

adenosine deaminase (ADA) deficiency and the X-linked lack of the gamma chain of the IL-2 receptor (218,242). Others include deficiency of the signal transduction proteins JAK3 and ZAP70, absence or decreased expression of CD3, deficiency of IL-2 production, and lack of HLA class I and HLA class II antigens. SCID can also be a component of one of several clinical syndromes, such as Omenn's syndrome, which includes histiocytic skin infiltrates, lymphadenopathy, eosinophilia, and severe T-cell defects (243,244), or cartilage hair hypoplasia, which consists of short-limbed dwarfism, fine sparse hair, and immunodeficiency. The immuno-deficiency in cartilage hair hypoplasia is usually mild to moderate (245,246), but cases of SCID have been reported in these patients (242,247).

As with XLA, prompt diagnosis is critical, as potentially life-saving treatment is available to a majority of these infants if delivered early enough. Treatments such as T-cell-depleted HLA-haploidentical bone marrow transplantation have markedly improved the prognosis for these infants, as will be noted in more detail below.

Clinical Features

The earliest clinical signs of SCID can occur as early as the first month of life, but infants generally present within the first 3–6 months. The presenting features of SCID most often involve chronic diarrhea, failure to thrive, refractory oral candidiasis, pneumonitis, and recurrent otitis media. Infection can occur with virtually any organism, including *Pseudomonas*, *Streptococci*, *E. coli*, and other gram-negative species, fungi, and parasites. Severe extensive viral infections are frequent. Sepsis and meningitis are not uncommon (248). Pneumonitis is frequently due to infection with opportunistic pathogens such as *Pneumocystis carinii*. A characteristic finding on physical exam, besides the stigmata of infection, is a lack of lymphoid tissue, including tonsils. Dermatitis is not uncommon and can frequently be due to graft-versus-host disease (GvHD) if transplacentally acquired maternal T cells are present. Histiocytic skin infiltrates are also seen with Omenn's syndrome. Thymic shadow is generally absent on chest roentgenogram in most patients with SCID.

Laboratory Findings

Upon an initial screening of a patient with stigmata of SCID, the most notable laboratory findings are marked lymphopenia; though an absolute lymphocyte count (ALC) of >1500 is generally considered normal for older individuals, an ALC of <3500 should be viewed as suspicious in an infant (249). IgG, IgA, and IgM are generally very low for age, although

IgG may appear normal in the neonatal period because of the presence of maternal antibody. T cells are usually absent, but B-cell numbers may be normal or elevated, particularly in boys with X-linked SCID (242,249). Some patients have been described whose circulating lymphocytes are almost entirely natural killer cells (250). Eosinophilia is a prominent finding in patients with Omenn's syndrome and can also be found in patients with GvHD secondary to transplacentally acquired maternal T cells (251).

Functional studies of the immune system are generally diagnostic. No functional antibody is present in the serum, and T-cell proliferative responses to mitogens and neoantigens are very low or absent in nearly all patients with SCID.

Treatment

Bone marrow transplantation (BMT) is the treatment of choice for patients with all forms of SCID. For those patients with an HLA-identical sibling, immune reconstitution can often be achieved in 2 weeks (252). Patients without an HLA-identical related donor can be transplanted using matched unrelated marrow, cord blood, or an HLA-haploidentical, T-cell-depleted marrow. The success rate for haploidentical marrow is as high as 75–80% in some types of SCID (253), and can approach 100% if the babies are diagnosed and treated shortly after birth. The depletion of mature T cells allows engraftment with a much lower risk of severe GvHD. Two methods of depleting mature T cells have been employed, one using monoclonal antibodies and the other using soybean lectin agglutination and sheep RBC rosette depletion. Success with and without pretransplantation chemoablation have been reported. Immunoreconstitution with T-cell-depleted marrow usually takes 3–4 months, to allow the stem cell to mature in the infant's rudimentary thymus (252–256).

From the time of suspected diagnosis until the time of successful immunoreconstitution, many precautions need to be taken to minimizing the risk of life-threatening infection. Children should remain in reverse isolation and receive prophylactic antibiotics such as TMP/SMZ and an antifungal agent such as nystatin. Only irradiated blood products should be transfused, to minimize the risk of transfusion-acquired GvHD. IVIG should also be administered to retain reasonably protective antibody levels. In many patients who have undergone successful BMT, IVIG is required on an ongoing basis, even after T-cell function has returned to normal. For patients with ADA deficiency, treatment with polyethylene glycol-modified ADA (PEG-ADA) (257) or gene therapy have become alternatives to BMT.

Deaths from SCID occur from either overwhelming infection or GvHD; bone marrow rejection also occurs. Risk of death can be minimized by recognizing the disease as early as possible (258), isolating the infants as noted above, and by arranging BMT as promptly as is prudent in each case.

DiGeorge Syndrome

First described in 1965 (259), the DiGeorge syndrome is a developmental anomaly involving the third and fourth pharyngeal pouches, leading to a spectrum of anatomical irregularities including characteristic facies, hypoplasia of the parathyroid glands, cardiac abnormalities, and hypoplastic thymic tissue. The syndrome can occur in "complete" and "partial" forms; patients with "partial DiGeorge syndrome" are generally immunocompetent (260,261).

Typical facies include micrognathia, short philtrum, hypertelorism, and low-set and/or malformed ears. Velopharyngeal incompetence may also be associated. Cardiac anomalies are generally midline defects, usually interrupted aortic arch or truncus arteriosis (261), with the former being most characteristic. The cardiac anomalies are the most common presenting component of this syndrome. However, because of lack of parathormone, infants often present with profound hypocalcemia and associated neonatal tetany during the first month of life. The combination of cardiac anomalies and hypocalcemia can also be seen in other infants who develop secondary hypocalcemia due to heart-lung bypass for cardiac surgery, and these patients need to be distinguished from those with DiGeorge syndrome. DiGeorge syndrome is considered to be a sporadic disease rather than genetic, though several chromosomal defects have been noted in patients with the DiGeorge syndrome, most commonly involving chromosome 22 (262).

It is the thymic aplasia or hypoplasia that leads to the characteristic immunodeficiency seen in the DiGeorge syndrome, though in a review of 18 patients with the syndrome, Bastien et al (263) reported only 4 patients with immunodeficiency, despite the fact that the thymus could not be identified in more than half. Patients with immunodeficiency are not necessarily lymphopenic, but all would show a decreased number of T cells of both helper ($CD3^+CD4^+$) and cytotoxic ($CD3^+CD8^+$) subsets and poor proliferative responses to mitogens is seen in the complete form of the disease. Lack of thymic shadow is often noted on chest roentgenogram, but is not predictive of the degree of immunodeficiency. Immunoglobulin levels are often normal in patients with the immunodeficiency associated with the DiGeorge syndrome, but occasionally are decreased. B-cell function, as evidenced by the ability to produce specific antibody, is absent in the immunodeficient patients, despite normal or increased numbers of B cells.

For patients without immunodeficiency, the prognosis for the Di-George syndrome is good if the cardiac anomalies are recognized and corrected in time and if the hypocalcemia is managed effectively. Complete DiGeorge syndrome, with absent T-cell function, is a medical emergency similar to SCID, and these patients must be treated in a comparable manner. A few patients have been reconstituted with matched related marrow. Haploidentical marrow is not an option because the infant does not have enough thymic tissue to mature the stem cells. Several children have been successfully reconstituted with fetal thymus or cultured thymic epithelium obtained from young children at the time of cardiac surgery.

Wiskott-Aldrich Syndrome

Wiskott-Aldrich syndrome (WAS) is an X-linked condition marked classically by the clinical triad of thrombocytopenia, eczema, and immunodeficiency. Of course, as with other such syndromes, great phenotypic variability can exist, and in a recent report by Sullivan et al., the full classic triad was found in only 30% of 154 patients reviewed (264).

Most patients initially present with bleeding difficulties with or without signs of recurrent infection. Draining otitis media is a classical finding, but pneumonia, diarrhea, sepsis, meningitis, and chronic viral infection (particularly HSV) can also be seen. Many patients with WAS develop autoimmune manifestations, most commonly autoimmune hemolytic anemia; ITP can also complicate the thrombocytopenia already present. These patients also have a significantly increased risk of lymphoreticular malignancies later in childhood or into adulthood if they survive (264).

Essentially all patients with WAS have thrombocytopenia, with 80% having platelet counts $<50,000/mm^3$; platelet size is consistently small, <5 fmol/platelet. Immunological findings are inconsistent. IgG, IgA, and IgM can be increased, decreased, or normal. IgE almost always is elevated. The most consistent abnormal finding is poor antibody responses, particularly to polysaccharide antigens. The most common T-cell abnormality is a low CD8+ count, but this only appears to be present in only about two-thirds of the patients in the report by Sullivan et al. While T-cell proliferative responses were low to all three mitogens, PHA, Con A, and pokeweed, in about one-fourth of patients, they were normal to all three mitogens in nearly half (264). More recently, Molina et al, have reported that there may be a more consistent finding in patients with WAS in that T-cell lines established from 7 boys with WAS either failed to proliferate to anti-CD3 monoclonal antibodies OKT3 and SPV-T3b, or showed a significantly decreased ability to proliferate. Normal T cells should respond vigorously to these antibodies (265). It should be noted that patients with

HIV disease can also present with an ITP-like syndrome, and this should be distinguished from WAS.

Several treatment options are available to patients with WAS. Great success has been obtained with HLA-matched sibling BMT. Unfortunately, unlike SCID, success has not been impressive with the use of HLA-haploidentical T-cell-depleted parental marrow for BMT. Matched unrelated donor transplants have been successful in a limited number of patients, and cord blood transplantation should make donors available to a greater number of patients. The rate of success for all transplants is best if the patient is transplanted before 5 years of age. For those patients in whom transplantation is not an option, splenectomy has led to normalization of platelet counts in many, with a significant reduction in severe bleeding episodes and increased life span. Unfortunately, splenectomy can also lead to an increased risk of sepsis in patients who are already immunocompromised (266) unless they are given prophylactic antibiotics. The gene for WASP (Wiskott-Aldrich-associated protein), a protein expressed in the cytoplasm of B and T cells (Table 5) has been identified, and as gene therapy becomes available, a more definitive treatment may be able to be offered to these affected men and boys.

Ataxia Telangiectasia

As the name implies, ataxia telangiectasia (AT) is a multisystem disorder composed of oculocutaneous telangiectasias, cerebellar ataxia, radiosensitivity with subsequent increased cancer risk, and variable immunodeficiency. Both the neurological and immunological components often present in the first 1 to $1\frac{1}{2}$ years of life (267,268). The telangiectasias do not generally present until later in childhood. The immune deficiency generally manifests itself with recurrent sinopulmonary infections caused by the standard bacterial pathogens, but disseminated viral infections including vaccine-associated poliomyelitis have been reported (269). Thymic hypoplasia is the rule in AT patients with immunodeficiency, with a subsequent lymphopenia. Seventy percent of these patients are IgA deficient (267), but abnormalities in other immunoglobulin classes and IgG subclasses are frequent. IgM has been reported as elevated (270), depressed (267), or normal (269).

The recent cloning of the AT gene (271), encoding a protein in cell cycle control, is of tremendous interest in that even heterozygous carriers of this autosomal recessively transmitted illness seem to be at an increased cancer risk due to radiosensitivity (271–273) and gene therapy might be offered for cancer prevention in these people (274).

D. Immunodeficiencies Affecting Primarily Granulocytes

Chronic Granulomatous Disease

Chronic granulomatous disease (CGD) is a disorder of phagocyte function due to a lack of superoxide generation leading to impaired bacteriocidal activity. Patients with CGD are prone to infection with catalase-positive organisms, since catalase-negative organisms are effectively able to generate their own peroxide. The essential defect is in the respiratory burst/ NADPH oxidase system, usually in a component of cytochrome b_{245}, the terminal link in the respiratory burst chain. CGD is found to be X-linked in approximately 60% of patients. It has been shown to be due to the absent or abnormal 91-kDa beta chain of the cytochrome B_{558} (gp91-phox) (275). In the remaining 40% the disease is autosomal recessive; in these patients the mothers cannot be shown to be carriers. One form is due to a deficiency of a 47-kDa cytosolic factor (NFC1, p47-phox) that is found in approximately 33%. A second autosomal form is due to a deficiency of a 67-kDa cytosolic factor (NFC2,-p67 phox) that is present in 5%, and the remaining 5% have abnormalities in the p22-phox cytochrome b_{558} (276–279).

Clinical Features

Infections in patients with CGD generally involve the lungs, lymph nodes, GI tract, and skin, as well as the musculoskeletal system and urinary tract, and usually begin in the first year of life. Muoy et al. (280) reported that approximately 70% of patients will develop infections before age one, 85% before their third, and 96% before their fifth birthdays. Infections can be either suppurative or granulomatous in nature.

Pneumonia, dermatitis, and/or lymphadenitis occur in the majority of patients, and the likelihood of fungal pneumonitis, particularly *Aspergillus*, should be considered because of its high mortality rate. Other organisms responsible for pneumonitis include *Staphylococcus*, *Enterobacteria*, atypical *Mycobacteria*, *Nocardia*, CMV, *Pneumocystis*, and *Pseudomonas cepacia* (275,280,281). Skin infections including pyoderma are frequent and are most commonly caused by *Staphylococcus* species, though pustulosis with other organismshas been reported. The offending organism in lymphadenitis is most commonly *S. aureus*, but infections with other organisms including gram-negative bacilli and BCG vaccine lymphadenitis can be seen (280).

Other sites of infection are also common in patients with CGD. The GI tract is frequently involved, with *Salmonella* infections being particularly severe; peritonitis is not uncommon. *S. aureus* and *Pseudomonas aeruginosa* cause hepatic abscesses requiring antibiotic therapy and frequent drainage, either surgically or through percutaneous aspiration. Perirectal abscesses can also occur.

Another commonly involved organ system is the musculoskeletal system; serious problems in CGD include osteomyelitis and septic arthritis, with, again, *S. aureus* and *Aspergillus* the leading causative agents. Unlike immunologically normal children who develop osteomyelitis, children with CGD often develop the infections in areas of bone other than the metaphyseal plates (282). Surgical drainage, as well as parenteral antibiotics, is generally necessary.

Inflammatory and granulomatous lesions can effect numerous organ systems. The most commonly involved sites are the GI tract in the forms of gastric outlet obstruction and esophageal narrowing, and the GU tract in the form of bladder granulomas leading to ureteral or urethral obstruction (283,284).

Laboratory Studies

The primary diagnostic test used to diagnose CGD is the nitroblue tetrazolium dye (NBT) reduction test, which involves the reduction of the NBT dye by normal oxidative products. Phagocytes of patients with CGD fail to reduce the dye; this is manifested by a failure of the dye to turn a dark blue hue. Though this is the most commonly used screening test for CGD, an abnormal bacteriocidal assay is the sine qua non of diagnosis (285). Recently, chemiluminescence measured by flow cytometry has supplanted the NBT test.

Blood counts in patients with CGD often reveal leukocytosis and anemia, though not invariably. Immunoglobulin levels can be normal or elevated (286). Studies of cellular immunity are typically normal. Erythrocyte sedimentation rate is elevated in patients with active disease, and this remains a useful marker for disease activity.

Treatment

The cornerstone of therapy of CGD has generally been prophylactic antibiotics and expectant treatment of breakthrough infections and obstructive lesions. Trimethoprim/sulfamethoxazole has remained the treatment of choice for prophylaxis because of its ability to penetrate into the white blood cells, with dicloxacillin an acceptable alternative for patients allergic to sulfa. Ketoconazole has been employed prophylactically to prevent fungal infections, but breakthrough episodes are frequent. Fungal infections often required amphotericin B for effective treatment, though over the past few years, itraconazole has been shown to be effective for prolonged treatment (287,288). The treatment of abscesses and osteomyelitis will most often require surgical intervention as well as antibiotics for effective resolution. In the 1970s and 1980s, granulocyte transfusions were employed as a means to treat infection in these patients with impaired bacteriocidal function, with some success. Osteomyelitis with *Aspergillus* remains a very recalcitrant clinical problem and often requires multimodal therapy (289).

The mainstay of treatment of obstructive, granulomatous lesions remains corticosteroids, which has been shown to be efficacious for lesions in both the GI and GU tracts (283). Cyclosporine has reportedly been effective in the treatment of granulomatous colitis (290).

Over the past few years, interferon-γ has been shown to be an effective agent in preventing infection in CGD patients, though the mechanism is still unclear. A multicenter study in 1991 reported that interferon-γ was more effective than prophylactic antibiotics in preventing serious infections in 128 patients with CGD (291). Children under 10 years of age were shown to benefit particularly, and it was effective in all genetic types of CGD. However, though the proposed mechanism of action of interferon-γ is an increase in phagocytic function, which has been demonstrated both in vivo and in vitro (292,293), increased function was not consistently shown in these patients. In 1992, Woodman et al. also failed to show increased respiratory burst activity in 18 of 19 patients with CGD treated with interferon-γ (294). Nevertheless, its clinical efficacy has been demonstrated and interferon-γ is now recommended as an option in patients with CGD, with or without the concomitant use of prophylactic antibiotics.

Leukocyte Adhesion Deficiency

First described in the 1970s, leukocyte adhesion deficiency (LAD) is a rare disorder leading to frequent, often severe bacterial infections (295,296). The primary defect is defective synthesis of CD18, a molecule which acts as the beta subunit of three related glycoproteins: Mac-1 (complement receptor 3, CD11a/CD18), lymphocyte function-associated antigen-1 (LFA-1, CD11b/CD18), and p150,95 (CD11c/CD18). These three glycoproteins ordinarily appear on the surfaces of leukocytes and function by aiding cellular adhesion. In LAD these molecules are not present, and so while leukocytes can be recruited, they are unable to accumulate at what would ordinarily be a site of inflammation. Phagocytosis is impaired because of a lack of the complement receptor, Mac-1, or CD18/CD11b.

The clinical syndrome can be divided into two phenotypes: moderate or partial deficiency and severe or complete deficiency. The differences between the phenotypes is distinguished by the severity and frequency of infection, though overwhelming infection can occur even in the moderate phenotype. In the neonatal period, patients with LAD can be distinguished by delayed separation of the umbilical cord, which will occur in many patients with the moderate or severe phenotype. Other infections which occur frequently in the first year of life and thereafter include recurrent skin infections, chronic gingivitis and periodontitis, recurrent otitis media, pneumonia, peritonitis, and anal abscesses. Poor wound healing is another hallmark of the disease. Infection can occur from virtually any bacterial pathogen, though *Staphylococcus aureus* and *Pseudomonas aeruginosa* are the most commonly implicated. Peritonitis can occur from enteric pathogens (295–297).

Leukocytosis, which can lead to a misleading diagnosis of hematopoietic disease, can be seen in most of these patients from the time of the earliest clinical signs, even when they appear well. The sedimentation rate increases during infections. Quantitative serum immunoglobulins are generally elevated, but antibody function is normal. Studies of T-cell number and function are normal, though natural killer function is decreased or absent. CGD is often considered in the differential diagnosis in these patients, but NBT test is normal; tests of leukocyte chemotaxis are abnormal, however. The diagnosis is confirmed by a lack of CD11a,b,c/CD18 on the surfaces of leukocytes as determined by flow cytometry (297).

For patients with the moderate phenotype of LAD, treatment is generally with prophylactic antibiotics and good dental hygiene. White blood cell transfusions can be life-saving in severe chronic infections that do not respond to antibiotics. Patients with complete deficiency are at high risk of developing severe, life-threatening infections and must be corrected by bone marrow transplantation (298,299).

References

1. Wagner AM, Hansen RC. Neonatal skin and skin disorders. In: Schachner LA, Hansen RC, eds. Pediatric Dermatology. 2d ed. New York: Churchill Livingstone, 1995:263–346.
2. Hurwitz S. Clinical Pediatric Dermatology. A Textbook of Skin Disorders of Childhood and Adolescence. 2d ed. Philadelphia: Saunders, 1993.
3. McCormack JJ, Boisits EK, Fisher LB. An in vitro comparison of the permeability of adult versus neonatal skin. In: Maibach HI, Boisits EK, eds. Neonatal Skin Structure and Function. New York: Marcel Dekker, 1982:149.
4. Schreiber RA, Walker WA. The gastrointestinal barrier: antigen uptake and perinatal immunity. Ann Allergy 1988; 61(part 2):3–12.
5. Bines JE, Walker WA. Growth factors and the development of neonatal host defense (review). Adv Exp Med Biol 1991; 310:31–39.
6. Cook GC. Infective gastroenteritis and its relationship to reduced gastric acidity. Scand J Gastroenterol 1985; 111(suppl):S17–S23.
7. Bullen JJ, Rogers HJ, Leigh L. Iron-binding proteins in milk and resistance to *Escherichia coli* infection in infants. Br Med J 1972; 1:69–75.

8. Hanson LÅ, Johansson BG. Immunological studies of milk. In: McKenzie H, ed. Milk Proteins, Chemistry and Molecular Biology. New York and London: Academic Press, 1970:45–123.

9. Tenuvuo J, Lehtonen O, Daltonen A. Antimicrobial factors in whole saliva of human infants. Infect Immunol 1986; 54:49–53.

10. Tenuvuo J, Pruitt KM. Relationship of the human salivary peroxidase system to oral health. J Oral Pathol 1984; 13:573–584.

11. Walker WA. Pathophysiology of intestinal uptake and absorption of antigens in food allergy. Ann Allergy 1987; 59(part 2):7–16.

12. Forstner G, Sturgess JM, Forstner J. Malfunction of intestinal mucus and mucus production. Adv Exp Med Biol 1976; 89:349–369.

13. Hyman PE, Clark DD, Everett SL. Gastric acid secretory function in preterm infants. J Pediatr 1985; 106:467–471.

14. Polin RA. Role of fibronectin in diseases of newborn infants and children. Rev Infect Dis 1990; 12:S428–S438.

15. Yoder M, Polin R. The immune system. In: Fanaroff AA, Martin RJ, eds. Neonatal-Perinatal Medicine: Diseases of the Fetus and Infant. St. Louis: Mosby, 1992:587–619.

16. McCafferty MH, Lepow M, Saba TM, Cho E, Meuwissen H, White J, Zuckerbrod SF. Normal fibronectin levels as a function of age in the pediatric population. Pediatr Res 1983; 17:482–485.

17. Valletta EA, Bonazzi L, Zuanazzi R, Del Col G, Stocchero L, Boner AL. Plasma fibronectin concentrations in healthy newborns and children. Eur J Pediatr 1988; 147:68–70.

18. Forestier F, Daffos F, Galactéros F, Bardakjian J, Rainaut M, Beuzard Y. Hematological values of 163 normal fetuses between 18 and 30 weeks of gestation. Pediatr Res 1986; 20:342–346.

19. Hill HR. Biochemical, structural, and functional abnormalities of polymorphonuclear leukocytes in the neonate. Pediatr Res 1987; 22:375–382.

20. Etzioni A. Neutrophil function in the newborn—a review. (review). Isr J Med Sci 1994; 30:328–330.

21. Christensen RD. Neutrophil kinetics in the fetus and neonate. Am J Pediatr Hematol Oncol 1989; 11:215–223.

22. McIntosh N, Kempson C, Tyler RM. Blood counts in extremely low birthweight infants. Arch Dis Child 1988; 63:74–76.

23. Schelonka RL, Yoder BA, des Jardins SE, Hall RB, Butler J. Peripheral leukocyte count and leukocyte indexes in healthy newborn term infants (see comments). J Pediatr 1994; 125:603–606.

24. Xanthou M. Leucocyte blood picture in healthy full-term and premature babies during neonatal period. Arch Dis Child 1979; 45:242–249.

25. Manroe BL, Weinberg AG, Rosenfeld CR, Browne R. The neonatal blood count in health and disease. I. Neutrophilic cells. J Pediatr 1979; 95:89–98.

26. Wheeler JG, Chauvenet AR, Johnson CA, Dillard R, Block SM, Boyle R, Abramson JS. Neutrophil storage pool depletion in septic, neutropenic neonates. Pediatr Infect Dis J 1984; 3:407–409.

27. Erdman SH, Christensen RD, Bradley PP, Rothstein G. Supply and release of storage neutrophils. A developmental study. Biol Neonate 1982; 41: 132–137.

28. Weinberg AG, Rosenfeld CR, Manroe BL, Browne R. Neonatal blood cell count in health and disease. II. Values for lymphocytes, monocytes, and eosinophils. J Pediatr 1985; 106:462–466.

29. Wright WC Jr, Ank B, Herbert J, Stiehm ER. Decreased bactericidal activity of leukocytes of stressed newborn infants. Pediatrics 1975; 56:579–584.

30. Masuda K, Kinoshita Y, Kobayashi Y. Heterogeneity of Fc receptor expression in chemotaxis and adherence of neonatal neutrophils. Pediatr Res 1989; 25:6–10.

31. Anderson DC, Rothlein R, Marlin SD, Krater SS, Smith CW. Impaired transendothelial migration by neonatal neutrophils: Abnormalities of Mac-1 (CD11b/CD18)-dependent adherence reactions. Blood 1990; 76:2613–2621.

32. McEvoy LT, Zakem-Cloud H, Tosi MF. Total cell content of CR3 (CD11b/CD18) and LFA-1 C (CD11a/CD18) in neonatal neutrophils: relationship to gestational age. Blood 1996; 87:3929–3933.

33. Jones DH, Schmalstieg FC, Dempsey K, Krater SS, Nannen DD, Smith CW, Anderson DC. Subcellular distribution and mobilization of Mac-1 (CD11b/CD18) in neonatal neutrophils. Blood 1990; 75:488–492.

34. Cairo MS, VandeVen C, Toy C, Suen Y, Mauss D, Sender L. GM-CSF primes and modulates neonatal PMN motility: up-regulation of C3bi (Mo1) expression with alteration in PMN adherence and aggregation. Am J Pediatr Hematol Oncol 1991; 13:249–257.

35. Yasui K, Masuda M, Matsuoka T, Yamazaki M, Komiyama A, Akabane T, Hasui M, Kobayashi Y, Murata K. Abnormal membrane fluidity as a cause of impaired functional dynamics of chemoattractant receptors on neonatal polymorphonuclear leukocytes: lack of modulation of the receptors by a membrane fluidizer. Pediatr Res 1988; 24:442–446.

36. Yin HS, Stossel TP. Control of cytoplasmic actin gelsol transformation by gelsolin, a calcium-dependent regulatory protein. Nature 1979; 281:583.

37. Harris MC, Shalit M, Southwick F. Diminished actin polymerization by neutrophils from newborn infants. Pediatr Res 1992; 33:27–31.

38. Miller ME. Phagocyte function in the neonate: Selected aspects. Pediatrics 1979; 64(suppl):709.

39. Kamran S, Usmani SS, Wapnir RA, Mehta R, Harper RG. In vitro effect of indomethacin on polymorphonuclear leukocyte function in preterm infants. Pediatr Res 1992; 33:32–35.

40. Tono-oko T, Nakayama M, Uehara H, Matsumoto S. Characteristics of impaired chemotactic function in cord blood leukocytes. Pediatr Res 1979; 13: 148–151.

41. Klein RB, Fischer TJ, Gard SE, Biberstein BS, Rich KC, Stiehm ER. Decreased mononuclear and polymorphonuclear chemotaxis in human newborns, infants, and young children. Pediatrics 1977; 60:467–472.

42. Yegin O. Chemotaxis in childhood. Pediatr Res 1983; 17:183–187.

43. Fontan G, Lorente F, Garcia Rodriguez MC, Ojeda JA. In vitro human neutrophil movement in umbilical cord blood. Clin Immunol Immunopathol 1981; 20:224–230.

44. Laurenti F, Ferro R, Marzetti G, Rossini M, Bucci G. Neutrophil chemotaxis in preterm infants with infections. J Pediatr 1980; 96:468–470.

45. Anderson DC. Abnormal mobility of neonatal polymorphonuclear leukocytes: relationship to impaired redistribution of surface adhesion sites by chemotactic factor or colchicine. J Clin Invest 1981; 68:863.

46. Jones DH. Subcellular distribution and mobilization of MAC-1 (CD11a/CD18) in neonatal neutrophils. Blood 1990; 75(2):488.

47. Sacchi F. Abnormality in actin polymerization associated with defective chemotaxis in neutrophils from neonates. Int Arch Allergy Appl Immunol 1987; 84:32.

48. Maeda M, van Schie RC, Yuksel B, Greenough A, Fanger MW, Guyre PM, Lydyard PM. Differential expression of Fc receptors for IgG by monocytes and granulocytes from neonates and adults. Clin Exp Immunol 1996; 103: 343–347.

49. Falconer AE, Carr R, Edwards SW. Impaired neutrophil phagocytosis in preterm neonates: lack of correlation with expression of immunoglobulin or complement receptors. Biol Neonate 1995; 68:264–269.

50. Forman ML, Stiehm ER. Impaired opsonic activity but normal phagocytosis in low-birth-weight infants. N Engl J Med 1969; 281:926.

51. Xanthou M. Phagocytosis and killing ability of *Candida albicans* by blood leucocytes of health term and preterm babies. Arch Dis Child 1975; 50:72.

52. Harris MC. Phagocytosis of group B streptococcus by neutrophils from newborn infants. Pediatrics Res 1983; 17:358.

53. Matoth Y. Phagocytic and ameboid activities of the leukocytes in the newborn infant. Pediatrics 1952; 9:748.

54. Shigeoka AO. Functional analysis of neutrophil granulocytes from healthy, infected and stressed neonates. J Pediatr 1979; 95:454.

55. Cocchi P, Marianelli L. Phagocytosis and intracellular killing of *Pseudomonas aeruginosa* in premature infants. Helv Paediatr Acta 1967; 1:110.

56. Anderson DC, Pickering LK, Feigin RD. Leukocyte function in normal and infected neonates. J Pediatr 1974; 85:420–425.

57. Mills EL, Thompson M, Bjorksten B, Filopovich D, Quie PG. The chemiluminescence response and bactericidal activity of polymorphonuclear neutrophils from newborns and their mothers. Pediatrics 1979; 63:429–434.

58. Driscoll MS, Thomas VL, Ramamurthy RS, Casto DT. Longitudinal evaluation of polymorphonuclear leukocyte chemiluminescence in premature infants. J Pediatrics 1990; 116:429–434.

59. Ambruso DR, Altenburger KM, Johnston RB. Defective oxidative metabolism in newborn neutrophils: discrepancy between superoxide anion and hydroxyl radical generation. Pediatrics 1979; 64:722–725.

60. Frenck RW, Buescher ES, Vadhan-Raj S. The effects of recombinant human granulocyte-macrophage colony stimulating factor on *in vitro* cord blood granulocyte function. Pediatr Res 1989; 26:43–48.

61. Bortolussi R, Howlett S, Rajaraman K, Halperin S. Deficient priming activity of newborn cord blood-derived polymorphonuclear neutrophilic granulocytes with lipopolysaccharide and tumor necrosis factor-alpha triggered with formyl-methionyl-leucyl-phenylalanine. Pediatr Res 1993; 34:243–248.

62. Qing G, Rajaraman K, Bortolussi R. Diminished priming of neonatal polymorphonuclear leukocytes by lipopolysaccharide is associated with reduced CD14 expression. Infect Immunol 1995; 63:248–252.

63. Dossett JH, Williams RC, Quie PG. Studies on interaction of bacteria, serum factors and polymorphonuclear leukocytes in mothers and newborns. Pediatrics 1969; 44:49.

64. Al-Hadithy H, Addison IE, Goldstone AH, Cawley JC, Shaw JC. Defective neutrophil function in low-birth-weight, premature infants. J Clin Pathol 1981; 34:366–370.

65. Becker ID, Robinson OM, Bazan TS, Lopez-Osuna M, Kretschmer RR. Bactericidal capacity of newborn phagocytes against Group B beta-hemolytic streptococci. Infect Immunol 1981; 34:535–539.

66. Oseas R, Lehrer RI. A micromethod for measuring neutrophil candidicidal activity in neonates. Pediatr Res 1978; 12:828–829.

67. Yoder MC, Hassan NF, Douglas SD. Mononuclear phagocyte system. In: Polin R, Fox W, eds. Fetal and Neonatal Physiology. Philadelphia: Saunders, 1992:1438–1461.

68. Speer CP, Gahr M, Wielenga JJ, Eber S. Phagocytosis-associated functions in neonatal monocyte-derived macrophages. Pediatr Res 1988; 24:213–216.

69. Raghunathan R, Miller ME, Everett S, Leake RD. Phagocyte chemotaxis in the perinatal period. J Clin Immunol 1982; 2:242–245.

70. Marwitz PA, Van Arkel Vigna E, Rijkers GT, Zegers BJ. Expression and modulation of cell surface determinants on human adult and neonatal monocytes. Clin Exp Immunol 1988; 72:260–266.

71. Speer CP. Phagocyte function. In: Ogra PL, ed. Neonatal Infections: Nutritional and Immunologic Interactions. Orlando, FL: Grune and Stratton, 1984: 21–36.

72. Schuit KE, Powell DA. Phagocytic dysfunction in monocytes of normal newborn infants. Pediatrics 1980; 65:501–504.

73. Marodi L, Leijh PC, van Furth R. Characteristics and functional capacities of human cord blood granulocytes and monocytes. Pediatr Res 1984; 18: 1127–1131.

74. Mardódi L, Káposzta R, Campbell DE, Polin RA, Csongor J, Johnston RB. Candidicidal mechanisms in the human neonate. Impaired IFN-γ activation of macrophages in newborn infants. J Immunol 1994; 153:5643–5649.

75. Stiehm ER, Sztein MB, Steeg PS, Mann D, Newland C, Blaese M, Oppenheim JJ. Deficient DR antigen expression on human cord blood monocytes; reversal with lymphokines. Clin Immunol Immunopathol 1984; 30:430–436.

76. Hoffman AA. Presentation of antigen by human newborn monocytes to maternal tetanus toxoid-specific T-cell blasts. J Clin Immunol 1981; 1:217.

77. Kurnick J. Long term maintenance of HLA-D restricted T cells specific for soluble antigens. Scand J Immunol 1980; 11:131.

78. Zlabinger GJ, Mannhalter JW, Eibl MM. Cord blood macrophages present bacterial antigen (*Escherichia coli*) to paternal T cells. Clin Immunol Immunopathol 1983; 28:405–412.

79. Wilmott RW, Harris MC, Haines KM, Douglas SD. Interleukin-1 activity from human cord blood monocytes. Diag Clin Immunol 1987; 5:201–204.

80. Peters AM, Bertram P, Gahr M, Speer CP. Reduced secretion of interleukin-1 and tumor necrosis factor-alpha by neonatal monocytes. Biol Neonate 1993; 63:157–162.

81. Schibler KR, Liechty KW, White WL, Rothstein G, Christensen RD. Defective production of interleukin-6 by monocytes: a possible mechanism underlying several host defense deficiencies of neonates. Pediatr Res 1992; 31: 18–21.

82. Yachie A, Takano N, Yokoi T, Kato M, Kashahara Y, Miyawaki T, Taniguchi N. The capacity of neonatal leukocytes to produce IL-6 on stimulation assessed by whole blood culture. Pediatr Res 1990; 27:227–233.

83. Schibler KR, Trautman MS, Liechty KW, White WL, Rothstein G, Christensen RD. Diminished transcription of interleukin-8 by monocytes from preterm neonates. J Leukocyte Biol 1993; 53:399–403.

84. Rowen JL, Smith CW, Edwards MS. Group B streptococci elicit leukotriene B4 and interleukin-8 from human monocytes: neonates exhibit a diminished response. J Infect Dis 1995; 172:420–426.

85. Winkelstein JA. The complement system in the fetus and newborn. In: Polin R, Fox W, eds. Fetal and Neonatal Physiology. Philadelphia: Saunders, 1992: 1470–1476.

86. Berger M. Complement deficiency and neutrophil dysfunction as risk factors for bacterial infection in newborns and the role of granulocyte transfusion in therapy. Rev Infect Dis 1990; 12:S401–S409.

87. Zilow G, Zilow EP, Burger R, Linderkamp O. Complement activation in newborn infants with early onset infection. Pediatr Res 1993; 34:199–203.

88. McCracken GH, Eichwald HF. Leukocyte function and the development of opsonic and complement activity in the neonate. Am J Dis Child 1971; 121: 120–126.

89. Anderson DC, Hughes BJ, Edwards MS, Buffone GJ, Baker CJ. Impaired chemotaxigenesis by type III group B streptococci in neonatal sera: relationship to diminished concentration of specific anticapsular antibody and abnormalties of serum complement. Pediatrics 1983; 17:496–502.

90. Gathings WE, Kubagawa H, Cooper MD. A distinctive pattern of B cell immaturity in perinatal humans. Immunol Rev 1981; 57:107–126.

91. Gathings WE, Lawton AR, Cooper MD. Immunofluorescent studies of the development of pre-B cells, B lymphocytes and immunoglobulin isotype diversity in humans. Eur J Immunol 1977; 7:804–810.

92. Kubagawa H, Gathings WE, Levitt D, Kearney JF, Cooper MD. Immunoglobulin isotype expression of normal pre-B cells as determined by immunofluorescence. J Clin Immunol 1982; 2:264–269.

93. Asma GEM, Langlois van den Bergh R, Vossen JM. Development of pre-B and B lymphocytes in the human fetus. Clin Exp Immunol 1984; 56: 407–414.

94. Bofill M, Janossy G, Janossa M, Burford GD, Seymour GJ, Wernet P, Keleman E. Human B cell development. II. Subpopulations in the human fetus. J Immunol 1985; 134:1531–1538.

95. Campana D, Janossy G, Bofill M, Trejdosiewicz LK, Ma D, Hoffbrand AV, Mason DY, Lebacq A-M, Forster HK. Human B cell development. I. Phenotypic differences of B lymphocytes in the bone marrow and peripheral lymphoid tissue. J Immunol 1985; 134:1524–1530.

96. Nahmias A, Stoll B, Hale E, Ibegbu C, Keyserling H, Innis-Whitehouse, W, Holmes R, Spira T, Czerkinsky C, Lee F. IgA-secreting cells in the blood of premature and term infants: normal development and effect of intrauterine infections. Adv Exp Med Biol 1991; 310:59–69.

97. Edwards JA, Durant BM, Jones DB, Evans PR, Smith JL. Differential expression of HLA Class II antigens in fetal human spleen: relationship of HLA-DP, DQ, and DR to immunoglobulin expression. J Immunol 1986; 137: 490–497.

98. Antin JH, Emerson SG, Martin P, Gadol N, Ault KA. Leu-1$^+$ (CD5$^+$) B cells. A major lymphoid subpopulation in human fetal spleen: phenotypic and functional studies. J Immunol 1986; 136:505–510.

99. Bastian JF, Ruedi JM, MacPherson GA, Golembeski HE, O'Connor RD, Thompson LF. Lymphocyte ecto-5'-nucleotidase activity in infancy: increasing activity in peripheral blood B cells precedes their ability to synthesize IgG *in vitro*. J Immunol 1984; 132:1767–1772.

100. Durandy A, de Saint Basile G, Lisowska-Grospierre B, Gauchat JF, Forveille M, Kroczek RA, Bonnefoy JY, Fischer A. Undetectable CD40 ligand expression on T cells and low B cell responses to CD40 binding agonists in human newborns. J Immunol 1995; 154:1560–1568.

101. Miyawaki T, Kubagawa H, Butler VP, Cooper MD. Ig isotypes produced by EBV-transformed B cells as a function of age and tissue distribution. J Immunol 1988; 140:3887–3892.

102. Konowalchuk J, Speirs JI, Perelmutter L. Immunoglobulin properties of Epstein-Barr virus transformed human umbilical cord and adult peripheral blood lymphocytes. Cell Immunol 1982; 67:190–196.

103. Miyawaki T, Moriya N, Nagaoki T, Tanguchi N. Maturation of B-cell differentiation ability and T-cell regulatory function in infancy and childhood. Immunol Rev 1981; 57:63–87.

104. Pittard WB, Miller KM, Sorensen RU. Perinatal influences on in vitro B lymphocyte differentiation in human neonates. Pediatr Res 1985; 19: 655–658.

105. Knutsen AP, Buckley RH. Immunoglobulin synthesis by cord and maternal blood mononuclear cells and their effect on synthesis by normal adult cells. In: Seligmann M, Hitzig W, eds. Primary Immunodeficiencies. Amsterdam: Elsevier North Holland Biomedical Press, 1980:13–22.

106. Miyagawa Y, Sugita K, Komiyama A, Akabane T. Delayed in vitro immunoglobulin production by cord lymphocytes. Pediatrics 1980; 65:497–500.

107. Hayward AR, Lawton AR. Induction of plasma cell differentiation of human fetal lymphocytes: evidence for functional immaturity of T and B cells. J Immunol 1977; 119:1213–1217.

108. Ito S, Lawton AR. Response of human B cells to *Staphylococcus aureus* Cowan I: T- independent proliferation and T-dependent differentiation to immunoglobulin secretion involve subsets separable by rosetting with mouse erythrocytes. J Immunol 1984; 133:1891–1895.

109. Miller KM, Pittard WB, Sorensen RU. Cord blood B cell differentiation. Clin Exp Immunol 1984; 56:415–424.

110. Punnonen J, Aversa GG, Vandekerckhove B, Roncarolo M, DeVries JE. Induction of isotype switching and Ig production by CD5+ and CD10+ human fetal B cells. J Immunol 1992; 148:3398–3404.

111. Rothberg RM. Immunoglobulin and specific antibody synthesis during during the first weeks of life of premature infants. J Pediatr 1969; 75:391–399.

112. Ballow M, Cates KL, Rowe JC, Goetz C, Desbonnet C. Development of the immune system in very low birth weight (less than 1500 g) premature infants: concentrations of plasma immunoglobulins and patterns of infections. Pediatr Res 1986; 9:899–904.

113. Buckley RH, Dees SC, O'Fallon WM. Serum immunoglobulins I. levels in normal children and in uncomplicated childhood allergy. Pediatrics 1968; 41:600–611.

114. Hanson LÅ, Carlsson B, Dahlgren U, Mellander L, Svanborg Eden C. The secretory IgA system in the neonatal period. Ciba Found Symp 1979; 77: 187–204.

115. Bridges RA, Condie RM, Zak SJ, Good RA. The morphologic basis of antibody formation development during the neonatal period. J Lab Clin Med 1959; 53:331–336.

116. Girard JP, de Kalbermatten A. Antibody activity in human duodenal fluid. Eur J Clin Invest 1970; 1:188–195.

117. Cohen AB, Goldberg S, London RL. Immunoglobulins in nasal secretions of infants. Clin Exp Immunol 1970; 6:735–760.

118. Hawworth JC, Dilling L. Concentration of γA-globulin in serum, saliva and nasopharyngeal secretions of infants and children. J Lab Clin Med 1966; 67: 922–933.

119. Burgio GR, Lanzaveccia A, Plebani A, Jaykar S, Ugazio AG. Ontogeny of secretory immunity: levels of secretory IgA and natural antibodies in saliva. Pediatr Res 1980; 14:1111–1114.

120. Burgio GR, Ugazio AG, Notarangelo LD. Immunology of the neonate. Curr Opin Immunol 1990; 2:770–777.

121. van Furth R, Schuit HR, Hijmans W. The immunological development of the human fetus. J Exp Med 1965; 122:1173–1186.

122. Gill TJ, Repetti CF, Metlay LA, Rabin BS, Taylor FH, Thompson DS, Cortese AL. Transplacental immunization of the human fetus to tetanus by immunization of the mother. J Clin Invest 1983; 72:987–996.

123. Mellander L, Carlsson B, Hanson L. Secretory IgA and IgM antibodies to E. coli O and poliovirus type I antigens occur in amniotic fluid, meconium and saliva from newborns. Clin Exp Immunol 1986; 63:555–561.

124. Halsey N, Galazka A. The efficacy of DTP and oral poliomyelitis immunization schedules initiated from birth to 12 weeks of age. Bull World Health Org 1985; 63:1151–1169.

125. Osborn JJ, Dancis J, Julia JF. Studies of the immunology of the human newborn infant. 1. Age and antibody production. Pediatrics 1952; 9:736–744.

126. Kurikka S, Kayhty H, Peltola H, Saarinen L, Eskola J, Makela PH. Neonatal immunization: response to *Haemophilus influenzae* type b-tetanus toxoid conjugate vaccine. Pediatrics 1995; 95:815–822.

127. Makela PH, Peltola H, Kayhty H, Jousimies H, Pettay O, Rouslahti E, Sivonen A, Renkonen OV. Polysaccharide vaccines of group A *Neisseria meningitidis* and *Haemophilis influenzae* type b: a field trial in Finland. J Infect Dis 1977; 190(suppl):57–62.

128. Anderson P, Smith DH, Ingram DL, Wilkins J, Wehrly PF, Howie VM. Antibody of polyribophosphate and *Haemophilus influenzae* type b in infants in children: effect of immunization of polyribophosphate. J Infect Dis 1977; 136(suppl):57–62.

129. Robbins JB, Parke JC, Schneerson R, Whisnant JK. Quantitative measurement of "natural" and immunization-induced *Haemophilus influenzae* type b capsular polysaccharide antibodies. Pediatr Res 1973; 7:103–110.

130. Cates KL, Goetz C, Rosenberg N, Pantschenko A, Rowe JC, Ballow M. Longitudinal development of specific and functional antibody in very low birth weight premature infants. Pediatr Res 1988; 23:14–22.

131. Holt PG. Postnatal maturation of immune competence during infancy and childhood. Pediatr Allergy Immunol 1995; 6:59–70.

132. Wilson CB, Lewis DB, English BK. T cell development in the fetus and neonate. Adv Exp Med Biol 1991; 310:17–27.

133. McDuffie M, Hayward AR. T-cell development. In: Polin R, Fox W, eds. Fetal and Neonatal Physiology. Philadelphia: Saunders, 1992:1427–1438.

134. Lobach DF, Haynes BF. Ontogeny of the human thymus during fetal development. Clin Immunol 1987; 7:81–97.

135. Hofman FM, Modlin RL, Bhoopat L, Taylor CR. Distribution of cells bearing the tac antigen during ontogeny of human lymphoid tissue. J Immunol 1985; 134:3751–3755.

136. Kay HEM, Doe J, Hockley A. Response of human foetal thymocytes to phytohaemagglutinin (PHA). Immunology 1970; 18:393–396.

137. Stites DP, Carr MC, Fudenberg HH. Ontogeny of cellular immunity in the human foetus: development of responses to phytohemagglutinin and to allogeneic cells. Cell Immunol 1974; 11:257–271.

138. Papiernik M. Correlation of lymphocyte transformation and morphology in the human fetal thymus. Blood 1970; 36:470–479.

139. Toivanen P, Uksila J, Leino A, Lassila O, Hirvonen T, Ruuskanen O. Development of mitogen responding T cells and natural killer cells in the human fetus. Immunol Rev 1981; 57:89–105.

140. Rayfield LS, Brent L, Rodeck CH. Development of cell-mediated lympholysis in human foetal blood lymphocytes. Clin Exp Immunol 1980; 42: 561–570.

141. Notarangelo LD, Panina P, Imberti L, Malfa P, Ugazio AG, Albertini A. Neonatal T4$^+$ Lymphocytes: analysis of the expression of 4B4 and 2H4 antigens. Clin Immunol Immunopathol 1988; 46:61–67.

142. Maccario R, Chirico G, Mingrat G, Arico M, Lanfranchi A, Montagna D, Moretta A, Rondini G. Expression of CD45R0 antigen on the surface of resting and activated neonatal T lymphocyte subsets. Biol Neonate 1993; 64: 346–353.

143. Miles EA, Warner JA, Lane AC, Jones AC, Colwell BM, Warner JO. Altered T lymphocyte phenotype at birth in babies born to atopic parents. Pediatr Allergy Immunol 1994; 5:202–208.

144. Morita CT, Parker CM, Brenner MB, Band H. TCR usage and functional capabilities of human gamma delta T cells at birth. J Immunol 1994; 153: 3979–3988.

145. Fuleihan R, Ahern D, Geha RS. Decreased expression of the ligand for CD40 in newborn lymphocytes. Eur J Immunol 1994; 24:1925–1928.

146. Brugnoni D, Airo P, Graf D, Marconi M, Lebowitz M, Plebani A, Giliani, S, Malacarne F, Cattaneo R, Ugazio AG. Ineffective expression of CD40 ligand on cord blood T cells may contribute to poor immunoglobulin production in the newborn. Eur J Immunol 1994; 24:1919–1924.

147. Zola H, Fusco M, Weedon H, MacArdle PJ, Ridings J, Roberton DM. Reduced expression of the interleukin-2-receptor γ chain on cord blood lymphocytes: relationship to functional immaturity of the neonatal immune response. Immunology 1996; 87:86–91.

148. Saito S, Morii T, Umekage H, Makita K, Nishikawa K, Narita N, Ichijo M, Morikawa H, Ishii N, Nakamura M, Sugamura K. Expression of the interleukin-2 receptor gamma chain on cord blood mononuclear cells. Blood 1996; 87:3344–3350.

149. Moretta A, Valtorta A, Chirico G, Chiara A, Bozzola M, De Amici M, Maccaria R. Lymphocyte subpopulations in preterm infants: high percentage of cells expressing P55 chain of Interleukin-2 receptor. Biol Neonate 1991; 59:213–219.

150. Gerli R, Bertotto A, Spinozzi F, Cernetti C, Battaglia A, Falchetti R, Grignani F, Rambotti P. Thymic hormone modulation of CD38 (T10) antigen on

human cord blood lymphocytes. Clin Immunol Immunopathol 1987; 45: 323–332.

151. Griffiths-Chu S, Patterson JAK, Berger CL, Edelson RL, Chu AC. Characterization of immature T cell subpopulations in neonatal blood. Blood 1984; 64:296–300.

152. Maccario R, Ferrari FA, Siena S, Vitiello MA, Martini A, Siccardi AG, Ugazio AG. Receptors for peanut agglutinin on a high percentage of human cord-blood lymphocytes: phenotype characterization of peanut-positive cells. Thymus 1981; 2:229–237.

153. Zola H, Fusco M, MacArdle PJ, Flego L, Robertson D. Expression of cytokine receptors by human cord blood lymphocytes: comparison with adult blood lymphocytes. Pediatr Res 1995; 38:397–403.

154. Yanase Y, Tango T, Okumura K, Tada T, Kawasaki T. Lymphocyte subsets identified by monoclonal antibodies in healthy children. Pediatr Res 1986; 20:1147–1151.

155. Erkeller-Yuksel FM, Deneys V, Yuksel B, Hannet I, Hulstaert F, Hamilton C, Mackinnon H, Turner-Stokes L, Munhyeshuli V, Vanlangendonck F, Bruyere Md, Bach BA, Lydyard PM. Age-related changes in human blood lymphocyte subpopulations. J Pediatr 1992; 120:216–222.

156. The European Collaborative Study. Age-related standards for T lymphocyte subsets based on uninfected children born to human immunodeficiency virus 1-infected women. Pediatr Infect Dis J 1992; 11:1018–1026.

157. Raes M, Alliet P, Gillis P, Zimmermann A, Kortleven J, Magerman K, Peeters V, Rummens JL. Lymphocyte subpopulations in healthy newborn infants: comparison of cord blood values with values five days after birth. J Pediatr 1993; 123:465–467.

158. Kontny U, Barrachina C, Habermehl P, Mannhardt W, Zepp F, Schofer O. Distribution of lymphocyte surface antigens in healthy neonates. Eur J Pediatr 1994; 153:257–259.

159. Slukvin II, Chernishov VP. Two-color flow cytometric analysis of natural killer and cytotoxic T-lymphocyte subsets in peripheral blood of normal human neonates. Biol Neonate 1992; 61:156–161.

160. Comans-Bitter WM, de Groot R, van den Beemd R, Neijens HJ, Hop WCJ, Groeneveld K, Hooikaas H, van Dongen JJM. Immunophenotyping of blood lymphocytes in childhood. J Pediatr 1997; 130:388–393.

161. Carr MC, Stites DP, Fudenberg HH. Cellular immune aspects of the human fetal-maternal relationship. I. *In vitro* response of cord blood lymphocytes to phytohemagglutinin. Cell Immunol 1972; 5:21–29.

162. Ceppellini R, Bonnard GD, Coppo F, Miggiano VC, Pospisil M, Curtoni ES, Pellegrino M. Mixed leukocyte cultures and HL-A antigens. I. Reactivity of young fetuses, newborns and mothers at delivery. Transplant Proc 1971; 3: 58–70.

163. Pirenne H, Aujard Y, Eliaafari A, Bourillon A, Oury JF, LeGac S, Blot P, Sterkers G. Comparison of T cell functional changes during childhood with

the ontogeny of CDw29 and CD45RA expression on CD4 $^+$ cells. Pediatr Res 1992; 32:81–86.

164. Stern DA, Hicks MJ, Martinez FD, Holberg CJ, Wright AL, Pinnas J, Halonen M, Taussig LM. Lymphocyte subpopulation number and function in infancy. Dev Immunol 1992; 2:175–179.

165. Montagna D, Moretta A, Marconi M, Mingrat G, Gasparoni A, Giarola M, Maccario R. In vivo activated cord blood lymphocytes express high affinity interleukin-2 receptor: evaluation of their responsiveness to in vitro stimulation with recombinant interleukin-2. Biol Neonate 1992; 62:385–394.

166. Gerli R, Bertotto A, Crupi S, Arcangeli C, Marinelli I, Spinozzi F, Gernetti C, Angelella P, Rambotti P. Activation of cord T lymphocytes. I. Evidence for a defective T cell mitogenesis induced through the CD2 molecule. J Immunol 1989; 142:2583–2589.

167. Bertotto A, Gerli R, Lanfrancone L, Crupi S, Arcangeli C, Cernetti C, Spinozzi F, Rambotti P. Activation of cord T lymphocytes. II. Cellular and molecular analysis of the defective response induced by anti-CD3 monoclonal antibody. Cell Immunol 1990; 127:247–259.

168. Papadogiannakis N, Johnson SA, Olding LB. Monocyte regulated hyporesponsiveness of human cord blood lymphocytes to OKT3 Mo-Ab-induced mitogenesis. Scand J Immunol 1986; 23:91–99.

169. Hassan J, Reen DJ. Interleukin-1 augments the diminished interleukin-2 mRNA expression and proliferative response of neonatal T lymphocytes to anti-CD2 antibodies. Scand J Immunol 1994; 39:597–601.

170. Bussel JB, Cunningham Rundles S, LaGamma EF, Shellabarger M. Analysis of lymphocyte proliferative response subpopulations in very low birth weight infants and during the first 8 weeks of life. Pediatr Res 1988; 23:457–462.

171. Leino A, Ruuskanen O, Kero P, Eskola J, Toivanen P. Depressed Phytohemagglutinin and concanavalin A responses in premature infants. Clin Immunol Immunopathol 1981; 19:260–267.

172. Noyes BE, Kurland G, Orenstein DM, Fricker FJ, Armitage JM. Experience with pediatric lung transplantation. J Pediatr 1994; 124:261–268.

173. Herrod HG, Cooke RJ, Valenski WR, Herman J, Dockter ME. Evaluation of lymphocyte phenotype and phytohemagglutinin response in healthy very low birth weight infants. Clin Immunol Immunopathol 1991; 60:268–277.

174. Kavelaars A, Zijlstra J, Bakker JM, Van Rees EP, Visser GH, Zegers BJ, Heijnen CJ. Increased dexamethasone sensitivity of neonatal leukocytes: different mechanisms of glucocorticoid inhibition of T cell proliferation in adult and neonatal cells. Eur J Immunol 1995; 25:1346–1351.

175. Olding LB, Oldstone MBA. Lymphocytes from human newborns abrogate mitosis of their mother's lymphocytes. Nature 1974; 249:161–162.

176. Unander AM, Olding LB. Ontogeny and postnatal persistence of a strong suppressor activity in man. J Immunol 1981; 127:1182–1186.

177. Miyawaki T, Moriya N, Nagaoki T, Kubo M, Yokoi T, Taniguchi N. Mode of action of humoral suppressor factor derived from pokeweed mitogen-

stimulated cord T cells on adult B cell differentiation. J Immunol 1981; 126: 282–285.

178. Rodriguez MA, Bankhurst AD, Ceuppens JL, Williams RC. Characterization of the suppressor cell activity in human cord blood lymphocytes. J Clin Invest 1981; 68:1577–1585.

179. Hayward AR, Merrill D. Requirement for OKT8+ suppressor cell proliferation for suppression by human newborn T cells. Clin Exp Immunol 1981; 45:468–474.

180. Yachie A, Miyawaki T, Nagaoki T, Yokoi T, Mukai M, Uwadana N, Taniguchi N. Regulation of B cell differentiation by T cell subsets defined with monoclonal OKT4 and OKT8 antibodies in human cord blood. J Immunol 1981; 127:1314–1317.

181. Papadogiannakis N, Johnsen S, Olding LB. Human fetal/neonatal suppressor activity: relation between OKT phenotypes and sensitivity to prostaglandin E_2 in maternal and neonatal lymphocytes. Am J Reprod Immunol 1985; 9: 105–110.

182. Jacoby DR, Oldstone MBA. Delineation of suppressor and helper activity within the OKT4-defined T lymphocyte subset in human newborns. J Immunol 1983; 131:1765–1770.

183. Cheng H, Delespesse G. Evaluation of the functional maturity of newborn T8+ suppressor cells and the resistance of newborn lymphocytes to suppression. Am J Reprod Immunol Microbiol 1986; 11:1–5.

184. Cheng H, Delespesse G. Human cord blood suppressor T lymphocytes. II. Characterization of inducer of suppressor cells. Am J Reprod Immunol Microbiol 1986; 11:39–43.

185. Morito T, Bankhurst AD, Williams RC. Studies of human cord blood and adult lymphocyte interactions with in vitro immunoglobulin production. J Clin Invest 1979; 64:990–995.

186. Dwyer JM, Johnson C. Comparative analysis of the suppression by cord blood mononuclear cells of adult and neonatal lymphocytes. Cell Immunol 1983; 81:81–87.

187. Papadogiannakis N, Johnsen S, Olding LB. Strong prostaglandin associated suppression of the proliferation of human maternal lymphocytes by neonatal lymphocytes linked to T verses T cell interactions and differential PGE_2 sensitivity. Clin Exp Immunol 1984; 61:125–134.

188. Johnsen S, Olding LB, Westberg NG, Wilhelmsson L. Strong suppression by mononuclear leukocytes from human newborns on maternal leukocytes: mediation by prostaglandins. Clin Immunol Immunopathol 1982; 23: 606–615.

189. Papadogiannakis N, Johnsen SA. Mitogenic action of phorbol ester TPA and calcium ionophore A23187 on human cord and maternal/adult peripheral lymphocytes: regulation by prostaglandin E_2. Clin Exp Immunol 1987; 70: 173–181.

190. Splawski JB, Lipsky PE. Cytokine regulation of immunoglobulin secretion by neonatal lymphocytes. J Clin Invest 1991; 88:667–677.

191. Bryson YJ, Winter HS, Gard SE, Fischer TJ, Stiehm ER. Deficiency of immune interferon production by leukocytes of normal newborns. Cell Immunol 1980; 55:191–200.
192. Miyawaki T, Seki H, Taga K, Sato H, Taniguchi N. Dissociated production of interleukin-2 and immune (gamma) interferon by phytohaemaglutinin stimulated lymphocytes in healthy infants. Clin Exp Immunol 1985; 59: 505–511.
193. Frenkel L, Bryson YJ. Ontogeny of phytohemagglutinin-induced gamma interferon by leukocytes of healthy infants and children: evidence for decreased production in infants less than 2 months of age. J Pediatr 1987; 111:97–100.
194. Lewis DB, Yu CC, Meyer J, English BK, Kahn SJ, Wilson CB. Cellular and molecular mechanisms for reduced interleukin 4 and interferon-gamma production by neonatal T cells. J Clin Invest 1991; 87:194–202.
195. Taylor S, Bryson YJ. Impaired production of gamma-interferon by newborn cells in vitro is due to a functionally immature macrophage. J Immunol 1985; 134:1493–1497.
196. Burchett SK, Corey L, Mohan KM, Westall J, Ashley R, Wilson CB. Diminished interferon-gamma and lymphocyte proliferation in neonatal and postpartum primary herpes simplex virus infection. J Infect Dis 1992; 165: 813–818.
197. Stephens S, Duffy SW, Page C. A longitudinal study of gamma-interferon production by peripheral blood mononuclear cells from breast- and bottle-fed infants. Clin Exp Immunol 1986; 65:396–400.
198. Wu CY, Demeure C, Kiniwa M, Gately M, Delespesse G. IL-12 induces the production of IFN-gamma by neonatal CD4 T cells. J Immunol 1993; 151: 1938–1949.
199. Watson W, Oen K, Ramdahin R, Harman C. Immunoglobulin and cytokine production by neonatal lymphocytes. Clin Exp Immunol 1991; 83:169–174.
200. Hassan J, Reen DJ. Reduced primary antigen-specific T-cell precursor frequencies in neonates is associated with deficient interleukin-2 production. Immunology 1996; 87:604–608.
201. Winter HS, Gard SE, Fischer TJ, Bryson YJ, Stiehm ER. Deficient lymphokine production of newborn lymphocytes. Pediatr Res 1983; 17:573–578.
202. Uksila J, Lassila O, Hirvonen T, Toivanen P. Natural killer cell function of human neonatal lymphocytes. J Immunol 1983; 130:153–156.
203. Ueno Y, Miyawaki T, Seki H, Matsuda A, Taga K, Sato H, Taniguchi N. Differential effects of recombinant human interferon-γ and interleukin 2 on natural killer cell activity of peripheral blood in early human development. J Immunol 1985; 135:180–184.
204. Phillips JH, Hori T, Nagler A, Bhat N, Spits H, Lanier LL. Ontogeny of human natural killer (NK) cells: fetal NK cells mediate cytolytic function and express cytoplasmic CD3ϵ,δ proteins. J Exp Med 1992; 175:1055–1066.
205. Antonelli P, Stewart W, Dupont B. Distribution of natural killer cell activity in peripheral blood, cord blood, thymus, lymph nodes, and spleen and the

effect of *in vitro* treatment with interferon preparation. Clin Immunol Immunopathol 1981; 19:161–169.

206. Kaplan J, Shope TC, Bollinger RO, Smith J. Human newborns are deficient in natural killer activity. J Clin Immunol 1982; 2:350–355.

207. Uksila J, Lassila O, Hirvonen T. Natural killer cell function of human neonatal lymphocytes. Clin Exp Immunol 1982; 48:649–654.

208. Lubens RG, Gard SE, Soderberg-Warner M, Stiehm ER. Lectin-dependent T-lymphocyte and natural killer cytotoxic deficiencies in human newborns. Cell Immunol 1982; 74:40–53.

209. Sancho L, de la Hera A, Casas J, Vaquer S, Martinez C, Alvarez-Mon M. Two different maturational stages of natural killer lymphocytes in human newborn infants. J Pediatr 1991; 119:446–454.

210. Abo T, Miller CA, Balch CM. Characterization of human granular lymphocyte subpopulations expressing HNK-1 (leu-7) and Leu-11 antigens in the blood and lymphoid tissues from fetuses, neonates, and adults. Eur J Immunol 1984; 14:616–623.

211. Sancho L, Martinez-A C, Nogales A, de la Hera A. Reconstitution of natural-killer-cell activity in the newborn by interleukin-2. N Engl J Med 1985; 314: 57–58.

212. Hallberg A, Malström P. Natural killer cell activity and antibody-dependent cellular cytotoxicity in newborn infants. Acta Paediatr Scand 1982; 71: 431–436.

213. Xanthou M, Mandyla-Sfagou H, Economou-Mavrou C, Matsaniotis N. Cytotoxicity of lymphocytes in the newborn. Arch Dis Child 1981; 56:377–381.

214. Montagna D, Maccario R, Ugazio AG, Mingrat G, Burgio GR. Natural cytotoxicity in the neonate: high levels of lymphokine activated killer (LAK) activity. Clin Exp Immunol 1988; 71:177–181.

215. Conley ME. Molecular genetic analysis of X-linked immunodeficiencies. In: Turhorst C, Malavasi F, Albertini A, eds. Generation of Antibody by Cells and Gene Immortalization. Vol. 7, Basal: Karger, 1993: 162–167.

216. Fischer A, Arnaiz-Villena A. Immunodeficiencies of genetic origin. Immunol Today 1995; 16:510–514.

217. Bruton OC. Agammaglobulinemia. Pediatrics 1952; 9:722–728.

218. WHO Scientific Group. Primary immunodeficiency diseases: report of a WHO scientific group. Clin Exp Immunol 1995; 99:1–24.

219. Pearl ER, Vogler LB, Okos AJ, Crist WM, Lawton AR, Cooper MD. B lymphocyte precursors in human bone marrow: an analysis of normal individuals and patients with antibody deficiency states. J Immunol 1978; 120: 1169–1175.

220. Tsukada S, Saffran DC, Rawlings DJ, Parolini O, Allen RC, Kilsak I, Sparkes RB, Kubagawa H, Mohandas T, Quan S, Belmont JW, Cooper MD, Conley ME, Witte ON. Deficient expression of a B cell cytoplasmic tyrosine kinase in human X-linked agammaglobulinemia. Cell 1993; 72:279–290.

221. Vetrie D, Vorechovsky I, Sideras P, Holland J, Davies A, Flinter F, Hammarstrom L, Kinnon C, Levinsky R, Bobrow M, Smith CIE, Bentley DR.

The gene involved in X-linked agammaglobulinaemia is a member of the src family of protein-tyrosine kinases. Nature 1993; 361:226–233.

222. Lederman HM, Winkelstein JA. X-linked agammaglobulinemia: an analysis of 96 patients. Medicine 1985; 64:145–156.

223. McKinney RE, Katz SL, Wilfert CM. Chronic enteroviral meningoencephalitis in agammaglobulinemic patients. Rev Infect Dis 1987; 9:334–356.

224. Wright PF, Milford HH, Kasselberg AG, Lowry SP, Wadlington WB, Karzon DT. Vaccine-associated poliomyelitis in a child with sex-linked agammaglobulinemia. J Pediatr 1977; 91:408–412.

225. Lavilla P, Gill A, Rodriguez MCG, Dupla ML, Pintado V, Fontan G. X-linked agammaglobulinemia and gastric adenocarcinoma. Cancer 1993; 72:1528–1531.

226. van der Meer JWM, Weening RS, Schellekens PTA, Van Munster IP, Nagengast FM. Colorectal cancer in patients with X-linked agammaglobulinemia. Lancet 1993; 341:1439–1440.

227. Siegal FP, Pernis B, Kunkel HG. Lymphocytes in human immunodeficiency states: a study of membrane associated immunoglobulins. Eur J Immunol 1971; 1:482–491.

228. Cooper MD, Lawton AR, Bockman DE. Agammaglobulinemia with B lymphocytes: specific defect of plasma-cell differentiation. Lancet 1971; ii:791–794.

229. Campana D, Farrant J, Inamdar N, Webster ADB, Janossy G. Phenotypic features and proliferative activity of B cell progenitors in X-linked agammaglobulinemia. J Immunol 1990; 145:1675–1680.

230. Crockard AD, Boyd NAM, McNeill TA, McCluskey DR. CD4 lymphocyte subset abnormalities associated with impaired delayed cutaneous hypersensitivity reactions in patients with X-linked agammaglobulinemia. Clin Exp Immunol 1992; 88:29–34.

231. Di Santo JP, Bonnefoy JY, Gauchat JF, Fischer A, de Saint Basile G. CD40 ligand mutations in X-linked immunodeficiency with hyper IgM. Nature 1993; 361:541–543.

232. Allen RC, Armitage RJ, Conley ME, Rosenblatt H, Jenkins NA, Copeland NG, Bedell MA, Edelhoff S, Disteche CM, Simoneaux DK, Fanslow WC, Belmont J, Spriggs MK. CD40 ligand gene defects responsible for X-linked hyper IgM syndrome. Science 1993; 259:990–993.

233. Conley ME, Larche M, Bonagura VR, Lawton AR, Buckley RH, Fu SM, Coustan-Smith E, Herrod HG, Campana D. Hyper IgM syndrome associated with defective CD40-mediated B cell activation. J Clin Invest 1994; 94:1404–1409.

234. Storb R, Thomas ED, Buckner CD, Appelbaum FR, Clift RA, Deeg HJ, Doney K, Hanson JA, Prentice RL, Sanders JE, Stewart P, Sullivan KM, Witherspoon RP. Marrow transplantation for aplastic anemia. Semin Hematol 1984; 21:27–35.

235. Tiller TL, Buckley RH. Transient hypogammaglobulinemia of infancy: review of the literature, clinical and immunologic features of 11 new cases, and long-term follow-up. J Pediatr 1978; 92:347–353.

236. Walker AM, Kemp AS, Hill DJ, Shelton MJ. Features of transient hypogammaglobulinemia in infants screened for immunologic abnormalities. Arch Dis Child 1994; 70:183–186.

237. McGeady SJ. Transient hypogammaglobulinemia of infancy: need to reconsider name and definition. J Pediatr 1987; 110:47–50.

238. Buckley RH, Sampson HA. The hyperimmunoglobulinemia E syndrome. In: Franklin EC, ed. Clinical Immunology Update. New York: Elsevier North-Holland, 1981:147–167.

239. Stone BD, Wheeler JG. Disseminated cryptococcal infection in a patient with hyperimmunoglobulinemia E syndrome. J Pediatr 1990; 117:92–95.

240. Paganelli R, Scala E, Capobianchi MR, Fanales-Belasio E, D'Offizi G, Fiorilli M, Aiuti F. Selective deficiency of interferon-gamma production in the hyper IgE syndrome. Relationship to in vitro IgE synthesis. Clin Exp Immunol 1991; 84:28–33.

241. King CL, Gallin JI, Malech HL, Abramson SL, Nutman TB. Regulation of immunoglobulin production in hyperimmunoglobulin E recurrent infection syndrome by interferon. Proc. Natl. Acad. Sci. USA 1989; 86:10085–10089.

242. Buckley RH, Schiff SE, Schiff RI, Roberts JL, Markert ML, Peters W, Williams LW, Ward FE. Haploidentical bone marrow stem cell transplantation in human severe combined immunodeficiency. Semin Hematol 1993; 30: 92–104.

243. Omenn GS. Familial reticuloendotheliosis with eosinophilia. N Engl J Med 1965; 273:427–432.

244. Businco L, Di Frazio A, Ziruolo MG, Boner AL, Valletta EA, Ruco LP, Vitolo D, Ensoli B, Paganelli R. Clinical and immunologic findings in four infants with Omenn's syndrome: a form of severe combined immunodeficiency with phenotypically normal T cells, elevated IgE, and eosinophilia. Clin Immunol Immunopathol 1987; 44:123–133.

245. Trojak JE, Polmar SH, Winkelstein JA, Hsu S, Francomano C, Pierce GF, Scillian JJ, Gale AN, McKusick VA. Immunologic studies of cartilage-hair hypoplasia in the Amish. Johns Hopkins Med J 1981; 148:157–164.

246. Polmar SH, Pierce GF. Cartilage hair hypoplasia: immunological aspects and their clinical implications. Clin Immunol Immunopathol 1986; 40:87–93.

247. Steele RW, Britton HA, Anderson CT, Kniker WT. Severe combined immunodeficiency with cartilage-hair hypoplasia: in vitro response to thymosin and attempted reconstitution. Pediatr Res 1976; 10:1003–1005.

248. Stephan JL, Vlekova V, Le Deist F, Blanche S, Donadieu J, de Saint-Basile G, Durandy A, Griscelli C, Fischer A. Severe combined immunodeficiency: a retrospective single-center study of clinical presentation and outcome in 117 patients. J Pediatr 1993; 123:564–572.

249. Conley ME, Buckley RH, Hong R, Guerra-Hanson C, Roifman CM, Brochstein JA, Pahwa S, Puck JM. X-linked severe combined immunodeficiency.

Diagnosis in males with sporadic severe combined immunodeficiency and clarification of clinical findings. J Clin Invest 1990; 85:1548–1554.

250. Sindel LJ, Buckley RH, Schiff SE, Ward FE, Mickey GH, Huang AT, Naspitz C, Koren H. Severe combined immunodeficiency with natural killer cell predominance: abrogation of graft-versus-host disease and immunologic reconstitution with HLA-identical bone marrow cells. J Allergy Clin Immunol 1984; 73:829–836.

251. Barrett MJ, Buckley RH, Schiff SE, Kidd PC, Ward FE. Accelerated development of immunity following transplantation of maternal stem cells into infants with severe combined immunodeficiency and transplacentally acquired lymphoid chimerism. Clin Exp Immunol 1988; 72:118–123.

252. Buckley RH. Advances in the correction of immunodeficiency by bone marrow transplantation. Pediatr Ann 1987; 16:412–421.

253. O'Reilly RJ, Keever C, Kernan NA, Brochstein J, Collins N, Flomenberg N, Laver J, Emanuel D, Dupont B, Castro-Malaspina H, Gulati S. HLA-nonidentical T cell depleted marrow transplants: A comparison of results in patients treated for leukemia and severe combined immunodeficiency disease. Transplant Proc 1987; 19:55–60.

254. Dror Y, Gallagher R, Wara DW, Colombe BW, Merino A, Benkerrou M, Cowan MJ. Immune reconstitution in severe combined immunodeficiency disease after lectin-treated, T cell depleted haplocompatible bone marrow transplantation. Blood 1993; 81:2021–2030.

255. Fischer A. Severe combined immunodeficiencies. Immunodefic Rev 1992; 3:83–100.

256. Buckley RH. Bone marrow transplantation in primary immunodeficiency. In: Rich RR, ed. Clinical Immunology: Principles and Practice. St. Louis: Mosby, 1995:1813–1830.

257. Hershfield MS, Buckley RH, Greenberg ML, Melton AL, Schiff RI, Hatem C, Kurtzberg J, Markert ML, Kobayashi RH, Kobayashi AL, Abuchowski A. Treatment of adenosine deaminase deficiency with polyethylene glycol-modified adenosine deaminase (PEG-ADA). N Engl J Med 1987; 316:589–596.

258. Hague RA, Rassam S, Morgan G, Cant AJ. Early diagnosis of severe combined immunodeficiency syndrome. Arch Dis Child 1994; 70:260–263.

259. DiGeorge AM. Discussions on a new concept of the cellular base of immunology. J Pediatr 1965; 67:907.

260. Lischner HW, Huff DS. T cell deficiency in DiGeorge syndrome. In: Bergsma D, Good RA, Finstad J, Paul NW, eds. Immunodeficiency in Man and Animals. Sunderland, MA: Sinauer Associates, 1975:16–21.

261. Conley ME, Beckwith JB, Mancer JFK, Tenckhoff L. The spectrum of DiGeorge syndrome. J Pediatr 1979; 94:883–890.

262. Greenberg F. DiGeorge syndrome: an historical review of clinical and cytogenetic features. J Med Genet 1993; 30:803–806.

263. Bastian J, Law S, Vogler LB, Lawton A, Herrod HG, Anderson SD, Horowitz SD, Hong R. Prediction of persistent immunodeficiency in the DiGeorge anomaly. J Pediatr 1989; 115:391–396.

264. Sullivan KE, Mullen CA, Blaese RM, Winkelstein JA. A multiinstitutional survey of the Wiskott-Aldrich syndrome. J Pediatr 1994; 125:876–885.

265. Molina IJ, Sancho J, Terhorst C, Rosen FS, Remold-O'Donnell E. T cells of patients with the Wiskott-Aldrich syndrome have a restricted defect in proliferative responses. J Immunol 1993; 151:4383–4390.

266. Mullen CA, Anderson KD, Blaese RM. Splenectomy and/or bone marrow transplantation in the management of the Wiskott-Aldrich syndrome: long-term follow-up of 62 cases. Blood 1993; 82:2961–2966.

267. Schlesinger I. Ataxia telangiectasia: a familial multisystem disorder. Conn Med 1989; 53:135–137.

268. Gatti RA, Boder E, Vinters HV, Sparkes RS, Norman A, Lange K. Ataxia-telangiectasia: an interdisciplinary approach to pathogenesis. Medicine 1991; 70:99–117.

269. Pohl KRE, Farley JD, Jan JE, Junker AK. Ataxia-telangiectasia in a child with vaccine-associated paralytic poliomyelitis. J Pediatr 1992; 121: 405–497.

270. Schwartzman JS, Sole D, Naspitz CK. Ataxia-telangiectasia: a clinical and laboratory review study of 14 cases. Allergol Immunopathol 1990; 18: 105–111.

271. Pippard EC, Hall AJ, Barker DJ, Bridges BA. Cancer in homozygotes and heterozygotes of ataxia-telangiectasia and xeroderma pigmentosum in Britain. Cancer Res 1988; 48:2929–2932.

272. Swift M, Sholman L, Perry M. Malignant neoplasms in the families of patients with ataxia-telangiectasia. Cancer Res 1976; 36:209–215.

273. Swift M, Morrell D, Massey RB, Chase CL. Incidence of cancer in 161 families affected by ataxia telangiectasia. N Engl J Med 1991; 325: 18831–1836.

274. Savitsky K, Bar-Shira A, Gilad S, Rotman G, Ziv Y, Vanagaite L, Tagle DA, Smith S, Uziel T, Sfez S, Ashkenazi M, Pecker I, Frydman M, Harnik R, Patanjali SR, Simmons A, Clines GA, Sartiel A, Gatti RA, Chessa L, Sanal O, Lavin MF, Jaspers NGJ, Taylor AMR, Arlett CF, Miki T, Weissman SM, Lovett M, Collins FS, Shiloh Y. A single ataxia telangiectasia gene with a product similar to PI-3 kinase. Science 1995; 268:1749–1753.

275. Baehner RL. Chronic granulomatous disease of childhood: clinical, pathological, biochemical, molecular and genetic aspects of the disease. Pediatr Pathol 1990; 10:143–153.

276. Weening RS, Corbeel L, de Boer M, Lutter R, van Zwieten R, Hamers MN, Roos D. Cytochrome b deficiency in an autosomal form of chronic granulomatous disease. J Clin Invest 1985; 75:915–920.

277. Volpp BD, Nauseef WN, Clark RA. Two cytosolic neutrophil oxidase components absent in autosomal recessive chronic granulomatous disease. Science 1988; 242:1295–1297.

278. Curnutte JT, Berkow RL, Roberts RL, Shurin SB, Scott PJ. Chronic granulomatous disease due to a defect in the cytosolic factor required for nicotinamide adenine dinucleotide phosphate oxidase activation. J Clin Invest 1988; 81:606–610.

279. Clark RA, Maclegh HL, Gallin JI, Nunoi H, Volpp BD, Pearson DW, Nauseef WM, Curnutte JT. Genetic variants of chronic granulomatous disease: prevalence of deficiencies of two cytosolic components of the NADPH oxidase system. N Engl J Med 1989; 321:647–652.

280. Muoy R, Fischer A, Vilmer E, Seger R, Griscelli C. Incidence, severity, and prevention of infections in chronic granulomatous disease. J Pediatr 1989; 114:555–560.

281. Curnutte JT. Chronic granulomatous disease: the solving of a clinical riddle at the molecular level. Clin Immunol Immunopathol 1993; 67:S2–S15.

282. Seger RA, Ezekowitz RAB. Treatment of chronic granulomatous disease. Immunodeficiency 1994; 5:113–130.

283. Danziger RN, Goren AT, Becker J, Greene JM, Douglas SD. Outpatient management with oral corticosteroid therapy for obstructive conditions in chronic granulomatous disease. J Pediatr 1993; 122:303–305.

284. Walther MM, Malech H, Berman A, Choyke P, Venzon DJ, Linehan WM, Gallin JI. The urological manifestations of chronic granulomatous disease. J Urol 1992; 147:1314–1318.

285. Borregaard N, Cross AR, Herlin T, Jones OT, Segal AW, Valerius NH. A variant form of X-linked chronic granulomatous disease with normal nitroblue tetrazolium slide test and cytochrome b. Eur J Clin Invest 1983; 13: 243–247.

286. Quie PG, Abramson JS. Disorders of the polymorphonuclear phagocyte system. In: Stiehm ER, ed. Immunological Diseases in Infants and Children. 3d ed. Philadelphia: Saunders, 1989:343–363.

287. Neijens JJ, Frenkel J, de Muink Keizer-Schrama SMPF, Dzolijic-Danilovic G, Meradij M, van Dongen JJM. Invasive *Aspergillus* infection in chronic granulomatous disease: treatment with itraconazole. J Pediatr 1989; 115: 1016–1019.

288. Spencer DA, John P, Ferryman SR, Weller PH, Darbyshire P. Successful treatment of invasive pulmonary aspergillosis in chronic granulomatous disease with orally administered itraconazole suspension. Crit Care Med 1994; 149:239–241.

289. Kline MW, Bocobo FC, Paul ME, Rosenblatt HM, Shearer WT. Successful medical therapy of *Aspergillus* osteomyelitis of the spine in an 11-year-old boy with chronic granulomatous disease. Pediatrics 1994; 93:830–835.

290. Rosh JR, Tang HB, Mayer L, Groisman G, Abraham SK, Prince A. Treatment of intractable gastrointestinal manifestations of chronic granulomatous disease with cyclosporin. J Pediatr 1996; 126:143–145.

291. International Chronic Granulomatous Disease Cooperative Study Group. A controlled trial of interferon gamma to prevent infection in chronic granulomatous disease. N Engl J Med 1991; 324:509.

292. Ezekowitz RAB, Dinauer MC, Jaffe HS, Orkin SH, Newburger PE. Partial correction of the phagocyte defect in patients with X-linked chronic granulomatous disease by subcutaneous interferon-gamma. N Engl J Med 1988; 319:146–151.

293. Sechler JMG, Malech HL, White CJ, Gallin JI. Recombinant human interferon-gamma reconstitutes defective phagocyte function in patients with chronic granulomatous disease of childhood. Proc Natl Acad Sci USA 1988; 85:4874–4878.

294. Woodman RC, Erickson RW, Rae J, Jaffe HS, Curnutte JT. Prolonged recombinant interferon-gamma therapy in chronic granulomatous disease: evidence against enhanced neutrophil oxidase activity. Blood 1992; 79: 1558–1562.

295. Anderson DC, Schmalsteig FC, Finegold MJ, Hughes BJ, Rothlein R, Miller LJ, Kohl S, Tosi MF, Jacobs RL, Waldrop TC, Goldman AS, Shearer WT, Springer TA. The severe and moderate phenotypes of heritable Mac-1, LFA-1deficiency: their quantitative definition and relation to leukocyte dysfunction and clinical features. J Infect Dis 1985; 152:668–689.

296. Ross GD. Clinical and laboratory features of patients with an inherited deficiency of neutrophil membrane complement receptor type 3 (CR3) and the related membrane antigens LFA-1 and p150,95. J Clin Immunol 1986; 6: 107–113.

297. Fischer A, Lisowska-Grospierre B, Anderson DC, Springer TA. Leukocyte adhesion deficiency: molecular basis and functional consequences. Immunodefic Rev 1988; 1:39–54.

298. Le Deist F, Blanche S, Keable H, Gaud C, Pham H, Descamp-Latscha B, Wahn V, Griscelli C, Fischer A. Successful HLA nonidentical bone marrow transplantation in three patients with leukocyte adhesion deficiency. Blood 1989; 74:512–516.

299. Fishbein JD, Bruggers CS, Friedman NJ, Graham MJ, Kurtzberg J. A seven-month-old infant with fever and neutrophilic leukocytosis. J Pediatr 1992; 120:819–824.

AUTHOR INDEX

Italic numbers give the page on which the complete reference is listed.

A

Aarli, J. A., 607, *630*
Aaronson, D. W., 887, *898*
Aaseth, J., 624, *635*
Abbate, R., 12, *23*
Abboud, R., 452, 460, *464*
Abboud, T., 188, *217*
Abdin, Z., 863, *892*
Abdul-Karim, R., 10, *21*
Abel, S. R., 173, *204*
Åberg, N., 660, *672, 678, 696*
Aberg, N., 768, 781, *802, 806*
Abernathy, R. S., 67, *71*
Abernathy-Carver, K. J., 875, *895*
Abo, T., 949, *984*
Abouleish, E., 181, *210*
Abous-Shala, N., 479, *485*
Abraham, G. E., 7, *20*
Abraham, R. A., 287, *308*, 323, 327, *329*
Abraham, S. K., 969, *989*
Abramovici, A., 191, *220*
Abrams, D. I., 584, *599*
Abramsky, O., 560, *564*
Abramson, J. S., 930, 968, *971, 989*

Abramson, S. B., 504, *515*
Abramson, S. L., 960, *986*
Abuchowski, A., 963, *987*
Aburto, H., 345, *364*
Acheson, F., 40, *54*
Ackerman, S. J., 875, *895*
ACOG Technical Bulletin, 558, 559, *564*
Adam, P. A. J., 381, *384*
Adams, E. J., 800, *811*
Adams, E. R., 190, *219*
Adams, J., 572, 588, *592*
Adams, K. F., 196, *224*
Adams, R. H., 10, *21*
Adams, R. W., *70*
Adamson, J. S., Jr., 194, *221*
Adamson, K., 40, 42, *54*
Adamsons, K., 179, *209*
Adcock, E. W., III, 14, *24*
Addis, G. J., 182, *212*
Addison, I. E., 933, *974*
Adelroth, E., 411, *462*
Ades, A. E., 580, *598*
Adinolfi, M., 108, *113*
Adkinson, N. F., 271, 272, *278*
Adler, A. F., 447, *463*

Barnett, M. A., *96*
Barno, A., 63, *92*
Baron, A. E., *521*
Baron, R. C., 67, *94*
Barquinero, J., 506, *516*
Barr, A., 190, *219*
Barr, L. W., 718, 725, 728, 730, *755*
Barr, M., 139, *154*
Barrachina, C., 946, *980*
Barrell, E., 843, *858*
Barrett, D. J., 619, *634*
Barrett, M. E., 128, *136*
Barrett, M. J., 963, *987*
Barrett, T. E., 479, *485*
Barrier, G., 188, *217*
Barriga, C., *98*
Barrington, R. A., 524, 532, *543*
Barron, B. A., 172, *203*
Barron, W. M., 453, *465*, 472, *484*, 503, *514*
Barrueto, L., 817, *851*
Barry, R. M., *95*
Barry, W., 843, *858*
Barsh, E., 435, *443*
Bar-Shira, A., 966, *988*
Barsi, I., 534, *547*
Bartecchi, C. E., 789, *809*
Bartels, H., 63, *69*
Bartfay-Szabo, A., 11, *21*
Barth, R., 267, *277*, 713, 714, 715, 716, 728, 732, *752*, *754*, 781, 783, 788, *806*, *811*
Bartlett, J. A., 582, 585, *598*
Barton, J. R., 51, *55*, 397, *400*, 487, 488, *496*
Barton, M., 40, 42, *54*, 766, 774, *804*
Barton, M. D., 179, *209*
Barton, P. L., *521*
Bartus, S., *95*, 531, *546*
Barzilai, 540, *550*
Bass, A. D., 194, *222*
Bassi, 716, *755*
Bastian, J., 939, 964, *976*, *988*
Bastian, L., 572, 588, *592*
Bastide, M., 559, *564*

Bataineh, A. S., 344, *364*
Batra, V. K., 190, *219*
Battaglia, A., 945, *979*
Battaglia, F. C., 14, *24*
Batter, V., 578, 579, 586, *596*
Batton, D. G., 174, 175, *207*
Bauchner, H., 123, 128, 130, *134*
Baudin, M., 146, *155*
Bauer, C. R., 494, *496*
Bauer, M., 585, *601*
Bauman, A., 678, *696*
Bavoux, F., 147, *155*
Bawdon, R. E., 191, *220*, 578, *597*
Bax, J., 628, *636*
Baxi, L. V., 176, *208*, 294, *310*
Baxter, B. D., 60, *91*
Baxter, G., 577, *595*
Baxter, H., 173, *204*
Baxter, J. D., 13, *24*
Baxter, R. C., 15, *24*
Bayard, F., 452, *465*, 528, *544*
Bayle, I. T., 18, *25*
Bayliss, D. A., 64, *70*
Bazan, T. S., 933, *974*
Bazaral, M., 659, *671*
Bazin, B., 572, 581, 584, *592*
Bazin, H., 692, *701*
Bazubagira, A., 575, 577, 586, *595*, *602*
Beach, J. E., 185, *214*
Beall, M. H., 183, *213*
Beard, R. W., 647, *652*
Beasley, R., 430, *442*
Beatty, P. G., 617, *633*
Beaty, T. H., 663, *673*
Beaudry, P. H., 716, 739, *755*
Beaufils, M., 12, *22*
Beautrais, A. L., 776, 777, *805*
Bebenek, K., 573, *593*
Bechtold, T., 65, *93*
Beck, E., 452, 460, *464*
Beck, G. J., 715, 717, *753*
Beck, H. I., 904, *919*
Beck, S. A., 886, *898*
Becker, I. D., 933, *974*
Becker, J., 968, 969, *989*

Author Index

K

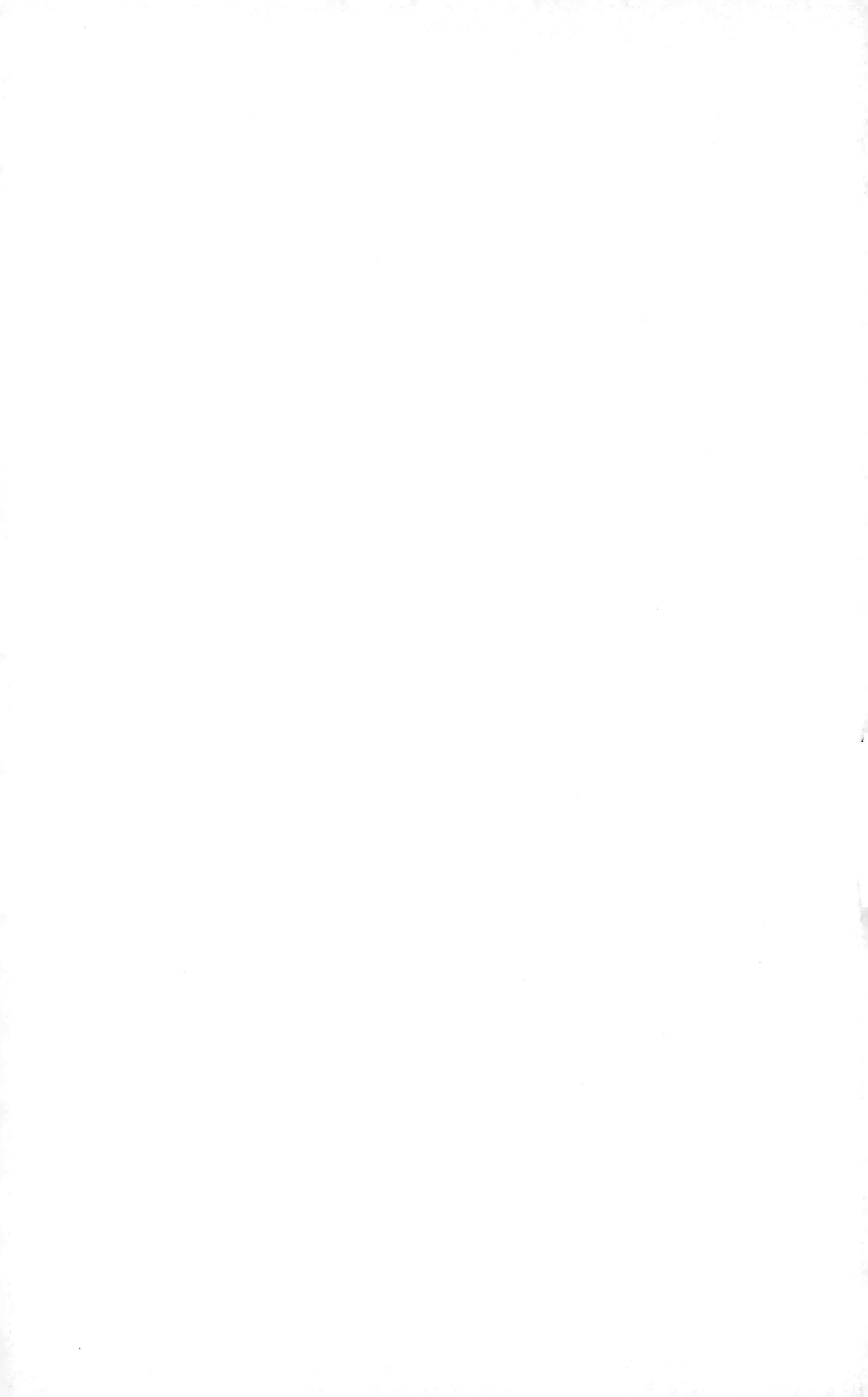